Nutritional Assessment

Sixth Edition

Robert D. Lee, DrPH, RD
Central Michigan University

David C. Nieman, DrPH, FACSM
Appalachian State University

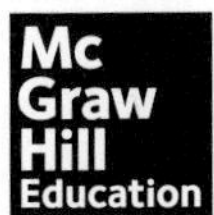

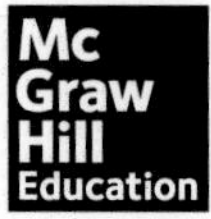

NUTRITIONAL ASSESSMENT, SIXTH EDITION
International Edition 2013

Published by McGraw-Hill Education, 2 Penn Plaza, New York, NY 10121.

10 09 08 07 06 05
20 19 18 17 16
CTP SLP

When ordering this title, use ISBN 978-007-132636-0 or MHID 007-132636-7

Printed in Singapore

www.mhhe.com

To the gifted and courageous women and men of nutritional science who came before us and upon whose shoulders each of us now stands.

Brief Contents

1 Introduction to Nutritional Assessment 1

2 Standards for Nutrient Intake 21

3 Measuring Diet 74

4 National Dietary and Nutrition Surveys 109

5 Computerized Dietary Analysis Systems 146

6 Anthropometry 166

7 Assessment of the Hospitalized Patient 221

8 Nutritional Assessment in Disease Prevention 256

9 Biochemical Assessment of Nutritional Status 317

10 Clinical Assessment of Nutritional Status 353

11 Counseling Theory and Technique 370

Appendix A Nutrition Assessment and Monitoring and Evaluation Terminology 387

Appendix B Nutrition Diagnostic Terminology 391

Appendix C Nutrition Intervention Terminology 393

Appendix D Food Record Recording Form 395

Appendix E Fruit and Vegetable Screener Developed by the U.S. National Cancer Institute 397

Appendix F MEDFICTS Dietary Assessment Questionnaire 401

Appendix G The National Institute of Health's The Diet History Questionnaire II 403

Appendix H The NHANES Food Frequency Questionnaire 412

Appendix I 2011 Behavioral Risk Factor Surveillance System Questionnaire 420

Appendix J Suppliers of Nutritional Assessment Equipment 428

Appendix K CDC Clinical Growth Charts 430

Appendix L Mean Body Weight, Height, and Body Mass Index, United States, 1960–2006 441

Appendix M Triceps Skinfold Norms from NHANES 2003–2006 457

Appendix N Subscapular Skinfold Norms from NHANES 2003–2006 461

Appendix O Means, Standard Deviations, and Percentiles of Sum of Triceps and Subscapular Skinfold Thickness (mm) by Age for Males and Females of 2 to 90 Years 465

Appendix P Means, Standard Deviations, and Percentiles of Upper-Arm Muscle Area (cm^2) by Age for Males and Females of 2 to 90 Years 467

Appendix Q Reference Values for Serum Total Cholesterol and Serum High-Density Lipoprotein, by Sex, Age, Race/Ethnicity, 1988–1994 469

Appendix R Example of a Form That Can Be Used for Self-Monitoring Eating Behavior 478

Appendix S Competency Checklist for Nutrition Counselors 479

CONTENTS

Preface ix

CHAPTER 1

INTRODUCTION TO NUTRITIONAL ASSESSMENT 1

Introduction 1
Good Nutrition Essential for Health 2
Deficiency Diseases Once Common 2
Chronic Diseases Now Epidemic 2
Nutritional Screening and Assessment 3
Nutritional Assessment Methods 3
Anthropometric Methods 3
Biochemical Methods 3
Clinical Methods 3
Dietary Methods 4
Importance of Nutritional Assessment 4
The Nutrition Care Process 4
The Nutrition Care Process Model 5
Nutritional Assessment in the Nutrition Care Process 6
Standardized Terminology in Nutritional Assessment 7
Nutrition Diagnosis in the Nutrition Care Process 8
Nutrition Intervention in the Nutrition Care Process 9
Nutritional Monitoring and Evaluation in the Nutrition Care Process 10
Opportunities in Nutritional Assessment 11
Meeting the *Healthy People 2020* Objectives 11
Health-Care Organizations 13
Diabetes Mellitus 13
Weight Management 13
Heart Disease and Cancer 15
Nutrition Monitoring 16
Nutritional Epidemiology 17

CHAPTER 2

STANDARDS FOR NUTRIENT INTAKE 21

Introduction 21
Early Dietary Standards and Recommendations 22
Observational Standards 22
Beginnings of Scientifically Based Dietary Standards 22
Recommended Dietary Allowances 23
Dietary Reference Intakes 24
Estimated Average Requirement 26
Recommended Dietary Allowance 27
Adequate Intake 33
Tolerable Upper Intake Level 34
Estimated Energy Requirement 35
Recommendations for Macronutrients 36
Uses of the DRIs 38
Nutrient Density 39
Nutrient Profiling 41
Indices of Diet Quality 41
Diet Quality Index 41
Healthy Eating Index 42
Dietary Guidelines 44
Early Dietary Guidelines 44
U.S. Dietary Goals 46
The Dietary Guidelines for Americans 47
The Surgeon General's Report on Nutrition and Health 50
Diet and Health 50
Other Dietary Guidelines 50
Nutrition Labeling of Food 50
U.S. Recommended Daily Allowances 50
The Nutrition Labeling and Education Act 50
Front-of-Package Labeling 54
Daily Values 55
Daily Reference Values 55
Reference Daily Intakes 57
Food Guides 57
Food Guide Pyramid 59
MyPyramid 60
MyPlate 60
The New American Plate 61
Food Exchange System 64

CHAPTER 3

MEASURING DIET 74

Introduction 74
Reasons for Measuring Diet 75
Approaches to Measuring Diet 75
Research Design Considerations 75
Characteristics of Study Participants 79
Available Resources 79

Techniques in Measuring Diet *80*
- 24-Hour Recall *80*
- Food Record, or Diary *81*
- Food Frequency Questionnaires *83*
  - *Willett Questionnaire 85*
  - *Block Questionnaires 86*
  - *Diet History Questionnaire 86*
  - *NHANES Food Frequency Questionnaire 86*
  - *Strengths and Limitations 88*
- Diet History *89*
- Duplicate Food Collections *90*
- Food Accounts *90*
- Food Balance Sheets *91*
- Telephone Interviews *92*
- Technological Innovations in Assessment *93*
- Surrogate Sources *94*

Considerations for Certain Groups *95*

Issues in Dietary Measurement *95*
- Validity *95*
  - *Use of Biological Markers 95*
  - *Energy Expenditure and Weight Maintenance 97*
- Reproducibility *98*

Estimating Portion Size *98*

CHAPTER 4

National Dietary and Nutrition Surveys *109*

Introduction *110*

Importance of National Dietary and Nutrition Surveys *110*

Nutritional Monitoring in the United States *110*

National Nutritional Monitoring and Related Research Program *111*

Role of the U.S. Department of Agriculture *112*
- Food Availability *112*
  - *ERS Food Availability (Per Capita) Data System 114*
- Continuing Survey of Food Intakes by Individuals *114*
- Diet and Health Knowledge Survey *115*
- Supplemental Children's Survey *115*
- Food Insecurity and Hunger *115*

Role of the U.S. Department of Health and Human Services *118*
- National Health Examination Surveys *119*
- Ten-State Nutrition Survey *119*
- National Health and Nutrition Examination Survey *120*
  - *First National Health and Nutrition Examination Survey (NHANES I) 120*
  - *Second National Health and Nutrition Examination Survey (NHANES II) 120*
  - *Hispanic Health and Nutrition Examination Survey (HHANES) 120*
  - *Third National Health and Nutrition Examination Survey (NHANES III) 120*
  - *NHANES: A Continuous and Integrated Survey 121*
- Other DHHS Surveys *125*
  - *Total Diet Study 126*
  - *Navajo Health and Nutrition Survey 127*
  - *Pregnancy Nutrition Surveillance System 127*
  - *Pediatric Nutrition Surveillance System 128*
  - *Health and Diet Survey 129*
  - *Behavioral Risk Factor Surveillance System 129*
  - *National Health Interview Survey 130*

Dietary Trends *131*
- Sources of Food Energy *131*
- Trends in Carbohydrates *134*
- Trends in Sweeteners *134*
- Trends in Dietary Fats and Oils *136*
- Trends in Dairy Products *136*
- Trends in Beverages *138*
- Trends in Red Meat, Poultry, and Fish *138*
- Trends in Fruits and Vegetables *138*
- Trends in Total Calories *139*

CHAPTER 5

Computerized Dietary Analysis Systems *146*

Introduction: Using Computers in Nutritional Assessment *146*

Factors to Consider in Selecting a Computerized Dietary Analysis System *147*
- Nutrient Database *147*
  - *USDA Nutrient Data Laboratory 147*
  - *USDA Nutrient Databases 147*
  - *Criteria for Developing High-Quality Databases 152*
- Program Operation *158*
- System Output *159*
- Computerized Dietary Analysis Systems *160*

Dietary Analysis on the Internet *161*

CHAPTER 6

Anthropometry *166*

Introduction *167*

What Is Anthropometry? *167*

Measuring Length, Stature, and Head Circumference *167*
- Length *167*
- Stature *168*
- Nonambulatory Persons *169*
- Head Circumference *169*

Measuring Weight *170*
- Infants *170*
- Children and Adults *170*
- Nonambulatory Persons *171*

CDC Growth Charts *171*
- Charts for Birth up to 24 Months *174*
- Charts for Ages 2 to 20 Years *175*

Weight Standards *176*
- Height-Weight Tables *177*
- Limitations of Height-Weight Tables *177*
- Strengths of Height-Weight Tables *179*

Measuring Frame Size *179*

Height-Weight Indices *180*
- Relative Weight *180*
- Power-Type Indices *181*

Body Fat Distribution *185*

Body Composition *186*

Cadaveric Studies *187*

Skinfold Measurements *188*
- Assumptions in Using Skinfold Measurements *188*
- Measurement Technique *188*
- Site Selection *190*
  - *Chest 190*
  - *Triceps 190*
  - *Subscapular 192*

Midaxillary 192
Suprailiac 193
Abdomen 193
Thigh 193
Medial Calf 194
Single-Site Skinfold Measurements *195*
Two-Site Skinfold Measurements *195*
Multiple-Site Skinfold Measurements *197*
What Is a Desirable Level of Fatness? *198*
Densitometry *199*
Underwater Weighing *199*
Equipment 200
Procedure 200
Weaknesses of Underwater Weighing 202
Air Displacement Plethysmography *202*
Total Body Water *204*
Total Body Potassium *205*
Neutron Activation Analysis *205*
Creatinine Excretion *206*
3-Methylhistidine *206*
Electrical Conductance *206*
Bioelectrical Impedance *207*
Total Body Electrical Conductivity *207*
Infrared Interactance *208*
Ultrasound *208*
Computed Tomography *208*
Magnetic Resonance Imaging *209*
Dual-Energy X-Ray Absorptiometry *209*

CHAPTER 7

ASSESSMENT OF THE HOSPITALIZED PATIENT *221*

Introduction *222*
Assessing Nutritional Status *222*
Nutritional Screening *222*
Nutritional Assessment *224*
History 225
Dietary Information 225
Physical Examination 225
Knee Height 226
Estimating Stature 227
Midarm Circumference 228
Calf Circumference 228
Recumbent Skinfold Measurements 229
Estimating Body Weight 231
Arm Muscle Area 233
Determining Energy Requirements *234*
Measuring Energy Expenditure *235*
Direct Calorimetry 235
Indirect Calorimetry 236
Doubly Labeled Water 237
Bicarbonate-Urea Method 238
Estimating Energy Needs *238*
Commonly Used Equations 238
Estimated Energy Requirement Equations 240
Energy Expenditure in Disease and Injury *241*
Energy Needs: Estimated or Measured? *244*
Determining Protein Requirements *244*
Protein Losses in Disease and Injury *244*
Estimating Protein Needs *244*
Mini Nutritional Assessment *246*
Malnutrition Universal Screening Tool *248*

CHAPTER 8

NUTRITIONAL ASSESSMENT IN DISEASE PREVENTION *256*

Introduction *257*
Coronary Heart Disease *257*
Coronary Heart Disease Risk Factors *258*
Serum Lipids and Lipoproteins *258*
Lipoproteins, Cholesterol, and Coronary Heart Disease *260*
Lipoprotein Ratios *262*
Triglyceride and Coronary Heart Disease *263*
Estimating CHD Risk *263*
National Cholesterol Education Program's Guidelines *266*
Assessing Risk for Coronary Heart Disease *266*
Therapeutic Lifestyle Changes *267*
Lowering Cholesterol in the Population *270*
Cardiovascular Disease in Youth *271*
Cardiovascular Disease Risk Reduction in Children and Adolescents *272*
Dietary Treatment in Coronary Heart Disease *276*
Saturated Fatty Acids *276*
Trans *Fatty Acids 277*
Dietary Cholesterol *277*
Total Calories *278*
Total and Unsaturated Fat *278*
Protein and Carbohydrate *278*
General Principles *279*
Issues in Measuring Lipid and Lipoprotein Levels *279*
Precision *279*
Accuracy *280*
Total Analytical Error *281*
Sources of Error in Cholesterol Measurement *281*
Fasting 282
Posture 282
Venous Occlusion 282
Anticoagulants 282
Recent Heart Attack and Stroke 282
Trauma and Acute Infections 282
Pregnancy 282
Hypertension *282*
Body Weight *285*
Sodium *286*
Alcohol *287*
Physical Activity *287*
Dietary Pattern *287*
Evaluating Blood Pressure in Children and Adolescents *288*
Osteoporosis *293*
Bones: Structure and Remodeling *294*
Osteoporosis: Classification and Risk Factors *294*
Diagnosing Osteoporosis *295*
Dual-Energy X-Ray Absorptiometry 295
Quantitative Ultrasound 296
Preventing Osteoporosis *299*
Diabetes Mellitus *300*
Types of Diabetes *301*
Diagnosis of Diabetes *302*
Oral Glucose Tolerance Test 303
Self-Monitoring of Blood Glucose 303
Glycated Hemoglobin 304
Medical Nutrition Therapy *305*

CHAPTER 9

Biochemical Assessment of Nutritional Status *317*

Introduction *317*
Use of Biochemical Measures *318*
Protein Status *318*
Creatinine Excretion and Creatinine-Height Index *319*
Nitrogen Balance *320*
Serum Proteins *320*
Albumin 320
Transferrin 321
Prealbumin 321
Retinol-Binding Protein 322
Iron Status *322*
Stages of Iron Depletion *322*
Serum Ferritin *324*
Soluble Transferrin Receptor *324*
Transferrin, Serum Iron, and Total Iron-Binding Capacity *324*
Erythrocyte Protoporphyrin *324*
Hemoglobin *325*
Hematocrit *325*
Mean Corpuscular Hemoglobin *325*
Mean Corpuscular Volume *325*
Assessing Iron Status *326*
Iron Overload *326*
Calcium Status *327*
Serum Calcium Fractions *327*
Urinary Calcium *328*
Zinc Status *329*
Plasma Zinc Concentrations *329*
Metallothionen and Zinc Status *329*
Hair Zinc *330*
Urinary Zinc *330*
Iodine Status *330*
Assessing Iodine Status *331*
Iodine Status in the United States *331*
Vitamin A Status *333*
Plasma Levels *333*
Relative Dose Response *334*
Conjunctival Impression Cytology *334*
Dark Adaptation *334*
Direct Measurement of Liver Stores *335*
Retinol Isotope Dilution *335*
Vitamin D Status *335*
Assessing Vitamin D Status *335*
Vitamin C Status *337*
Serum and Leukocyte Vitamin C *339*
Vitamin B_6 Status *339*
Plasma and Erythrocyte Pyridoxal 5′-Phosphate *339*
Plasma Pyridoxal *340*
Urinary 4-pyridoxic Acid *340*
Methionine Load Test *340*
Folate Status *340*
Vitamin B_{12} Status *341*
Biochemical Indicators of B_{12} Status *343*
Blood Chemistry Tests *343*
Alanine Aminotransferase *343*
Albumin and Total Protein *344*
Alkaline Phosphatase *345*
Aspartate Aminotransferase *345*
Bilirubin *345*
Blood Urea Nitrogen *345*
Calcium *345*
Carbon Dioxide *345*
Chloride *345*
Cholesterol *346*
Creatinine *346*
Glucose *346*
Lactic Dehydrogenase *346*
Phosphorus *346*
Potassium *346*
Sodium *346*
Triglyceride *346*

CHAPTER 10

Clinical Assessment of Nutritional Status *353*

Introduction *353*
Medical History *354*
Dietary History *355*
Subjective Global Assessment *356*
Elements of the History *356*
Elements of the Physical Examination *356*
Protein-Energy Malnutrition *359*
Clinical Signs *359*
Classifying Protein-Energy Malnutrition *361*
HIV Infection *362*
Eating Disorders *365*

CHAPTER 11

Counseling Theory and Technique *370*

Introduction *370*
Communication *371*
Verbal Communication *371*
Nonverbal Communication *372*
Effective Communication *372*
Listening *373*
Interviewing *374*
Interviewing Skills *374*
Obtaining Information *374*
Counseling Theories *375*
Person-Centered Approach *375*
Behavior Modification *376*
Antecedents and Consequences 376
Self-monitoring 376
Goals and Self-contracts 377
Modeling 377
Reinforcers 378
Behavior Modification Techniques Summarized 378
Rational-Emotive Therapy *378*
Reality Therapy *380*
Initiating and Maintaining Dietary Change: A Practical Plan *381*
Motivation *381*
Characteristics of Effective Counselors *381*
Initial Assessment *381*
Initiating Dietary Change *382*
Maintaining Dietary Change *382*
Relapse Prevention *383*
Knowing One's Limits *383*

Glossary *482*

Index *493*

PREFACE

The ability to accurately assess nutritional status has become critically important in recent decades, as knowledge of and interest in the relationships between diet and health have increased. Nutrition researchers must be able to measure food and nutrient intake with accuracy and precision in order to identify causal relationships between diet and disease risk. Periodic monitoring of a nation's health and nutritional status is necessary to develop effective programs targeting specific health and nutrition concerns, such as atherogenic serum lipid and lipoprotein levels, hypertension, diabetes, food insecurity and hunger, maternal and infant health, and obesity. Awareness of these health and nutrition concerns has led the government to establish such programs as the National Cholesterol Education Program; the National Diabetes Education Program; the Supplemental Nutrition Assistance Program; the Special Supplemental Food Program for Women, Infants, and Children; and Sisters Together: Move More, Eat Better. Periodic nutritional and health monitoring provides empirical data to determine the cost effectiveness of such programs in attempts to preserve effective ones from changing political agendas and governmental budgetary priorities. Dietitians and physicians rely on objective measures of nutritional status before administering nutritional support to a critically ill patient and to determine that patient's responsiveness to treatment. The public is increasingly interested in the health implications of nutritional supplement use and of knowing how much of which supplements can actually improve health and reduce disease risk.

The sixth edition of *Nutritional Assessment* addresses these and many other topics, including computerized dietary analysis systems, national surveys of dietary intake and nutritional status, assessment techniques and standards for the hospitalized patient, nutritional assessment in the prevention of such diseases as coronary heart disease, osteoporosis, and diabetes, clinical assessment, and proper counseling techniques. The sixth edition builds on the strengths of the previous five editions and is primarily a textbook for students of dietetics and public health nutrition. It is also intended to be a valuable reference for health professionals who interact on a regular basis with patients who have diet-related medical problems.

ORGANIZATION

We recommend that study of *Nutritional Assessment* follow the progression of the 11 chapters in the order in which they are presented. Chapter 1 gives a thorough introduction to the topic of nutritional assessment and the Nutrition Care Process, exploring various definitions and concepts. Chapter 2 reviews the wide assortment of standards for nutrient intake, such as the Dietary Reference Intakes, the Food Exchange System, the MyPlate graphic, and the *Dietary Guidelines for Americans,* and it gives practical guidelines for their use.

Methods for measuring diet and the strengths and weaknesses of each technique are outlined in Chapter 3. Results from the U.S. Department of Agriculture's monitoring of food insecurity and hunger, the National Health and Nutrition Examination Survey, the Behavioral Risk Factor Surveillance System, and other diet and nutrition surveys are interpreted in Chapter 4, and statistics on the trends in food availability are summarized. Chapter 5 reviews the use of computerized dietary analysis systems in nutritional assessment and gives guidelines for evaluating the operating features, nutrient databases, and overall strengths and weaknesses of any commercially available program.

Chapters 6 and 7 survey anthropometric techniques for both healthy and hospitalized people, with complete descriptions of how to measure body skinfolds and circumferences and then make appropriate decisions on classification. Nutritional assessment, as it relates to prevention of coronary heart disease, hypertension, osteoporosis, and diabetes, is reviewed in Chapter 8. Numerous laboratory tests are interpreted, and biochemical methods for assessing protein, iron, calcium, vitamin D, and other nutrient status are discussed in Chapter 9. Chapter 10 gives an overview of the clinical assessment of nutritional status. Chapter 11 reviews the major theories and techniques of both individual and group counseling methods.

New to This Edition

The numerous revisions and additions to the sixth edition of *Nutritional Assessment* make it the most comprehensive and up-to-date textbook available on the subject. Included in this edition are updates to the U.S. Department of Agriculture's nutrient databases, recent advances in computerized dietary analysis systems, and information on the increased availability of online dietary analysis systems such as the National Cancer Institute's Internet-based automated self-administered 24-hour dietary recall. The coverage of surveys conducted by the U.S. Department of Health and Human Services such as the Pregnancy Nutrition Surveillance System, the Pediatric Nutrition Surveillance System, the Total Diet Study, and the Behavioral Risk Factor Surveillance System has been expanded. Data and graphics on food and nutrient intake and the prevalence of overweight, obesity, hypertension, and food insecurity have been thoroughly updated. Discussion of plasma-based markers of coronary heart disease risk, lifestyle modifications to prevent and manage hypertension, the diagnosis and prevention of osteoporosis, and the diagnostic criteria for diabetes has been expanded and updated.

Student Learning Outcomes have been added to the beginning of each chapter to outline the concepts to be learned.

The food composition tables (Appendix I in the fifth edition) have been removed and substituted with online tables from *Home and Garden Bulletin #72* (Gebhardt, Susan E., and Robin G. Thomas. 2002. Nutritive Value of Foods. U.S. Department of Agriculture, Agricultural Research Service, Home and Garden Bulletin 72). The online food composition tables will allow the student to perform manual calculations of the nutrient content of their diet using a concise database.

Chapter 1

- Expanded and detailed coverage of the Nutrition Care Process in nutritional assessment, monitoring, and evaluation.
- Updated tables and figures reflecting the most recent data from the National Center for Health Statistics and the National Health and Nutrition Examination Survey.
- New information on the *Healthy People 2020 Objectives*.
- The recently updated American Cancer Society Guidelines on Nutrition and Physical Activity for Cancer Prevention are included.

Chapter 2

- Updated DRI tables for vitamin D and calcium.
- Revised coverage of nutrient density.
- Discussion of the *2010 Dietary Guidelines for Americans*.
- Coverage of the MyPlate graphic.

Chapter 3

- Discussion of the ASA24, the National Cancer Institute's Internet-based automated self-administered 24-hour dietary recall.
- Coverage of the new Diet History Questionnaire II from the National Cancer Institute.
- Updated coverage of the DHQ*Web, an automated, Web-based food frequency questionnaire.
- Introduction of the NHANES Food Frequency Questionnaire.
- Updated coverage of technological innovations in dietary measurement.
- New information and figures on estimating portion sizes.

Chapter 4

- Updated discussion of per capita food availability data.
- New information on Loss-Adjusted Food Availability data.
- Updated data from the USDA on food security.
- Updated discussion of the NHANES Mobile Examination Center.
- More than 20 new or revised figures illustrating U.S. dietary practices.
- Updated discussion of dietary trends in the United States.

Chapter 5

- Revised list of terms and acronyms with definitions used by the Nutrient Data Laboratory (NDL).
- Complete update on the USDA National Nutrient Database for Standard Reference, Release 24.
- New information on the Choose My Plate SuperTracker (www.choosemyplate.gov/SuperTracker).
- Updated information on computerized dietary analysis systems.

Chapter 6

- New information on the updated CDC growth charts from birth to 2 years of age.
- Updated prevalence data on overweight and obesity from NHANES.

- Updated information on the relationship between body weight and disease risk.
- New information on the global prevalence of overweight and obesity.

Chapter 7

- Updated discussion on nutritional screening of the hospitalized patient.
- Discussion of the Mini Nutritional Assessment and the new Mini Nutrition Assessment–Short Form.
- New discussion of the Malnutrition Universal Screening Tool.

Chapter 8

- Update on questions regarding the causal relationship between serum HDL-C and coronary heart disease.
- Expanded coverage of the primordial and primary prevention of coronary heart disease in youth.
- Discussion of the NHLBI's report, *The Expert Panel on Integrated Guidelines for Cardiovascular Health and Risk Reduction in Children and Adolescents.*
- Discussion of new guidelines for universal lipid and lipoprotein screening in youth.
- Updated figures on the prevalence of dyslipidemia and hypertension.
- New tables on food sources of calcium and treatment recommendations for promoting bone health.
- Updated diagnostic criteria for gestational diabetes from the American Diabetes Association.
- Updated criteria for diagnosing diabetes from the American Diabetes Association which now include glycated hemoglobin or HbA_{1C}.
- Updates to the medical nutrition therapy of diabetes.

Chapter 9

- Eleven new figures on biochemical indicators of vitamin and mineral status.
- Updated information on the assessment of protein status.
- New information on assessing iron status including measurement of serum soluble transferrin receptor and use of the body iron model.
- New section on the iodine status of the U.S. population.
- New information on using retinol isotope dilution for assessing vitamin A status.
- Updated discussion on assessing folate status.
- New information on assessing vitamin B_{12} status.
- New section on assessing vitamin D status.

Appendices

- International Dietetics & Nutrition Terminology for nutritional assessment and monitoring, nutrition diagnosis, and nutrition intervention have been added.
- Addition of the Diet History Questionnaire II and NHANES Food Frequency Questionnaires.
- Updated anthropometric reference data from NHANES.

Nutritional Assessment Website (www.mhhe.com/lee-nieman6)

This website provides readers with a convenient and authoritative online source for additional information and resources on nutritional assessment. Following the organization of the book's chapters, it contains links to private and governmental websites related to nutritional assessment, sources of data from national health and nutrition surveys, and links to suppliers of nutritional assessment equipment. It serves to update readers on new information and developments in the field of nutritional assessment as they become available. For instructors, a password-protected testbank and PPT lecture outlines are available.

Features

Chapter Outline and Student Learning Outcomes

Each chapter begins with an outline of the contents of the chapter and a set of student learning outcomes. Reading these before beginning the chapter gives the student an idea of the material to be covered and the key concepts contained in the chapter, and serve as useful review tools when the student is studying for exams.

Figures and Tables

There are more than 100 tables in the text, supplemented with 160 graphs, illustrations, and photographs, and nearly 70 text boxes. Figures in Chapter 4, for example, illustrate trends in food and nutrient intake based on data from the National Health and Nutrition Examination Survey and the U.S. Department of Agriculture's monitoring of food available for consumption from the U.S. food supply. Chapters 6 and 7 contain numerous photographs illustrating the exact procedures involved in skinfold measurement and other anthropometric techniques used in assessing nutritional status.

Summaries

A summary at the end of each chapter highlights all important chapter information and will be especially helpful when the student reviews for exams.

References

A complete list of up-to-date references is included at the end of each chapter. This list provides the student and instructor with extensive sources for continued study.

Assessment Activities

Most chapters end with two or three practical assessment activities to help the student better understand the concepts presented in the chapter. For example, some activities are analyzing diet using software on a personal computer, obtaining information on food composition from online databases, accessing nutritional monitoring data from government websites, practicing anthropometry and one-on-one dietary counseling, and interpreting serum lipid and lipoprotein results.

Appendixes

Appendixes A, B, and C contain the International Dietetics & Nutrition Terminology for nutritional assessment and monitoring, nutrition diagnosis, and nutrition intervention. Various recording forms and questionnaires used in measuring diet are presented in Appendixes D through I, including the first several pages of the Diet History Questionnaire II and the NHANES Food Frequency Questionnaire, and sections of the 2011 Behavioral Risk Factor Surveillance System Questionnaire. Appendix J lists suppliers of nutritional assessment equipment. Appendix K provides the CDC clinical growth charts for children and adolescents, including the recently revised charts for infants and children from birth to 2 years of age. Various anthropometric standards are tabled in Appendixes L through P. Appendix Q provides reference data for serum lipid and lipoprotein levels for children, adolescents, and adults. Appendix R contains a form for self-monitoring dietary intake, and Appendix S has a checklist for counseling competencies.

Glossary

Throughout the text, important terms are shown in boldface type. Concise definitions for more than 360 terms can be found in the glossary.

ACKNOWLEDGMENTS

We would like to express our sincere gratitude to the editorial and production team at McGraw-Hill. We are particularly indebted to our wives, Sandra and Cathy, for their encouragement, support, and patience. We wish to thank those professors who served as critical reviewers of the sixth edition. Their suggestions have been most helpful, and we are grateful for their contributions. They are

Judith Anglin
California State University, Long Beach
Catherine Anstrom
Olivet Nazarene University
Janet Beary
Washington State University
Brenda Eissenstat
The Pennsylvania State University
Chengshun Fang
University of Delaware
Linda Fleming
University of Bridgeport
Holly F. Huye
The University of Southern Mississippi
Colette Joanson-Sand
University of New Hampshire
Kristine Jordan
University of Utah
Rebecca Pobocik
Bowling Green State University
Maureen Timlin
Southeast Missouri State University
Claire Zizza
Auburn University

Robert D. Lee
David C. Nieman

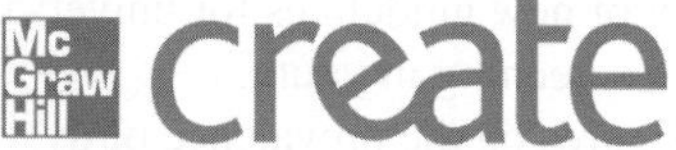

McGraw-Hill Create™

Craft your teaching resources to match the way you teach! With McGraw-Hill Create, you can easily rearrange chapters, combine material from other content sources, and quickly upload content you have written like your course syllabus or teaching notes. Find the content you need in Create by searching through thousands of leading McGraw-Hill textbooks. Arrange your book to fit your teaching style. Create even allows you to personalize your book's appearance by selecting the cover and adding your name, school, and course information. Order a Create book and you'll receive a complimentary print review copy in 3–5 business days or a complimentary electronic review copy (eComp) via email in minutes. Go to www.mcgrawhillcreate.com today and register to experience how McGraw-Hill Create empowers you to teach *your* students *your* way.

Electronic Textbook Option

This text is offered through CourseSmart for both instructors and students. CourseSmart is an online resource where students can purchase the complete text online at almost half the cost of a traditional text. Purchasing the eTextbook allows students to take advantage of CourseSmart's web tools for learning, which include full text search, notes and highlighting, and email tools for sharing notes between classmates. To learn more about CourseSmart options, contact your sales representative or visit www.CourseSmart.com.

CHAPTER

Introduction to Nutritional Assessment 1

Chapter Outline

Introduction
Good Nutrition Essential for Health
Nutritional Screening and Assessment
Nutrition Care Process
Opportunities in Nutritional Assessment
Summary
References

Student Learning Outcomes

After studying this chapter, the student will be able to:

1. Describe the factors that contributed to a change in the leading causes of death during the twentieth century.
2. Name the leading causes of death in the United States in which diet or excessive alcohol consumption play a role.
3. Distinguish between nutritional screening and nutritional assessment.
4. Name the four methods used to collect nutritional assessment data.
5. Explain the Nutrition Care Process Model.
6. Discuss the role of nutritional assessment in the Nutrition Care Process.
7. Discuss the role of nutritional assessment in the prevention and treatment of disease.

Introduction

Throughout most of human history, agriculture has been a labor-intensive process with relatively small yields of a limited number of crops. Hunger, nutrient deficiency, and starvation were common, and infectious diseases were the leading causes of death. Beginning in the late 19th century and early 20th century, improvements in plant breeding, the mechanization of agriculture, and the widespread use of fertilizers and pesticides resulted in dramatic increases in crop yields per unit of land. Food became much more available and less expensive, and by the middle of the 20th century developed nations went from a dismal era of food scarcity to one of food excess. Nutrient deficiency diseases have become much less common and chronic diseases related to excess consumption of food, tobacco and alcohol use, and a lack of physical activity are now the leading causes of death and disability throughout the world. During the same time, improvements in sanitation, convenient access to safe drinking water, vaccine and antibiotic development, and improvements in health care have dramatically reduced the **incidence** and **prevalence** of infectious diseases and dramatically increased **life expectancy** in developed countries. However, many developing countries experience a double burden of death from chronic diseases and infectious diseases.[1,2]

These changes have resulted in an **epidemic** of chronic diseases, many of which are directly linked to excess consumption of high-fat foods and alcoholic beverages, inadequate consumption of foods high in complex carbohydrates and fiber, and a sedentary lifestyle. This situation, along with heightened public and professional interest in the role of nutrition in health and disease, has created an increased need for health professionals proficient in nutritional assessment. The ability to identify persons at nutritional risk, describe and label an existing nutrition problem, and then plan and implement a nutrition intervention addressing the nutrition problem has made nutritional assessment an essential element of health care and a necessary skill for health professionals concerned about making health care more cost-effective.

Good Nutrition Essential for Health

Good nutrition is critical for the well-being of any society and to each individual within that society. The variety, quality, quantity, cost, and accessibility of food and the patterns of food consumption can profoundly affect health.

Scurvy, for example, was among the first diseases recognized as being caused by a nutritional deficiency. One of the earliest descriptions of scurvy was made in 1250 by French writer Joinville, who observed it among the troops of Louis IX at the siege of Cairo. When Vasco da Gama sailed to the East Indies around the Cape of Good Hope in 1497, more than 60% of his crew died of scurvy.[3] In 1747, James Lind, a British naval surgeon, conducted the first controlled human dietary experiment showing that consumption of citrus fruits cures scurvy.[4]

Deficiency Diseases Once Common

Up until the middle of the twentieth century, scurvy and other **deficiency diseases,** such as **rickets, pellagra, beriberi, xerophthalmia,** and iodine-deficiency diseases such as **goiter** and **cretinism** (caused by inadequate dietary vitamin D, niacin, thiamin, vitamin A, and iodine, respectively), were commonly seen in the United States and throughout the world and posed a significant threat to human health.[3,4]

Infectious disease and malnutrition remain serious problems in developing nations. According to the World Health Organization, infectious diseases are responsible for 68% of deaths in children less than five years of age, and malnutrition is an underlying or contributing cause of 33% of deaths in this age group.[5] Sanitation measures, improved health care, vaccine development, and mass immunization programs have dramatically reduced the incidence of infectious disease in developed nations. An abundant food supply, **fortification** of some foods with important nutrients, **enrichment** to replace certain nutrients lost in food processing, and better methods of determining the nutrient content of foods have made nutrient-deficiency diseases relatively uncommon in developed nations. Despite these gains, deficiencies of certain nutrients, food insecurity, and hunger remain problems faced by many families and individuals in developed nations throughout the world, including the United States and Canada.[6]

Chronic Diseases Now Epidemic

Despite the many advances of nutritional science, nutrition-related diseases not only continue to exist but also result in a heavy toll of disease and death. In recent decades, however, they have taken a form different from the nutrient-deficiency diseases common in the early 1900s. Diseases of dietary excess and imbalance now rank among the leading causes of illness and death in North America and play a prominent role in the epidemic of chronic disease that all nations are currently experiencing.[5] Table 1.1 ranks the 15 leading causes of death in the United States in 2010. Five of these are causes in which diet plays a prominent role: diseases of the heart (e.g., coronary heart disease), malignant neoplasms (i.e., cancers), cerebrovascular diseases (i.e., stroke), diabetes mellitus, and hypertension (including hypertensive renal

Table 1.1 Estimated Deaths and Percent of Total Deaths for the 15 Leading Causes of Death, United States, 2010

Rank	Cause of Death	Number of Deaths	Percent of Total Deaths
	All causes	2,436,652	100.0
1*	Diseases of the heart	598,607	25.6
2*	Malignant neoplasms	568,668	23.3
3	Chronic lung disease	137,082	5.6
4*	Cerebrovascular disease	128,603	5.3
5†	Unintentional injuries	117,176	4.8
6	Alzheimer's disease	78,889	3.2
7*	Diabetes mellitus	68,504	2.8
8	Influenza, pneumonia	53,582	2.2
9	Nephritis, nephrosis	48,714	2.0
10†	Suicide	36,547	1.5
11	Septicemia	35,587	1.5
12†	Chronic liver disease	30,444	1.2
13*	Hypertension	25,651	1.1
14	Parkinson's disease	20,552	0.8
15†	Homicide	16,591	0.7
	All other causes	471,455	19.3

Data from the National Center for Health Statistics

*Causes of death in which diet plays a role.

†Causes of death in which excessive alcohol consumption plays a role.

disease). Four of the leading causes of death are linked to excessive alcohol consumption: unintentional injuries (what are commonly referred to as accidents), suicide, chronic liver disease (including cirrhosis), and homicide.

Overweight and obesity are major contributing factors to coronary heart disease, certain types of cancer, type 2 diabetes, and hypertension. In the United States, 72% of men and 64% of women are overweight or obese (have a body mass index $\geq$ 25.0 kg/m^2), with 34% of adults being obese (have a body mass index $\geq$ 30.0 kg/m^2). In Canada, 61% of men and 44% of women are overweight or obese, with 24% being obese.[6,7] Hypertension is a major risk factor for coronary heart disease, stroke, congestive heart failure, and kidney disease. In the United States, 34% of adults have hypertension and an additional 36% of Americans have prehypertension (a blood pressure higher than normal but not high enough to be classified as hypertension). In Canada, 19% of adults aged 20 to 79 years have hypertension.[8]

The continuing presence of nutrition-related disease makes it essential that health professionals be able to determine the nutritional status of individuals. Nutritional assessment is critical in determining whether a person is at nutritional risk, what the nutritional problem is, and how best to treat it and to monitor the person's response to the treatment. Nutritional assessment is the first of the four steps in the nutrition care process.[9–12]

NUTRITIONAL SCREENING AND ASSESSMENT

Nutritional screening can be defined as "a process to identify an individual who is malnourished or who is at risk for malnutrition to determine if a detailed nutrition assessment is indicated."[13] If nutritional screening identifies a person at nutritional risk, a more thorough assessment of the individual's nutritional status can be performed. Nutritional screening can be done by any member of the health-care team such as a dietitian, dietetic technician, dietary manager, nurse, or physician. Nutritional screening and how it fits into the nutritional care process are discussed in greater detail in Chapter 7, and examples of screening instruments are shown there.

Nutritional assessment is defined by the American Society for Parenteral and Enteral Nutrition as "a comprehensive approach to diagnosing nutrition problems that uses a combination of the following: medical, nutrition, and medication histories; physical examination; anthropometric measurement; and laboratory data."[13] The Academy of Nutrition and Dietetics defines nutritional assessment as "a systematic method for obtaining, verifying, and interpreting data needed to identify nutrition-related problems, their causes, and their significance."[9] It involves initial data collection and continuous reassessment and analysis of data, which are compared to certain criteria such as the Dietary Reference Intakes or other nutrient intake recommendations.[9]

Nutritional Assessment Methods

Four different methods are used to collect data used in assessing a person's nutritional status: anthropometric, biochemical or laboratory, clinical, and dietary. The reader may find the mnemonic "ABCD" helpful in remembering these four different methods.

Anthropometric Methods

Anthropometry is the measurement of the physical dimensions and gross composition of the body. Examples of anthropometry include measurements of height, weight, and head circumference and the use of measurements of **skinfold thickness, body density** (underwater weighing), **air-displacement plethysmography, magnetic resonance imaging,** and **bioelectrical impedance** to estimate the percentage of fat and lean tissue in the body. These results often are compared with standard values obtained from measurements of large numbers of subjects. Anthropometry will be covered in Chapters 6 and 8. At the end of most chapters are suggested exercises, called assessment activities, that allow you to apply the concepts covered. In the assessment activities of Chapter 6, you will try your hand at skinfold measurements to estimate percent body fat and compare several methods of determining body composition.

Biochemical Methods

In nutritional assessment, biochemical or laboratory methods includes measuring a nutrient or its metabolite in blood, feces, or urine or measuring a variety of other components in blood and other tissues that have a relationship to nutritional status. The quantity of **albumin** and other **serum proteins** frequently is regarded as an indicator of the body's protein status, and **hemoglobin** and serum ferritin levels reflect iron status. Serum lipid and lipoprotein levels, which are influenced by diet and other lifestyle factors, reflect coronary heart disease risk.

Biochemical methods are covered in Chapters 7 through 9. An assessment activity in Chapter 8 suggests that you have your blood drawn and tested at a clinical laboratory and compare your results with recommended values. Assessment activities in Chapters 7 and 9 guide you through the application of key concepts as you evaluate biochemical and other data from patient records.

Clinical Methods

The patient's personal and family history, medical and health history, and physical examination are clinical methods used to detect **signs** and **symptoms** of **malnutrition.** Symptoms are disease manifestations that the patient is usually aware of and often complains about. Signs are observations made by a qualified examiner during physical examination. Enlargement of the salivary glands and loss of tooth enamel are clinical signs of frequent vomiting sometimes seen in patients with bulimia nervosa. Examining a patient for loss of subcutaneous fat and muscle in the neck, shoulders, and upper arms, a clinical sign of inadequate calorie intake, is included in **Subjective Global Assessment,** a clinical approach for assessing nutritional status that relies on information collected by the clinician through observation and interviews at the patient's bedside. Clinical signs and symptoms in nutritional assessment will be discussed in Chapter 10.

Dietary Methods

Dietary methods generally involve surveys measuring the quantity of the individual foods and beverages consumed during the course of one to several days or assessing the pattern of food use during the previous several months. These can provide data on intake of nutrients or specific classes of foods. Chapters 2 through 4 cover dietary methods. One of the assessment activities in Chapter 3 involves collecting a 24-hour dietary recall from a classmate and analyzing his or her nutrient intake using food composition tables.

Included among dietary methods is the use of computers to analyze dietary intake. A number of online dietary and physical activity assessment tools are available, as are numerous software programs for computers that allow nutritionists and dietitians to quickly analyze the nutrient composition of dietary intake. These online systems and software programs vary widely in price and certain features, such as the number and types of different foods and nutrients that each contains. Chapter 5 covers selection and use of nutritional analysis software and online systems. The assessment activity in Chapter 5 involves computerized analysis of the 24-hour recall and 3-day food record collected as part of the assessment activities in Chapter 3.

Importance of Nutritional Assessment

The use of nutritional assessment to identify diet-related disease has increased in importance in recent years because of our greater knowledge of the relationship between nutrition and health and our expanded ability to alter the nutritional state.

Evidence related to the role of diet in maternal and child health indicates that well-nourished mothers produce healthier children.[15,16] Sufficient intake of energy and nutrients, including appropriate body weight before pregnancy and adequate weight gain during pregnancy, improves infant birth weight and reduces infant **morbidity** and **mortality.** Consequently, nutritional assessment has become an integral part of maternity care at the beginning of pregnancy and periodically throughout pregnancy and lactation.[15,17] Nutrition also can have a profound influence on health, affecting growth and development of infants, children, and adolescents; immunity against disease; morbidity and mortality from illness or surgery; and risk of such diseases as cancer, coronary heart disease, and diabetes.[17–19]

Interventions to alter a person's nutritional state can take many forms. In certain situations, nutrient mixes can be delivered into the stomach or small intestine through feeding tubes **(enteral nutrition)** or administered directly into veins **(parenteral nutrition)** to improve nutritional status. Thus, nutritional assessment is important in identifying persons at nutritional risk, in determining what type of nutrition intervention, if any, may be appropriate to alter nutritional status, and in monitoring the effects of nutrition intervention.

The Nutrition Care Process

The Nutrition Care Process (NCP) is "a systematic problem-solving method" in which dietetic practitioners use critical-thinking skills to make evidence-based decisions addressing the nutrition-related problems of those they serve, whether it be patients, clients, groups, or communities of any age or health condition (collectively referred to as "patients/clients").[9–12] Developed by the Academy of Nutrition and Dietetics (formerly known as the American Dietetic Association), the NCP establishes a consistent, *standardized process* for the delivery of nutrition-related care to patients/clients that is safe, effective, and of high quality. In addition, the Academy of Nutrition and Dietetics has created a set of standardized phrases or "terms" that are organized into categories or "domains," with each phrase having its own unique alphanumeric code for identification and documentation purposes. These phrases or terms were developed to allow dietetic practitioners to clearly describe, document, and evaluate the nutrition-related care they provide to their patients/clients. The terms facilitate clear and specific communication among practitioners and with other members of the health-care team.[9,12] This standardized terminology is described in greater detail later in this chapter.

It is important to note that while the NCP is intended to help standardize the process of delivering nutrition-related care, is not intended to standardize the actual nutrition care that different patients/clients receive.[9,10] The nutrition-related problems experienced by different patients/clients are highly variable, depending on numerous individual characteristics and circumstances that are unique to each patient/client and that will require an intervention that is uniquely suited to the condition of each individual patient/client. The NCP is designed to improve the consistency and quality of nutrition-related care that patients/clients receive and to ensure that the outcomes or results of that care are more predictable.[9,10]

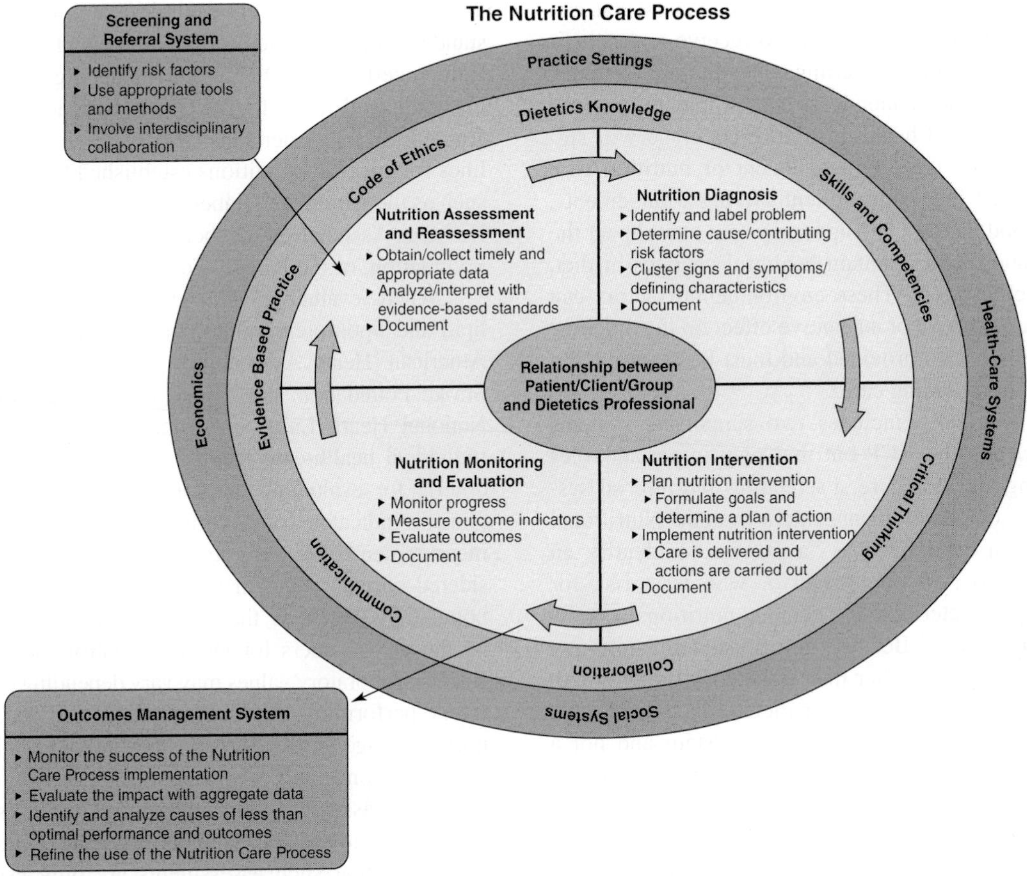

Figure 1.1 **The four distinct but interrelated and connected steps of the Nutrition Care Process and Model.**

The Nutrition Care Process and Model, *International Dietetics and Nutrition Terminology (IDNT) Reference Manual: Standardized Language for the Nutrition Care Process,* Third Edition. Copyright © 2011Academy of Nutrition and Dietetics (formerly the American Dietetic Association). Reproduced with permission.

There are four steps in the NCP: nutritional assessment, nutrition diagnosis, nutrition intervention, and nutritional monitoring and evaluation.[9,10] Nutritional assessment, the first step, involves collecting, verifying, recording, and interpreting a variety of data that are relevant to the nutritional status of the patient or client. These data, also referred to as **nutrition care indicators,** allow the practitioner to determine whether a nutrition problem exists and to make informed decisions about the nature, cause, and significance of nutrition-related problems that do exist.[10] Thus, nutritional assessment is essential to and an initial step in the delivery of cost-effective and high-quality nutrition care.

The Nutrition Care Process Model

The NCP is graphically represented by the Nutrition Care Process Model shown in Figure 1.1. At the very center of the NCP is the relationship between the dietetic professional and the patient/client, illustrating that the nutrition care provided is to be patient/client-centered. The practitioner should interact with the patient/client in a respectful, empathetic, nonjudgmental, and culturally sensitive manner and demonstrate good listening skills. This will help ensure that the patient/client is actively involved in setting the goals and outcomes of any intervention and that these are patient-focused, reasonable, achievable, incremental, and measurable.

The inner ring in Figure 1.1 lists the four steps of the NCP: nutritional assessment, nutrition diagnosis, nutrition intervention, and nutritional monitoring and evaluation. Nutritional assessment is the initial step in the NCP, and its purpose is to establish a foundation for progressing through the remaining three steps. The strengths and abilities that the practitioner brings to the process are listed in the middle ring: unique dietetics knowledge, skills and competencies, critical-thinking skills, collaboration, communication, evidence-based practice, and a code of ethics. Evidence-based practice involves incorporating the most current available scientific information in the nutrition-related care provided. Adherence to a professional code of ethics ensures that patients/clients are cared for in a manner conforming to strict social, professional, and moral standards of conduct.[9,10]

The outer ring lists environmental factors that can impact the patient/client's ability to receive and benefit from the NCP: practice settings, health-care systems, social systems, and economics. For example, the patient/client's income and health insurance coverage will significantly impact the type and extent of nutrition care that is provided. The patient/client's living arrangements, access to food, and social-support system can impact the ability to adopt and maintain healthful changes in diet, physical activity, etc. These environmental factors can have either a positive or a negative effect on the outcome of the nutrition care provided and must be assessed and considered in providing care.

The model also includes two supporting systems that are *outside* the NCP but that play important roles in providing nutrition care: a screening and referral system and an outcomes management system. Nutritional screening can be defined as "a process to identify an individual who is malnourished or who is at risk for malnutrition to determine if a detailed nutritional assessment is indicated."[13] Because nutritional screening may be done by someone other than a dietetics professional, such as a registered dietitian or dietetic technician, this is considered an external supportive system and not a step within the NCP.[10] If nutritional screening identifies a person at nutritional risk, a more thorough assessment of the individual's nutritional status should be performed. Nutritional screening is discussed in greater detail in Chapter 7, and examples of screening instruments are shown there. The outcomes management system evaluates the effectiveness and efficiency of the process by collecting and analyzing relevant data in a timely manner in order to adjust and improve the performance of the process.[10]

Nutritional Assessment in the Nutrition Care Process

Nutritional assessment begins once the nutritional screening indicates that the patient/client is at risk of malnutrition or may benefit from nutrition-related care. This in-depth assessment involves collecting a variety of relevant data, reviewing the data for factors affecting nutritional and health status, clustering or grouping various data points in order to establish a nutrition diagnosis, and then identifying nutrition care criteria against which the data will be compared for purposes of analysis. The NCP groups these nutrition care criteria into two categories: (1) a nutrition prescription or goal established by the nutrition practitioner in consultation with the medical team, and (2) reference standards for food and nutrient intake. A nutrition prescription or goal for a patient whose nutrition diagnosis is inadequate energy intake would include a level of energy intake that is considered appropriate for the patient's height, activity, and age and that would be expected to return the patient to a healthy body weight over time. Examples of reference standards for food and nutrient intake include the Dietary Reference Intakes (DRIs), the Dietary Reference Values for Food and Energy for the United Kingdom, the Dietary Guidelines for Americans, and clinical practice guidelines for specific conditions established by organizations such as the American Diabetes Association, the Canadian Diabetes Association, Diabetes UK, the National Kidney Foundation, or the Kidney Foundation of Canada.

When evaluating biochemical measures such as lipid and lipoprotein values, standards established by the American Heart Association, the Canadian Heart and Stroke Foundation, the British Heart Foundation, or the National Heart, Lung, and Blood Institute can be used. Individual health-care facilities generally have their own criteria for evaluating anthropometric, biochemical, and clinical indicators of nutritional status. Anthropometric measurements can be compared against what are considered normal values or ranges typically seen in healthy populations, such as the pediatric growth charts issued by the U.S. Centers for Disease Control and Prevention. Because laboratory values may vary depending on the laboratory performing the assay, as discussed in Chapter 8, normal ranges provided by the individual laboratory should be consulted.[9,10]

When assessing food and nutrient intake using information provided by the patient/client, it is important to remember that such assessments are only *estimates* of actual consumption because they are based on subjective information provided by the patient or a member of the patient's family. One exception to this is when the patient's sole source of nutrition is enteral and/or parenteral nutrition support, which can be objectively and accurately measured. Data on food and nutrient intake can then be compared to the patient/client's nutrition prescription or goal or to some reference standard such as the DRIs. When using the DRIs, it is important to note that they are intended for healthy populations and that clinical judgment is necessary when applying them to those who are ill or injured. In addition, an intake less than the Recommended Dietary Allowance or Adequate Intake does not necessarily mean that a nutrient deficiency exists. Finally, a thorough assessment of nutritional status must also include evaluation of anthropometric, biochemical, and clinical data, consideration of the patient's history, and relevant information collected by other members of the health-care team.[9–12]

If a nutrition problem exists, the data collected during the nutritional assessment and its analysis serve as the foundation for establishing the nutrition diagnosis, which is the second step in the NCP. Nutritional assessment is not a one-time, isolated event occurring at the beginning of a patient's nutrition-related care. It is more than simply the initial step of the NCP. It is a continuous, ongoing, nonlinear, data collection process spanning the entire duration of the patient/client's care and serving as

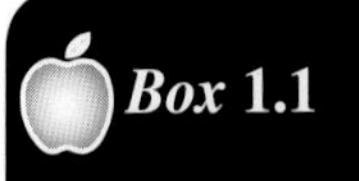

Box 1.1 The Categories or Domains of Nutrition Assessment Data and Nutrition Monitoring and Evaluation Data with Some Examples of the Types of Data Found Within Each Domain*

1. **Food/Nutrition-Related History**

   Food and nutrient intake: includes such factors as composition and adequacy of food and nutrient intake, and meal and snack patterns.

   Food and nutrient administration: includes current and previous diets and/or food modifications, eating environment, and enteral and parenteral nutrition administration.

   Medication and herbal supplement use: includes prescription and over-the-counter medications, including herbal preparations and complementary medicine products used.

   Knowledge, beliefs, attitudes: includes understanding of nutrition-related concepts and conviction of the truth and feelings/emotions toward some nutrition-related statement or phenomenon, along with readiness to change nutrition-related behaviors.

   Behavior: includes patient/client activities and actions which influence achievement of nutrition-related goals.

   Factors affecting access to food and food/nutrition-related supplies: includes factors that affect intake and availability of a sufficient quantity of safe, healthful food and water as well as food/nutrition-related supplies.

   Physical activity and function: includes physical activity, cognitive and physical ability to engage in specific tasks, e.g., breastfeeding and self-feeding.

   Nutrition-related patient/client-centered measures: includes the patient/client's perception of his or her nutrition intervention and its impact on life.

2. **Anthropometric Measures:** includes height, weight, body mass index (BMI), growth pattern indices/percentile ranks, and weight history.
3. **Biochemical Data, Medical Tests, and Procedures:** includes laboratory data (e.g., electrolytes, glucose, and lipid panel) and tests (e.g., gastric emptying time, resting metabolic rate).
4. **Nutrition-Focused Physical Findings:** includes findings from an evaluation of body systems, muscle and subcutaneous fat wasting, oral health, such as swallow/breathe ability, appetite, and affect.
5. **Client History***

   Personal history: includes general patient/client information such as age, gender, race/ethnicity, language, education, and role in the family.

   Patient/client/family medical/health history: includes patient/client or family disease states, conditions, and illnesses that may have a nutritional impact.

   Social history: includes items such as socioeconomic status, housing situation, medical care support, and involvement in social groups.

*The domains and types of nutrition assessment data and nutrition monitoring and evaluation data are the same except for the fifth domain, Client History. In nutrition monitoring and evaluation there are no nutrition care indicators associated with the domain Client History.

Source: *International Dietetics and Nutrition Terminology (IDNT) Reference Manual: Standardized Language for the Nutrition Care Process,* Third Edition.

the basis for the reassessment and reanalysis of relevant data in the fourth step of the NCP, nutritional monitoring and evaluation.[9,10]

Standardized Terminology in Nutritional Assessment

In the NCP, numerous types of data or nutrition care indicators are used to assess, describe, and document a patient's nutritional status and to monitor and evaluate the outcomes of the nutritional intervention. These indicators are organized into five categories or domains as shown in Box 1.1. When the nutritional assessment identifies a nutrition problem in a patient (that is, the patient's nutrition care indicator deviates in a clinically significant way from what would be expected or considered normal), a standardized term is used so that the problem can be specifically identified, clearly described, and easily documented. The Academy of Nutrition and Dietetics has developed approximately 170 standardized terms or phrases to be used for this purpose. These are listed in Appendix A. Because nutritional assessment and nutritional monitoring and evaluation share common elements (as discussed in greater detail below), most of the terms used in nutritional assessment listed in Appendix A are also used in monitoring, evaluating, and documenting the patient's response to any nutrition intervention he or she is receiving.[9] Similar sets of standardized terms have been developed for use when making nutrition diagnoses and planning and implementing any nutrition intervention. The standardized nutrition diagnostic terminology is shown in Appendix B, and the nutrition intervention terminology is shown in Appendix C. An example of how these standardized terms are used in nutritional assessment to identify and describe the type and severity of a problem is given in Box 1.2.

Because of the large amount of data that could potentially be considered for analysis, critical-thinking skills are necessary to enable the practitioner to limit the selection of data for analysis to only the data that are clinically relevant to the unique circumstances of the patient/client. Likewise, critical-thinking skills are

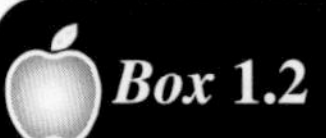

Box 1.2 How Standardized Language Is Used in Nutritional Assessment to Describe the Type and Severity of a Nutrition Problem

You are assigned to provide nutrition care to Mr. Anderson, a 54-year-old male admitted to your facility who has a medical diagnosis of essential hypertension. You begin your care with the first step in the Nutrition Care Process (NCP), assessing the patient's nutritional status. The first domain in the NCP standardized terminology for nutritional assessment shown in Appendix A is "Food/Nutrition-Related History" represented by the acronym "FH." As shown in the appendix, this domain considers the "composition and adequacy of food and nutrient intake, and meal and snack patterns."[9] Notice that the FH domain has the greatest number of nutrition care indicators of any of the five domains, and that these indicators are grouped into eight categories, with each category given a number (i.e., food and nutrient intake; food and nutrient administration; medication and herbal supplement use; knowledge/beliefs/attitudes; behavior; factors affecting access to food and food/nutrition-related supplies; physical activity and function; nutrition-related patient/client-centered measures). Under each of the eight categories in the FH domain are listed a number of nutrition care indicators, each assigned a unique alphanumeric code.

As you evaluate the Mr. Anderson's food/nutrition-related history (FH), you assess, among other things, his fluid/beverage intake (FH-1.2.1) and his food intake (FH-1.2.2) by administering a 24-hour recall (discussed in Chapter 3) and seeking additional detail by asking him to describe his usual diet over the course of a typical week. Because of his medical diagnosis and your knowledge of the relationship between sodium and potassium intake and risk of hypertension, you're particularly interested in his mineral/element intake (FH-1.6.2), especially his sodium intake (FH-1.6.2.7) and his potassium intake (FH-1.6.2.5).

As a result of your assessment of his usual diet, you discover that Mr. Anderson routinely eats breakfasts and lunches at fast-food restaurants and that he generally doesn't consider how much salt is in the foods he selects. When at home in the evenings, he frequently consumes canned soups, frozen entrees heated in a microwave oven, frozen pizzas that are baked in an oven, and a variety of other processed foods. Additionally, he reports that he seldom eats vegetables or fruits or other foods that are rich in potassium.

Based on his reported beverage and food intake and your analysis of information using diet analysis software (discussed in Chapter 5), your conservative estimate of Mr. Anderson's intake of sodium (FH-1.6.2.7) ranges between 3000 mg and 4500 mg per day. This is two to three times greater than 1500 mg per day, which, according to the *Dietary Guidelines for Americans* (discussed in Chapter 2), is the maximum recommended amount of sodium for someone who is 51 years of age or older or for anyone who has hypertension. In addition, you estimate that his usual potassium intake (FH-1.6.2.5) is 2500 mg per day, roughly half of the Adequate Intake (discussed in Chapter 2) of 4700 mg of potassium per day for adults. In this instance, the *Dietary Guidelines for Americans* and the Adequate Intake (one of the Dietary Reference Intakes) serve as appropriate reference standards for food and nutrient intake against which to compare or evaluate the nutrition care indicators sodium and potassium.

necessary in the appropriate interpretation of the collected data. The set of data that is considered relevant and how those data are interpreted will vary from one patient to another, depending on the patient's status.[9] To guide practitioners in the proper selection, measurement, application, and interpretation of nutrition care indicators, the Academy of Nutrition and Dietetics has developed a set of "Nutrition Assessment and Nutrition Monitoring and Evaluation Reference Sheets," which are available from the Academy.[9]

Nutrition Diagnosis in the Nutrition Care Process

The purpose of the second step in the NCP is to establish a nutrition diagnosis that specifically identifies and describes a nutrition problem that a dietetic practitioner is responsible for independently treating.[9] It is important to note that a nutrition diagnosis is different from a medical diagnosis. The medical diagnosis refers to the process of determining the existence of a disease and identifying or classifying the disease based on various criteria, such as the patient's **signs** and **symptoms,** the results of diagnostic tests, and relevant data from the nutritional assessment. The medical diagnosis then allows the medical practitioner (e.g., physician, physician assistant, nurse practitioner) to make medical decisions about treating the disease and predicting the likely outcome of the disease. In contrast, the nutrition diagnosis is the "identification and labeling of a specific nutrition problem that food and nutrition professionals are responsible for treating independently."[9] The nutrition diagnosis and subsequent intervention focus on specific nutrition and dietary issues and food-related behaviors that may cause a disease or be a consequence of a disease. In other words, the dietetic practitioner establishes the nutrition diagnosis by identifying and labeling a nutrition problem which he or she is legally and professionally responsible for treating by working collaboratively with the patient and with other members of the health-care team to improve the patient's nutritional status.[9,11] Data from the nutritional assessment are the basis for establishing the nutrition diagnosis and for setting reasonable and measurable outcomes that can be expected from any subsequent intervention in the third step of the NCP.

As part of its process of establishing a standardized language for dietetic practitioners, the Academy of Nutrition and Dietetics has identified 70 nutrition diagnostic terms that specifically and clearly identify those nutrition diagnoses or problems that dietetic practitioners can independently treat. Each term has its own unique alphanumeric code for identification and documentation purposes. These nutrition diagnostic terms and their codes are shown in Appendix B. The terms are grouped into three categories or domains: intake, clinical, and behavioral/environmental. The intake domain includes those nutrition problems related to *inadequate*, *excessive,* or *inappropriate intake* of energy, nutrients, fluids, or bioactive substances through oral diet or nutrition support (i.e., enteral or parenteral nutrition). For example, excessive energy intake is represented by the code NI-1.5 and excessive fat intake is represented by the code NI-5.6.2. The clinical domain includes those nutritional findings or problems related to medical or physical conditions such as swallowing difficulty (code NC-1.1), a food–medication interaction (code NC-2.3), or unintentional weight loss (code NC-3.2). The behavioral/environmental domain includes those nutrition findings related to knowledge, attitudes/beliefs, physical environment, food safety, or access to food, water, or nutrition-related supplies. For example, a food-related knowledge deficit is represented by the code NB-1.1, and limited access to food or water is coded NB-3.2.[9]

In addition to this set of nutrition diagnostic terms for identifying and labeling nutrition problems, there is a nutrition diagnosis reference sheet for each nutrition diagnosis. Each reference sheet gives the nutrition diagnosis label, defines the nutrition diagnosis, lists common etiologies (causes) of the diagnosis, and lists signs and symptoms that often accompany the diagnosis.

During documentation, the nutrition diagnosis is summarized in a single, structured sentence or nutrition diagnosis statement having three distinct components: the problem (P), the etiology (E), and the signs and symptoms (S). Also known as a PES statement, it identifies the problem using the appropriate diagnostic term, addresses the etiology or root cause or contributing risk factors of the problem, and lists signs and symptoms and other data from the nutritional assessment that provide evidence to support the nutrition diagnosis.

The problem or diagnostic term describes the alteration in the patient's nutritional status that the dietetic practitioner is responsible for independently treating. It allows the practitioner to identify reasonable and measurable outcomes for an intervention and to monitor and evaluate changes in the patient's nutritional status. The etiology is the factors that are causally related to the problem or contribute to it. Clearly identifying the etiology will allow the practitioner to design a nutrition intervention intended to resolve the underlying cause of the nutrition problem, if possible. Evidence substantiating the nutrition diagnosis is relevant data from the nutritional assessment, the signs (objective data) reported by a physician or other qualified member of the health-care team, and the symptoms (subjective data) reported by the patient.

The PES statement is to be written following a specific format beginning with the nutrition diagnostic label, followed by the etiology, and ending with the signs and symptoms. These three components of the PES statement are linked together with the words "related to" and "as evidenced by." The format is: (the nutrition diagnostic label) related to (the etiology) as evidenced by (the signs and symptoms). For example, consider a 61-year-old male who has had a poor appetite and an unintentional weight loss of 15% during the past three months since he had a medical diagnosis of colon cancer, underwent a partial resection of his colon, and began receiving chemotherapy. The weight loss is based on the patient's weight history as documented in the medical record. The patient complains that since beginning chemotherapy, "food has tasted funny" and consequently he doesn't eat as much as usual. Dysgeusia, a distorted sense of taste, is a common drug–nutrient interaction associated with the chemotherapy agents he is receiving, and this often leads to inadequate oral intake. An assessment of the patient's usual diet for the past three months shows that his usual energy intake is approximately 60% of his estimated needs, clearly indicating inadequate oral intake (nutrition diagnostic code NI-2.1). An example of a PES statement for this patient would be: "Inadequate oral intake related to chemotherapy-associated dysgeusia as evidenced by oral intake at 60% of estimated needs." In this instance, the nutrition diagnostic label is inadequate oral intake, the etiology is the chemotherapy-associated dysgeusia, and the signs and symptoms are an oral intake at 60% of the patient's estimated needs. Another example of how standardized language is used to establish a nutrition diagnosis and how a PES statement is written is given in Box 1.3.

Nutrition Intervention in the Nutrition Care Process

The purpose of nutrition intervention is to resolve or improve the patient/client's nutrition problem by planning and implementing appropriate strategies that will change nutritional intake, nutrition-related knowledge and behavior, environmental conditions impacting diet, or access to supportive care and services.[9] The selection of the intervention is driven by the nutrition diagnosis and its etiology. The objectives and goals of the intervention serve as the basis for measuring the outcome of the intervention and monitoring the patient/client's progress.[9,11]

Nutrition intervention has two basic components: planning and implementation. During planning, multiple nutrition diagnoses must be prioritized based on

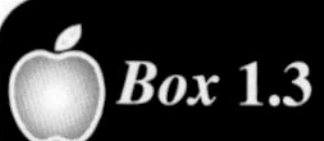

Box 1.3 How Standardized Language Is Used to Establish a Nutrition Diagnosis and to Write a PES Statement

Consider the case of Mr. Anderson, the 54-year-old male who has a medical diagnosis of essential hypertension and who was previously discussed in Box 1.2. Based on your evaluation of what he says he typically eats throughout the week, you estimate that Mr. Anderson's sodium intake ranges between 3000 mg and 4500 mg per day, which is two to three times greater than the *Dietary Guidelines for Americans* recommendation of no more than 1500 mg per day. You also estimate that his potassium intake is approximately 2500 mg per day which is considerably less than the Adequate Intake of 4700 mg per day for adults. Based on these estimates of Mr. Anderson's sodium and potassium intake, you are ready to proceed to the next step in the NCP, establishing a nutrition diagnosis.

You conclude that the most pressing nutritional problems needing to be addressed at this time are Mr. Anderson's excessive sodium intake and his inadequate potassium intake. Appendix B lists the nutrition diagnostic terminology, which is divided into three domains: intake, clinical, and behavioral-environmental.[9] The nutrition diagnostic term for excessive sodium intake is NI-5.10.2.7 and the term for inadequate intake of potassium is NI-5.10.1.5. The PES statement addressing Mr. Anderson's sodium intake would be: "Excessive sodium intake related to daily consumption of fast food and processed foods as evidenced by an estimated sodium intake of 3000–4500 mg per day compared to recommended 1500 mg per day." The PES statement addressing Mr. Anderson's potassium intake would be: "Inadequate potassium intake related to infrequent consumption of potassium-rich foods as evidenced by an estimated potassium intake of 2500 mg per day compared to recommended 4700 mg per day."

the severity of the nutrition problem, the intervention's potential impact on the problem, and the patient's needs and perceptions. Ideally, the intervention should target the etiology or root cause of the nutrition problem, although in some instances it may not be possible for the dietetic practitioner to change the etiology, in which case the signs and symptoms may have to be targeted. When determining the patient's recommended intake of energy, nutrients, and foods, the most current and appropriate reference standards and dietary guidelines should be used and modified, if necessary, based on the patient's nutrition diagnosis and health condition. These intake recommendations, along with a brief description of the patient's health condition and the nutrition diagnosis, are concisely summarized in a statement known as the nutrition prescription. Once the nutrition prescription is written, the specific strategies and goals of the intervention can be established. The intervention strategies should be based on the best available evidence and consistent with institutional policies and procedures. The goals of the intervention should be patient-focused, reasonable, achievable, measurable, and incremental, and, whenever possible, established in collaboration with the patient. During implementation, the dietetic practitioner communicates the plan to all relevant parties and carries it out. Relevant data on the patient's nutritional status are collected and used to monitor and evaluate the intervention's effectiveness and the patient's progress and, when warranted, to change the intervention to improve its safety and effectiveness.[9,11]

The Academy of Nutrition and Dietetics has established a standardized set of nutrition intervention terms, which are shown in Appendix C. These terms are grouped into four domains: food and/or nutrient delivery, nutrition education, nutrition counseling, and coordination of nutrition care.[9] The food and/or nutrient delivery domain includes those interventions that involve providing food and nutrition to the patient through meals, snacks, supplements, and enteral/parenteral nutrition support. The nutrition education domain includes those interventions that involve instructing or training the patient in a skill or providing knowledge that allows the patient to make better food choices that improve or maintain health. Nutrition counseling involves those interventions assisting the patient in setting priorities, establishing goals, and creating action plans that allow the patient to assume more responsibility for his or her own care. Coordination of nutrition care involves connecting the patient with other institutions or agencies that can assist the patient in managing his or her nutrition-related problems.[9,11] In addition, the Academy has developed a set of nutrition intervention reference sheets to guide practitioners in providing nutrition interventions that are consistent across the profession and that conform to the best available scientific evidence.

Nutritional Monitoring and Evaluation in the Nutrition Care Process

The purpose of the fourth step in the NCP, nutritional monitoring and evaluation, is to determine whether and to what extent the goals and objectives of the intervention are being met. In the NCP, nutritional monitoring and evaluation begins by identifying specific and measurable nutrition care indicators of the patient's behavior and/or nutritional status that are the desired results of the patient's nutrition care. These nutrition care indicators should be carefully selected so that they are relevant to the nutrition diagnosis, the etiology of the nutrition problem, the patient's signs and symptoms, and the goals and objectives of the intervention. In many instances the nutrition care indicators selected for monitoring and evaluation will be the same as those used in the initial assessment of the patient's nutritional status. The practitioner then monitors, measures, and evaluates changes in these nutrition care indicators to determine whether the patient's behavior and/or nutritional status are improved in response to the intervention.[9] The practitioner monitors the patient's knowledge, beliefs, and behaviors for evidence indicating whether the nutrition intervention is meeting its intended goals and objectives. Measurements of specific nutrition care indicators provide objective data on whether intervention outcomes are being met. The practitioner then evaluates the intervention's overall impact on the patient's behavior or status by comparing the current findings to those obtained earlier—for example, during the initial assessment of the patient's nutritional status.[9] Practitioners will find the "Nutrition Assessment and Nutrition Monitoring and Evaluation Reference Sheets" helpful in the proper selection, measurement, application, and interpretation of nutrition care indicators. These are available from the Academy of Nutrition and Dietetics.[9]

The definition of nutritional monitoring used in the NCP is somewhat different from that used when discussing national surveys of diet and health, which are covered in Chapter 4. When discussing these surveys of population groups, the term *nutritional monitoring* is defined as "an ongoing description of nutrition conditions in the population, with particular attention to subgroups defined in socioeconomic terms, for purposes of planning, analyzing the effects of policies and programs on nutrition problems, and predicting future trends."[14]

In the NCP, nutritional monitoring and evaluation is similar to nutritional assessment in several ways. In both steps, the types of data collected and their evaluation are similar, and the domains and types of nutritional assessment data shown in Box 1.1 are the same as those used in nutritional monitoring except for the fifth domain, client history. In nutrition monitoring and evaluation there are no nutrition care indicators associated with the client history domain. In both steps, the practitioner collects and records the data and then evaluates the data by comparing them to appropriate nutrition care criteria, such as the nutrition prescription or goal or some reference standard for food and nutrient intake. Nutritional assessment and nutritional monitoring and evaluation share the same set of standardized terms shown in Appendix A. However, important differences exist between the two steps. In nutritional assessment, the purpose of data collection and analysis is to establish the nutrition diagnosis if a nutrition problem exists and to develop any necessary intervention, whereas in nutritional monitoring the purpose of collecting and analyzing data is to evaluate the outcomes of the intervention. Generally, more nutrition care indicators are measured and evaluated during nutritional assessment than during nutritional monitoring and evaluation, because some data that are useful for initially assessing nutritional status may not be relevant as nutrition care indicators when determining the effectiveness of the nutrition intervention.[9]

Opportunities in Nutritional Assessment

Numerous opportunities currently exist for applying nutritional assessment skills. As our understanding of the relationships between nutrition and health increases, these opportunities will only increase. Following are some examples of areas in which nutritional assessment is making a significant contribution to health care.

Meeting the *Healthy People 2020* Objectives

The *Healthy People 2020* Objectives outline a comprehensive, nationwide health promotion and disease prevention agenda designed to improve the health of all people in the United States during the second decade of the twenty-first century.[20] Like the preceding *Healthy People 2010* initiative, *Healthy People 2020* is committed to a single, fundamental purpose: promoting health and preventing illness, disability, and premature death.[21] The 2020 objectives focus on four overarching goals: attain high-quality, longer lives free of preventable disease, disability, injury, and premature death; achieve health equity, eliminate disparities, and improve the health of all groups; create social and physical environments that promote good health for all; and promote quality of life, healthy development, and healthy behaviors across all life stages.[21] There are approximately 1200 objectives organized into 42 topic areas, with each topic area representing an important public health concern. The 42 topic areas are shown in Box 1.4. Of the approximately 1200 objectives, 22 are listed in the nutrition and weight status topic area, as shown in Box 1.5. Numerous other nutrition-related objectives are listed under other topic areas, such as cancer, diabetes, food safety, heart disease and stroke, physical activity, and maternal, infant, and child health.

For example, meeting objective NWS-10 (Reduce the proportion of children and adolescents who are considered obese) requires health professionals skillful in anthropometry and able to intelligently use the CDC growth charts or other appropriate methods for assessing body mass index or body composition. The ability to evaluate dietary intake and interpret laboratory data and physical signs and symptoms reflecting iron status would be important in evaluating progress on objectives NWS-21 and NWS-22. Objective NWS-18 (Reduce consumption of saturated fat in the population aged 2 years and older) requires a working knowledge of dietary survey methods to initially assess fat intake and to monitor long-term adherence to the objective.

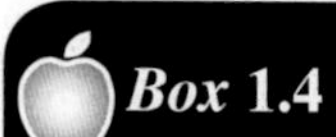

Box 1.4 *Healthy People 2020* Topic Areas

1. Access to health services
2. Adolescent health
3. Arthritis, osteoporosis, and chronic back pain
4. Blood disorders and blood safety
5. Cancer
6. Chronic kidney disease
7. Dementias, including Alzheimer's disease
8. Diabetes
9. Disability and health
10. Early and middle childhood
11. Educational and community-based programs
12. Environmental health
13. Family planning
14. Genomics
15. Global health
16. Health communication and information technology
17. Healthcare-associated infections
18. Health-related quality of life and well-being
19. Hearing, sensory, and communication disorders
20. Heart disease and stroke
21. HIV
22. Immunization and infectious disease
23. Injury and violence prevention
24. Lesbian, gay, bisexual, and transgender health
25. Maternal, infant, and child health
26. Medical product safety
27. Mental health and mental disorders
28. Nutrition and weight status
29. Occupational safety and health
30. Older adults
31. Oral health
32. Physical activity
33. Preparedness
34. Public health infrastructure
35. Respiratory diseases
36. Sexually transmitted diseases
37. Sleep health
38. Social determinants of health
39. Substance abuse
40. Tobacco use
41. Vision

From U.S. Department of Health and Human Services. 2010. *Healthy People 2020.* Office of Disease Prevention and Health Promotion. www.healthypeople.gov.

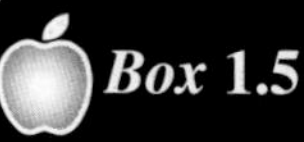

Box 1.5 *Healthy People 2020* Objectives for the Nutrition and Weight Status (NWS) Topic Area*

NWS–1: Increase the number of States with nutrition standards for foods and beverages provided to preschool-aged children in child care.

NWS–2: Increase the proportion of schools that offer nutritious foods and beverages outside of school meals.

NWS–3: Increase the number of States that have State-level policies that incentivize food retail outlets to provide foods that are encouraged by the Dietary Guidelines for Americans.

NWS–4: Increase the proportion of Americans who have access to a food retail outlet that sells a variety of foods that are encouraged by the Dietary Guidelines for Americans.

NWS–5: Increase the proportion of primary care physicians who regularly measure the body mass index of their patients.

NWS–6: Increase the proportion of physician office visits that include counseling or education related to nutrition or weight.

NWS–7: Increase the proportion of work sites that offer nutrition or weight management classes or counseling.

NWS–8: Increase the proportion of adults who are at a healthy weight.

NWS–9: Reduce the proportion of adults who are obese.

NWS–10: Reduce the proportion of children and adolescents who are considered obese.

NWS–11: Prevent inappropriate weight gain in youth and adults.

NWS–12: Eliminate very low food security among children.

NWS–13: Reduce household food insecurity and in so doing reduce hunger.

NWS–14: Increase the contribution of fruits to the diets of the population aged 2 years and older.

NWS–15: Increase the variety and contribution of vegetables to the diets of the population aged 2 years and older.

NWS–16: Increase the contribution of whole grains to the diets of the population aged 2 years and older.

NWS–17: Reduce consumption of calories from solid fats and added sugars in the population aged 2 years and older.

NWS–18: Reduce consumption of saturated fat in the population aged 2 years and older.

NWS–19: Reduce consumption of sodium in the population aged 2 years and older.

NWS–20: Increase consumption of calcium in the population aged 2 years and older.

NWS–21: Reduce iron deficiency among young children and females of childbearing age.

NWS–22: Reduce iron deficiency among pregnant females.

*NWS = nutrition and weight status

From U.S. Department of Health and Human Services. 2010. *Healthy People 2020.* Office of Disease Prevention and Health Promotion. www.healthypeople.gov.

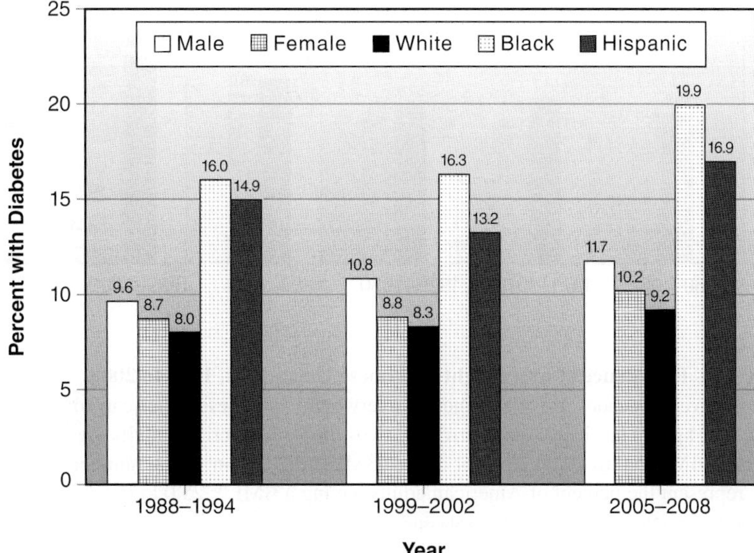

Figure 1.2 Percent of U.S. adults with diabetes by sex, race, and ethnicity, 1988–2008.

The values represent both physician-diagnosed diabetes and undiagnosed diabetes. Undiagnosed diabetes is defined as a fasting blood glucose ≥ 126 mg/dL or a hemoglobin Alc ≥ 6.5% and no reported physician diagnosis.

Data from the National Center for Health Statistics.

Health-Care Organizations

Health-care organizations such as physicians' offices, urgent-care clinics, emergency rooms, acute-care hospitals, and long-term care facilities offer many opportunities for health professionals trained in nutritional assessment. Inadequate food and nutrient intake are commonly seen in chronically ill patients, and one manifestation of this is **protein-energy malnutrition (PEM),** which is a loss of lean body mass resulting from inadequate consumption of energy and/or protein or resulting from the increased energy and nutrient requirements of certain diseases.[23]

Although the relationship between malnutrition and treatment outcome often is obscured by other factors that can affect the outcome of a patient's hospital stay (for example, the nature and severity of the disease process), several researchers have reported that patients with PEM tend to have a longer hospital stay, a higher incidence of complications, and a higher mortality rate.[22–26]

Identifying patients at nutritional risk is a major activity necessary for providing cost-effective medical treatment and helping contain health-care costs. Good medical practice and economic considerations make it imperative that hospital patients be nutritionally assessed and that steps be taken, if necessary, to improve their nutritional status. Evaluation of a patient's weight, height, midarm muscle area, and triceps skinfold thickness and values from various laboratory tests can be valuable aids in assessing protein and energy nutriture. Some researchers believe that rapid, nonpurposeful weight loss is the single best predictor of malnutrition currently available. These and other assessment techniques for hospitalized patients will be discussed in detail in Chapter 8.

Diabetes Mellitus

Diabetes is an increasingly common chronic disease in both developed and developing countries.[1,2] According to data from the National Center for Health Statistics, the prevalence of diabetes has increased in the United States in recent decades and among all U.S. adults is estimated to be 11%. As shown in Figure 1.2, there are marked differences in the prevalence of diabetes, depending on one's race or ethnicity. Nutritional assessment has been an important component in diagnosing and managing diabetes in recent decades and plays a major role in the American Diabetes Association's nutrition recommendations and principles for people with diabetes.[27] Goals for the person with diabetes are based on dietary history, nutrient intake, and clinical data. A thorough knowledge of the patient gained through nutritional assessment will assist the dietitian—the primary provider of nutrition therapy—in guiding the patient to a successful treatment outcome. The role of nutritional assessment in managing diabetes is discussed further in Chapter 8.

Weight Management

The *Dietary Guidelines for Americans*[6] defines a "healthy weight" range for most adults as a body mass index, or BMI (weight in kilograms divided by height in meters

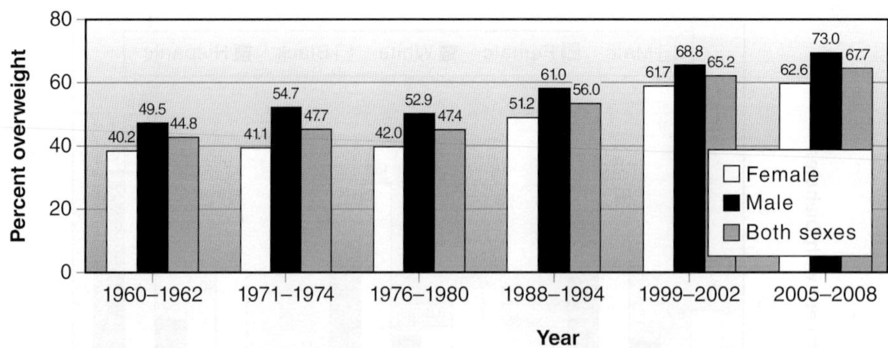

Figure 1.3 Prevalence of overweight and obese U.S. adults, 1960 to 2008.
In the past several decades, the prevalence of overweight and obese American adults (BMI $\geq$ 25.0 kg/m^2) has increased. Currently, two-thirds of American adults are either overweight (BMI 25.0 to 29.9 kg/m^2) or obese (BMI $\geq$ 30.0 kg/m^2). The numbers at the top of the bars represent the percent of American adults having a BMI $\geq$ 25.0 kg/m^2.
Source: Data from the National Center for Health Statistics.

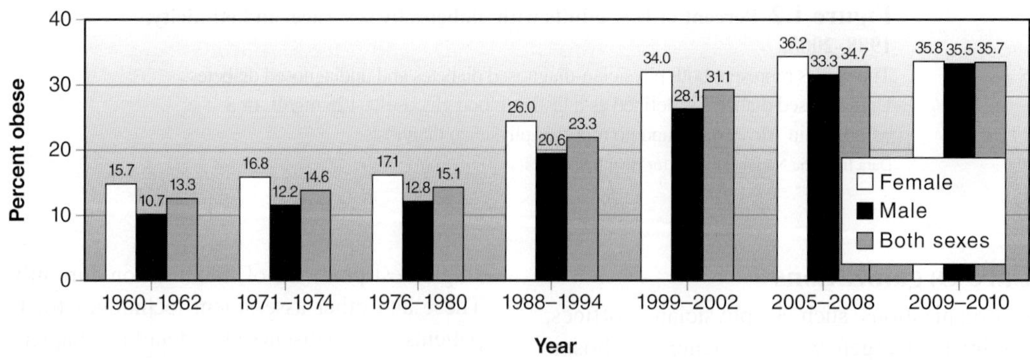

Figure 1.4 Prevalence of obesity among U.S. adults, 1960 to 2010.
The prevalence of obesity among American adults (BMI $\geq$ 30.0 kg/m^2) has increased, particularly between 1988 and 2002. More recent data show that the rate of increase has slowed considerably. Still, obesity remains a major public health problem, affecting more than one-third of American adults. The numbers at the top of the bars represent the percent of American adults having a BMI $\geq$ 30.0 kg/m^2.
Source: Data from the National Center for Health Statistics.

squared), of 18.5 kg/m^2 to 24.9 kg/m^2. **Overweight** is defined as a BMI range of 25.0 kg/m^2 to 29.9 kg/m^2, while **obesity** is defined as a BMI $\geq$ 30.0 kg/m^2. Based on these definitions, 73.0% of U.S. adult males and 62.6% of U.S. adult females are considered either overweight or obese (i.e., they have a BMI > 25.0 kg/m^2), while 33.3% of U.S. adult males and 36.2% of U.S. adult females are considered obese (i.e., they have a BMI $\geq$ 30.0 kg/m^2). Figure 1.3 shows how the prevalence of U.S. adults who are either overweight or obese (i.e., a BMI $\geq$ 25.0 kg/m^2) has increased since the early 1960s. Figure 1.4 shows the change in prevalence of obesity (i.e., a BMI $\geq$ 30.0 kg/m^2) between 1960 and 2010. Since the early 1960s the prevalence of obesity has also increased among U.S. children and adolescents, as shown in Figure 1.5. In persons 2 to 20 years of age, obesity is now defined as a BMI greater than or equal to the 95th percentile of BMI for sex and age using the pediatric growth charts developed by the U.S. Centers for Disease Control and Prevention, which are discussed in detail in Chapter 6.

National surveys conducted in Canada during the past three decades have shown a steady increase in the prevalence of overweight and obesity.[28–31] Between 1985 and 2003, the prevalence of obesity (BMI $\geq$ 30.0 kg/m^2) among Canadian adults nearly tripled, from 5.6% to 15.3%. In a survey conducted between 2002 and 2003, the prevalence of overweight (BMI 25.0 kg/m^2 to 29.9 kg/m^2) among Canadian males and females age 20 years and older was estimated to be 41.1% and 26.1%, respectively.[29] A survey conducted between 2007 and 2009 showed the prevalence of obesity (BMI $\geq$ 30.0 kg/m^2) among Canadian males and females age 20 to 74 years of age to be 24.3% and 23.9%, respectively.[31]

The increasing prevalence of overweight and obesity is not limited to the people of developed nations such

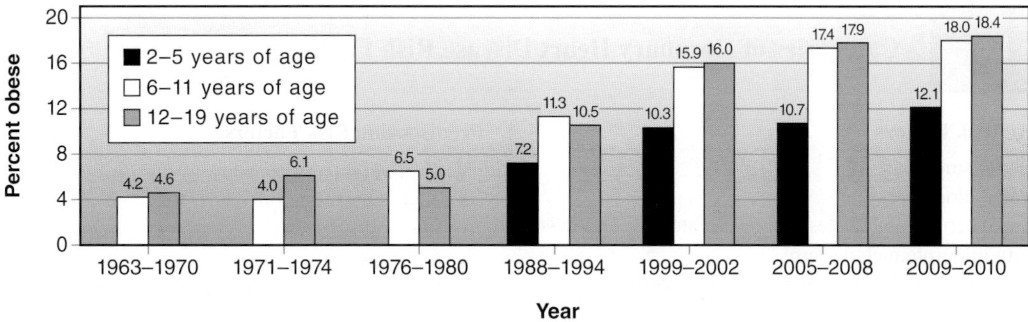

Figure 1.5 Prevalence of obesity among U.S. children and adolescents, 1963–2010.
In the past several decades, the prevalence of obesity has increased among U.S. children and adolescents. In persons 2 to 20 years of age, obesity is defined as a BMI greater than or equal to the 95th percentile of BMI for sex and age using the pediatric growth charts developed by the U.S. Centers for Disease Control and Prevention, or a BMI of 30 kg/m^2, whichever is smaller. Obesity prevalence data for persons 2–5 years old are not available prior to the 1988–1994 survey period.
Source: Data from the National Center for Health Statistics.

as the United States, Canada, and the European Union. The urban populations of many developing nations are experiencing a marked increase in the prevalence of overweight, obesity, and diet-related diseases such as cardiovascular disease and type 2 diabetes, paradoxically, while malnutrition, hunger, and starvation continue to plague the rural populations of these countries.[1] The term **globesity** has been coined to identify what many epidemiologists consider to be a global epidemic of obesity. While the term *epidemic* is typically used to describe a marked increase in the number of cases of an infectious or communicable disease over a certain period of time, the term can appropriately be used in the case of noncommunicable diseases or other adverse health conditions such as overweight and obesity, motor vehicle crashes, domestic violence, and firearm deaths. The World Health Organization estimates that by 2020 two-thirds of the global burden of disease will be due to noncommunicable diseases—such as cardiovascular diseases, type 2 diabetes, and obesity—that are linked to such dietary factors as increased consumption of fats, refined and processed foods, and foods of animal origin, and lifestyle factors such as tobacco smoking and physical inactivity.[32,33]

One of the *Healthy People 2020* objectives is to increase the proportion of U.S. adults who are at a healthy weight from the current proportion of approximately 30.8% who are at a healthy weight to the target of 33.9%, which is a 10% improvement.

National surveys provide important nutritional assessment data, such as prevalence of overweight and obesity in a particular population. Dietary methods can be valuable in initially assessing the quantity and quality of caloric intake and in monitoring dietary intake throughout treatment for obesity. Anthropometry is important in monitoring changes in percent body fat to help ensure that decrements in weight primarily come from body fat stores and that losses of lean body mass (mostly viscera and skeletal muscle) are minimized. Techniques for monitoring changes in percent body fat will be discussed in Chapter 6.

Heart Disease and Cancer

Heart disease and cancer are the first and second leading causes of death in the United States, respectively. Together they accounted for 48.9% of all deaths in 2010. Dietary factors playing a major role in heart disease are consumption of saturated fat, trans fat, and dietary cholesterol, and an imbalance between energy intake and energy expenditure leading to obesity.

Categories of coronary heart disease (CHD) risk factors are shown in Box 1.6. The "causative risk factors" are the major causal risk factors for CHD. When these are modified, CHD risk is reduced.[34,35] They can account for as much as 90% of the increased CHD risk in persons having these risk factors when compared with nonsmokers who have optimally low levels of blood pressure and total cholesterol, relatively high levels of high-density lipoprotein cholesterol, and no diabetes.[34,35] The "conditional risk factors" are correlated with CHD risk, but there are insufficient data from large, prospective studies to accurately quantify the extent to which these factors increase CHD risk.

The "predisposing risk factors" contribute to the development of CHD by intensifying or worsening the effects of the causative and conditional risk factors. According to the American Heart Association, two of these, obesity (particularly abdominal obesity) and physical inactivity are considered major risk factors because they are so strongly related to increased risk of CHD. Abdominal obesity is a particularly strong risk factor in postmenopausal women. Here it is defined as a

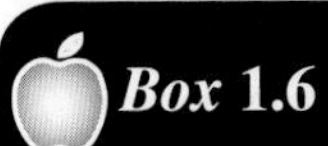

Box 1.6 Categories of Coronary Heart Disease Risk Factors*

Causative Risk Factors

- Cigarette smoking
- Elevated blood pressure
- Elevated serum total cholesterol or elevated serum low-density lipoprotein cholesterol
- Low serum high-density lipoprotein cholesterol
- Diabetes
- Advancing age

Conditional Risk Factors

- Serum triglycerides†
- Small low-density lipoprotein particles†
- Serum lipoprotein (a)†
- Serum homocysteine†
- Factors promoting blood coagulation†
- Inflammatory markers

Predisposing Risk Factors

- Overweight and obesity‡
- Abdominal obesity‡
- Physical inactivity‡
- Male sex
- Family history of premature coronary heart disease
- Socioeconomic factors
- Behavioral factors (e.g., mental depression)
- Insulin resistance

*A more detailed discussion of this box can be found in Chapter 8.
†These are considered conditional risk factors when serum levels are high.
‡Obesity and physical inactivity are considered major risk factors by the American Heart Association.

Adapted from Smith SC, Greenland P, Grundy SM. 2000. Prevention Conference V: Beyond secondary prevention: Identifying the high-risk patient for primary prevention: Executive summary. *Circulation* 101:111–116.

waist circumference > 102 cm (> 40 in.) in males and > 88 cm (> 35 in.) in females. Several of these factors (e.g., elevated blood pressure, diabetes, overweight and obesity, and serum levels of total and LDL-cholesterol, triglycerides, and homocysteine) are related to diet.

Despite a decline of more than 50% in the **age-adjusted death rate** since the 1970s, heart disease remains the leading cause of death in the United States and accounts for approximately 26% of all deaths. Because dietary therapy is the cornerstone of lowering serum low-density lipoprotein cholesterol, nutritional assessment skills are vitally important in its management. Proficiency in measuring diet, for example, would enable a dietitian to assess a client's consumption of saturated fat, *trans* fatty acids, and dietary cholesterol and suggest appropriate dietary changes. Chapter 3 includes a discussion of a questionnaire for assessing adherence to a cholesterol-lowering diet. Chapter 8 covers nutritional assessment in preventing heart disease.

Cancer is largely a preventable disease that results in more than a half-million deaths annually, which is more than 23% of all deaths in the United States.[36] Among Americans less than 85 years of age, cancer is the leading cause of death, although heart disease remains the leading cause of death when all Americans are grouped together.[36] Roughly two-thirds of all cancer deaths in the United States are linked to tobacco use, obesity, physical inactivity, and certain dietary choices, all of which can be modified by both individual and societal action. The percentage of cancer deaths attributable to dietary factors is estimated to be one-third.

The American Cancer Society guidelines on nutrition and physical activity for cancer prevention are shown in Box 1.7.[37] Methods for assessing dietary levels of fruits, vegetables, cereals, legumes, meats and other animal products, and alcoholic beverages will be necessary in applying these guidelines, as will anthropometric skills.

Nutrition Monitoring

When discussing national surveys of diet and health, which are covered in Chapter 4, nutrition monitoring is defined as "those activities necessary to provide timely information about the contributions of food and nutrient consumption and nutritional status to the health of the U.S. population."[14] As previously discussed, this definition of the term *nutrition monitoring* is different from when it is used within the context of the nutrition care process. A milestone in nutrition monitoring in the United States was passage of the National Nutrition Monitoring and Related Research Act of 1990. Key provisions of the act were development of a 10-year comprehensive plan for coordinating the activities of more than 20 different federal agencies involved in nutrition monitoring and assurance of the collaboration and coordination of nutrition monitoring at federal, state, and local levels.[14] This included all data collection and analysis activities associated with health and nutrition status measurements, food composition measurements, dietary knowledge, attitude assessment, and surveillance of the food supply. Considerable nutritional assessment expertise is required for conducting such surveys as the National Health and Nutrition Examination Survey and the Behavioral Risk Factor Surveillance System. These will be discussed in Chapter 4.

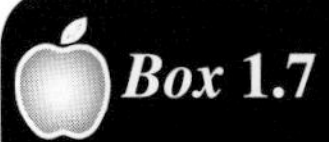

Box 1.7 American Cancer Society Guidelines on Nutrition and Physical Activity for Cancer Prevention

ACS Recommendations for Individual Choices

Achieve and maintain a healthy weight throughout life.

- Be as lean as possible throughout life without being underweight.
- Avoid excess weight gain at all ages. For those who are currently overweight or obese, losing even a small amount of weight has health benefits and is a good place to start.
- Engage in regular physical activity and limit consumption of high-calorie foods and beverages as key strategies for maintaining a healthy weight.

Adopt a physically active lifestyle.

- Adults should engage in at least 150 minutes of moderate intensity or 75 minutes of vigorous intensity activity each week, or an equivalent combination, preferably spread throughout the week.
- Children and adolescents should engage in at least 1 hour of moderate or vigorous intensity activity each day, with vigorous intensity activity occurring at least 3 days each week.
- Limit sedentary behavior such as sitting, lying down, watching television, or other forms of screen-based entertainment.
- Doing some physical activity above usual activities, no matter what one's level of activity, can have many health benefits.

Consume a healthy diet, with an emphasis on plant foods.

- Choose foods and beverages in amounts that help achieve and maintain a healthy weight.
- Limit consumption of processed meat and red meat.
- Eat at least 2.5 cups of vegetables and fruits each day.
- Choose whole grains instead of refined grain products.

If you drink alcoholic beverages, limit consumption.

- Drink no more than 1 drink per day for women or 2 per day for men.

ACS Recommendations for Community Action

Public, private, and community organizations should work collaboratively at national, state, and local levels to implement policy and environmental changes that:

- Increase access to affordable, healthy foods in communities, worksites, and schools, and decrease access to and marketing of foods and beverages of low nutritional value, particularly to youth.
- Provide safe, enjoyable, and accessible environments for physical activity in schools and worksites, and for transportation and recreation in communities.

Source: Adapted from Kushi LH, Doyle C, McCullough M, Rock CL, Demark-Wahnefried W, Bandera EV, Gapstur S, Patel AV, Andrews K, Gansler T, American Cancer Society 2010 Nutrition and Physical Activity Guidelines Advisory Committee. 2012. American Cancer Society Guidelines on Nutrition and Physical Activity for Cancer Prevention. *CA: A Cancer Journal for Clinicians* 62:30–67.

Nutritional Epidemiology

Practically all nutrition research undertaken by universities, private industry, and government involves some aspect of nutritional assessment. An understanding of the theory behind assessment techniques, an awareness of the strengths and weaknesses of assessment methods, and proficiency in their use are essential skills for anyone currently involved in or contemplating a career in **nutritional epidemiology.**

For example, to arrive at valid conclusions about the relationships between the intake of antioxidant nutrients, such as β-carotene, and risk of cancer or heart disease, nutritional epidemiologists need to know which methods best assess β-carotene nutriture and how to appropriately use those methods. Failing to do so, they would likely arrive at erroneous conclusions and disseminate inaccurate information about diet-health relationships. Methods for measuring diet are discussed in Chapter 3, and measurement of vitamin A status is presented in Chapter 9.

Epidemiologists examining the prevention and treatment of **osteoporosis** must understand, among other things, the strengths and weaknesses of various techniques to assess changes in bone mineralization. Such techniques will be discussed in Chapter 8. Researchers investigating the influence of diet and/or exercise on weight loss and changes in percent body fat use a variety of dietary and anthropometric methods to monitor caloric intake and changes in weight and body composition.

Studying the relationship between diet and disease risk is complicated by the difficulty of measuring the diet of humans, the considerable variety of foods people consume, the many nutrients and food components found in food, incomplete data on the nutrient composition of food, and the many other factors besides diet that influence disease risk. Consequently, there is considerable need for improved methods of measuring diet and assessing the body's vitamin and mineral status, as well as a need for better data on the nutrient composition of foods.

Summary

1. The relationship between nutrition and health has long been recognized. Scientific evidence confirming this relationship began accumulating as early as the mid-eighteenth century, when James Lind showed that consumption of citrus fruits cured scurvy.
2. Before the middle of the twentieth century, infectious disease was the leading cause of death worldwide, and nutrient deficiency diseases and starvation were common. Because of advances in public health, medicine, and agriculture, chronic diseases such as coronary heart disease, cancer, and stroke now surpass infectious diseases as the leading causes of death throughout the world and hunger and nutrient deficiencies remain problematic but are less common.
3. Although many factors contribute to the high incidence of chronic disease, diet plays an important role in 5 of the 15 leading causes of death in the United States, and excessive alcohol consumption is a prominent factor in 4 of the 15. The increasing prevalence of overweight and obesity is a particularly troubling global trend, even in developing nations where malnutrition, hunger, and starvation are, paradoxically, also common. Epidemiologists have coined the term *globesity* to identify what many regard as a global epidemic of obesity.
4. The continuing presence of nutrition-related disease makes it important that health professionals be able to assess nutritional status to identify who might benefit from nutrition intervention and which interventions would be appropriate.
5. Nutritional screening allows persons who are at nutritional risk to be identified, so that a more thorough evaluation of the individual's nutritional status can be performed. Nutritional assessment is an attempt to evaluate the nutritional status of individuals or populations through measurements of food and nutrient intake and nutrition-related health. Nutritional assessment techniques can be classified according to four types: anthropometric, biochemical or laboratory, clinical, and dietary. Use of the mnemonic "ABCD" can help in remembering these four types.
6. Our expanded ability to alter the nutritional state of a patient and our increased knowledge of the relationship between nutrition and health has made nutritional assessment an important tool in health care.
7. The Nutrition Care Process is a standardized problem-solving approach in which practitioners use critical-thinking skills to make evidence-based decisions addressing the nutrition-related problems of their clients/patients.
8. Nutritional assessment is the first step in the Nutrition Care Process and is critical to providing cost-effective and high-quality nutrition care in any health-care organization.
9. Objectives related to nutrition and health have a prominent place in the *Healthy People 2020* objectives. Skill in applying nutritional assessment techniques will play a major part in the health professional's efforts to help achieve those objectives.
10. Nutritional assessment is now a major component of the American Diabetes Association's nutrition recommendations and principles for people with diabetes.
11. Nutritional assessment also plays a significant role in identifying diet-related risk factors for heart disease and cancer and in monitoring efforts to reduce risk.
12. Nutritional assessment is central to current government efforts to monitor and improve the nutritional status of its citizens. It is also a skill essential for nutritional epidemiologists and other nutrition researchers investigating links between diet and health.

References

1. Yach D, Hawkes C, Gould CL, Hofman KJ. 2004. The global burden of chronic diseases: Overcoming impediments to prevention and control. *Journal of the American Medical Association* 291:2616–2622.
2. Stein AD, Martorell R. 2006. The emergence of diet-related chronic diseases in developing countries. In Bowman BA, Russell RM (eds.), *Present knowledge in nutrition,* 9th ed., 891–905. Washington, DC: International Life Science Institute.

3. Todhunter EN. 1976. Chronology of some events in the development and application of the science of nutrition. *Nutrition Reviews* 34:353–65.
4. Todhunter EN. 1962. Development of knowledge in nutrition. *Journal of the American Dietetic Association* 41:335–40.
5. Black RE, Cousens S, Johnson HL, Lawn JE, et al. 2010. Global, regional and national causes of child mortality in 2008: A systemic analysis. *Lancet.* Published online May 12, 2010. DOI:10.1016/S0140-6736(10)60549-1.
6. U.S. Department of Health and Human Services and U.S. Department of Agriculture. 2010. *Dietary Guidelines for Americans, 2010.* Washington, DC: U.S. Government Printing Office.
7. Shields M, Carroll MD, Ogden CL. 2011. *Adult Obesity Prevalence in Canada and the United States.* NCHS Data Brief no. 56. Hyattsville, MD: National Center for Health Statistics.
8. Shi Y, de Groh M, Morrison H, Robinson C, Vardy L. 2011. Dietary sodium intake among Canadian adults with and without hypertension. *Chronic Diseases in Canada* 31:79–87.
9. American Dietetic Association. 2011. *International Dietetics and Nutrition Terminology (IDNT) Reference Manual: Standardized Language for the Nutrition Care Process.* 3rd ed. Chicago: American Dietetic Association.
10. Lacey K, Pritchett E. 2003. Nutrition care process and model: ADA adopts road map to quality care and outcomes management. *Journal of the American Dietetic Association* 103:1061–1072.
11. Writing Group of the Nutrition Care Process/Standardized Language Committee. 2008. Nutrition care process and model part I: The 2008 update. *Journal of the American Dietetic Association* 108:1113–1117.
12. Writing Group of the Nutrition Care Process/Standardized Language Committee. 2008. Nutrition care process part II: Using the International Dietetics and Nutrition Terminology to document the nutrition care process. *Journal of the American Dietetic Association* 108:1287–1293.
13. Mueller C, Compher C, Druyan ME. 2011. ASPEN clinical guidelines: Nutrition screening, assessment, and intervention in adults. *Journal of Parenteral and Enteral Nutrition* 35:16–24.
14. Briefel RR. 2006. Nutrition monitoring in the United States. In Bowman BA, Russell RM (eds.), *Present knowledge in nutrition,* 9th ed., 838–58. Washington, DC: International Life Science Institute.
15. Turner RE. 2006. Nutrition during pregnancy. In Shils ME, Shike M, Ross AC, Cabellero B, Cousins RJ (eds.), *Modern Nutrition in Health and Disease,* 10th ed., 771–783. Philadelphia: Lippincott Williams & Wilkins.
16. Institute of Medicine. 2009. *Weight Gain During Pregnancy: Reexamining the Guidelines.* Washington, DC: National Academies Press.
17. Picciano MF, McDonald SS. 2006. Lactation. In Shils ME, Shike M, Ross AC, Cabellero B, Cousins RJ (eds.), *Modern nutrition in health and disease,* 10th ed., 784–796. Philadelphia: Lippincott Williams & Wilkins.
18. Heird WC, Cooper A. 2006. Infancy and childhood. In Shils ME, Shike M, Ross AC, Cabellero B, Cousins RJ (eds.), *Modern Nutrition in Health and Disease,* 10th ed., 797–817. Philadelphia: Lippincott Williams & Wilkins.
19. Treuth MS, Griffin IJ. 2006. Adolescence. In Shils ME, Shike M, Ross AC, Cabellero B, Cousins RJ (eds.), *Modern nutrition in health and disease,* 10th ed., 818–829. Philadelphia: Lippincott Williams & Wilkins.
20. U.S. Department of Health and Human Services. 2010. *Healthy People 2020.* Office of Disease Prevention and Health Promotion. www.healthypeople.gov.
21. Koh HK. 2010. A 2020 vision for healthy people. *New England Journal of Medicine* 362:1653–1656.
22. Torun B. 2006. Protein-energy malnutrition. In Shils ME, Shike M, Ross AC, Cabellero B, Cousins RJ (eds.), *Modern nutrition in health and disease,* 10th ed., 881–908. Philadelphia: Lippincott Williams & Wilkins.
23. Hensrud DD. 1999. Nutrition screening and assessment. *Medical Clinics of North America* 83:1526–1546.
24. Jeejeebhoy KN. 1998. Nutritional assessment. *Gastroenterology Clinics of North America* 27:347–369.
25. Pirlich M, Schutz T, Kemps M, Luhman N, Burmester GR, Baumann G. 2003. Prevalence of malnutrition in hospitalized medical patients: Impact of underlying disease. *Digestive Diseases* 21:245–251.
26. Donini LM, De Bernardini L, De Felice MR, Savina C, Coletti C, Cannella C. 2004. Effect of nutritional status on clinical outcome in a population of geriatric rehabilitation patients. *Aging Clinical and Experimental Research* 16:132–138.
27. American Diabetes Association. 2008. Nutrition recommendations and interventions for diabetes: A position statement of the American Diabetes Association. *Diabetes Care* 31(Suppl 1):S61–S78.
28. Katzmarzyk PT. 2002. The Canadian obesity epidemic, 1985–1998. *Canadian Medical Association Journal* 166:1039–1040.
29. Sanmartin C, Ng E, Blackwell D, Gentleman J, Martinez M, Simile C. 2004. *Joint Canada/United States Survey of Health, 2002–03.* Ottawa: Statistics Canada.
30. Katzmarzyk PT, Mason C. 2006. Prevalence of class I, II and III obesity in Canada. *Canadian Medical Association Journal* 174:156–157.
31. Shields M, Carroll MD, Ogden CL. 2011. *Adult Obesity Prevalence in Canada and the United States.* NCHS Data Brief no 56. Hyattsville, MD: National Center for Health Statistics.
32. Evans A, Tolonen H, Hense HW, Ferrario M, Sans S, Kuulasmaa K, for the WHO MONICA Project.

2001. Trends in coronary risk factors in the WHO MONICA Project. *International Journal of Epidemiology* 30 (Suppl 1): S35–S40.

33. Chopra M, Galbraith S, Darnton-Hill I. 2002. A global response to a global problem: The epidemic of overnutrition. *Bulletin of the World Health Organization* 80:952–958.
34. Smith SC, Greenland P, Grundy SM. 2000. Prevention Conference V: Beyond secondary prevention: Identifying the high-risk patient for primary prevention: Executive summary. *Circulation* 101:111–116.
35. U.S. Department of Health and Human Services. 2002. *Third Report of the National Cholesterol Education Program Expert Panel on Detection, Evaluation, and Treatment of High Blood Cholesterol in Adults.* Washington, DC: National Institutes of Health, National Heart, Lung, and Blood Institute.
36. Siegel R, Naishadham D, Jemal A. 2012. Cancer statistics 2012. *CA: A Cancer Journal for Clinicians* 62:10–29.
37. Kushi LH, Doyle C, McCullough M, Rock CL, Demark-Wahnefried W, Bandera EV, Gapstur S, Patel AV, Andrews K, Gansler T, American Cancer Society 2010 Nutrition and Physical Activity Guidelines Advisory Committee. 2012. American Cancer Society Guidelines on Nutrition and Physical Activity for Cancer Prevention. *CA: A Cancer Journal for Clinicians* 62:30–67.

CHAPTER

STANDARDS FOR NUTRIENT INTAKE 2

CHAPTER OUTLINE

Introduction

Early Dietary Standards and Recommendations

Recommended Dietary Allowances

Dietary Reference Intakes

Nutrient Density

Indices of Diet Quality

Dietary Guidelines

Nutrition Labeling of Food

Food Guides

Food Guide Pyramid

MyPlate

Food Exchange System

Summary

References

Assessment Activity 2.1: Using Standards to Evaluate Nutrient Intake

Assessment Activity 2.2: Food Exchange System

STUDENT LEARNING OUTCOMES

After studying this chapter, the student will be able to:

1. Compare and contrast the factors that influenced the development of early and more recent dietary standards.
2. Differentiate between observational and scientifically based dietary standards.
3. Discuss the development of the dietary reference intakes.
4. Name the characteristics of nutrient-dense foods.
5. Describe how the Healthy Eating Index-2005 is used to score dietary intake.
6. Discuss the key differences between the latest edition of the *Dietary Guidelines for Americans* and earlier editions.
7. Identify the purposes of the Nutrition Labeling and Education Act of 1990.
8. Demonstrate an understanding of the key aspects of the Nutrition Facts label.
9. Explain the Institute of Medicine's recent recommendations for the design of front-of-package labels.

INTRODUCTION

This chapter discusses a variety of recommendations and standards that can be used for evaluating the food and nutrient intake of groups and individuals. Prominent among these are the Dietary Reference Intakes, the *Dietary Guidelines for Americans,* regulations governing the nutrition labeling of food, the USDA's MyPlate graphic, and various other graphics developed to pictorially communicate recommendations for food intake and principles of good nutrition. Although most of these standards originally were designed to serve as standards for nutritional adequacy, to aid in diet planning, or to improve nutritional status, they are also useful as standards for evaluating the amounts and proportions of macronutrients, micronutrients, and various food components consumed by individuals and groups.

The primary impetus in the development of early dietary standards was the public's need for simple guidance on how to achieve nutritional adequacy from low-cost, readily available foods. During the millennia of human history prior to the mechanization of food production (which, historically speaking, is a relatively recent phenomenon), obtaining food was very labor intensive and subject to failure because of such conditions as drought and flooding, crop damage from pests, communicable diseases in humans, poverty, civil strife, and war. During this era hunger, nutrient deficiency, and starvation were common, and tragically, these conditions continue to plague sizeable numbers of people, particularly in developing nations. However, more recently the most pressing problem has been the increasing prevalence of chronic disease due in large part to the disproportionate consumption of total fats, saturated and *trans* fats, refined sugars, refined grains, sodium, and heavily processed foods, and the imbalance between energy intake and energy expenditure. Consequently, the focus of more recently developed dietary standards has shifted to what some refer to as our "food toxic environment," which contributes to the high prevalence of chronic disease such as obesity, heart disease, cancer, stroke, and type 2 diabetes.

Recognition of diet's role in health and disease has led to numerous efforts in the past several decades to formulate dietary guidelines and goals to promote health and prevent disease. A clear consensus has developed among most dietary guidelines and goals: dietary patterns are important factors in several of the leading causes of death, and dietary modifications can, in a number of instances, reduce one's risk of premature disease and death. Nutritional assessment is pivotal to improving dietary intake, thus reducing disease risk and improving health.

Early Dietary Standards and Recommendations

The earliest formal dietary standard was established in the British Merchant Seaman's Act of 1835. The act made the provision of lemon juice (known as "lime juice") compulsory in the rations of British merchant sailors. This action followed the 1753 treatise by British naval surgeon James Lind (1716–1794) stating that citrus fruits cure scurvy and the introduction in 1796 of lemon juice for the British Navy.[1] Throughout the remainder of the nineteenth century, dietary standards for protein, carbohydrates, and fat were proposed by scientists in Europe, the United Kingdom, and North America. These dietary standards had two things in common. First, the catalyst for their development was the occurrence of starvation and the diseases associated with it, resulting from economic dislocation and unemployment.[1,2] Second, they were, for the most part, **observational standards** because they were based on *observed* intakes rather than *measured* needs.[1]

Observational Standards

Carl Voit (1831–1908), a distinguished German physiologist of the late 1800s, made extensive observations of the amounts and kinds of foods eaten by German laborers and soldiers. Based on his observations, Voit concluded that the nutritional needs of a 70-**kilogram (kg)** male of his day doing moderate work would be met by a diet containing 118 g of protein, 500 g of carbohydrate, and 56 g of fat—a total of approximately 3000 **kilocalories (kcal).**[3] In 1895, Wilber Olin Atwater (1844–1907), a notable American physiologist and nutrition researcher who studied in Germany under Voit, observed the dietary habits of Americans. He recommended that men weighing 70 kg (154 lb) consume 3400 kcal and 125 g of protein each day.[2,3] For men engaged in more strenuous occupations, Voit and Atwater recommended 145 g and 150 g of protein per day, respectively. Rather than representing the actual physiological needs of the body, these recommendations were based on observations of what people eat when guided by their appetites and financial resources.[3]

One notable exception to the observational nature of dietary standards of the nineteenth century was the work of Edward Smith (1819–1874), a British physician, public health advocate, social reformer, and scientist who advocated better living conditions for Britain's lower classes, including prisoners. Smith conducted a dietary survey of unemployed British workers to determine what kind of diet would maintain health at the lowest cost.[2] His suggested allowances for protein, carbohydrate, and fat were based on actual laboratory measurements of caloric need and nitrogen excretion, as well as clinical observations that included absence of edema and anemia, "firmness of muscle, elasticity of spirits, capability for exertion."[1] Smith recommended approximately 3000 kcal of energy and 81 g of protein per day and believed that a diet adequate in calories and protein also would provide sufficient quantities of other necessary nutrients.[1,2]

Beginnings of Scientifically Based Dietary Standards

Advances in the early twentieth century in the ability to more accurately estimate actual energy and nutrient needs led to recommendations based on physiologic requirements for protein, carbohydrate, and fat. At the same time, tremendous strides were made in understanding the role of vitamins and minerals in human nutrition. This led to a reassessment and scaling down of protein recommendations in standards established during the 1920s and 1930s by the United Kingdom, the United States, and the League of Nations. There was also an effort to include recommendations for vitamins and minerals and to make allowances for nutritional needs during pregnancy, lactation, and growth.[2]

Concern about limited resources worldwide and food shortages in European countries during World War I led the British Royal Society to appoint a committee to establish a standard for human energy needs. After reviewing the energy expenditure data of several scientists, the Royal Society Committee accepted the results of calorimetry research conducted by the nutrition scientist Graham Lusk (1866–1932) as applicable to the population of the United Kingdom. Lusk recommended 3000 kcal/day as an average energy requirement for adult males, with an appropriate adjustment for the needs of women and children. This standard also was used in estimating food requirements for the United Kingdom, France, and Italy as a basis for American food exports to these countries during World War I. In addition, the Royal Society Committee recommended that daily protein intake for adult males not fall below 70 g to 80 g, with no less than 25% of calories coming from fat. The committee made no specific recommendation for vitamins and minerals, but it recommended that "processed" foods should not be allowed to constitute a large proportion of the diet and that all diets should include a "certain proportion" of fresh fruits and green vegetables.[1]

The economic depression following the stock market crash in 1929 was the impetus for several dietary standards developed by the United Kingdom, the League of Nations, and the United States. Foremost among these was the standard proposed by Dr. Hazel Katherine Stiebeling (1896–1989) of the USDA in 1933 (see Figure 2.1). Hers was the first dietary standard to make deliberate recommendations for minerals and vitamins and maintenance of health rather than maintenance of work capacity.[2,4] In addition to energy and protein, the desirable amounts of calcium, phosphorus, iron, and vitamins A and C were stated. In 1939, these recommendations were expanded to include thiamin and riboflavin.[1,4]

Beginning in 1935, the League of Nations Technical Commission issued a series of dietary recommendations that were less concerned with defining requirements of food constituents than with outlining desirable allowances of the "protective" foods that had been lacking in so many diets.[1] Consumption of such foods as fruits, leafy vegetables, milk, eggs, fish, and meat was encouraged. These were among what outstanding American biochemist E.V. McCollum termed "protective foods," because of his early observations that they tend to protect against nutritional deficiencies. The recommendations also raised questions about the use of refined sugar, milled grain, and other foods low in vitamins and minerals.[2]

In 1938 the Canadian Council on Nutrition adopted the *Dietary Standard for Canada,* the first set of dietary standards intended specifically for use in Canada. Based in part on the recommendations of the League of Nations and on information collected by the Canadian Council on Nutrition, it initially included recommendations for calories, protein, fat, calcium, iron, iodine, ascorbic acid, and vitamin D. The *Dietary Standard for Canada* was revised in 1950, 1963, and 1975. In 1983 Health Canada published the *Recommended Nutrient Intakes (RNIs) for Canadians.* As the links between diet and chronic disease risk became increasingly apparent, Canadian researchers realized the need for dietary recommendations that not only ensured adequate intake of all essential nutrients, but also reduced the risk of chronic conditions such as atherosclerotic heart disease, cancer, obesity, hypertension, osteoporosis, and dental caries (tooth decay). In 1990, Health Canada published *Nutrition Recommendations: The Report of the Scientific Review Committee.* In addition to the RNIs, which were intended to ensure adequate nutrient intake to prevent deficiency, the report recommended an energy intake consistent with maintaining a healthy body weight, restricting total fat to no more than 30% of energy and saturated fat to no more than 10% of energy, reducing sodium in the diet, ensuring adequate intake of potassium, consuming alcoholic and caffeinated beverages in moderation, and that community water supplies be fluoridated to the level of 1 mg/liter.

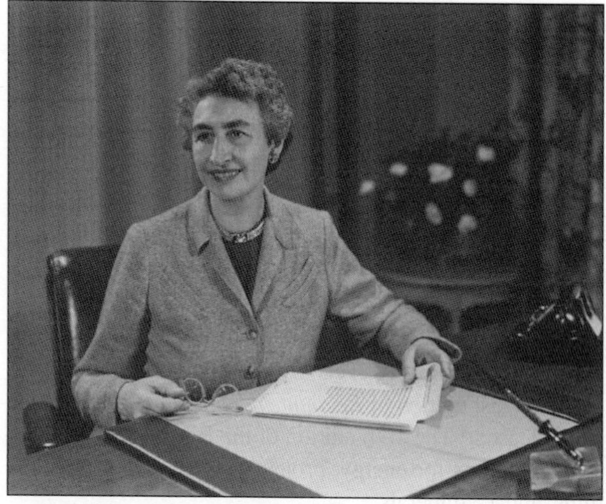

Figure 2.1 **Hazel K. Stiebeling (1896–1989)**
Stiebeling served in the U.S. Department of Agriculture from 1930 to 1963 as a research scientist and administrator. She was a pioneer in studying the food consumption patterns and dietary intakes of families in the United States and was instrumental in the development of the first edition of the Recommended Dietary Allowances.
Photo courtesy of Special Collections, National Agricultural Library, USDA.

Recommended Dietary Allowances

In 1940, the U.S. federal government established the Committee of Food and Nutrition under the National Research Council of the National Academy of Sciences in Washington, DC. In 1941, this committee was established on a permanent basis and renamed the Food and Nutrition Board.[2] The role of the committee was to advise government agencies on problems relating to food and nutrition of the people and on nutrition problems in connection with national defense.[5] In 1941, the committee prepared the first Recommended Dietary Allowances (RDAs), as shown in Table 2.1, "to serve as a guide for planning adequate nutrition for the civilian population of the United States."[7] The RDAs first appeared in print in 1941 in an article in the *Journal of the American Dietetic Association.*[7] However, it was not until 1943 that the first officially published edition of the RDAs appeared in book form.[2,4] To reflect advances in nutritional science, the RDAs were revised approximately every 5 years until 1989, when the 10th and last edition of *Recommended Dietary Allowances* was released.[8] The 10th edition of the RDAs provided recommendations for energy, protein, 3 electrolytes, 13 vitamins, and 12 minerals.

In essence, the RDAs have served as recommendations for nutrient intakes for 18 life stage and gender groups (life stage considers age and, when appropriate, pregnancy and lactation). The RDAs have accounted for individual differences in nutrient requirements and have included a fairly large margin of safety (i.e., they were set at a level considerably greater than the average requirement necessary to prevent deficiency disease).[9] They have been defined as "the levels of intake of essential nutrients that, on the basis of scientific knowledge, are judged by the Food and Nutrition Board to be adequate to meet the known nutrient needs of practically all healthy persons."[8] The first edition of *Recommended Dietary Allowances* was published with the objective of "providing standards to serve as a goal for good nutrition" and to serve as a guide for advising "on nutrition problems in connection with national defense."[8] However, since their inception, the RDAs have been used for a variety of other purposes for which they were not originally intended. These include use in labeling food, evaluating dietary survey data, planning and procuring food supplies for groups, planning food and nutrition information and education programs, and serving as a nutritional benchmark in the Food Stamp Program (renamed the Supplemental Nutrition Assistance Program or SNAP in October 2008); the Special Supplemental Food Program for Women, Infants, and Children (WIC); and the National School Lunch Program.

For more than 5 decades, the RDAs served as the premier nutrient standard, not only for the United States but also for many other countries throughout the developed and developing world. However, as knowledge of human nutrition increased and as nutritional concerns changed over time, limitations in the RDAs became apparent. For example, an underlying intent of the RDAs was to prevent deficiency disease. In recent decades, as chronic degenerative diseases have supplanted infectious and nutrient-deficiency diseases as the leading causes of death, there has been growing interest in the role of diet and nutrition in decreasing chronic disease risk, conditions that the RDAs fail to adequately address. For example, the RDAs provided no recommendations for carbohydrate, dietary fibers, total fat, saturated fat, or cholesterol. There were no nutrient recommendations for older persons and no recommendations for food components that are not traditionally defined as nutrients (e.g., phytochemicals, aspartame, caffeine, and alcohol).[10] In addition, the recommended nutrient intake levels of the RDAs were generally limited to amounts obtainable through diet alone, and there was no guidance on the safe and effective use of vitamin, mineral, and other nutrient supplements, despite considerable public interest in use of such supplements.

Consequently, there arose a need for a more comprehensive set of nutritional and dietary standards that adequately addressed more contemporary nutritional concerns. In response, the Food and Nutrition Board, working in conjunction with scientists from the Canadian Institute of Nutrition and Health Canada, developed a new and expanded set of nutrient intakes known as the Dietary Reference Intakes.[10–15]

Dietary Reference Intakes

The Dietary Reference Intakes (DRIs) are defined as "reference values that are quantitative estimates of nutrient intakes to be used for planning and assessing diets for apparently healthy people."[12] As shown in Box 2.1, they include four nutrient-based reference values—the Estimated Average Requirement, the Recommended Dietary Allowance, the Adequate Intake, and the Tolerable Upper Intake Level—and a recommendation for dietary energy intake known as the Estimated Energy Requirement. The DRIs attempt to address the weaknesses of the RDAs and to expand on the original Recommended Dietary Allowances by adding three new reference values and a recommendation for dietary energy intake.

The initiative to develop the DRIs formally began in June 1993, when the Food and Nutrition Board (FNB) organized a symposium and public hearing entitled "Should the Recommended Dietary Allowances Be Revised?"[9,10] This was followed by several symposia at nutrition-related professional meetings, at which the FNB discussed its tentative plans and invited input from interested nutrition professionals. From these activities arose a clear consensus that a more comprehensive set of nutritional and dietary standards was needed.

During this time period, Health Canada and Canadian scientists were reviewing the need to revise the Recommended Nutrient Intakes.[16] In April 1995, at a symposium cosponsored by the Canadian National Institute of Nutrition and Health Canada, Canadian scientists reached a consensus that the Canadian government should investigate working with the FNB in developing a set of nutrient-based recommendations that will

Table 2.1 The 1941 Recommended Dietary Allowances for Specific Nutrients*

	Kilocalories	Protein (*Grams*)	Calcium (*Grams*)	Iron (*Milligrams*)	Vitamin A† (*IU*‡)	Thiamin (*Milligrams*)	Ascorbic Acid (*Milligrams*)	Riboflavin (*Milligrams*)	Nicotinic Acid (Milligrams)	Vitamin D (*IU*)
Man (70 kg)										
Moderately active	3000	70	0.8	12	5000	1.8	75	2.7	18	§
Very active	4500	70	0.8	12	5000	2.3	75	3.3	23	
Sedentary	2500	70	0.8	12	5000	1.5	75	2.2	15	
Woman (56 kg)										
Moderately active	2500	60	0.8	12	5000	1.5	70	2.2	15	§
Very active	3000	60	0.8	12	5000	1.8	70	2.7	18	
Sedentary	2100	60	0.8	12	5000	1.2	70	1.8	12	
Pregnancy (latter half)	2500	85	1.5	15	6000	1.8	100	2.5	18	400–800
Lactation	3000	100	2.0	15	8000	2.3	150	3.0	23	400–800
Children up to 12 Years										
Under 1 year‖	100 per kg	3–4 per kg	1.0	6	1500	0.4	30	0.6	4	400–800
1–3 years¶	1200	40	1.0	7	2000	0.6	35	0.9	6	§
4–6 years	1600	50	1.0	8	2500	0.8	50	1.2	8	
7–9 years	2000	60	1.0	10	3500	1.0	60	1.5	10	
10–12 years	2500	70	1.2	12	4500	1.2	75	1.8	12	
Children over 12 Years										
Girls: 14–15 years	2800	80	1.3	15	5000	1.4	80	2.0	14	§
6–20 years	2400	75	1.0	15	5000	1.2	80	1.8	12	
Boys: 13–15 years	3200	85	1.4	15	5000	1.6	90	2.4	16	§
16–20 years	3800	100	1.4	15	6000	2.0	100	3.0	20	

This table was originally published in the *Journal of the American Dietetic Association,* Volume 17, June/July 1941, pages 565–567. Copyright Elsevier 2012.

*These are tentative allowances toward which to aim in planning practical dietaries. These allowances can be met by a good diet of natural foods that will also provide other minerals and vitamins, the requirements for which are less well known.

†Requirements may be less than the amounts stated if provided as vitamin A and greater if the source is chiefly the pro-vitamin carotene.

‡IU = International Units.

§Vitamin D is undoubtedly necessary for older children and adults. When not available from sunshine, it should be provided probably up to the minimal amounts recommended for infants.

‖Needs of infants increase from month to month. The amounts given are for infants approximately 6 to 18 months of age. The amounts of protein and calcium needed are less if from breast milk.

¶Allowances are based on the middle year for each group (as 2, 5, 8, etc.) and for moderate activity.

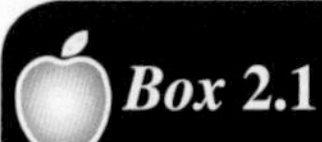

Box 2.1 The Dietary Reference Intakes

Estimated Average Requirement (EAR): The daily dietary intake level that is estimated to meet the nutrient requirement of 50% of healthy individuals in a particular life stage and gender group.

Recommended Dietary Allowance (RDA): The average daily dietary intake level that is sufficient to meet the nutrient requirement of nearly all (97% to 98%) healthy individuals in a particular life stage gender group.

Adequate Intake (AI): The recommended daily dietary intake level that is assumed to be adequate and that is based on experimentally determined approximations of nutrient intake by a group (or groups) of healthy people. The AI is an observational standard that is used when insufficient data is available to determine an RDA.

Tolerable Upper Intake Level (UL): The highest level of daily nutrient intake that is likely to pose no risk of adverse health affects to almost all apparently healthy individuals in the general population. As intake increases above the UL, the risk of adverse (toxic) effects increases.

Estimated Energy Requirement (EER): The average dietary energy intake that is predicted to maintain energy balance in a healthy adult of a defined age, gender, weight, height, and level of physical activity, consistent with good health. In children and in pregnant and lactating women, the EER includes the needs associated with the deposition of tissues or the secretion of milk consistent with good health.

Adapted from Panel on Macronutrients, Panel on the Definition of Dietary Fiber, Subcommittee on Upper Reference Levels of Nutrients, Subcommittee on Interpretation and Uses of Dietary Reference Intakes, Standing Committee on the Scientific Evaluation of Dietary Reference Intakes. 2002. *Dietary Reference Intakes for Energy, Carbohydrate, Fiber, Fat, Fatty Acids, Cholesterol, Protein, and Amino Acids.* Washington, DC: National Academy Press.

serve, where appropriate, the needs of both countries. In December 1995, the FNB began a close collaboration with the Canadian government and appointed a Standing Committee on the Scientific Evaluation of Dietary Reference Intakes (DRI Committee) composed of scientists from Canada and the United States to conduct and oversee the project. Consequently, the DRIs not only supersede the 10th edition of the *Recommended Dietary Allowances*[8] but also the Canadian Recommended Nutrient Intakes, which were last published in 1990.

The DRI Committee began its work by grouping the various nutrients and food components into eight categories and assigning each nutrient group to a panel of experts on those nutrients. The DRI Committee also formed two subcommittees: a Subcommittee on Upper Reference Levels of Nutrients to assist each panel in the development of the Tolerable Upper Intake Levels and a Subcommittee on Interpretation and Uses of Dietary Reference Intakes to determine appropriate examples for using the DRIs.[10–15] Box 2.2 shows the tasks of each panel.

The first DRI report was released in August 1997 and covered calcium, phosphorus, magnesium, vitamin D, and fluoride.[10] Subsequent reports have provided recommendations for the remaining vitamins and elements as well as for electrolytes, water, energy, physical activity, dietary fiber, and the macronutrients.[11–15] In 2011 the DRIs for calcium and vitamin D were updated in response to concerns that calcium intake might be inadequate in some groups and that calcium supplementation use was increasing, particularly among older persons, and the uncertainty about what levels of calcium intake were optimal or excessive. In recent years there has been increasing interest in the potential role of vitamin D in a variety of health outcomes, such as increasing immunity and preventing cancer, diabetes, and preeclampsia during pregnancy.[16] In addition, the DRI Committee has released three reports that provide guidance on applying the DRIs in dietary assessment, dietary planning, and the nutrition labeling and fortification of foods.[17–19] Table 2.2 shows the Estimated Average Requirements (EARs) for the 22 different life stage and gender groups, which are shown in the column at the extreme left of the table. Tables 2.3 and 2.4 show the Recommended Dietary Allowances (RDAs) and the Adequate Intakes (AIs) for vitamins and elements, respectively. In these two tables, the values in bold type are RDAs, and those values in ordinary type and followed by an asterisk are AIs. Tables 2.5 and 2.6 show the Tolerable Upper Intake Levels (ULs) for vitamins and elements, respectively. The DRIs use different life stage and gender groups for the ULs than those used for the RDAs, AIs, and the EARs. A link to the updated DRI tables is available on the *Nutritional Assessment* website at www.mhhe.com/lee-nieman6.

Estimated Average Requirement

The Estimated Average Requirement (EAR) is defined as "the daily intake value that is estimated to meet the requirement, as defined by the specified indicator of adequacy, in half of the apparently healthy individuals in a life stage or gender group."[12] The EAR serves as the basis for setting the Recommended Dietary Allowance (RDA). If an EAR cannot be established, then an RDA cannot be set. The currently established EARs are shown in Table 2.2.

Because of individual biological variation in nutrient absorption and metabolism, some individuals have a relatively low (lower than average) requirement for a nutrient,

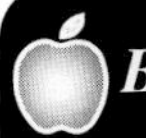

Box 2.2 Tasks of the DRI Panels

- Review the scientific literature for each nutrient or food component under consideration for each of the sex, age, and condition groups.
- Consider the roles of each nutrient or food component in decreasing risk of chronic and other diseases and conditions.
- Interpret the current nutrient or food component intake data for each of the sex, age, and condition groups in North America.
- Develop criteria or indicators of adequacy for each nutrient or food component and provide substantive rationale for each criterion or indicator.
- Establish the Estimated Average Requirement (EAR) for each nutrient or food component (assuming that sufficient data are available) and the Recommended Dietary Allowance (RDA) for each life stage and gender group. If data are insufficient for establishing the EAR/RDA, set the Adequate Intake (AI).
- Establish an Estimated Energy Requirement (EER) at four levels of energy expenditure for each of the sex, age, and condition groups in North America, recommend physical activity levels (PAL) for children and adults to decrease chronic disease risk, and establish Acceptable Macronutrient Distribution Ranges (AMDRs) for carbohydrate, total fat, *n*-6 and *n*-3 polyunsaturated fatty acids, and protein for children and adults.
- Participate with the Subcommittee on Upper Reference Levels of Nutrients in estimating the level of nutrient or food component intake above which there is increased risk of toxicity or an adverse reaction—the Tolerable Upper Intake Level (UL).
- Participate with the Subcommittee on Interpretation and Uses of the DRIs in developing practical information and guidance on appropriately using the DRIs.

Adapted from Standing Committee on the Scientific Evaluation of Dietary Reference Intakes, Food and Nutrition Board, Institute of Medicine. 1997. *Dietary Reference Intakes for Calcium, Phosphorus, Magnesium, Vitamin D, and Fluoride.* Washington, DC: National Academy Press, and from Panel on Macronutrients, Panel on the Definition of Dietary Fiber, Subcommittee on Upper Reference Levels of Nutrients, Subcommittee on Interpretation and Uses of Dietary Reference Intakes, Standing Committee on the Scientific Evaluation of Dietary Reference Intakes. 2002. *Dietary Reference Intakes for Energy, Carbohydrate, Fiber, Fat, Fatty Acids, Cholesterol, Protein, and Amino Acids.* Washington, DC: National Academy Press.

while others have a relatively high (higher than average) requirement. If the requirement of nutrient X in a given life stage and gender group (e.g., 19- to 30-year-old females who are neither pregnant nor lactating) were plotted as shown in Figure 2.2, a normal, or Gaussian, distribution might result, creating a bell-shaped curve. Although it is usually assumed that nutrient requirements are normally distributed, this is not always the case. In some instances, the nutrient requirements of a particular group may not be known because of insufficient data or, in the case of infants, because it would be unethical to perform the types of studies on infants that would be necessary to determine their nutrient requirements.[10–16] The EARs are sometimes, of necessity, based on scanty data or data drawn from studies with design limitations.[10–16] As seen in Figure 2.2, some individuals have a requirement for nutrient X that is much less than average, but the proportion of these people in a particular life stage and gender group is small, as indicated by the height of the curve above the horizontal axis. Likewise, the proportion having a requirement much greater than average is also small.

The DRI Committee defines requirement as "the lowest continuing intake level of a nutrient that, for a specified indicator of adequacy, will maintain a defined level of nutriture in an individual."[10–16] When setting the EAR, a specific criterion (or criteria) of adequacy must first be selected based on a thorough review of the scientific literature.[10–16] The DRI reports clearly identify the criterion or criteria used in establishing the EAR for each nutrient.[10–15] In some instances, the criterion differs for individuals at different life stages. Criteria used in establishing the EAR include the amount needed to prevent classic deficiency diseases, amounts of the nutrient or its metabolites measured in various tissues during depletion-repletion studies or during induced deficiency states in healthy adult volunteers, and the amount needed to adequately maintain a certain metabolic pathway that is dependent on the nutrient in question. When necessary because of insufficient data on the nutrient requirements of children, adolescents, and pregnant or lactating females, the DRI Committee may choose, when appropriate, to adjust the adult EAR on the basis of differences in reference weights of younger persons or to account for the increased nutrient requirements of the fetus and placenta and for milk production.[10–16] When selecting the criterion to be used, reduction of chronic degenerative disease risk is considered. But despite the intense interest in dietary modification of chronic disease risk, data related to the effects of nutrient intakes on morbidity and mortality from chronic disease in the United States and Canada are limited.

Recommended Dietary Allowance

The Recommended Dietary Allowance (RDA) is defined as "the average daily dietary intake level that is sufficient to meet the nutrient requirement of nearly all (97% to 98%) apparently healthy individuals in a particular life stage and gender group."[12] This is essentially the same definition as that used in the 10th edition of the *Recommended Dietary Allowances.*[8]

TABLE 2.2 Dietary Reference Intakes (DRIs): Estimated Average Requirements
Food and Nutrition Board, Institute of Medicine, National Academies

Life Stage Group	Calcium (mg/d)	CHO (g/d)	Protein (g/kg/d)	Vit A (μg/d)[a]	Vit C (mg/d)	Vit D (μg/d)	Vit E (mg/d)[b]	Thiamin (mg/d)	Riboflavin (mg/d)	Niacin (mg/d)[c]	Vit B_6 (mg/d)	Folate (μg/d)[d]	Vit B_{12} (μg/d)	Copper (μg/d)	Iodine (μg/d)	Iron (mg/d)	Magnesium (mg/d)	Molybdenum (μg/d)	Phosphorus (mg/d)	Selenium (μg/d)	Zinc (mg/d)
Infants																					
0 to 6 mo																					
6 to 12 mo			1.0													6.9					2.5
Children																					
1–3 y	500	100	0.87	210	13	10	5	0.4	0.4	5	0.4	120	0.7	260	65	3.0	65	13	380	17	2.5
4–8 y	800	100	0.76	275	22	10	6	0.5	0.5	6	0.5	160	1.0	340	65	4.1	110	17	405	23	4.0
Males																					
9–13 y	1,100	100	0.76	445	39	10	9	0.7	0.8	9	0.8	250	1.5	540	73	5.9	200	26	1,055	35	7.0
14–18 y	1,100	100	0.73	630	63	10	12	1.0	1.1	12	1.1	330	2.0	685	95	7.7	340	33	1,055	45	8.5
19–30 y	800	100	0.66	625	75	10	12	1.0	1.1	12	1.1	320	2.0	700	95	6	330	34	580	45	9.4
31–50 y	800	100	0.66	625	75	10	12	1.0	1.1	12	1.1	320	2.0	700	95	6	350	34	580	45	9.4
51–70 y	800	100	0.66	625	75	10	12	1.0	1.1	12	1.4	320	2.0	700	95	6	350	34	580	45	9.4
> 70 y	1,000	100	0.66	625	75	10	12	1.0	1.1	12	1.4	320	2.0	700	95	6	350	34	580	45	9.4
Females																					
9–13 y	1,100	100	0.76	420	39	10	9	0.7	0.8	9	0.8	250	1.5	540	73	5.7	200	26	1,055	35	7.0
14–18 y	1,100	100	0.71	485	56	10	12	0.9	0.9	11	1.0	330	2.0	685	95	7.9	300	33	1,055	45	7.3
19–30 y	800	100	0.66	500	60	10	12	0.9	0.9	11	1.1	320	2.0	700	95	8.1	255	34	580	45	6.8
31–50 y	800	100	0.66	500	60	10	12	0.9	0.9	11	1.1	320	2.0	700	95	8.1	265	34	580	45	6.8
51–70 y	1,000	100	0.66	500	60	10	12	0.9	0.9	11	1.3	320	2.0	700	95	5	265	34	580	45	6.8
> 70 y	1,000	100	0.66	500	60	10	12	0.9	0.9	11	1.3	320	2.0	700	95	5	265	34	580	45	6.8
Pregnancy																					
14–18 y	1,000	135	0.88	530	66	10	12	1.2	1.2	14	1.6	520	2.2	785	160	23	335	40	1,055	49	10.5
19–30 y	800	135	0.88	550	70	10	12	1.2	1.2	14	1.6	520	2.2	800	160	22	290	40	580	49	9.5
31–50 y	800	135	0.88	550	70	10	12	1.2	1.2	14	1.6	520	2.2	800	160	22	300	40	580	49	9.5
Lactation																					
14–18 y	1,000	160	1.05	885	96	10	16	1.2	1.3	13	1.7	450	2.4	985	209	7	300	35	1,055	59	10.9
19–30 y	800	160	1.05	900	100	10	16	1.2	1.3	13	1.7	450	2.4	1,000	209	6.5	255	36	580	59	10.4
31–50 y	800	160	1.05	900	100	10	16	1.2	1.3	13	1.7	450	2.4	1,000	209	6.5	265	36	580	59	10.4

Sources: Dietary Reference Intakes for Calcium, Phosphorous, Magnesium, Vitamin D, and Fluoride (1997); *Dietary Reference Intakes for Thiamin, Riboflavin, Niacin, Vitamin B_6, Folate, Vitamin B_{12}, Pantothenic Acid, Biotin, and Choline* (1998); *Dietary Reference Intakes for Vitamin C, Vitamin E, Selenium, and Carotenoids* (2000); *Dietary Reference Intakes for Vitamin A, Vitamin K, Arsenic, Boron, Chromium, Copper, Iodine, Iron, Manganese, Molybdenum, Nickel, Silicon, Vanadium, and Zinc* (2001); *Dietary Reference Intakes for Energy, Carbohydrate, Fiber, Fat, Fatty Acids, Cholesterol, Protein, and Amino Acids* (2002/2005); and *Dietary Reference Intakes for Calcium and Vitamin D* (2011). These reports may be accessed via www.nap.edu.

Note: An Estimated Average Requirement (EAR) is the average daily nutrient intake level estimated to meet the requirements of half of the healthy individuals in a group. EARs have not been established for vitamin K, pantothenic acid, biotin, choline, chromium, fluoride, manganese, or other nutrients not yet evaluated via the DRI process.

[a]As retinol activity equivalents (RAEs). 1 RAE = 1 μg retinol, 12 μg β-carotene, 24 μg α-carotene, or 24 μg β-cryptoxanthin. The RAE for dietary provitamin A carotenoids is two-fold greater than retinol equivalents (RE), whereas the RAE for preformed vitamin A is the same as RE.

[b]As α-tocopherol. α-Tocopherol includes *RRR*-α-tocopherol, the only form of α-tocopherol that occurs naturally in foods, and the *2R*-stereoisomeric forms of α-tocopherol (*RRR-, RSR-, RRS-*, and *RSS*-α-tocopherol) that occur in fortified foods and supplements. It does not include the *2S*-stereoisomeric forms of α-tocopherol (*SRR-, SSR-, SRS-*, and *SSS*-α-tocopherol), also found in fortified foods and supplements.

[c]As niacin equivalents (NE). 1 mg of niacin = 60 mg of tryptophan.

[d]As dietary folate equivalents (DFE). 1 DFE = 1 μg food folate = 0.6 μg of folic acid from fortified food or as a supplement consumed with food = 0.5 μg of a supplement taken on an empty stomach.

TABLE 2.3 Dietary Reference Intakes (DRIs): Recommended Dietary Allowances and Adequate Intakes, Vitamins

Food and Nutrition Board, Institute of Medicine, National Academies

Life Stage Group	Vitamin A (μg/d)[a]	Vitamin C (mg/d)	Vitamin D (μg/d)[b,c]	Vitamin E (mg/d)[d]	Vitamin K (μg/d)	Thiamin (mg/d)	Riboflavin (mg/d)	Niacin (mg/d)[e]	Vitamin B_6 (mg/d)	Folate (μg/d)[f]	Vitamin B_{12} (μg/d)	Pantothenic Acid (mg/d)	Biotin (μg/d)	Choline (mg/d)[g]
Infants														
0 to 6 mo	400*	40*	10*	4*	2.0*	0.2*	0.3*	2*	0.1*	65*	0.4*	1.7*	5*	125*
6 to 12 mo	500*	50*	10*	5*	2.5*	0.3*	0.4*	4*	0.3*	80*	0.5*	1.8*	6*	150*
Children														
1–3 y	**300**	**15**	**15**	**6**	30*	**0.5**	**0.5**	**6**	**0.5**	**150**	**0.9**	2*	8*	200*
4–8 y	**400**	**25**	**15**	**7**	55*	**0.6**	**0.6**	**8**	**0.6**	**200**	**1.2**	3*	12*	250*
Males														
9–13 y	**600**	**45**	**15**	**11**	60*	**0.9**	**0.9**	**12**	**1.0**	**300**	**1.8**	4*	20*	375*
14–18 y	**900**	**75**	**15**	**15**	75*	**1.2**	**1.3**	**16**	**1.3**	**400**	**2.4**	5*	25*	550*
19–30 y	**900**	**90**	**15**	**15**	120*	**1.2**	**1.3**	**16**	**1.3**	**400**	**2.4**	5*	30*	550*
31–50 y	**900**	**90**	**15**	**15**	120*	**1.2**	**1.3**	**16**	**1.3**	**400**	**2.4**	5*	30*	550*
51–70 y	**900**	**90**	**15**	**15**	120*	**1.2**	**1.3**	**16**	**1.7**	**400**	**2.4**[h]	5*	30*	550*
> 70 y	**900**	**90**	**20**	**15**	120*	**1.2**	**1.3**	**16**	**1.7**	**400**	**2.4**[h]	5*	30*	550*
Females														
9–13 y	**600**	**45**	**15**	**11**	60*	**0.9**	**0.9**	**12**	**1.0**	**300**	**1.8**	4*	20*	375*
14–18 y	**700**	**65**	**15**	**15**	75*	**1.0**	**1.0**	**14**	**1.2**	**400**[i]	**2.4**	5*	25*	400*
19–30 y	**700**	**75**	**15**	**15**	90*	**1.1**	**1.1**	**14**	**1.3**	**400**[i]	**2.4**	5*	30*	425*
31–50 y	**700**	**75**	**15**	**15**	90*	**1.1**	**1.1**	**14**	**1.3**	**400**[i]	**2.4**	5*	30*	425*
51–70 y	**700**	**75**	**15**	**15**	90*	**1.1**	**1.1**	**14**	**1.5**	**400**	**2.4**[h]	5*	30*	425*
> 70 y	**700**	**75**	**20**	**15**	90*	**1.1**	**1.1**	**14**	**1.5**	**400**	**2.4**[h]	5*	30*	425*
Pregnancy														
14–18 y	**750**	**80**	**15**	**15**	75*	**1.4**	**1.4**	**18**	**1.9**	**600**[j]	**2.6**	6*	30*	450*
19–30 y	**770**	**85**	**15**	**15**	90*	**1.4**	**1.4**	**18**	**1.9**	**600**[j]	**2.6**	6*	30*	450*
31–50 y	**770**	**85**	**15**	**15**	90*	**1.4**	**1.4**	**18**	**1.9**	**600**[j]	**2.6**	6*	30*	450*
Lactation														
14–18 y	**1,200**	**115**	**15**	**19**	75*	**1.4**	**1.6**	**17**	**2.0**	**500**	**2.8**	7*	35*	550*
19–30 y	**1,300**	**120**	**15**	**19**	90*	**1.4**	**1.6**	**17**	**2.0**	**500**	**2.8**	7*	35*	550*
31–50 y	**1,300**	**120**	**15**	**19**	90*	**1.4**	**1.6**	**17**	**2.0**	**500**	**2.8**	7*	35*	550*

Sources: Dietary Reference Intakes for Calcium, Phosphorous, Magnesium, Vitamin D, and Fluoride (1997); *Dietary Reference Intakes for Thiamin, Riboflavin, Niacin, Vitamin B_6, Folate, Vitamin B_{12}, Pantothenic Acid, Biotin, and Choline* (1998); *Dietary Reference Intakes for Vitamin C, Vitamin E, Selenium, and Carotenoids* (2000); *Dietary Reference Intakes for Vitamin A, Vitamin K, Arsenic, Boron, Chromium, Copper, Iodine, Iron, Manganese, Molybdenum, Nickel, Silicon, Vanadium, and Zinc* (2001); *Dietary Reference Intakes for Water, Potassium, Sodium, Chloride, and Sulfate* (2005); and *Dietary Reference Intakes for Calcium and Vitamin D* (2011). These reports may be accessed via www.nap.edu.

Note: This table (taken from the DRI reports, see www.nap.edu) presents Recommended Dietary Allowances (RDAs) in **bold type** and Adequate Intakes (AIs) in ordinary type followed by an asterisk (*). An RDA is the average daily dietary intake level; sufficient to meet the nutrient requirements of nearly all (97–98 percent) healthy individuals in a group. It is calculated from an Estimated Average Requirement (EAR). If sufficient scientific evidence is not available to establish an EAR, and thus calculate an RDA, an AI is usually developed. For healthy breastfed infants, an AI is the mean intake. The AI for other life stage and gender groups is believed to cover the needs of all healthy individuals in the groups, but lack of data or uncertainty in the data prevent being able to specify with confidence the percentage of individuals covered by this intake.

[a] As retinol activity equivalents (RAEs). 1 RAE = 1 μg retinol, 12 μg β-carotene, 24 μg α-carotene, or 24 μg β-cryptoxanthin. The RAE for dietary provitamin A carotenoids is two-fold greater than retinol equivalents (RE), whereas the RAE for preformed vitamin A is the same as RE.

[b] As cholecalciferol. 1 μg cholecalciferol = 40 IU vitamin D.

[c] Under the assumption of minimal sunlight.

[d] As α-tocopherol. α-Tocopherol includes *RRR*-α-tocopherol, the only form of α-tocopherol that occurs naturally in foods, and the *2R*-stereoisomeric forms of α-tocopherol (*RRR-*, *RSR-*, *RRS-*, and *RSS*-α-tocopherol) that occur in fortified foods and supplements. It does not include the *2S*-stereoisomeric forms of α-tocopherol (*SRR-*, *SSR-*, *SRS-*, and *SSS*-α-tocopherol), also found in fortified foods and supplements.

[e] As niacin equivalents (NE). 1 mg of niacin = 60 mg of tryptophan; 0–6 months = preformed niacin (not NE).

[f] As dietary folate equivalents (DFE). 1 DFE = 1 μg food folate = 0.6 μg of folic acid from fortified food or as a supplement consumed with food = 0.5 μg of a supplement taken on an empty stomach.

[g] Although AIs have been set for choline, there are few data to assess whether a dietary supply of choline is needed at all stages of the life cycle, and it may be that the choline requirement can be met by endogenous synthesis at some of these stages.

[h] Because 10 to 30 percent of older people may malabsorb food-bound B_{12}, it is advisable for those older than 50 years to meet their RDA mainly by consuming foods fortified with B_{12} or a supplement containing B_{12}.

[i] In view of evidence linking folate intake with neural tube defects in the fetus, it is recommended that all women capable of becoming pregnant consume 400 μg from supplements or fortified foods in addition to intake of food folate from a varied diet.

[j] It is assumed that women will continue consuming 400 μg from supplements or fortified food until their pregnancy is confirmed and they enter prenatal care, which ordinarily occurs after the end of the periconceptional period—the critical time for formation of the neural tube.

TABLE 2.4 Dietary Reference Intakes (DRIs): Recommended Dietary Allowances and Adequate Intakes, Elements

Food and Nutrition Board, Institute of Medicine, National Academies

Life Stage Group	Calcium (mg/d)	Chromium (μg/d)	Copper (μg/d)	Fluoride (mg/d)	Iodine (μg/d)	Iron (mg/d)	Magnesium (mg/d)	Manganese (mg/d)	Molybdenum (μg/d)	Phosphorus (mg/d)	Selenium (μg/d)	Zinc (mg/d)	Potassium (g/d)	Sodium (g/d)	Chloride (g/d)
Infants															
0 to 6 mo	200*	0.2*	200*	0.01*	110*	0.27*	30*	0.003*	2*	100*	15*	2*	0.4*	0.12*	0.18*
6 to 12 mo	260*	5.5*	220*	0.5*	130*	**11**	75*	0.6*	3*	275*	20*	**3**	0.7*	0.37*	0.57*
Children															
1–3 y	**700**	11*	**340**	0.7*	**90**	**7**	**80**	1.2*	**17**	**460**	**20**	**3**	3.0*	1.0*	1.5*
4–8 y	**1,000**	15*	**440**	1*	**90**	**10**	**130**	1.5*	**22**	**500**	**30**	**5**	3.8*	1.2*	1.9*
Males															
9–13 y	**1,300**	25*	**700**	2*	**120**	**8**	**240**	1.9*	**34**	**1,250**	**40**	**8**	4.5*	1.5*	2.3*
14–18 y	**1,300**	35*	**890**	3*	**150**	**11**	**410**	2.2*	**43**	**1,250**	**55**	**11**	4.7*	1.5*	2.3*
19–30 y	**1,000**	35*	**900**	4*	**150**	**8**	**400**	2.3*	**45**	**700**	**55**	**11**	4.7*	1.5*	2.3*
31–50 y	**1,000**	35*	**900**	4*	**150**	**8**	**420**	2.3*	**45**	**700**	**55**	**11**	4.7*	1.5*	2.3*
51–70 y	**1,000**	30*	**900**	4*	**150**	**8**	**420**	2.3*	**45**	**700**	**55**	**11**	4.7*	1.3*	2.0*
> 70 y	**1,200**	30*	**900**	4*	**150**	**8**	**420**	2.3*	**45**	**700**	**55**	**11**	4.7*	1.2*	1.8*
Females															
9–13 y	**1,300**	21*	**700**	2*	**120**	**8**	**240**	1.6*	**34**	**1,250**	**40**	**8**	4.5*	1.5*	2.3*
14–18 y	**1,300**	24*	**890**	3*	**150**	**15**	**360**	1.6*	**43**	**1,250**	**55**	**9**	4.7*	1.5*	2.3*
19–30 y	**1,000**	25*	**900**	3*	**150**	**18**	**310**	1.8*	**45**	**700**	**55**	**8**	4.7*	1.5*	2.3*
31–50 y	**1,000**	25*	**900**	3*	**150**	**18**	**320**	1.8*	**45**	**700**	**55**	**8**	4.7*	1.5*	2.3*
51–70 y	**1,200**	20*	**900**	3*	**150**	**8**	**320**	1.8*	**45**	**700**	**55**	**8**	4.7*	1.3*	2.0*
> 70 y	**1,200**	20*	**900**	3*	**150**	**8**	**320**	1.8*	**45**	**700**	**55**	**8**	4.7*	1.2*	1.8*
Pregnancy															
14–18 y	**1,300**	29*	**1,000**	3*	**220**	**27**	**400**	2.0*	**50**	**1,250**	**60**	**12**	4.7*	1.5*	2.3*
19–30 y	**1,000**	30*	**1,000**	3*	**220**	**27**	**350**	2.0*	**50**	**700**	**60**	**11**	4.7*	1.5*	2.3*
31–50 y	**1,000**	30*	**1,000**	3*	**220**	**27**	**360**	2.0*	**50**	**700**	**60**	**11**	4.7*	1.5*	2.3*
Lactation															
14–18 y	**1,300**	44*	**1,300**	3*	**290**	**10**	**360**	2.6*	**50**	**1,250**	**70**	**13**	5.1*	1.5*	2.3*
19–30 y	**1,000**	45*	**1,300**	3*	**290**	**9**	**310**	2.6*	**50**	**700**	**70**	**12**	5.1*	1.5*	2.3*
31–50 y	**1,000**	45*	**1,300**	3*	**290**	**9**	**320**	2.6*	**50**	**700**	**70**	**12**	5.1*	1.5*	2.3*

Note: This table (taken from the DRI reports, see www.nap.edu) presents Recommended Dietary Allowances (RDAs) in **bold type** and Adequate Intakes (AIs) in ordinary type followed by an asterisk (*). An RDA is the average daily dietary intake level; sufficient to meet the nutrient requirements of nearly all (97–98 percent) healthy individuals in a group. It is calculated from an Estimated Average Requirement (EAR). If sufficient scientific evidence is not available to establish an EAR, and thus calculate an RDA, an AI is usually developed. For healthy breastfed infants, an AI is the mean intake. The AI for other life stage and gender groups is believed to cover the needs of all healthy individuals in the groups, but lack of data or uncertainty in the data prevent being able to specify with confidence the percentage of individuals covered by this intake.

Sources: Dietary Reference Intakes for Calcium, Phosphorous, Magnesium, Vitamin D, and Fluoride (1997); *Dietary Reference Intakes for Thiamin, Riboflavin, Niacin, Vitamin B_6, Folate, Vitamin B_{12}, Pantothenic Acid, Biotin, and Choline* (1998); *Dietary Reference Intakes for Vitamin C, Vitamin E, Selenium, and Carotenoids* (2000); *Dietary Reference Intakes for Vitamin A, Vitamin K, Arsenic, Boron, Chromium, Copper, Iodine, Iron, Manganese, Molybdenum, Nickel, Silicon, Vanadium, and Zinc* (2001); *Dietary Reference Intakes for Water, Potassium, Sodium, Chloride, and Sulfate* (2005); and *Dietary Reference Intakes for Calcium and Vitamin D* (2011). These reports may be accessed via www.nap.edu.

TABLE 2.5 Dietary Reference Intakes (DRIs): Tolerable Upper Intake Levels, Vitamins

Food and Nutrition Board, Institute of Medicine, National Academies

Life Stage Group	Vitamin A (μg/d)[a]	Vitamin C (mg/d)	Vitamin D (μg/d)	Vitamin E (mg/d)[b,c]	Vitamin K	Thiamin	Riboflavin	Niacin (mg/d)[c]	Vitamin B_6 (mg/d)	Folate (μg/d)[c]	Vitamin B_{12}	Pantothenic Acid	Biotin	Choline (g/d)	Carotenoids[d]
Infants															
0 to 6 mo	600	ND[e]	25	ND	ND	ND	ND	ND	ND	ND	ND	ND	ND	ND	ND
6 to 12 mo	600	ND	38	ND	ND	ND	ND	ND	ND	ND	ND	ND	ND	ND	ND
Children															
1–3 y	600	400	63	200	ND	ND	ND	10	30	300	ND	ND	ND	1.0	ND
4–8 y	900	650	75	300	ND	ND	ND	15	40	400	ND	ND	ND	1.0	ND
Males															
9–13 y	1,700	1,200	100	600	ND	ND	ND	20	60	600	ND	ND	ND	2.0	ND
14–18 y	2,800	1,800	100	800	ND	ND	ND	30	80	800	ND	ND	ND	3.0	ND
19–30 y	3,000	2,000	100	1,000	ND	ND	ND	35	100	1,000	ND	ND	ND	3.5	ND
31–50 y	3,000	2,000	100	1,000	ND	ND	ND	35	100	1,000	ND	ND	ND	3.5	ND
51–70 y	3,000	2,000	100	1,000	ND	ND	ND	35	100	1,000	ND	ND	ND	3.5	ND
> 70 y	3,000	2,000	100	1,000	ND	ND	ND	35	100	1,000	ND	ND	ND	3.5	ND
Females															
9–13 y	1,700	1,200	100	600	ND	ND	ND	20	60	600	ND	ND	ND	2.0	ND
14–18 y	2,800	1,800	100	800	ND	ND	ND	30	80	800	ND	ND	ND	3.0	ND
19–30 y	3,000	2,000	100	1,000	ND	ND	ND	35	100	1,000	ND	ND	ND	3.5	ND
31–50 y	3,000	2,000	100	1,000	ND	ND	ND	35	100	1,000	ND	ND	ND	3.5	ND
51–70 y	3,000	2,000	100	1,000	ND	ND	ND	35	100	1,000	ND	ND	ND	3.5	ND
> 70 y	3,000	2,000	100	1,000	ND	ND	ND	35	100	1,000	ND	ND	ND	3.5	ND
Pregnancy															
14–18 y	2,800	1,800	100	800	ND	ND	ND	30	80	800	ND	ND	ND	3.0	ND
19–30 y	3,000	2,000	100	1,000	ND	ND	ND	35	100	1,000	ND	ND	ND	3.5	ND
31–50 y	3,000	2,000	100	1,000	ND	ND	ND	35	100	1,000	ND	ND	ND	3.5	ND
Lactation															
14–18 y	2,800	1,800	100	800	ND	ND	ND	30	80	800	ND	ND	ND	3.0	ND
19–30 y	3,000	2,000	100	1,000	ND	ND	ND	35	100	1,000	ND	ND	ND	3.5	ND
31–50 y	3,000	2,000	100	1,000	ND	ND	ND	35	100	1,000	ND	ND	ND	3.5	ND

Sources: Dietary Reference Intakes for Calcium, Phosphorous, Magnesium, Vitamin D, and Fluoride (1997); *Dietary Reference Intakes for Thiamin, Riboflavin, Niacin, Vitamin B_6, Folate, Vitamin B_{12}, Pantothenic Acid, Biotin, and Choline* (1998); *Dietary Reference Intakes for Vitamin C, Vitamine E, Selenium, and Carotenoids* (2000); *Dietary Reference Intakes for Vitamin A, Vitamin K, Arsenic, Boron, Chromium, Copper, Iodine, Iron, Manganese, Molybdenum, Nickel, Silicon, Vanadium, and Zinc* (2001); and *Dietary Reference Intakes for Calcium and Vitamin D* (2011). These reports may be accessed via www.nap.edu.

Note: A Tolerable Upper Intake Level (UL) is the highest level of daily nutrient intake that is likely to pose no risk of adverse health effects to almost all individuals in the general population. Unless otherwise specified, the UL represents total intake from food, water, and supplements. Due to a lack of suitable data, ULs could not be established for vitamin K, thiamin, riboflavin, vitamin B_{12}, pantothenic acid, biotin, and carotenoids. In the absence of a UL, extra caution may be warranted in consuming levels above recommended intakes. Members of the general population should be advised not to routinely exceed the UL. The UL is not meant to apply to individuals who are treated with the nutrient under medical supervision or to individuals with predisposing conditions that modify their sensitivity to the nutrient.

[a]As preformed vitamin A only.

[b]As α-tocopherol; applies to any form of supplemental α-tocopherol.

[c]The ULs for vitamin E, niacin, and folate apply to synthetic forms obtained from supplements, fortified foods, or a combination of the two.

[d]β-Carotene supplements are advised only to serve as a provitamin A source for individuals at risk of vitamin A deficiency.

[e]ND = Not determinable due to lack of data of adverse effects in this age group and concern with regard to lack of ability to handle excess amounts. Source of intake should be from food only to prevent high levels of intake.

TABLE 2.6 Dietary Reference Intakes (DRIs): Tolerable Upper Intake Levels, Elements

Food and Nutrition Board, Institute of Medicine, National Academies

Life Stage Group	Arsenic[a]	Boron (mg/d)	Calcium (mg/d)	Chromium	Copper (μg/d)	Fluoride (mg/d)	Iodine (μg/d)	Iron (mg/d)	Magnesium (mg/d)[b]	Manganese (mg/d)	Molybdenum (μg/d)	Nickel (mg/d)	Phosphorus (g/d)	Selenium (μg/d)	Silicon[c]	Vanadium (mg/d)[d]	Zinc (mg/d)	Sodium (g/d)	Chloride (g/d)
Infants																			
0 to 6 mo	ND[e]	ND	1,000	ND	ND	0.7	ND	40	ND	ND	ND	ND	ND	45	ND	ND	4	ND	ND
6 to 12 mo	ND	ND	1,500	ND	ND	0.9	ND	40	ND	ND	ND	ND	ND	60	ND	ND	5	ND	ND
Children																			
1–3 y	ND	3	2,500	ND	1,000	1.3	200	40	65	2	300	0.2	3	90	ND	ND	7	1.5	2.3
4–8 y	ND	6	2,500	ND	3,000	2.2	300	40	110	3	600	0.3	3	150	ND	ND	12	1.9	2.9
Males																			
9–13 y	ND	11	3,000	ND	5,000	10	600	40	350	6	1,100	0.6	4	280	ND	ND	23	2.2	3.4
14–18 y	ND	17	3,000	ND	8,000	10	900	45	350	9	1,700	1.0	4	400	ND	ND	34	2.3	3.6
19–30 y	ND	20	2,500	ND	10,000	10	1,100	45	350	11	2,000	1.0	4	400	ND	1.8	40	2.3	3.6
31–50 y	ND	20	2,500	ND	10,000	10	1,100	45	350	11	2,000	1.0	4	400	ND	1.8	40	2.3	3.6
51–70 y	ND	20	2,000	ND	10,000	10	1,100	45	350	11	2,000	1.0	4	400	ND	1.8	40	2.3	3.6
> 70 y	ND	20	2,000	ND	10,000	10	1,100	45	350	11	2,000	1.0	3	400	ND	1.8	40	2.3	3.6
Females																			
9–13 y	ND	11	3,000	ND	5,000	10	600	40	350	6	1,100	0.6	4	280	ND	ND	23	2.2	3.4
14–18 y	ND	17	3,000	ND	8,000	10	900	45	350	9	1,700	1.0	4	400	ND	ND	34	2.3	3.6
19–30 y	ND	20	2,500	ND	10,000	10	1,100	45	350	11	2,000	1.0	4	400	ND	1.8	40	2.3	3.6
31–50 y	ND	20	2,500	ND	10,000	10	1,100	45	350	11	2,000	1.0	4	400	ND	1.8	40	2.3	3.6
51–70 y	ND	20	2,000	ND	10,000	10	1,100	45	350	11	2,000	1.0	4	400	ND	1.8	40	2.3	3.6
> 70 y	ND	20	2,000	ND	10,000	10	1,100	45	350	11	2,000	1.0	3	400	ND	1.8	40	2.3	3.6
Pregnancy																			
14–18 y	ND	17	3,000	ND	8,000	10	900	45	350	9	1,700	1.0	3.5	400	ND	ND	34	2.3	3.6
19–30 y	ND	20	2,500	ND	10,000	10	1,100	45	350	11	2,000	1.0	3.5	400	ND	ND	40	2.3	3.6
61–50 y	ND	20	2,500	ND	10,000	10	1,100	45	350	11	2,000	1.0	3.5	400	ND	ND	40	2.3	3.6
Lactation																			
14–18 y	ND	17	3,000	ND	8,000	10	900	45	350	9	1,700	1.0	4	400	ND	ND	34	2.3	3.6
19–30 y	ND	20	2,500	ND	10,000	10	1,100	45	350	11	2,000	1.0	4	400	ND	ND	40	2.3	3.6
31–50 y	ND	20	2,500	ND	10,000	10	1,100	45	350	11	2,000	1.0	4	400	ND	ND	40	2.3	3.6

Sources: Dietary Reference Intakes for Calcium, Phosphorous, Magnesium, Vitamin D, and Fluoride (1997); *Dietary Reference Intakes for Thiamin, Riboflavin, Niacin, Vitamin B_6, Folate, Vitamin B_{12}, Pantothenic Acid, Biotin, and Choline* (1998); *Dietary Reference Intakes for Vitamin C, Vitamin E, Selenium, and Carotenoids* (2000); *Dietary Reference Intakes for Vitamin A, Vitamin K, Arsenic, Boron, Chromium, Copper, Iodine, Iron, Manganese, Molybdenum, Nickel, Silicon, Vanadium, and Zinc* (2001); *Dietary Reference Intakes for Water, Potassium, Sodium, Chloride, and Sulfate* (2005); and *Dietary Reference Intakes for Calcium and Vitamin D* (2011). These reports may be accessed via www.nap.edu.

Note: A Tolerable Upper Intake Level (UL) is the highest level of daily nutrient intake that is likely to pose no risk of adverse health effects to almost all individuals in the general population. Unless otherwise specified, the UL represents total intake from food, water, and supplements. Due to a lack of suitable data, ULs could not be established for vitamin K, thiamin, riboflavin, vitamin B_{12}, pantothenic acid, biotin, and carotenoids. In the absence of a UL, extra caution may be warranted in consuming levels above recommended intakes. Members of the general population should be advised not to routinely exceed the UL. The UL is not meant to apply to individuals who are treated with the nutrient under medical supervision or to individuals with predisposing conditions that modify their sensitivity to the nutrient.

[a]Although the UL was not determined for arsenic, there is no justification for adding arsenic to food or supplements.

[b]The ULs for magnesium represent intake from a pharmacological agent only and do not include intake from food and water.

[c]Although silicon has not been shown to cause adverse effects in humans, there is no justification for adding silicon to supplements.

[d]Although vanadium in food has not been shown to cause adverse effects in humans, there is no justification for adding vanadium to food and vanadium supplements should be used with caution. The UL is based on adverse effects in laboratory animals and this data could be used to set a UL for adults but not children and adolescents.

[e]ND = Not determinable due to lack of data of adverse effects in this age group and concern with regard to lack of ability to handle excess amounts. Source of intake should be from food only to prevent high levels of intake.

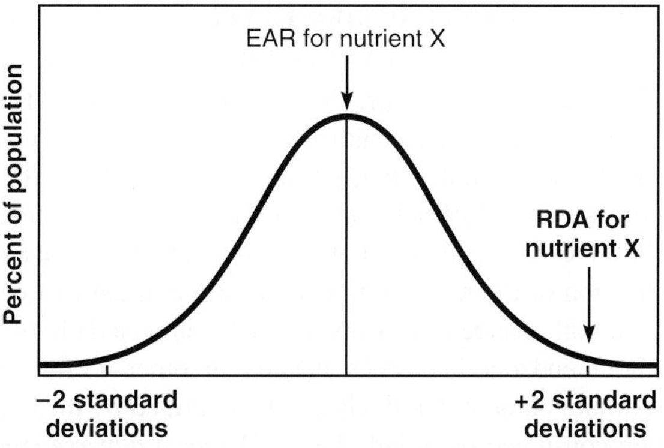

Figure 2.2 The distribution of the requirement for nutrient X for a life stage and gender group.
The Estimated Average Requirement (EAR) and the Recommended Dietary Allowance (RDA) are shown. The nutrient requirement level that is 2 standard deviations greater than the EAR is generally selected for the RDA.

Source: Adapted from Otten JJ, Hellwig JP, Meyers LD. 2006. *Dietary Reference Intakes: The Essential Guide to Nutrient Requirements.* Washington, DC: National Academy Press.

The RDA for a particular nutrient can be set only if the EAR for that nutrient is established. If the requirement for the nutrient among individuals in the life stage and gender group is normally distributed and if data about the variability in requirements are sufficient to calculate the **standard deviation (SD)** of the EAR (SD_{EAR}), the RDA is set at 2 standard deviations above the EAR, as illustrated in Figure 2.2. This is shown mathematically by the following equation:

$$RDA = EAR + 2\ SD_{EAR}$$

Obviously, if the RDA were set at the EAR, the RDA would meet the needs of only half the individuals in a life stage and gender group—those individuals having a requirement equal to or less than the EAR. The requirement for nutrient X for the other half of individuals in the group—those with a requirement greater than the EAR—would not be met. Thus, to meet the needs of nearly all apparently healthy individuals in a particular life stage and gender group, the RDA is set at 2 standard deviations above the EAR. The standard deviation indicates the degree of variation from the mean; in this case, it indicates how different the nutrient requirements of individual group members are from the group mean. At 2 standard deviations above the mean, the requirement for nutrient X would be met for nearly 98% of individuals in a life stage and gender group.

If data about variability in nutrient requirements are insufficient to calculate a standard deviation, a **coefficient of variation (CV)** for the EAR (CV_{EAR}) of 10% is generally assumed and used in place of the standard deviation.[10–16] The coefficient of variation is the standard deviation divided by the mean, as shown in the following equations:

$$CV_{EAR} = SD_{EAR} \div EAR,$$

$$SD_{EAR} = CV_{EAR} \times EAR$$

In this situation, the RDA can be calculated as follows:

$$RDA = EAR + 2(CV_{EAR} \times EAR), \text{ or}$$

$$RDA = EAR + 2(0.1 \times EAR), \text{ or}$$

$$RDA = 1.2 \times EAR$$

If the nutrient requirement for a particular group is known to be skewed, other approaches can be used to find the intake level sufficient to meet the nutrient requirement of 97% to 98% of healthy persons in a particular life stage and gender group in order to set the RDA.[10–16]

A safety margin also is built into the RDA of a nutrient to compensate for its incomplete use by the body and to account for variations in the levels of the nutrient provided by various food sources. Adjustment also is made in some RDAs to account for the consumption of certain dietary components that are subsequently converted within the body to an essential nutrient. For example, the amino acid tryptophan can be converted to niacin within the body.[11] Examples of RDAs that have been included as part of the DRIs were shown in bold type in Tables 2.3 and 2.4.

Adequate Intake

If insufficient data are available to calculate an EAR, and thus an RDA cannot be set for a particular nutrient, a separate reference intake, known as Adequate Intake (AI), is used instead of the RDA. Adequate Intake is defined as "a value based on experimentally derived intake levels or approximations of observed mean nutrient intakes by a group (or groups) of healthy people."[10–16] For example, as was shown in Tables 2.3 and 2.4, most nutrient intake levels for infants (birth to 12 months of age) are expressed as AIs instead of RDAs because the types of studies necessary to determine the nutrient requirements of infants (e.g., depletion-repletion studies) cannot ethically be done. The AIs for infants from birth to 6 months of age were calculated based on the mean nutrient intakes of healthy, full-term infants 2 to 6 months of age who were exclusively breast-fed.[10–16] By weighing these infants before and after breast-feeding, researchers determined that the average volume of milk intake was 780 ml/day. Based on the nutritional composition of human milk, researchers could then determine the average nutritional intake of these infants. For infants 7 to 12 months of age, the AIs are based on the average nutrient intakes of 7- to 12-month-old infants fed a combination of human milk and typical complementary weaning foods used in North America.

As shown in Tables 2.3 and 2.4, the recommended intakes for vitamin D, vitamin K, pantothenic acid, biotin, choline, calcium, chromium, fluoride, manganese, potassium, sodium, and chloride are expressed as AIs for all life stages and gender groups. This is because there are insufficient data on the requirements of these nutrients, resulting in an inability to establish an EAR and an RDA. As future research provides additional data on the requirements for these nutrients, an EAR and RDA can be set.

It is important to note that the AI is an observational standard—it is based on observed or experimentally derived approximations of average nutrient intake that appear to maintain a defined nutritional state or criterion of adequacy in a group of people.[10–16] Defined nutritional states include normal growth, maintenance of normal circulating nutrient values, and other indicators of nutritional well-being and general health. Because it is set using presumably healthy groups of individuals, the AI is expected to meet or exceed the actual nutrient requirement in practically all healthy members of a specific life stage and gender group. Like the RDA, the AI is intended to serve as a goal for the nutrient intake of healthy individuals. When nutrient requirements are altered due to injury, disease, or some other special health need, the RDA and AI should serve as the basis for an individual's nutrient recommendations, which, depending on the situation, may then need to be adjusted by a registered dietitian or qualified health professional to accommodate the individual's increased or decreased nutrient needs.[10–16] Unlike the RDA, however, the AI is used when data on nutrient requirements are lacking, and consequently greater uncertainty surrounds the AI.[10–16] Its use indicates a need for additional research on the requirements for that particular nutrient or food component.

Tolerable Upper Intake Level

The Tolerable Upper Intake Level (UL) is defined as "the highest average daily nutrient intake level that is likely to pose no risk of adverse health effects in almost all individuals in the specified life stage group."[10–16] Examples of these were shown in Tables 2.5 and 2.6. The UL is not intended to be a recommended level of nutrient intake but, rather, an indication of the maximum amount of a nutrient that can, with a high degree of probability, be taken on a daily basis without endangering one's health—in other words, the maximum amount that likely can be *tolerated* by the body when consumed on a daily basis. The term *adverse effect* is defined as "any significant alteration in the structure or function of the human organism" or any "impairment of a physiologically important function that could lead to a health effect that is adverse."[10] To determine the UL, the DRI Committee uses a risk assessment model, which is discussed at length in the DRI reports.[10–16]

The UL was created in response to concerns about the potential for excessive nutrient intakes resulting from recent increases in consumption of nutrient-fortified foods and dietary supplements. Just as inadequate nutrient intake can adversely affect health (e.g., result in nutrient-deficiency disease), so can excessive nutrient intake. As illustrated in Figure 2.3, when a nutrient's level of intake is low, risk of inadequacy increases, as indicated by the curve on the left side of the figure. At a very low intake level, the curve is at its highest point, signifying that risk of inadequacy is 100% (indicated as 1.0 in Figure 2.3). When nutrient intake is very high, there is increased risk of excess nutrient intake (what

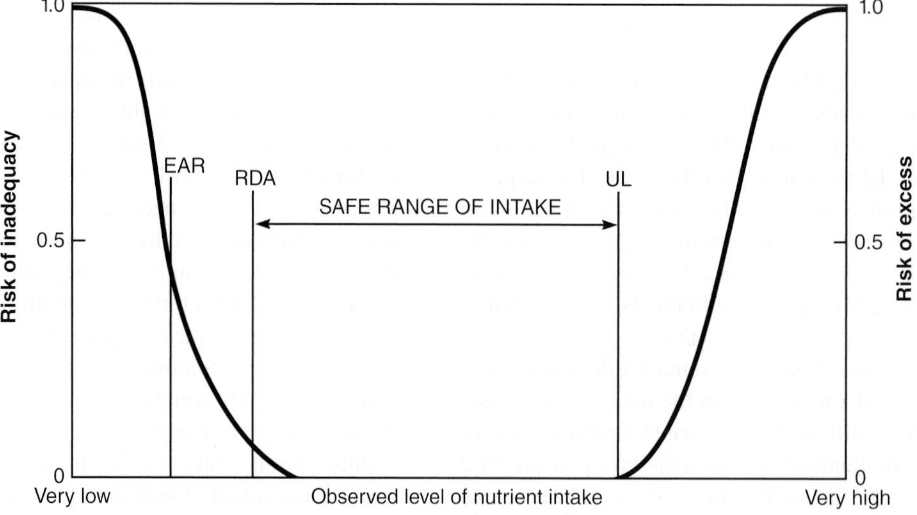

Figure 2.3 The risk of inadequate or excess intake varies according to the level of nutrient intake. When nutrient intake is very low, the risk of inadequacy is high. When nutrient intake is very high, the risk of excessive intake is high. Between the RDA and UL is a safe range of intake associated with a very low probability of either inadequate or excessive nutrient intake. EAR = Estimated Average Requirement; RDA = Recommended Dietary Allowance; UL = Tolerable Upper Intake Level.

Source: Adapted from Otten JJ, Hellwig JP, Meyers LD. 2006. *Dietary Reference Intakes: The essential guide to nutrient requirements.* Washington, DC: National Academy Press.

the DRI Committee calls "risk of adverse effects"), as indicated by the curve on the right side of the figure. An intake level at the UL is unlikely to pose a risk of excessive nutrient intake for most (but not necessarily all) individuals in a specific group. However, as nutrient intake increases above the UL, the risk of adverse health effects increases. When nutrient intake is at the EAR, risk of inadequacy is considered 50% (indicated as 0.5 in Figure 2.3). At the RDA, 97% to 98% of healthy individuals will have their requirement met. Between the RDA and UL is a safe range of intake associated with a very low probability of either inadequate or excessive nutrient intake. However, setting a UL does not suggest that a nutrient intake level greater than the RDA or AI is of any benefit to an individual.

Figure 2.3 does not show the AI because it is an observational standard and set without being able to estimate the requirement. However, the AI is intended to meet or exceed the actual nutrient requirement in practically all healthy members of a specific life stage and gender group and, thus, should be fairly close to the RDA for that nutrient and life stage and gender group, if the RDA is known. Once additional research provides data on the distribution of the requirement for a nutrient and the AI can be replaced with an EAR and RDA, it is likely that the RDA will be slightly less than, if not greater than, the RDA.[10–16]

Prior to the development of the DRIs, the Recommended Dietary Allowances failed to provide any guidance on the safe use of nutritional supplements and addressed the issue of supplement use only by recommending that the RDAs be met by consuming a diet "... composed of a *variety* of foods that are derived from diverse food groups rather than by supplementation or fortification. . . ."[8] It is important to note that this remains an excellent recommendation for a variety of reasons. For example, given the complexity of nutrients and other components in food (some of which we know little or nothing about) it is clear that we cannot solely rely on nutritional supplements as a source of these nutrients and other components and must depend primarily on food to obtain them.[12] However, there is need for information on the maximum amounts of supplemental nutrients that can be safely consumed, given the recent proliferation of nutrient-fortified foods in the marketplace, the increased interest in and use of nutritional and dietary supplements by North Americans, and a growing body of scientific evidence demonstrating that in some instances nutrient intakes in excess of the amounts typically obtained solely from diets can reduce chronic disease risk. The ULs help provide this information and fill an important niche. The ULs are not intended to apply to persons receiving nutrient or other dietary supplements under medical supervision.[12]

If adverse effects of excess nutrient consumption are associated with total nutrient intake, the ULs are based on total nutrient intake from food, water, and supplements. If adverse effects are associated only with intakes from supplements or fortified foods, the ULs are based on nutrient intakes from those sources.[12] For many nutrients, there are insufficient data available to set a UL. But the absence of a UL does not imply that a high intake of that nutrient is risk-free. On the contrary, it may suggest that greater caution is warranted when intakes exceed the RDA or AI.[12]

Estimated Energy Requirement

The Estimated Energy Requirement (EER) is the average dietary energy intake that is predicted to maintain energy balance in a healthy person of a defined age, gender, weight, height, and level of physical activity consistent with good health.[14] For infants, children, and adolescents the EER includes the energy needed for a desirable level of physical activity and for optimal growth, maturation, and development at an age- and gender-appropriate rate that is consistent with good health, including maintenance of a healthy body weight and appropriate body composition. For females who are pregnant or lactating, the EER includes the energy needed for physical activity, for maternal and fetal development, and for lactation at a rate that is consistent with good health.[14]

The EER is calculated using prediction equations developed by the DRI Committee for healthy-weight individuals age 0 to 100 years based on the 24-hour total energy expenditures of more than 1200 subjects measured using the doubly labeled water technique.[14] The doubly labeled water method (described in Chapter 7) is considered the most accurate approach for determining total energy expenditure (TEE) in free-living individuals (i.e., research subjects who are not restricted to a laboratory and who are able to go about their normal daily routines unencumbered by breathing equipment or any other laboratory apparatus). Using the measured 24-hour total energy expenditure data obtained from these healthy-weight subjects, the DRI Committee developed a series of regression equations that best predict the energy requirement of healthy-weight individuals using such variables as age, gender, life stage (pregnant or lactating), body weight, height, and physical activity level. A separate set of prediction equations were developed for adults (age 19 years and older) who are overweight or obese and for children and adolescents (age 3 to 18 years) who are at risk of overweight or who are overweight.[14] The equations for calculating EER are discussed at length in Chapter 7.

There is no Recommended Dietary Allowance or Tolerable Upper Intake Level for energy. By definition, the RDA is generally set at 2 standard deviations greater than the EAR for a given nutrient (e.g., vitamins, elements, and protein) and an energy intake 2 standard deviations greater than the average energy requirement would result in weight gain. Likewise, the UL is set at a nutrient intake level in excess of even the RDA, and an energy intake at such a high level would result in an undesirable and potentially unhealthy weight gain.[14]

Recommendations for Macronutrients

The DRI Committee has developed recommendations for the consumption of macronutrients and various food components. Table 2.7 shows the RDAs (values in bold type) and AIs (values in ordinary type followed by an asterisk) for **total water,** carbohydrate, **total fiber,** total fat, linoleic acid, α-linolenic acid, and protein for the 22 different life stage and gender groups.[14,15] Total water includes drinking water, water in other beverages, and water (moisture) in foods.[15] The values for carbohydrates are based on the minimum amount of glucose needed by the brain and are typically exceeded in order for a person to meet the energy needs of the body while consuming an acceptable proportion of energy from fats and protein.[14]

The AI for total fiber in Table 2.7 is based on research findings showing that risk of coronary heart disease is reduced in adults consuming 14 g of total fiber/1000 kilocalories (kcal). Except for infants, the AI for total fiber was set by multiplying the recommendation for total fiber (i.e., 14 g of total fiber/1000 kcal) by the median

TABLE 2.7 Dietary Reference Intakes (DRIs): Recommended Dietary Allowances and Adequate Intakes, Total Water and Macronutrients

Food and Nutrition Board, Institute of Medicine, National Academies

Life Stage Group	Total Water[a] (L/d)	Carbohydrate (g/d)	Total Fiber (g/d)	Fat (g/d)	Linoleic Acid (g/d)	α-Linolenic Acid (g/d)	Protein[b] (g/d)
Infants							
0 to 6 mo	0.7*	60*	ND	31*	4.4*	0.5*	9.1*
6 to 12 mo	0.8*	95*	ND	30*	4.6*	0.5*	**11.0**
Children							
1–3 y	1.3*	**130**	19*	ND[c]	7*	0.7*	**13**
4–8 y	1.7*	**130**	25*	ND	10*	0.9*	**19**
Males							
9–13 y	2.4*	**130**	31*	ND	12*	1.2*	**34**
14–18 y	3.3*	**130**	38*	ND	16*	1.6*	**52**
19–30 y	3.7*	**130**	38*	ND	17*	1.6*	**56**
31–50 y	3.7*	**130**	38*	ND	17*	1.6*	**56**
51–70 y	3.7*	**130**	30*	ND	14*	1.6*	**56**
> 70 y	3.7*	**130**	30*	ND	14*	1.6*	**56**
Females							
9–13 y	2.1*	**130**	26*	ND	10*	1.0*	**34**
14–18 y	2.3*	**130**	26*	ND	11*	1.1*	**46**
19–30 y	2.7*	**130**	25*	ND	12*	1.1*	**46**
31–50 y	2.7*	**130**	25*	ND	12*	1.1*	**46**
51–70 y	2.7*	**130**	21*	ND	11*	1.1*	**46**
> 70 y	2.7*	**130**	21*	ND	11*	1.1*	**46**
Pregnancy							
14–18 y	3.0*	**175**	28*	ND	13*	1.4*	**71**
19–30 y	3.0*	**175**	28*	ND	13*	1.4*	**71**
31–50 y	3.0*	**175**	28*	ND	13*	1.4*	**71**
Lactation							
14–18	3.8*	**210**	29*	ND	13*	1.3*	**71**
19–30 y	3.8*	**210**	29*	ND	13*	1.3*	**71**
31–50 y	3.8*	**210**	29*	ND	13*	1.3*	**71**

Source: Dietary Reference Intakes for Energy, Carbohydrate, Fiber, Fat, Fatty Acids, Cholesterol, Protein, and Amino Acids (2002/2005) and *Dietary Reference Intakes for Water, Potassium, Sodium, Chloride, and Sulfate* (2005). The report may be accessed via www.nap.edu.

Note: This table (taken from the DRI reports, see www.nap.edu) presents Recommended Dietary Allowances (RDA) in **bold type** and Adequate Intakes (AI) in ordinary type followed by an asterisk (*). An RDA is the average daily dietary intake level; sufficient to meet the nutrient requirements of nearly all (97–98 percent) healthy individuals in a group. It is calculated from an Estimated Average Requirement (EAR). If sufficient scientific evidence is not available to establish an EAR, and thus calculate an RDA, an AI is usually developed. For healthy breastfed infants, an AI is the mean intake. The AI for other life stage and gender groups is believed to cover the needs of all healthy individuals in the groups, but lack of data or uncertainty in the data prevent being able to specify with confidence the percentage of individuals covered by this intake.

[a]Total water includes all water contained in food, beverages, and drinking water.

[b]Based on g protein per kg of body weight for the reference body weight, e.g., for adults 0.8 g/kg body weight for the reference body weight.

[c]Not determined.

energy intake for each of the life stage and gender groups.[14] Human milk, which contains no **dietary fiber,** is considered the optimal source of nourishment for infants throughout at least the first year of life and is recommended as the only source of nourishment for the first four to six months of life. As solid foods are gradually introduced during the second six months of life, dietary fiber intake will increase. However, there are no data on dietary fiber intake for infants and no functional criteria for fiber status available upon which to establish an AI for total fiber for infants. Total fiber is defined as the sum of dietary fiber and **functional fiber.**[14] Dietary fibers are nondigestible carbohydrates and lignin that are naturally present in plant foods and that are consumed in their natural, intact state (i.e, in an unmodified form) as part of an unrefined food. Functional fibers are nondigestible carbohydrates that have beneficial physiological effects in humans but that have been isolated or extracted (i.e., removed) from foods and then added as an ingredient to food or taken as a dietary supplement. Although functional fibers are predominantly of plant origin, a few are of animal origin, such as the animal-derived connective tissues chitin and chitosan, which are found in the exoskeletons of arthropods such as crabs and lobsters. In essence, what distinguishes functional fiber from dietary fiber is the source of the fiber. Functional fibers have been removed from their original source and then added to another food or are consumed as a nutritional supplement. Dietary fibers are naturally present in plant foods that are eaten.[14] For example, the pectin consumed when an apple is eaten would be considered a dietary fiber. When the pectin is industrially extracted from fruits and then added as a gelling agent to jams, it is considered a functional fiber.[14]

Except for infants, no RDA or AI have been established for total fat because there are insufficient data available to determine a level of total fat intake associated with risk of inadequacy or prevention of chronic disease. There is no UL established for total fat because no level has been identified that is associated with an averse effect.[14] The AI for total fat for infants birth to 6 months is set at the mean intake of fat by infants of this age who are exclusively breast-fed. The AI for total fat for infants 7 to 12 months of age is based on the mean fat intake of infants of this age who are fed human milk and age-appropriate complementary foods.[14] Linoleic acid (an *n*-6 fatty acid) and α-linolenic acid (an *n*-3 fatty acid) are necessary for optimal health, and an insufficient intake of either can result in adverse clinical symptoms such as a scaly skin rash, neurological abnormalities, and poor growth. Because neither linoleic acid nor α-linolenic acid are synthesized by the human body and because both are necessary for optimal health, they are considered essential fatty acids and an AI has been established for each.[14] For infants birth to 6 months of age, the AIs for linoleic acid and α-linolenic acid are set at the mean intakes of these fatty acids by infants of this age who are exclusively breast-fed. The AIs for linoleic acid and α-linolenic acid for infants 7 to 12 months of age are based on the mean intakes of these fatty acids by infants of this age who are fed human milk and age-appropriate complementary foods.[14] For the remaining life stage and gender groups, the AIs for linoleic acid and α-linolenic acid are set at the median intake of these fatty acids in the diets of Americans who have no apparent deficiency of these essential fatty acids.[14] The AI for protein for infants birth to 6 months of age is set at the mean protein intake of infants of this age who are exclusively breast-fed. The RDA for protein (grams of protein per day) for the remaining life stage and gender groups are shown in Table 2.7.[14] Although there were insufficient data available to establish a UL for protein, the DRI Committee has cautioned against the consumption of any single amino acids at levels greater than those normally found in foods.[14]

Acceptable Macronutrient Distribution Ranges (AMDRs) provide guidance to individuals on the consumption of total fat, *n*-6 polyunsaturated fatty acids (linoleic acid), *n*-3 polyunsaturated fatty acids (α-linolenic acid), carbohydrate, and protein to ensure adequate intake and to decrease risk of chronic disease. The AMDRs, shown in Table 2.8, are expressed in terms of percent of

TABLE 2.8 Dietary Reference Intakes (DRIs): Acceptable Macronutrient Distribution Ranges
Food and Nutrition Board, Institute of Medicine, National Academies

	Range (percent of energy)		
Macronutrient	**Children, 1–3 y**	**Children, 4–18 y**	**Adults**
Fat	30–40	25–35	20–35
n-6 polyunsaturated fatty acids[a] (linoleic acid)	5–10	5–10	5–10
n-3 polyunsaturated fatty acids[a] (α-linolenic acid)	0.6–1.2	0.6–1.2	0.6–1.2
Carbohydrate	45–65	45–65	45–65
Protein	5–20	10–30	10–35

Source: Dietary Reference Intakes for Energy, Carbohydrate, Fiber, Fat, Fatty Acids, Cholesterol, Protein, and Amino Acids (2002/2005). The report may be accessed via www.nap.edu.

[a]Approximately 10 percent of the total can come from longer-chain *n*-3 or *n*-6 fatty acids.

Table 2.9 Dietary Reference Intakes (DRIs): Acceptable Macronutrient Distribution Ranges
Food and Nutrition Board, Institute of Medicine, National Academies

Macronutrient	Recommendation
Dietary cholesterol	As low as possible while consuming a nutritionally adequate diet
Trans fatty acids	As low as possible while consuming a nutritionally adequate diet
Saturated fatty acids	As low as possible while consuming a nutritionally adequate diet
Added sugars[a]	Limit to no more than 25% of total energy

Source: Dietary Reference Intakes for Energy, Carbohydrate, Fiber, Fat, Fatty Acids, Cholesterol, Protein, and Amino Acids (2002/2005). The report may be accessed via www.nap.edu.

[a]Not a recommended intake. A daily intake of added sugars that individuals should aim for to achieve a healthful diet was not set.

energy from each of these macronutrients for three different age ranges: 1 to 3 years of age, 4 to 18 years of age, and 19 years of age and older. No other distinctions are made with regard to life stage or gender.[14] Additional macronutrient recommendations for the prevention of chronic disease are shown in Table 2.9. These recommendations address concerns related to the health implications of diets containing excessive quantities of dietary cholesterol, *trans* fatty acids, saturated fatty acids, and added sugars. It is important to note that while it is suggested that consumption of added sugars be *limited to no more than 25% of total energy,* this is not a recommended level of intake. The daily intake of added sugars that an individual should have to achieve a healthful diet has not been set.

Uses of the DRIs

The suggested uses of the DRIs fall into two broad categories: assessing nutrient intakes and planning for nutrient intakes. Each of the two categories is further divided into uses pertaining to individuals and uses pertaining to groups. The uses of the DRIs for assessing and planning the intakes of apparently healthy individuals and groups are outlined in Boxes 2.3 and 2.4, respectively.

The DRIs are not intended to serve as the only means of assessing the nutritional adequacy of an individual's diet. An individual's actual nutrient requirement can vary widely from the group average (the EAR), and without various biochemical and physiologic measures it is impossible to determine whether an individual's actual nutrient requirement is close to the group EAR, greater than the EAR, or less than the EAR. In addition, intake of most nutrients varies considerably from one day to the next, requiring many days of measurement to estimate *usual* nutrient intake, as discussed in Chapter 3. Consequently, when assessing the adequacy of an individual's diet, use of multiple nutritional assessment methods—dietary, anthropometric, biochemical, and clinical—must be considered.

If an individual's usual intake of a nutrient is equal to or greater than the RDA or AI, it is unlikely that intake is inadequate. When usual intake is less than the EAR, there is a high likelihood that intake is inadequate. However, if usual intake falls between the EAR and RDA, the likelihood of inadequate intake will be difficult to determine, and in such instances use of other assessment techniques is important in determining nutrient adequacy.[17] If an individual's usual intake of a nutrient is less than the UL, there is little risk of excessive intake. Risk of adverse health effects from excessive intake increases when usual intake rises above the UL.[17] When planning a healthy individual's diet, the RDAs and AIs are intended to serve as a goal for average daily nutrient intake over time (over several days to several weeks, depending on the turnover rate of the nutrient in question).[18]

Assessing the adequacy of a group's nutrient intake involves comparing the distribution of usual intakes among group members with the distribution of the requirement for the nutrient.[17] A "cutpoint approach" is typically used to estimate the percentage of group members whose usual intakes are less than the EAR. The RDA is not intended to be used for estimating the prevalence of inadequate intakes in groups.[17] In the absence of an EAR, it may be necessary to use the AI to assess the adequacy of a group's intake, but greater care must be exercised than when using the EAR, given the fact that the AI is an observational standard.[17] The proportion of the population with usual intakes above the UL is likely to be at some risk of adverse effects due to overconsumption, while the proportion below the UL is likely to be at no risk.[17]

Data from the third National Health and Nutrition Examination Survey (discussed in Chapter 4) indicate that approximately 11% of nonsmoking adult females and 21% of nonsmoking adult males have a usual vitamin C intake (from food and supplements) less than the EAR for vitamin C.[12] Estimating the prevalence of inadequate nutrient intakes in a population requires accurate, quantitative information on usual nutrient intake by the group. Both the U.S. Department of Health and Human Services and the U.S. Department of Agriculture participate in the National Health and Nutrition Examination Survey, or NHANES, which provides data on the food and nutrient intake of Americans as well as data on various health determinants such as height, weight, blood pressure, blood cholesterol levels, and so on. NHANES and the other nutritional monitoring activities of these two agencies are discussed in Chapter 4.

The EAR is used in planning or making recommendations for the nutrient intake of groups. The group's mean nutrient intake should be high enough so that only a small percentage of group members have an intake less than the

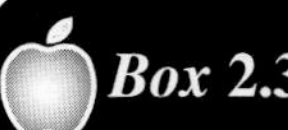

Box 2.3 Uses of DRIs for Assessing Intakes of Individuals and Groups

FOR AN INDIVIDUAL

EAR: Use to examine the probability that usual intake is inadequate.

RDA: Usual intake at or above this level has a low probability of inadequacy.

AI: Usual intake at or above this level has a low probability of inadequacy.

UL: Usual intake above this level may place an individual at risk of adverse effects from excessive nutrient intake.

FOR A GROUP

EAR: Use to estimate the prevalence of inadequate intakes within a group.

RDA: Do not use to assess intakes of groups.

AI: Mean usual intake at or above this level implies a low prevalence of inadequate intakes.[a]

UL: Use to estimate the percentage of the population at potential risk of adverse effects from excessive nutrient intake.

EAR = Estimated Average Requirement

RDA = Recommended Dietary Allowance

AI = Adequate Intake

UL = Tolerable Upper Intake Level

[a]When the AI for a nutrient is not based on mean intakes of healthy populations, this assessment is made with less confidence.

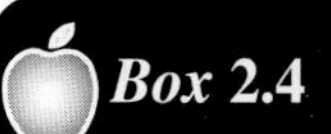

Box 2.4 Uses of DRIs for Planning Intakes of Apparently Healthy Individuals and Groups

FOR AN INDIVIDUAL

EAR[a]: Do not use as an intake goal for the individual.

RDA: Plan for this intake; usual intake at or above this level has a low probability of inadequacy.

AI: Plan for this intake; usual intake at or above this level has a low probability of inadequacy.

UL: Plan for usual intake below this level to avoid potential risk of adverse effects from excessive nutrient intake.

FOR A GROUP

EAR[a]: Use to plan for an acceptably low prevalence of inadequate intakes within a group.

RDA: Do not use to plan intakes of groups.

AI[b]: Plan for mean intake at this level; mean usual intake at or above this level implies a low prevalence of inadequate intakes.

UL: Use in planning to minimize the proportion of the population at potential risk of excessive nutrient intake.

[a]In the case of energy, an EER is provided. The EER is the dietary energy intake that is predicted (with variance) to maintain energy balance in a healthy adult of a defined age, gender, weight, height, and level of physical activity. In children and in pregnant and lactating women, the EER includes the needs associated with deposition of tissues or secretion of milk at rates consistent with good health. For individuals, the EER represents the midpoint of a range within which an individual's energy requirements are likely to vary. As such, it is below the needs of half the individuals with the specified characteristics, and it exceeds the needs of the other half. Body weight should be monitored and energy intake adjusted accordingly.

[b]The AI should be used with less confidence if it has not been established as a mean intake of a healthy group.

EAR but not so high that too many group members have intakes above the UL. If the prevalence of nutrient inadequacy is too high, an appropriate intervention should be undertaken to increase intakes by those at greatest risk of inadequacy while maintaining an acceptably low prevalence of group members with intake above the UL.

NUTRIENT DENSITY

Nutrient density refers to a food's vitamin and mineral content relative to its energy content.[20–22] A nutrient-dense food is a good source of vitamins, minerals, and other food components that may have positive health effects but is relatively low in energy. Nutrient-dense foods are lean or low in solids fats (fats that are solid at room temperature and that are major sources of saturated and *trans* fats) and are low in added sugars and refined starches, all of which add kilocalories but few essential nutrients or dietary fiber. Nutrient-dense foods also minimize or exclude added salt or other components that are high in sodium.[23]

Box 2.5 compares high-nutrient-dense foods with low-nutrient-dense foods. Although the low-nutrient-dense foods share similarities with the high-nutrient-dense foods, they differ in that they are higher in kilocalories because of fats and sugars, most of which are added during processing, during preparation, or at the

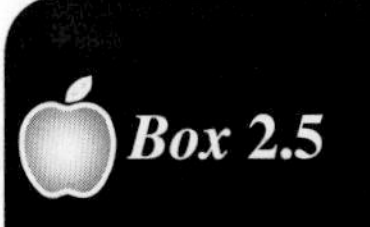

Box 2.5 **Foods having a high nutrient density (the left column) are good sources of essential nutrients but are relatively low in kilocalories compared to similar foods having a low nutrient density (the right column), which are relatively high in kilocalories because of the fats and sugars added during processing or preparation.**

High-Nutrient-Dense Foods	Low-Nutrient-Dense Foods
Broccoli, steamed, served with lemon wedges	Broccoli, batter dipped, deep-fat fried
Potato, baked	Potato, French fried
Turkey breast, skinless, broiled	Hamburger patty, fried
Salad dressing, low-calorie	Salad dressing, regular
Milk, nonfat, plain	Milk, whole, plain
Orange juice, unsweetened, calcium-fortified	Soft-drink, orange-flavored, sugar-sweetened
Yogurt, nonfat, unsweetened	Yogurt, fruit-flavored, sweetened

table. For example, broccoli that is served with a cheese sauce or is dipped in batter and deep-fat fried will have many of the same vitamins and minerals as the steamed broccoli, but the cheese sauce or deep-fat frying will add extra kilocalories that many people want to avoid to prevent unnecessary weight gain. Furthermore, a person can eat a liberal amount of the steamed broccoli served with lemon wedges without consuming excessive energy.

Figure 2.4 illustrates the difference in the number of calories in a food that is not nutrient-dense as opposed to a nutrient-dense form of the food. For example, a regular ground beef patty (75% lean) that weighs 3 ounces after cooking contains 236 calories, whereas a cooked 3-ounce extra lean beef patty (90% lean) contains 184 calories. By choosing the extra lean beef instead of the regular ground beef, a person would consume less beef fat, amounting to 52 fewer calories. Breaded fried chicken strips weighing 3 ounces contain 246 calories, whereas a 3-ounce baked chicken breast contains only 138 calories. In this instance, a relatively simple change in the method of preparation and cooking the chicken has eliminated 108 calories that were added by the breading and frying fat. According to the *Dietary Guidelines for Americans,* nutrient-dense foods include all vegetables, fruits, whole

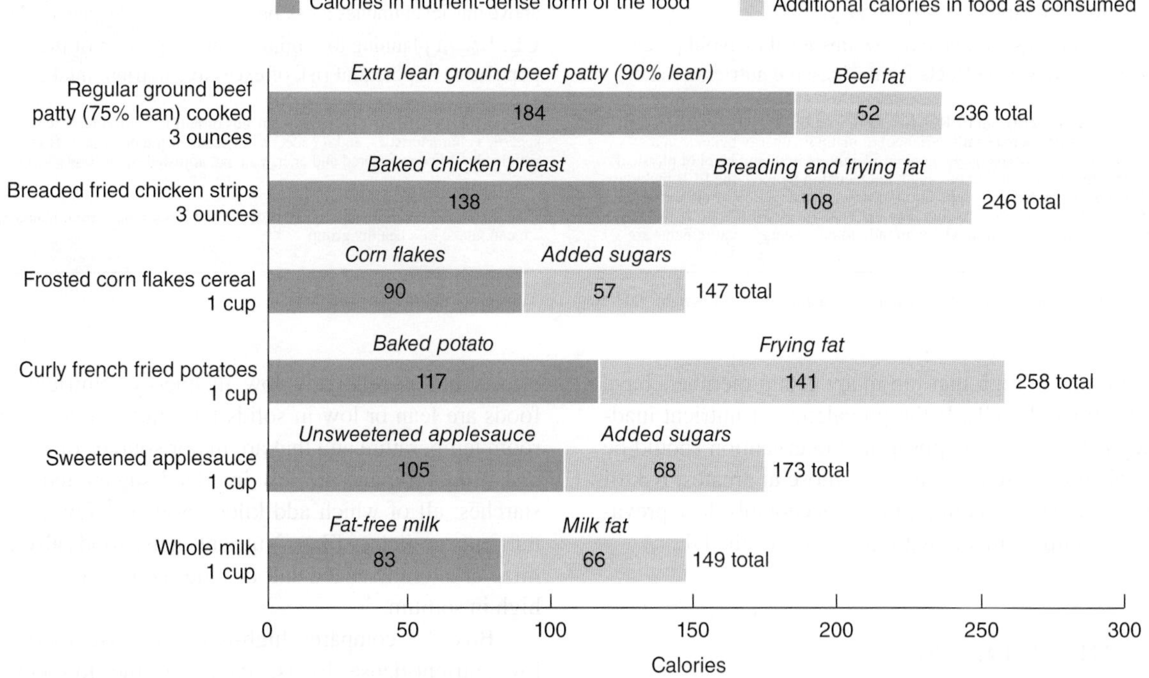

Figure 2.4 **Examples of the calories in food choices that are not in nutrient-dense forms and the calories in nutrient-dense forms of these foods.**

Source: U.S. Department of Health and Human Services and U.S. Department of Agriculture. 2010. *Dietary Guidelines for Americans, 2010.* Washington, DC: U.S. Government Printing Office. www.dietaryguidelines.gov.

grains, fat-free or low-fat milk and milk products, beans and peas, nuts and seeds, eggs, seafood, and lean poultry and meats that are prepared without added solid fats, sugars, refined grains, and salt and other sources of sodium.[23]

Nutrient density is not a new concept. Forty years ago it was initially defined as the ratio of the amount of a nutrient in a food to the energy provided by the same food, and was expressed as the amount of a nutrient per 1000 kcal.[24] A basic premise of nutrient density was that if the quantity of nutrients per 1000 kcal was great enough, the nutrient needs of a person would be met when his or her energy needs were met. In recent years there has been renewed interest in nutrient density as a useful approach to help people plan diets that maintain adequate nutrient intake while minimizing consumption of unnecessary kilocalories and reducing the intake of sodium, solid fats, dietary cholesterol, added sugars, and refined grains.[23] A key recommendation of the most recent edition of the *Dietary Guidelines for Americans* is that individuals choose nutrient-dense foods, a recommendation that is widely supported by health professionals and nutrition organizations.[23,25] The diets of many North Americans are energy dense but nutrient poor.[22] Nutrient density addresses the issue that many people need to manage their body weight by controlling their energy intake while ensuring that they consume adequate nutrients and reduce their consumption of those food components that should be limited.[23] There is consistent scientific evidence that dietary patterns emphasizing nutrient-dense foods improve weight loss and weight management among adults and decrease the risk of developing type 2 diabetes among adults.[26]

Nutrient Profiling

Using the concept of nutrient density to select nutritious foods and to plan healthy diets is hindered by the fact that there is no valid or scientific method for defining the nutrient density of foods and no specific standard or criteria for consistently identifying nutrient-dense foods.[25,27] Nutrient profiling can be used to address this problem. Nutrient profiling is the science of ranking or classifying foods based on their nutrient composition.[25,27,28] In recent years, numerous nutrient profiling models (sometimes referred to as nutrition quality indices) have been developed by a variety of groups, including food manufacturers, food retailers, government agencies, nonprofit organizations, and groups of experts not related to the food industry.[29,30] Nutrient profiling models use a mathematical formula or algorithm to calculate a score using a certain set of nutrient values to include as variables in the algorithm. Some models include those nutrients and food components that should be consumed more frequently, other models use only those nutrients and food components that should be consumed less frequently, while other models use a combination of both.[25,30] The algorithms of some models are not available to the public or scientific community but are proprietary (i.e., copyrighted, patented, or kept a trade secret), whereas the algorithms of other models are freely available to the public and scientific community.[31] Unfortunately, few of the models have been studied to determine whether they actually improve the food choices of consumers to result in measurable improvements in health.[28] In recent years there has been considerable interest in using nutrient profiling models as one approach for rating the nutritional value of foods in front-of-package labeling systems.[29,31] Front-of-package labeling systems are discussed later in this chapter within the context of the nutrition labeling of food.

INDICES OF DIET QUALITY

Numerous indices of diet quality have been proposed and reported in the scientific literature.[32–34] How these indices define diet quality varies considerably, depending on the attributes selected by the creator of the particular index and by the era in which the index was developed. For example, earlier indices tend to define a high-quality diet as one supplying adequate protein and selected micronutrients for a given energy level. More recent indices define diet quality in terms of proportionality (eating more servings of certain food groups and fewer of others), moderation (limiting intake of foods and beverages contributing to excess intake of fat, dietary cholesterol, added sugars, sodium, and alcohol), and variety (thus increasing exposure to a wide range of nutritive and other food components).[32–34] Reflecting the nutritional era in which they were developed, earlier indices tend to focus on prevention of deficiency diseases, while more recent ones tend to address risk of chronic disease.

Diet quality indices are typically based on one of three approaches to assessing diet: comparing intake of certain nutrients and food components to a standard, comparing intake of foods or food groups to a standard, or evaluating both nutrient intake and foods or food groups.[32–34] The Diet Quality Index and the Healthy Eating Index evaluate intake of various nutrients and food components and assess consumption of foods and food groups.

Diet Quality Index

The Diet Quality Index (DQI) is an instrument used to assess the overall diet quality of groups and to evaluate risk for chronic disease related to dietary pattern.[32,35] It was originally published in 1994 and was based on 8 dietary recommendations from the National Academy of Sciences publication *Diet and Health: Implications for Reducing Chronic Disease Risk.*[36] It was revised in 1999 to reflect the development of the Food Guide Pyramid in 1992, revisions in the *Dietary Guidelines for Americans,* and the creation of the Dietary Reference

TABLE 2.10 Diet Quality Index Components and Scoring Guidelines*

Component	Scoring Criteria	
Total fat ≤ 30% of energy intake	≤ 30%	10 points
	31% to 40%	5 points
	> 40%	0 points
Saturated fat ≤ 10% of energy intake	≤ 10%	10 points
	11% to 13%	5 points
	> 13%	0 points
Dietary cholesterol < 300 mg per day	≤ 300 mg	10 points
	300 to 400 mg	5 points
	> 400 mg	0 points
2–4 servings of fruit per day	10–0 points, proportional to percent of recommended number of servings*	
3–5 servings of vegetables per day	10–0 points, proportional to percent of recommended number of servings	
6–11 servings of grains per day	10–0 points, proportional to percent of recommended number of servings	
Calcium intake as a percentage of Adequate Intake for life stage and gender group	10–0 points, proportional to percentage of Adequate Intake for life stage and gender group	
Iron intake as percent of Recommended Dietary Allowance for life stage and gender group	10–0 points, proportional to percentage of Recommended Dietary Allowance for life stage and gender group	
Dietary diversity score	10–0 points, proportional to consumption of foods across 23 food group categories	
Dietary moderation score	10–0 points, based on intake of added sugars, discretionary fat,† sodium, and alcohol in excess of recommended levels of intake	

Adapted from Haines PS, Siega-Riz AM, Popkin BM. 1999. The Diet Quality Index Revised: A measurement instrument for populations. *Journal of the American Dietetic Association* 99:697–704.

*Serving recommendations based on energy intake according to the Food Guide Pyramid.

†Discretionary fat is defined as all excess fat from the five major food groups beyond that which would be consumed if only the lowest fat forms of a given food were eaten. It includes fats added to food in preparation or at the table, including margarine, cheese, oil, meat drippings, and chocolate.

Intakes. Table 2.10 shows the revised Diet Quality Index (what its creators call the Diet Quality Index Revised). The Diet Quality Index scores diet on the basis of 10 indicators of diet quality. The first three indicators reflect macronutrient intake, the next three reflect the 1992 Food Guide Pyramid's recommendations for fruit, vegetable, and grain consumption, and the two recommendations for calcium and iron are based on the Dietary Reference Intakes. The last two indicators address the importance of consuming foods from a variety of food groups and having a moderate intake of sugar, discretionary fat, sodium, and alcoholic beverages.[32] Each of the 10 components contributes a maximum of 10 points to the total DQI score, which has a maximum of 100 points. The higher the score, the higher the diet quality.

The DQI has been shown to be a useful instrument in evaluating dietary patterns. Healthier maternal dietary patterns during gestation as measured by the DQI were shown to be associated with offspring having a reduced risk of neural tube defects and orofacial clefts.[37] In an intervention designed to promote and evaluate dietary change among older cancer survivors enrolled in a home-based intervention trial, the DQI was shown to be an effective instrument in developing an intervention to improve the diet quality as well as in evaluating overall diet quality.[38]

Healthy Eating Index

The Healthy Eating Index (HEI) is an instrument developed by researchers at the U.S. Department of Agriculture for assessing how well the diets of Americans adhere to U.S. federal dietary guidance.[39] When originally developed in 1995, it was designed to determine adherence to the Food Guide Pyramid's serving recommendations. It was revised in 2005 following the release of the 2005 edition of the *Dietary Guidelines for Americans* (discussed later in this chapter), which made several important changes in federal dietary guidance. Among these were encouraging adequate consumption of whole grains, whole fruit instead of fruit juice, and vegetables, particularly dark green and orange vegetables, and encouraging moderate consumption of sodium, saturated fat, and calories from alcoholic beverages and foods containing solid fats and added sugars. The current version, known as the Healthy Eating Index-2005 (HEI-2005), is used by the U.S. Department of Agriculture to assess diet quality as defined by the current *Dietary Guidelines for Americans.*[40] The HEI-2005 can also be used to monitor changes in food consumption patterns, to evaluate menus and diet plans, to identify target areas for nutrition education and health promotion programs, and to evaluate those programs. It is the only index issued by the U.S. federal government and computed on a regular basis for gauging the overall diet quality of Americans.

Table 2.11 compares the original HEI developed in 1995 with the revised HEI-2005. The various components are grouped into two categories: adequacy and moderation. The "adequacy components" were established to ensure adequacy of nutrient intake while the "moderation components" are those whose intake should be limited. The original HEI used 10 components to determine adherence to the Food Guide Pyramid's serving recommendations for the five major food groups (total fruit, total vegetables, total grains, milk, and meat and beans), total sodium intake, saturated fat and total fat as a percent of energy, cholesterol intake, and variety.[39]

TABLE 2.11 Original Healthy Eating Index (HEI) and Healthy Eating Index-2005 (HEI-2005) Components and Standards for Scoring

Component	Score				
	0	5	8	10	20
	Points				
Original HEI					
Adequacy					
Total Fruit	0 ←			→ 2–4 servings (approx. 1–2 cups[1])	
Total Vegetables	0 ←			→ 3–5 servings (approx. 1.5–2.5 cups[1])	
Total Grains	0 ←			→ 6–11 servings (approx. 6–11 oz eq[1])	
Milk	0 ←			→ 2–3 servings (approx. 2–3 cups[2])	
Meat (and beans)	0 ←			→ 2–3 servings (approx. 5.5–7.0 oz eq[1])	
Variety	≤ 6 ←			→ ≥ 16 different foods in 3 days	
Moderation					
Sodium	≥ 4.8 ←			→ ≤ 2.4 g	
Saturated Fat	≥ 15 ←			→ ≤ 10% energy	
Total Fat	≥ 45 ←			→ ≤ 30% energy	
Cholesterol	≥ 450 ←			→ ≤ 300 mg	
HEI-2005					
Adequacy					
Total Fruit[3]	0 ←	→ ≥ 8.4 cup eq/1000 kcal			
Whole Fruit[4]	0 ←	→ ≥ 0.4 cup eq/1000 kcal			
Total Vegetables	0 ←	→ ≥ 1.1 cup eq/1000 kcal			
Dark Green and Orange Vegetables and Legumes[5]	0 ←	→ ≥ 0.4 cup eq/1000 kcal			
Total Grains	0 ←	→ ≥ 3.0 oz eq/1000 kcal			
Whole Grains	0 ←	→ ≥ 1.5oz eq/1000 kcal			
Milk[6]	0 ←			→ ≥ 1.3 cup eq/1000 kcal	
Meat and Beans[7]	0 ←			→ ≥ 2.5 oz eq/1000 kcal	
Oils[8]	0 ←			→ ≥ 12 g/1000 kcal	
Moderation					
Saturated Fat	≥ 15 ←		→ 10 ←	→ ≤ 7% of energy	
Sodium	≥ 20 ←		→ 1.1 ←	→ ≤ **0.7** g/1000 kcal	
Calories from Solid Fats, Alcoholic Beverages, and Added Sugars	≥ 50 ←		→ ≤ 20% of energy		

Source: Adapted from Guenther PM, Reedy J, Krebs-Smith SM, Reeve BB, Basiotis PP. 2007. *Development and Evaluation of the Healthy Eating Index-2005, Technical Report.* Center for Nutrition Policy and Promotion, U.S. Department of Agriculture, and Guenther PM, Reedy J, Krebs-Smith SM. 2008. Development of the Healthy Eating Index-2005. *Journal of the American Dietetic Association* 108:1896–1901.

[1]According to sex and age.

[2]According to age.

[3]Includes 100% fruit juice.

[4]Includes all forms except juice.

[5]Includes legumes only after meat and beans standard is met.

[6]Includes all milk products, such as fluid milk, yogurt and cheese, and soy beverages.

[7]Includes legumes only if the meat and beans standard is otherwise not met.

[8]Includes nonhydrogenated vegetable oils and oils in fish, nuts, and seeds.

Scores for each of the 10 components range from 0 to 10, with a maximum total score of 100 points, and were assigned in terms of absolute amounts that varied according to energy level.[39] In the case of total fruit, the minimum score of 0 was assigned if intake of total fruit was 0 servings per day while the maximum score of 10 was assigned when 2 to 4 servings (approximately 1 to 2 cups) were consumed per day. Those who had a low energy requirement could receive the maximum score when 2 servings were consumed while those with a high energy requirement would have to consume 4 servings per day to get the maximum score. The original HEI provided a single, summary score with a high score implying a "good" diet and a low score suggesting a "poor" diet.[39] Greater intakes of the adequacy components result in higher scores while lower intakes of the moderation components result in higher scores.

The HEI-2005 includes 12 components with the first 9 assessing how adequate the subject's diet is in terms of total fruit (including 100% juice), whole fruit (excluding juice), total vegetables, dark green and orange vegetables and legumes, total grains, whole grains, milk, meat and beans, and oils (nonhydrogenated vegetable oils and oils in fish, nuts, and seeds). The last three components focus on the extent to which intake of saturated fat, sodium, and calories from solid fat, alcoholic beverages, and added sugars are limited. In the HEI-2005 two different components assess the adequacy of fruit intake: total fruit, which includes 100% fruit juice and whole fruit, which excludes fruit juice. Unlike the original HEI, the HEI-2005 represents intake of foods and nutrients on a density basis, that is, as amounts per 1000 kilocalories of intake. For example, the maximum score is given when total fruit intake is equivalent to ≥ 0.8 cup/1000 kilocalories and when whole fruit intake is equivalent to ≥ 0.4 cup/1000 kilocalories. By representing intake of foods and nutrients on a density basis, many of the recommendations are similar across energy levels.[40] For the first six components listed in Table 2.11 for the HEI-2005, the maximum scores are 5 points and the maximum scores for milk, meat and beans, oils, saturated fat, and sodium are 10 points. The maximum score for calories from solid fat, alcoholic beverages, and added sugars is set at 20 because of the priority the 2005 *Dietary Guidelines for Americans* give to encouraging the selection of foods that are low in fat and low in added sugars and because foods containing solid fat, alcoholic beverages, and added sugars are currently consumed in amounts that far exceed current recommendations.[40] The HEI-2005 can provide a single, total score indicating overall diet quality, which can vary between 0 and 100 (the higher the score, the more adherent the diet is to the federal dietary recommendations). Scores can also be generated for each component or for groups of components to examine intakes of individual components or groups of components.

Using dietary intake data collected from 8272 Americans age 2 years and older who participated in the 2003–2004 National Health and Nutrition Examination Survey (discussed in Chapter 4), researchers at the U.S. Department of Agriculture evaluated the diet quality of all participants grouped together and also compared the diet quality of low-income participants with those having a higher income.[41] As shown in Table 2.12, when evaluating the diets of all participants grouped together (age 2 and older, all incomes), all the HEI-2005 component scores were below the maximum possible except for total grains and meat and beans. Scores were particularly low (less than half the maximum) for dark green and orange vegetables and legumes and for whole grains (indicating a lower than recommended intake of these foods) and for sodium and calories from solid fats, alcoholic beverages, and added sugars (indicating a higher than recommended intake).[30] Compared to higher-income participants, low-income participants had significantly lower component scores for total vegetables, dark green and orange vegetables and legumes, and whole grains (indicating a lower than recommended intake of these foods) and a higher component score for sodium (indicating a lower intake of sodium and better adherence to the recommendation to limit sodium intake). There was no significant difference in total HEI-2005 scores for children ages 2 to 18 years old by family income level, and children in both income groups had component scores that were below the maximum for all components except for total grains. The only difference between these two groups was that children from low-income families had a higher component score for total vegetables, which may be due to the fact that children from low-income families are more likely to participate in the National School Lunch Program.[41] The researchers concluded that the diets of all Americans, regardless of income level, could be improved by increasing intake of nutrient-dense foods including fruits, vegetables, whole grains, and fat-free and low-fat milk and limiting the intake of foods containing solid fats, saturated fats, added sugars, and sodium.[41]

Dietary Guidelines

Dietary guidelines or goals can be defined as statements from authoritative scientific bodies translating nutritional recommendations into practical advice to consumers about their eating habits. Rather than merely ensuring adequate nutrient intake, *they are primarily intended to address the more common and pressing nutrition-related health problems, such as heart disease, certain cancers, stroke, hypertension, and diabetes.* They often are expressed as nonquantitative changes from the present average national diet or from people's typical eating habits. Examples of guidelines are "consume a variety of nutrient dense foods and beverages within and among the basic food groups while choosing foods that limit the intake of saturated and *trans* fats, cholesterol, added sugars, salt, and alcohol" and "choose fiber-rich fruits, vegetables, and whole grains often." Table 2.13 contrasts the DRIs with dietary guidelines.

Early Dietary Guidelines

Informal dietary guidelines have existed since time immemorial in the form of cultural practices, taboos, and religious teachings. The first formal set of dietary guidelines of modern times, however, was developed by nutrition professors from Sweden, Finland, Norway, and Denmark

TABLE 2.12 Estimated Mean Healthy Eating Index-2005 Total and Component Scores, All and Low-Income Populations, United States, 2003–2004

Component (maximum score)	Age 2 and older All incomes (n = 8272) *Score (CI)*[1]	Age 2 and older Low income[2] (n = 3293) *Score (CI)*	Age 2 and older Higher income (n = 4979) *Score (CI)*	Age 2–18 years Low income[3] (n = 2148) *Score (CI)*	Age 2–18 years Higher income (n = 1405) *Score (CI)*
Total Fruit (5)	2.9 (2.6, 3.1)	2.9 (2.5, 3.2)	2.9 (2.5, 3.2)	3.3 (2.9, 3.7)	3.1 (2.8, 3.4)
Whole Fruit (5)	3.1 (2.8, 3.5)	2.8 (2.4, 3.2)	3.2 (2.8, 3.7)	2.7 (2.2, 3.2)	2.8 (2.3, 3.3)
Total Vegetables (5)	3.2 (3.2, 3.3)	3.0 (2.9, 3.2)*	3.3 (3.2, 3.4)*	2.5 (2.4, 2.6)*	2.2 (2.1, 2.4)*
Dark Green and Orange Vegetables and Legumes (5)	1.2 (1.1, 1.3)	1.0 (0.9, 1.1)*	1.2 (1.1, 1.4)*	0.6 (0.5, 0.8)	0.6 (0.4, 0.7)
Total Grains (5)	5.0 (5.0, 5.0)	5.0 (5.0, 5.0)	5.0 (5.0, 5.0)	5.0 (5.0, 5.0)	5.0 (5.0, 5.0)
Whole Grains (5)	0.9 (0.8, 1.0)	0.8 (0.7, 0.9)*	0.9 (0.9, 1.0)*	0.7 (0.6, 0.9)	0.7 (0.7, 0.8)
Milk (10)	6.2 (5.9, 6.6)	6.3 (5.9, 6.7)	6.2 (5.8, 6.7)	8.4 (7.8, 8.9)	8.5 (7.9, 9.1)
Meat and Beans (10)	10.0 (10.0, 10.0)	9.9 (9.4, 10.0)	10.0 (10.0, 10.0)	8.4 (7.8, 8.9)	8.1 (7.6, 8.7)
Oils (10)	7.3 (7.0, 7.6)	7.1 (6.6, 7.6)	7.4 (7.0, 7.8)	6.8 (6.2, 7.5)	6.8 (6.4, 7.1)
Saturated Fat (10)	5.9 (5.6, 6.1)	5.9 (5.5, 6.3)	5.8 (5.5, 6.1)	4.9 (4.2, 5.6)	5.6 (5.0, 6.1)
Sodium (10)	4.0 (3.8, 4.1)	4.4 (4.2, 4.7)*	3.8 (3.6, 4.0)*	4.6 (4.3, 4.9)	4.2 (3.9, 4.5)
Calories from Solid Fats, Alcoholic Beverages, and Added Sugars (20)	7.8 (7.3, 8.4)	7.4 (6.6, 8.2)	8.0 (7.5, 8.5)	8.3 (7.5, 9.1)	7.8 (6.9, 8.7)
Total HEI-2005 score (100)	57.5 (56.0, 59.0)	56.5 (54.3, 58.8)	57.8 (56.2, 59.4)	56.4 (53.9, 58.9)	55.4 (52.6, 58.2)

Source: From Guenther PM, Juan WY, Lino M, Hiza HA, Fungwe T, Lucas R. 2008. Diet quality of low-income and higher income Americans in 2003–04 as measured by the Healthy Eating Index-2005. *Nutrition Insight* 42. Center for Nutrition Policy and Promotion, U.S. Department of Agriculture.

[1]95% confidence interval.

[2]Household income <130% of the federal poverty level.

[3]Household income <185% of the federal poverty level.

*Significant difference between income levels ($p < 0.05$).

TABLE 2.13 The Dietary Reference Intakes (DRIs) and Dietary Guidelines Contrasted

DRIs	Dietary Guidelines
Developed earlier	Developed more recently
Only one set per country	Multiple (sometimes incongruent) sets possible in a country
Expressed in quantitative terms as weight of nutrient per day	Often expressed as nonquantitative change from present average national diet
Primarily intended to ensure adequate nutrient intake	Primarily intended to help reduce risk of developing chronic degenerative disease
More firmly established scientifically	More provisional, based more on epidemiologic data
More concerned with micronutrients	Primarily deal with macronutrients but may also address micronutrient intake
Specific recommendations for each life stage and gender group	Generally the same advice for all in the defined target group
Expressed in technical language	Technical language avoided, better understood by the public

Adapted from Truswell AS. 1999. Dietary goals and guidelines: National and international perspectives. In Shils ME, Olson JA, Shike M, Ross AC, eds. *Modern nutrition in health and disease*, 9th ed. Baltimore: Williams & Wilkins.

and published in 1968.[42] Several factors influenced the creation of this set of guidelines for the Nordic countries (Sweden, Finland, Norway, Denmark, and Iceland).[42] Dietary surveys showed that the proportion of calories from fat in the Swedish diet had increased from an average of about 29% at the end of the nineteenth century to 42% by the mid-1960s. There was concern over the high intakes of saturated fat, calories, and refined sugars and low intakes of fruits, vegetables, cereal products, lean meats, and nonfat dairy products. Swedish health authorities were concerned about the association between such dietary practices and obesity, coronary heart disease, hypertension, stroke, and tooth decay.

The Swedish guidelines called for a reduced energy intake (when appropriate) to prevent overweight; decreased consumption of total fat, saturated fat, sugar, and sugar-containing products; increased consumption of vegetables, fruits, potatoes, nonfat milk, fish, lean meat, and cereal products; and regular physical activity, especially for those with sedentary occupations.[42]

These dietary trends were recognized in other Western nations, such as Australia, New Zealand, The Netherlands, the United Kingdom, Germany, and Canada, which, in the early 1970s, issued dietary guidelines of their own.[43]

During this time, a similar situation existed in the United States. Scientists were concerned about trends in the eating habits of Americans. Data from the USDA showed that the distribution of calories from carbohydrate and fat had changed significantly between 1909 and the 1970s. Based on the *disappearance* of food from the marketplace (see Chapter 4), the USDA concluded that the percent of calories provided by fats had increased from 32% to about 43%, while calories provided by carbohydrate had declined from 57% to 46%. The percent of calories from fats obtained from meat and dairy products had risen sharply, while carbohydrate from fruits, vegetables, and grains had fallen precipitously.[36] At the same time, there was increasingly convincing evidence linking dietary habits to the major causes of death in America: heart disease, cancer, and stroke. Although scientists recognized that heredity, age, and numerous environmental factors besides diet were involved in the causation of these diseases, diet was one factor over which people had a certain amount of control. This led private agencies, such as the American Medical Association, the American Heart Association, and the American Health Foundation, to publish dietary guidelines.

U.S. Dietary Goals

In February 1977, the report *Dietary Goals for the United States* was issued by the U.S. Senate Select Committee on Nutrition and Human Needs.[43] This was the first of several government reports setting prudent dietary guidelines for Americans.

In its introduction, the Senate Select Committee made this statement:

> The overconsumption of foods high in fat, generally, and saturated fat in particular, as well as cholesterol, refined and processed sugars, salt and/or alcohol has been associated with the development of one or more of six to ten leading causes of death: heart disease, some cancers, stroke and hypertension, diabetes, arteriosclerosis and cirrhosis of the liver.[43]

The committee then submitted seven goals, listed in Box 2.6. The Dietary Goals were to be accomplished through the changes in food selection and preparation listed in Box 2.7.

The reaction to *Dietary Goals for the United States* from U.S. nutrition scientists and professionals was swift,

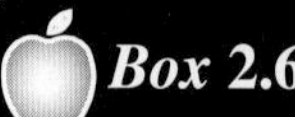

Box 2.6 Dietary Goals for the United States

1. To avoid overweight, consume only as much energy (calories) as is expended; if overweight, decrease energy intake and increase energy expenditure.
2. Increase the consumption of complex carbohydrates and "naturally occurring" sugars from about 28% of energy intake to about 48% of energy intake.
3. Reduce the consumption of refined and processed sugars by about 45% to account for about 10% of total energy intake.
4. Reduce overall fat consumption from approximately 40% to about 30% of energy intake.
5. Reduce saturated fat consumption to account for about 10% of total energy intake and balance that with polyunsaturated and monounsaturated fats, which should account for about 10% of energy intake each.
6. Reduce cholesterol consumption to about 300 milligrams per day.
7. Limit the intake of sodium by reducing the intake of salt to about 5 grams a day.

From Select Committee on Nutrition and Human Needs. 1977. *Dietary goals for the United States*. Washington, DC: U.S. Senate.

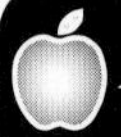

Box 2.7 Recommendations from Dietary Goals for the United States

1. Increase consumption of fruits, vegetables, and whole grains.
2. Decrease consumption of refined and other processed sugars and foods high in such sugars.
3. Decrease consumption of foods high in total fat and partially replace saturated fats, whether obtained from animal or vegetable sources, with polyunsaturated fats.
4. Decrease consumption of animal fat and choose meats, poultry, and fish, which will reduce saturated fat intake.
5. Except for young children, substitute low-fat and nonfat milk for whole milk and low-fat dairy products for high-fat dairy products.
6. Decrease consumption of butterfat, eggs, and other high-cholesterol sources. Some consideration should be given to easing the cholesterol goal for premenopausal women, young children, and the elderly to obtain the nutritional benefit of eggs in the diet.
7. Decrease consumption of salt and foods high in salt content.

From Select Committee on Nutrition and Human Needs. 1977. *Dietary goals for the United States*. Washington, DC: U.S. Senate.

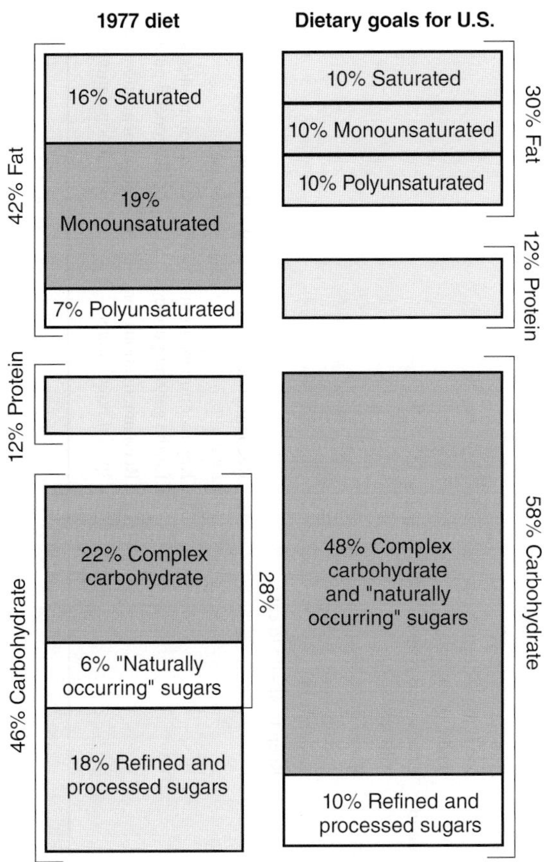

Figure 2.5 The *Dietary Goals for the United States*, established in 1977 (outlined in the column on the right) compared with the diet of the typical American adult of that time (outlined in the column on the left).

strong, and polarized.[31] *Nutrition Today* published opinions about the goals from some leading nutrition scientists and professionals.[33,34] Some felt the goals were "hastily conceived and based on fragmentary evidence," "premature . . . because the diet has not yet been tested," "blatant sensationalism," "speculation," and "a nutritional debacle." One professional declared that the "Senate Select Committee has perpetrated a hoax." Other scientists believed the goals were "long overdue," "a giant step forward in improving the health of our citizens," "a valid criticism of our current diet," and "a significant achievement" and deserved "the broadest support from all who are concerned with the health and well-being of American citizens." Who was right? Time would tell.

It was immediately clear, however, that, to meet the goals, Americans would need to change the way they ate. Figure 2.5 compares the 1977 U.S. Dietary Goals with the diet of that time and highlights the necessary changes.

The Dietary Guidelines for Americans

In 1980 the U.S. Department of Agriculture and U.S. Department of Health and Human Services jointly published the first edition of *Dietary Guidelines for Americans*.[46] Since then, the *Dietary Guidelines for Americans* (DGAs) have been revised every 5 years, with editions in 1985, 1990, 1995, 2000, 2005, and 2010. Since their inception, the DGAs have remained relatively consistent in terms of their recommendations for variety, proportionality, and moderation in healthful eating and in their focus on preventing chronic disease. Their ultimate goal has always been to "improve the health of our Nation's current and future generations by facilitating and promoting healthy eating and physical activity choices so that these behaviors become the norm among all individuals."[23] A basic premise of each edition has been that nutrient needs should be met primarily by consuming naturally occurring foods as opposed to relying on fortified foods or dietary supplements. Because of its remarkably complex nature, food provides a vast array of nutrients, food components, and phytochemicals that have beneficial effects on health. However, the DGAs recognize that in some instances, fortified foods and dietary supplements may be useful.[23,26]

Over the course of seven editions spanning three decades, the *Dietary Guidelines for Americans* have evolved considerably. As shown in Table 2.14, the first edition, published in 1980, had seven guidelines. This number was increased to 10 guidelines in the 2000 edition. The 2005 edition had a total of 41 recommendations grouped in nine "focus areas." There were 23 key recommendations intended for the general population as well as 18 key recommendations for specific population groups such as women who are pregnant or breastfeeding, children and adolescents, and older persons. The 2010 edition has a total of 29 recommendations grouped under 5 "major themes." There are 23 key recommendations for the general public and 6 additional recommendations for specific population groups. This greater number of recommendations reflects the increased specificity of the DGAs. Box 2.8 summarizes 23 recommendations from 4 of the 5 themes in the 2010 DGAs. For example, in Table 2.14, the directional recommendation "avoid too much fat, saturated fat, and cholesterol" published in the 1980 and 1985 editions is addressed by several recommendations in the 2010 edition (as seen in Box 2.8), including two recommendations giving specific numerical values for limiting intake of saturated fat and dietary cholesterol. This increased specificity is necessary, in large part, because several U.S. government nutrition assistance programs are required to adhere to the DGAs. Among these are the Child and Adult Care Food Program, Congregate Nutrition Services, Home-Delivered Nutrition Services, and the National School Lunch Program.[47] The greater specificity makes it easier to determine whether these nutrition assistance programs are in compliance with the DGAs.

Originally the *Dietary Guidelines for Americans* were targeted to the general public, but beginning with the 2005 edition they became more technical in nature and oriented toward policy makers, nutrition educators,

TABLE 2.14 *Dietary Guidelines for Americans*, **1980 to 2010**

1980 7 Guidelines	1985 7 Guidelines	1990 7 Guidelines	1995 7 Guidelines	2000 10 Guidelines	2005 9 Focus Areas	2010 5 Major Themes
Eat a variety of foods.	Eat a variety of foods.	Eat a variety of foods.	Eat a variety of foods.	Let the Pyramid guide your food choices.	Adequate nutrients within caloric needs	Balancing calories to manage weight
Maintain ideal weight.	Maintain desirable weight.	Maintain healthy weight.	Balance the food you eat with physical activity—maintain or improve your weight.	Aim for a healthy weight.	Weight management	Foods and food components to reduce
				Be physically active each day.	Physical activity	Foods and nutrients to increase
					Food groups to encourage	
Avoid too much fat, saturated fat, and cholesterol.	Avoid too much fat, saturated fat, and cholesterol.	Choose a diet low in fat, saturated fat, and cholesterol.	Choose a diet low in fat, saturated fat, and cholesterol.	Choose a diet that is low in saturated fat and cholesterol and moderate in total fat.	Fats	Building healthier eating patterns
					Carbohydrates	Helping Americans make healthy choices
Eat foods with adequate starch and fiber.	Eat foods with adequate starch and fiber.	Choose a diet with plenty of vegetables, fruits, and grain products.	Choose a diet with plenty of grain products, vegetables, and fruits.	Choose a variety of grains daily, especially whole grains.	Sodium and potassium	
					Alcoholic beverages	
				Choose a variety of fruits and vegetables daily.	Food safety	
Avoid too much sugar.	Avoid too much sugar.	Use sugars only in moderation.	Choose a diet moderate in sugars.	Choose beverages and foods to moderate your intake of sugars.		
Avoid too much sodium.	Avoid too much sodium.	Use salt and sodium only in moderation.	Choose a diet moderate in salt and sodium.	Choose and prepare foods with less salt.		
If you drink alcohol, do so in moderation.	If you drink alcoholic beverages, do so in moderation.	If you drink alcoholic beverages, do so in moderation.	If you drink alcoholic beverages, do so in moderation.	If you drink alcoholic beverages, do so in moderation.		
				Keep food safe to eat.		
					41 Recommendations in total 23 Key recommendations for the general public 18 Recommendations for special populations	29 Recommendations in total 23 Key recommendations for the general public 6 Recommendations for special populations

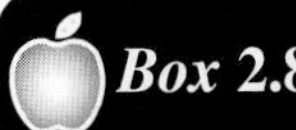

Box 2.8 *Dietary Guidelines for Americans, 2010,* Seventh Edition

Balancing Calories To Manage Weight

- Prevent and/or reduce overweight and obesity through improved eating and physical activity behaviors.
- Control total calorie intake to manage body weight. For people who are overweight or obese, this will mean consuming fewer calories from foods and beverages.
- Increase physical activity and reduce time spent in sedentary behaviors.
- Maintain appropriate calorie balance during each stage of life—childhood, adolescence, adulthood, pregnancy and breastfeeding, and older age.

Foods And Food Components To Reduce

- Reduce daily sodium intake to less than 2300 milligrams (mg) and further reduce intake to 1500 mg among persons who are 51 and older and those of any age who are African American or have hypertension, diabetes, or chronic kidney disease. The 1500 mg recommendation applies to about half of the U.S. population, including children, and the majority of adults.
- Consume less than 10 percent of calories from saturated fatty acids by replacing them with monounsaturated and polyunsaturated fatty acids.
- Consume less than 300 mg per day of dietary cholesterol.
- Keep *trans* fatty acid consumption as low as possible by limiting foods that contain synthetic sources of *trans* fats, such as partially hydrogenated oils, and by limiting other solid fats.
- Reduce the intake of calories from solid fats and added sugars.
- Limit the consumption of foods that contain refined grains, especially refined grain foods that contain solid fats, added sugars, and sodium.
- If alcohol is consumed, it should be consumed in moderation—up to one drink per day for women and two drinks per day for men—and only by adults of legal drinking age.

Foods And Nutrients To Increase

Individuals should meet the following recommendations as part of a healthy eating pattern while staying within their calorie needs.

- Increase vegetable and fruit intake.
- Eat a variety of vegetables, especially dark-green and red and orange vegetables and beans and peas.
- Consume at least half of all grains as whole grains. Increase whole-grain intake by replacing refined grains with whole grains.
- Increase intake of fat-free or low-fat milk and milk products, such as milk, yogurt, cheese, or fortified soy beverages.
- Choose a variety of protein foods, which include seafood, lean meat and poultry, eggs, beans and peas, soy products, and unsalted nuts and seeds.
- Increase the amount and variety of seafood consumed by choosing seafood in place of some meat and poultry.
- Replace protein foods that are higher in solid fats with choices that are lower in solid fats and calories and/or are sources of oils.
- Use oils to replace solid fats where possible.
- Choose foods that provide more potassium, dietary fiber, calcium, and vitamin D, which are nutrients of concern in American diets. These foods include vegetables, fruits, whole grains, and milk and milk products.

Building Healthy Eating Patterns

- Select an eating pattern that meets nutrient needs over time at an appropriate calorie level.
- Account for all foods and beverages consumed and assess how they fit within a total healthy eating pattern.
- Follow food safety recommendations when preparing and eating foods to reduce the risk of foodborne illnesses.

Recommendations for Specific Population Groups

Women capable of becoming pregnant

- Choose foods that supply heme iron, which is more readily absorbed by the body, additional iron sources, and enhancers of iron absorption such as vitamin C-rich foods.
- Consume 400 micrograms (mcg) per day of synthetic folic acid (from fortified foods and/or supplements) in addition to food forms of folate from a varied diet.

Women who are pregnant or breastfeeding

- Consume 8 to 12 ounces of seafood per week from a variety of seafood types.
- Due to their high methyl mercury content, limit white (albacore) tuna to 6 ounces per week and do not eat the following four types of fish: tilefish, shark, swordfish, and king mackerel.
- If pregnant, take an iron supplement, as recommended by an obstetrician or other health care provider.

Individuals ages 50 years and older

- Consume foods fortified with vitamin B12, such as fortified cereals, or dietary supplements.

Source: U.S. Department of Health and Human Services and U.S. Department of Agriculture. 2010. *Dietary Guidelines for Americans, 2010.* Washington, DC: U.S. Government Printing Office.

nutritionists, and health-care providers for use in developing educational materials and in designing and implementing nutrition-related programs, including federal food, nutrition education, and information programs. The recommendations shown in Box 2.8 are based on sound scientific evidence collected through a thorough review of the best available scientific research and are considered authoritative statements to be used in developing federal nutrition policy. Because they are interrelated and mutually dependent, they should be used together when planning healthful diets.

Traditionally the DGAs were intended to apply to healthy persons age 2 years and older, but given the high prevalence of overweight, obesity, coronary heart disease, hypertension, and type 2 diabetes in America, the 2010 edition now intends them to be applied to those who are at increased risk of chronic disease as well as to those who are healthy. While making it clear that ultimately, individuals make their own food and physical activity choices, the 2010 edition points out that individuals' ability to make healthy choices is influenced by the food environment and the physical environment and that substantive and sustainable improvements in the nation's health will require improvements in the food and physical environments.[23] To achieve this, small and large businesses, communities and organizations, policy makers, health professionals, and educators will all have to work together in partnership to develop the programs and policies to encourage and support healthy eating and active living by individuals and families.

The Surgeon General's Report on Nutrition and Health

In 1988, *The Surgeon General's Report on Nutrition and Health* was issued.[48] This was a landmark publication summarizing the scientific evidence linking specific dietary factors to health maintenance and disease prevention and presenting recommendations for dietary change to improve the health of the American people.[49] The report recognized that what we eat can affect our risk for several of the leading causes of death and identified, as of primary importance, the need to reduce consumption of fat, especially saturated fat. It served as an authoritative source of information on which to base nutrition policy decisions and distinguished recommendations appropriate for the general public from those for special populations.[50]

Diet and Health

In 1989, the book *Diet and Health: Implications for Reducing Chronic Disease Risk* was published by the Committee on Diet and Health of the National Research Council.[36] It represented the view that dietary recommendations should go beyond the prevention of nutrient deficiencies to the prevention of chronic disease. From their extensive review of the scientific literature, the committee members concluded that, in addition to genetic and environmental factors, "dietary patterns are important factors in the **etiology** of several major chronic diseases and that dietary modifications can reduce such risks." The influence of diet is "very strong" for coronary heart disease and hypertension and "highly suggestive" for certain cancers (esophagus, stomach, large bowel, breast, lung, and prostate). The committee stated that dietary habits also play a role in dental caries, chronic liver disease, and obesity, which increases the risk of **type 2 diabetes mellitus.** Of particular concern was the need for Americans to reduce consumption of fats, saturated fats, and cholesterol and increase intake of fruits, vegetables, legumes, and whole-grain cereals.

Other Dietary Guidelines

Since the U.S. Dietary Goals were issued in 1977, numerous scientific organizations and professional groups have studied the impact of American dietary practices on health and disease and have issued their own dietary guidelines. Only those considered most important have been discussed here.[23,36,43,48,51–53] Some of the more important ones are summarized in Table 2.15.

Although the various dietary recommendations shown in Table 2.15 span more than three decades, there is a remarkable degree of similarity in their major tenets. Although some of the recommendations require special emphasis or modification because of certain health conditions or the unique needs of minorities, children, women, and the elderly, the available evidence suggests that all the major recommendations apply across population groups.

Nutrition Labeling of Food

Nutrition labeling of food in the United States began in 1973, when the U.S. Food and Drug Administration (FDA) established the U.S. Recommended Daily Allowances (U.S. RDAs) and instituted specific regulations for food labeling. In 1990, food labeling regulations in the United States were extensively revised by the Nutrition Labeling and Education Act of 1990. It should be noted that the U.S. Recommended Daily Allowances (U.S. RDAs) are not the same as the Recommended Dietary Allowances (RDAs).

U.S. Recommended Daily Allowances

In 1973, the FDA issued regulations requiring the nutrition labeling of any food containing one or more added nutrients or whose label or advertising included claims about the food's nutritional properties or its usefulness in the daily diet. Nutrition labeling was voluntary for almost all other foods. The *U.S. Recommended Daily Allowances (U.S. RDAs)* were nutrient standards developed by the FDA at that time for use in regulating the nutrition labeling of food. They replaced the Minimum Daily Requirement, which had been in use since 1940 for labeling vitamin and mineral supplements, breakfast cereals, and some special foods.

The Nutrition Labeling and Education Act

Between 1973 and 1993, there was growing awareness that the major nutritional problem facing North Americans was overconsumption of foods rich in total

TABLE 2.15 Summary of Major Dietary Recommendations

Nutrient or Food Component	U.S. Dietary Goals, 1977	*Surgeon General's Report on Nutrition and Health*, 1988	Diet and Health, NRC, 1989	ACS Guidelines on Nutrition and Physical Activity for Cancer Prevention, 2012	National Cholesterol Education Program, Adult Treatment Panel III, 2002	American Diabetes Association, 2008*	*Dietary Guidelines for Americans*, USDA/USDHHS, 2010
Total fat (% of kcal)	≤ 30%	Reduce intake	≤ 30%	Limit consumption of processed meat, red meat	25% to 35%	Must be individualized	20% to 35%
Saturated fatty acids (% of kcal)	≤ 10%	Reduce intake	≤ 10%	NC	< 7%	< 10% (< 7% if LDL-C is elevated)	< 10%
Polyunsaturated fatty acids (% of kcal)	≤ 10%	NS	≤ 10%	NC	Up to 10%	Must be individualized	Most fats should be polyunsaturated and monounsaturated
Monounsaturated fatty acids (% of kcal)	≤ 10%	NS	NS	NC	Up to 20%	Must be individualized	
Trans fatty acids	NC	NC	NS	NC	Keep intake low	Minimize intake	Keep consumption as low as possible
Dietary cholesterol (mg/day)	250 to 300 mg	Reduce intake	< 300 mg	NC	< 200 mg	< 300 mg (< 200 mg if LDL-C is elevated)	< 300 mg
Added sugars	Limit	Limit intake	Consume in moderation	Choose whole grains instead of refined grain products	NC	Eat sugars in the context of a healthy diet	Choose foods and beverages with little added sugars
Carbohydrate (% of kcal)	> 55%	Increase consumption	≥ 55%	Eat at least 2.5 cups of vegetables and fruits each day	50% to 60%	Choose whole grains, fruits, vegetables, and nonfat dairy foods	Choose fiber-rich fruits, vegetables, and whole grains often
Dietary fiber	Increase	Increase consumption	NS		20 g to 30 g/day	Choose a variety of fiber-containing foods	
Sodium (mg/day)	≤ 2000 mg	Reduce intake	< 2400 mg	NC	< 2400 mg	< 2400 mg	< 2300 mg
Alcohol consumption	Moderate alcohol consumption, if any	Consume in moderation, if at all	Consume in moderation, if at all	If you drink alcoholic beverages, limit consumption	Moderate intake; Men: ≤ 2 drinks/d Women: ≤ 1 drink/d	Moderate intake: Men: ≤ 2 drinks/d Women: ≤ 1 drink/d	If alcohol is consumed, do so in moderation
Maintain healthy weight, be physically active	Yes	Achieve and maintain a desirable body weight	Achieve and maintain a desirable body weight	Achieve and maintain a healthy weight throughout life Adopt a physically active lifestyle	Balance energy intake and expenditure to maintain healthy body weight or to prevent weight gain	Reduced energy intake, physical activity, and modest weight loss improve insulin sensitivity	Be physically active and control calorie intake to manage body weight
Other	Reduce additives and processed foods	Foods rich in calcium and iron: fluoridated water for some people	Adequate fluoride and calcium intake: moderate protein intake; avoid excess supplement use	Organizations should work together to create environments that support the adoption and maintenance of healthy behaviors	Daily potassium intake ≥ 3500 mg/d	Chromium and magnesium supplementation only when medically needed	Follow food safety recommendations when preparing and eating foods

Note: NRC = National Research Council; ACS = American Cancer Society; AHA = American Heart Association; USDA = U.S. Department of Agriculture; USDHHS = U.S. Department of Health and Human Services. NC = No comment; NS = Not specified.

*Many of these recommendations must be individualized to suit the personal lifestyle and treatment goals of the individual with diabetes. See Chapter 8 for additional details.

fat, saturated fat, and cholesterol and low in complex carbohydrates. There were also major breakthroughs in our knowledge of essential nutrient requirements (for example, the RDAs had been revised three times during this time). Despite these advances, the U.S. RDAs had not been updated, and food labeling regulations remained virtually unchanged. During the same period, the public and various professional and consumer interest groups called for food labels that were easily understood, that were truthful, and that reflected awareness of the relationship between diet and health. In 1990, the FDA's Nutrition Labeling and Education Act (NLEA) was passed, mandating nutrition labeling for almost all processed foods regulated by the FDA and authorizing appropriate health claims on the labels of such products. It brought about the most extensive food labeling reform in U.S. history. The NLEA also called for activities to educate consumers about nutrition information on the label and the importance of using that information in maintaining healthful dietary practices. The NLEA's final regulations were published in the 6 January 1993 *Federal Register.* 8 August 1994 was the final deadline for manufacturers to comply. The USDA's Food Safety and Inspection Service, responsible for the inspection of meat and poultry, issued parallel regulations that governed the labeling of meat and poultry.

The NLEA requires virtually all processed foods to carry nutrition information on the label (Figure 2.6). Foods exempted from the regulations include plain coffee and tea, some spices and flavorings, and other foods having insignificant nutritional value; ready-to-eat food prepared primarily on-site, such as deli and bakery items; foods in very small packages; restaurant food; bulk food that is not resold; and foods produced by businesses with food sales of less than $50,000 per year or total sales less than $500,000 per year unless the food item contains a nutrition claim. Nutrition labeling is voluntary for most raw foods. The 20 most frequently eaten raw fruits, vegetables, and fish are included in the FDA's voluntary point-of-purchase nutrition information program. The 45 major cuts of meat and poultry are covered under the USDA's voluntary point-of-purchase program.

The nutrients and food components required on the label were selected because of their relationship to current health concerns, and the order in which they are listed reflects their public health significance. Box 2.9 shows the mandatory and voluntary nutrients and dietary components in the order they must appear on food labels. The mandatory nutrients and dietary components are required on all food labels. Listing of the voluntary ones is optional. If a food is fortified or enriched with any of the voluntary nutrients or dietary components, or if a health or nutrient content claim is made about any of them, the pertinent nutrition information then becomes mandatory. Total calories, total fat, total carbohydrate, protein, sodium, vitamins A and C, calcium, and iron were carryovers from the previous label. Saturated fat, *trans* fat, cholesterol, sugars, dietary fiber, and calories from fat were added by the new regulations. Niacin, thiamin, and riboflavin are now voluntary nutrients.

Serving sizes listed on the label are specified by the FDA, are uniform across all product lines so consumers can more easily compare brands, and are closer to the amounts people actually eat. Using data from USDA food consumption surveys, the FDA determined the amounts of various foods that people customarily consume per eating occasion. These are called **reference amounts** and are expressed in metric units. The serving size listed on food labels is the amount in common household measures closest to the reference amount. It is important to note that serving sizes as defined by the FDA do not always agree with the serving sizes used by the exchange system.

A list of all ingredients must appear on all processed and packaged foods. When appropriate, ingredient lists must include any FDA-certified color additives, the sources of any protein hydrolysates, a declaration that caseinate is a milk derivative when caseinate is found in foods claiming to be nondairy, and a declaration of the total percentage of juice in any beverage claiming to contain juice.

An important feature of the NLEA is that it regulates nutrient content claims and health claims on food labels or other labeling of food, such as advertisements. Nutrient content claims are those describing the amount of nutrients in foods, such as "cholesterol free," "low fat," "light," or "lean." Examples of these are shown in Table 2.16. In addition to the nutrient claims shown in Table 2.16 are those using the word *reduced* or *less.* A food making the claim "reduced or less sodium" has to contain at least 25% less sodium per serving than an appropriate food used for comparison purposes. For example, potato chips labeled "low sodium" must contain at least 25% less sodium than comparable potato chips (the "reference food").

The FDA defines a health claim as any claim on the package label or other labeling of a food that characterizes the relationship of any nutrient or other substance in the food to a disease or health-related condition. According to FDA regulations, health claims are allowed only under certain circumstances and must be scientifically based and standardized. Allowable health claims are shown in Box 2.10. The NLEA stipulates that foods bearing health claims must not contain any nutrient or substance in an amount that increases the risk of a disease or a health condition. Foods bearing health claims must contain 20% or less of the Daily Value of fat, saturated fat, cholesterol, and sodium per serving. For example, whole milk (which is high in calcium) may not bear a calcium-osteoporosis claim because its fat content exceeds 20% of the Daily Value for fat. Skim and 1% fat milk easily qualify for the calcium-osteoporosis claim. According to FDA regulation, claims that a substance will prevent a disease are drug claims. Health claims on food labels are limited to

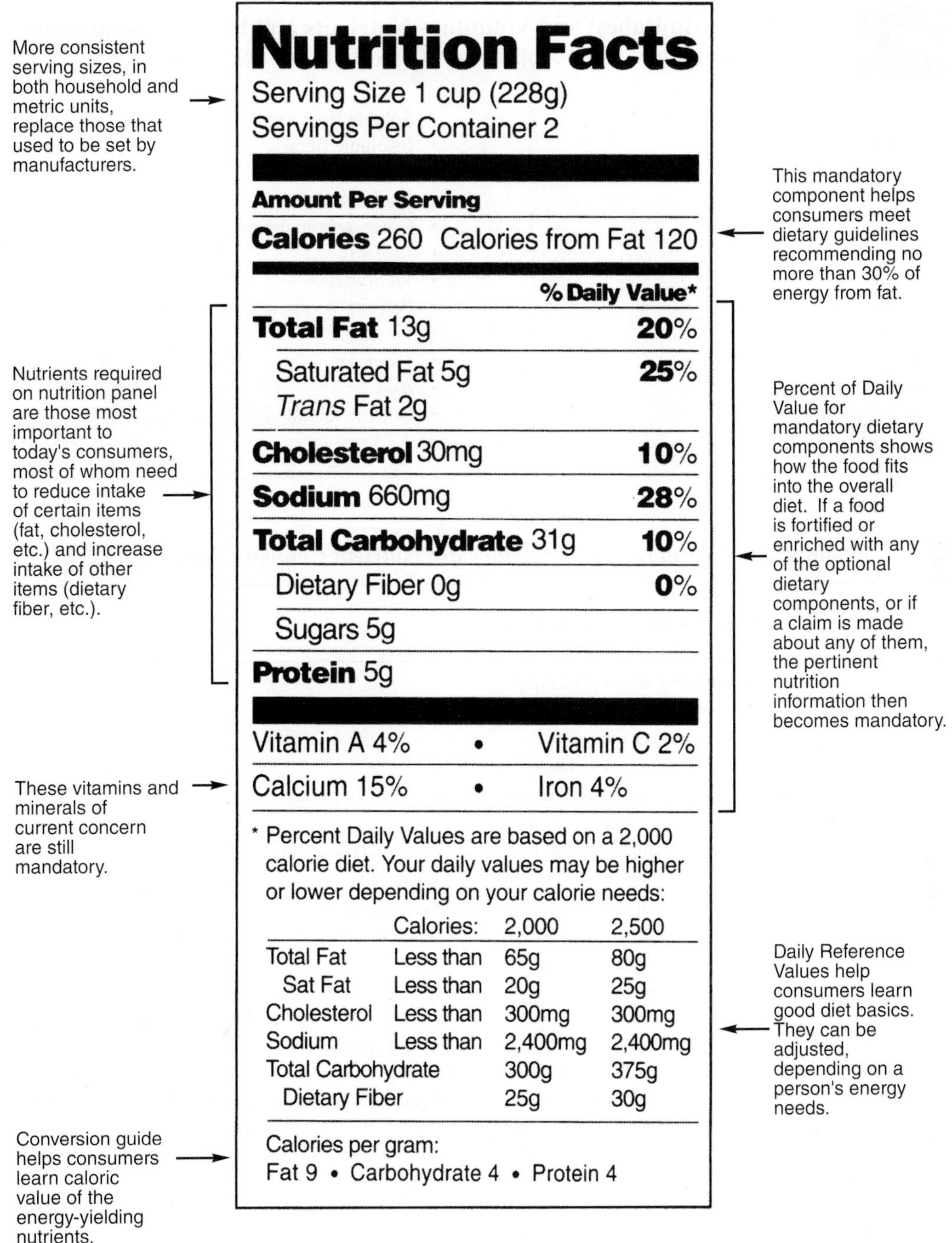

Figure 2.6 Key concepts of the Nutrition Facts label.

saying that a food "may" or "might" reduce the risk of a disease or health condition.

As shown in Figure 2.7, the Nutrition Facts label of foods for children under age 2 years (except infant formula, which has special labeling rules under the Infant Formula Act of 1980) may not carry information about saturated fat, polyunsaturated fat, monounsaturated fat, cholesterol, calories from fat, or calories from saturated fat. This is to prevent parents from wrongly assuming that infants and toddlers should restrict their fat intake, when, in fact, they should not. Fat is important during these years to ensure adequate growth and development. The labels of foods for children under age 4 years may not include the Percent of Daily Values for total fat, saturated fat, cholesterol, sodium, potassium, total carbohydrate, and dietary fiber because the FDA has not established Daily Values for these nutrients in this age category. However, the label may carry the Percent of Daily Values for protein, vitamins, and minerals, which the FDA has established.

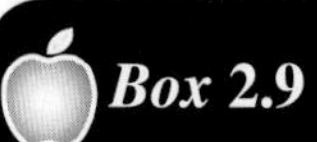

Box 2.9 Mandatory (in Italics) and Voluntary Nutrients and Dietary Components in the Order They Must Appear on the Nutrition Facts Label

- *Total calories*
- *Calories from fat*
- Calories from saturated fat
- *Total fat*
- *Saturated fat*
- *Trans fat*
- Polyunsaturated fat
- Monounsaturated fat
- *Cholesterol*
- *Sodium*
- Potassium
- *Total carbohydrate*
- *Dietary fiber*
- Soluble fiber
- Insoluble fiber
- *Sugars*
- Sugar alcohols
- Other carbohydrates
- *Protein*
- *Vitamin A*
- Percent of vitamin A as beta-carotene
- *Vitamin C*
- *Calcium*
- *Iron*
- Other essential vitamins and minerals

TABLE 2.16 Examples and Meanings of Some Allowable Nutrient Content Claims

Example of Nutrient Content Claim	Meaning of Nutrient Content Claim
Sugar free	Less than 0.5 g sugars per serving
Calorie free	Less than 5 kcal per serving
Low calorie	40 kcal or less per serving
Fat free	Less than 0.5 g fat per serving
Saturated fat free	Less than 0.5 g saturated fat and less than 0.5 g *trans* fat per serving
Low fat	3 g or less per serving
Low saturated fat	1 g or less of saturated fat and less than 0.5 g *trans* fat per serving
Trans fat free	Less than 0.5 g *trans* fat and less than 0.5 g saturated fat per serving
Cholesterol free	Less than 2 mg of cholesterol and 2 g or less of both saturated fat and *trans* fat
Low cholesterol	20 mg or less of cholesterol and 2 g or less of both saturated fat and *trans* fat
Sodium free	Less than 5 mg sodium per serving
Low sodium	140 mg or less per serving
Very low sodium	35 mg or less per serving
Lean meat or poultry	Less than 10 g total fat, less than 4.5 g of saturated and *trans* fat combined, and less than 95 mg cholesterol per serving and per 100 g for individual foods
Extra lean meat or poultry	Less than 5 g total fat, less than 2 g saturated and *trans* fat combined, and less than 95 mg cholesterol per serving and per 100 g for individual foods
High, rich in	20% or more of Daily Value to describe protein, vitamins, minerals, dietary fiber, or potassium per serving
Good source of More, added	10% to 19% or more of Daily Value per serving
	Contains a nutrient that is at least 10% percent of Daily Value more than the reference food, regardless of whether the food is altered (fortified or enriched)
Light, lite	One-third fewer calories or half the fat of the reference food; if the food derives 50% or more of its calories from fat, the reduction must be 50% of the fat; can also mean that sodium content has been reduced by at least 50%

Source: U.S. Food and Drug Administration, Center for Food Safety and Applied Nutrition.

Front-of-Package Labeling

A relatively new approach to nutrition labeling is to use front-of-package (FOP) labeling systems displaying symbols or icons, typically printed on the front of the label, to summarize key nutritional aspects or characteristics of foods.[29] Some FOP systems are based on a nutrition profiling model (discussed earlier in this chapter). Some show the percent daily value for select nutrients or food components, whereas others highlight that the food is a good source of a particular food group, such as whole grains or vegetables. A recent review of 20 different FOP systems representative of those in the marketplace found wide variation in the criteria used for ranking foods and some cases where various systems conflicted with each other.[29] Some FOP systems cannot be evaluated because the evaluation criteria they use are not publicly available.

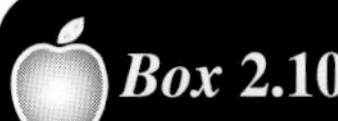

Box 2.10 Nutrient–Disease Relationship Claims Allowed on the Nutrition Facts Label

- Calcium and risk of osteoporosis
- Sodium and risk of hypertension
- Dietary saturated fat and cholesterol and risk of coronary heart disease
- Dietary fat and risk of cancer
- Fiber-containing grain products, fruits, and vegetables and risk of cancer
- Fruits, vegetables, and grain products that contain fiber, particularly soluble fiber and risk of coronary heart disease
- Fruits and vegetables and risk of cancer
- Folic acid and risk of neural tube defects
- Sugar alcohols and risk of dental caries
- Soluble fiber and risk of coronary heart disease
- Soy protein and risk of coronary heart disease
- Plant sterol and stanol esters and risk of coronary heart disease

Source: U.S. Food and Drug Administration, Center for Food Safety and Applied Nutrition.

The large number of widely different FOP systems and the lack of transparency in how the nutritional value of foods are rated contributes to confusion among consumers.[54,55] Although such systems ostensibly are intended to help consumers easily identify nutritious foods, concerns have been raised about the use of FOP systems in marketing foods that are of questionable nutritional value.[54,55] For example, some FOP systems selectively focus on a product's vitamin and mineral fortification while ignoring its high content of salt and added sugars. Concerns have been raised that some FOP systems and health claims made by manufacturers have violated Food and Drug Administration regulations prohibiting food labeling from bearing statements that are "false and misleading in any particular."[54] One FOP system developed by a group of several food manufacturers was voluntarily withdrawn after the Connecticut attorney general began an investigation into whether the system violated that state's consumer protection law.[56]

The need for a scientifically based FOP system that not only informs consumers but encourages healthier food choices and purchasing behaviors prompted the U.S. Congress to direct the Centers for Disease Control and Prevention and the Food and Drug Administration (FDA) to work with the Institute of Medicine (IOM) to examine some of the existing FOP systems and develop recommendations for an FOP nutrition rating system and symbols.[29,31] This led to a recommendation for the development of a "single, standardized system that is easily understood by most age groups"—focusing on those nutrients or food components "most strongly associated with diet-related health risks affecting the greatest number of Americans"—and that is regulated by the FDA.[31] The IOM recommended that one, standard symbol be used to display calories per serving and to assign zero to three nutritional "points" for the content of saturated fat, *trans* fat, and added sugars.[31] The symbol should appear on all grocery products, appearing in a consistent location across all products. The criteria for scoring foods should be freely available to the public (nonproprietary) and consistent with and linked to the Nutrition Facts panel.[31]

Daily Values

The **Daily Values** are dietary reference values intended to help consumers use food label information to plan healthy diets. They serve as the basis for quantifying the amounts of various nutrients and food components on food labels. They are to be used for regulatory purposes only and are not intended to serve as recommended intakes. The basis for calculating the Daily Values are two separate sets of nutrient reference values: the **Daily Reference Values (DRVs)** and the **Reference Daily Intakes (RDIs).**

Daily Reference Values

The DRVs are reference values for nutrients and food components for which no set of standards (e.g., the RDAs or U.S. RDAs) previously existed. Table 2.17 shows the DRVs for 2000-kcal and 2500-kcal diets. For labeling purposes, 2000 kcal is the reference for calculating Percent of Daily Values, although some labels may also include DRVs for a higher energy intake, such as 2500 kcal. The DRVs include values for total fat, saturated fatty acids, cholesterol, total carbohydrate, dietary fiber, sodium, potassium, and protein. Some of the DRVs are based on recommendations to increase or maintain intake of the particular food component (carbohydrate, dietary fiber, and potassium), whereas other DRVs reflect levels that are limitations on intake (total fat, saturated fat, cholesterol, and sodium).

Four of the seven food components for which DRVs have been established require a specific energy intake to quantify reference values. Those for total fat, saturated fat, and carbohydrate are based on intake levels of approximately 30%, 10%, and 60% of total energy, respectively. The DRV for protein is based on 10% of energy from protein for adults and children 4 years of age and older. The reference value for dietary fiber is based on an intake of approximately 11.5 g per 1000 kcal. The DRV for cholesterol is based on recommendations that individuals, regardless of energy intake, limit

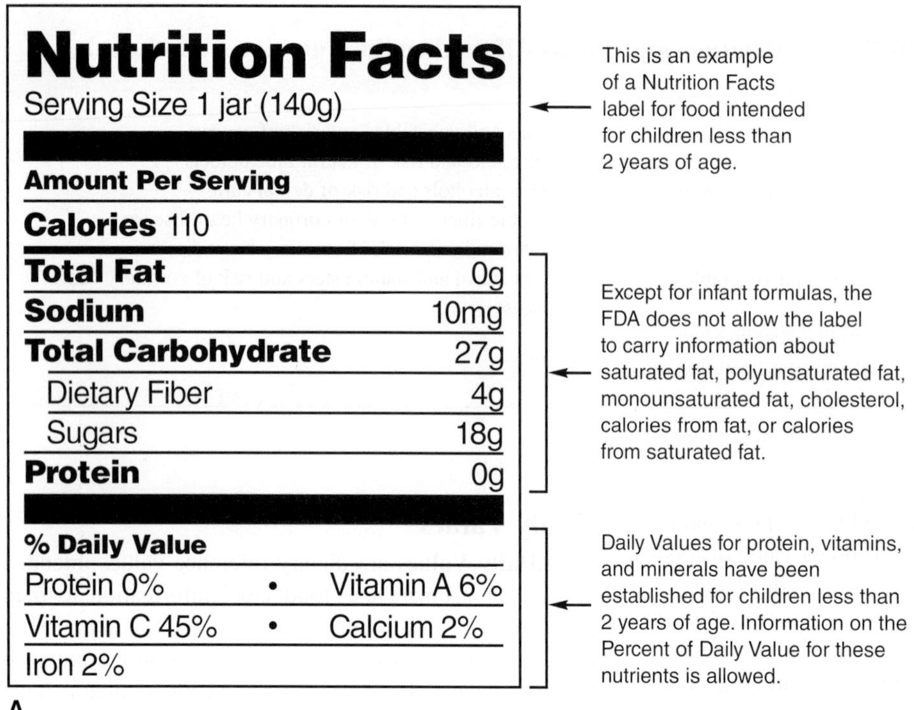

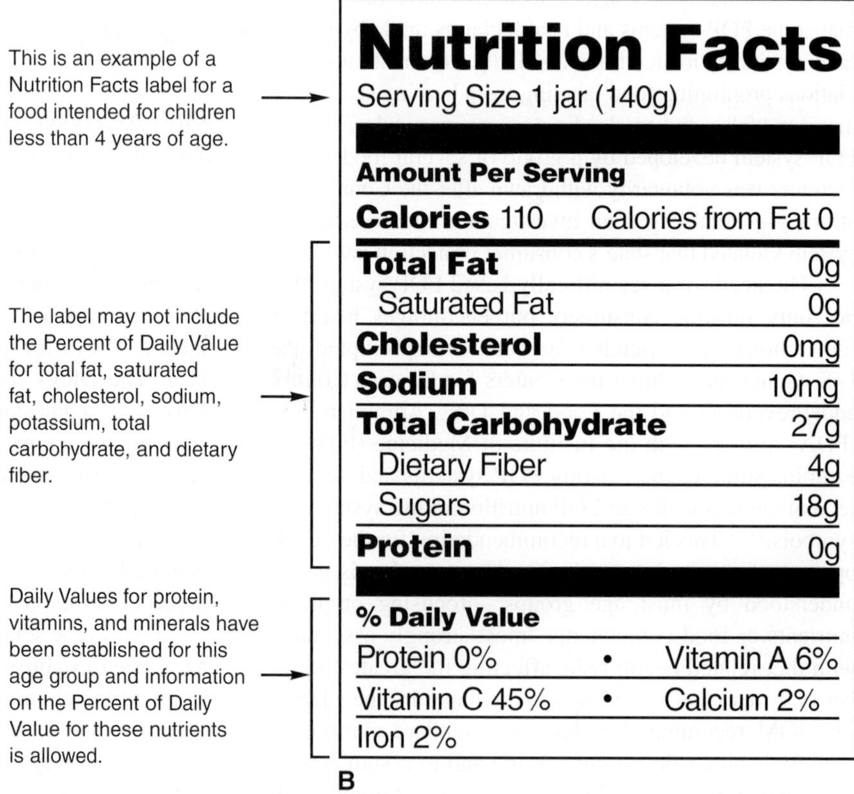

Figure 2.7 **Examples of mandatory differences in the Nutrition Facts labels for foods designed for children less than 2 years of age (A) and for foods intended for children less than 4 years of age (B).**

TABLE 2.17 The Food and Drug Administration's Daily Reference Values (DRVs) for 2000-kcal and 2500-kcal diets

	Daily Reference Value	
Food Component	**2000 kcal**	**2500 kcal**
Fat	< 65 g	< 80 g
Saturated fatty acids	< 20 g	< 25 g
Cholesterol	< 300 mg	< 300 mg
Total carbohydrate	300 g	375 g
Fiber	25 g	30 g
Sodium	< 2400 mg	< 2400
Potassium	3500 mg	3500 mg
Protein*	50 g	63 g

*The DRV for protein applies only to children older than 4 years and adults. The RDIs for protein for infants, children 1 to 4 years, pregnant females, and nursing females are 14 g, 16 g, 60 g, and 65 g, respectively.

their consumption to less than 300 mg/day. The value for sodium resulted from recommendations that all persons limit their *salt* intake to less than 6 g/day, which is a sodium intake of less than 2.4 g/day. The DRV for potassium is 3500 mg, a level associated with decreased risk of hypertension.

Reference Daily Intakes

The RDIs serve as reference values for vitamins and minerals and are the U.S. RDAs (discussed in the section "U.S. Recommended Daily Allowances") with a new name. The RDIs are shown in Table 2.18. In 1990, the FDA proposed updating the U.S. RDAs but was temporarily prevented from doing so by Congress. Part of the rationale for changing the name of the U.S. RDAs to RDIs was to decrease confusion over the terms "RDA" and "U.S. RDA." The FDA plans to update the RDIs in the near future, so that they will be more representative of our contemporary understanding of nutrient requirements.

FOOD GUIDES

A food guide is a nutrition education tool translating scientific knowledge and dietary standards and recommendations into an understandable and practical form for use by those who have little or no training in nutrition.[40,57] Food guides are problem oriented and address specific nutritional problems identified within the targeted population. Typically, foods are classified into basic groups according to similarity of nutrient content or some other criteria. If a certain number of servings from each group is consumed, a balanced and adequate diet is thought likely to result.

TABLE 2.18 The Food and Drug Administration's Reference Daily Intakes (RDIs)*

Nutrient	Amount
Vitamin A	5000 IU†
Vitamin C	60 mg
Thiamin	1.5 mg
Riboflavin	1.7 mg
Niacin	20 mg
Calcium	1000 mg
Iron	18 mg
Vitamin D	400 IU
Vitamin E	30 IU
Vitamin B_6	2.0 mg
Folic acid	400 μg
Vitamin B_{12}	6 μg
Phosphorus	1000 mg
Iodine	150 μg
Magnesium	400 mg
Zinc	15 mg
Copper	2 mg
Biotin	300 μg
Pantothenic acid	10 mg

*Based on the National Academy of Sciences' 1986 Recommended Dietary Allowances.

†IU = international units.

The USDA has been at the forefront of food guide development in the United States. The major food guides developed by the USDA from 1916 through development of the Food Guide Pyramid are outlined in Table 2.19. The USDA's first food guides are credited to Caroline Hunt (1865–1927), a nutrition specialist in USDA's Bureau of Home Economics.[57] In 1916, she developed *Food for Young Children,* followed in 1917 by *How to Select Foods.* In these, foods were categorized into five groups—milk and meat; cereals; vegetables and fruits; fats and fat foods; and sugars and sugary foods. These "buying guides" were designed to ensure adequate energy intake from fat, carbohydrate, and protein while encouraging sufficient variety for minerals and some of the newly discovered body-regulating substances we now know as vitamins. The financial constraints imposed by the economic depression of the early 1930s led to the development of food guides providing advice to families for purchasing foods at various cost levels. Hazel Stiebeling (1896–1989), a food economist in USDA's Bureau of Home Economics, led in the development of these buying guides. She emphasized a balance between high-energy foods (e.g., fats and sweets) and "protective" or nutrient-dense foods supplying essential nutrients. Among the protective foods are milk, which supplies calcium, and fruits and vegetables, which supply vitamins A and C.[57]

Table 2.19 Major USDA Food Guides (1916–1995), Showing Food Groups and Numbers of Servings*

Food Guide	Number of Food Groups	Protein-Rich Foods: Milk	Protein-Rich Foods: Meat	Breads	Vegetables	Fruits	Other: Fats	Other: Sugars
Caroline Hunt buying guides (1916)	5	Meats and other protein-rich foods 10% of energy from milk 10% of energy from other foods 1 c milk + 2–3 svgs of other foods based on 3-oz svg		Cereals and other starchy foods 20% of energy 9 svgs based on 1 oz or ¾ c dry cereal	Vegetables and fruits 30% of energy 5 svgs based on average 8-oz svg		Fatty foods 20% of energy 9 svgs based on 1-Tbsp svg	Sugars 10% of energy 10 svgs based on 1-Tbsp svg
H. K. Stiebeling buying guide (1930s)	12	Milk 2 c	Lean meat, poultry, fish 9–10 svgs/wk Dry, mature beans, peas, nuts 1 svg/wk Eggs 1	Flours, cereals as desired	Leafy green, yellow 11–12 svgs per wk Potato, sweet potato 1 svg Other vegetables and fruit 3 svgs	Tomato and citrus 1 svg	Butter Other fats	Sugars
Basic Seven foundation diet (1940s)	7	Milk and milk products 2 or more svgs svg = 1 c	Meat, poultry, fish, eggs, dried beans, peas, nuts 1–2 svgs	Breads, flour, and cereals every day	Leafy green, yellow 1 or more svgs Potato and other fruits and vegetables 2 or more svgs	Citrus, tomato, cabbage, salad greens 1 or more svgs	Butter, fortified margarine some daily	
Basic Four foundation diet (1956–1970s)	4	Milk group 2 or more svgs	Meat group 2 or more svgs 2–3 oz svgs	Bread, cereal 4 or more svgs 1 oz dry, 1 slice ½–¾ c cooked	Vegetable-fruit group 4 svgs include dark green/yellow vegetables frequently ½ c or typical portion			
Hassle-Free foundation diet (1979)	5	Milk-cheese group 2 svgs 1 c, 1½ oz cheese	Meat, poultry, fish, and bean group 2 svgs 2- to 3-oz svg	Bread-cereal group 4 or more svgs 1 oz dry, 1 slice ½–¾ c cooked	Vegetable-fruit group 4 svgs include vitamin C source daily and dark-green/yellow vegetables frequently ½ c or typical portion		Fats, sweets, alcohol group use dependent on calorie needs	
Food Guide Pyramid total diet (1984)	6	Milk, yogurt, cheese 2–3 svgs 1 c, 1½ oz cheese	Meat, poultry, fish eggs, dry beans, nuts 2–3 svgs 5–7 oz total/day	Breads, cereals rice pasta 6–11 svgs whole-grain and enriched 1 slice, ½ c cooked	Vegetable 3–5 svgs dark green deep yellow starchy/legumes other ½ c raw ½ c cooked	Fruit 2–4 svgs citrus other ½ c or average	Fats, oils, sweets total fat not to exceed 30% of energy sweets vary according to energy need	

Source: U.S. Department of Agriculture, Center for Nutrition Policy and Promotion.

*Number of servings are daily unless noted otherwise; svg = serving.

Hunt's and Stiebeling's buying guides gave way to food guides promoting "foundation diets." These food guides recommended a minimum number of servings from different food groups, which provided a foundation diet supplying a major portion of the RDAs. It was assumed that, to meet their energy needs, most people would consume more food than the guide specified. This extra food would provide not only necessary energy but additional nutrients as well. It was further assumed that such a diet would meet requirements for all essential nutrients, not just those included in the RDAs.[45,46] During the mid-1940s, the USDA developed the "Basic Seven," which was widely used for many years. Its complexity and lack of specific serving sizes led to the development of the "Basic Four" in 1956.[57,58] The assumption underlying development of the Four Food Groups was that eating the specified numbers of servings from the different food groups would supply approximately 1200 kcal, approximately 100% of the RDAs for vitamins A and C and calcium, and at least 80% of the RDAs for the remaining five nutrients of the 1953 revision of the RDAs.[58] Vitamins A and C and calcium were given priority status because they were shown to be **shortfall nutrients** (nutrients whose intakes were below recommended levels among a significant part of the population).[58]

In 1979, the USDA issued the Hassle-Free Guide to a Better Diet. This was a revision of the Four Food Groups that gave more attention to micronutrients in food groups and included a fifth food group: fats, sweets, and alcohol. The purpose of including this fifth group was to help consumers recognize fats, sweets, and alcohol as empty calories and to draw attention to the need for considering them in meal planning, since no servings from this group were recommended. The Hassle-Free guide highlighted the need to use fat, sugars, and alcohol moderately and gave special attention to calories and dietary fiber.[57]

Publication of the *Dietary Goals for the United States* in 1977 (review Figure 2.4 and Box 2.6) was a turning point for dietary guidance and food guides. Following this landmark event, the USDA and USDHHS published the *Dietary Guidelines for Americans* in 1980, with revisions following every 5 years. In 1980, the USDA began working on a new food guide to replace the Basic Four. This led to development of the food guide shown in Table 2.20. Three key messages of this guide were variety (eating a selection of foods of various types that together meet nutritional needs); proportionality (eating appropriate amounts of various types of foods to meet nutritional needs); and moderation (avoiding too much of food components in the total diet that have been linked to diseases).[57] Despite dissemination of the food guide in several publications developed by the USDA and other groups (including the 1990 edition of *Dietary Guidelines for Americans*), the perception remained among the public and professionals that the USDA was still using the Basic Four developed in the 1950s.[57,58] This led the USDA to develop a separate publication explaining the food guide and containing an appealing illustration conveying the key messages of the guide.

TABLE 2.20 Daily Food Guide Developed by the USDA to Replace the Basic Four

Food Group	Suggested Servings*
Vegetables	3–5
Fruits	2–4
Breads, cereals, rice, and pasta	6–11
Milk, yogurt, and cheese	2–3
Meats, poultry, fish, dry beans and peas, eggs, and nuts	2–3

From USDA/USDHHS. 1990. *Nutrition and your health: Dietary guidelines for Americans,* 3rd ed. Washington, DC: U.S. Government Printing Office.

*Eat a variety of foods daily, choosing different foods from each group. Most people should have at least the lower number of servings suggested from each food group. Some people may need more because of their body size and activity levels. Young children should have a variety of foods but may need small servings.

FOOD GUIDE PYRAMID

The Food Guide Pyramid was released in 1992 and designed to serve as a graphic outline of what constituted a healthy diet and to convey the concepts of variety, proportionality, and moderation. As shown in Figure 2.8, five food groups (cereals and grains, vegetables, fruits, dairy products, and protein-rich foods) were arranged horizontally, with cereals and grains at the base of the pyramid to indicate that foods from this group should compose the largest portion of the diet. At the apex of the pyramid were fats, oils, and sweets, to indicate that these were to be consumed sparingly. The recommended number of servings from each of the five groups was expressed as a range: persons consuming the number of servings at the low end of the range would consume approximately 1600 kcal per day, while those consuming the number of servings at the high end of the range would consume approximately 2800 kcal per day.

The Food Guide Pyramid has been criticized by some as representing "a mix of well-supported findings, educated guesses, and political compromises with powerful economic interests such as the dairy and meat industries."[59] Some felt that the recommended number of servings of meat (two to three per day) may be unhealthy and that the Food Guide Pyramid ignored important differences in types of fat, such as saturated and *trans* fatty acids, as opposed to monounsaturated fatty acids.[59] Others objected to the USDA's approach to grouping foods—for example, grouping nonfat dairy products (skim milk or nonfat yogurt, for example) with higher-fat dairy products, such as ice cream and many cheeses, or grouping legumes with meat, many of which are high in fat. The USDA's failure to emphasize sources of calcium other

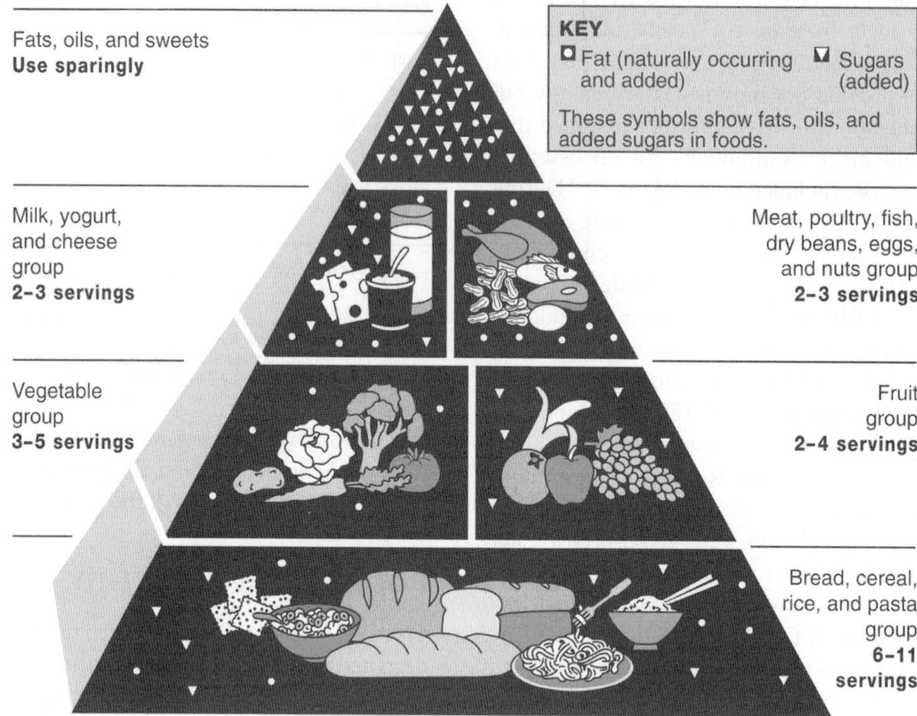

Figure 2.8 **The U.S. Department of Agriculture's Food Guide Pyramid.**

than dairy products was regarded by some as insensitive to individuals of African, Asian, or Hispanic descent, who are more likely to experience lactose malabsorption than are those of Northern European descent. In response to these and other concerns, alternative pyramids were developed. Among these were the Mediterranean Pyramid, the Vegetarian Pyramid, and a variety of Asian Pyramids.[59]

MyPyramid

In 2005 the USDA released an updated and revised food guide graphic called "MyPyramid" that replaced the Food Guide Pyramid released in 1992. The USDA's stated motives for developing the MyPyramid graphic was to increase consumer use of its food guidance system, better motivate consumers to make healthier food choices, more effectively address the increasing prevalence of overweight and obesity in America, and ensure that its food guidance system reflected recent advances in nutritional science. The new graphic was accompanied by an online system of interactive, consumer-friendly tools that provided advice on diet and physical activity that was specific and tailored to the needs of the individual user. With access to a computer and the Internet, an individual could develop a detailed set of dietary recommendations suitable for one's age, sex, and physical activity level.

In general, MyPyramid was part of an overall food guidance system from the federal government that emphasized the need for a more individualized approach to improving diet and lifestyle. MyPyramid supported accumulating scientific evidence that individuals could dramatically improve their overall health by making modest dietary improvements and by incorporating regular physical activity into their daily lives.

MyPlate

In June 2011, the USDA released the MyPlate graphic as part of the federal government's efforts to develop a comprehensive approach to effectively communicate the 2010 *Dietary Guidelines for Americans* (DGAs). Shown in Figure 2.9, MyPlate uses a familiar mealtime symbol as a simple visual cue and reminder to eat healthfully at mealtimes by incorporating healthier choices among the food groups, with particular emphasis on increasing intake of vegetables and fruits.[60] The graphic was deliberately designed to be simple in order to grab consumers' attention and be recognized by a wide variety of audiences. It is intended not to provide a specific message but to serve as a beginning point for the efforts of educators to help people of all age groups, cultures, and learning

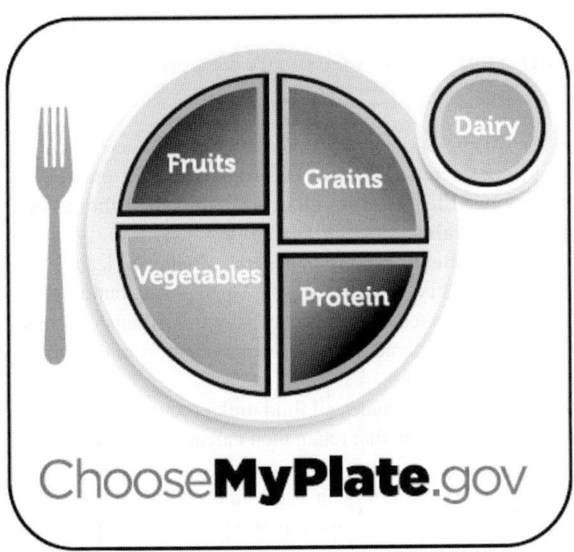

Figure 2.9 In 2011 the U.S. Department of Agriculture released the MyPlate graphic, which provides a visual representation of the advice contained in the 2010 *Dietary Guidelines for Americans.*

Source: USDA Center for Nutrition Policy and Promotion.

levels better understand how to make healthier choices at mealtimes. It is also intended to serve as a reminder of healthful eating, reinforcing what has been conveyed through educational efforts.[61]

The graphic and accompanying educational materials are the result of a multiyear research and development program by the USDA in response to what many in the nutrition community felt was a need for a new image to refocus attention on healthy eating that would replace the Pyramids. From this research program, two apparently opposing needs emerged: a need to simplify nutrition messaging and the need for more information. It also became apparent that no single message or graphic would be sufficient to meet the needs of all consumers and that a comprehensive and layered approach would be necessary to effectively communicate the 2010 DGAs. After studying the responses of consumers to several different potential images, researchers decided that a plate graphic best conveyed a positive yet simple visual message emphasizing the need to increase consumption of vegetables and fruits and to eat healthfully. To meet consumers' desire for more information, a variety of new educational resources are available to the public and to educators to be used in conjunction with the MyPlate graphic.[60,61]

To help consumers understand their energy, food, and nutrient requirements, the USDA has developed an innovative online feature called SuperTracker, which is discussed in Chapter 5 and can be accessed at www.choosemyplate.gov/SuperTracker. One feature of SuperTracker provides meal plans and sample menus based on an individual's recommended energy level, which is based on the individual's age, sex, height, weight, and physical activity level, and so forth. Box 2.11 outlines 12 meal plans from SuperTracker based on varying energy requirements. For example, a 40-year-old female who gets 30 to 60 minutes of moderate physical activity per day, is 66 inches tall, and weighs 135 pounds needs approximately 2200 calories per day. Under this diet plan, SuperTracker recommends 7 ounces of grains with an emphasis on whole grains; 3 cups of vegetables with an emphasis on dark green and orange varieties; 2 cups per day of a variety of fruits; 6 ounces of low-fat or lean meats, poultry, fish, beans, peas, nuts, and seeds; 3 cups of low-fat or fat-free milk, yogurt, and other milk products; 6 teaspoons of oils; and 266 discretionary or empty calories from added sugars or solid fats. SuperTracker encourages users to obtain most of their fat from nuts, vegetable oils, and fish; to limit consumption of solid fats like butter, margarine, shortening, and lard; to read the Nutrition Facts food label in order to keep their intake of saturated fats, *trans* fats, and sodium low; and to choose foods and beverages that are low in added sugars.

The New American Plate

The concept of using a graphic image of vegetables, fruits, and other plant products covering half or more of a dinner plate is not unique to MyPlate. The New American Plate, shown in Figure 2.10, is a food guide based on the recommendations of the research report *Food, Nutrition, and the Prevention of Cancer: A Global Perspective,* which was published by the American Institute for Cancer Research (AICR) and its affiliate, the World Cancer Research Fund located in the United Kingdom. The report (available at http://www.aicr.org), first published in 1997 and updated in 2007, is an exhaustive review of the scientific literature relating to the influence of diet and nutrition on the risk of cancer. The report's key finding is that 30% to 40% of all cancers could be prevented by eating healthfully and being physically active. The New American Plate encourages healthful eating by illustrating that plant foods such as vegetables, fruits, whole grains, and beans should cover two-thirds (or more) of one's plate. Animal foods such as fish, poultry, lean meats, or low-fat dairy products should cover one-third (or less) of the plate. The report encourages variety, moderation, and proportionality and emphasizes eating more plant foods and moderate amounts of lean meats and low-fat dairy products. There is overwhelming scientific evidence that diets emphasizing nutrient-dense plant foods increase a person's daily consumption of vitamins, minerals, dietary fiber, and phytochemicals and tend to be lower in calories. Such diets are associated with a substantially lower risk of cancer and obesity. Furthermore, eating smaller portions of low-fat dairy products and lean meats, especially fish and chicken, is also linked to lower risk of cancer and

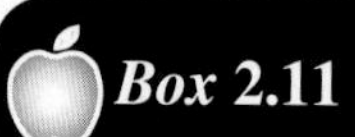

Box 2.11 USDA Meal Planning Guide for 12 Different Levels of Energy Expenditure

Food Intake Patterns

The suggested amounts of food to consume from the basic food groups, subgroups, and oils to meet recommended nutrient intakes at 12 different calorie levels. Nutrient and energy contributions from each group are calculated according to the nutrient-dense forms of foods in each group (e.g., lean meats and fat-free milk). The table also shows the discretionary calorie allowance that can be accommodated within each calorie level, in addition to the suggested amounts of nutrient-dense forms of foods in each group.

1. **Calorie Levels** are set across a wide range to accommodate the needs of different individuals. The attached table "Estimated Daily Calorie Needs" can be used to help assign individuals to the food intake pattern at a particular calorie level.
2. **Fruit Group** includes all fresh, frozen, canned, and dried fruits and fruit juices. In general, 1 cup of fruit or 100% fruit juice, or 1/2 cup of dried fruit can be considered as 1 cup from the fruit group.
3. **Vegetable Group** includes all fresh, frozen, canned, and dried vegetables and vegetable juices. In general, 1 cup of raw or cooked vegetables or vegetable juice, or 2 cups of raw leafy greens can be considered as 1 cup from the vegetable group.
4. **Grains Group** includes all foods made from wheat, rice, oats, cornmeal, barley, such as bread, pasta, oatmeal, breakfast cereals, tortillas, and grits. In general, 1 slice of bread, 1 cup of ready-to-eat cereal, or 1/2 cup of cooked rice, pasta, or cooked cereal can be considered as 1 ounce equivalent from the grains group. **At least half of all grains consumed should be whole grains.**
5. **Meat & Beans Group** in general, 1 ounce of lean meat, poultry, or fish, 1 egg, 1 Tbsp. peanut butter, 1/4 cup cooked dry beans, or 1/2 ounce of nuts or seeds can be considered as 1 ounce equivalent from the meat and beans group.
6. **Milk Group** includes all fluid milk products and foods made from milk that retain their calcium content, such as yogurt and cheese. Foods made from milk that have little to no calcium, such as cream cheese, cream, and butter, are not part of the group. Most milk group choices should be fat-free or low-fat. In general, 1 cup of milk or yogurt, 1 1/2 ounces of natural cheese, or 2 ounces of processed cheese can be considered as 1 cup from the milk group.
7. **Oils** include fats from many different plants and from fish that are liquid at room temperature, such as canola, corn, olive, soybean, and sunflower oil. Some foods are naturally high in oils, like nuts, olives, some fish, and avocados. Foods that are mainly oil include mayonnaise, certain salad dressings, and soft margarine.
8. **Discretionary Calorie Allowance** is the remaining amount of calories in a food intake pattern after accounting for the calories needed for all food groups—using forms of foods that are fat-free or low-fat and with no added sugars.

Daily Amount of Food from Each Group

Calorie Level[1]	1,000	1,200	1,400	1,600	1,800	2,000	2,200	2,400	2,600	2,800	3,000	3,200
Fruits[2]	1 cup	1 cups	1.5 cups	1.5 cups	1.5 cups	2 cups	2 cups	2 cups	2 cups	2.5 cups	2.5 cups	2.5 cups
Vegetables[3]	1 cup	1.5 cups	1.5 cups	2 cups	2.5 cups	2.5 cups	3 cups	3 cups	3.5 cups	3.5 cups	4 cups	4 cups
Grains[4]	3 oz-eq	4 oz-eq	5 oz-eq	5 oz-eq	6 oz-eq	6 oz-eq	7 oz-eq	8 oz-eq	9 oz-eq	10 oz-eq	10 oz-eq	10 oz-eq
Meat and Beans[5]	2 oz-eq	3 oz-eq	4 oz-eq	5 oz-eq	5 oz-eq	5.5 oz-eq	6 oz-eq	6.5 oz-eq	6.5 oz-eq	7 oz-eq	7 oz-eq	7 oz-eq
Milk[6]	2 cups	2 cups	2 cups	3 cups	3 cups	3 cups	3 cups	3 cups	3 cups	3 cups	3 cups	3 cups
Oils[7]	3 tsp	4 tsp	4 tsp	5 tsp	5 tsp	6 tsp	6 tsp	7 tsp	8 tsp	8 tsp	10 tsp	11 tsp
Discretionary Calorie Allowance[8]	165	171	171	132	195	267	290	362	410	426	512	648

Vegetable Subgroup Amounts Are Per Week

Calorie Level	1,000	1,200	1,400	1,600	1,800	2,000	2,200	2,400	2,600	2,800	3,000	3,200
Dark green veg.	1 c/wk	1.5 c/wk	1.5 c/wk	2 c/wk	3 c/wk	3 c/wk	3 c/wk	3 c/wk	3 c/wk	3 c/wk	3 c/wk	3 c/wk
Orange veg.	.5 c/wk	1 c/wk	1 c/wk	1.5 c/wk	2 c/wk	2 c/wk	2 c/wk	2 c/wk	2.5 c/wk	2.5 c/wk	2.5 c/wk	2.5 c/wk
Legumes	.5 c/wk	1 c/wk	1 c/wk	2.5 c/wk	3 c/wk	3 c/wk	3 c/wk	3 c/wk	3.5 c/wk	3.5 c/wk	3.5 c/wk	3.5 c/wk
Starchy veg.	1.5 c/wk	2.5 c/wk	2.5 c/wk	2.5 c/wk	3 c/wk	3 c/wk	6 c/wk	6 c/wk	7 c/wk	7 c/wk	9 c/wk	9 c/wk
Other veg.	3.5 c/wk	4.5 c/wk	4.5 c/wk	5.5 c/wk	6.5 c/wk	6.5 c/wk	7 c/wk	7 c/wk	8.5 c/wk	8.5 c/wk	10 c/wk	10 c/wk

continued

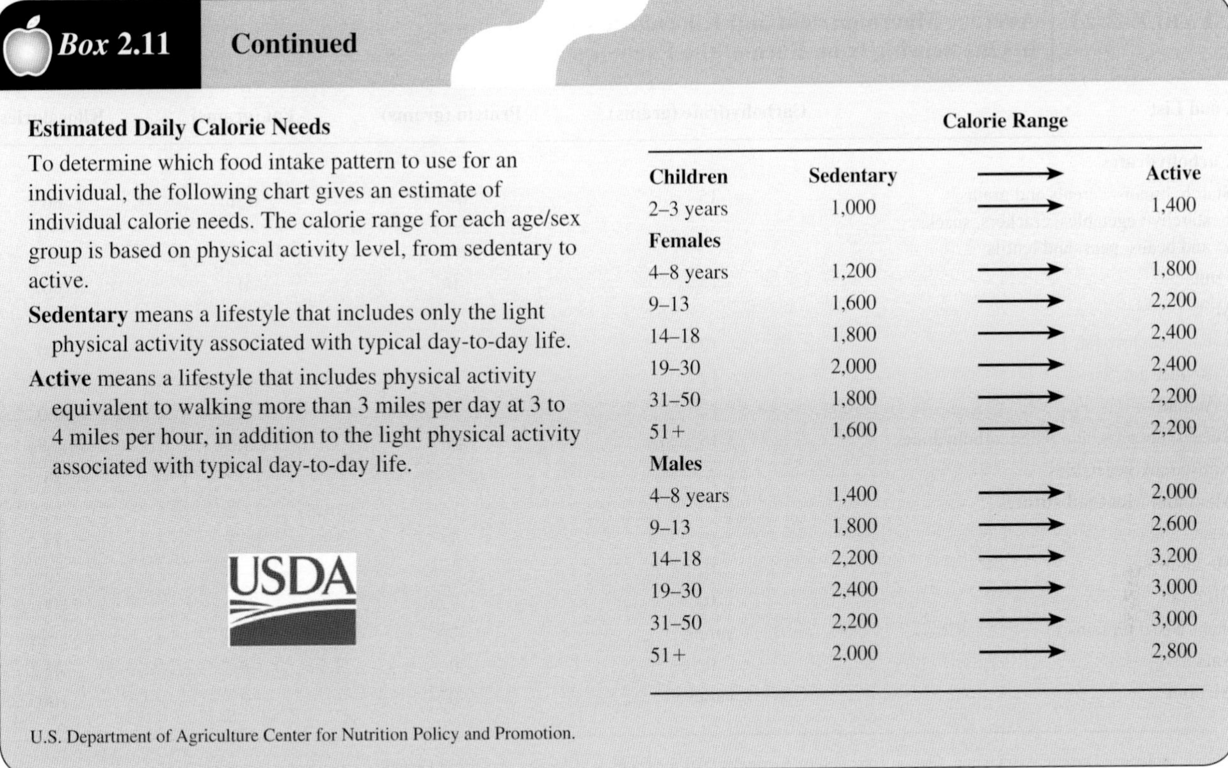

Box 2.11 Continued

Estimated Daily Calorie Needs

To determine which food intake pattern to use for an individual, the following chart gives an estimate of individual calorie needs. The calorie range for each age/sex group is based on physical activity level, from sedentary to active.

Sedentary means a lifestyle that includes only the light physical activity associated with typical day-to-day life.

Active means a lifestyle that includes physical activity equivalent to walking more than 3 miles per day at 3 to 4 miles per hour, in addition to the light physical activity associated with typical day-to-day life.

USDA

	Calorie Range		
Children	**Sedentary**	→	**Active**
2–3 years	1,000	→	1,400
Females			
4–8 years	1,200	→	1,800
9–13	1,600	→	2,200
14–18	1,800	→	2,400
19–30	2,000	→	2,400
31–50	1,800	→	2,200
51+	1,600	→	2,200
Males			
4–8 years	1,400	→	2,000
9–13	1,800	→	2,600
14–18	2,200	→	3,200
19–30	2,400	→	3,000
31–50	2,200	→	3,000
51+	2,000	→	2,800

U.S. Department of Agriculture Center for Nutrition Policy and Promotion.

obesity. A key recommendation from the AICR is to eat at least five servings of vegetables and fruits each day. This one dietary change alone has the potential to prevent at least 20% of all cancers. A standard serving of vegetables is one-half cup of cooked vegetables or one cup of raw vegetables such as salad. An example of a serving of fruit is a medium-size apple, orange, pear, or banana or one-half cup of chopped fruit. It is important to eat a variety of vegetables, including dark green, leafy vegetables and those that are deep orange in color. A variety of whole fruits (as opposed to juice) should be eaten as well, including citrus fruits and those that are good sources of vitamin C. In addition, the AICR recommends eating at least seven servings per day of other

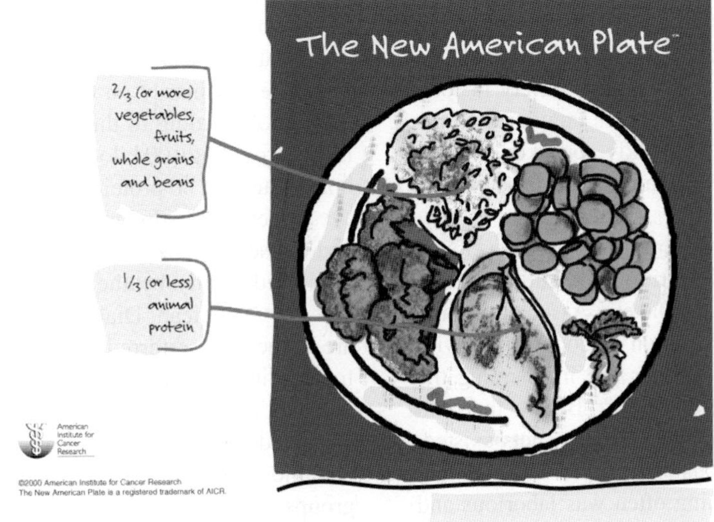

Figure 2.10 The New American Plate emphasizes the kinds of foods that can significantly reduce risks for disease and promote a healthy body weight.

Reprinted with permission from the American Institute for Cancer Research®, www.aicr.org.

TABLE 2.21 Average Macronutrient and Kilocalorie Content in One Serving from Each of the Exchange Lists

Food List	Carbohydrate (grams)	Protein (grams)	Fat (grams)	Kilocalories
Carbohydrates				
Starch: breads, cereals and grains, starchy vegetables, crackers, snacks, and beans, peas, and lentils	15	0–3	0–1	80
Fruits	15	0	0	60
Milk				
Fat-free, low-fat, 1%	12	8	0–3	100
Reduce-fat, 2%	12	8	5	120
Whole	12	8	8	160
Sweets, desserts, and other carbohydrates	15	varies	varies	varies
Nonstarchy vegetables	5	2	0	25
Meat and Meat Substitutes				
Lean	0	7	0–3	45
Medium-fat	0	7	4–7	75
High-fat	0	7	8+	100
Plant-based proteins	varies	7	varies	varies
Fats	0	0	5	45
Alcohol	varies	0	0	100

Source: American Dietetic Association. *Choose Your Foods: Exchange Lists for Diabetes.* Chicago: American Dietetic Association. Copyright © 2008 Academy of Nutrition and Dietetics (formerly the American Dietetic Association). Reproduced with permission.

plant-based foods such as brown rice, whole-wheat pasta, whole-wheat bread, crushed buckwheat (kasha), millet, lentils, black-eyed peas, and various beans such as black, pinto, kidney, navy, and garbanzo.

Food Exchange System

The **food exchange system** is a method of planning meals that simplifies controlling energy consumption (particularly from carbohydrate), helps ensure adequate nutrient intake, and allows considerable variety in food selection. Also, once a person becomes familiar with the system, he or she can use it to quickly approximate kilocalorie and macronutrient levels in individual foods or an entire meal.

The food exchange system originally was developed in 1950 by the Academy of Nutrition and Dietetics (formerly known as the American Dietetic Association) and the American Diabetes Association in cooperation with the U.S. Public Health Service for use in planning the diets of persons who have diabetes.[62] Before then, no standardized method for planning diabetic diets existed, and many health professionals and people with diabetes complained that meal planning often was laborious and difficult to adapt to individual food preferences.

The system categorizes foods and beverages according to their carbohydrate, protein, fat, alcohol, and energy content and lists them in four categories—carbohydrates, meat and meat substitutes, fat, and alcoholic beverages—as shown in Table 2.21. The carbohydrate group includes foods that supply most of their energy in the form of carbohydrate: starchy foods, fruits, milk and other dairy products, other carbohydrates, and nonstarchy vegetables. The milk and dairy products are further divided into three categories on the basis of their fat and energy content. The meat and meat substitutes include foods that serve as good protein sources, supply variable amounts of fat, and no carbohydrate except for the plant-based meat substitutes. The meat and meat substitutes are further divided into four categories, primarily on the basis of their fat and energy content. According to this system, an alcoholic beverage is one providing 100 kilocalories, variable amounts of carbohydrate, and no protein or fat.

A detailed listing of foods within each of the groups and the serving size for each food are given in materials published jointly by the American Dietetic Association and the American Diabetes Association.[63] These lists are sometimes referred to as "exchange lists" because foods within each of the groups on the list provide, on average, a similar number of kilocalories and grams of carbohydrate, protein, and fat, as shown in Table 2.21. Common examples of exchanges from some of the groups are given in Table 2.22. When planning a meal, foods within a group can be "exchanged," or traded, for any other food within that group without varying the approximate amount of carbohydrate, protein, fat, and energy supplied by the meal, as long as the serving size

TABLE 2.22 The Exchange Lists for Meal Planning

Starch List

One starch exchange contains 15 g carbohydrate, 3 g protein, 0 to 1 g fat, and 80 calories. Foods that are considered starches include cereals, grains, pasta, breads, crackers, starchy vegetables, and cooked dried beans, peas, and lentils (cooked dried beans, peas, and lentils are also found on the meat and meat substitute list). In general, one starch exchange is:

- 1/2 cup of cooked cereal, grain, or starchy vegetable
- 1/3 cup of cooked rice or pasta
- 1 ounce of bread, such as one slice of bread

Bread	
Bagel, large (about 4 oz)	1/4 (1 oz)
Bread, whole-wheat, white, pumpernickel, rye	1 slice (1 oz)
Hot dog or hamburger bun	1/2 (1 oz)
Pita, 6 inches across	1/2 (1 oz)
Tortilla, corn or flour, 6 inches across	1 (1 oz)
Grains and Cereals	
Cereal, unsweetened, ready-to-eat	3/4 cup
Oatmeal, cooked	1/2 cup
Pasta, cooked	1/2 cup
Rice, white or brown	1/3 cup
Starchy Vegetables	
Corn, canned	1/2 cup
Peas, green	1/2 cup
Potato, baked with skin, large	1/4 (3 oz)
Potato, boiled	1/2 cup (3 oz)
Snacks and Crackers	
Crackers, saltine	6
Crackers, regular or crispbreads	2–5 (3/4 oz)
Popcorn, lower fat or no added fat	3 cups
Rice cakes, 4 inches across	2
Matzoh	3/4 oz
Beans, Peas, and Lentils	
Beans, cooked (black, garbanzo, kidney, pinto, etc.)	1/2 cup
Lentils, cooked	1/2 cup
Peas, cooked (black-eyed, split)	1/2 cup
Refried beans, canned	1/2 cup

Fruit List

One fruit exchange contains 15 g carbohydrate, 0 g protein, 0 g fat, and 60 calories. Fresh, frozen, canned, and dried fruits and fruit juices are on this list. In general, one fruit exchange is:

- 1 small piece of fresh fruit (4 oz)
- 1/2 cup of fresh or canned fruit or fruit juice ("unsweetened" or "no sugar added")
- 2 tablespoons of dried fruit

Apple, unpeeled, small	1 (4 oz)
Banana, regular size	1/2 (4 oz)
Grapefruit, large	1/2 (11 oz)
Orange, small	1 (6 1/2 oz)
Strawberries	1 1/4 cup whole berries
Watermelon	1 1/4 cup cubed
Juice, apple, grapefruit, orange, pineapple	1/2 cup
Juice, grape, prune	1/3 cup

continued

TABLE 2.22 The Exchange Lists for Meal Planning—*continued*

Milk

One exchange of milk contains 12 g carbohydrate and 8 g protein with the number of grams of fat and the number of calories varying, as shown in Table 2.21. In general one milk exchange is:

- 1 cup or 8 fluid oz

Yogurt, plain or artificially sweetened, fat-free or low-fat	2/3 cup (6 oz)
Evaporated milk, fat-free or low-fat	1/2 cup

Nonstarchy Vegetables

One exchange of a nonstarchy vegetable (those containing small amounts of carbohydrate) provides 5 g carbohydrate, 2 g protein, 0 g fat, and 25 calories. One exchange of a nonstarchy vegetable is:

- 1/2 cup cooked vegetables or vegetable juice
- 1 cup raw vegetables

Beans, green
Broccoli
Brussels sprouts
Cabbage
Carrots
Celery
Cucumber
Greens, collard, kale, mustard
Onions
Peppers
Radish
Tomato

Meat and Meat Substitutes

One exchange of meat contains 0 g carbohydrate, 7 g protein, with the number of grams of fat and the number of calories varying, as shown in Table 2.21. One exchange of a meat substitute provides 7 g protein with variable amounts of carbohydrate, fat, and energy, as shown in Table 2.21. One exchange of a meat or a meat substitute is:

- 1 oz cooked or canned meat, poultry, or fish
- 1/4 cup cooked cheese, ricotta cheese
- 1 oz cheese
- 2 egg whites
- 1 whole egg

Fats

One exchange of fat contains 0 g carbohydrate, 0 g protein, 5 g fat, and 45 calories. One fat exchange is:

- 1 teaspoon of oil
- 1 1/2 teaspoon of nut butters
- 1 teaspoon stick butter, margarine, shortening, or lard
- 1 tablespoon cream cheese, regular
- 1 slice bacon
- 8 large black olives
- 10 large green olives

Source: American Dietetic Association. *Choose Your Foods: Exchange Lists for Diabetes.* Chicago: American Dietetic Association.

of the food adheres to that specified in the exchange list. At breakfast, for example, a person could exchange one slice of bread for 3/4 cup of unsweetened, ready-to-eat cereal because each of these foods is considered one exchange from the starch group, and as such, each has the same amount of macronutrients and the same number of kilocalories. The American Dietetic Association and the American Diabetes Association have also developed exchange lists for foods commonly eaten by various ethnic and regional groups.

TABLE 2.23 Sample Meal Patterns Using the Exchange Lists for Meal Planning

1500-Kilocalorie Diet with Two Snacks

	Breakfast	Lunch	Snack	Dinner	Snack
Starch	2	2	½	2	½
Meat, medium-fat	1	2	1	2	
Vegetable		1		1	
Fruit	1	1		1	
Milk, skim	½	½			½
Fat	1	1		1	

		Kcal	Carbohydrate	Protein	Fat
Total		1510	178 g	79 g	45 g
Percent of energy			50%	22%	28%

2000-Kilocalorie Diet with Two Snacks

	Breakfast	Lunch	Snack	Dinner	Snack
Starch	2	2	½	3	½
Meat, medium-fat	1	2	1	2	1
Vegetable		1		2	
Fruit	2	2		2	
Milk, skim	1	1		1	
Fat	1	1		1	

		Kcal	Carbohydrate	Protein	Fat
Total		2005	261 g	103 g	50 g
Percent of energy			55%	22%	23%

2500-Kilocalorie Diet with Two Snacks

	Breakfast	Lunch	Snack	Dinner	Snack
Starch	3	3	1	4	1
Meat, medium-fat	1	3	1	3	1
Vegetable		2		2	
Fruit	2	2		2	
Milk, skim	1	1		1	
Fat	1	1		1	

		Kcal	Carbohydrate	Protein	Fat
Total		2500	326 g	131 g	60 g
Percent of energy			55%	22%	23%

Ideally, when diabetes is diagnosed in a patient, a dietitian works with the patient to design a meal plan individualized to the patient's dietary preferences, daily schedule, medications, body weight, serum lipid levels, and exercise habits. This meal plan is sometimes expressed in terms of the number of foods from the exchange lists. Many weight management programs and meal plans for people with diabetes are based on the exchange system because it simplifies the task of counting calories. An outstanding feature of the exchange system is that, rather than specifying a particular food, it gives a person an almost unlimited variety of foods from which to choose in planning meals. A person following one of the meal patterns in Table 2.23 can select a number of different foods from the starch list to get his or her exchanges from that list. The same is true for the protein, fruit, milk, and fat selections. The important thing is to select the specified *number* of exchanges and the correct *serving size* from each exchange list.[63]

Summary

1. A number of tools and methods are available for nutrition professionals to use in evaluating dietary intakes of individuals and groups. Included among these are standards of recommended nutrient intake, measurements of nutrient density, dietary guidelines or goals, and food guides.
2. With a few exceptions, dietary standards up until the twentieth century were observational and lacked a firm scientific base. Advances in metabolic, vitamin, and mineral research during the early twentieth century led to the establishment of scientifically based estimates of human nutrient requirements by the League of Nations and several European countries, Canada, and the United States.
3. One of the earliest and most familiar of the dietary standards is the Recommended Dietary Allowance (RDA), developed by the Food and Nutrition Board of the National Research Council. The RDAs provided specific nutrient recommendations for healthy persons in each life stage and gender group. They were originally developed in 1941 and revised about every 5 years. Their primary focus was prevention of micronutrient deficiency. The last edition of the RDAs was published in 1989.
4. Limitations in the RDAs became apparent as nutritional science advanced and as the primary nutrition concern of North America changed from nutrient deficiency to food and nutrient overconsumption, with an attendant increase in chronic disease risk. In addition, the RDAs had no recommendations for carbohydrate, fiber, fat, cholesterol, and food components not traditionally regarded as nutrients (e.g., phytochemicals). They failed to address the role of nutrition in reducing chronic disease risk and gave no guidance on use of nutritional supplements.
5. In response to the RDAs' limitations, scientists from the Food and Nutrition Board, the Canadian Institute of Nutrition, and Health Canada developed a new set of nutrient reference values, known as the Dietary Reference Intakes (DRIs). The DRIs include four reference values: Estimated Average Requirement (EAR), Adequate Intake (AI), Tolerable Upper Intake Level (UL), and Recommended Dietary Allowance (RDA). In addition, the DRIs include an Estimated Energy Requirement and Acceptable Macronutrient Distribution Ranges that suggest the percent of kilocalories to be obtained from total fat, essential fatty acids, carbohydrate, and protein.
6. EAR is the daily dietary intake level estimated to meet the nutrient requirement of 50% of healthy individuals in a particular life stage and gender group. The EAR is the basis for establishing the RDA, which, as traditionally defined, is an intake level sufficient to meet the nutrient requirement of nearly all healthy individuals in a particular life stage and gender group.
7. If there are insufficient data to establish an EAR, then the AI is used instead of the RDA. The AI is actually an observational standard and is defined as a recommended intake level that is assumed to be adequate and that is based on experimentally determined approximations of nutrient intake by a group (or groups) of healthy people. The UL is the highest level of daily nutrient intake that is likely to pose no risk of adverse health effects to almost all apparently healthy individuals in the general population.
8. The suggested uses of the DRIs are clearly delineated and fall into two broad categories: assessing nutrient intakes of individuals and groups and planning for nutrient intakes of individuals and groups. The DRIs address health promotion and the prevention of both chronic and deficiency disease. They also provide guidance on using nutritional supplements. They are intended to be used in conjunction with other nutritional assessment approaches, rather than as the only means of assessing nutrient adequacy.
9. A nutrient-dense food is a good source of vitamins, minerals, and other food components that may have positive health effects, but is relatively low in energy. Nutrient-dense foods are lean or low in solids fats and are low in added sugars and refined starches, all of which add kilocalories but few essential nutrients or little dietary fiber. Nutrient-dense foods also minimize or exclude added salt or other components that are high in sodium.
10. Dietary guidelines, or goals, are dietary standards primarily intended to address the more common and pressing nutrition-related health problems of chronic disease. They often are expressed as nonquantitative change from the present average national diet or from people's typical eating habits.
11. Since the late 1960s, numerous dietary guidelines have been issued by governments and various health organizations. Overall, they have consistently called for maintenance of healthy body weight, decreased consumption of saturated fat, *trans* fat,

and added sugars, increased consumption of complex carbohydrates, and use of alcoholic beverages in moderation, if at all.

12. Nutrition labeling in the United States began in 1973, when the Food and Drug Administration established the U.S. Recommended Daily Allowances (U.S. RDAs). In 1990, Congress passed the Nutrition Labeling and Education Act, which made sweeping changes in nutrition labeling regulations, replaced the U.S. RDAs with the Reference Daily Intakes (RDIs), and established the Daily Reference Values (DRVs). The RDIs and DRVs are collectively referred to as the Daily Values.
13. Food guides are nutrition education tools that translate dietary standards and recommendations into understandable and practical forms for use by those who have little or no training in nutrition. Generally, foods are classified into groups according to their similarity in nutrient content. If a certain amount of food from each group is consumed, a balanced and adequate diet is thought likely to result. A familiar example of a food guide is MyPlate.
14. The food exchange system simplifies meal planning for persons limiting energy consumption and helps ensure adequate nutrient intake. Originally developed to facilitate meal planning for persons with diabetes, it is easily adapted to personal food preferences and is useful for quickly approximating kilocalorie and macronutrient levels in foods. The specified serving sizes of foods within each exchange list are approximately equal in their contribution of energy and macronutrients.

REFERENCES

1. Leitch I. 1942. The evolution of dietary standards. *Nutrition Abstracts and Reviews* 11:509–521.
2. Harper AE. 1985. Origin of recommended dietary allowances: An historic overview. *American Journal of Clinical Nutrition* 41:140–148.
3. McCollum EV. 1957. *A history of nutrition.* Boston: Houghton Mifflin.
4. Harper AE. 2003. Contributions of women scientists in the U.S. to the development of Recommended Dietary Allowances. *Journal of Nutrition* 133:3698–3702.
5. Roberts LJ. 1958. Beginnings of the Recommended Dietary Allowances. *Journal of the American Dietetic Association* 34:903–908.
6. Otten JJ, Hellwig JP, Meyers LD, editors. 2006. *Dietary Reference Intakes: The essential guide to nutrient requirements.* Washington, DC: National Academy Press.
7. Committee on Food and Nutrition, National Research Council. 1941. Recommended allowances for the various dietary essentials. *Journal of the American Dietetic Association* 17:565–567.
8. Food and Nutrition Board, National Research Council. 1989. *Recommended Dietary Allowances,* 10th ed. Washington, DC: National Academy Press.
9. Food and Nutrition Board, Institute of Medicine. 1994. *How should the Recommended Dietary Allowances be revised?* Washington, DC: National Academy Press.
10. Standing Committee on the Scientific Evaluation of Dietary Reference Intakes, Food and Nutrition Board, Institute of Medicine. 1997. *Dietary Reference Intakes for calcium, phosphorus, magnesium, vitamin D, and fluoride.* Washington, DC: National Academy Press.
11. Standing Committee on the Scientific Evaluation of Dietary Reference Intakes, Food and Nutrition Board, Institute of Medicine. 1998. *Dietary Reference Intakes for thiamin, riboflavin, niacin, vitamin B6, folate, vitamin B12, pantothenic acid, biotin, and choline.* Washington, DC: National Academy Press.
12. Standing Committee on the Scientific Evaluation of Dietary Reference Intakes, Food and Nutrition Board, Institute of Medicine. 2000. *Dietary Reference Intakes for vitamin C, vitamin E, selenium, and carotenoids.* Washington, DC: National Academy Press.
13. Panel on Micronutrients, Subcommittee on Upper Reference Levels of Nutrients and of Interpretation and Uses of Dietary Reference Intakes, Standing Committee on the Scientific Evaluation of Dietary Reference Intakes. 2001. *Dietary Reference Intakes for vitamin A, vitamin K, arsenic, boron, chromium, copper, iodine, iron, manganese, molybdenum, nickel, silicon, vanadium, and zinc.* Washington, DC: National Academy Press.
14. Panel on Macronutrients, Panel on the Definition of Dietary Fiber, Subcommittee on Upper Reference Levels of Nutrients, Subcommittee on Interpretation and Uses of Dietary Reference Intakes, Standing Committee on the Scientific Evaluation of Dietary Reference Intakes. 2002. *Dietary Reference Intakes for energy, carbohydrate, fiber, fat, fatty acids, cholesterol, protein, and amino acids.* Washington, DC: National Academy Press.

15. Panel on Dietary Reference Intakes for Electrolytes and Water, Standing Committee on the Scientific Evaluation of Dietary Reference Intakes, Food and Nutrition Board. 2004. *Dietary Reference Intakes for water, potassium, sodium, chloride, and sulfate.* Washington, DC: National Academy Press.

16. Committee to Review Dietary Reference Intakes for Vitamin D and Calcium, Food and Nutrition Board. Ross AC, Taylor CL, Yaktine AL, Del Valle HB, editors. 2011. *Dietary Reference Intakes for calcium and vitamin D.* Washington, DC: National Academy Press.

17. Subcommittee on Interpretation and Uses of Dietary Reference Intakes, Standing Committee on the Scientific Evaluation of Dietary References Intakes, Food and Nutrition Board. 2000. *Dietary Reference Intakes: Applications in dietary assessment.* Washington, DC: National Academy Press.

18. Subcommittee on Interpretation and Uses of Dietary Reference Intakes, Standing Committee on the Scientific Evaluation of Dietary References Intakes. 2003. *Dietary Reference Intakes: Applications in dietary planning.* Washington, DC: National Academy Press.

19. Committee on Use of Dietary Reference Intakes in Nutrition Labeling, Food and Nutrition Board. 2003. *Dietary Reference Intakes: Guiding principles for nutrition labeling and fortification.* Washington, DC: National Academy Press.

20. Backstrand JR. 2003. Quantitative approaches to nutrient density for public health nutrition. *Public Health Nutrition* 6:829–837.

21. Drewnowski A. 2009. Defining nutrient density: Development and validation of the Nutrient Rich Foods index. *Journal of the American College of Nutrition* 28:421S–426S.

22. Kennedy E, Racsa P, Dallal G, Lichtenstein AH, Goldberg J, Jacques P, Hyatt R. 2008. Alternative approaches to the calculation of nutrient density. *Nutrition Reviews* 66:703–709.

23. U.S. Department of Health and Human Services and U.S. Department of Agriculture. 2010. *Dietary Guidelines for Americans, 2010.* Washington, DC: U.S. Government Printing Office.

24. Hansen RG, Wyse BW. 1980. Expression of nutrient allowances per 1,000 kilocalories. *Journal of the American Dietetic Association* 76:223–227.

25. Nicklas TA. 2009. Nutrient profiling: The new environment. *Journal of the American College of Nutrition* 28:416S–420S.

26. Dietary Guidelines Advisory Committee. 2010. *Report of the Dietary Guidelines Advisory Committee on the Dietary Guidelines for Americans, 2010.* Washington, DC: U.S. Department of Agriculture, Agricultural Research Service.

27. Drenowski A, Fulgoni V. 2008. Nutrient profiling of foods: Creating a nutrient-rich food index. *Nutrition Today* 66:23–39.

28. Chiuve SE, Sampson L, Willett WC. 2011. The association between a nutritional quality index and risk of chronic disease. *American Journal of Preventive Medicine* 40:505–513.

29. Institute of Medicine. 2010. *Examination of front-of-package nutrition rating systems and symbols: Phase I report.* Washington, DC: National Academies Press.

30. Fulgoni VL, Keast DR, Drewnowski A. 2009. Development and validation of the Nutrient-Rich Foods index: A tool to measure nutritional quality of foods. *Journal of Nutrition* 139:1549–1554.

31. Institute of Medicine. 2012. *Front-of-package nutrition rating systems and symbols: Promoting healthier choices.* Washington, DC: National Academies Press.

32. Haines PS, Siega-Riz AM, Popkin BM. 1999. The Diet Quality Index Revised: A measurement instrument for populations. *Journal of the American Dietetic Association* 99:697–704.

33. Waijers PMCM, Feskens EJM, Ocke MC. 2007. A critical review of predefined diet quality scores. *British Journal of Nutrition* 97:219–231.

34. Fransen HP, Ocke MC. 2008. Indices of diet quality. *Current Opinion in Clinical Nutrition and Metabolic Care* 11:559–565.

35. Patterson RE, Haines PS, Popkin BM. 1994. Diet Quality Index: Capturing a multidimensional behavior. *Journal of the American Dietetic Association* 94:57–64.

36. Food and Nutrition Board, National Research Council. 1989. *Diet and health: Implications for reducing chronic disease risk.* Washington, DC: National Academy Press.

37. Carmichael SL, Yang W, Feldkamp ML, Munger RG, Siega-Riz AM, Botto LS, Shaw G. 2012. Reduced risks of neural tube defects and orofacial clefts with higher diet quality. *Archives of Pediatric and Adolescent Medicine* 166:121–126.

38. Snyder DC, Sloane R, Haines PS, Miller P, Clipp EC, Morey MC, Pieper C, Cohen H, Demark-Wahnefried W. 2007. The Diet Quality Index-Revised: A tool to promote and evaluate dietary change among older cancer survivors enrolled in a home-based intervention trial. *Journal of the American Dietetic Association* 107:1519–1529.

39. Kennedy ET, Ohls J, Carlson S, Fleming K. 1995. The Healthy Eating Index: Design and applications. Journal of the American Dietetic Association 95:1103–1108.

40. Guenther PM, Reedy J, Krebs-Smith SM, Reeve BB, Basiotis PP. 2007. Development and evaluation of the Healthy Eating Index–2005, Technical Report. Washington, DC: Center for Nutrition Policy and Promotion, U.S. Department of Agriculture.

41. Guenther PM, Juan WY, Lino M, Hiza HA, Fungwe T, Lucas R. 2008. Diet quality of low-income and higher income Americans in 2003–04 as measured by the Health Eating Index–2005. *Nutrition Insight* 42. Washington, DC: Center for Nutrition Policy and Promotion, U.S. Department of Agriculture.

42. Truswell AS. 1987. Evolution of dietary recommendations, goals, and guidelines. *American Journal of Clinical Nutrition* 45:1060–1072.

43. Select Committee on Nutrition and Human Needs, U.S. Senate. 1977. *Dietary goals for the United States*. Washington, DC: U.S. Government Printing Office.
44. Twenty commentaries. 1977. *Nutrition Today* 12(6):10–27.
45. Additional commentaries. 1978. *Nutrition Today* 13(1):30–32.
46. U.S. Department of Agriculture/ U.S. Department of Health and Human Services. 1980. *Nutrition and your health: Dietary Guidelines for Americans*. Washington, DC: U.S. Government Printing Office.
47. Watts ML, Hager MH, Toner CD, Weber JA. 2011. The art of translating nutrition science into dietary guidance: History and evolution of the Dietary Guidelines for Americans. *Nutrition Reviews* 69:404–412.
48. U.S. Department of Health and Human Services. 1988. *The surgeon general's report on nutrition and health*. Washington, DC: U.S. Government Printing Office.
49. Nestle M. 1988. The surgeon general's report on nutrition and health: New federal dietary guidance policy. *Journal of Nutrition Education* 20:252–254.
50. McGinnis JM, Nestle M. 1989. The surgeon general's report on nutrition and health: Policy implications and implementation strategies. *American Journal of Clinical Nutrition* 49:23–28.
51. Kushi LH, Doyle C, McCullough M, Rock CL, Demark-Wahnefried W, Bandera EV, Gapstur S, Patel AV, Andrews K, Gansler T. 2012. American Cancer Society guidelines on nutrition and physical activity for cancer prevention. *CA: A Cancer Journal* 62:30–67.
52. National Cholesterol Education Program. 2001. *Third report of the expert panel on detection, evaluation, and treatment of high blood cholesterol in adults*. Bethesda, MD: U.S. Department of Health and Human Services, Public Health Service; National Institutes of Health; National Heart, Lung, and Blood Institute.
53. American Diabetes Association. 2008. Nutrition recommendations and interventions for diabetes. *Diabetes Care* 31(Suppl. 1):S61–S78.
54. Nestle M, Ludwig DS. 2010. Front-of-package food labels: Public health or propaganda? *Journal of the American Medical Association* 303:771–772.
55. Brownell KD, Koplan JP. 2011. Front-of-package nutrition labeling: An abuse of trust by the food industry? *New England Journal of Medicine* 364:2373–2375.
56. Neuman W. 2009. Food label program to suspend operations. *New York Times*, October 24, B1.
57. Welsh S, Davis C, Shaw A. 1992. A brief history of food guides in the United States. *Nutrition Today* 27(6):6–11.
58. Welsh SO, Davis C, Shaw A. 1993. *USDA's Food Guide: Background and development*. Hyattsville, MD: U.S. Department of Agriculture, Human Nutrition Information Service.
59. Willett WC. 1994. Diet and health: What should we eat? *Science* 264:532–37.
60. Post R, Haven J, Maniscalco S. 2012. Putting MyPlate to work for nutrition educators. *Journal of Nutrition Education and Behavior* 44:98–99.
61. U.S. Department of Agriculture. 2011. *Development of 2010 Dietary Guidelines for Americans consumer messages and new food icon: Executive summary of formative research*. Alexandria, VA: USDA Center for Nutrition Policy and Promotion.
62. Caso EK. 1950. Calculation of diabetic diets. *Journal of the American Dietetic Association* 26:575–583.
63. American Dietetic Association. 2008. *Choose your foods: Exchange lists for diabetes*. Chicago: American Dietetic Association.

ASSESSMENT ACTIVITY 2.1

Using Standards to Evaluate Nutrient Intake

Nutrient standards are indispensable in establishing a benchmark from which to assess adequacy of nutrient intake. This assessment activity will help you become familiar with the Dietary Reference Intakes (DRIs) and the recommendations established by the U.S. Food and Drug Administration (FDA) for food labeling purposes: the Daily Reference Values (DRVs) and the Reference Daily Intakes (RDIs). The activity asks you to use these standards to assess the intake levels of eight nutrients and to compare results from these standards.

Table 2.24 shows mean intakes for eight nutrients by U.S. females age 20 to 29 years from the What We Eat in America, National Health and Nutrition Examination Survey (NHANES) conducted during 2007 and 2008. What We Eat in America, NHANES (discussed in detail in Chapter 4) is a national food survey conducted as a partnership between the U.S. Department of Health and Human Services and the U.S. Department of Agriculture. The data were averaged from 24-hour dietary recalls.

1. Locate the recommended intakes of the eight nutrients for females from the appropriate DRI table found in this chapter and either the Daily Reference Value or Reference Daily Intake from Table 2.17 or Table 2.18. When using the Daily Reference Values from Table 2.17, assume a 2000 kcal intake. Record these in Table 2.24 in the appropriate "Standard" columns.

TABLE 2.24 Mean Intakes of Selected Nutrients and Energy of U.S. Females 20–29 Years Old and How They Compare with the Dietary Reference Intakes, Daily Reference Values, and Reference Daily Intakes

		Dietary Reference Intakes		Daily Reference Values/ Reference Daily Intakes	
Nutrient	**Mean Intake***	**Standard**	**Percent of Standard**	**Standard**	**Percent of Standard**
Folate	460 μg	______	______	______	______
Vitamin C	81 mg	______	______	______	______
Vitamin D	4.6 μg	______	______	______	______
Calcium	869 mg	______	______	______	______
Magnesium	246 mg	______	______	______	______
Iron	12.6 mg	______	______	______	______
Potassium	2094 mg	______	______	______	______
Sodium	3009 mg	______	______	______	______

*From What We Eat in America, NHANES 2007–2008.

2. Calculate how intakes compare with each standard by using the following formula. Enter the percent of standard value in the appropriate "Percent of Standard" columns in Table 2.24.

$$\text{Percent of standard} = \frac{\text{Intake of nutrient}}{\text{Recommended level of intake for that nutrient}}$$

3. Which of the average nutrient intakes are greater than recommended? Which are lower than recommended?

4. Note that recommended nutrient levels vary between the DRIs and the standards established by the FDA. Neither of the standards established by the FDA have been updated since they were established more than three decades ago as part of the Nutrition Labeling and Education Act of 1990. Some leading nutrition researchers have called for the FDA to periodically update the DRVs and RDIs to reflect advances in our understanding of nutrition and nutrient requirements. Discuss why this may or may not be a good suggestion.

ASSESSMENT ACTIVITY 2.2

Food Exchange System

Using the food exchange system to plan meals and assess macronutrient intake is quite easy once you become accustomed to the technique and familiar with the exchange lists. Begin this assessment activity by planning an evening meal and snack for two days using the meal pattern in the far left column of Table 2.25. To manage energy intake and promote dental health, it is probably best for most people to limit eating to meal times and avoid snacking. However, persons taking insulin often need midafternoon and late-evening snacks to maintain adequate blood sugar levels.

1. In the spaces provided under "Meal Plan 1" and "Meal Plan 2," write foods from the exchange lists (see Table 2.22) and their serving sizes that would match the meal pattern. An example of three exchanges from the starch list is a small baked potato, ½ cup of green peas, and a small, plain roll. One strength of the exchange system is that it allows almost unlimited variety and can be easily adapted to personal or cultural eating practices.

2. Once you become familiar with the exchange lists, you can use them to rapidly approximate energy and macronutrient levels in individual foods or entire meals. The far left column of Table 2.26 lists a typical American breakfast. Using Table 2.21 (which gives the average kilocalorie and macronutrient content of the six exchanges) and Table 2.22 (which details the food exchange lists), enter in the appropriate columns the quantities of energy, carbohydrate, protein, and fat for each food and then total them.

TABLE 2.25 Planning Meals and Snacks Using an Exchange List Meal Pattern

Meal Pattern	Meal Plan 1	Meal Plan 2
Evening Meal		
Starch—3 exchanges	______	______
	______	______
	______	______
Lean meat and substitutes—2 exchanges	______	______
	______	______
Vegetables—2 exchanges	______	______
	______	______
Fruit—1 exchange	______	______
Fat—2 exchanges	______	______
	______	______
Evening Snack		
Starch—1/2 exchange	______	______
Low-fat milk—1/2 exchange	______	______

Table 2.26 Estimating Energy and Macronutrient Levels in Foods Using the Exchange Lists

Food	Energy (kcal)	Carbohydrate (g)	Protein (g)	Fat (g)
Bran Chex, 1½ cup	______	______	______	______
Milk, 2% fat, 1 cup	______	______	______	______
Banana, 1/2	______	______	______	______
Orange, 1 medium	______	______	______	______
Bagel, 1/2	______	______	______	______
Cream cheese, 1 Tbsp.	______	______	______	______
Totals	______	______	______	______

CHAPTER 3 MEASURING DIET

OUTLINE

Introduction
Reasons for Measuring Diet
Approaches to Measuring Diet
Techniques in Measuring Diet
Considerations for Certain Groups
Issues in Dietary Measurement
Estimating Portion Size
Summary
References
Assessment Activity 3.1: Collecting a 24-Hour Recall
Assessment Activity 3.2: Completing a 3-Day Food Record
Assessment Activity 3.3: Diet History Questionnaire
Assessment Activity 3.4: The Automated Self-Administered 24-Hour Recall (ASA24)

STUDENT LEARNING OUTCOMES

After studying this chapter, the student will be able to:

1. Discuss why measuring diet is important in assessing nutritional status and in nutritional epidemiology.
2. Explain how research design considerations, characteristics of study participants, and available resources influence the selection of the dietary measurement method.
3. Describe the strengths and limitations of the methods for measuring dietary intake.
4. Discuss the strengths and limitations of using telephone interviews to obtain 24-hour recalls.
5. Discuss how technology is changing how dietary intake data are collected.
6. Describe the use of biologic markers in measuring food and nutrient intake.
7. Explain how estimation or measurement of energy requirements and energy expenditure can be used in validating dietary measurement methods.

INTRODUCTION

Measurement of nutrient intake is probably the most widely used indirect indicator of nutritional status. It is used routinely in national nutrition monitoring surveys, epidemiologic studies, nutrition studies of free-living participants (those living outside a controlled setting), and various federal and state health and nutrition program evaluations. To the uninitiated, measurement of nutrient intake may appear to be straightforward and fairly easy. However, estimating an individual's usual dietary and nutrient intake is difficult. The task is complicated by weaknesses of data-gathering techniques, human behavior, the natural tendency of an individual's nutrient intake to vary considerably from day to day, and the limitations of nutrient composition tables and databases. Despite these weaknesses, nutrient intake data are valuable in assessing nutritional status when used in conjunction with anthropometric, biochemical, and clinical data.

This chapter discusses the reasons for measuring diet and different ways of approaching the topic. Techniques for measuring diet are described along with their strengths and weaknesses. The issues of accuracy and validity are examined, and the number of days of individual dietary intake required to characterize the usual nutrient intake of groups and individuals is discussed.

In some instances, data on the kinds and amounts of food eaten by groups or individuals are important because they allow the estimation of nutrient intake. However, conversion of dietary intake data to nutrient intake data requires information on the nutrient content of foods. This is provided by food composition tables and nutrient databases, which are subject to certain limitations and potential sources of error.

Reasons for Measuring Diet

Assessing dietary status includes considering the types and amounts of foods consumed and the intake of the nutrients and other components contained in foods. When food consumption data are combined with information on the nutrient composition of food, the intake of particular nutrients and other food components can be estimated.[1]

Why measure diet? The ultimate reason is to improve human health.[2,3] Nutritional problems are at the root of the leading causes of death, particularly in developed nations. Food and nutrient intake data are critical for investigating the relationships between diet and these diseases, identifying groups at risk for nutrient deficiency or excess, and formulating food and nutrition policies for disease reduction and health promotion. In general, however, there are four major uses of dietary intake data: assessing and monitoring food and nutrient intake, formulating and evaluating government health and agricultural policy, conducting epidemiologic research, and using the data for commercial purposes.[4] These are outlined in Box 3.1.

Planning national and international food and nutrition programs depends on estimates of per capita (per person) food, energy, and nutrient consumption. Although per capita consumption cannot easily be measured directly, estimates of food disappearance (or availability) (discussed in detail in Chapter 4) are frequently used indirect indicators of consumption. Food consumption data are used in formulating public and private agricultural policies for the production, distribution, and consumption of food.

Repeated surveys estimating food disappearance, such as those conducted by the U.S. Department of Agriculture (USDA), suggest important trends in overall patterns of food consumption over time. Among these are changes in the American diet since the early 1900s in sources of energy, composition of foods, consumption of specific food groups, and eating patterns (such as snacking and eating away from home), all of which can have profound health, social, and economic implications. Dietary assessment is used in determining the extent of malnutrition in a population, developing nutrition intervention and consumer education programs, constructing food guides, devising low-cost food plans, and providing a basis for food and nutrition legislation. Comparisons of dietary practices and nutritional intake with the distribution of disease have demonstrated important links between diet and disease and have shown how dietary changes can modulate disease risk and enhance health.

Approaches to Measuring Diet

Various methods for collecting food consumption data are available. It is important to note, however, that no single best method exists, and diet measurement will always be accompanied by some degree of error.[5] Each method has its own advantages and disadvantages. Despite these disadvantages and the inevitability of error, properly collected and analyzed, dietary intake data have considerable value, as summarized in Box 3.1. Being informed about the strengths and weaknesses of the methods available will better enable researchers and others to scrutinize nutrition research and to draw their own conclusions about a study's results. It will also allow researchers to choose the approach best suited for the task and enable them to use the methods in ways that improve data quality. Selecting the appropriate measurement method, correctly applying it, and using proper data analysis techniques can make the difference between data showing a diet-disease relationship and data showing no relationship where one may actually exist. Choosing the appropriate method for measuring diet depends on such considerations as the research design, characteristics of the study participants, and available resources.

Research Design Considerations

Let's consider five types of research designs: ecological, cross-sectional, case-control, prospective cohort, and experimental. **Ecological** or **correlational studies** compare the level of some factor (e.g., saturated fat intake) with the level of another factor (e.g., coronary heart disease mortality) in the same population. They are useful only for generating hypotheses regarding associations between suspected risk factors and disease outcome and are incapable of testing hypotheses to determine whether a cause-and-effect relationship exists between two variables. It is important to keep in mind that correlation is not necessarily causation. The data used in ecological studies often are only a rough estimate of dietary intake derived from food disappearance studies (discussed in Chapter 4) and are not based on actual dietary intake

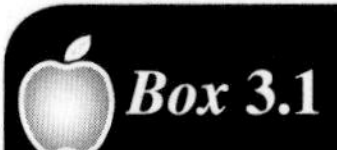

Box 3.1 Reasons for Measuring Diet

Assessing and Monitoring Food and Nutrient Intake	
Ensuring adequacy of the food supply	Data from national surveys and food disappearance indicate the adequacy of food, energy, and nutrient supply
Estimating the adequacy of dietary intakes of individuals and groups	Individual nutrient intake data combined with anthropometric, biochemical, and clinical measures allow assessment of nutritional status
	The proportion of group members having adequate or inadequate intake of a particular nutrient can be determined when the average group intake and the distribution of that intake are known
Monitoring trends in food and nutrient consumption	Trends in percent of energy from fat, carbohydrate, and protein per person can be derived from dietary surveys and food disappearance data
Estimating exposure to food additives and contaminants	The FDA's Total Diet Study monitors average intakes of pesticides, toxins, industrial chemicals, and radioactive substances to determine whether they constitute a health risk
Formulating and Evaluating Government Health and Agricultural Policy	
Planning food production and distribution	Data indicating a marginal or an inadequate supply of energy and/or nutrients can provide direction for planning food production, regulating food imports and exports, and setting priorities for food aid
	Food consumption data allow certain groups or income levels to be targeted for food assistance programs, such as WIC, food stamps, and the school lunch program
Establishing food and nutrition regulations	National and individual consumption data allow identification of potential problems to be addressed by food regulations (e.g., labeling) and programs for food enrichment or fortification
Establishing programs for nutrition education and disease risk reduction	The National Cholesterol Education Program is in part a response to dietary studies indicating that many Americans consume too much total fat, saturated fat, and cholesterol
	National survey data showing increasing average body weights for Americans indicate the need for a national strategy for weight management
Evaluating the success and cost-effectiveness of nutrition education and disease risk reduction programs	The decline in the average serum total cholesterol of Americans suggests that cholesterol-lowering campaigns have been successful
Conducting Epidemiologic Research	
Studying the relationships between diet and health	The purpose of many studies is to investigate the relationship between dietary and nutritional intake and health and disease—for example, the relationships between diet and coronary heart disease, cancer, hypertension, and anemia
Identifying groups at risk of developing diseases because of their diet and/or nutrient intake	Nutrient consumption data show that women of childbearing age often have low folate intake, which increases the risk of their children being born with neural tube defects
Commercial Purposes	Data from national nutrition surveys are used by food manufacturers to develop advertising campaigns or new food products

Adapted from Sabry JH. 1988. Purposes of food consumption surveys. In *Manual on methodology for food consumption studies*, Cameron ME, Van Staveren WA, eds. New York: Oxford University Press. (See also references 5 and 6.)

measurements obtained by the methods discussed in this chapter. Much of these data are readily available from national and international agencies. Using such data, early researchers into the causes of coronary heart disease (CHD) showed that saturated fat consumption is positively correlated with risk of CHD. This association led to more definitive studies that demonstrated a cause-and-effect relationship between high saturated fat intake and increased risk of CHD. An example of an ecological study is shown in Figure 3.1, which illustrates the relationship between per capita (per person) meat consumption in various countries and the annual incidence of cases of colon cancer in women. Such research does not establish that a cause-and-effect relationship exists between meat consumption and risk of colon cancer in woman, but it does suggest that this is a question worth investigating further using a research method better capable of testing hypotheses.

Cross-sectional studies provide a "snapshot" of the health of a population at a specific point in time. Figure 3.2 illustrates data collected by NHANES between 2005 and 2008 that show how the prevalence of hypertension

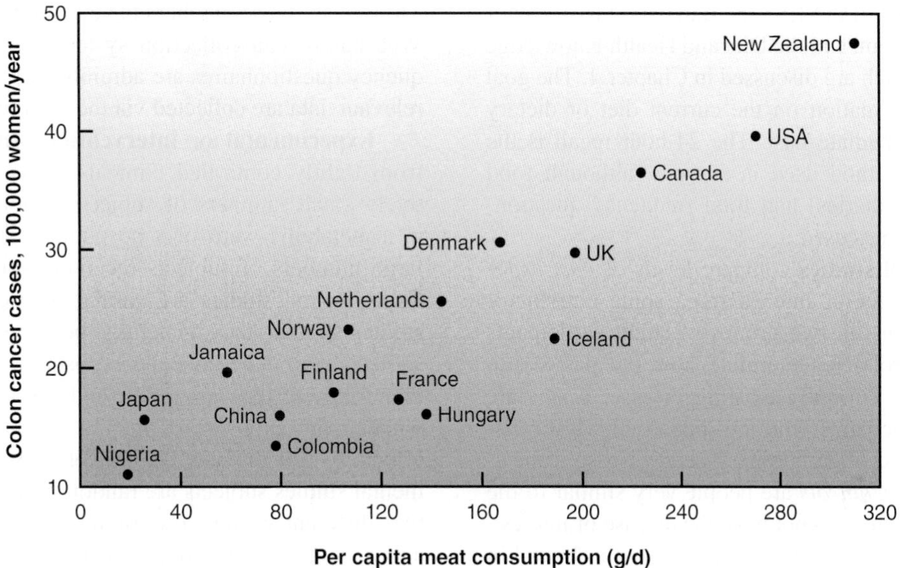

Figure 3.1 In this ecological study, an association was shown between per capita meat consumption and annual incidence of colon cancer per 100,000 women in various countries. Although useful at generating hypotheses, ecological studies are not capable of testing hypotheses.

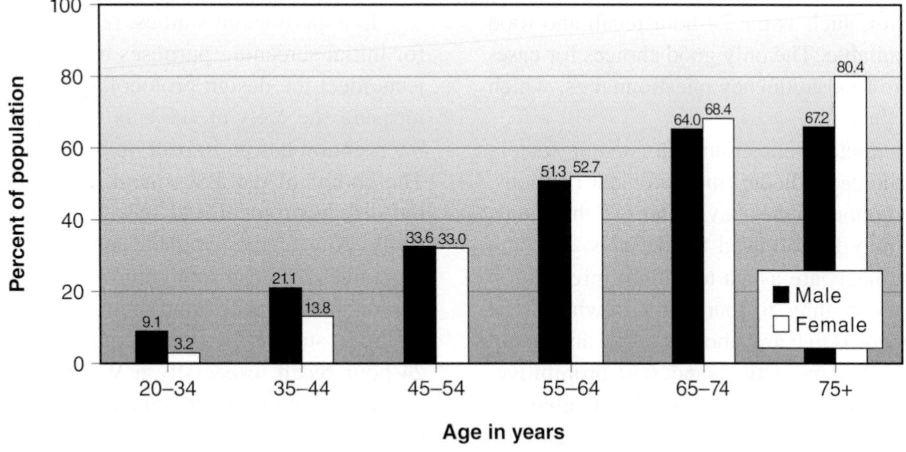

Figure 3.2 Cross-sectional data collected by the National Health and Nutrition Examination Survey between 2005 and 2008 show how the prevalence of hypertension increases as Americans age.

Source: Data from the National Center for Health Statistics.

(here defined as a systolic blood pressure ≥140 mm Hg or a diastolic blood pressure ≥90 mm Hg) increases as Americans age. Various health and dietary measurements are performed on a relatively small group of people that is representative of the larger general population. The much smaller "sample" is selected from the "population" using statistical sampling techniques to ensure that it is representative of the larger population. Analysis of the data collected from the sample allow conclusions to be drawn about the health and dietary habits of the population from which the sample has been taken. Examples of surveys include the National Health and Nutrition Examination Survey, the National Health Interview Survey (NHANES), the Behavioral Risk Factor Surveillance System, and the Diet and Health Knowledge Survey, all of which are discussed in Chapter 4. The goal is to collect information on the current diet or dietary habits in the immediate past. The 24-hour recall is the most common method used in surveys, although food records (or food diaries) and food frequency questionnaires are sometimes used.

Case-control studies compare levels of *past exposure* to some factor of interest (e.g., some nutrient or dietary component) in two groups of study participants (cases and controls) to determine how the past exposure relates to a currently existing disease. *Cases* are those study participants who are diagnosed with a disease being studied (e.g., coronary heart disease, cancer, or osteoporosis). *Controls* are people very similar to the cases except that they do not have the disease of interest. The investigators then look *retrospectively* (backward in time) to measure each group's level of exposure to the factor of interest to determine whether differences in the level of exposure are related to the reasons cases have the disease and controls do not. Thus, case-control studies require methods that measure dietary intake in the recent past (e.g., the year before diagnosis) or in the distant past (e.g., 10 years ago or in childhood). Methods that focus on current behavior, such as the 24-hour recall and food records, are not suitable. The only good choices for case-control studies are food frequency questionnaires, which assess diet in the past.

Time and budgetary constraints are major factors influencing the choice of dietary measurement methods, particularly with cohort studies having tens of thousands of subjects who may be followed for decades. In some cohort studies, subjects are asked to submit information about their diets every three to four years, in which case relying on food records that are labor intensive and costly to analyze would be impractical and cost-prohibitive. Traditionally, 24-hour recalls have been labor intensive to collect and analyze, but technology has changed that. The National Cancer Institute has recently developed an Internet-based automated self-administered 24-hour dietary recall (ASA24) application to collect and code dietary intake data.[6–8] Based on the USDA's Automated Multiple-Pass Method of collecting a 24-hour recall (discussed later in this chapter), the ASA24 allows subjects to report foods consumed by either typing the name of the food into a text box or browsing through a list of foods and clicking on the desired option. Subjects are then asked to provide information on portion size for each food reported.[7] The self-administered food frequency questionnaire has generally been the dietary assessment method of choice for studies involving large numbers of subjects. Traditionally, these have been paper-and-pencil questionnaires, designed to be optically scanned, that are mailed to subjects, completed at home, and then mailed back to the researchers for data entry and processing. More recently, researchers have been moving to entirely Web-based data collection systems in which food frequency questionnaires are administered online and other relevant data are collected via the Internet.[6]

Experimental or **intervention studies** can range from tightly controlled clinical studies involving relatively small numbers of subjects, who may be housed in a metabolic ward of a hospital, to studies involving large numbers of subjects receiving some intervention. Experimental studies are similar to prospective cohort studies in that they generally begin with disease-free subjects who undergo some exposure of interest and are then followed forward in time and observed to determine whether the exposure of interest (or lack of exposure) affects risk of disease. Unlike cohort studies, in experimental studies subjects are randomly assigned to at least two different groups, one or more experimental group and a control group. The experimental group receives the exposure of interest (the intervention), which could be a special diet, a pharmaceutical agent, or a nutritional supplement. The control group receives a placebo (an ineffectual treatment), which allows it to serve as a comparison group because it is treated in the same way as the experimental group(s) with the exception that the control group does not receive the exposure of interest.

In experimental studies, researchers may assess diet for initial screening purposes to determine whether subjects meet the design protocol, or they may periodically measure the diets of subjects to determine whether the intervention has an impact on diet and nutritional status. The choice of the assessment methodology depends on the design protocol and the number of subjects in the study. Any of the available methods would be suitable for studies having a small number of subjects. Large population studies necessitate more efficient data collection methods, such as the food frequency questionnaire or the 24-hour recall, especially a Web-based food frequency questionnaire or an automated self-administered 24-hour recall.[6,9]

Prospective cohort studies or simply **cohort studies** compare *future exposure* to various factors in a large group or *cohort* of study participants in an attempt to determine how exposure to the factors relates to diseases that may develop. Consequently, cohort studies require methods that measure current diet or dietary habits in the immediate past, such as 24-hour recalls, food records, and food frequency questionnaires.[6]

The Framingham Heart Study is an example of a longitudinal study. Initiated in 1949, the original cohort consisted of more than 5000 30- to 62-year-old residents of Framingham, Massachusetts. Since joining the study, the participants have undergone regular examinations and dietary assessments in an attempt to identify factors contributing to the subsequent development of coronary heart disease and high blood pressure. Only 2% of the study participants have been lost to follow-up, and approximately one-half of the original participants are still alive. This and other prospective studies have shown that reducing fat intake, controlling body weight and blood pressure, avoiding smoking, and exercising regularly can reduce risk for coronary heart disease and stroke.

Sometimes the goal of dietary assessment is to quickly screen a group of people for probable dietary risk. In these instances, a brief questionnaire identifying people with a high intake of fat, cholesterol, or sodium or a low intake of dietary fiber, fruits, or vegetables can be administered. Two such instruments—the "fat screener," developed by researchers at the National Cancer Institute, and the MEDFICTS questionnaire—are discussed in the section on food frequency questionnaires. The food frequency questionnaire and the 24-hour recall are also suitable for this purpose.[6]

A recent case-control study investigated whether the quality of the diets of mothers in the year prior to pregnancy was associated with the risk of neural tube defects (e.g., spina bifida or anencephaly) and orofacial clefts (e.g., cleft lip or cleft palate) in their offspring.[5] Using a food frequency questionnaire, researchers evaluated the diets of 936 mothers who had given birth to an infant with a neural tube defect and 2475 mothers who had given birth to an infant with an orofacial cleft. These were the cases. The same food frequency questionnaire was used to evaluate the diets of 6147 mothers who shared many characteristics with the cases but who did not give birth to an infant with one of the malformations being studied. These were the controls. Using data from the food frequency questionnaires, the quality of the mothers' diets was scored using the Diet Quality Index (discussed in Chapter 2). The data analysis showed that mothers having the highest scores on the Diet Quality Index (those in the top quartile) were much less likely to have an offspring with a malformation compared to mothers having the lowest scores (in the bottom quartile).[5]

Characteristics of Study Participants

Factors influencing the selection of a dietary measurement technique include literacy, memory, commitment, age, ability to communicate, and culture of the participants. If some study participants are likely to be unable to read and/or write, the best methods would be a 24-hour recall or a food frequency questionnaire administered by a member of the research team. The food record, the automated self-administered 24-hour recall, or the self-administered food frequency questionnaire would not be recommended. The 24-hour recall and food frequency questionnaire require the ability to remember past eating habits. Food records, the automated self-administered 24-hour recall, and the self-administered food frequency questionnaire require the training and active participation of the study participants. In the case of the food record, the level of effort required can also lead participants to change their dietary patterns during the recording period. Consequently, there is concern about response rates, the comparability of recording skills among participants, and the quality of dietary intake results.[1,6]

The ability to communicate may be limited in study participants who are very young, elderly, developmentally disabled, victims of stroke or Alzheimer's disease, or deceased. In these instances, dietary intake data may have to be collected from another person familiar with the study participant, such as a parent, spouse, child, or sibling. This other person is known as a **surrogate source.** Surrogate sources are discussed later in this chapter in the section "Surrogate Sources." A food inventory method can be useful for older persons living at home. Direct observation of eating habits of persons in institutional care facilities can also be done.[1] The eating habits of children have been assessed using the 24-hour recall, food records, and food frequency questionnaires. Assessing the diets of younger children may require information from surrogates or use of the "consensus recall method," in which the child and both parents give combined responses on a 24-hour recall. This approach has been shown to give more accurate information than a recall from either parent alone.[1]

Assessing the diets of ethnic populations requires modification of existing methods. If participants are interviewed, it is preferable that these be done by persons of the same ethnic or cultural background, so that dietary information can be gathered more effectively. Nutrient analyses of ethnic foods and dishes will likely require changes in food composition databases. Food frequency questionnaires will have to be modified to include food common to the ethnic group being studied.[1,6]

Available Resources

Some methods for measuring diet are more expensive and labor intensive to administer than others. Before a study begins, the budget must be carefully considered, so that the costs entailed will match the available resources. Except in the case of the automated self-administered 24-hour recall, the 24-hour recall must be administered by a trained interviewer. If the food record is used, study participants should be trained to properly record their diets. Considerable labor is required to enter data from conventional 24-hour recalls and food records into a computer for analysis. Food frequency questionnaires can be self-administered, and responses can be marked on a form, which is then optically scanned. Data can then be downloaded into a computer for analysis, thus saving considerable time, effort, and expense. Food records and 24-hour recalls tend to be more feasible methods to use in research with smaller numbers of participants. Food frequency questionnaires, on the other hand, are often preferred by researchers studying large numbers of people.

Techniques in Measuring Diet

Measurement of dietary intake usually is conducted for one of three purposes: to compare average nutrient intakes of different groups, to rank individuals within a group, and to estimate an individual's usual intake. Dietary measurement techniques can be categorized as daily food consumption methods (food record and 24-hour recall) and recalled "usual" or average food consumption methods (diet history and food frequency questionnaire).[1,6] These techniques have also been categorized as meal-based (food record and 24-hour recall) and list-based (food frequency questionnaire).[5]

24-Hour Recall

In the traditional dietary recall method, a trained interviewer asks the respondent to recall in detail all the food and drink consumed during a period of time in the recent past. The interviewer then records this information for later coding and analysis. (In coding, a number is assigned to each kind of food, allowing it to be identified easily for computer analysis.) In most instances, the time period is the previous 24 hours. Thus, the method is most commonly known as the **24-hour recall.**[1,6] Occasionally, however, the time period is the previous 48 hours, the past 7 days, or, in rare instances, even the preceding month. However, memories of intake may fade rather quickly beyond the most recent day or two, so that loss in accuracy may exceed gain in representativeness.[1,6]

In addition to recording responses, the interviewer helps the respondent remember all that was consumed during the period in question and assists the respondent in estimating portion sizes of foods consumed. A common technique of the 24-hour recall is to begin by asking what the respondent first ate or drank on last awakening. The recall proceeds from the morning of the present day to the current moment. The interviewer then begins at the point exactly 24 hours in the past and works forward to the time of awakening. Some researchers ask respondents to recall their diet from midnight to midnight of the previous day. Asking the respondent about his or her activities during the day and inquiring how they might have been associated with eating or drinking can help in recalling food intake. An inquiry about the previous evening's activities, for example, will stimulate the respondent's memory and may help him or her recall the snack eaten while watching a favorite television program.

After the interview, the recall is checked for omissions and/or mistakes. A respondent may have to be contacted later by telephone or mail to clarify an entry or to obtain information such as brand names, preparation methods, and serving sizes. The recall can then be analyzed using a computerized diet analysis program.

The 24-hour recall has several strengths. It is inexpensive, it is quick to administer (20 minutes or less), and it can provide detailed information on specific foods, especially if brand names can be recalled.[1,6] It requires only short-term memory. It is well accepted by respondents because they are not asked to keep records, and their expenditure of time and effort is relatively low. Thus, probability sampling within populations and individuals is possible. The method is considered by some to be more objective than the dietary history and food frequency questionnaire, and its administration does not alter the usual diet.[1,6–8]

Recalls have several limitations. Respondents may withhold or alter information about what they ate because of poor memory or embarrassment or to please or impress the interviewer and researchers. Respondents tend to underreport binge eating, consumption of alcoholic beverages, and consumption of foods perceived as unhealthful. Respondents also tend to overreport consumption of name-brand foods, expensive cuts of meat, and foods considered healthful.[1,6] Foods eaten but not reported are known as **missing foods,** while foods not eaten but reported are known as **phantom foods.** Several researchers report that, when respondents' actual food consumption is low, they have a tendency to overestimate the amount recalled, and, when their actual consumption is high, they underestimate the amount recalled. Some researchers call this phenomenon the "flat-slope syndrome."[10,11] Energy intake often is underestimated if drinks, sauces, and dressings are not reported.

Underreporting can be limited by using a *multiple-pass 24-hour recall method,* in which the interviewer and respondent review the previous day's eating episodes several times to obtain detailed and accurate information about food intake.[1,6] In one version of the method, a *quick list* of foods eaten in the previous 24 hours is initially compiled. In the second pass, a *detailed description* of foods on the quick list is obtained. The respondent is asked to clarify the description and preparation methods of foods on the quick list. For example, if a respondent reports eating breakfast cereal, the interviewer will ask whether milk was used on the cereal and, if so, what kind of milk and how much was used. In the third pass, called the *review,* the interviewer reviews the data collected, probes for additional eating occasions, and clarifies food portion sizes using household dishes and measures (e.g., cups, bowls, glasses, spoons), geometric shapes (e.g., circles, triangles, rectangles), and food labels.

A computer-assisted, five-step, multiple-pass 24-hour recall system is the primary instrument for measuring dietary intake in the National Health and Nutrition Examination Survey (NHANES), which is discussed in Chapter 4.[6] This computer-assisted interview system was developed by the USDA and is known as the USDA Automated Multiple-Pass Method (AMPM). In the first pass, a quick list of foods is obtained. In the second pass, information about the meal, time, and place where foods are eaten is recorded. Information about foods that may have been forgotten is collected in the third pass. Additional food details are collected and a final review is completed in the fourth and fifth passes.[6] A 24-hour recall using this method typically takes 30 to 45 minutes to complete.[6] Use of the AMPM, thorough training and retention of interviewers, and use of other quality-control measures should assure collection of accurate data from this national survey.[6]

Another technological advancement in dietary assessment methodology has been the creation of an Internet-based automated self-administered 24-hour dietary recall application known as the ASA24. Developed by the National Cancer Institute, the ASA24 uses technology drawn from the USDA's Automated Multiple-Pass Method to provide a Web-based tool to researchers, educators, and the public for collecting multiple automated self-administered 24-hour recalls.[6–8] During the first pass of the interview, respondents are asked to report each eating occasion and time of consumption, with queries about where the meals or snacks were eaten, whether the food was eaten while alone or in the presence of others, and whether there was television and/or computer use while eating. The ASA24 allows subjects to report foods consumed by either typing the name of the food into a text box or browsing through a list of food and drink terms derived from the National Health and Nutrition Examination Survey (discussed in Chapter 4). Respondents are asked detailed questions about food preparation, portion size, and additions to foods and beverages so that food codes from USDA's Food and Nutrient Database for Dietary Studies (discussed in Chapter 5) can be assigned. Respondents are able to modify food and drink choices at multiple points during the interview and are asked to provide information about the use of dietary supplements. The system uses a variety of images of foods on plates, in bowls, and in beverage containers to help respondents estimate portion sizes. The ASA24 has visual cues with an optional animated guide and optional audio cues to instruct respondents, enabling the system to be used by low-literacy individuals and those with speech and hearing impairments, and is available in either Spanish or English. A "child friendly" version for use by school-age children is under development. It will use a shorter list of foods and beverages from which to choose and will also ask fewer detailed questions about food preparation.[6–8] The ASA24 can be accessed at the website of the National Cancer Institute at http://riskfactor.cancer.gov/tools/instruments/.

The primary limitation of the 24-hour recall is that data on a *single day's diet,* no matter how accurate, are a very poor descriptor of an individual's *usual* nutrient intake because of day-to-day or **intraindividual variability.**[1,6] Even if several 24-hour recalls are collected from one person, it may be impossible to measure intake of infrequently eaten foods, such as liver. However, a sufficiently large number of 24-hour recalls may provide a reasonable estimate of the mean nutrient intake of a group.[1,6] Depending on the purpose for which data are used, multiple 24-hour recalls performed on an individual and spaced over various seasons may provide a reasonable estimate of that person's usual nutrient intake.[6] Two separate multiple-pass 24-hour recalls are obtained from most NHANES participants using the USDA's AMPM. The first recall is obtained by a trained staff member in a face-to-face interview with the respondent. The second recall is obtained 3 to 10 days later by telephone, which research shows is a feasible and valid method for obtaining 24-hour recalls.[6]

The necessary number of days of data collection depends on several factors: whether estimates of usual intake are for individuals or groups, the nutrients of interest, sample size, and degree of intraindividual and interindividual variability. Twenty-four-hour recalls can provide reasonably accurate data about the preceding day's dietary intake, but reports of diet for the preceding week or month do not accurately characterize dietary intake during those periods.[1,6] Box 3.2 summarizes the strengths and limitations of the 24-hour recall method.

Food Record, or Diary

In this method, the respondent records, at the time of consumption, the identity and amounts of all foods and beverages consumed for a period of time, usually ranging from 1 to 7 days. An example of a food record form is given in Appendix D. Food and beverage consumption can be quantified by estimating portion sizes, using household measures, or weighing the food or beverage on scales. In many instances, household measures such as cups, tablespoons, and teaspoons or measurements made with a ruler are used to quantify portion size. Certain items, such as eggs, apples, or 12-oz cans of soft drinks, may be thought of as units and simply counted. This method is sometimes referred to as the **estimated food record** because portion sizes are estimated (that is, in terms of coffee cups, dippers, bowls, glasses, and so on), or household measures are used. When food is weighed, the record may be referred to as a **weighed food record.** Box 3.3 compares these two methods. The use of food scales is preferred by European nutrition researchers, who consider it more accurate than using household measures, as is typically done by North American researchers. The degree of accuracy from household measures appears acceptable for most research purposes, especially considering the fact that some respondents may find it burdensome to accurately record their diet if they have to weigh everything they eat and drink.

The food record does not depend on memory because the respondent ideally records food and beverage consumption (including snacks) at the time of eating. In addition, it can provide detailed food intake data and important information about eating habits (for example, when, where, and with whom meals are eaten and the respondent's mood when choosing certain foods). Data from a multiple-day food record also is more representative of usual intake than are single-day data from either a 24-hour recall or a 1-day food record. However, multiple food records from nonconsecutive, random days (including weekends) covering different seasons are necessary to arrive at useful estimates of usual intake.[1,6]

Food records have several limitations. They require a literate and cooperative respondent who is able and willing to expend the time and effort necessary to record

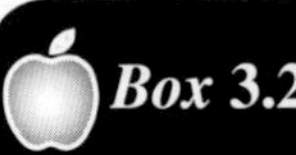

Box 3.2 Strengths and Limitations of the 24-Hour Recall

STRENGTHS

- Requires less than 20 minutes to administer
- Inexpensive
- Easy to administer
- Can provide detailed information on types of food consumed
- Low respondent burden
- Probability sampling possible
- Can be used to estimate nutrient intake of groups
- Multiple recalls can be used to estimate nutrient intake of individuals
- More objective than dietary history
- Does not alter usual diet
- Useful in clinical settings

LIMITATIONS

- One recall is seldom representative of a person's usual intake
- Underreporting/overreporting occurs
- Relies on memory
- Omissions of dressings, sauces, and beverages can lead to low estimates of energy intake
- May be a tendency to overreport intake at low levels and underreport intake at high levels of consumption
- Data entry can be very labor intensive

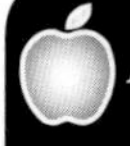

Box 3.3 Comparison of the Estimated Food Record and the Weighed Food Record

ESTIMATED FOOD RECORD

- Amounts of food and leftovers are measured in household measures (cups, tablespoons, teaspoons) or estimated using such measures as coffee cups, bowls, glasses, and dippers
- The researchers then quantify these measures by volume and weight
- Considered less accurate than the weighed food record
- Considered an acceptable method for collecting group intake data
- Puts less burden on the respondent than the weighed food record and thus cooperation rates are likely to be higher, especially over long recording periods
- As effective in ranking subjects into thirds and fifths as weighed records

WEIGHED FOOD RECORD

- Food and leftovers are weighed using scales or computerized techniques supplied by researchers
- Considered more accurate than the estimated food record
- Preferred by some researchers for gathering data on individuals
- Requires a greater degree of subject cooperation than the estimated food record and thus is likely to have a greater impact on eating habits than the estimated food record
- Cost of scales may be prohibitive in some instances

Adapted from Bingham SA, Nelson M, Paul AA, et al. 1988. Methods for data collection at an individual level. In Cameron ME, Van Staveren WA (eds.), *Manual on methodology for food consumption studies*. New York: Oxford University Press.

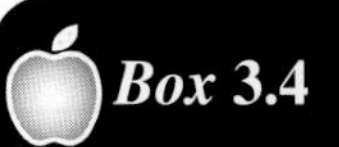

Box 3.4 Strengths and Limitations of the Food Record

STRENGTHS	LIMITATIONS
Does not depend on memory	Requires high degree of cooperation
Can provide detailed intake data	Response burden can result in low response rates when used in large national surveys
Can provide data about eating habits	Subject must be literate
Multiple-day data more representative of usual intake	Takes more time to obtain data
Reasonably valid up to 5 days	Act of recording may alter diet
	Analysis is labor intensive and expensive

dietary intake. However, such a respondent may not be representative of the general population. The act of recording food intake after several days can lead even motivated respondents to reduce the number of foods and snacks eaten and to decrease the complexity of their diets to simplify the recording process.[1,6] When asked directly about recording their food intake, 30% to 50% of respondents have reported changing their eating habits while keeping a food record.[6] Thus, the food record may significantly underreport energy and nutrient intakes.[1,6] Box 3.4 summarizes the strengths and limitations of the food record.

Food Frequency Questionnaires

Food frequency questionnaires assess energy and/or nutrient intake by determining how frequently a person consumes a limited number of foods that are major sources of nutrients or of a particular dietary component in question. The questionnaires consist of a list of approximately 150 or fewer individual foods or food groups that are important contributors to the population's intake of energy and nutrients. Respondents indicate how many times a day, week, month, or year that they usually consume the foods.[1,6] In some food frequency questionnaires, a choice of portion size is not given. These generally use "standard" portion sizes (the amounts customarily eaten per serving for various age/sex groups) drawn from large-population data. An example of this format is given in Figure 3.3A. It simply asks how many times a year, month, week, or day a person eats dark bread or ice cream. This is sometimes referred to as a **simple,** or **nonquantitative food frequency questionnaire** format. The **semiquantitative food frequency questionnaire,** shown in Figure 3.3B, gives respondents an idea of portion size. It asks how many times a year, month, week, or day a person eats a slice of dark bread or a 1/2 cup serving of ice cream. In addition to asking the frequency of consumption, the **quantitative food frequency questionnaire,** shown in Figure 3.3C, asks the respondent to describe the size of his or her usual serving as small, medium, or large relative to a standard serving. Respondents mark their answers on an answer sheet, which can then be optically scanned, so that their responses can be directly downloaded into a computer for analysis, thus saving the researchers considerable time and money. This feature makes food frequency questionnaires a cost-effective approach for measuring diet in large epidemiologic studies that can have tens of thousands of subjects.

Food frequency questionnaires known as "screeners" have been developed to assess intake of calcium, dietary fiber, fruits and vegetables, and percent energy from fat. Screeners are particularly useful in situations that do not require assessment of the total diet or quantitative accuracy in dietary estimates and in situations in which financial resources are limited. They are commonly used in epidemiologic research investigating the relationship between diet and such conditions as cancer and cardiovascular disease but are not considered substitutes for more definitive approaches to measuring diet, such as multiple 24-hour recalls.[1,6,12,13] Figure 3.4 shows a self-administered, machine-readable screener developed by the U.S. National Cancer Institute's Risk Factor Monitoring and Methods Branch (http://www.riskfactor.cancer.gov) to estimate an individual's usual intake of percent energy from fat. The foods asked about on the instrument were selected because they were the most important predictors of variability in percent energy from fat among adults in USDA's 1989–91 Continuing Survey of Food Intakes of Individuals (discussed in Chapter 4). Procedures for scoring the screener are available at the Risk Factor Monitoring and Methods Branch website (http://www.riskfactor.cancer.gov).

The U.S. National Cancer Institute has also developed a variety of screeners for assessing intake of fruits and vegetables, fiber and whole grains, added sugars, dairy products, red meats and processed meats, and calcium, and percentage of energy from total fats. An example of a fruit and vegetable screener developed by the National Cancer Institute is shown in Appendix E. This self-administered, machine-readable instrument was

A Food Item	Average Use During Past Year < 1 month	1–3 month	1–4 week	5–7 week	2–4 day	5+ day
coffee						
dark bread						
ice cream						

B Food Item	Average Use During Past Year < 1 month	1–3 month	1 week	2–4 week	5–6 week	1 day	2–3 day	4–5 day	6+ day
coffee (1 cup)									
dark bread (1 slice)									
ice cream (1/2 cup)									

C Food Item	Medium Serving	Your Serving Size S	M	L	How Often? Day	Week	Month	Year	Never
coffee	(1 cup)								
dark bread	(1 slice)								
ice cream	(1/2 cup)								

Figure 3.3 Examples of three food frequency questionnaire formats: (A) the simple, or nonquantitative, format; (B) the semiquantitative format; (C) the quantitative format.

designed to assess consumption of fruits and vegetables in the past month and can be completed in about 14 minutes. When compared to estimates of fruit and vegetable intake based on four telephone-administered 24-hour recalls, this screener and a similar one were shown to have potential for estimating median intake of fruits and vegetables but were less useful for accurately ranking the intakes of individuals.[13] Additional information on this screener and scoring procedures are available at the Risk Factor Monitoring and Methods Branch website (www.riskfactor.cancer.gov).

A questionnaire developed to quickly estimate how frequently foods high in total fat, saturated fatty acids, and cholesterol are eaten is shown in Appendix E. It is called the MEDFICTS Dietary Assessment Questionnaire (**M**eats, **E**ggs, **D**airy, **F**ried foods, **I**n baked goods, **C**onvenience foods, **T**able fats, **S**nacks) and is recommended by the National Cholesterol Education Program as a simple approach to assess a person's intake of total fat, saturated fat, and dietary cholesterol.[14]

MEDFICTS focuses on foods that are major contributors of total fat, saturated fat, and cholesterol commonly eaten by North Americans. Within each of the questionnaire's eight categories, foods are placed into either a high-fat, high-cholesterol group (Group 1) or a low-fat, low-cholesterol group (Group 2). Group 1 foods are major contributors of dietary fat and cholesterol, and to the right of these groups is a series of boxes with numbers representing points under each box. Group 2 foods are minor contributors of fat and cholesterol. No points are given for Group 2 foods except if a respondent indicates a large portion size for Group 2 meats, in which case six points are given. In completing the questionnaire, the respondent simply checks the boxes representing his or her frequency of weekly consumption and typical serving size for each food group. The points for weekly consumption (shown below each box) are multiplied by the points for serving size and totaled in the score column. The points from each side of the questionnaire are totaled and compared with the key. A total score of 70 or more indicates a need for dietary change to reduce intake of total fat, saturated fat, and dietary cholesterol. A score between 40 and 69 suggests that the respondent is following a "heart-healthy diet" as defined by the National Cholesterol Education Program.[14] A score less than 40 suggests adherence to the National Cholesterol Education Program's therapeutic lifestyle changes diet, which is discussed in Chapter 8 and outlined in the *Third Report of the Expert Panel on Detection, Evaluation, and Treatment of High Blood Cholesterol in Adults.*[1] Studies suggest that the MEDFICTS does a good job of estimating intake of total

National Cancer Institute Quick Food Scan

1. Think about your eating habits over the past 12 months. About how often did you eat or drink each of the following foods? Remember breakfast, lunch, dinner, snacks, and eating out. Blacken in only one bubble for each food.

Type of Food	Never	Less than Once Per Month	1–3 Times Per Month	1–2 Times Per Week	3–4 Times Per Week	5–6 Times Per Week	1 Time Per Day	2 or More Times Per Day
Cold cereal	○	○	○	○	○	○	○	○
Skim milk, on cereal or to drink	○	○	○	○	○	○	○	○
Eggs, fried or scrambled in margarine, butter, or oil	○	○	○	○	○	○	○	○
Sausage or bacon, regular-fat	○	○	○	○	○	○	○	○
Margarine or butter on bread, rolls, pancakes	○	○	○	○	○	○	○	○
Orange juice or grapefruit juice	○	○	○	○	○	○	○	○
Fruit (not juices)	○	○	○	○	○	○	○	○
Beef or pork hot dogs, regular-fat	○	○	○	○	○	○	○	○
Cheese or cheese spread, regular-fat	○	○	○	○	○	○	○	○
French fries, home fries, or hash brown potatoes	○	○	○	○	○	○	○	○
Margarine or butter on vegetables, including potatoes	○	○	○	○	○	○	○	○
Mayonnaise, regular-fat	○	○	○	○	○	○	○	○
Salad dressings, regular-fat	○	○	○	○	○	○	○	○
Rice	○	○	○	○	○	○	○	○
Margarine, butter, or oil on rice or pasta	○	○	○	○	○	○	○	○

2. Over the past 12 months, when you prepared foods with margarine or ate margarine, how often did you use a reduced-fat margarine?

○	○	○	○	○	○
Didn't use Margarine	Almost never	About 1/4 of the time	About 1/2 of the time	About 3/4 of the time	Almost always or always

3. Overall, when you think about the foods you ate over the past 12 months, would you say your diet was high, medium, or low in fat?

○	○	○
High	Medium	Low

Figure 3.4 A short food frequency questionnaire known as a "screener" developed by the National Cancer Institute to estimate an individual's usual intake of percent of energy from fat.

Source: National Cancer Institute, Risk Factor Monitoring and Methods Branch (www.riskfactor.cancer.gov).

fat, saturated fat, and cholesterol, compared with intake estimates based on multiple food records.[15,16]

Numerous food frequency questionnaires have been developed and tested. Three of the more common ones used in nutritional epidemiology research are those developed by Walter Willett and coworkers at Harvard University School of Public Health, Gladys Block and Amy Subar, Frances Thompson, and coworkers at the National Cancer Institute.

Willett Questionnaire

Beginning in 1979, a team of Harvard University nutritionists and epidemiologists headed by Walter C. Willett developed a series of self-administered semiquantitative food frequency questionnaires to conduct epidemiologic research on the relationships between nutrient and food intake and risk of chronic disease. Over the years, their original 61-item questionnaire was modified several times.[17–19] A more recently developed 131-item questionnaire was designed to classify individuals according to levels of average daily intake of nutrients and certain foods and food components during the past year.[20] Its format is similar to that shown in Figure 3.3B. It is self-administered and machine readable, thus making it convenient for use in large epidemiologic studies. Foods included in the questionnaire are those that are major sources of the nutrients, foods, and food components of interest to the researchers. Open-ended questions are also included to identify specific brands of margarine, ready-to-eat cereals, cooking oils, vitamin/mineral supplements, and other foods eaten at least once per week.[20] For each item on the questionnaire, respondents are given nine choices ranging from less than once per month to six or more times per day. Nutrient values are calculated by multiplying nutrient content of each item by frequency of use.

The Willett questionnaire has been designed to be self-administered by nurses and other health professionals in such epidemiologic studies as the Nurses' Health Study and the Health Professionals Follow-up Study with populations of more than 120,000 female nurses and nearly 50,000 male health professionals, respectively.[45,46] A similar food frequency questionnaire is being used successfully in the Iowa Women's Health Study, a prospective cohort study involving a socioeconomically diverse group of older women living in Iowa.[21]

Researchers at Harvard University Medical School and Brigham and Women's Hospital in Boston have adapted the Willett food frequency questionnaire for assessing the diets of children and adolescents ages 9 to 18. Known as the Youth/Adolescent Questionnaire (YAQ), it is self-administered and includes a list of 151 foods. According to reproducibility studies, it has a reasonable ability to assess the eating habits of children and adolescents.

Block Questionnaires

Over the past 3 decades, Dr. Gladys Block has developed a series of self-administered, scannable quantitative food frequency questionnaires and screeners that are based on an earlier food frequency questionnaire known as the Block Health Habits and History Questionnaire (HHHQ), which was developed by Block and coworkers at the National Cancer Institute in 1992.[6] The HHHQ was designed to collect data on diet and well-established risk factors for cancer and total mortality, and it has proven useful in assessing total dietary intake.[6] In 1993, Block founded the firm NutritionQuest (NutritionQuest.com) that develops and markets a number of products and services to health professionals and researchers. Included among these are a series of food frequency questionnaires for children, adolescents, and adults, food screeners for adults, and physical activity surveys and screeners for adolescents and adults. All of NutritionQuest's questionnaires and screeners are available in "paper-and-pencil" format and electronic format. With the paper-and-pencil format, the respondent completes a printed questionnaire, which is then mailed to NutritionQuest for processing and the results are then returned to the researchers. With the electronic format, respondents complete the questionnaire or screener online or the questionnaire can be downloaded onto a computer and completed "off-line" and then submitted electronically for analysis. The food frequency questionnaires from NutritionQuest are variable in length, ranging from 70 to 110 food items and are available in English and Spanish. There are screeners for fat, sugar, fruits, vegetables, soy products, dietary fiber, vitamin D, and folic acid, which range in length from seven to 50 questions. Block questionnaires have been used in a number of research projects including studies conducted by the National Aeronautic and Space Administration (NASA) and the National Institutes of Health.

Diet History Questionnaire

The Diet History Questionnaire (DHQ) is a freely available, self-administered, food frequency questionnaire developed by staff at the U.S. National Cancer Institute's Risk Factor Monitoring and Methods Branch. It can be used by researchers, clinicians, or teachers without permission. The original DHQ I had 124 food items and included information about portion sizes and dietary supplement use. It took about one hour to complete and was designed, based on cognitive research findings, to be easy to use.[22,23] The DHQ II has an updated list of 134 food items based on more recent dietary data from national surveys and has eight questions about dietary supplement uses. The DHQ II is available in four versions: assessment of the past year's dietary intake with questions about portion sizes (the standard version), past-year assessment without portion sizes, past-month assessment with portion sizes, and past-month assessment without portion sizes.[24] The DHQ II is available in a paper-based form and in an identical Web-based form referred to as DHQ*Web. The paper-based DHQ II and its analysis software are available for downloading at no charge from the website of the National Cancer Institute. The DHQ*Web is an automated, electronic food frequency questionnaire allowing respondents to log in at any time and to complete the questionnaire in one sitting or to save their responses, log out, and then to return to the questionnaire later to begin where they left off. The software prompts respondents to correct or modify any missing or inconsistent entries and to completely answer all questions before proceeding to the next question. The first several pages of the DHQ II are shown in Appendix G. The entire questionnaire can be downloaded from the National Cancer Institute's website at http://riskfactor.cancer.gov/dhq2. The DHQ II software provides quantitative data on the intake of 176 nutrients, dietary constituents, and food groups, as shown in Table 3.1. Data on Food Guide Pyramid servings are also available. New foods and nutrients can be added to the database, and other modifications can be made in the DHQ software with relative ease.[24]

NHANES Food Frequency Questionnaire

The NHANES Food Frequency Questionnaire (NHANES FFQ) is a recently developed food frequency questionnaire that is based on the Diet History Questionnaire and

TABLE 3.1 Nutrients and Food Components Analyzed by the Diet History Questionnaire II

Energy
Total fat
Carbohydrate
Protein
Alcohol

Cholesterol
Saturated fatty acids
Monounsaturated fatty acids
Polyunsaturated fatty acids
SFA 4:0 (Butanoic)
SFA 6:0 (Hexanoic)
SFA 8:0 (Octanoic)
SFA 10:0 (Decanoic)
SFA 12:0 (Dodecanoic)
SFA 14:0 (Tetradecanoic)
SFA 16:0 (Hexadecanoic)
SFA 18:0 (Octadecanoic)
MFA 16:1 (Hexadecenoic)
MFA 18:1 (Octadecenoic)
MFA 20:1 (Eicosenoic)
MFA 22:1 (Docosenoic)
PFA 18:2 (Octadecadienoic)
PFA 18:3 (Octadecatrienoic)
PFA 18:4 (Octadecatetraenoic)
PFA 20:4 (Eicosatetraenoic)
PFA 20:5 (Eicosapentaenoic)
PFA 22:5 (Docosapentaenoic)
PFA 22:6 (Docosahexaenoic)
SFA 17:0 (margaric acid)
SFA 20:0 (arachidic acid)
SFA 22:0 (behenic acid)
MUFA 14:1 (myristoleic acid)
Trans 18:1 (trans-octadecenoic acid)
Trans 18:2 (trans-octadecadienoic acid)
Trans 16:1 (trans-hexadecenoic acid)
Total trans fatty acids
Omega-3 fatty acids

Dietary fiber
Total sugars
Fructose
Galactose
Glucose
Lactose
Maltose
Sucrose
Starch
Total dietary fiber
Soluble dietary fiber
Insoluble dietary fiber
Sucrose polyester
Sucralose
Available carbohydrate
Glycemic load
Erythritol
Inositol
Lactitol
Maltitol
Mannitol
Pinitol
Sorbitol
Xylitol

Total protein
Nitrogen
Animal protein
Vegetable protein
Tryptophan
Threonine
Isoleucine
Leucine
Lysine
Methionine
Cystine
Phenylalanine
Tyrosine
Valine
Arginine
Histidine
Alanine
Aspartic acid
Glutamin acid
Glycine
Proline
Serine
3-Methylhistidine

Retinol
Vitamin E (alpha-tocopherol)
Vitamin K
Vitamin C
Thiamin
Riboflavin
Niacin
Vitamin B_6
Total folate
Vitamin B_{12}
Folate (DFE)
Food folate
Folic acid
Vitamin A
Vitamin D
Total vitamin A activity (IU)
Total vitamin A activity (RE)
Niacin equivalents
Pantothenic acid
Vitamin E (IU)

Calcium
Phosphorus
Magnesium
Iron
Zinc
Copper
Selenium
Sodium
Potassium
Manganese

Beta-carotene
Alpha-carotene
Beta-cryptoxanthin
Lutein + zeaxanthin
Lycopene
Beta-carotene equivalents
Total alpha-tocopherol equivalents
Beta-tocopherol
Gamma-tocopherol
Delta-tocopherol
Natural alpha-tocopherol
Synthetic alpha-tocopherol

Caffeine
Aspartame
Saccharin
Phytic acid
Oxalic acid
Ash
Water
Daidzein
Genistein
Glycitein
Coumestrol
Biochanin A
Formononetin
Acesulfame potassium
Choline
Betaine

Source: National Cancer Institute, Risk Factor Monitoring and Methods. http://riskfactor.cancer.gov/dhq2/.

is used in the National Health and Nutrition Examination Survey (NHANES). Formerly called the Food Propensity Questionnaire, the NHANES FFQ was developed by researchers at the National Cancer Institute to collect food intake data that are used with data collected from two 24-hour recalls to estimate *usual* dietary intakes in the National Health and Nutrition Examination Survey (discussed in Chapter 4) and in other surveys. Researchers at the National Cancer Institute have developed a statistical method for estimating usual dietary intake by combining data from two 24-hour recalls with data collected by the NHANES FFQ and other data about a subject's gender, age, and race.[26,27]

The 24-hour recall, the primary dietary data collection instrument used in NHANES, is capable of collecting a considerable amount of detail about when, with what, and how much a person eats and drinks for each day that the recall is obtained. But because the diet of an individual varies greatly from one day to the next (known as intraindividual variability, as discussed earlier in this chapter), the 24-hour recall is incapable of adequately measuring the usual intake of foods that are not consumed nearly every day. Measuring the intake of these infrequently consumed foods requires multiple 24-hour recalls, which is impractical given the respondent burden and the expense involved in obtaining a large number of recalls. A strength of the FFQ is that it provides good data on the probability of an individual's intake of foods, including those that are infrequently consumed, because it asks how often a person consumes those foods and beverages over a relatively long period of time, usually over the course of a year. A shortcoming of the FFQ is that it does not provide good data about how much of the food and beverage a person consumes. By knowing how frequently a food or beverage is consumed over the course of a year and by knowing how much of the food or beverage is consumed (or is likely to be consumed) each day or every time it is consumed, researchers can estimate usual food and nutrient intake with reasonable accuracy.[25–27] The NHANES FFQ is designed to collect information about frequency of food intake during the past year but does not ask about portion size, which reduces the respondent burden compared to that of a quantitative food frequency questionnaire. Studies suggest that the National Cancer Institute's statistical approach of combining data from two 24-hour recalls with data from the NHANES FFQ and other data on a subject's gender, age, and race can be effective in estimating the usual dietary intake of infrequently consumed foods.[26,27] The entire questionnaire can be downloaded from the National Cancer Institute's website at http://riskfactor.cancer.gov/dhq2. The first several pages of the NHANES FFQ are shown in Appendix H.

Strengths and Limitations

Food frequency questionnaires have several strengths. They place a modest demand on the time and energy of respondents and generate estimates of food and nutrient intake that may be more representative of usual intake than a few days of diet records. They are relatively quick to administer. Approximately 30 minutes are required to complete the diet section of the Block Dietary Questionnaire and about 60 minutes are needed to complete the DHQ. They can be self-administered, machine read, or administered online and thus are relatively economical to use in large-scale studies.[6,19,23,28,29] However, data quality may be better when the questionnaire is administered by a trained interviewer. Estimates of nutrient and food intake from repeat administrations of food frequency questionnaires generally compare favorably, showing reasonable reproducibility (see the section "Reproducibility" later in this chapter).[6,17–20]

There are questions about how well food frequency questionnaires estimate the actual average nutrient intakes of individuals and groups—what is called validity. Studies comparing nutrient or food intake estimates obtained from food frequency questionnaires with estimates obtained from "criterion methods," such as multiple food records or 24-hour recalls, suggest that food frequency questionnaires are appropriate for estimating mean intakes of energy and some nutrients for groups and for ranking persons as having a low, average, or high consumption of energy and certain nutrients.[1,6,17–23] Some investigators, however, challenge these conclusions.[30,31] In one epidemiologic study designed to assess dietary measurement error using the Diet and Health Questionnaire, energy expenditure based on doubly labeled water was compared to reported energy intake, and urinary nitrogen excretion was used as an objective measurement of protein intake.[32] The researchers found that male and female subjects underreported their energy intakes an average of 31% to 36% and 34% to 38%, respectively, and underreported their protein intakes an average of 30% to 34% and 27% to 32%, respectively.[32]

Food frequency questionnaires have definite limitations. Because the food list is limited to approximately 100 to 150 foods and food groups, these must be representative of the most common foods consumed by respondents in the sample. Short questionnaires are faster and easier to administer but lack comprehensiveness. Long questionnaires may do a better job of assessing nutrient intake but also require respondents to make an almost overwhelming number of decisions. Longer food frequency questionnaires have the disadvantage of being tedious to complete. Individual foods listed on the questionnaire are more likely to be remembered than foods grouped under such headings as "any other fruit" or "any other vegetable" unless a trained interviewer carefully probes the respondent. Grouping foods under broad categories precludes the ability to collect information about specific food items.[30] Portion sizes allow limited choices as well, and they must be the most typical of what is usually eaten. Questionnaires lacking portion size selections or having poorly chosen ones may identify only individuals at the extremes of the nutrient-intake distribution. However, the usefulness of such portion size information is questioned by research suggesting that defined portion sizes may not be meaningful to some respondents.[33] However, frequency is a more important determinant of nutrient intake than portion size.[34] Another limitation is reliance on the ability of the respondent to describe his or her diet.[1,6]

It is important that food frequency questionnaires be culturally sensitive. Failure to include foods commonly eaten by groups with unique dietary habits may result in underestimates of nutrient intake, particularly if the foods are major sources of certain nutrients or food components. The Block and Willett questionnaires address this shortcoming by providing space for respondents to write in foods that they at least occasionally eat but that are not included in the food list. Food lists also must be periodically updated to keep pace with the thousands of new food products entering the marketplace each year.

Despite these limitations, the food frequency questionnaire is used in NHANES and in other large population surveys to collect data on how frequently food is consumed, especially those foods consumed infrequently, for use in statistical models to estimate usual food intake. The food frequency questionnaire is considered by some as the method of choice for research on relationships between diet and disease, on both the macronutrient and the micronutrient levels, especially in large prospective cohort studies involving tens of thousands of subjects. Box 3.5 summarizes the strengths and limitations of food frequency questionnaires.

Diet History

Diet history is used to assess an individual's usual dietary intake over an extended period of time, such as the past month or year.[1,6] Traditionally, the diet history approach has been associated with the method of assessing a respondent's usual diet developed by B. S. Burke during the 1940s.[35]

Burke's original method involved four steps: (1) collect general information about the respondent's health habits, (2) question the respondent about his or her usual eating pattern, (3) perform a cross-check on the data given in step 2, and (4) have the respondent complete a 3-day food record.[35]

A trained nutritionist begins the interview by asking questions about the number of meals eaten per day; appetite; food dislikes; presence or absence of nausea and vomiting; use of nutritional supplements; cigarette smoking; habits related to sleep, rest, work, and exercise; and so on. This allows the interviewer to become acquainted with the respondent in ways that may be helpful in obtaining further information. This is followed by a 24-hour recall, in which the interviewer also inquires about the respondent's usual pattern of eating during and between meals, beginning with the first food or drink of the day. The interviewer records the respondent's description of his or her usual food intake, including types of food eaten, serving sizes, frequency and timing, and significant seasonal variations.

With the respondent's stated usual dietary practices recorded, the interviewer then cross-checks the data by asking specific questions about the respondent's dietary preferences and habits. For example, the respondent may have said that he or she drinks an 8-oz glass of milk every morning. The interviewer then should inquire about the participant's milk-drinking habits to clarify and verify the information given about the respondent's milk intake. Finally, the participant is asked to complete a 3-day food record, which serves as an additional means of checking the usual intake. Burke admits that this is the least helpful part of the method, and it generally is omitted by the few researchers who currently use this method.

The strengths of the diet history approach are that it assesses the respondent's usual nutrient intake, including seasonal changes, and data on all nutrients can be obtained.[1,6] The method is one of the preferred methods for obtaining estimates of usual nutrient intake.[1,6] Estimates of protein intake by the method correlate well with measures of nitrogen excretion. If what is needed for research purposes is a list of items that is typical of an individual's diet rather than a specific list of items eaten during a certain period of time, the diet history appears adequate to determine the typical diet. Most people are able to report what they typically eat, even if they cannot report exactly what they ate during a specific period of time.[33]

Among the method's limitations are that 1 to 2 hours are required to conduct the interview, highly trained interviewers are needed, coding is difficult and expensive, and nutrient intake tends to be overestimated.[1,6,35] The method also requires a cooperative respondent with the ability to recall his or her usual diet.

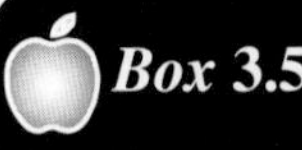

Box 3.5 Strengths and Limitations of Food Frequency Questionnaires

STRENGTHS

- Can be self-administered
- Machine readable
- Modest demand on respondents
- Relatively inexpensive for large sample sizes
- May be more representative of usual intake than a few days of diet records
- Design can be based on large population data
- Considered by some as the method of choice for research on diet-disease relationships

LIMITATIONS

- May not represent usual foods or portion sizes chosen by respondents
- Intake data can be compromised when multiple foods are grouped within single listings
- Depend on ability of subject to describe diet

Box 3.6 summarizes the strengths and limitations of the diet history method.

Duplicate Food Collections

Collection of food consumption data generally is not an end in itself but, rather, a means of eventually arriving at an estimate of nutrient intake. The limitations of using food consumption data to arrive at nutrient intake are the incompleteness of food composition tables, mistakes in coding and entering data, and nutrient losses during food storage and preparation that may not be accounted for in food composition tables.[1,3] A more direct method of calculating nutrient intake that avoids these particular problems is **duplicate food collections.**

When performing duplicate food collections, participants place in collection containers identical portions of all foods and beverages consumed during a specified period.[36] This then is chemically analyzed at a laboratory for nutrient content. To prevent bacterial decomposition of the duplicate samples, they should be kept refrigerated and delivered to the laboratory daily.

This method has the strength of potentially providing a more accurate determination of actual nutrient intake, compared with calculations based on food composition data. Values in composition tables may not be representative of nutrient levels in the particular foods that respondents consume because of seasonal or regional differences, agricultural practices, and losses during marketing and preparation. A participant may have eaten a food that was introduced recently into the marketplace that is not listed in a food composition table or database. Among the method's limitations are the necessity of preparing the additional amount of food to be collected and the work involved in measuring or weighing exactly duplicate portions of food and beverage. In a 1-year dietary intake study conducted by researchers at the USDA Human Nutrition Research Center in Beltsville, Maryland, respondents kept daily food records throughout the 1-year period and provided duplicate food collections for 1 week during each of the four seasons of the year.[36,37] The participants' mean calculated nutrient intake was 12.9% less during the 4 weeks when duplicate food collections were done. Reductions were greatest for foods rich in fat and protein—often the most expensive foods. The respondents may have felt guilty about "wasting" food that went into the collection jar or were concerned about the food's expense, despite receiving payment for their participation in the study. Thus, intakes during food collection periods may not be representative of habitual nutrient intake.

Box 3.7 summarizes the strengths and limitations of the duplicate food collection method.

Food Accounts

Food accounts are used to measure dietary intake within households and institutions where congregate feeding is practiced, such as penal institutions, nursing homes, military bases, and boarding schools.[38] The method

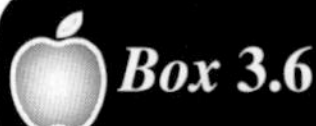

Box 3.6 Strengths and Limitations of the Diet History Method

Strengths	Limitations
Assesses usual nutrient intake	Lengthy interview process
Can detect seasonal changes	Requires highly trained interviewers
Data on all nutrients can be obtained	Difficult and expensive to code
Can correlate well with biochemical measures	May tend to overestimate nutrient intake
	Requires cooperative respondent with ability to recall usual diet

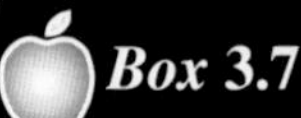

Box 3.7 Strengths and Limitations of the Duplicate Food Collection Method

Strengths	Limitations
Can provide more accurate measurements of actual nutrient intake than calculations based on food composition tables	Expense and effort of preparing more food
	Effort and time to collect duplicate samples
	May underestimate usual intake

accounts for all food on hand in the home or institution at the beginning of the survey period, all that is purchased or grown throughout the period, and all that remains by the end of the survey. Inventories establish amounts of food on hand at the beginning and ending of the survey period, and invoices or other accounting methods provide records of food purchased or obtained from a farm or garden. Trained personnel make site visits at the beginning and ending of the survey period and as necessary throughout the period to assist in recordkeeping. The daily mean consumption per person is calculated for each food item from the total amount of food consumed during the survey period and the number of people in the household or institution.[38]

When used to measure household food consumption, the usual survey period is 2 to 4 weeks. To capture seasonal variations, some researchers may record consumption over different seasons for shorter periods. In addition to the amounts of different foods consumed by family members, it is necessary to account for the number of people present at each meal, the number of meals eaten away from home, and the number served to visitors.[38]

The strengths of the method are that the survey can include a large sample size, food consumption can be monitored for a relatively long period of time, and data on the annual mean consumption and general food patterns and habits of the population can be obtained. The likelihood that the method will alter the diet is less than with the food record method. The method is also relatively economical because personnel need only make periodic visits for supervising and controlling the recording.[38]

Included among the limitations of the method are its inability to account for food that is given to animals, thrown away due to spoilage, or discarded as plate waste or for other reasons. Because respondent literacy and cooperation are necessary, families or institutions willing to keep food accounts may not be representative of the population of interest. Accuracy may suffer due to forgetfulness or lack of faithfulness in maintaining food accounts. The method provides information only on the mean daily consumption of the whole family; it does not indicate how food is distributed among the various family members. Thus, it is only appropriate for measuring food consumption of groups.[38]

Box 3.8 summarizes the strengths and limitations of the food account method.

Food Balance Sheets

The **food balance sheet** is a method of indirectly estimating the amounts of food consumed by a country's population at a certain time. It provides data on food *disappearance* (sometimes referred to as *food availability*) rather than actual food consumption. It is calculated using beginning and ending inventories, figures on food production, imports and exports, and adjustments for nonhuman food consumption (for example, cattle feed, pet food, seed, and industrial use). Food disappearance can be thought of as the amount of food that "disappears" from the food distribution system. Much of this is purchased by consumers at supermarkets; however, a considerable amount is lost due to spoilage.

Mean per capita annual amounts are calculated by dividing total disappearance of food by the country's population.[38] This method has been valuable for detecting trends in the amount of food that disappears from the food distribution system within a country over time and thus has been used to roughly indicate likely trends in consumption as well. It is useful for promoting agricultural production in various parts of the world and for encouraging a more even distribution of food among different countries.[38] Because these data are collected in a roughly similar manner in countries around the world, they are useful in epidemiologic research across countries. Food disappearance data will be discussed in greater detail in Chapter 4 in connection with national surveys.

The strengths of the method are that it can give a total view of the food supplies of a country, can be used in drawing conclusions about general food habits and dietary trends within a country, and is valuable in planning international nutrition policy and formulating food

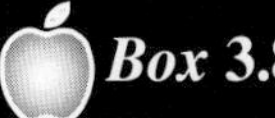

Box 3.8 Strengths and Limitations of the Food Account Method

STRENGTHS	LIMITATIONS
Suitable for use with large sample sizes	Does not account for food losses
Can be used over relatively long periods	Respondent literacy and cooperation necessary
Gives data on dietary patterns and habits of families and other groups	Not appropriate for measuring individual food consumption
Less likely to lead to alterations in diet than some other methods	
Relatively economical	

programs.[38] In some instances, information on food disappearance may be the only accessible data representing a country's food consumption practices.

The method has a number of limitations. The accuracy of data depends on available statistics, the quality of which can vary greatly, depending on a country's level of development. The data represent only the total amount of food that reportedly leaves the food distribution system, apparently for consumption. Note that it is not an estimate of what was actually consumed. It also does not show how food was distributed among individuals or groups within a particular country. The method also does not account for food that is wasted or fed to animals (for example, pets).[38]

Box 3.9 summarizes the strengths and limitations of the food balance sheet.

Telephone Interviews

Telephone interviewing has, in recent years, become an accepted and widely used method for collecting dietary intake data. Investigators have used the technique to administer 24-hour recalls and food frequency questionnaires, particularly to follow up on face-to-face interviews. In NHANES, two computer-assisted, multiple-pass 24-hour recalls are obtained from each participant; the first is collected during an in-person interview, and the second is obtained by telephone 3 to 10 days later.[4] Telephone interviews are now the USDA's principal method of collecting dietary intake data.[39,40] Preadolescent children were shown to be able to provide 24-hour recall data during telephone interviews that compared favorably with written records of their intake unobtrusively collected by parents.[41] Recalls obtained by telephone interview showed good agreement with the observed intake of both college students and elderly participants.[42] Telephone reporting has been shown to be an acceptable method of collecting food record data, whether the data are reported directly to an individual or left on a recording device, such as a telephone answering machine.

Telephone interviews have several strengths. Cost of the method has been reported to be approximately one-fourth to one-half that of comparable personal interviews. They also have the potential of easing the time, logistical, and personnel constraints associated with nutrition surveys.[39,42,43] Telephone surveys have higher response rates than mail surveys.[43] The respondent burden may be somewhat lower with this method, compared with personal interviews. In an era of pervasive suspicion of strangers resulting from rising crime rates, some respondents may find this method more conducive to personal safety than interviews within their homes.

The use of telephone interviewing has been complicated in recent years by the growth of call-screening technologies and heightened privacy concerns resulting from an increased number of telemarketing calls and by changes in personal communication technologies, most notably the dramatic increase in the percentage of cellular-telephone-only households. Between 2003 and 2009, the percentage of cellular-telephone-only households increased by more than 700% from 2.9% to 24.5%. Compared to those who still have landlines, persons living in cellular-telephone-only households are more likely to be renters, minorities, male respondents, or those living at or near the federal poverty level. People 18 to 34 years of age are especially likely to be living in a cellular-telephone-only household.[43] This can result in lower response rates and undercoverage bias. A further complication is the fact that approximately 2% of U.S. households have no telephone service of any type. To improve the quality and validity of data collected by surveys that have traditionally relied on data collected by telephone interviews, surveys are increasingly turning to multiple modes of collecting data, including contacting more subjects via cellular phone and using mail to follow up with nonrespondents.[43]

Twenty-four-hour recall or food frequency data collected over the telephone is subject to the same limitations as that collected in personal interviews. The problem of estimating portion sizes can be addressed by providing respondents with measuring cups, spoons, rulers, two-dimensional and three-dimensional measuring guides, and photographic atlases of food portion sizes.[6–8,18,44] NHANES participants are given a set of measuring

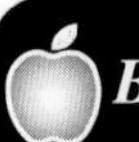

Box 3.9 Strengths and Limitations of the Food Balance Sheet

Strengths	Limitations
Can give a total view of a country's food supplies	Accuracy of data may be questionable
Indicates food habits and dietary trends	Only represents food available for consumption
Used to plan international nutrition policies and food programs	Does not represent food actually consumed
May be the only data available on a country's food consumption practices	Does not indicate how food was distributed
	Does not account for wasted food

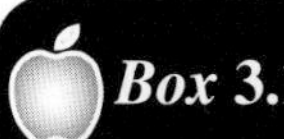

Box 3.10 Strengths and Limitations of Telephone Interviews

STRENGTHS

One-quarter to one-half the cost of a comparable personal interview

Fewer time, logistical, and personnel constraints

Lower respondent burden

Gives respondent more personal security

LIMITATIONS

Subject to many of the same disadvantages of collecting 24-hour recall and food record data

Estimating portion sizes in recalls may be difficult unless steps are taken to address the problem

guides after the first 24-hour recall is obtained during the in-person interview and are instructed on how to use them when the second 24-hour recall is obtained during a subsequent telephone interview.[6–8] The tendency of 24-hour recalls to underestimate energy and nutrient intake can be ameliorated by using the multiple-pass 24-hour recall method.[6–8,45]

Box 3.10 summarizes the strengths and limitations of telephone interviews.

Technological Innovations in Assessment

An area of active research and development in dietary assessment methodology is the use of technology to improve dietary measurement by reducing respondent burden, increasing the validity of dietary intake data, and reducing costs.[9,46,47] Examples of technological innovations previously mentioned in this chapter include the Automated Multiple-Pass Method (AMPM) 24-hour recall, the Internet-based automated self-administered 24-hour dietary recall (ASA24), and the Web-based version of the food frequency questionnaire known as DHQ*Web. In the early 1990s, researchers at the USDA's Western Human Nutrition Research Center developed a dietary measurement system utilizing an electronic scale interfaced with a handheld computer.[48–50] Called the Nutrition Evaluation Scale System, the respondent entered into the computer the identity of foods to be eaten, and the computer then guided the respondent through the steps of weighing the foods and any leftovers after the meal. The software has been shown to be user-friendly, using icons, sounds, and on-screen prompts to guide respondents through the process of entering data. The identity and weights of foods consumed are saved in the computer's memory. These data then can be transferred to another computer for review by a dietitian and eventual analysis using a food composition database.

More recently, there has been considerable interest in using digital images to simplify the process of recording, identifying, and quantifying meals and snacks.[51–55] This could be thought of as a digital image food record, an example of which is shown in Figure 3.5. One common approach being investigated is to have a respondent use a digital camera to capture images of foods and beverages before and after eating. These images are then electronically sent to researchers who analyze them to identify and quantify the foods in the images. Some researchers are using mobile phones equipped with high-resolution digital cameras to capture images that can be automatically sent to researchers for analysis.[51–53] Others are investigating the use of proprietary devices specifically designed to capture images.[54,55] One system uses a miniature camera attached to a lanyard that can be worn around the neck to capture images of food that can then be provided to researchers.[54] Another uses a handheld personal digital assistant with an integrated camera and mobile telephone card that respondents can use to capture images of foods and beverages, which are then sent to researchers for analysis.[55]

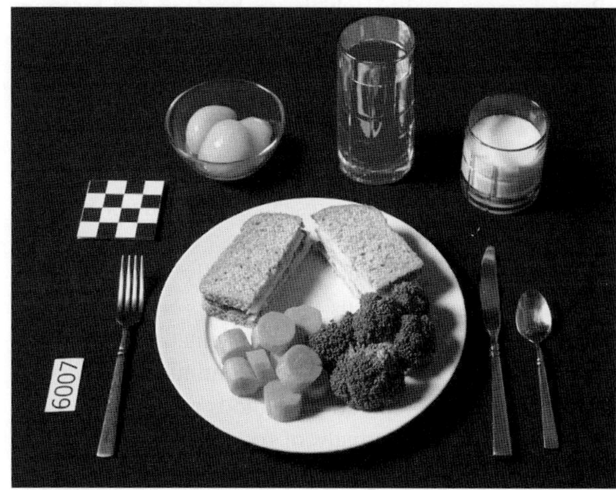

Figure 3.5
Digital images of a meal such as this one can be taken by respondents and electronically sent to researchers who can analyze the images to identify and quantify the foods and beverages in the meal. The fiducial marker in the left side of the image assists researchers in accurately estimating portion sizes of food items.
The McGraw-Hill Companies, Inc. / Jesselyn Zbytowski, photographer.

Advantages of these systems include a relatively low respondent burden and the potential for image analysis software to automatically record, identify, and quantify the volume of foods and beverages in the image. However, if there is uncertainly about the identity and volume of the food, the technology allows the respondent to fairly easily provide detailed information that might be requested by researchers. A lower respondent burden may lead to fewer alterations in diet that inevitably result from maintaining several days of food records. Research suggests that this technology may be particularly valuable for use by adolescents, who are generally adept at using technology but have poor compliance when asked to report their food intake using more traditional diet measurement techniques.[52] These systems are limited by their higher cost relative to the more traditional methods and image quality, which can be degraded by room lighting and poor camera resolution and focus. There is also the need for an object of known dimensions and markings (referred to as a *fiducial marker*) to be in the image as a size reference in order to accurately estimate portion size. Fiducial markers can include a checkered tablecloth provided by the researchers, a dinner plate of known diameter, or some other object of known dimension. Distinguishing between visually similar foods (such as skim milk versus whole milk, or premium ice cream versus ice milk) can be problematic. Some form of written or verbal records will continue to be necessary to document preparation methods and identify visually similar foods. Estimates of food consumption based on the analysis of photographs and digital images of the meals of respondents have been compared with weighed food records made on the same meals. When performed by trained observers, these estimates compared favorably to the weighed food records, supporting the validity of digital images as methods for measuring food intake and estimating food portion size.[55–57]

Box 3.11 summarizes the strengths and limitations of the digital imaging methods.

Surrogate Sources

There are times when a respondent may not be able to provide the dietary intake data that investigators desire. In some instances, a respondent may have a problem with hearing, speech, or memory due to disease, trauma, or advanced age. This is especially a problem with elderly respondents participating in case-control studies. In such instances, obtaining information from **surrogate sources** may improve information quality and provide data otherwise unavailable from deceased or incompetent participants. Potential surrogate respondents include the respondent's spouse or partner, children, other close relatives, and friends.[1,6,58]

Several investigators have studied the use of surrogate sources of dietary intake. A review of these studies demonstrates that "surrogate respondents can provide dietary information, but that incomplete responses must be anticipated."[58] In some cases, surrogate respondents provide more valid data than the respondents themselves. Surrogate sources often can provide good information on specific foods or nutrients. The availability of data from surrogate respondents varies with the surrogate's relationship to the participant, the surrogate's sex (e.g., females provide more accurate data about the eating habits of males than males do about the eating habits of females), and the number of shared meals. There may be considerable difference in the quality of surrogate data between spouses or partners of deceased participants and spouses or partners of living participants.[6]

Surrogate sources are good in studies in which there is rapid mortality of study participants, in which there is concern about biased recall from participants, or in which participants have problems with memory impairment or difficulty communicating because of such causes as stroke or Alzheimer's disease. In some instances, data from surrogates are good enough for ranking persons in quintiles (one of five levels) in terms of their nutrient intake (i.e., as having an intake that is very low, low, average, high, or very high). In any event, surrogate sources must be carefully selected and data closely scrutinized because misclassification of dietary intake can occur easily when relying on surrogate sources alone.[1,6,58]

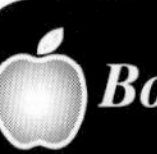

Box 3.11 Strengths and Limitations of Digital Imaging Methods

Strengths	Limitations
Digital imaging method has good validity	Large initial expense is involved, but this may be offset by lower long-term costs
Recording food intake takes less time than 24-hour recalls or food records	Periodic revalidations are recommended
Respondent burden is less	Unable to distinguish visually similar foods or document preparation methods
Methods appear to be acceptable to subjects	Subject to technical problems caused by sophisticated equipment
Eating habits may be less affected by recording	

CONSIDERATIONS FOR CERTAIN GROUPS

Adaptations in dietary measurement can be made for certain groups, such as young persons, the reading-impaired, individuals having problems recalling their diet, persons who are visually or hearing-impaired, and the obese. These considerations, summarized in Box 3.12, facilitate collection of intake data from persons who otherwise might have difficulty participating in surveys.

ISSUES IN DIETARY MEASUREMENT

Validity

Validity is the ability of an instrument to actually measure what it is intended to measure.[1,6] In most instances, investigators are interested in knowing what a respondent's *usual intake* is or has been. Thus, validating an instrument involves comparing estimates of intake obtained by that instrument with a respondent's usual intake. Because it is difficult if not impossible to know a person's true usual intake, investigators must turn to *relative,* or *criterion, validity*. Relative, or criterion, validity is defined as the comparison of a new instrument with another instrument (a so-called gold standard), which has a greater degree of *demonstrated,* or *face, validity*.[1,6] However, if the two instruments fail to compare favorably, the question must be asked, "Which instrument (if any) gives the best estimate of usual intake?" The failure of one instrument to compare favorably with another may not lie in the instrument's being validated; it actually may have given the best estimate of usual intake. The fault may lie in the criterion instrument.

The validity of food frequency questionnaires has been examined by comparing estimates of food and nutrient intake obtained from food frequency questionnaires with estimates obtained from multiple food records or 24-hour recalls, which are thought to give a more detailed and quantitative estimate of dietary intake over an extended period.[1,6] Researchers at Harvard University, for example, collected four 1-week weighed-diet records over the course of a year from 173 participants.[17] These served as an estimate of usual intake during the 1-year period and the criterion against which intake data from the food frequency questionnaire were compared. Results of the study showed that a simple self-administered food frequency questionnaire can provide useful information about individual nutrient intakes over a 1-year period. To study the questionnaire's ability to assess diet in the recent past, the researchers administered it to the same group of participants 3 to 4 years after the weighed food records were collected, and they concluded that the questionnaire was useful in estimating nutrient intake 4 years in the past.[18] A number of other validation studies have been done as well.[1,6,20,21] Nutrient estimates derived from food frequency questionnaires compared favorably with those derived from criterion methods, suggesting that food frequency questionnaires can be appropriate to use in epidemiologic research. Overall, these studies support the use of food frequency questionnaires for estimating a group's average intake for energy and some nutrients. They also suggest that the method is appropriate for ranking individuals in terms of nutrient intake (e.g., categorizing individuals as having a low, average, or high intake of some nutrient).[1,6,17] Other investigators, however, question the use of food frequency questionnaires in epidemiologic research.[30,31]

The validity of a food frequency questionnaire depends in large part on items included in the food list and assumptions about portion size and nutrient content of the various groups.[1,6] Another important consideration in validation studies is the appropriateness of the criterion instrument. Given the weaknesses of food records and 24-hour recalls in characterizing usual intake, how appropriate are they to use as a truth measure against which to judge another instrument, such as the food frequency questionnaire? If, in a validation study, data from food frequency questionnaires compare unfavorably to data from a criterion method, is it necessarily the fault of the food frequency questionnaire? A proposal for circumventing this dilemma is to include a biological marker as a *third* criterion method in the validation process.[6,34] Biological markers are discussed in the section "Use of Biological Markers."

Some investigators have compared estimates of dietary intake using various methods with respondents' *actual* intake, which the investigators observed surreptitiously.[10,11] Usually, the respondents ate all or at least most of their meals in a cafeteria or residential metabolic research facility where their food intake could be observed. Different assessment methods then could be used to measure respondents' intake during the period when their diet was observed. Among these were the 24-hour recall, food records, and food frequency questionnaires. However, such comparisons over relatively short periods of time in monitored or controlled situations fail to adequately validate a method intended to assess the usual, self-selected diets of free-living persons.[1,6,11]

Use of Biological Markers

Another approach to validating dietary measurement methods is to compare intake data with certain biological markers associated with dietary intake.[1,6,19,34,62,63] Biological markers offer the advantages of being easily accessible (urine, feces, blood, tissue samples) and providing a validity check of dietary intake independent of respondents' accuracy and truthfulness. A major problem, however, is that many factors other than dietary intake can affect nutrient concentrations in tissues, even in well-fed persons.[1,6,19] Although many biological markers have

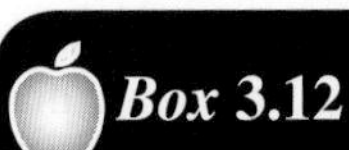

Box 3.12 Considerations When Measuring Diet in Certain Groups

Group	Considerations
Young persons	Dietary intake data on children under 8 years of age are best obtained from the person responsible for meals. For information on food eaten away from home, interview the child in the presence of the parent or guardian. Data on meals eaten at school, kindergarten, or day care center can be obtained from those responsible for their meals. Reliable data on intake in the previous 24 hours can be obtained from children 8 years of age and older.
Persons with recall problems	There appears to be no firm evidence that memory of past diet is impaired during aging despite popular belief to the contrary. The ability to recall past diet may be more a function of how much attention is paid to what is eaten.[1,6] Diet recall can be helped through the use of checklists and visual aids, such as food models and photographs.[1,6] Information obtained from surrogates (spouse, sibling, or caregiver) can improve the quality of data.[6,58] Reproducibility of recall of diet many years in the past by older persons has been shown to be good but is reduced by older age, cognitive impairment, and male sex.[1,6]
Persons with impaired vision or hearing	Intake measurement instructions can be communicated to the visually impaired through large-print materials, tape recordings, radio, telephone, personal interview, and Braille. Some visually impaired persons have video equipment that will enlarge print to a readable size. Data can be collected through personal interview, by telephone or tape recorder, or over specially equipped computer systems. Communication of instructions to and collection of data from hearing-impaired persons is easily done with self-explanatory and well-prepared printed materials. Use of an interpreter of sign language and visual aids, such as food models or photographs, can be helpful. Verbal responses to an interviewer can facilitate collection of data.
Persons who cannot read well	Personal and telephone interviews, digital imaging methods, and computerized or web-based systems with visual and audio prompts can all be used in collecting dietary intake data from the reading-impaired. Persons with limited reading ability may be able to use printed materials having an appropriate vocabulary. Food models, photographs, and digital images are especially helpful.
The obese	Several studies have questioned the validity of reported energy intake in obese persons, indicating a tendency to underreport energy intake using the dietary history and food records.[59–61]

Source: Adapted from Cameron ME, Van Staveren WA. 1988. *Manual on methodology for food consumption studies.* New York: Oxford University Press, and other indicated sources.

potential for use, only a limited number have been investigated. Among these are urinary nitrogen, sodium, and potassium; plasma levels of carotenoids, vitamin E, and vitamin C; fatty acids in adipose tissue; changes in serum triglyceride; and assessment of energy expenditure and body weight.[6,19,34,62,63]

Analysis of nitrogen in multiple 24-hour urine samples, a well-known biological marker, has been used to verify protein intake in dietary surveys.[6,19,34,64,65] If acceptable agreement exists between urinary nitrogen excretion and estimated protein intake, it can be assumed that intake of other nutrients is fairly well represented.

Use of this method depends on several assumptions: that respondents are in nitrogen balance (there is no accumulation of protein for growth or repair or unusual losses due to starvation or injury); that estimates of extrarenal nitrogen excretion sufficiently cover losses through the feces, hair, skin, and other routes; and that all urine has been collected over the course of the collection period.[66]

Urinary sodium is a useful measure of dietary sodium intake, especially because amounts used at the table and in cooking are difficult to assess. Fecal sodium losses are minimal, and in temperate climates it is assumed that amounts in sweat are negligible. Differences in urinary sodium and estimated dietary intakes have been shown to be as low as 5%. Although fecal losses of potassium are greater and more variable than with sodium, urinary potassium has been used for validating dietary potassium intake.[19,65,66]

A potential problem with measurements of nitrogen, sodium, and potassium in 24-hour urine samples is the necessity of obtaining a *complete* 24-hour urine sample—a requirement some participants have difficulty adhering to. One approach to checking on the completeness of 24-hour urine samples is use of the para-amino-benzoic acid (PABA) marker. Participants take one PABA tablet three times a day with their meals. The PABA is excreted in the urine. A 24-hour urine collection containing less than 85% of the PABA marker is considered unsatisfactory, either because the participant did not take all the PABA tablets or one or more urine specimens was omitted from the collection.[65,66]

Plasma levels of total carotenoids, α-carotene, β-carotene, lycopene, vitamin C, and vitamin E have been shown to compare favorably with intakes of these substances based on administration of a food frequency questionnaire.[64,67] Changes in plasma triglyceride levels have been shown useful in estimating total fat intake.[62,63] This measurement is based on the observation that as intake of total fat (except for *trans* fatty acids) increases, plasma triglyceride decreases and, to a lesser extent, plasma high-density lipoprotein cholesterol increases.

Linoleic acid in adipose tissue can be used as an index of dietary intake of linoleic acid over the past 2 to 3 years, whereas the linoleic acid content of erythrocytes (red blood cells) can be an index of dietary linoleic acid during the past 6 to 8 weeks.[62] A small piece of adipose tissue can be easily removed from beneath the skin and measured for linoleic acid. This can be an independent way of estimating intake of specific fatty acids that are not endogenously synthesized. Such measurements have been shown to compare favorably with estimates of usual intake based on 2 weeks of weighed food records and a food frequency questionnaire.[19,62]

Energy Expenditure and Weight Maintenance

Another approach to validating dietary measurement methods is to compare reported energy intake with body weight and energy expenditure calculated from an equation or measured using the doubly labeled water method. Self-reported energy intake has been compared with energy expenditure determined through use of the doubly labeled water method (discussed in greater detail in Chapter 8). Briefly, participants drink a known amount of water labeled with deuterium (^2H) and oxygen-18 ($^2H_2{}^{18}O$).[61,68,69] They provide periodic samples of urine or saliva over the next 2 weeks or so, which allows monitoring of the body's elimination of deuterium and oxygen-18. Knowledge of the rates at which these isotopes are eliminated allows researchers to calculate energy expenditure in free-living participants with considerable accuracy and precision, despite certain limitations discussed in Chapter 8.

During a 10-day field exercise in the Canadian Arctic, the self-reported energy intake of 20 infantry soldiers was 39% less than their actual energy expenditure measured by doubly labeled water.[70] Researchers from the Ontario Cancer Institute and the University of British Columbia studied the accuracy of reported energy intakes from 7 consecutive days of food records obtained from a subset of 29 women participating in the Canadian Diet and Breast Cancer Prevention Trial. The mean body mass index (BMI, weight in kilograms divided by height in meters squared, or kg/m^2) of the subjects was 23.1 ± 2.5 (mean ± standard deviation) and thus essentially within what is considered a healthy range for BMI. Reported energy intakes averaged 20% less than mean total energy expenditure determined by doubly labeled water.[71] Researchers from Maastricht University compared total energy expenditure measured by doubly labeled water with reported energy estimates from 7-day food records completed by 30 adult males. The subjects had a mean BMI (kg/m^2) of 34 ± 4 (mean ± standard deviation) and thus were considered obese. Reported energy intakes averaged 37% less than mean total energy expenditure. The researchers estimated that, during the week that subjects kept food records, their energy consumption averaged 26% less than the previous week, when subjects were not recording their intake. These results suggest that, not only do subjects underreport energy intake, but they also are likely to eat less food during the recording period.[61,72]

Researchers from the University of Vermont compared total energy expenditure measured by doubly labeled water with estimates of energy intake based on four multiple-pass 24-hour recalls obtained over a 2-week period in a group of 35 low-income adult females. Underreporting of energy intake averaged 17%. However, underreporting was greater in subjects who were obese and in those who had lower literacy (difficulty reading and spelling), compared with nonobese subjects and those who had a higher degree of literacy.[73] In another study, energy intake was measured in 118 fourth- and fifth-graders who kept 8-day food records with the help of parents and nutritionists. Average daily energy intake was found to range from 17% to 33% less than total energy expenditure measured by doubly labeled water.[74]

Researchers at the USDA Beltsville Human Nutrition Research Center compared self-reported energy intakes with the amount of energy the participants actually required to maintain their body weight to within ± 0.9 kg. The data, collected from 266 research participants over a 14-year period, showed that only 11% of self-reported energy intakes were accurate to within ± 100 kcal and that 81% of participants underreported their energy intake by 700 kcal ± 379 kcal (mean ± standard deviation).[75]

Another approach to check for underreporting is to compare reported usual energy intake with **resting energy expenditure** (REE), calculated using various equations, such as those shown in Table 3.2 and the Estimated Energy Requirement (EER) equations discussed in Chapter 7. If a subject's reported usual energy intake is <1.2 times his or her calculated REE, underreporting of energy, and therefore nutrient, intake is highly likely.[76] Using data from the third National Health and Nutrition Examination Survey, researchers at the National Center for Health Statistics compared reported energy intakes of nearly 8000 adult survey participants with their calculated resting energy expenditure.[77] About 18% of males and 28% of females were classified as underreporters. Underreporting was highest in females and in persons who were older, overweight, or trying to lose weight. Researchers at the USDA Western Human Nutrition Research Center compared reported energy intakes from 7-day food records with energy intake necessary to maintain a stable body weight in 22 adult females of widely varying body weight.[78] The subjects completed a variety of behavioral questionnaires that measured hunger, restrained eating, emotional eating (excessive eating in response to anger, fear, or anxiety), anxiety, and depression. Cognitive performance tests were also administered to the subjects. These assessed mental acuity, the ability to sustain or focus attention, short-term memory, and manual dexterity. Underreporting of energy by nonobese females (mean BMI 21.3 kg/m^2) was estimated at 10%, while that of obese subjects (mean BMI 34.2 kg/m^2) was nearly 20%. In the obese group, the presence of emotional factors related to depression were linked to greater likelihood of underreporting.

The observation that underreporting of food intake is common led researchers at the Beltsville Human Nutrition Research Center to propose the hypothesis of the "uncertainty principle of food-intake measurements: the degree of deviation of reported from real intake is proportional to the degree of attention focused on the intake."[75] Although the task of maintaining food records resulted in an 18% underestimate of energy intake, collection of duplicate food portions resulted in a decline of an additional 13%.[75] Thus, although the collection of dietary data is critical to our understanding of nutrition, *dietary intake data must be interpreted with considerable caution,* whether self-reported or obtained by observers of whose presence respondents are aware.[75,79]

Despite the difficulty of accurately measuring usual dietary intake, our ability to quantify the degree of misreporting and to identify some of the characteristics of subjects related to misreporting represents progress toward the goal of accurately measuring diet. The potential now exists for "targeting specific areas of dietary assessment techniques to prevent or at least to minimize the effect of each factor on collection of valid data."[80]

TABLE 3.2 Equations for Calculating Resting Energy Expenditure*

World Health Organization		
Females	3–9 years old	22.5 W + 499
	10–17 years old	12.2 W + 746
	18–29 years old	14.7 W + 496
	30–60 years old	8.7 W + 829
	> 60 years old	10.5 W + 596
Males	3–9 years old	22.7 W + 495
	10–17 years old	17.5 W + 651
	18–29 years old	15.3 W + 679
	30–60 years old	11.6 W + 879
	> 60 years old	13.5 W + 487
Harris-Benedict (Values Rounded for Simplicity)		
Females	REE = 655 + 9.6W + 1.9S − 4.7A	
Males	REE = 66 + 13.8W + 5S − 6.8A	

*REE = resting energy expenditure; W = body weight in kg; S = stature in cm; A = age in years.

Reproducibility

Reproducibility, or **reliability,** can be defined as the ability of a method to produce the same estimate on two or more occasions, assuming that nothing has changed in the interim. Reproducibility is concerned only with whether a method is capable of providing the *same or similar answer* two or more times and does not necessarily indicate whether the answer is *correct.* Reproducibility studies can partially answer the validity question; a method cannot give a correct answer every time unless it gives approximately the same answer each time. Problems in instrument design, respondent instructions, or quality control also can be uncovered by reproducibility studies.

Estimating Portion Size

Accurate estimation of portion size is an important element in self-reports of dietary intake. Research shows that without training, individuals have difficulty

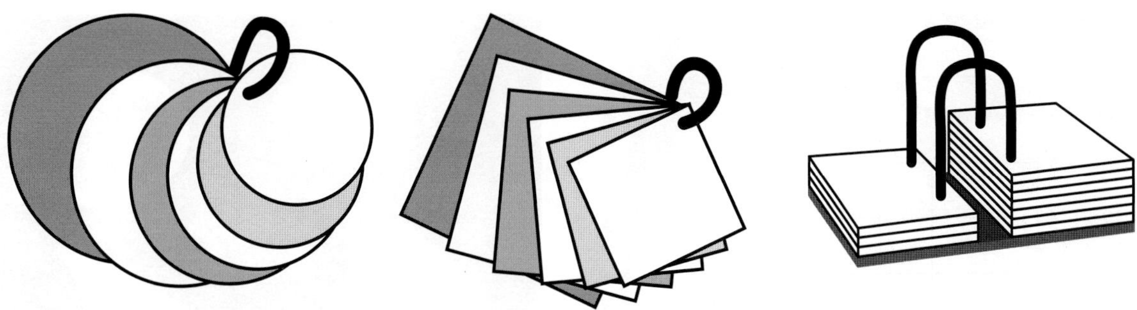

Figure 3.6 Simple geometric shapes representing foods are sometimes used to help survey participants estimate food portion size. Each piece has a known dimension (surface area or thickness) and is made from poster board or other materials.

accurately estimating the portion sizes of foods eaten and that this is particularly the case with children.[6,7] A variety of approaches have been developed to help respondents estimate portion sizes. Among the simplest and least costly are "food models" composed of two-dimensional geometric shapes of various sizes cut out of poster board, as shown in Figure 3.6. Circles of various diameters can be used to help estimate the diameter of round foods, such as apples, oranges, tomato slices, hamburger patties, hamburger buns, and cookies. Square and rectangular pieces are useful in estimating the length and width of bread, cake, some cuts of meat, and cheese. Pie-shaped pieces of various radii can be used in estimating portion sizes of pie, round cake, watermelon, and pizza. Pieces of polyurethane foam 3 to 4 inches square and of varying thicknesses can be used to help respondents estimate the thickness of foods, providing a third dimension. Individual pieces can be used, or several can be stacked to achieve the desired thickness. An alternate approach is to have a number of pieces of cardboard cut 3 to 4 inches square, which can then be stacked to aid in estimating the thickness of food. Polystyrene balls of various diameters are useful in estimating sizes of round food objects. Bowls, plates, measuring cups and spoons, and drinking cups of various sizes also can be used to help respondents estimate serving sizes of soup, breakfast cereal, salad, beverages, sugar, and margarine. An increasingly common approach is using photographs or digital images to facilitate portion size estimation.[7,44,80–82] Photographs of actual foods illustrating three different serving sizes on a plate can be used, as shown in Figure 3.7. The plates used in Figure 3.7 are all the same size and are used to provide a sense of scale. Researchers at the USDA have developed a *Food Model Booklet* that contains a collection of life-size, two-dimensional images representing different shapes and sizes of foods, including life-size images of plates, bowls, cups, and glasses.[44] Figure 3.8 is an image from the *Food Model Booklet* showing a life-size dinner plate with four different-size amorphous mounds representing different portion sizes of foods that mound on a plate, such as

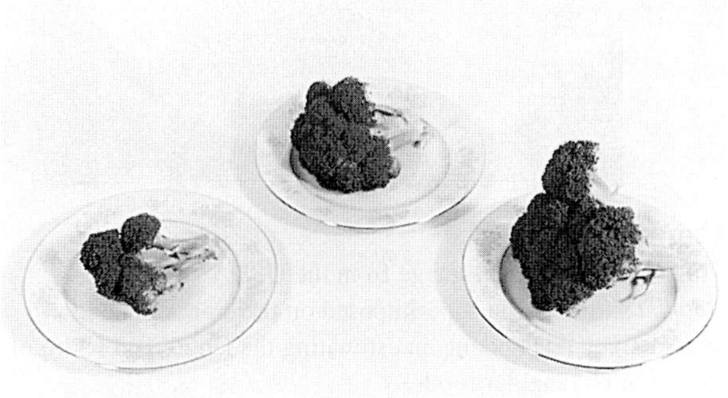

Figure 3.7
Some investigators use photographs to help respondents more accurately estimate food portion size.

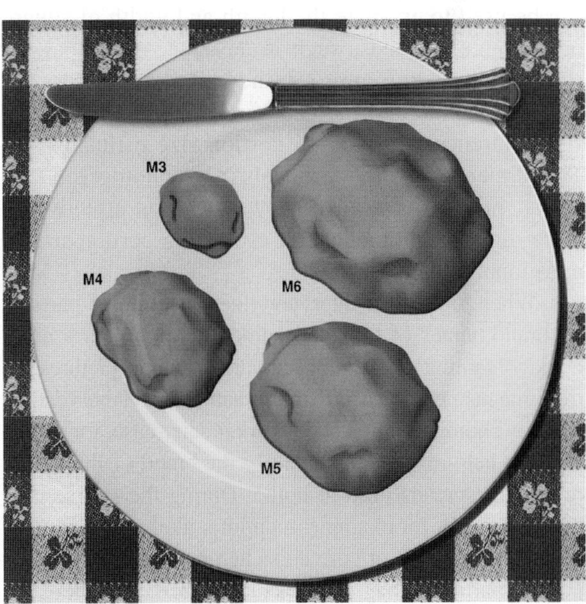

Figure 3.8
This two-dimensional image from the USDA's *Food Model Booklet* shows a life-size dinner plate with four different size amorphous mounds representing different portion sizes of foods that mound on a plate. The knife lying across the top of the plate provides a size reference.
Source: Photo courtesy of the USDA.

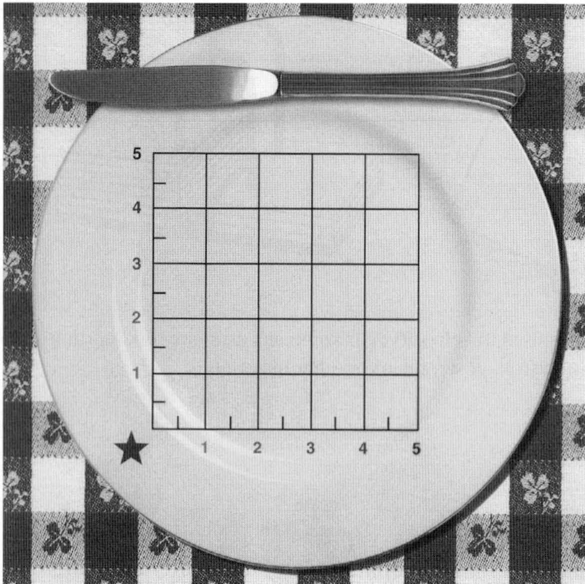

Figure 3.9
This two-dimensional image from the USDA's *Food Model Booklet* shows a grid superimposed on the dinner plate to assist survey respondents in estimating the length and width of square or rectangular foods.
Source: Photo courtesy of the USDA.

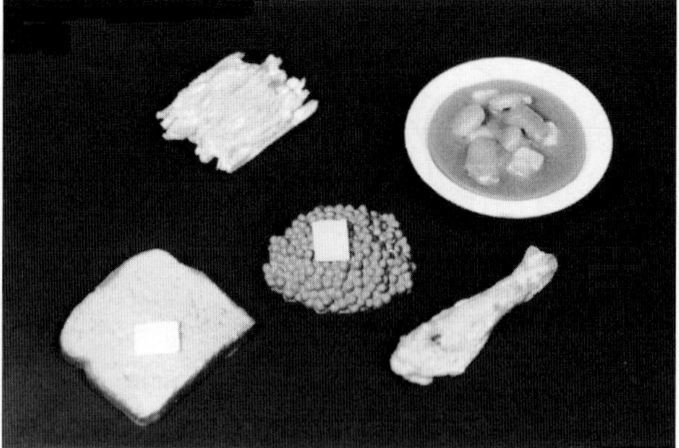

Figure 3.10
Lifelike food models can be used to improve accuracy in estimating food portion sizes.

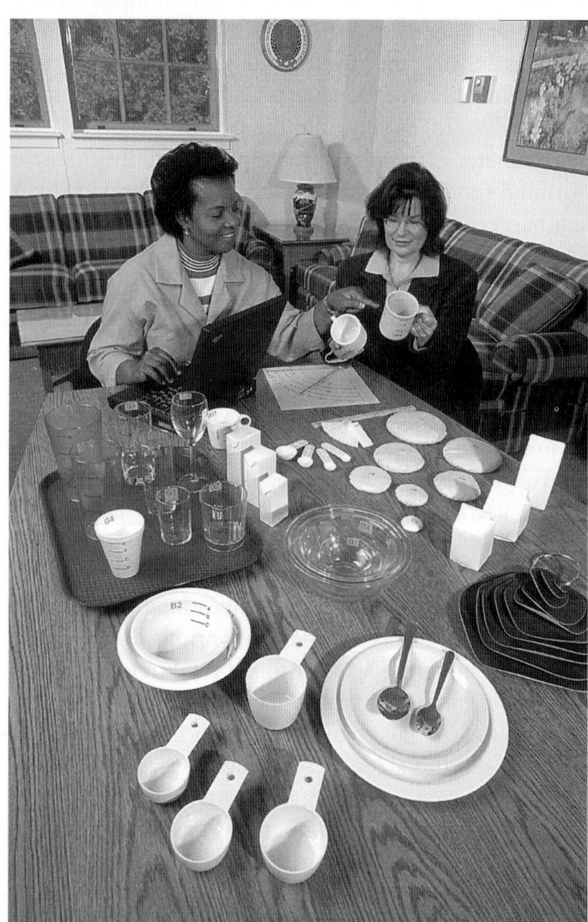

Figure 3.11
Using serving size aids during an in-home interview, USDA nutritionist Grace Omolewa-Tomobi, left, helps a study participant with her 24-hour recall of food portions.
Source: Photo by Stephen Ausmus, courtesy of USDA.

casseroles, mashed potatoes, or rice. The knife lying across the top of the plate provides a size reference. The grid superimposed on the dinner plate in Figure 3.9 can be used to estimate the length and width of square or rectangular foods, such as lasagna, meat loaf, or sheet cake. As in Figure 3.8, the knife lying across the top of the plate and the checkered tablecloth serve as size references to improve portion size estimates.[44,45] Two-dimensional food models and photographs or digital images have been shown to be as effective as three-dimensional models for estimating portion size in nutritional research.[6,7,81,82]

When, during an interview, identification of particular brand names of foods consumed is important, a notebook containing photographs of various foods, pictures cut from magazine advertisements, or actual food labels can be used. A photograph of a supermarket dairy case, for example, can help respondents identify the brand of margarine or similar spreads used at home. During the course of a 24-hour recall, for example, a child is likely to remember the brand of potato or corn chips he or she ate but perhaps not the particular bag size. Including in the notebook an assortment of snack food wrappers (for candy, chips, and chewing gum of various brands and sizes) can be helpful in collecting accurate intake data. Lifelike food models, such as those shown in Figure 3.10, also can be used to help respondents estimate food portion sizes. In addition, glasses, bowls, and cups of various sizes; household spoons; measuring spoons; and measuring cups can be used as aids in helping respondents estimate portion size, as shown in Figure 3.11.

The 24-hour recall is the principle dietary assessment method used in the National Health and Nutrition Examination Survey (discussed in Chapter 4) and most participants provide two 24-hour recalls, both using the Automated Multiple-Pass Method (AMPM). The first recall is administered in person and a variety of plates, bowls, cups, glasses, and three-dimensional forms are used to assist participants in estimating the portion sizes of foods, as shown in Figure 3.11. During this initial face-to-face interview the participant is given a copy of the *Food Model Booklet* and instructed in its use. The second 24-hour recall is administered over the telephone at a later, randomly selected time, also using the AMPM. During the second 24-hour recall, the participant can use the *Food Model Booklet* to help in accurately estimating the portion sizes of foods.

SUMMARY

1. The ultimate reason for measuring diet is to improve human health. Other reasons include assessing and monitoring food and nutrient intake, formulating and evaluating government health and agricultural policy, conducting epidemiologic research, and using the data for commercial purposes.
2. No single best method exists for measuring dietary intake. Each method possesses certain advantages and disadvantages. The method used depends on research design considerations, characteristics of the study participants, available resources, and whether the intent is to estimate average group intake, rank individuals within a group, or estimate an individual's usual intake.
3. In the 24-hour recall method, a trained interviewer may ask the respondent to remember all foods and beverages consumed during the past 24 hours. The Automated Multiple-Pass Method and the Internet-based automated self-administered 24-hour recall have simplified and improved the collecting of dietary data using the 24-hour recall. The 24-hour recall is quickly administered, has a low respondent burden, but does not give data representative of an individual's usual intake.
4. When keeping a food record, or diary, the respondent records, at the time of consumption, the identity and amounts of all foods and beverages consumed during a 1- to 7-day period. Foods can be either quantified using household measures or weighed, in which case the method is called weighed food recording. This method does not rely on memory, can provide detailed intake data, requires a high degree of respondent cooperation, and may result in alterations of diet.
5. A food frequency questionnaire assesses nutrient intake by determining the frequency of consumption of a limited number of foods known to be major sources of the dietary components of interest. Respondents indicate how many times a day, week, month, or year the foods usually are consumed. Relatively high-quality data can be gathered on large groups of respondents; data may be more representative of usual intake than a few days of diet records; respondents must be able to describe their diets; and foods and portion sizes included in questionnaires must be carefully chosen. An Internet-based food frequency questionnaire, the DHQ*Web, can be completed online, simplifying the collection and submission of questionnaire data.
6. Collection of duplicate food portions is a more direct method of assessing nutrient intake that avoids some of the problems associated with coding and entering data and the limitations of food composition tables, such as nutrient losses during food storage and preparation. Respondents collect identical portions of all foods and beverages consumed during a specified period, which are then analyzed for nutrient content. Respondent concern about the expense of duplicate portions can alter eating habits, resulting in underestimates of nutrient intake.
7. Food accounts estimate dietary intake within households and institutions where congregate feeding is practiced. The food inventory at the end of the survey period is subtracted from the sum of the beginning inventory and food obtained during the study period. Daily mean consumption per person is calculated by dividing total food consumed by number of meals served. This is a relatively economical method of assessing dietary intake of large groups. It does not account for food losses or meals eaten outside the group and cannot provide estimates of individual food intake.
8. The food balance sheet provides data on food disappearance (or availability) rather than actual food consumption. Mean per capita annual amounts are calculated by dividing total food disappearance

by the country's population. It detects trends in food availability within a country over time and generates data that are useful in epidemiologic research across countries. The data represent only food that disappeared from the food distribution system and may be of questionable accuracy.

9. The high cost of research has led to innovations in the collection of dietary intake data. Included among these are telephone interviewing, analyzing images of meals submitted by respondents, and Internet-based administration of 24-hour recalls and food frequency questionnaires. Some of these methods have the potential for reducing respondent burden and increasing the validity of dietary intake data and the cost-effectiveness of collecting such data.

10. Surrogate sources are necessary when intake data are needed from persons unwilling or unable to provide them. Potential surrogate respondents include the spouse, partner, children, other close relatives, and friends of the respondent.

11. Validity is the ability of an instrument to measure what it is intended to measure. Validating a method involves comparing measurements of intake obtained by that method with estimates obtained using another method that is thought to have a greater degree of demonstrated, or face, validity. Some biological markers can provide a validity check of dietary intake independent of respondents' accuracy and truthfulness.

12. Reproducibility, or reliability, is the ability of a method to produce the same estimate on two or more occasions, assuming that nothing has changed in the interim. Reproducibility studies are important in partially answering the validity question; a method cannot give a correct answer every time unless it gives approximately the same answer each time.

13. Estimates of portion sizes can be sources of error in measuring dietary intake. A number of tools have been developed to assist respondents in accurately reporting amounts of foods consumed. These include photographs of food, geometric shapes of various sizes, measuring devices, and lifelike plastic food models.

References

1. Van Saveren WA, Ocké MC. 2006. Estimation of dietary intake. In Bowman BA, Russell RM (eds.), *Present knowledge in nutrition,* 9th ed. Washington, DC: ILSI Press, 795–806.
2. Stamler J. 1994. Assessing diets to improve world health: Nutritional research on disease causation in populations. *American Journal of Clinical Nutrition* 59(suppl):146S–156S.
3. Sabry JH. 1988. Purposes of food consumption surveys. In Cameron ME, Van Staveren WA (eds.), *Manual on methodology for food consumption studies.* New York: Oxford University Press.
4. Carroll RJ, Freedman LS, Hartman AM. 1996. Use of semiquantitative food frequency questionnaires to estimate the distribution of usual intake. *American Journal of Epidemiology* 143:392–404.
5. Carmichael SL, Yang W, Feldkamp ML, Munger RG, Siega-Riz AM, Botto LD, Shaw G. 2012. Reduced risks of neural tube defects and orofacial clefts with higher diet quality. *Archives of Pediatric and Adolescent Medicine* 166:121–126.
6. Thompson FE, Subar AF. 2008. Dietary assessment methodology. In Coulston AM, Boushey CJ (eds.), *Nutrition in the prevention and treatment of disease,* 2nd ed. San Diego: Academic Press, 3–39.
7. Subar AF, Crafts J, Zimmerman TP, Wilson M, Mittl B, Islam NG, McNutt S, Potischman N, Buday R, Hull SG, Baranowski T, Guenther PM, Willis G, Tapia R, Thompson FE. 2010. Assessment of the accuracy of portion size reports using computer-based food photographs aids in the development of an automated self-administered 24-hour recall. *Journal of the American Dietetic Association* 110:55–64.
8. Zimmerman TP, Hull SG, McNutt S, Mittl B, Islam N, Guenther PM, Thompson FE, Potischman NA, Subar AF. 2009. Challenges in converting an interviewer-administered food probe database to self-administration in the National Cancer Institute Automated Self-Administered 24-Hour Recall (ASA24). *Journal of Food Composition and Analysis* 22(Suppl. 1):S48–S51.
9. Ngo J, Engelen A, Molag M, Roesle J, Garcia-Segovia P. 2009. A review of the use of information and communication technologies for dietary assessment. *British Journal of Nutrition* 101:S102–S112.
10. Johnson RK, Driscoll P, Goran MI. 1996. Comparison of multiple-pass 24-hour recall estimates of energy intake with total energy expenditure determined by the doubly labeled water method in young children. *Journal of the American Dietetic Association* 96:1140–1144.
11. McNutt S, Hall J, Cranston B, Soto P, Hults S. 2000. The 24-hour

dietary recall data collection and coding methodology implemented for the 1999–2000 National Health and Nutrition Examination Survey. *FASEB Journal* 14:A759.

12. Yaroch AL, Resnicow K, Khan LK. 2000. Validity and reliability of qualitative dietary fat index questionnaires: A review. *Journal of the American Dietetic Association* 100:240–244.
13. Thompson FE, Subar AF, Smith AF, Midthune D, Radimer KL, Kahle LL, Kipnis V. 2002. Fruit and vegetable assessment: Performance of 2 new short instruments and a food frequency questionnaire. *Journal of the American Dietetic Association* 102:1764–1772.
14. National Institutes of Health. 2001. *Third report of the Expert Panel on Detection, Evaluation, and Treatment of High Blood Cholesterol in Adults.* Washington, DC: National Institutes of Health, National Heart, Lung, and Blood Institute.
15. Kris-Etherton P, Eissenstat B, Jaax S, Srinath U, Scott L, Rader J, Pearson T. 2001. Validation for MEDFICTS: A dietary assessment instrument for evaluating adherence to total and saturated fat recommendations of the National Cholesterol Education Program step 1 and step 2 diets. *Journal of the American Dietetic Association* 101:81–86.
16. Srinath U, Shacklock F, Scott LW, Jaax S, Kris-Etherton PM. 1993. Development of MEDFICTS: A dietary assessment instrument for evaluating fat, saturated fat, and cholesterol intake. *Journal of the American Dietetic Association* 93:A105.
17. Willett WC, Sampson L, Stampfer MJ, Rosner B, Bain C, Witschi J, Hennekens CH, Speizer FE. 1985. Reproducibility and validity of a semiquantitative food frequency questionnaire. *American Journal of Epidemiology* 122:51–65.
18. Feskanich D, Rimm EB, Giovannucci EL, Colditz GA, Stampfer MJ, Litin LB, Willett WC. 1993. Reproducibility and validity of food intake measurements from a semiquantitative food frequency questionnaire. *Journal of the American Dietetic Association* 93:790–796.
19. Willett WC. 1998. *Nutritional epidemiology*, 2nd ed. New York: Oxford University Press.
20. Rimm EB, Giovannucci EL, Stampfer MJ, Colditz GA, Litin LB, Willett WC. 1992. Reproducibility and validity of an expanded self-administered semiquantitative food frequency questionnaire among male health professionals. *American Journal of Epidemiology* 135:1114–1126.
21. Munger RG, Folsom AR, Kushi LH, Kaye SA, Sellers TA. 1992. Dietary assessment of older Iowa women with a food frequency questionnaire: Nutrient intake, reproducibility, and comparison with 24-hour dietary recall interviews. *American Journal of Epidemiology* 136:192–200.
22. Thompson FE, Subar AF, Brown CC, Smith AF, Sharbaugh CO, Jobe JB, Mittl B, Gibson JT, Ziegler RG. 2002. Cognitive research enhances accuracy of food frequency questionnaire reports: Results of an experimental validation study. *Journal of the American Dietetic Association* 102:212–218, 223–225.
23. Subar AF, Thompson FE, Kipnis V, Midthune D, Hurwitz P, McNutt S, McIntosh A, Rosenfeld S. 2001. Comparative validation of the Block, Willett, and National Cancer Institute food frequency questionnaires: The Eating at America's Table Study. *American Journal of Epidemiology* 154:1089–1099.
24. National Cancer Institute, Risk Factor Monitoring and Methods. http://riskfactor.cancer.gov/dhq2/.
25. Subar AF, Dodd KW, Guenther PM, Kipnis V, Midthune D, McDowell M, Tooze JA, Freedman LS, Krebs-Smith SM. 2006. The food propensity questionnaire: Concept, development, and validation for use as a covariate in a model to estimate usual food intake. *Journal of the American Dietetic Association* 106:1556–1563.
26. Tooze JA, Midthune D, Dodd KW, Freedman LS, Krebs-Smith SM, Subar AF, Guenther PM, Carroll RJ, Kipnis V. 2006. A new statistical method for estimating the usual intake of episodically consumed foods with application to their distribution. *Journal of the American Dietetic Association* 106:1575–1587.
27. Tooze JA, Kipnis V, Buckman DW, Carroll RJ, Freedman LS, Guenther PM, Krebs-Smith SM, Subar AF, Dodd KW. 2010. A mixed-effects model approach for estimating the distribution of usual intake of nutrients: The NCI method. *Statistics in Medicine* 29:2857–2868.
28. Byers T. 2001. Food frequency dietary assessment: How bad is good enough? *American Journal of Epidemiology* 154:1087–1088.
29. Willett W. 2001. Invited commentary: A further look at dietary questionnaire validation. *American Journal of Epidemiology* 154:1100–1102.
30. Briefel RR, Flegal KM, Winn DM, Loria CM, Johnson CL, Sempos CT. 1992. Assessing the nation's diet: Limitations of the food frequency questionnaire. *Journal of the American Dietetic Association* 92:959–962.
31. Schaefer EJ, Augustin JL, Schaefer MM, Rasmussen H, Ordovas JM, Dallal GE, Dwyer JT. 2000. Lack of efficacy of a food-frequency questionnaire in assessing dietary macronutrient intakes in subjects consuming diets of known composition. *American Journal of Clinical Nutrition* 71:746–751.
32. Subar AF, Kipnis V, Troiano RP, Midthune D, Schoeller DA, Bingham S, et al. 2003. Using intake biomarkers to evaluate the extent of dietary misreporting in a large sample of adults: The OPEN Study. *American Journal of Epidemiology* 158:1–13.
33. Smith AF. 1991. Cognitive processes in long-term dietary recall. *Vital and Health Statistics* 6(4). Hyattsville, MD: National Center for Health Statistics.
34. Willett WC. 1994. Future directions in the development of

food-frequency questionnaires. *American Journal of Clinical Nutrition* 59(suppl):171S–174S.

35. Burke BS. 1947. The dietary history as a tool in research. *Journal of the American Dietetic Association* 23:1041–1046.
36. Kim WW, Mertz W, Judd JT, Marshall MW, Kelsay JL, Prather ES. 1984. Effect of making duplicate food collections on nutrient intakes calculated from diet records. *American Journal of Clinical Nutrition* 40:1333–1337.
37. Mertz W. 1992. Food intake measurements: Is there a "gold standard"? *Journal of the American Dietetic Association* 82:1463–1465.
38. Pekkarinen M. 1970. Methodology in the collection of food consumption data. *World Review of Nutrition and Dietetics* 12:145–171.
39. Casey PH, Goolsby SLP, Lensig SY, Perloff BP, Bogle ML. 1999. The use of telephone interview methodology to obtain 24-hour dietary recalls. *Journal of the American Dietetic Association* 99:1406–1411.
40. Tran KM, Johnson RK, Soultanakis RP, Matthews DE. 2000. In-person vs. telephone administered multiple-pass 24-hour recalls in women: Validation with doubly labeled water. *Journal of the American Dietetic Association* 100:777–780, 783.
41. Van Horn LV, Gernhofer N, Moag-Stahlberg A, Ferris R, Hartmuller G, Lasser VI, Stumbo P, Craddick S, Ballew C. 1990. Dietary assessment in children using electronic methods: Telephones and tape recorders. *Journal of the American Dietetic Association* 90:412–416.
42. Dubois S, Boivin JF. 1990. Accuracy of telephone dietary recalls in elderly subjects. *Journal of the American Dietetic Association* 90:1680–1687.
43. Hu SS, Pierannunzi C, Balluz L. 2011. Integrating a multimode design into a national random-digit-dialed telephone survey. *Preventing Chronic Disease* 8(6):A145. http://www.cdc.gov/pcd/issues/2011/nov/10_0230.htm.
44. McBride J. 2001. Was it a slab, a slice, or a sliver? *Agricultural Research* 49(3):4–7.
45. Bliss RM. 2004. Researchers produce innovation in dietary recall. *Agricultural Research* 52(6):10–12.
46. Long JD, Littlefield LA, Estep G, Martin H, Rogers TJ, Boswell C, Shriver BJ, Roman-Shriver CR. 2010. Evidence review of technology and dietary assessment. *Worldviews on Evidence-Based Nursing* 7:191–204.
47. Thompson FE, Subar AF, Loria CM, Reedy JL, Baranowski T. 2010. Need for technological innovation in dietary assessment. *Journal of the American Dietetic Association* 110:48–51.
48. Fong AKH, Kretsch MJ. 1990. Nutrition evaluation scale system reduces time and labor in recording quantitative dietary intake. *Journal of the American Dietetic Association* 90:664–670.
49. Kretsch MJ, Fong AKH. 1990. Validation of a new computerized technique for quantitating individual dietary intake: The Nutrition Evaluation Scale System (NESSy) vs. the weighed food record. *American Journal of Clinical Nutrition* 51:477–484.
50. Weiss R, Fong AKH, Kretsch MJ. 2003. Adapting ProNutra to interactively track food weights from an electronic scale using ProNESSy. *Journal of Food Composition and Analysis* 16:305–311.
51. Weiss R, Stumbo PJ, Divakaran A. 2010. Automatic food documentation and volume computation using digital imaging and electronic transmission. *Journal of the American Dietetic Association* 101:42–44.
52. Boushey CJ, Kerr DA, Wright J, Lutes KD, Ebert DS, Delp EJ. 2009. Use of technology in children's dietary assessment. *European Journal of Clinical Nutrition* 63:S50–S57.
53. Six BL, Schap TE, Zhu FM, Mariappan A, Bosch M, Delp EJ, Ebert DS, Kerr DA, Boushey CJ. 2010. Evidence-based development of a mobile telephone food record. *Journal of the American Dietetic Association* 110:74–79.
54. Sun M, Fernstrom JD, Jia W, Hackworth SA, Yao N, Li Y, Li C, Fernstrom MH, Sclabassi RJ. 2010. A wearable electronic system for objective dietary assessment. *Journal of the American Dietetic Association* 110:45–47.
55. Wang D, Kogashiwa M, Kira S. 2007. Development of a new instrument for evaluating individual's dietary intakes. *Journal of the American Dietetic Association* 106:1588–1593.
56. Williamson DA, Allen HR, Martin PD, Alfonso AJ, Gerald B, Hunt A. 2003. Comparison of digital photography to weighed and visual estimation of portion sizes. *Journal of the American Dietetic Association* 103:1139–1145.
57. Wang DH, Kogashiwa M, Ohta S, Kira S. 2002. Validity and reliability of a dietary assessment method: The application of a digital camera with a mobile phone card attachment. *Journal of Nutritional Science and Vitaminology* 48:498–504.
58. Samet JM. 1989. Surrogate measures of dietary intake. *American Journal of Clinical Nutrition* 50:1139–1144.
59. Sudo N, Perry C, Reicks M. 2010. Adequacy of dietary intake information obtained from mailed food records differed by weight status and not education level of midlife women. *Journal of the American Dietetic Association* 101:95–100.
60. Scagliusi FB, Ferriolli E, Laureano C, Cunha CSF, Gualano B, Lourenco BH, Lancha AH. 2009. Characteristics of women who frequently under report their energy intake: A doubly labeled water study. *European Journal of Clinical Nutrition* 63:1192–1199.
61. Trabulsi J, Schoeller DA. 2001. Evaluation of dietary assessment instruments against doubly labeled water, a biomarker of habitual energy intake. *American Journal of Physiology—Endocrinology and Metabolism* 281:E891–E899.
62. Hodson L, Skeaff CM, Fielding BA. 2008. Fatty acid composition of adipose tissue and blood in humans and its use as a biomarker of dietary intake. *Progress in Lipid Research* 27:348–380.
63. Overby NC, Serra-Majem L, Andersen LF. 2009. Dietary assessment methods on n-3 fatty acid intakes: A systematic review. *British Journal of Nutrition* 102:S56–S63.
64. Satia-Abouta J, Patterson RE, King IB, Stratton KL, Shattuck AL, Kristal AR, Potter JD, Thornquist

MD, White E. 2003. Reliability and validity of self-report of vitamin and mineral supplement use in the Vitamins and Lifestyle Study. *American Journal of Epidemiology* 157:944–954.

65. Day NE, McKeown, Yong MY, Welch A, Bingham S. 2001. Epidemiological assessment of diet: A comparison of a 7-day diary with a food frequency questionnaire using urinary markers of nitrogen, potassium, and sodium. *International Journal of Epidemiology* 30:309–317.
66. Bingham SA. 1994. The use of 24-h urine samples and energy expenditure to validate dietary assessments. *American Journal of Clinical Nutrition* 59(suppl):227S–231S.
67. McNaughton SA, Marks GC, Gaffney P, Williams G, Green A. 2005. Validation of a foodfrequency questionnaire of carotenoid and vitamin E intake using weighed food records and plasma biomarkers: The method of triads model. *European Journal of Clinical Nutrition* 59:211–218.
68. Speakman JR. 1998. The history and theory of doubly labeled water technique. *American Journal of Clinical Nutrition* 68(suppl):932S–938S.
69. Burrows TL, Martin RJ, Collins CE. 2010. A systematic review of the validity of dietary assessment methods in children when compared with the method of doubly labeled water. *Journal of the American Dietetic Association* 101:1501–1510.
70. Jones PJH, Jacobs I, Morris A, Duchmarme MB. 1993. Adequacy of food rations in soldiers during an Arctic exercise measured by doubly labeled water. *Journal of Applied Physiology* 75:1790–1797.
71. Martin LJ, Su W, Jones PJ, Lockwood GA, Tritchler DL, Boyd NF. 1996. Comparison of energy intakes determined by food records and doubly labeled water in women participating in a dietary-intervention trial. *American Journal of Clinical Nutrition* 63:483–490.
72. Goris AHC, Westerterp-Plantenga MS, Westerterp KR. 2000. Undereating and underrecording of habitual food intake in obese men: Selective underreporting of fat intake. *American Journal of Clinical Nutrition* 71:130–134.
73. Johnson RK, Soultanakis RP, Matthews DE. 1998. Literacy and body fatness are associated with underreporting of energy intake in US low-income women using the multiple-pass 24-hour recall: A doubly labeled water study. *Journal of the American Dietetic Association* 98:1136–1140.
74. Champagne CM, Baker NB, DeLany JP, Harsha DW, Bray GA. 1998. Assessment of energy intake underreporting by doubly labeled water and observations on reported energy intake in children. *Journal of the American Dietetic Association* 98:426–430, 433.
75. Mertz W, Tsui JC, Judd JT, Reiser S, Hallfirsch J, Morris ER, Steele PD, Lashley E. 1991. What are people really eating? The relation between energy intake derived from estimated diet records and intake determined to maintain body weight. *American Journal of Clinical Nutrition* 54:291–295.
76. Goldberg GR, Black AE, Jebb SA, Cole TJ, Murgatroyd PR, Coward WA, Prentice AM. 1991. Critical evaluation of energy intake data using fundamental principles of energy physiology. I. Derivation of cut-off limits to identify underrecording. *European Journal of Clinical Nutrition* 45:569–581.
77. Briefel RR, Sempos CT, McDowell MA, Chien S, Alaimo K. 1997. Dietary methods research in the third National Health and Nutrition Examination Survey: Underreporting of energy intake. *American Journal of Clinical Nutrition* 65(suppl):1203S–1209S.
78. Kretsch MJ, Fong AKH, Green MW. 1999. Behavioral and body size correlates of energy intake underreporting by obese and normal-weight women. *Journal of the American Dietetic Association* 99:300–306.
79. Schoeller DA. 1999. Recent advances from application of doubly labeled water to measurement of human energy expenditure. *Journal of Nutrition* 129:1765–1768.
80. Kubena KS. 2000. Accuracy in dietary assessment: On the road to good science. *Journal of the American Dietetic Association* 100:775–776.
81. Posner BM, Smigelski C, Duggal A, Morgan JL, Cobb J, Cupples A. 1992. Validation of two dimensional models for estimating portion size in nutrition research. *Journal of the American Dietetic Association* 92:738–741.
82. Toobert DJ, Strycker LA, Hampson SE, Westling E, Christiansen SM, Hurley TG, Herbert JR. 2011. Computerized portion-size estimation compared to multiple 24-hour dietary recalls for measurement of fat, fruit, and vegetable intake in overweight adults. *Journal of the American Dietetic Association* 111:1578–1583.

ASSESSMENT ACTIVITY 3.1

Collecting a 24-Hour Recall

The 24-hour recall is probably the most commonly used technique for measuring diet. Consequently, it is important that health professionals involved in nutritional assessment understand, practice, and master this technique. In this assessment activity, you will collect a 24-hour recall from a classmate and calculate that person's intake of kilocalories, protein, carbohydrate, total fat, calcium, and iron from a food composition table. Be sure to have a classmate collect a 24-hour recall from you, too. This will provide you with additional experience with recalls. You also will need your own 24-hour recall for an assessment activity in Chapter 5.

24-Hour Recording Form for Assessment Activity 3.1

Name of person interviewed ______________________ **Date** ____________ **Day of week** ____________

Food/Drink	Type/How Prepared	Quantity	Kilocalories	Protein	Carbohydrate	Total Fat	Calcium	Iron
Total								

This assessment activity also will help you become more familiar with using food composition tables. Experience in using food composition tables is valuable. Sometimes it is faster and easier to refer to a food composition table for a nutrient value than to use a computer. Familiarity with food composition tables will also make that task easier.

1. For this assessment activity, we suggest you use a photocopy of the form provided on page 106. It not only provides space for recording the names and quantities of foods and beverages consumed, but it also allows you to easily record values for energy and nutrients for reported foods.
2. Familiarize yourself with the form *before* beginning your interview. Enter the name of the person being interviewed and the day and date.
3. After completing the recall form, manually calculate the intakes of kilocalories, protein, carbohydrate, total fat, calcium, and iron, using the food composition table in Appendix I. If you cannot find a particular food or beverage in the food composition table, use a similar food or beverage or refer to another food composition table.
4. As you do this assignment, think about the following questions:
   How representative of your respondent's usual dietary intake is this one day of intake data?
   Did you have any difficulty finding any foods in the food composition table?
   If you had to substitute one food for another, how do you think that substitution affected the total nutrient values?

ASSESSMENT ACTIVITY 3.2

Completing a 3-Day Food Record

Obtaining dietary intake data that are representative of the usual intake of *individuals* requires data from multiple days. According to research conducted by the USDA, estimating usual intake of energy (kilocalories) requires an average of approximately 30 days of intake data. Vitamin A requires approximately 400 days of data. Fewer days of data are required when characterizing the average intake of groups.

Although this assessment activity will not even come close to giving you the data necessary to estimate your usual nutrient intake, it will give you an idea of what is involved in collecting multiple-day intake data. In this assignment, you will complete a 3-day food record on yourself using the food diary recording form in Appendix C or one provided by your professor. You may want to analyze your food record using the diet analysis software available from the publisher or at your school's computer lab.

1. Familiarize yourself with the form in Appendix C and accompanying instructions *before* beginning your diary.
2. Record your food and beverage intake for two weekdays (Monday through Friday) and one weekend day (Saturday or Sunday). Because most people eat differently on weekend days than on weekdays, this will make your record more representative of your usual intake throughout the entire week.
3. Do not alter your normal diet during the recording period. Provide responses that are as accurate as possible. Record your food and beverage intake as soon after eating as possible.
4. You may save your completed food record for later analysis using diet analysis software.

ASSESSMENT ACTIVITY 3.3

Diet History Questionnaire

Compared with other techniques for measuring diet, food frequency questionnaires are a recent development. There is considerable interest in food frequency questionnaires as a relatively simple and inexpensive approach to characterizing the usual food and nutrient intake of individuals. A food frequency questionnaire developed by researchers at the U.S. National Cancer Institute (NCI) and used in several epidemiologic studies sponsored by the NCI is the Diet History Questionnaire (DHQ). The DHQ is explained in greater detail in this chapter. Several pages of the DHQ are shown in Appendix H, and the entire questionnaire can be downloaded from the website of the NCI. In addition, a Web-based version of the

DHQ named the DHQ*Web is available for use by the public at no cost and can be accessed through the website of the NCI. A link to this website is available at the *Nutritional Assessment* website at www.mhhe.com/hper/nutrition. The software for analyzing the DHQ, along with supporting documentation, are also available from the NCI's website, which can be accessed using a link available throught the *Nutritional Assessment* website.

Instructors may wish to administer the DHQ to students and use the software to process the questionnaires to develop nutrient intake data for discussion purposes. Instructors can also have their students complete the DHQ online using the DHQ*Web version of the questionnaire. Data from either the paper-and-pencil or Web-based versions can then be compared with national averages. Output from multiple groups of students from different disciplines could be compared to see if significant differences in food and nutrient intake exist along different groups of students.

Assessment Activity 3.4

The Automated Self-Administered 24-Hour Recall (ASA24)

The Automated Self-Administered 24-hour Recall (ASA24) is an Internet-based automated self-administered 24-hour dietary recall application developed by the National Cancer Institute. The ASA24 uses technology drawn from the USDA's Automated Multiple-Pass Method to provide a Web-based tool to researchers, educators, and the public for collecting multiple automated self-administered 24-hour recalls. Anyone interested in seeing how the ASA24 works can enter a 24-hour recall at a demonstration website for respondents. The demonstration version will not save any recall data or provide any dietary analyses. The full version of ASA24 is available only to registered users at a researcher website, which allows researchers, clinicians, and teachers to register a study and obtain dietary analyses. For example, a teacher could register students in a nutritional assessment course who would be given the assignment of entering two or more 24-hour recalls over a specified period of time. This activity would provide real-life experience in the administration of 24-hour recalls and an exposure to how technology is changing the collection of dietary intake data. The ASA24 website can be found at http://riskfactor.cancer.gov/tools/instruments/asa24/.

CHAPTER

4

NATIONAL DIETARY AND NUTRITION SURVEYS

OUTLINE

Introduction

Importance of National Dietary and Nutrition Surveys

Nutritional Monitoring in the United States

National Nutritional Monitoring and Related Research Program

Role of the U.S. Department of Agriculture

Role of the U.S. Department of Health and Human Services

Dietary Trends

Summary

References

Assessment Activity 4.1: Accessing Data from the Behavioral Risk Factor Surveillance System Website

Assessment Activity 4.2: What's in the Foods You Eat?

STUDENT LEARNING OUTCOMES

After studying this chapter, the student will be able to:

1. Discuss the goals and objectives of the National Nutrition Monitoring and Related Research Program.
2. Compare and contrast the roles of the two U.S. federal agencies primarily involved in nutritional monitoring activities in the United States.
3. Distinguish between nutritional monitoring activities conducted by the USDHHS and those conducted by the USDA, when presented with a list of surveys.
4. Discuss the USDA's role in collecting data on food availability, individual food and nutrient consumption, and attitudes and knowledge about diet and health.
5. Discuss the USDHHS's role in collecting data on individual food and nutrient consumption, health status, and exposure to pesticide residues, industrial chemicals, and radionuclides.
6. Describe the concept of the Mobile Examination Center and how it is used in conducting NHANES.
7. Name the methods used to collect dietary intake data in NHANES.
8. Compare and contrast estimates of food consumption based on annual per capita food availability data and data collected by direct survey methods.
9. Discuss the role and significance of the survey What We Eat in America, NHANES.
10. Demonstrate the ability to access online sources of diet and health survey data.

Introduction

Nutritional monitoring is an important activity for any government serious about promoting its citizens' health. The principle goal of nutritional monitoring is to accurately measure the dietary and nutritional status of a population and the quality, quantity, and safety of the food it consumes.[1] Data on the nutritional and health status of a population that are generated by nutritional monitoring are used for many purposes. They can identify nutritional problems of the country as a whole (e.g., excessive fat and cholesterol consumption) and groups at nutritional risk (e.g., low calcium intake by adolescent females). These data are used to justify changes in government policy and the spending of billions of dollars for planning and implementing programs related to food, nutrition, and health promotion, such as the Special Supplemental Nutrition Program for Women, Infants, and Children (WIC) and the National Cholesterol Education Program. They are important in evaluating the cost-effectiveness of such programs, particularly when voters and legislators express concern about escalating budget deficits, controlling the high cost of government, cutting taxes, or limiting government involvement in issues related to diet and health. These data are also critical to research into the relationships between nutrition and health. This chapter discusses nutritional monitoring in the United States and the most important surveys comprising the federal government's nutrition and health surveillance activities. It also discusses the major findings of these surveys.

Importance of National Dietary and Nutrition Surveys

National dietary and nutrition surveys have a number of important functions. They can show how food supplies are distributed according to such demographic factors as region, income, sex, race, and ethnicity. Survey data are important in monitoring nutritional status of a country's population. By observing trends in the health and dietary practices of a population, relationships between diet and health can be elucidated. They identify groups that are at nutritional risk and that may benefit from food assistance programs. They are important for developing the Thrifty Food Plan, which forms the basis for determining benefit levels for participants of the Food Stamp Program. They are also used for evaluating the effectiveness of various USDA food assistance programs. For example, a before-and-after comparison of food consumption practices by Food Stamp Program participants revealed that the program allowed families to purchase more nutritious foods and increased the market for surplus agricultural products. After analyzing nutritional and health survey data, the U.S. Government Accountability Office or GAO reported that women participating in the WIC program had a 25% reduction in low birth weight births (under 2500 g, or 5.5 lb) and a 44% reduction in very low birth weight births (under 1500 g, or 3.3 lb) compared with similar women not participating in the WIC program.[2] The Government Accountability Office estimated that, for each tax dollar spent on WIC benefits, nearly $3.00 were saved within the first year by federal, state, and local governments and private insurance companies in reduced health care costs and special education. These and other uses of data from nutrition and health surveys are summarized in Box 4.1.

Data from dietary surveys can be used to track food consumption trends over time, examine current dietary practices of specific groups of people, and monitor average intakes of pesticides, toxic substances, radioactive substances, and industrial chemicals. Studies of nutritional status allow monitoring of the general health of a population through health and medical histories, dietary interviews, physical examinations, and laboratory measurements.[3]

Dietary and nutrition surveys are important to government agencies that supervise their country's agriculture and food industries. Data from surveys provide a sound basis for developing policies and programs related to agricultural production, marketing agricultural products, projecting supply and demand, and determining the adequacy of the available food supply.[4] These data provide early warning of impending food shortages and can indicate how such crises may be prevented or alleviated.[5] They have been used to develop the *Dietary Guidelines for Americans* and the nutrition and related health objectives included in *Healthy People 2020.*

Using food balance sheets (see Chapter 3), a government can estimate the "disappearance" of food from its food distribution system and thus arrive at an indirect and rough estimate of food consumption by its citizens. Data on food disappearance or "availability" do not measure actual food consumption, only what enters and leaves the food distribution system. However, these data allow comparisons among different countries and the creation of a world food picture. These comparisons, in turn, can serve as the basis for the formulation of international policies designed to improve the world food and nutrition situation and prevent imbalances in dietary standards among countries.[6]

Nutritional Monitoring in the United States

Nutritional monitoring can be defined as "the assessment of dietary or nutritional status at intermittent times with the aim of detecting changes in the dietary or nutritional status of a population."[7] It involves data collection and data analysis in five general areas:

- Nutritional and health status measurements
- Food consumption measurements

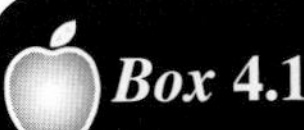

Box 4.1 Uses of Data from Nutrition and Health Surveys

PUBLIC POLICY

Monitoring Surveillance

- Identify high-risk groups and geographic areas with nutrition-related problems to facilitate implementation of public health intervention programs and food assistance programs
- Evaluate changes in agricultural policy that may affect the nutritional quality and healthfulness of the U.S. food supply
- Assess progress toward achieving the nutrition objectives in *Healthy People 2010*
- Evaluate the effectiveness of nutritional initiatives of military feeding systems
- Report health and nutrition data from state-based programs to comply with federal administrative program requirements
- Monitor food production and marketing

Nutrition-Related Programs

- Nutrition education and dietary guidance *(Dietary Guidelines for Americans)*
- Food assistance programs
- Nutrition intervention programs
- Public health programs

Regulatory

- Food labeling
- Food fortification
- Food safety

SCIENTIFIC RESEARCH

- Nutrient requirements (Dietary Reference Intakes)
- Diet-health relationships
- Knowledge and attitudes and their relationship to dietary and health behavior
- Nutritional monitoring research—national and international
- Food composition analysis
- Economic aspects of food consumption
- Nutrition education research

From various surveys conducted by the U.S. Department of Health and Human Services and the U.S. Department of Agriculture.

- Food composition measurement and nutrient data banks
- Dietary knowledge, behavior, and attitude assessments
- Food supply and demand determinations[1]

Since about the middle of the twentieth century, the U.S. government has sought to obtain objective data on which to base decisions regarding nutrition-related public policies. Initially, this was done by the U.S. Department of Agriculture (USDA), which collected food disappearance data and began conducting national household food consumption surveys. In the latter part of the twentieth century, the USDA abandoned household food consumption surveys and began conducting a cross-sectional survey of food intakes of individuals that eventually became known as the Continuing Survey of Food Intakes by Individuals. In the 1960s, the U.S. Department of Health and Human Services (DHHS) began conducting their own cross-sectional surveys of the health and nutritional status of the U.S. population, which evolved into the National Health and Nutrition Examination Surveys.[8] Some nutritional monitoring activities are conducted at the state level, providing state-specific data on nutritional and health status that may not be available from national surveys. Many of these state activities are supported and coordinated by federal agencies, such as the USDA and DHHS.

NATIONAL NUTRITIONAL MONITORING AND RELATED RESEARCH PROGRAM

As early as 1971, Congress, the nutrition community, various private groups, and expert panels expressed concern about problems with the federal government's nutritional monitoring program and the lack of coordination between the USDA and DHHS. Issues were raised about the frequency and costs of data collected by the two agencies, delays in reporting data, the low response rates seen in some surveys, and, in certain instances, the poor quality of data.[1,8–10] Problems in the two agencies' nutritional monitoring activities were addressed by a number of reports by the National Research Council, the Federation of American Societies for Experimental Biology, and the Government Accountability Office (a research arm of Congress that audits government programs and highlights areas of waste and fraud). These reports called for the agencies to develop better methods for collecting dietary intake data, to use standardized data collection techniques that allow data to be compared across the different surveys, and to improve coverage of groups at nutritional risk, such as pregnant and lactating women, infants, preschool children, adolescents, and older persons.[1]

Recognition of the need to improve nutrition monitoring led to passage of the National Nutrition Monitoring and Related Research Act of 1990 (PL 101–445). This legislation required the secretaries of the USDA and DHHS to prepare and implement a comprehensive 10-year plan for integrating the nutritional monitoring activities of the two agencies. This 10-year coordinated effort was called the National Nutrition Monitoring and Related Research Program (NNMRRP).[1,11] The legislation also calls for the creation of an Interagency Board for Nutrition Monitoring and Related Research and a National Nutrition Monitoring Advisory Council.

The NNMRRP coordinates the nutrition monitoring activities of numerous federal agencies under the joint direction of the USDA and DHHS. The program encompasses a group of more than 50 surveys and surveillance activities assessing the health and nutritional status of the U.S. population.[12] The program's goal is to "establish a comprehensive nutrition monitoring and related research program for the federal government by collecting quality data that are continuous, coordinated, timely, and reliable; using comparable methods for data collection and reporting of results; and efficiently and effectively disseminating and exchanging information with data users."[11] Critical to the success of reaching this goal are three overall national objectives and three objectives addressing state and local nutrition monitoring efforts. The three national objectives are (1) to achieve continuous and coordinated data collection, (2) to improve the comparability and quality of data collected by the USDA and DHHS, and (3) to improve the research base for nutrition monitoring. The three state and local objectives are (1) to develop and strengthen state and local capacities for continuous and coordinated data collection; (2) to improve methodologies to enhance comparability of NNMRRP data across federal, state, and local levels; and (3) to improve the quality of state and local nutrition monitoring data.[1,11] The NNMRRP also addresses the need for better nutrition monitoring information about selected population subgroups, more efficient and effective data dissemination to users, and better ways to meet the needs of data users.

To facilitate data dissemination, the National Nutrition Monitoring and Related Research Act of 1990 requires periodic publication of reports on the dietary, nutritional, and health-related status of the U.S. population. For example, every year the National Center for Health Statistics publishes *Health: United States*. This outstanding publication highlights and updates nutrition monitoring data, information, and research in a user-friendly format, using colorful graphics, extensive data tables, and brief narratives. To improve communication among data users, *The Directory of Federal and State Nutrition Monitoring and Related Research Activities* is periodically published by the Interagency Board for Nutrition Monitoring and Related Research. The directory contains information about federal and state nutrition monitoring activities, the sponsoring agency, contact persons, and the survey's purpose, date, target population, and design.[13] Both of these publications can be downloaded from the website of the National Center for Health Statistics (http://www.cdc.gov/nchs).

Data collected through surveys are made available in a variety of forms, such as journal articles, government publications, CD-ROMs, and electronic files available for download from various government websites, such as those of the USDA's Food Surveys Research Group and the DHHS's National Center for Health Statistics. Links to these and other websites related to nutrition monitoring can be found at the *Nutritional Assessment* website at www.mhhe.com/lee-nieman6.

Role of the U.S. Department of Agriculture

The earliest efforts at nutritional monitoring in the United States were carried out by the USDA.[1,4,14] In the late 1800s and early 1900s, USDA researchers used the food inventory method to collect data on the amounts and costs of food consumed by a relatively small, nonrepresentative group of households. Between 1935 and 1948, the USDA conducted three nationwide, nonrepresentative surveys of food consumption at the household level. Beginning in 1955, the USDA began a series of four nationally representative surveys of food consumption at the household level. The first of these was the 1955 Household Food Consumption Survey (HFCS). This was followed by the 1965–66 HFCS, the 1977–78 Nationwide Food Consumption Survey (NFCS), and the 1987–88 NFCS; these three surveys also measured food intake by individual household members. Following the 1987–88 NFCS, the USDA discontinued the NFCS and its efforts to measure household food consumption and focused entirely on assessing individual food intake through the Continuing Survey of Food Intakes by Individuals (CSFII) and evaluating the dietary knowledge and attitudes of CSFII respondents through the Diet and Health Knowledge Survey. In 1998, the USDA initiated the Supplemental Children's Survey to the CSFII to provide a sample of sufficient size in order to adequately estimate exposure to pesticide residues in the diets of children. The USDA also collects data on the amounts of food passing through the wholesale and retail food distribution system (called food availability data) and evaluates food security in America.

Food Availability

Since about the middle of the twentieth century, the USDA has been developing annual estimates of the amount of food that is *available for consumption* from the U.S. food distribution system. Known as food availability data or per capita food availability, these data are based on the measurement of the amount of food moving through the domestic food production and distribution system from farms to all outlets: supermarkets, restaurants, and fast-food outlets.[15,16] Per capita (per person) food availability is calculated by dividing the total amount of food available for consumption by the total number of people in the U.S. population.[16] These estimates have also been referred to as food disappearance data because they estimate the amount of food that disappears into the food marketing system.[15,16] It is important to note that food availability is not a direct measure of actual food consumption but, rather, an estimate of the amount of food that has left the wholesale and retail food distribution system, which includes foods eaten at home and away from home. Food availability data serve as a proxy or substitute for actual consumption and can only estimate the amount of food leaving the food distribution system. It is reasonable to assume that most, but not all, of the food leaving the food distribution system is consumed by people. Unless adjusted for losses due to food being discarded due to spoilage, or wasted or fed to animals, food availability data typically overstate the amount of foods and nutrients that people actually consume.[16,17]

Factors that led the USDA to begin compiling food availability data included a need to track food surpluses during World War I, legislation in the early 1930s to ensure an adequate food supply for domestic consumption during the Great Depression, and concerns about potential food shortages during the droughts of 1934 and 1936. Food availability data are valuable for monitoring the ability of the food supply to meet the nutritional needs of the U.S. population, for examining historical trends in food and nutrient consumption, and for evaluating changes in the American diet, especially in response to technological changes in agriculture and food processing. These data are helpful for determining whether federal enrichment and fortification standards are being met, monitoring how the food and agriculture industries are responding to the public's health concerns, and providing data for the development of dietary recommendations.[16] The USDA issued its first estimates of per capita food availability in 1941 to assess food requirements and supplies as America's entry into World War II was imminent. In 1949 the USDA was able to compile and publish data on per capita food availability for as far back as 1909, the first year for which reliable data were available.[4] Since then, estimates of per capita availability of major foods have been published annually with only a few exceptions. Historical series on per capita food availability were developed to analyze long-term trends, shifts in demand, and nutrients provided by foods.

Food availability data are derived using the **balance sheet approach** (discussed in Chapter 3) to track more than 250 agricultural commodities that are the major sources of food energy and nutrients for Americans. As shown in Figure 4.1, annual data on food exports, food not meant for human consumption (for example, livestock feed, seed, and food used for industrial purposes), military procurement, and year-end inventories are subtracted from data on beginning year inventories, total food production, and imports to arrive at an estimate of food available for domestic consumption.[3,4] This estimate then is divided by the U.S. population count to derive per capita availability of food. Per capita availability of energy and a number of nutrients is then calculated using food composition tables.[3,4] Food availability data reflect changes in overall patterns of food availability over time and have been the only source of information on food and nutrient trends since the beginning of the twentieth century.[3,7,14,15] When used in conjunction with similar data developed in other countries, epidemiologists have been able to study the relationships between diet and disease. For example, scientists have investigated how different levels of dietary fat and cholesterol intake across countries relate to coronary heart disease death rates in those countries.[3] Food availability data also serve as a rough check on the reasonableness of results from household food consumption surveys.[4] Because data on per capita food availability are obtained directly from food producers and distributors instead of from individual consumers, they are not subject to the error in reporting that often is seen in consumer survey data. There are drawbacks to this approach, and per capita food availability data must be interpreted with care.[4,15,16] The estimates are largely based on data collected for purposes other than estimating food and nutrient intake and can vary considerably in adequacy, accuracy, and accessibility. They do not provide information relating to food consumption on a regional, household, or individual basis. Additionally, unless adjusted for losses, the estimates fail to account

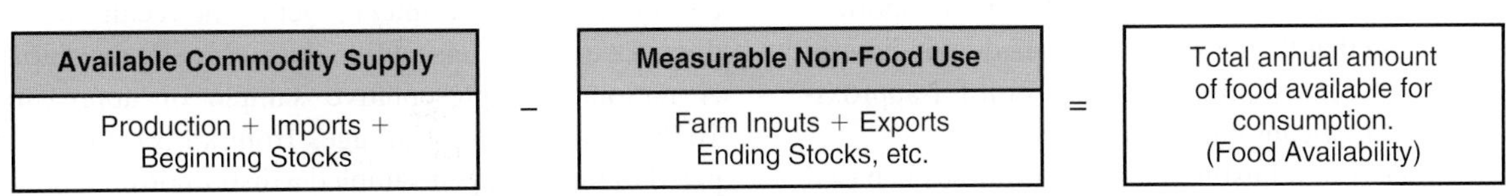

Figure 4.1 How the food balance sheet approach is used to arrive at data on unadjusted food availability.

Source: Gerrior S, Bente L, Hiza H. 2004. Nutrient content of the U.S. food supply, 1909–2000. *Home Economics Research Report No. 56.* Washington, DC: U.S. Department of Agriculture, Center for Nutrition Policy and Promotion.

for food losses at the primary level (from farm to retail), losses at the retail level (for example, food at the supermarket that spoils or reaches its expiration date and is discarded), or losses at the consumer level, including at restaurants, at fast-food outlets, and in households (for example, disposal of inedible parts, spoiled food, plate waste, and food fed to pets and other animals).[16,17]

ERS Food Availability (Per Capita) Data System

The USDA's Economic Research Service (ERS) (www.ers.usda.gov) collects food availability data and makes them available to users through the ERS Food Availability (Per Capita) Data System, which contains three related but separate series or sets of food availability data: Food Availability data, Loss-Adjusted Food Availability data, and Nutrient Availability data.[17] The Food Availability data series, which is the core set of data, is the only data set on the amount of food available for consumption in the United States, providing data extending as far back in time as 1909. In compiling these data, the ERS calculates the amounts of several hundred foods available for human consumption in the United States and provides estimates of per capita availability. For example, users can obtain data on pounds of red meat and poultry or gallons of fluid milk and cream available for domestic consumption per capita per year. Units of measurement depend on whether the commodity is a solid or a liquid. As shown in Figure 4.1, this series is compiled using data on production, imports, exports, beginning and ending stocks and nonfood uses. Per capita estimates are arrived at by dividing the total amount of food available by the U.S. population for that year.[17]

In the mid-1990s the ERS began an effort to make food availability data more useful by adjusting them for losses at the primary, retail, and consumer levels and converting the adjusted data into daily individual intake amounts and numbers of servings, which better represent what consumers actually eat.[17] Referred to as the Loss-Adjusted Food Availability data series, they are available in Excel spreadsheets from the ERS website beginning with data from 1970, the first year in the loss-adjusted data series. The spreadsheets provide estimated loss-adjusted data for per capita availability in pounds per year, calories available per day, and servings expressed as MyPyramid equivalents available per day. These estimates can then be compared with various dietary and nutrient intake standards to determine, for example, whether Americans are meeting the *Dietary Guidelines for Americans* for different food groups.[17] It is important to keep in mind that the loss-adjusted data do not directly measure actual consumption, but are useful for approximating what Americans eat on a daily basis.[17]

The process of adjusting the data for losses is based on several assumptions and limited research and documentation, which may result in the losses being understated or overstated. Food loss is difficult to measure, especially at the consumer level, given the fact that participants in household surveys on food waste often change their behavior during the survey period, failing to acknowledge or report the amount of food they typically discard or waste.[16,17]

The USDA Center for Nutrition Policy and Promotion (www.cnpp.usda.gov) is responsible for calculating nutrient availability data using the unadjusted food availability data from the ERS and data on the nutrient composition of foods from the USDA Nutrient Database for Standard Reference (discussed in Chapter 5). Nutrient availability data are provided in Excel spreadsheets from the ERS website for calories per capita per day of food energy and 27 nutrients and dietary components (for example, protein, carbohydrates, fats, vitamins, and minerals) in the U.S. food supply. Because these data are based on unadjusted food availability data, they likely overstate actual nutrient intake.[17] Per capita food and nutrient availability data are summarized in the "Dietary Trends" section of this chapter.

Continuing Survey of Food Intakes by Individuals

In 1985, the USDA began a national survey of individual dietary intake known as the *Continuing Survey of Food Intakes by Individuals (CSFII),* which was conducted during three time intervals, 1985–86, 1989–91, and 1994–96.[7,14] The CSFII replaced the NFCS as the USDA's primary survey for estimating individual food and nutrient intake.[1,14] The CSFII provided timely information on U.S. diets; allowed further study of the dietary habits of certain population groups thought to be at nutritional risk (e.g., low-income people); provided data on "usual" diets by measuring several days of data collected over the course of a year; and demonstrated how diets vary over time for individuals and groups of people.

In the 1985–86 CSFII, dietary intake data were collected using six 24-hour recalls that were obtained at approximately 2-month intervals. This not only provided data somewhat more representative of usual dietary intake but also diminished seasonal influence on dietary intake because data were collected throughout the year. In the 1989–91 CSFII, data were collected using one 24-hour recall and a 2-day food diary.

In the 1994–96 CSFII, popularly known as the "What We Eat in America" survey, data were collected using two multiple-pass 24-hour recalls administered in the home by trained interviewers. The recalls were conducted on 2 nonconsecutive days, 3 to 10 days apart.[7,14] A nationally representative sample of approximately 16,000 individuals of all ages from all 50 states participated in the survey. It sampled a disproportionately larger number of low-income people, young children, and older persons to better ascertain their dietary practices. This is known as "oversampling."

In 2002 the CSFII and the National Health and Nutrition Examination Survey (NHANES) were integrated, as discussed later in this chapter. Under the integrated framework, the USDA is responsible for the survey's dietary data collection methodology, maintenance of the database used to code and process the data, and data review and processing.[18]

Diet and Health Knowledge Survey

The Diet and Health Knowledge Survey (DHKS) measured the attitudes and knowledge of Americans about diet and health. It was initiated during the 1989–91 CSFII and conducted again during the 1994–96 CSFII, but has not been conducted since then. The DHKS provided information about Americans' perceptions about the adequacy of their own food and nutrient intakes, the personal importance they placed on dietary guidance messages, their self-appraised weight status, the importance they placed on factors related to buying food, and the beliefs they held that influenced dietary behavior.[14] For example, 56% of respondents in the 1994–96 CSFII/DHKS reported that they thought their diet was "about right" in calcium. However, nearly two-thirds of these persons had a mean calcium intake less than the 1989 RDA for calcium. Among those adults reporting that their weight was "about right," 45% of adult males and 17% of adult females had a body mass index that placed them in the "overweight" or "obese" category, based on self-reported height and weight.

The DHKS was conducted after the CSFII was completed. For example, approximately 2 weeks after the second 24-hour recall was collected in the 1994–96 CSFII, a group of nearly 6000 persons ages 20 years and older were randomly selected by a computerized process from among all adults who had provided 2 days of dietary intake data. These persons were then contacted by telephone and asked to answer a series of questions on knowledge and attitudes about dietary guidance and health. Administering the DHKS shortly after the completion of the CSFII allowed individuals' attitudes and knowledge about healthy eating to be linked with their food choices and nutrient intakes.

The future of the DHKS has been uncertain after the integration of the CSFII and NHANES in 2002. Although some questions about health and diet behavior are included in the integrated survey, the DHKS has not been totally included in the current survey.

Supplemental Children's Survey

The purpose of the Supplemental Children's Survey was to collect dietary intake data from a representative group of children of sufficient size in order to estimate exposure to pesticide residues in the diets of American children. Between December 1997 and November 1998, two 24-hour recalls were collected from roughly 5000 children up to age 9 years. The recalls were obtained through in-person interviews on 2 nonconsecutive days. For infants and children under 6 years of age, a parent or knowledgeable caregiver was asked to provide the data. For children 6 to 9 years of age, the child was interviewed with adult assistance. In addition to the in-home 24-hour recall, interviewers contacted schools, baby-sitters, and day care providers for information about food eaten away from home.

The Supplemental Children's Survey was a response to concerns about pesticide residues in the diets of infants and children and the lack of good data to accurately assess youngsters' exposure to pesticide residues in the foods they were eating. Concerns about children's exposure to pesticides were heightened by a 1993 report of the National Academy of Sciences entitled "Pesticides in the Diets of Infants and Children." This report was instrumental in passage of the Food Quality Protection Act of 1996, which required the USDA to provide the Environmental Protection Agency with statistically valid information on the food consumption patterns of American infants and children, so that children's exposure to pesticide residues could be estimated with reasonable accuracy.

Food Insecurity and Hunger

Although hunger in North America does not compare in severity to that experienced by many in developing countries, it is a problem nevertheless. Hunger in North America has been a long-term concern of public health nutritionists on the continent and among some of the more enlightened and compassionate legislators and policy makers. However, it was only in the 1990s that the U.S. government actually developed a comprehensive national measure of the severity of food insecurity and hunger in the United States.[17] One of the mandates of the National Nutrition Monitoring and Related Research Program (NNMRRP) was that the USDA's Food and Nutrition Service and the DHHS's National Center for Health Statistics jointly develop "a standardized mechanism and instrument(s) for defining and obtaining data on the prevalence of 'food insecurity' or 'food insufficiency' in the U.S. and methodologies that can be used across the NNMRRP and at state and local levels." In response to this mandate, the USDA led a several-year collaborative effort to draft, pilot-test, and refine an instrument to measure the prevalence and severity of food insecurity and hunger in America, building on the prior work of several nongovernmental organizations.[5]

The USDA determines food security or food insecurity using responses to 18 questions (shown in Box 4.2) about conditions and behaviors known to characterize households having difficulty meeting basic food needs. Each question asks whether the condition or behavior occurred during the previous 12 months and whether the

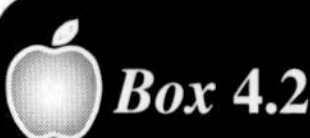

Box 4.2 Questions Used by U.S. Department of Agriculture to Assess the Food Security of U.S. Households

1. "We worried whether our food would run out before we got money to buy more." Was that often, sometimes, or never true for you in the last 12 months?
2. "The food that we bought just didn't last and we didn't have money to get more." Was that often, sometimes, or never true for you in the last 12 months?
3. "We couldn't afford to eat balanced meals." Was that often, sometimes, or never true for you in the last 12 months?
4. In the last 12 months, did you or other adults in the household ever cut the size of your meals or skip meals because there wasn't enough money for food? (Yes/No)
5. (If yes to Question 4) How often did this happen—almost every month, some months but not every month, or in only 1 or 2 months?
6. In the last 12 months, did you ever eat less than you felt you should because there wasn't enough money for food? (Yes/No)
7. In the last 12 months, were you ever hungry, but didn't eat, because there wasn't enough money for food? (Yes/No)
8. In the last 12 months, did you lose weight because there wasn't enough money for food? (Yes/No)
9. In the last 12 months did you or other adults in your household ever not eat for a whole day because there wasn't enough money for food? (Yes/No)
10. (If yes to Question 9) How often did this happen—almost every month, some months but not every month, or in only 1 or 2 months?

(Questions 11–18 were asked only if the household included children age 0–17)

11. "We relied on only a few kinds of low-cost food to feed our children because we were running out of money to buy food." Was that often, sometimes, or never true for you in the last 12 months?
12. "We couldn't feed our children a balanced meal, because we couldn't afford that." Was that often, sometimes, or never true for you in the last 12 months?
13. "The children were not eating enough because we just couldn't afford enough food." Was that often, sometimes, or never true for you in the last 12 months?
14. In the last 12 months, did you ever cut the size of any of the children's meals because there wasn't enough money for food? (Yes/No)
15. In the last 12 months, were the children ever hungry but you just couldn't afford more food? (Yes/No)
16. In the last 12 months, did any of the children ever skip a meal because there wasn't enough money for food? (Yes/No)
17. (If yes to Question 16) How often did this happen—almost every month, some months but not every month, or in only 1 or 2 months?
18. In the last 12 months, did any of the children ever not eat for a whole day because there wasn't enough money for food? (Yes/No)

Source: Coleman-Jensen A, Nord M, Andrews M, Carlson S. 2011. Household food security in the United States in 2010. *Economic Research Report No. 125.* Economic Research Service, U.S. Department of Agriculture.

reason for the condition or behavior was a lack of money or other resources to obtain food.[19] For example, an interviewer would read the following statement: "We worried whether our food would run out before we got money to buy more." The interviewer would then ask whether, in the last 12 months, this was often, sometimes, or never true in the household. Or the interviewer would ask the following question: "In the last 12 months were you ever hungry, but didn't eat, because there wasn't enough money for food?"

Since 1995, the U.S. Bureau of the Census has administered this instrument as part of its annual Current Population Survey (CPS), thus providing statistically valid, nationally representative data on the prevalence and severity of food insecurity in America.[5,19] In 2006, the USDA introduced new terms to categorize the ranges of severity of food security and insecurity to ensure that the terms were objective, measurable, and scientifically sound and that they conveyed useful and relevant information to policy officials and to the public.[19] The change in terminology (outlined in Table 4.1) was made upon the recommendation of an independent panel of experts convened by the National Academy of Sciences at the USDA's request.[19,20] It is important to note that while the terms were changed, there was no change in the methods used to assess household food security and insecurity. As shown in Table 4.1, two general categories have consistently been used to describe the food security condition of U.S. households: "food security," and "food insecurity," and these categories did not change in 2006. Prior to 2006, households reporting food insecurity were further categorized as having "food insecurity without hunger" or as having "food insecurity with hunger." Beginning in 2006, these two categories were changed to "low food security" and "very low food security," respectively. Box 4.3 defines these key terms.

While data on the prevalence of hunger is of considerable interest and value for policy and program design, the expert panel noted that the USDA's methodology did not measure "resource-constrained hunger" (i.e., physiological

TABLE 4.1 Terms to Categorize the Ranges of Food Security and Insecurity Used by the USDA before 2006 and since 2006

General Categories (these did not change in 2006)	Detailed Categories: Name of category before 2006	Detailed Categories: Name of category since 2006	Detailed Categories: Description of conditions in the household
Food security	Food security	**High food security**	No reported indications of food access problems or limitations.
		Marginal food security	One or two reported indications—typically of anxiety over food sufficiency or shortage of food in the house. Little or no indication of changes in diets or food intake.
Food insecurity	Food insecurity without hunger	**Low food security**	Reports of reduced quality, variety, or desirability of diet. Little or no indication of reduced food intake.
	Food insecurity with hunger	**Very low food security**	Reports of multiple indications of disrupted eating patterns and reduced food intake.

Source: Economic Research Service, U.S. Department of Agriculture.

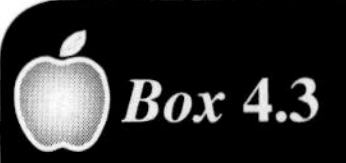

Box 4.3 Definitions of Food Security, Food Insecurity, Low Food Security, Very Low Food Security, and Hunger

FOOD SECURITY

Access by all people at all times to enough food for an active, healthy life. Food security includes at a minimum: (1) the ready availability of nutritionally adequate and safe foods, and (2) an assured ability to acquire acceptable foods in socially acceptable ways (e.g., without resorting to emergency food supplies, scavenging, stealing, or other coping strategies).

FOOD INSECURITY

Limited or uncertain availability of nutritionally adequate and safe food or limited or uncertain ability to acquire acceptable foods in socially acceptable ways.

LOW FOOD SECURITY

Households classified as having low food security report multiple indications of food access problems, but typically report few, if any, indications of reduced food intake. These households reduced the quality, variety, and desirability of their diets, but the quantity of food intake and normal eating patterns were not substantially disrupted.

VERY LOW FOOD SECURITY

Households classified as having very low food security report that the food intake of one or more members was reduced and eating patterns were disrupted because of insufficient money or other resources for food. In most but not all of these households, one or more household members were hungry at some time during the year and did not eat because there was not enough money for food.

HUNGER

A potential consequence of food insecurity that, because of prolonged, involuntary lack of food, results in discomfort, illness, weakness, or pain that goes beyond the usual uneasy sensation.

Sources: Nord M, Andrews M, Carlson S. 2008. Household food security in the United States, 2007. *Economic Research Report No. 66.* Economic Research Service, U.S. Department of Agriculture. http://www.ers.usda.gov/Publications/ERR66, and Wunderlich GS, Norwood JL (eds.). 2006. *Food insecurity and hunger in the United States: An assessment of the measure.* Committee on National Statistics, Division of Behavioral and Social Sciences and Education, National Research Council. Washington, DC: National Academies Press.

hunger resulting from food insecurity). The expert panel suggested that the term "hunger" should refer to a "potential consequence of food insecurity that, because of prolonged, involuntary lack of food, results in discomfort, illness, weakness, or pain that goes beyond the usual uneasy sensation."[19,20] To measure hunger in this sense would require collection of more detailed and extensive information on physiological experiences of individual household members than could be accomplished effectively in the context of the CPS. The panel recommended, therefore, that new methods be developed to measure hunger and that a national assessment of hunger be conducted using an appropriate survey of individuals rather than a survey of households.[20]

The USDA estimates that in 2011, 85.5% of all American households were food-secure and that 14.5% of all American households were food-insecure, as shown in Figure 4.2 and Table 4.2. Of the food-insecure households, 9.1% reported low food security and 5.4% reported very low food security. Figure 4.3 shows the prevalence of food security and insecurity in U.S. households with children in 2010. Of these households, 79.8% were classified as food-secure in 2010 and 20.2% were classified as food-insecure. In 10.4% of these food-insecure households, only the adults reported having experienced food insecurity. In 8.8% of households with children, both adults and children reported having experienced food insecurity, and in 1.0% of those households both adults and children reported having experienced very low food security. As shown in Table 4.2, the prevalence of food insecurity in households with a female head and no spouse is nearly three times greater than in households headed by a married couple. Food insecurity among black non-Hispanic and Hispanic households is more than twice as great compared to white non-Hispanic households.[19]

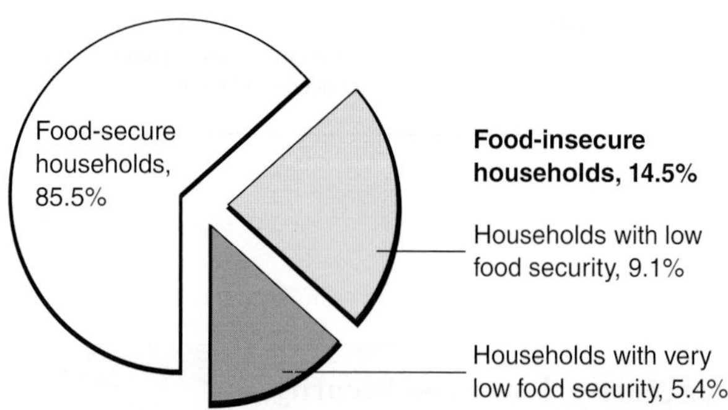

Figure 4.2 Food security of U.S. households in 2010. Nearly 86% of U.S. households were classified as food-secure in 2010. Of the 14.5% of households classified as food-insecure, 9.1% had low food security and 5.4% had very low food security.

Source: Data from the Economic Research Service, USDA.

Role of the U.S. Department of Health and Human Services

The U.S. Department of Health and Human Services (DHHS) has been involved in nutritional and health-related monitoring since the late 1950s, at which time it was known as the Department of Health, Education, and Welfare. Its current name was adopted in 1979. The DHHS's involvement in nutritional monitoring began in response to the National Health Survey Act of 1956, which mandated a continuing survey of the U.S. population for statistical data on amount, distribution, and effects of illness and disability in the United States. To comply with the 1956 act, DHHS conducted a series of three National Health Examination Surveys. These were followed by the landmark Ten-State Nutrition Survey and then the National Health and Nutrition Examination Surveys, including the Hispanic Health and Nutrition

Table 4.2 Prevalence of Food Security, Food Insecurity, Low Food Security, and Very Low Food Security among U.S. Households by Selected Characteristics, by Percent, 2010

		Food Insecure		
Category	**Food Secure**	**All**	**Low Food Security**	**Very Low Food Security**
All households	85.5	14.5	9.1	5.4
Households with children < 18 years old	79.8	20.2	14.5	5.7
Households, married-couple families	86.2	13.8	10.2	3.6
Households, female head, no spouse	64.9	35.1	24.3	10.8
Households, male head, no spouse	74.6	25.4	18.7	6.7
Households, white non-Hispanic	89.2	10.8	6.6	4.2
Households, black non-Hispanic	74.9	25.1	16.0	9.1
Households, Hispanic	73.8	26.2	17.8	8.4

Source: Data from the USDA Economic Research Service.

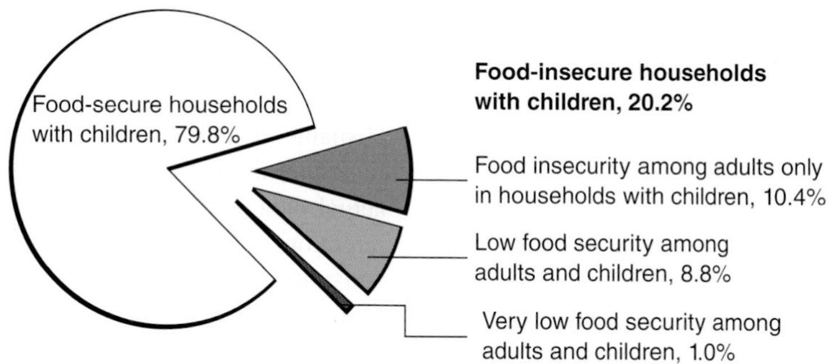

Figure 4.3 Food security of U.S. households with children in them in 2010.

Of U.S. households that had children in them, 79.8% were classified as food-secure in 2010 and 20.2% of U.S. households with children were classified as food-insecure. In 10.4% of these food-insecure households, only the adults reported having experienced food insecurity. In 8.8% of households with children in them, both adults and children reported having experienced food insecurity and in 1.0% both adults and children reported having experienced very low food security.

Source: Data from the Economic Research Service, USDA.

Examination Survey. In addition to these, the DHHS is responsible for a number of other surveys related to diet and nutrition, health, knowledge and attitudes, and food labeling. Included among these are the Adult Nutrition Surveillance System, the National Health Interview Survey, the Pediatric Nutrition Surveillance System, the Total Diet Study, the Health and Diet Study, the Behavioral Risk Factor Surveillance System, and the Food Label and Package Survey.

National Health Examination Surveys

The National Health Examination Surveys (NHES) were a series of three health surveys conducted by the National Center for Health Statistics of the DHHS. NHES I was conducted from 1960 to 1962 and examined the prevalence of selected chronic diseases and health conditions in nearly 7000 Americans 18 to 79 years of age.[21] Using a variety of physical and physiologic measurements, such as blood pressure, serum cholesterol, skinfold measurements, height and weight, and electrocardiography, NHES I was able to focus on such conditions as coronary heart disease, arthritis, rheumatism, and diabetes.[21]

NHES II was conducted from 1963 to 1965 and sampled more than 7000 children 6 to 11 years old. From 1966 to 1970, NHES III studied nearly 7000 persons 12 to 17 years old. A primary task of NHES II and NHES III was to measure growth and development in American children and adolescents. This provided much of the data used by the National Center for Health Statistics in formulating its original growth charts, which have been updated using data from NHANES III (described in Chapter 6 and shown in Appendix K).

Ten-State Nutrition Survey

The Ten-State Nutrition Survey was the nation's first comprehensive survey to assess the nutritional status of a large segment of the U.S. population.[8] During the 1960s, concerns about hunger and malnutrition in America escalated, leading legislators, health professionals, and private citizens to investigate the problem. Their reports revealed "chronic hunger and malnutrition in every part of the United States"[22] and described the situation as "shocking" and having reached "emergency proportions."[8] Congress responded by mandating the Department of Health, Education, and Welfare to conduct a "comprehensive survey of the incidence and location of serious hunger and malnutrition and health problems incident thereto in the United States."[8]

The Ten-State Nutrition Survey targeted geographic areas having high proportions of low-income persons, inner-city residents, and migrant workers. Between 1968 and 1970, data were collected in the following 10 states: California, Kentucky, Louisiana, Massachusetts, Michigan, New York (including New York City), South Carolina, Texas, Washington, and West Virginia.[8]

Although the survey helped reveal the extent and severity of hunger and malnutrition in America, groups surveyed were not representative of the general U.S. population, and consequently its findings could not be extrapolated to the overall population. The survey also demonstrated the difficulty and complexity of assessing nutritional status and recognized the need for additional data on the nutritional status of the U.S. population and the need for a continuing program of national nutritional surveillance. This led to the addition of a nutritional assessment component to the National Health

Examination Survey and the beginning of the National Health and Nutrition Examination Survey.[8]

National Health and Nutrition Examination Survey

The **National Health and Nutrition Examination Surveys (NHANES)** were originally conducted by the National Center for Health Statistics (NCHS), an agency of the DHHS. Since January 2002 the CSFII has been integrated into NHANES, and the operation of NHANES has been a joint effort of DHHS and USDA. Its purpose is to monitor the overall nutritional status of the U.S. population through detailed interviews and comprehensive examinations. Interviews include dietary, demographic, socioeconomic, and health-related questions. Examinations consist of a medical and dental examination, physiologic measurements, and laboratory tests.[12,23,24]

First National Health and Nutrition Examination Survey (NHANES I)

NHANES I, conducted from 1971 to 1975, was designed to assess general health status, with particular emphasis on nutritional status and health of the teeth, skin, and eyes. Its target population was a representative sample of approximately 29,000 noninstitutionalized civilian Americans ages 1 to 74 years. The nutrition component of NHANES I consisted of four major parts: dietary intake based on a 24-hour recall and food frequency questionnaire; biochemical levels of various nutrients based on assays of whole blood, serum, and urine samples; clinical signs of nutrient-deficiency disease; and anthropometric measurements. Although NHANES I originally was designed to provide data on the population's health and nutritional status at the time of the survey (in other words, a **cross-sectional survey**), the NHANES I Epidemiologic Follow-up Study, conducted in 1982–84, allowed subjects to be reexamined to assess the influence of nutritional status on development of disease and death.

Second National Health and Nutrition Examination Survey (NHANES II)

NHANES II was conducted from 1976 to 1980. It targeted nearly 28,000 noninstitutionalized civilian Americans 6 months to 74 years of age, of which more than 25,000 (91%) were interviewed and more than 20,000 (73%) were examined. Examination components included dietary interviews, anthropometric measurements, a variety of biochemical assays on whole blood, serum, and urine, glucose tolerance tests, blood pressure measurement, electrocardiography, and radiography of the chest and cervical and lumbar spine.[7]

Hispanic Health and Nutrition Examination Survey (HHANES)

HHANES was the largest and most comprehensive Hispanic health survey ever conducted in the United States. Planning for the survey began in 1979, and the actual data were collected from 1982 to 1984 under the direction of the NCHS.[25] The survey collected health and nutritional data on the three largest subgroups of Hispanics living in the 48 contiguous states: nearly 9500 Mexican Americans residing in five southwestern states (Arizona, California, Colorado, New Mexico, and Texas); more than 2000 Cuban Americans living in Dade County, Florida; and more than 3500 Puerto Ricans residing in the New York City metropolitan area (selected counties in New York, New Jersey, and Connecticut).[25,26] Response rates ranged from 79% to 89% for interviews and from 61% to 75% for physical examinations. Because HHANES was not designed as a national Hispanic survey, its results do not necessarily apply to all Hispanics living in the United States. However, the sampled population included about 76% of the Hispanic-origin population of the United States as of 1980.[25]

Rather than providing a comprehensive picture of the health status or total health care needs of Hispanics, HHANES was designed to obtain basic data on certain chronic conditions and baseline health and nutritional information. As in NHANES, HHANES used five data-collecting techniques: interviews, physical examinations, diagnostic testing, anthropometrics, and laboratory tests.[25,27,28] Interviews were conducted at the homes of survey participants, followed by examinations at a mobile examination center, which consisted of three connected semitrailers, which were specially designed and equipped for testing.[27] The nutritional component included an evaluation of iron status and anemia, serum vitamin A levels, and food consumption as related to diabetes, digestive diseases, overweight, dental health, and alcohol consumption.[25]

Third National Health and Nutrition Examination Survey (NHANES III)

Data collection for NHANES III began October 1988 and ended October 1994.[12,24,29] The survey was conducted in two phases of equal length and sample size. A total of approximately 40,000 noninstitutionalized Americans ages 2 months and older were asked to complete an extensive examination and interview. The response rates for the interview and examination were 86% and 78%, respectively.[12] Four population groups were specially targeted for examination: children ages 2 months to 5 years, persons 60 years of age and older, black Americans, and Mexican Americans.[24] A disproportionately large number of persons in these four groups were examined to appropriately assess their nutritional and health status.

In planning for the survey in 1985, the NCHS intended it to provide several types of data: prevalence estimates of compromised nutritional status and trends in nutrition-related risk factors; data on the relationships among diet, nutritional status, and health; prevalence estimates of overweight and obesity in the U.S. population; and anthropometric data on children and adolescents, allowing revision of the original NCHS growth charts (see Chapter 6 and Appendix K), which were based on data collected before 1976.[30] Four areas received special emphasis: child health, health of older Americans, occupational health, and environmental health.

NHANES: A Continuous and Integrated Survey

In response to the recommendations of the National Nutrition Monitoring and Related Research Act of 1990, major changes have taken place in the operation of NHANES. In 1999 NHANES became a continuous, annual survey rather than one conducted periodically. Each year about 6000 persons from 15 counties across the United States are interviewed, and of these, approximately 5000 are examined in the NHANES mobile examination centers, which are discussed later in this section. All NHANES data collection methods are automated, and interview and examination data are recorded online, which results in rapid entry and transmittal of data.[18] Automated edit checks, quality control measures, and questionnaire sequencing have reduced data entry errors and improved interviewer performance. Every year, data are collected from a representative sample of the U.S. population, from newborns to older persons, and released in 2-year cycles, whereas previously it took as long as 6 years before a representative population sample was assessed. Results are now reported in a more timely manner; before this change, researchers sometimes had to wait as long as 10 years before gaining access to data that were representative of the entire U.S. population.

Another major change was the integration of the USDA Continuing Survey of Food Intakes by Individuals (CSFII) and NHANES in January 2002. Under the integrated framework, USDA is responsible for establishing the dietary data collection methodology, maintaining the database on food composition, and coding and processing all dietary intake data, and DHHS is responsible for the sample design and collecting all data.[18] Data from the integrated survey, sometimes referred to as *What We Eat in America, NHANES,* are available from the website of the National Center for Health Statistics, www.cdc.gov/nchs. By working cooperatively and combining the expertise of their respective staff, the two agencies provide more comprehensive and more accurate information on the health and nutrition characteristics of the U.S. population in a cost-effective and timely manner.

The Food and Drug Administration (FDA) uses data from NHANES to evaluate the need to change fortification regulations for the nation's food supply and to develop and evaluate the effectiveness of new regulations to improve food safety.[31] NHANES data are used in developing and evaluating public education efforts, such as the National Cholesterol Education Program and the National High Blood Pressure Education Program. Many of the health objectives for the year 2010, including several in the nutrition priority area, rely on data from NHANES. The goals of NHANES are listed in Box 4.4.

Initial health interviews are conducted in the respondents' homes by specially trained staff members. Anthropometric measurements, physical examinations, testing, blood and urine collections, additional interviews, and the initial 24-hour recalls are performed in specially designed and equipped mobile examination centers (MECs), which travel to survey locations throughout the country. Each MEC consists of four trailers, each approximately 48 ft long by 8 ft wide, providing about 1570 sq ft of space. Several days before a survey is to begin at a particular location, the trailers are transported to the survey site, aligned, and leveled (as shown in Figure 4.4), and all connections of the passageways, electricity, water, and sewer are made. Each MEC contains a laboratory; examination rooms for physical, dental, vision, hearing, bone density, and X-ray examinations and anthropometric measurements; a computer room; and other rooms for conducting interviews and collecting specimens.[24]

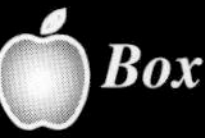

***Box* 4.4 Goals of NHANES**

1. To estimate the number and percent of persons in the U.S. population and designated subgroups with selected diseases and risk factors
2. To monitor trends in the prevalence, awareness, treatment, and control of selected diseases
3. To monitor trends in risk behaviors and environmental exposures
4. To analyze risk factors for selected diseases
5. To study the relationship among diet, nutrition, and health
6. To explore emerging public health issues and new technologies
7. To establish a national probability sample of genetic material for future genetic testing

Source: National Center for Health Statistics.

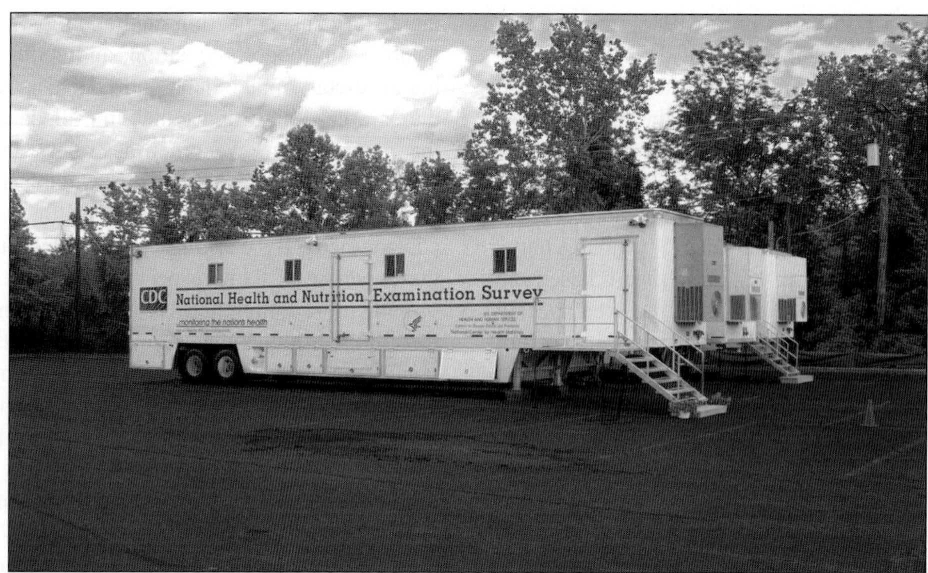

Figure 4.4 **One of the Mobile Examination Centers (MEC) used in the National Health and Nutrition Examination Survey (NHANES).**

Source: Photo courtesy of the National Center for Health Statistics, U.S. Centers for Disease Control and Prevention.

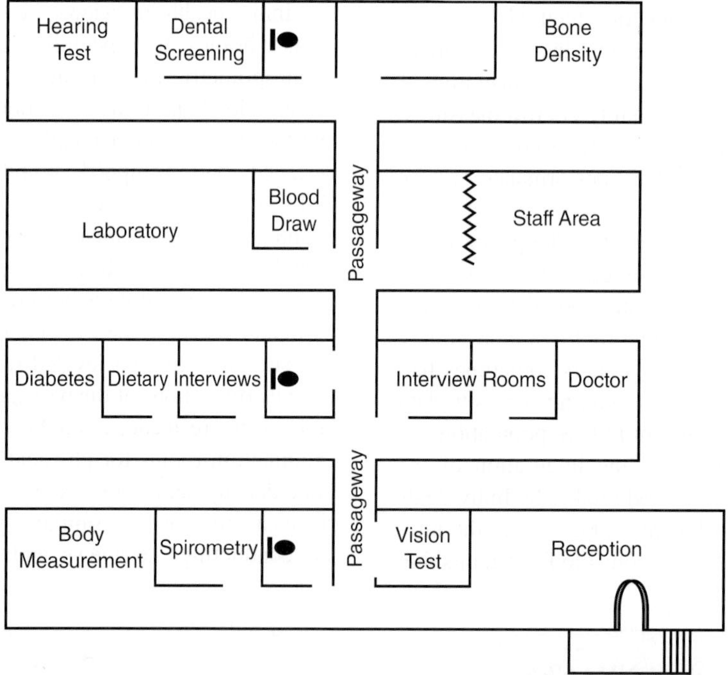

Figure 4.5 **Floor plan of the Mobile Examination Centers used in the National Health and Nutrition Examination Survey (NHANES).**

Source: National Center for Health Statistics.

The floor plan of the MEC is shown in Figure 4.5. There are three MECs and two separate examination teams. At any given time, two MECs are set up and fully operational, and one MEC is in the process of being moved from one survey site to another, parked, set up, and made ready by the time an examination team arrives. A link to the National Center for Health Statistics' narrated slide show tour of the MEC can be found at the Nutritional Assessment website at www.mhhe.com/lee-nieman6.

The primary dietary assessment methods for NHANES are the 24-hour recall and a self-administered food frequency questionnaire (both are discussed in

Chapter 3). Data from the 24-hour recalls are combined with data from the self-administered food frequency questionnaire to arrive at an estimate of usual nutrient intake. Two separate automated multiple-pass 24-hour recalls are obtained using the USDA's computer-assisted interview system. The automated system uses a standardized interview format and automated probes to obtain detailed information about foods, including brand names, food preparation methods, and ingredients used in food preparation, particularly ingredients that contribute fat and sodium.[23] Information recorded in the 24-hour recalls include the time foods are consumed, food names, type of meal or snack, and where the foods are consumed. The first recall is obtained by a trained staff member in a face-to-face interview in the MEC, as shown in Figure 4.6. The second recall is obtained 3 to 10 days later by telephone. After the health examination in the MEC, the self-administered food frequency questionnaire is mailed to the respondent, who completes it at home and sends it back to the NHANES staff by return mail.[23] In addition, during the home interview, some respondents are asked to complete a food frequency questionnaire that evaluates consumption of milk and dairy products, green leafy vegetables, dried beans, fish and shellfish, and alcoholic beverages.[23]

During the household interview, respondents are asked about their use of vitamin, mineral, and other nutritional supplements (both over-the-counter and prescription), botanicals, ergogenic aids, memory aids, and weight loss aids as well as analgesics, antacids, and prescribed medications. There are also questions about participation in food programs such as the food stamp program, the Special Supplemental Nutrition Program for Women, Infants, and Children (WIC program), and the school lunch and breakfast programs. Other diet-related questions address issues such as weight loss methods, use of special diets, infant feeding practices, use of salt at the table, consumption of water and alcoholic beverages, and habits regarding the trimming of skin and fat from poultry and other meats. Older respondents are asked whether, during the past 12 months, they received meals from a community program or center or had meals delivered to their homes by programs such as Meals on Wheels. NHANES also studies the impact of food insecurity on dietary intake, nutritional status, and health. At the household level, questions are asked about the number of days per month on which there is no food or no money to buy food and the reasons for the problem. Individuals are asked the frequency of and reasons for skipping meals and going without food and are asked whether any members receive emergency food aid from a food bank, soup kitchen, food pantry, or church. Table 4.3 summarizes the nutrition-related information collected in NHANES by respondent age and information type.

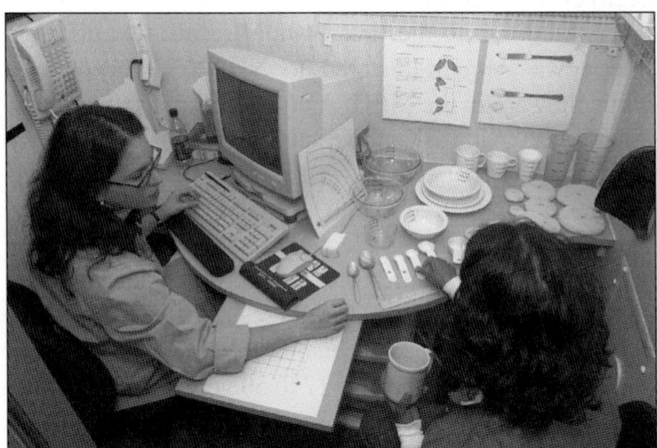

Figure 4.6
The first of the two automated multiple-pass 24-hour recalls collected from NHANES respondents is completed by a trained interviewer in the Mobile Examination Center (MEC). Two-dimensional and three-dimensional aids are used to help respondents more accurately estimate portion sizes. A variety of spoons, measuring spoons, bowls, plates, cups, and tumblers are used in the interview.

Source: Photo courtesy of the National Center for Health Statistics, U.S. Centers for Disease Control and Prevention.

TABLE 4.3 Nutrition-Related Information Collected in NHANES by Respondent Age and Information Type

Information	Age
24-hour dietary recall	All ages
Food security*	All ages
Food program participation*	All ages
Drinking water source* and quantity	All ages
Vitamin and mineral supplement usage	All ages
Salt use frequency and type	All ages
Breakfast practices	1 year and over
Dietary changes for health reasons	1 year and over
Infant feeding practices, including breast-feeding	Birth to 5 years
Food frequency	12 years and over
Alcohol use	12 years and over
Antacids use	17 years and over
Lifetime milk frequency	20 years and over
Self- (or proxy-) reported height and weight	All ages
Self- (or proxy-) assessed weight status	All ages
Birth weight	Birth to 11 years
Weight loss practices and reasons	1 year and over
Desired weight	12 years and over
Weight history	25 years and over

Source: National Center for Health Statistics.
*Also collected at the household (family) level.

Each of the two examination teams consists of a group of 16 persons who work and travel together: two dietary interviewers, a physician, a dentist, an ultrasonographer, four X-ray technicians, a phlebotomist, three medical technologists, a health interviewer, a home examiner, and a coordinator. Two locally hired staff supplement the team at each site. Most of the staff, especially the interviewers, are fluent in both Spanish and English. Although the interviewing staff are not required to have academic credentials, most are experienced interviewers who represent a cross section of society. A large staff of interviewers conduct the household interviews. In each location, local health and government officials are notified of the upcoming survey. Households in the survey receive an advance letter and booklet to introduce the survey.

Participants are provided with transportation to and from the MEC. Participants receive reimbursement for completing the 4-hour examination and an additional sum if they arrive at the MEC on time and, if requested, are fasting. Those unable to go to the MEC are given a less extensive examination in their homes. All participants receive a thorough physical examination, various anthropometric measurements, a dietary interview, and a private health interview and have their blood drawn for multiple analyses. Depending on the participant's age, additional examination components are performed. In general, the older the participant, the more extensive the examination. Table 4.4 shows the components of the NHANES examination by age range. A large number of analyses are performed on blood and urine samples obtained from respondents, as shown in Table 4.5. For example, Table 4.5 shows that blood lipid measurements are performed on the blood samples of all respondents 3 years of age and older and that various hematology and nutritional biochemistry assays are performed on samples drawn from respondents as young as 1 year of age. Data on blood glucose, insulin, C-peptide, and glycohemoglobin (hemoglobin A1c) from respondents 12 years of age and older are used to estimate the prevalence of diabetes and impaired glucose tolerance and to develop early intervention and prevention programs and to assess their effectiveness. The extensive environmental health profile includes numerous blood and urine assays for heavy metals, pesticides, industrial chemicals, pollutants, and phytoestrogens.

NHANES uses a variety of measures to assess health and nutritional status, as illustrated in Figure 4.7. In addition to the numerous assays performed on respondents' blood and urine samples, several anthropometric measures are performed on participants, as shown in Table 4.6. Anthropometric data are used to examine the relationships between body measures and body composition and activity, dietary patterns, and risk factors for cardiovascular disease, diabetes, and hypertension. They also allow growth and development in children to be monitored and provide nationally representative data on selected body measures and estimates of the prevalence of overweight and obesity. The recent increase in the prevalence of overweight and obesity among all sex, age, and racial and ethnic groups has been called an epidemic. NHANES is unique in collecting nationally representative measured data on body measures and composition. Body measures data from NHANES are used to provide representative reference data, set health objectives, and monitor trends. Anthropometry data have been collected with comparable methods since the first National Health Examination Survey, conducted between 1960 and 1962.

TABLE 4.4 Components of NHANES Examination by Age Range

Component	Age Range
Audiometry	20–69 years
Balance, vestibular testing	40–69 years
BIA	8–49 years
Blood pressure, pulse	8 years and older
CV fitness	12–49 years
Dermatology exam	12–59 years
DXA	8 years and older
LED	40 years and older
Muscular strength	50 years and older
Oral health	2 years and older
Physical exam	All ages
Physical functioning	50 years and older
Vision	12 years and older

Abbreviations: BIA, bioelectrical impedance analysis; CV, cardiovascular; DXA, dual-energy X-ray absorptiometry; LED, lower extremity disease.
Source: National Center for Health Statistics.

In addition to the first 24-hour recall, two different interviews are administered to NHANES respondents while they are in the MEC. A computer-assisted personal interview (CAPI) asks about current health status, physical activity, urinary incontinence (persons 20 to 59 years of age), reproductive health (females age 12 years and older), and tobacco and alcohol use (persons 20 years of age and older). A more private audio computer-assisted personal self-interview (ACASI) seeks information about alcohol and tobacco use (persons 12 to 19 years of age), use of illegal drugs (persons 12 to 59 years of age), sexual behavior (persons 14 to 59 years of age), and instances of misconduct such as shoplifting, vandalism, cruelty to animals, and lying (persons 12 to 19 years of age).

After the MEC examination, persons 6 years of age and older are asked to wear the physical activity monitor at home for one week. This small ($2.0 \times 1.6 \times 0.6$ in. in size), lightweight (1.5 oz) electronic instrument, technically referred to as a single-axis accelerometer, is worn around the waist 24 hours a day. Several times per second, it measures and records the amount and intensity of body motion. After one week of wearing the activity

TABLE 4.5 Components of NHANES Laboratory Tests by Age Range

Blood Lipids	
Total cholesterol	3 years and older
HDL-cholesterol	3 years and older
LDL-cholesterol	3 years and older
Triglycerides	3 years and older
Nutritional Biochemistry/Hematology	
Complete blood count	1 year and older
Erythrocyte protoporphyrin	1 year and older
Serum folate	3 years and older
Red blood cell folate	3 years and older
Serum iron	1 year and older
Total iron binding capacity	1 year and older
Serum ferritin	1 year and older
Transferrin saturation	1 year and older
Serum vitamin A	3 years and older
Serum vitamin E	3 years and older
Serum carotenoids	3 years and older
Retinyl esters	3 years and older
Plasma homocysteine	3 years and older
Selenium	3 years and older
Methyl malonic acid	3 years and older
Serum vitamin B_{12}	3 years and older
Diabetes Profile	
Glucose	12 years and older
Insulin	12 years and older
C-peptide	12 years and older
Glycohemoglobin	12 years and older
Infectious Disease Profile	
Cryptosporidium	6–49 years
Helicobacter pylori	3 years and older
Hepatitis viruses	2 years and older
Markers of Immunization Status	
Measles	6–49 years
Rubella	6–49 years
Varicella	6–49 years
Kidney Disease Profile	
Serum creatinine	12 years and older
Blood urea nitrogen	12 years and older
Albumin (urine)	6 years and older
Creatinine (urine)	6 years and older
Environmental Health Profile	
Lead	1 year and older
Cadmium	1 year and older
Mercury (blood and hair)	1–5 years
Mercury (blood and hair)	16–49 years, females
Persistent pesticides	12 years and older
Polychlorinated biphenyls (PCBs)	12 years and older
Dioxins	12 years and older
Furans	12 years and older
Phytoestrogens (blood)	12 years and older
Phytoestrogens (urine)	6 years and older
Persistent organochlorines	6 years and older
Nonpersistent pesticides (urine)	6 years and older
Heavy metals (urine)	6 years and older
Phthalates (urine)	6 years and older
Polyaromatic hydrocarbons (urine)	6 years and older
Sexually Transmitted Diseases Profile	
Chlamydia trachomatis	14–39 years
Neisseria gonorrhoeae	14–39 years
Herpes simplex 1 and 2	14–49 years
Human immunodeficiency virus	18–49 years
Human papillomavirus	14–59 years
Vaginal swab, self-administered	14–59 years (females)
Miscellaneous Laboratory Assays	
Cotinine	3 years and older
C-reactive protein	3 years and older
Fibrinogen	40 years and older
Latex allergy	12–59 years
Pregnancy test	12–59 years (females)
Prostate specific antigen (PSA)	40 years and older (males)
Standard biochemical profile	12 years and older

Note: Tests are on blood (whole, serum, or plasma) unless otherwise specified.
Abbreviations: HDL, high-density lipoprotein; LDL, low-density lipoprotein;
Source: National Center for Health Statistics.

monitor, subjects use a prepaid return envelope to mail it back to NHANES staff, who then download the data from the activity monitor into a computer to calculate physical activity and energy expenditure. Three to 10 days after the MEC examination, the second 24-hour recall is obtained by telephone. In addition, a self-administered food propensity questionnaire is mailed to respondents, who are asked to complete it and mail it back to NHANES staff.

Other DHHS Surveys

Other surveys that provide important data on health and on food and nutrient intake include the Total Diet Study, the Navajo Health and Nutrition Survey, the Pregnancy Nutrition Surveillance System, the Pediatric Nutrition Surveillance System, the Health and Diet Survey, the Behavioral Risk Factor Surveillance System, and the National Health Interview Survey.

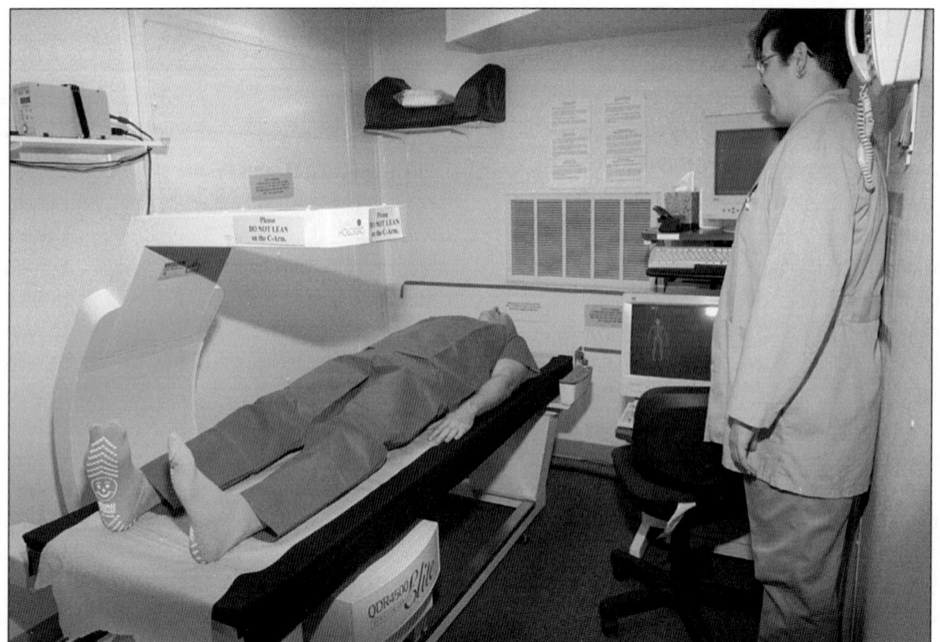

Figure 4.7
The use of dual-energy X-ray absorptiometry (DXA) for measuring bone mineral density to assess body composition is one example of the many different examination components used in the National Health and Nutrition Examination Survey (NHANES).
Source: Photo courtesy of the National Center for Health Statistics, U.S. Centers for Disease Control and Prevention.

TABLE 4.6 Anthropometric Measures Performed in NHANES by Age Group

	0–2 Months	2–24 Months	24–48 Months	4–8 Years	8 Years and Older
Head circumference	X	X*			
Weight	X	X	X	X	X
Upper leg length					X
Calf circumference					X
Recumbent length	X	X	X		
Standing height			X	X	X
Upper arm length		X	X	X	X
Arm circumference		X	X	X	X
Waist circumference			X	X	X
Thigh circumference					X
Triceps skinfold		X	X	X	X
Subscapular skinfold		X	X	X	X

*Through six months of age.
Source: National Center for Health Statistics.

Total Diet Study

The Total Diet Study (TDS) is an ongoing program conducted by the U.S. Food and Drug Administration that provides national estimates of average dietary intakes for pesticide residues, industrial chemicals, elements, radionuclides, and folate for the total U.S. population and 14 age/sex subgroups.[11,32] The analytes measured in the TDS are listed in Table 4.7. Sometimes referred to as the Market Basket Study, the TDS was originally established in 1961 as a program to monitor radioactive contaminants following atmospheric testing of thermonuclear weapons. Four times a year, the FDA purchases foods in grocery stores in selected cities in four geographic regions of the United States (West, North Central, South, and Northeast). These foods are among a group of approximately 280 core foods in the U.S. diet (i.e., foods that are among the most

TABLE 4.7	Analytes Measured in the Total Diet Study	
Pesticides	Pentachlorophenol	Substituted ureas
Organochlorine	Pyrethroids	Benomyl
Organophosphorus	Organosulfur	Carbendazim
N-methylcarbamates	Ethylenethiourea	Thiabendazole
Chlorophenoxy acids		
Industrial Chemicals	Polychlorinated biphenyls	Volatile organic compounds
Elements	Lead	Phosphorus
Arsenic	Magnesium	Potassium
Cadmium	Manganese	Selenium
Calcium	Mercury	Sodium
Copper	Nickel	Zinc
Iron		
Radionuclides	Cobalt-60	Ruthenium-103
Americium-241	Iodine-131	Ruthenium-106
Barium-140	Lanthanum-140	Strontium-90
Cesium-134	Potassium-60	Thorium-232
Cesiu-137	Radium-226	
Other	Folate	

Source: U.S. Food and Drug Administration, Center for Food Safety and Applied Nutrition.

commonly eaten by Americans). In each one of the four regions, foods are purchased in three different cities. The foods in these sample collections (also referred to as "market baskets") are then shipped to a central FDA laboratory, prepared as they would be if consumed as part of a meal, and then analyzed. Data from these analyses are then combined with food consumption data from NHANES to arrive at estimates of daily intakes of these substances. The Total Diet Study allows the FDA to monitor the exposure of Americans to these substances, some of which are harmful if consumed in excess. If necessary, the FDA can take action to limit the use of pesticides, additives, and industrial chemicals in agriculture and food processing to maintain the public's exposure to these substances within desirable ranges.[11,32]

The Canadian Total Diet Study, a similar program conducted by Health Canada, monitors the dietary intakes of contaminants such as lead, mercury, arsenic, cadmium, polychlorinated biphenyls (PCBs), dioxins, industrial chemicals, and pesticides in a sample of about 210 different foods commonly consumed by the people of Canada.[33] Since 1969, Health Canada has periodically conducted the Total Diet Study to estimate the levels of chemicals to which Canadians in 16 different age-sex groups are exposed through the food supply. Also referred to as the Market Basket Study, it is conducted in several major Canadian cities over a period of several years. In each city, the 210 individual foods are purchased from three or four different supermarkets and sent to Kemptville College, located outside Ottawa, Ontario. The foods are then prepared as they would be in the typical household kitchen, and analyzed. Data from these analyses are combined with food intake data to arrive at estimates of daily intakes of the contaminants.[33]

Navajo Health and Nutrition Survey

The Navajo Health and Nutrition Survey was a reservation-wide, population-based survey planned by the Indian Health Service to establish prevalence data on nutrition-related chronic diseases and to generate a valid description of the health and nutritional status and dietary behaviors of the Navajo people in general and for selected subgroups within that population.[11,34] A total of 985 people 12 years of age and older from 459 households participated in the survey. Data collection took place over a 5-month period during 1991 to 1992. Information was collected on dietary intake, food frequency, anthropometric measurements, lipid profiles, blood pressure, and full blood chemistries, including oral glucose tolerance tests.[11] The survey showed that obesity is a major problem among the Navajo, that 40% of Navajos age 45 years and older have diabetes (a third of these individuals are unaware of their condition), and that another 18% have impaired glucose tolerance and are, therefore, at risk of developing type 2 diabetes.[34] Among the Navajo, risk factors for cardiovascular disease are common, vegetable and fruit consumption is low, consumption of fats is high, and there is a lack of clinical services, particularly for managing diabetes and hypertension. Although reproductive health issues related to traditionally high parity (e.g., iron deficiency anemia) are problems among Navajo women, they do not appear to be as important as the high prevalence of obesity, diabetes, and coronary heart disease risk factors seen in Navajo women. The survey illustrates some of the critical health and nutrition concerns facing Native North American people and the need to better address those concerns.[34]

Pregnancy Nutrition Surveillance System

The Pregnancy Nutrition Surveillance System (PNSS), conducted by the U.S. Centers for Disease Control and Prevention (CDC), is designed to monitor the prevalence of nutrition-related problems and behavioral risk factors that are related to infant mortality and low birth weight among high-risk prenatal populations. These factors include overweight, underweight, smoking, alcohol consumption, anemia, lack of prenatal care, and adolescent pregnancy. The program was begun in 1979 when five states (Arizona, California, Kentucky, Louisiana, and Oregon) began working with the CDC in monitoring the prevalence of nutrition problems among infants born to high-risk pregnant women. In 2009, 31 states, the

District of Columbia, one U.S. territory, and five Native American Tribal Organizations contributed data representing approximately 1,300,000 women. The system also is studying the relationship of nutritional status to weight gain during pregnancy and birth outcome. Data are collected from the Special Supplemental Nutrition Program for Women, Infants, and Children (WIC) and the Title V Maternal and Child Health Program (MCH).[11,35]

Pediatric Nutrition Surveillance System

The Pediatric Nutrition Surveillance System (PedNSS), conducted by the CDC, is an ongoing child-based public health surveillance system whose goal is to collect, analyze, and disseminate data to guide public health policy and action.[11,36] Data from PedNSS are used for priority setting and for planning, implementing, monitoring, and evaluating specific public health programs to improve the health and nutritional status of U.S. children. Data from the Ten-State Nutrition Survey (1968–1970) showed that the nutritional status of children from low-income families was unsatisfactory. Of particular concern were findings from the survey showing inadequate intakes of calories, calcium, iron, and vitamins A and C by low-income black and Hispanic children. In response, the CDC began working with five states (Arizona, Kentucky, Louisiana, Tennessee, and Washington) in 1973 to develop a system to continuously monitor the nutritional status of selected high-risk population groups, which was the beginning of PedNSS. In 2009, 47 states, two U.S. territories, six Native American Tribal Organizations, and the District of Columbia contributed data representing approximately 8,940,000 children < 5 years of age.[36] The data are routinely collected by health, nutrition, and food assistance programs, such as Special Supplemental Nutrition Program for Women, Infants, and Children (WIC), the Early and Periodic Screening, Diagnosis, and Treatment (EPSDT) Program, the Title V Maternal and Child Health Program, and Head Start. Examples of data collected by the PedNSS are shown in Figure 4.8 and Figure 4.9. Figure 4.8 shows trends in the prevalence of low birth weight (LBW) (a birth weight < 2500 grams or < 5.5 pounds) by race and ethnicity from 2001–2010. American Indians, Alaska Natives, and Hispanics experience the lowest prevalence of LBW, whereas non-Hispanic blacks have the highest prevalence at approximately 13%. The average for all groups is approximately 9%, which is considerably higher than the year 2020 goal of reducing the prevalence of LBW to 7.8% or less.[36] Figure 4.9 shows the prevalence of obesity and overweight among children 2 to 5 years of age by race and ethnicity.

Non-Hispanic blacks and Asian/Pacific Islanders have the lowest prevalence of obesity and overweight, and American Indians/Alaska Natives and Hispanics experience the highest prevalence. In persons 2 to 20 years of age, obesity is defined as a BMI-for-age ≥ 95th percentile, and overweight is defined as a BMI-for-age ≥ 85th but to < 95th percentile using the 2000 CDC Growth Charts (as discussed in Chapter 6).[36]

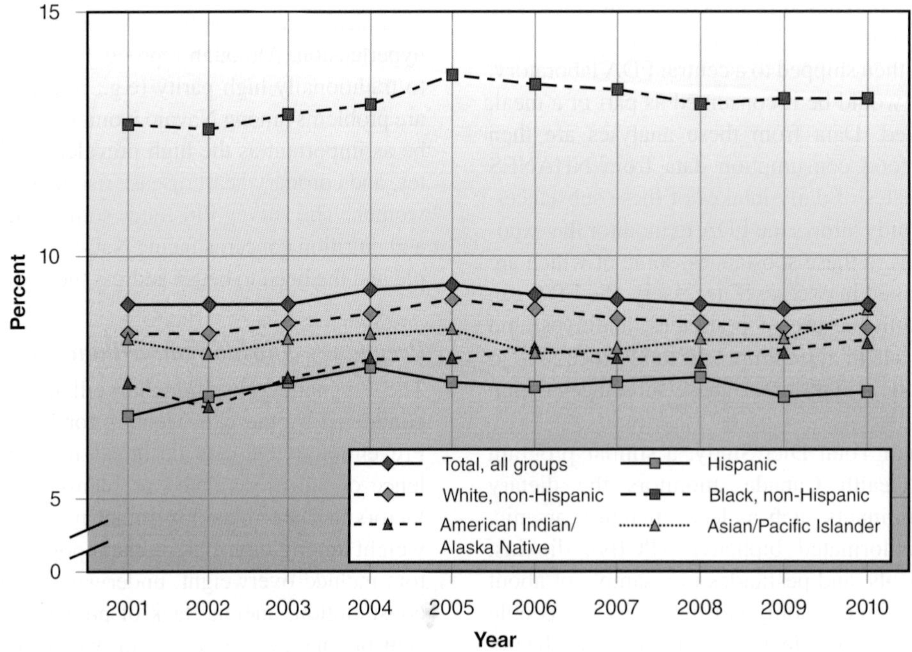

Figure 4.8 Trends in the prevalence of low birth weight, by race and ethnicity, 2001–2010.

Low birth weight is defined as a birth weight <2500 g or <5.5 lb.

Source: Pediatric Nutrition Surveillance System, U.S. Centers for Disease Control and Prevention.

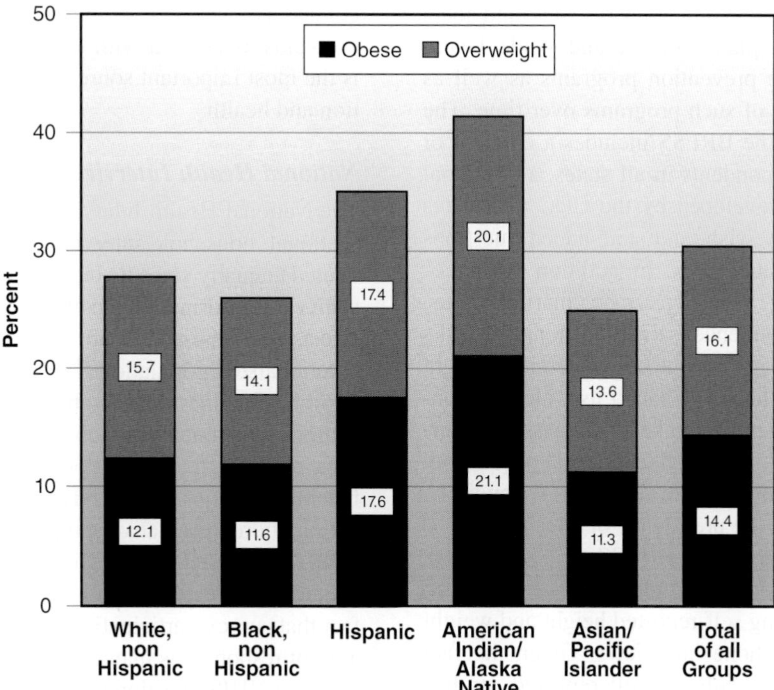

Figure 4.9 Prevalence of obesity and overweight among U.S. children age 2 to 5 years, by race and ethnicity, 2010.

Obesity is defined as a BMI-for-age ≥ 95th percentile and overweight is defined as a BMI-for-age ≥ 85th to < 95th percentile using the 2000 CDC Growth Charts, as discussed in Chapter 6.

Source: Pediatric Nutrition Surveillance System, U.S. Centers for Disease Control and Prevention.

Health and Diet Survey

The Health and Diet Survey is a random-digit dialed telephone survey of a nationally representative sample of American households conducted periodically by the U.S. Food and Drug Administration's Center for Food Safety and Applied Nutrition. Each survey contains a core set of questions relating to health and nutrition and additional questions that provide timely information on current health and diet issues or special topics. Participants are asked about topics that include knowledge and perceptions about sodium, cholesterol, fats, and food labels; self-reported health-related behaviors, such as dieting, sodium avoidance, and efforts to lower blood pressure and blood cholesterol levels; and beliefs about the relationships between diet and cancer, high blood pressure, and heart disease. Survey data are used to evaluate the effectiveness of public education initiatives of various federal agencies, such as the National Cholesterol Education Program. Between the 2004 survey and the 2008 survey, the percent of the U.S. population correctly identifying *trans* fat as a coronary heart disease risk factor almost doubled, going from 32% to 62%.[37]

Behavioral Risk Factor Surveillance System

The Behavioral Risk Factor Surveillance System (BRFSS) was established in 1984 by the Centers for Disease Control and Prevention and is the world's largest ongoing health surveillance system.[38] The BRFSS is a state-based telephone survey of the civilian, noninstitutionalized adult population intended to provide data on the prevalence of personal health practices identified as risk factors for one or more of the 10 leading causes of death. The BRFSS is administered by state health departments each month in all 50 states, the District of Columbia, Puerto Rico, the Virgin Islands, and Guam. Data can be analyzed by an individual state as well as by smaller geographic areas within states known as metropolitan and micropolitan statistical areas (MMSAs). A metropolitan statistical area is a group of counties that contains at least one urbanized area of 50,000 or more inhabitants, and a micropolitan statistical area is a group of counties that contains at least one urban cluster of at least 10,000 but less than 50,000 inhabitants.[38] In contrast, NHANES and other national surveys do not provide data that are specific to a particular state or region within a state.

Data from the BRFSS are used by state and local health departments to plan, initiate, and guide health promotion and disease prevention programs as well as to monitor the success of such programs over time. The questionnaire used in the BRFSS includes a core set of questions asked of respondents in all states, an optional module of questions developed by the CDC that states can elect to use if they wish, and state-added questions developed by individual states. In addition to demographic questions (e.g., sex, age, race, marital status, income, county of residence), the questionnaire asks about health status, health care access, exercise, weight control, diabetes, oral health, tobacco use, alcohol consumption, fruit and vegetable intake, awareness of hypertension and cholesterol, and the like. Several pages from a recent BRFSS questionnaire are shown in Appendix I.

Figure 4.10 shows the prevalence of obesity in 2010 based on data collected by the BRFSS. In Figure 4.10, obesity is defined as a body mass index (BMI) ≥ 30 kg/m^2, which is calculated using self-reported height and weight data collected by telephone interviews. Given the fact that overweight participants in self-reported studies tend to underestimate their weight and that all participants tend to overestimate their height, it is reasonable to assume that the data illustrated in Figure 4.10 underestimate the true prevalence of obesity. Figure 4.11 shows the percentage of U.S. adults who, during a telephone interview, reported that they had been told by a physician that they had diabetes. These data in the figure were also collected by the BRFSS and are self-reported. Despite the problems associated with self-reported data, the BRFSS is the most important source of state-based data on nutrition and health.

National Health Interview Survey

The National Health Interview Survey (NHIS) is a cross-sectional, household interview survey that has been conducted annually since its inception in 1957. It is the major source of information on the amount, distribution, and effects of illness and disability in the U.S. civilian noninstitutionalized population.[39] NHIS data are used to monitor trends in illness and disability, to track progress toward achieving national health objectives, to conduct epidemiologic research, to establish policy analysis, and to evaluate federal health programs. NHIS data are collected from a nationally representative sample of approximately 35,000 to 40,000 households containing about 75,000 to 100,000 persons. The response rate is greater than 90% despite the fact that survey participation is voluntary. The confidentiality of responses is mandated by federal law.

The NHIS questionnaire has two components: a core set of questions and a set of supplemental questions. The core set of questions remains essentially unchanged from year to year and contains questions that are directed to the family unit, to one adult randomly selected from the household, and to one child, if any, randomly selected from the household. The supplemental set of questions collects data on emerging public health concerns as they arise. Data are collected through a personal household interview conducted by interviewers employed and trained

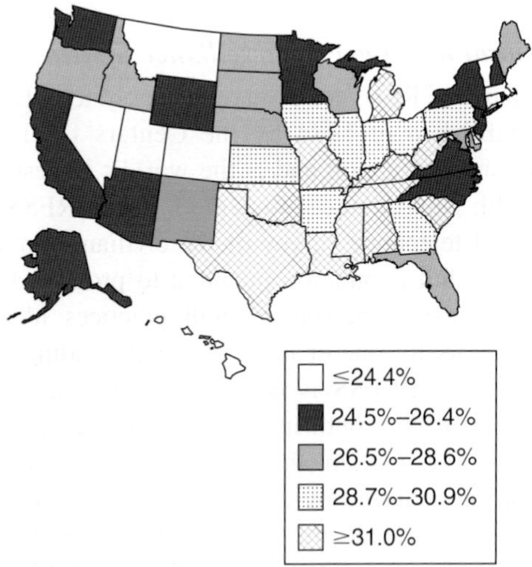

Figure 4.10 Prevalence of self-reported obesity among U.S. adults in 2010, by state.
In this figure, obesity is defined as a body mass index (BMI) ≥ 30 kg/m^2, and the prevalence estimates were calculated using self-reported weights and heights as collected by telephone interview by the Behavioral Risk Factor Surveillance System.

Source: Behavioral Risk Factor Surveillance System, Centers for Disease Control and Prevention.

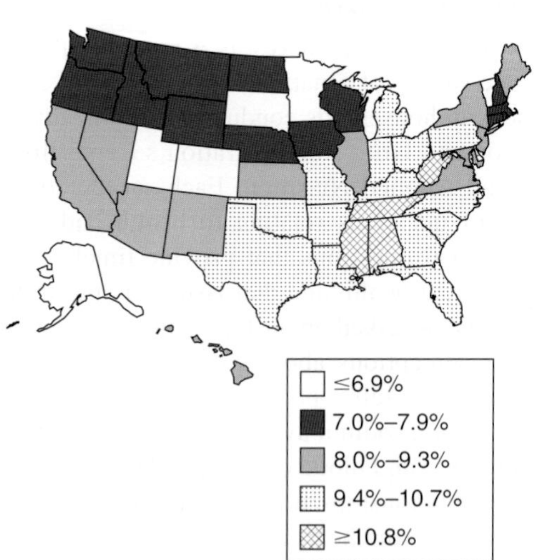

Figure 4.11 Prevalence of self-reported diabetes among U.S. adults in 2010, by state.
This figure shows the percentage of U.S. adults who, during a telephone interview in 2010, reported that they had been told by a physician that they had diabetes.

Source: Behavioral Risk Factor Surveillance System, Centers for Disease Control and Prevention.

by the U.S. Bureau of the Census according to procedures specified by NCHS. The interviewers are employees who are selected through an examination and testing process and who are thoroughly trained in basic interviewing procedures. The current NHIS interview employs computer-assisted personal interviewer (CAPI) technology using a laptop computer, with interviewers entering responses directly into the computer during the interview. This procedure makes data collection faster, easier, more accurate, and more cost-effective; speeds the analysis of the data by NCHS statisticians; and makes survey results more readily available to policy analysts and epidemiologists.[39]

DIETARY TRENDS

Data on per-capita food availability (also referred to as food disappearance) and consumption at the individual level have revealed a number of significant changes in the American diet.[15–17,40,41] These include changes in the sources of food energy; average amounts of energy consumed by Americans; use of specific food groups, including alcoholic and nonalcoholic beverages, and changes in eating patterns; such as snacking and eating away from home. In the following sections, some of the data presented are based on food availability, whereas other data are derived from surveys that measured actual food consumption (or at least attempted to). Food availability data are useful to nutrition policy makers, educators, researchers, and health-conscious consumers because they measure the capacity of the food supply to satisfy the nutritional needs of the population and they identify sources of nutrients and food components in the food supply. Food availability attempts to measure the flow of raw and semiprocessed commodities through the U.S. food marketing system. These data represent the amount of food that is available for consumption and, consequently, are not a direct measure of food and nutrient consumption and are not based on the quantity of food ingested, as are data from surveys such as What We Eat in America, NHANES. For this reason, food availability is a supply measure, not an intake measure.[40] As mentioned earlier in this chapter, the USDA's Economic Research Service (ERS) maintains the Food Availability (Per Capita) Data System, which contains three related but separate series or sets of food availability data: Food Availability data, Loss-Adjusted Food Availability data, and Nutrient Availability data.[17] Data from the Food Availability data series, the core set of food availability data that provides estimates beginning as early as the year 1909, are not adjusted to account for food lost from spoilage, trimming, cooking, or plate waste or food fed to animals and, consequently, overstate actual food and nutrient consumption. The Loss-Adjusted Food Availability data, which provide estimates beginning from 1970 to the present, are adjusted for food losses at the primary, retail, and consumer levels and, consequently, better represent what consumers actually eat. Despite the limitations of food availability data, they are useful indicators of trends in U.S. food and nutrient availability that now span more than 100 years.[40]

Sources of Food Energy

The distribution of food energy from carbohydrate, fat, and protein has changed since the USDA's Economic Research Service first began compiling food availability data. This is shown in Figure 4.12. From 1909

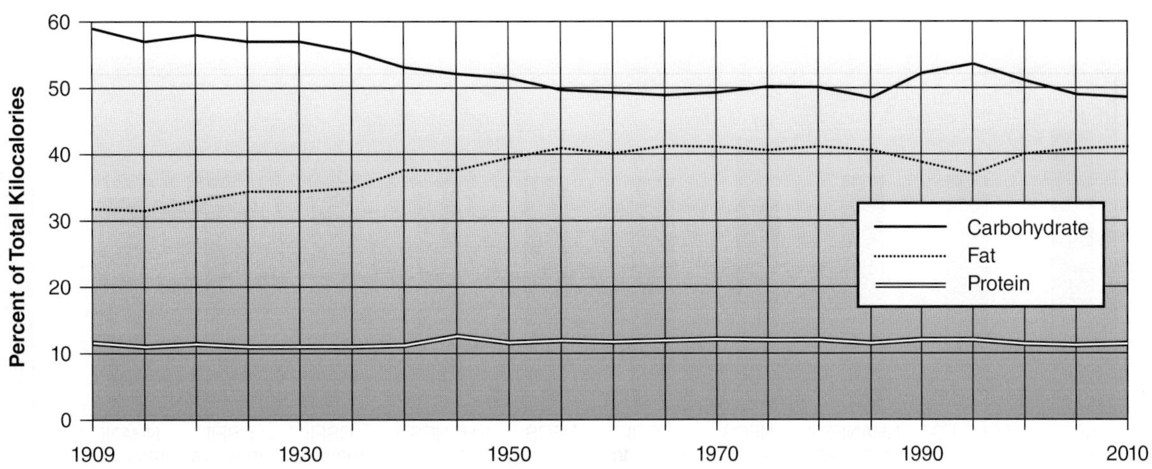

Figure 4.12 Percent of food energy (percent of total kilocalories) contributed by carbohydrate, fat, and protein from 1909 to 2010, based on food availability data from the U.S. Department of Agriculture.

The data used to develop this chart have not been adjusted for losses due to spoilage, trimming, waste, etc., and overstate actual food consumption.

Source: Data from the Economic Research Service, U.S. Department of Agriculture.

to 2010, energy available from protein remained essentially unchanged at 11% to 12% of total kilocalories. Percentage of kilocalories available from carbohydrate declined from 59% in 1909 to 49% in 2010. Fat availability ranged from approximately 32% in 1909 to about 41% in 2010.

Data from NHANES 2007–2008 for percent of energy from protein, carbohydrate, total fat, saturated fat, and alcohol are shown in Figure 4.13. According to surveys conducted between 1965 and 2008 that measured actual food of individuals, the percentage of kilocalories from fat has ranged from a high of 42.1% to a low of 32.7%, as shown in Figure 4.14. Although the percentages in Figure 4.14 seem somewhat inconsistent from one survey to the next, the figure does suggest that the mean percent of kilocalories from fat in the diets of American adults has gradually declined in recent years.

It is important to note that factors other than changes in food consumption practices over time influence the reported percentages of kilocalories from fat in the

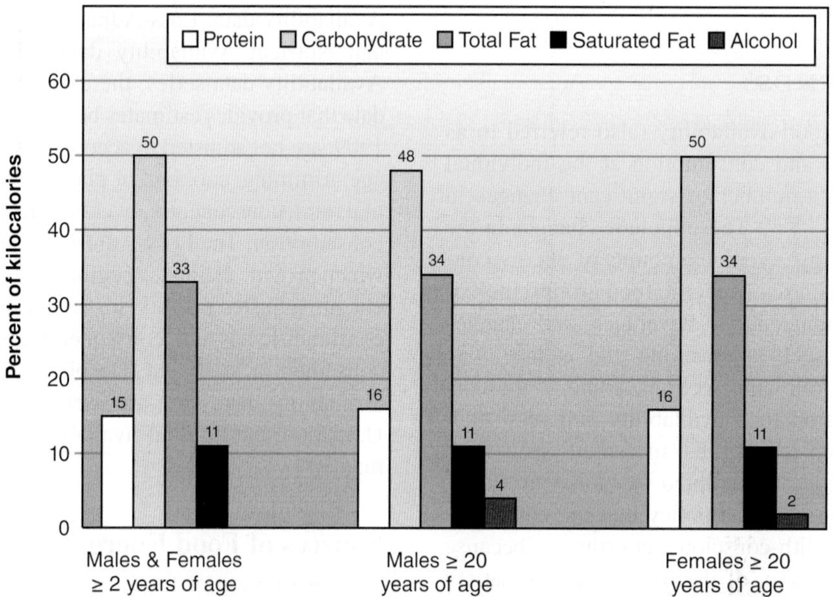

Figure 4.13 The percent of kilocalories from protein, carbohydrate, total fat, saturated fat, and alcohol by age and sex, United States, from What We Eat in America, National Health and Nutrition Examination Survey (NHANES) 2007–2008.

Data on alcohol are shown only for persons ≥ 20 years of age.

Source: Data from the Agricultural Research Service, U.S. Department of Agriculture.

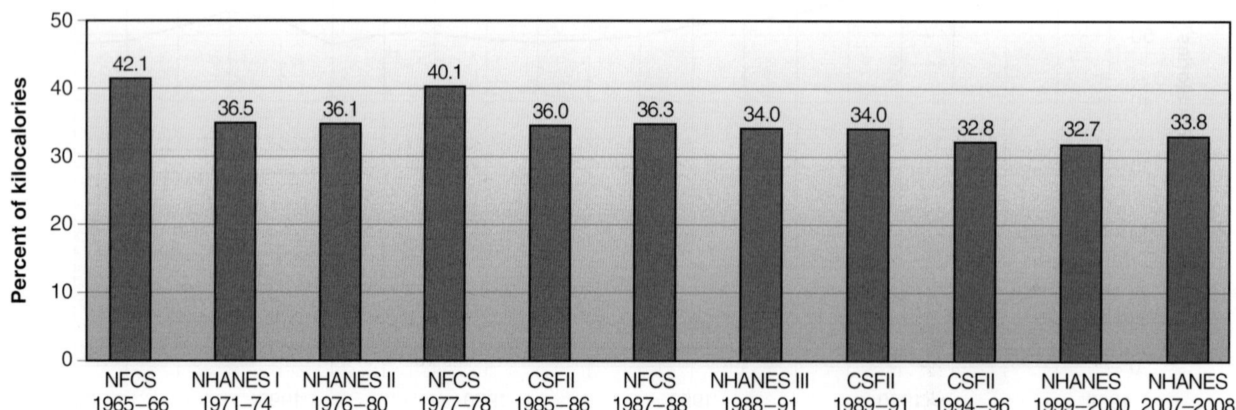

Figure 4.14 Percent of kilocalories from fat in the diets of American adults for selected years, 1965–2008.

Although these percentages seem somewhat inconsistent from one survey to the next, the data suggest that mean percentage of kilocalories from fat has gradually declined in recent years. This is particularly evident in the figure's last three surveys, which have benefited from improvements in food intake data collection methodology.

Source: Data from the USDHHS National Center for Health Statistics and the USDA Foods Survey Research Group.

various surveys represented in Figure 4.14. Among these are differences in how surveys collect dietary intake data, changes in the public's perceptions regarding certain "sensitive food items," ways in which foods are coded, and changes in nutrient content databases. Not all of the surveys represented in Figure 4.14 used the same methods to collect dietary intake data. Research on food intake methodology and advances in technology have led to considerable change and improvement in the way dietary intake data are collected. For example, compared with NHANES II, there was a greater percentage of 24-hour recalls collected for weekend days in NHANES III. In NHANES II, the 24-hour recalls were collected on paper forms and manually coded by dietary interviewers, whereas NHANES now uses a computer-assisted, five-step, automated multiple-pass 24-hour recall system and obtains two 24-hour recalls on virtually every respondent. In addition, the interviewers systematically probe for detailed information about all foods consumed and items added at the table. Over the years there have been improvements in the ways that food intake data have been collected and in the nutrient composition databases used. The USDA Automated Multiple Pass Method for collecting 24-hour recalls now used in NHANES has likely improved the quality of data collected in more recent surveys compared with the data collected by surveys of previous years.

As mentioned in Chapter 3, underreporting of food intake by as much as 25% frequently occurs, particularly in females, overweight persons, and those who are weight conscious. In NHANES, this is addressed by comparing a participant's reported energy intake with his or her calculated resting energy expenditure. If the reported usual energy intake is < 1.2 times the participant's calculated resting energy expenditure, underreporting of energy intake, and therefore, nutrient intake, is probable. The stigma or status attached to consuming certain foods and beverages (so-called sensitive items) can result in either underreporting or overreporting of these foods. For example, changes in public attitudes toward moderate alcohol consumption can influence a respondent's honesty in reporting his or her alcoholic beverage consumption. Given the efforts made to ensure the collection of high-quality data, recent estimates of food and nutrient intake from NHANES are probably among the best available to date.

Percentage of energy from carbohydrate for males and females are shown in Figure 4.15. Females tend to have a greater carbohydrate intake than males, as do children and adolescents compared with older persons. Data from What We Eat in America, NHANES indicate marked discrepancies between the average intakes for Americans and several recommendations made by the *Dietary Guidelines for Americans* and other nutrient intake standards, such as the Dietary Reference Intakes, in terms of sources of food energy, sodium, potassium, and food groups such as whole grains, vegetables, fruits, dairy, and seafood. Figure 4.16 shows that intakes of several food groups and key nutrients are less than the goals set by the *Dietary Guidelines* and other nutrient intake standards, while several exceed the recommended limits. Particularly problematic is intake of calories from solid fats and added sugars, abbreviated "SoFAS" by the *Dietary Guidelines for Americans.* Figure 4.16 shows that calories from solid fats and added sugars are nearly three times the recommended level.

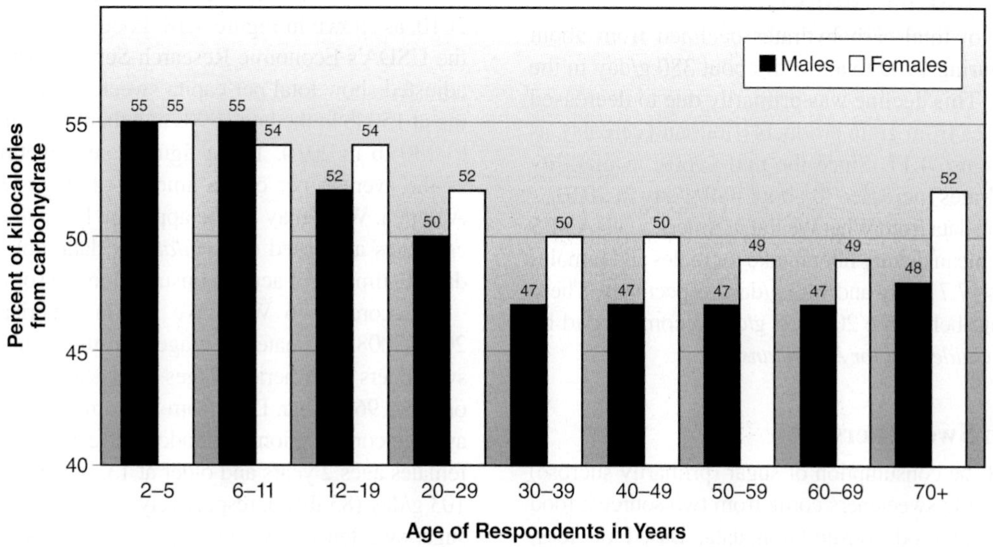

Figure 4.15 The percent of kilocalories from carbohydrate for males and females by age in years, United States, from *What We Eat in America,* NHANES 2007–2008.

Source: Data from the Agricultural Research Service, U.S. Department of Agriculture.

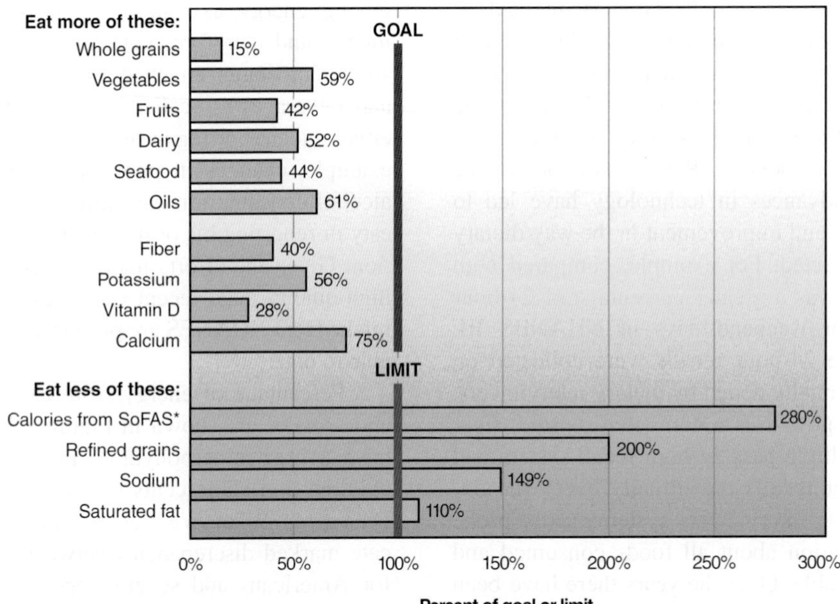

Figure 4.16 How the typical American diet compares to recommended intake levels or limits.
The horizontal bars show average intakes for all individuals as a percent of the recommended intake level or limit. Recommended intakes for food groups and limits for refined grains and solid fats and added sugars (SoFAS) are based on amounts in the USDA 2000-calorie food pattern. Recommended intakes for fiber, potassium, vitamin D, and calcium are based on the highest adequate intake (AI) or recommended dietary allowance (RDA) for ages 14 to 70 years. Limits for sodium are based on the tolerable upper intake level (UL) and for saturated fat on 10% of calories.

*SoFAS = solid fats and added sugars.

Source: U.S. Department of Health and Human Services and U.S. Department of Agriculture. 2010. *Dietary Guidelines for Americans, 2010.* Washington, DC: U.S. Government Printing Office. www.dietaryguidelines.gov.

Trends in Carbohydrates

Availability of total carbohydrates declined from about 500 g/day during 1909 to a low of about 380 g/day in the early 1960s. This decline was primarily due to decreased use of starches from grain products (flour and cereals), as shown in Figure 4.17. Since the mid-1960s, availability of carbohydrates increased to about 480 g/day in 2010.

Based on data from What We Eat in America, NHANES 2007–2008, mean dietary fiber intake for males and females of all ages is 17.7 g/day and 14.3 g/day, respectively. These values remain below the 20 to 35 g/day recommended by the *Dietary Guidelines for Americans.*

Trends in Sweeteners

Estimates of the consumption of sugar (primarily sucrose) and other caloric sweeteners come from two sources: food availability and food consumption data. Based on loss-adjusted per capita food availability data, the annual per capita availability of total sweeteners held relatively steady during the 1970s at about 85 lb, peaked at about 106 lb in the late 1990s, and then decreased slightly to about 95 lb by 2010, as shown in Figure 4.18. Food availability data from the USDA's Economic Research Service that are *not* loss-adjusted show total per capita sweetener availability peaking at 150 lb in the late 1990s and then declining somewhat to 130 lb in 2010. These figures are sometimes reported as the average per capita amount of sugars *consumed* in America. What may not be apparent, however, is that these estimates are based on *availability* data, not *consumption* data. Estimates of actual consumption are somewhat less.

According to What We Eat in America, NHANES 2007–2008, estimated average consumption of all added sweeteners for Americans ages 2 years and older is 82 g/day, or about 96 lb/year. Data from the same survey estimate the average consumption of all added sweeteners for males and females ages 2 years and older at 133 g/day (107 lb/yr) and 103 g/day (83 lb/yr), respectively. As shown in Figure 4.19, sugar-sweetened beverages (e.g., regular soft drinks, fruits drinks, energy drinks, and other beverages sweetened with a caloric sweetener) are the major contributors of added sweeteners in the diets of Americans ages 2 years and older.[42]

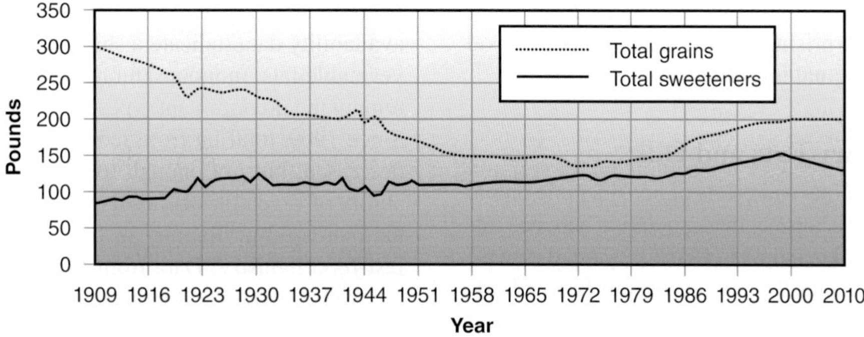

Figure 4.17 Annual per capita availability of total grain products and total sugars and caloric sweeteners from the U.S. food supply, 1909–2010.

Source: Data from the Economic Research Service, U.S. Department of Agriculture.

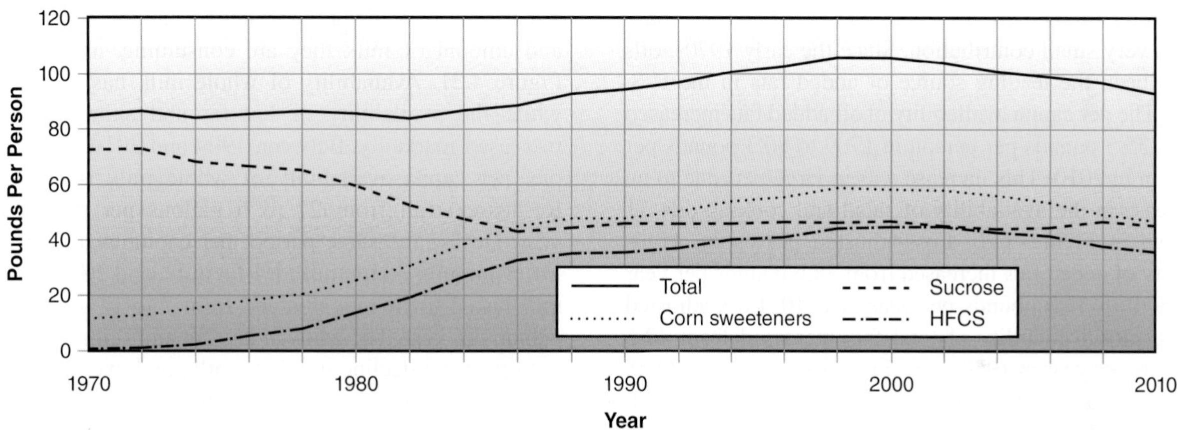

Figure 4.18 Changes in loss-adjusted per capita food availability for total caloric sweeteners, sucrose (cane and beet sugars), all corn sweeteners, and high-fructose corn sweetener (HFCS) in pounds per person from 1970 to 2010.

Source: Food Availability (Per Capita) Data System, Economic Research Service, USDA.

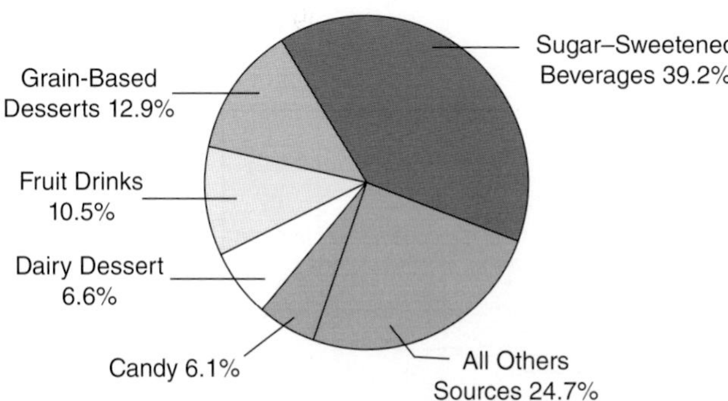

Figure 4.19 The percentage of total intake of added sweeteners by food category for persons 2 years of age and older, based on data from What We Eat in America, NHANES 2007–2008.

Of any food category, sugar-sweetened beverages are the single largest source of added sweeteners in the U.S. diet.

Source: Data from the Agricultural Research Service, USDA. HYPERLINK "http://www.ars.usda.gov/ba/bhnrc/fsrg" www.ars.usda.gov/ba/bhnrc/fsrg

How much sugar and sweeteners do Americans, on the average, actually consume each year? The recent estimate of 130 lb based on availability data that are unadjusted for losses is an overestimation. Based on unadjusted availability data, this value fails to account for waste, spoilage, and nonfood uses of sugars (for example, in the production of alcoholic beverages). Unadjusted data on per capita availability of sugar and other sweeteners are based on shipments of sweeteners by refiners and importers to buyers such as food industries, wholesalers, and retailers. They are valuable for indicating trends in total sweetener use and use of specific sweeteners in the food supply. Actual per capita sugar consumption is much closer to the 95 lb per year estimate based on loss-adjusted food availability and the 96 pound per year estimate based on data from NHANES, which is an estimate of what people actually consume. However, despite the limitations involved in attempting to measure individual dietary intake and the difficulty of adjusting per capita food availability data for losses, estimates from these two methods are surprisingly close and are likely good approximations of actual intake.

Trends in Dietary Fats and Oils

The consumption of fats and oils is of considerable public health significance because of the association between saturated fatty acid intake and risk of coronary heart disease (as discussed in Chapter 9) and because all fats and oils are energy dense, providing 9 kilocalories per gram, and when consumed in excessive amounts have the potential to contribute to obesity. Figure 4.20 shows trends in the annual per capita availability (unadjusted for losses due to waste and spoilage) of the leading types of added fats and oils in the United States from 1909 to 2010. In 1909, butter and vegetable shortening were the leading forms of added fats in the U.S. diet, with margarine and oils making a very small contribution. Since the early 1970s, oils have been the leading source of added fats in the U.S. diet. The per capita availability of all added fats increased from 35.5 pounds per person in 1909 to 80.3 pounds per person in 2010. This increase was in large part due to an increase in the availability of salad and cooking oils, as shown in Figure 4.20. Loss-adjusted per capita availability of added fats increased from 38.6 pounds per year in 1970 to 53.0 pounds per year in 2010. Loss-adjusted per capita availability of total fats increased from 42.6 pounds per year in 1970 to 63.5 pounds per year in 2010. Between 1909 and 2010, the per capita availability of all fats (naturally occurring in foods and added), unadjusted for losses, increased from 122 grams per day to 178 grams per day. Between 1909 and 2010, the per capita availability of saturated fat, unadjusted for losses, remained remarkably flat at 52 to 54 grams per day. During the same interval, however, the per capita availability of monounsaturated fats increased from 47 grams per day to 77 grams per day, while polyunsaturated fats increased from 13 grams per day to 39 grams per day. Although availability data indicate a shift away from animal fats to vegetable fats, monounsaturated and saturated fatty acids remain the predominant types of fat in the American diet. Since 1909, total fat from red meat, butter, and lard have decreased, but not enough to offset the increased availability of vegetable oils used in cooking and on salads and the increased availability of fried foods produced by the fast-food industry. Data from What We Eat in America, NHANES 2007–2008 indicate that saturated fats contribute an average of 11% of total calories in the diet, a value greater than that recommended by the *Dietary Guidelines for Americans,* which is less than 10% of total calories from saturated fats.

Trends in Dairy Products

Americans have made substantial changes in the types and amount of milk they are consuming, as shown in Figure 4.21. Availability of whole milk has decreased, while the availability of low-fat and skim milk has increased markedly. Between 1909 and 2010, for example, per capita availability of whole milk (unadjusted for losses) fell from 27 to 6 gallons per person per year. During the same period, per capita availability of lower-fat milk (skim milk, 1% fat milk, and 2% fat milk), unadjusted for losses, doubled from 7 to 14 gallons per person per year. The gains in low-fat and skim milk have not offset the decline in whole milk, and overall, annual per capita availability of all fluid milk has declined from 34 gallons in 1909 to 22 gallons in 2010. Figure 4.22 illustrates changes in the annual per capita availability of eggs (left Y axis) and cheese (right Y axis) per person per year in the United States from 1909 to 2010 (unadjusted for losses). Between 1909 and 2010, the annual per capita availability of all eggs (those in the shell and those used in the processing of food) declined somewhat from 284 eggs per person per year to 243 eggs per person per year,

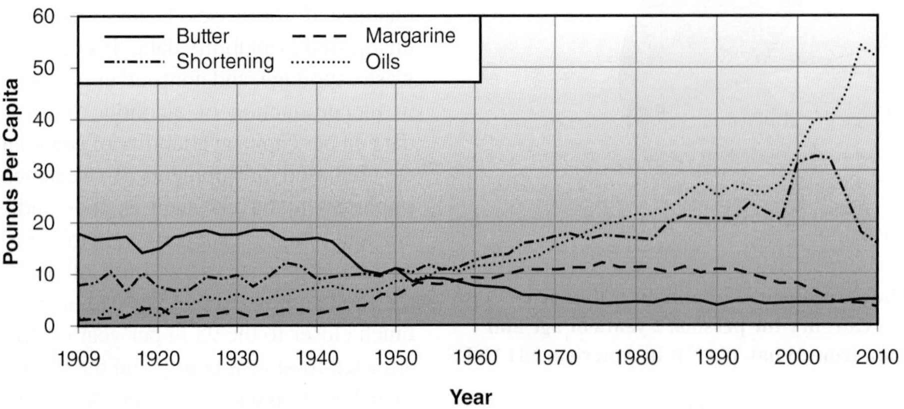

Figure 4.20 Trends in the annual per capita availability of the leading types of added fats and oils in the United States, 1909 to 2010.

Source: Food Availability (Per Capita) Data System, Economic Research Service, USDA.

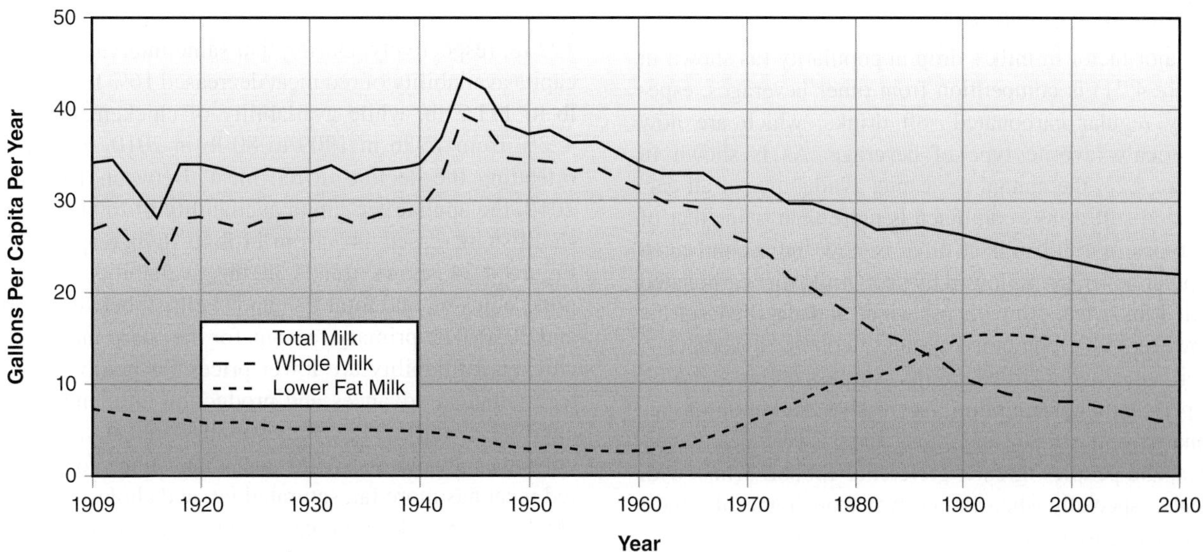

Figure 4.21 Trends in the annual per capita availability of total fluid milk, whole milk, and lower fat milk in gallons per person per year in the United States, 1909 to 2010.
Lower fat milk includes skim (fat-free) milk, 1% fat milk, and 2% fat milk combined. During the past century, per capita availability of lower fat milks has increased somewhat but not nearly enough to offset the steep decline in the availability of whole milk. Availability of total fluid milk in 2010 was one-third less than it was in 1909 and approximately one-half of what it was in 1944 when availability was at its peak.
Source: Food Availability (Per Capita) Data System, Economic Research Service, USDA.

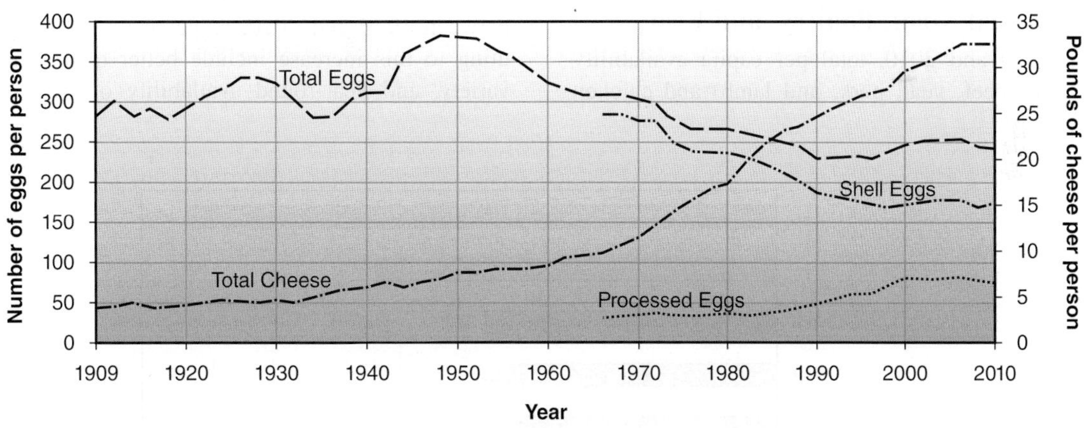

Figure 4.22 Trends in the annual per capita availability of eggs and cheese per person per year in the United States, 1909 to 2010, unadjusted for losses.
The availability of all eggs (those in the shell and those used in the processing of food) declined somewhat from 284 eggs per person per year in 1909 to 243 eggs per person per year in 2010. Between 1966 and 2010, availability of eggs in the shell declined from 284 eggs to 173 eggs per person per year while the number of eggs used in food processing increased from 30 to 73 eggs per person per year. Between 1909 and 2010, the annual per capita availability of cheese increased nearly 10-fold from 3.8 pounds per person per year to 32.8 pounds per person per year.
Source: Food Availability (Per Capita) Data System, Economic Research Service, USDA.

respectively. In 1966 the USDA began collecting separate data on shell eggs and processed eggs. Between 1966 and 2010, availability of eggs in the shell declined from 284 eggs to 173 eggs per person per year while the number of eggs used in food processing increased from 30 to 73 eggs per person per year. The increased availability of processed eggs is primarily due to the greater consumption of fast foods and convenience foods prepared with processed eggs, many of which are eaten outside the home. In addition, concerns about consuming too much dietary cholesterol have led to increased popularity of commercially available cholesterol-free egg substitutes made from egg whites. Between 1909 and 2010, the annual per capita availability of cheese (unadjusted for losses) increased nearly 10-fold from 3.8 pounds per person per year to 32.8 pounds per person per year.

Trends in Beverages

A major factor in milk's drop in popularity (as shown in Figure 4.21) is competition from other beverages, especially regular carbonated soft drinks, which are now America's favorite type of beverage. As is shown in Figure 4.23, the annual per capita availability of all carbonated soft drinks combined is more than twice that of all types of fluid milk. Coffee is now the second most popular beverage, followed by beer, milk, diet carbonated soft drinks, tea, fruit juices, wine, and distilled spirits. However, as a combined group, alcoholic beverages—beer, wine, and distilled spirits—surpass coffee and milk in per capita consumption. Aggressive marketing of carbonated soft drinks and other sugar-sweetened beverages, and peoples' greater preference for soft drinks with meals, especially when eating away from home, also have contributed to declining milk consumption.

Between 1984 and 2008, total per capita availability of all carbonated soft drinks increased 20 percent from 39 gallons per person per year to 47 gallons, respectively. During the same interval, availability of diet soft drinks increased 58 percent from 9 gallons per person per year to 15 gallons, and the availability of regular soft drinks increased 9 percent from 30 to 32 gallons per person per year.[43]

Trends in Red Meat, Poultry, and Fish

Between 1909 and 2010, total per capita availability of red meat (beef, veal, pork, and lamb) and chicken (unadjusted for losses) increased 30% from 149 lb to 192 lb, respectively. During that same interval, total per capita availability of red meat decreased 16% from 133.5 lb to 111.7 lb, while availability of chicken increased 423% from 15 lb in 1909 to 80 lb in 2010, more than offsetting the decline in red meat. Between 1909 and 2010, the annual per capita availability of total fish and shellfish increased 44% from 11 lb to 16 lb, respectively. Figure 4.24 shows trends in the availability of beef, pork, chicken, and total fish and shellfish between 1909 and 2010. The primary reasons for the sharp increase in chicken availability are lower prices for poultry due to technological advances and production efficiencies and aggressive marketing by the poultry industry. Greater consumer awareness of the fact that, ounce for ounce, red meat has more fat, saturated fat, and cholesterol than chicken and fish, and concerns about the link between red meat consumption and risk of coronary heart disease, have likely contributed to the overall decline in availability of red meat and the greater availability of chicken and fish.[17,40]

Trends in Fruits and Vegetables

As shown in Figure 4.25, total per capita availability of fruits and vegetables increased 21% and 11% between 1970 and 2010, respectively. Factors contributing to this increase include better quality, increased variety, and year-round availability of fresh produce.

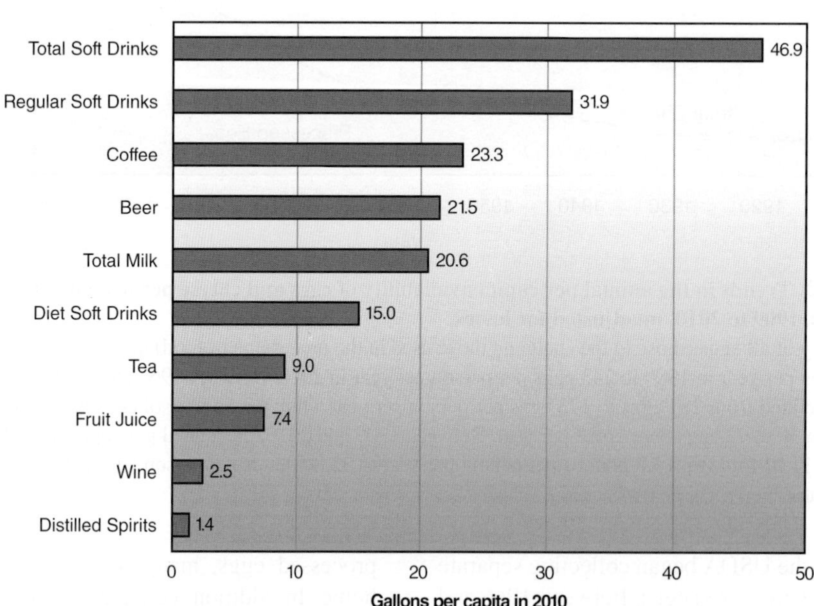

Figure 4.23 Annual per capita availability of beverages in the United States in gallons in 2010, unadjusted for losses.

By a wide margin, soft drinks are the most popular beverages in the United States, exceeding by more than twofold the availability of total milk. When all alcoholic beverages are combined in one group, they become the second most popular beverage in the United States.

Source: Food Availability (Per Capita) Data System, Economic Research Service, USDA.

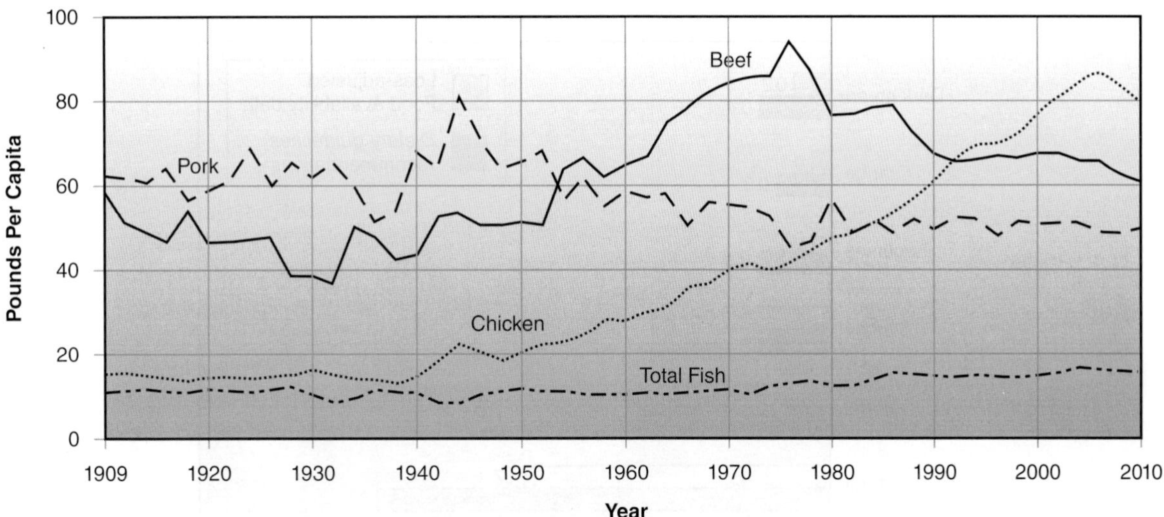

Figure 4.24 Trends in the annual per capita availability of beef, pork, chicken, and total fish and shellfish per person per year in the United States, 1909 to 2010, unadjusted for losses.
While the availability of beef and pork fluctuated between 1909 and 2010, overall, the availability of beef remained essentially unchanged in 2010 from what it was in 1909, while availability of pork declined slightly during this interval. Most notably, there was a more than fourfold increase in the availability of chicken during this period. Total fish and shellfish availability increased slightly.
Source: Food Availability (Per Capita) Data System, Economic Research Service, USDA.

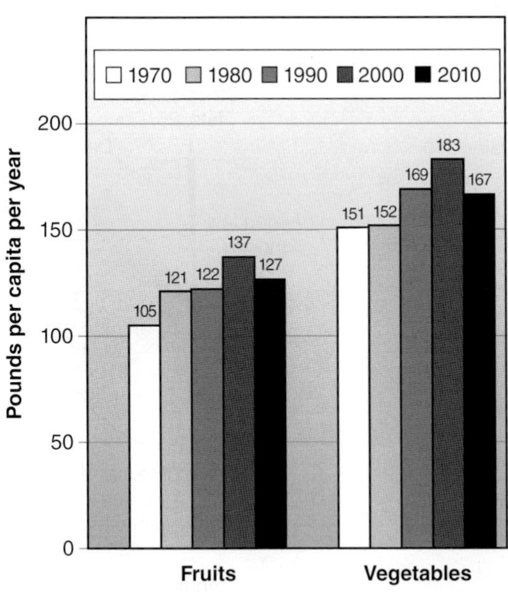

Figure 4.25 Trends in the annual per capita availability of fruits and vegetables in pounds per person in the United States, 1970–2010, adjusted for losses.
Between 1970 and 2010, the annual per capita availability of fruits and vegetables (adjusted for losses), increased overall.
Source: Food Availability (Per Capita) Data System, Economic Research Service, USDA.

Public awareness of the health benefits of fruit and vegetable consumption may also be a factor. Much of the increase in vegetables occurred since 1982, when the U.S. National Academy of Sciences published its landmark report "Diet, Nutrition, and Cancer," which emphasized the importance of increased fruit and vegetable consumption as part of a comprehensive program to reduce cancer risk. This increased availability has been tempered by the fact that the price of fruits and vegetables has increased more than many other food items. Availability data also indicate changes in the kinds of fruits and vegetables Americans are purchasing. For example, in recent years per capita availability of iceberg lettuce has declined, while that of romaine and leaf lettuces has increased. Specialty lettuces not tracked by the USDA, such as radicchio, frisee, and arugula, have also gained in popularity. Much of the recent increase in fruits has been contributed by the greater availability of apples, bananas, and grapes, while the increase in vegetables has been due to greater availability of tomatoes, onions, and leaf lettuces.[17,40]

Despite the increased loss-adjusted per capita availability of vegetables shown in Figure 4.25, these estimates of the amount of vegetables available for consumption remain less than what is recommended by the *Dietary Guidelines for Americans,* as is shown in Figure 4.26. Except in the case of starchy vegetables such as potatoes, the availability of vegetables in the United States is less than recommended by the *Dietary Guidelines,* especially for legumes and orange vegetables.[17]

Trends in Total Calories

As shown in Figure 4.27, the average, daily per capita number of calories available for consumption, adjusted for losses, from 2057 calories in 1970 to 2674 calories in

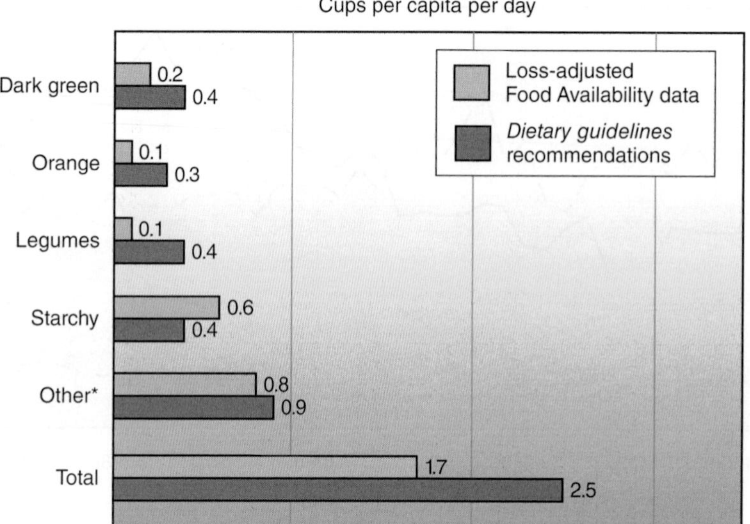

Figure 4.26 Per capita loss adjusted food availability data for vegetables compared with the *Dietary Guidelines'* recommendations for vegetable consumption for someone following a 2000 calorie per day diet.
Except in the case of starchy vegetables such as potatoes, the loss adjusted availability of vegetables in the United States is less than the amounts recommended by the *Dietary Guidelines for Americans,* especially for legumes and orange vegetables.

*Other vegetables include asparagus, broccoli, green beans, tomatoes, etc.

Source: Food Availability (Per Capita) Data System, Economic Research Service, USDA.

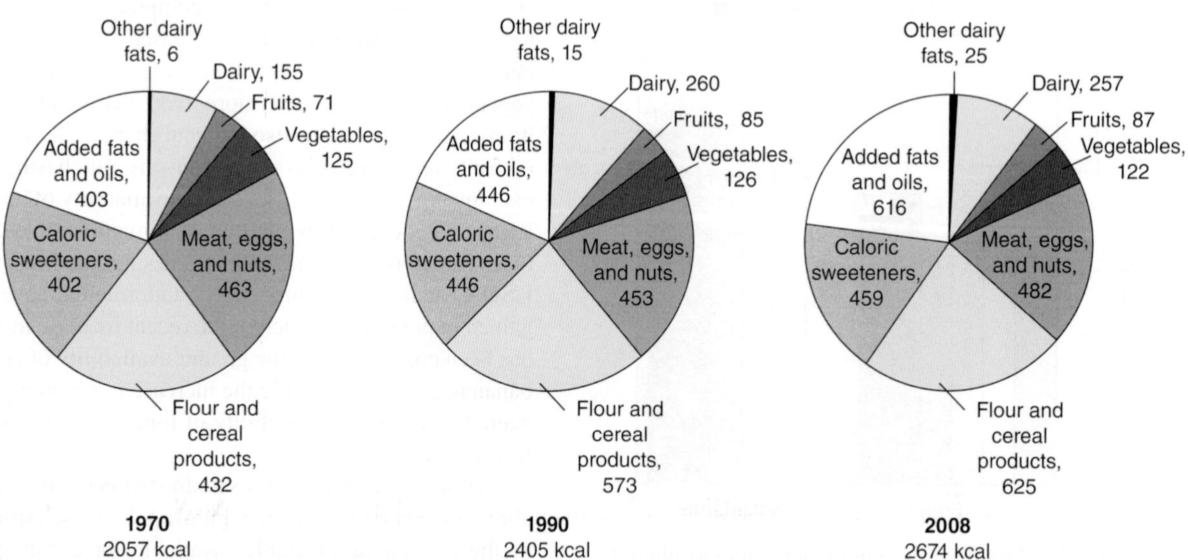

Figure 4.27 Between 1970 and 2008, the average daily per capita number of calories available for consumption (adjusted for losses) has increased by 30%.
The data are from the Food Availability (Per Capita) Data System, Economic Research Service, USDA.

Source: Adapted from Dietary Guidelines Advisory Committee. 2010. *Report of the Dietary Guidelines Advisory Committee on the Dietary Guidelines for Americans, 2010.* U.S. Department of Agriculture, Agricultural Research Service, Washington, DC.

2008, which is a 30% increase. Between 1970 and 2008, the loss-adjusted per capita number of calories availability from added fats and oils (not including fats naturally occurring in dairy products and meats) increased 53 percent from 403 calories per person per day in 1970 to 616 calories per person per day in 2008. The availability of calories from all dairy products increased 75% from 161 calories in 1970 to 282 calories in 2008.

SUMMARY

1. National dietary and nutrition survey data are important in monitoring the nutritional status of a country's population, revealing the relationships between diet and health, identifying groups at nutritional risk and those who may benefit from food assistance programs, and evaluating the cost-effectiveness of food assistance and health education programs. These data are used to track food consumption trends and to monitor intakes of pesticides and other toxic substances.
2. Survey data provide a sound basis for agricultural policy and program development. They provide an early warning of impending food shortages and indicate how such crises may be prevented or alleviated. Food balance sheets estimate the amount of food that is available for consumption from the food distribution system.
3. Nutritional monitoring is the assessment of dietary or nutritional status at intermittent times to detect changes in the dietary or nutritional status of a population. In the United States, this has been conducted by two federal agencies: the U.S. Department of Agriculture (USDA) and the U.S. Department of Health and Human Services (DHHS).
4. Passage of the National Nutrition Monitoring and Related Research Act of 1990 required the USDA and DHHS to coordinate the nutritional monitoring activities of numerous federal agencies, which encompassed a wide variety of surveys and surveillance activities assessing the health and nutritional status of the U.S. population.
5. The USDA has been involved in collecting data on food availability, individual food consumption, and household food consumption. Since 1909, the USDA has used the balance sheet approach to estimate the annual per capita amount of food available for consumption. Availability (or food disappearance) is not an actual measure of food consumption. Loss-adjusted food availability data are modified to account for losses resulting from spoilage, disposal of inedible parts, trimming, cooking, food fed to pets and other animals, or wasted. It is useful for examining food trends, making international comparisons, and studying the relationships between diet and disease.
6. The USDA began assessing individual food intake with the Household Food Consumption Survey, which was later renamed the Nationwide Food Consumption Survey (NFCS) and was conducted during 1977–78 and 1987–88. The Continuing Survey of Food Intakes by Individuals replaced the NFCS. It provided timely information on U.S. diets, studied the dietary habits of persons at nutritional risk, provided data on "usual" diets by collecting several days of data over the course of a year, and demonstrated how diets varied over time.
7. Other nutritional monitoring activities of the USDA include development of food composition and nutrient databases, reporting of food and nutrient availability data, and the Supplemental Children's Survey. The Supplemental Children's Survey measures children's food consumption, so that pesticide residue exposure in children can be calculated.
8. Surveys conducted by the DHHS include the National Health and Nutrition Examination Survey (NHANES), Hispanic Health and Nutrition Examination Survey (HHANES), Total Diet Study, Navajo Health and Nutrition Survey, Pregnancy Nutrition Surveillance System, Pediatric Nutrition Surveillance System, the Health and Diet Survey, and the Behavioral Risk Factor Surveillance System.
9. The NHANES monitors overall nutritional status of the U.S. population through detailed interviews (using dietary, demographic, socioeconomic, and health-related questions) and comprehensive physical examinations, including medical and dental examinations, anthropometric measurements, and diagnostic and laboratory tests.
10. The HHANES was the largest and most comprehensive Hispanic health survey ever carried out in the United States. It collected health and nutritional data on the three largest subgroups of Hispanics living in the 48 continental states: Mexican Americans residing in five southwestern states, Cuban Americans living in Dade County, Florida, and Puerto Ricans residing in the New York City metropolitan area.
11. In response to the National Nutrition Monitoring and Related Research Act of 1990, NHANES became a continuous, annual survey in 1999. In 2002, the USDA's Continuing Survey of Food Intakes by Individuals and NHANES were integrated. Under the integrated framework, USDA is responsible for dietary data collection methodology, the food composition database, and

the coding and processing of all dietary intake data. DHHS is responsible for the sample design and data collection. Food and nutrient intake data from the integrated survey are referred to as *What We Eat in America, NHANES.*

12. Food availability data show that the percent of kilocalories from protein has held fairly steady at 11% to 12% since 1909 to the present. During the same period, the percent of kilocalories available from carbohydrate has decreased, while the percent of energy available from fat has increased.

13. Consumption of carbohydrate has declined because Americans now eat fewer grain and flour products and potatoes. Consumption of all sweeteners by Americans has increased in recent decades, and the estimated average intake of sweeteners based on data from NHANES and loss-adjusted per capita food availability is approximately 95 lb per person per year. Based on data from NHANES, dietary fiber intake is estimated to average about 14 and 18 g/day for females and males, respectively.

14. The availability of kilocalories from fat has increased since the early 1900s because of increased consumption of polyunsaturated and monounsaturated fats. The percent of kilocalories from saturated fat remained relatively constant throughout the twentieth century.

15. Overall, Americans are drinking less milk and more sugar-sweetened beverages. Reasons for this include the popularity of soft drinks in restaurants and fast-food outlets, more meals eaten away from home, concern about saturated fat intake in dairy products, and the heavy advertising of sugar-sweetened beverages. When Americans do drink milk, they are now more likely to drink low-fat or skim milk than whole milk.

16. The annual per capita availability of red meat (beef, pork, veal, and lamb) has decreased between 1909 to the present. During the same interval, the availability of chicken has increased markedly as Americans have shown an increased preference for poultry because of its lower price and greater convenience.

17. Since 1970, the annual per capita loss-adjusted availability of fruits and vegetables has increased. During the same interval, the total number of calories available for consumption by Americans has increased 30% from 2057 calories in 1970 to 2674 calories in 2008.

References

1. U.S. General Accounting Office. 1994. *Nutrition monitoring: Progress in developing a coordinated program.* Washington, DC: United States General Accounting Office. GAO/PEMD-94-23.
2. U.S. General Accounting Office. 1992. *Early intervention: Federal investments like WIC can produce savings.* Washington, DC: United States General Accounting Office. GAO/HRD-92-18.
3. National Research Council. 1989. *Diet and health: Implications for reducing chronic disease risk.* Washington, DC: National Academy Press.
4. Pao EM, Sykes KE, Cypel YS. 1989. *USDA methodological research for large-scale dietary intake surveys, 1975–88.* Washington, DC: U.S. Department of Agriculture, Human Nutrition Information Service.
5. Pelletier DL, Olson CM, Frongillo EA. 2006. Food insecurity, hunger, and undernutrition. In Bowman BA, Russell RM (eds.), *Present knowledge in nutrition,* 9th ed. Washington, DC: ILSI Press, 906–922.
6. Borrel A, Young H. 2006. Public nutrition in complex emergencies. In Bowman BA, Russell RM (eds.), *Present knowledge in nutrition,* 9th ed. Washington, DC: ILSI Press, 923–938.
7. Life Science Research Office, Federation of American Societies for Experimental Biology. 1989. *Nutrition monitoring in the United States: An update report on nutrition monitoring.* Washington, DC: U.S. Government Printing Office.
8. Moshfegh AL. 1994. The National Nutrition Monitoring and Related Research Program: Progress and activities. *Journal of Nutrition* 124:1843S–1845S.
9. Kuczmarski MF, Moshfegh A, Briefel R. 1994. Update on nutrition monitoring activities in the United States. *Journal of the American Dietetic Association* 94:753–760.
10. Woteki CE, Briefel RR, Klein CJ, Jacques PF, Kris-Etherton PM, Mares-Perlman JA, Meyers LD. 2002. Nutrition monitoring: Summary of a statement from an American Society for Nutritional Sciences working group. *Journal of Nutrition* 132:3782–3783.

11. U.S. Department of Health and Human Services, U.S. Department of Agriculture. 1993. Ten-year comprehensive plan for the national nutrition monitoring and related research program; notice. *Federal Register* 58(111):32751–32806.
12. Briefel RR. 1994. Assessment of the U.S. diet in national nutrition surveys: National collaborative efforts and NHANES. *American Journal of Clinical Nutrition* 59(suppl):164S–167S.
13. Interagency Board for Nutrition Monitoring and Related Research. Bialostosky K, ed. 2000. *Nutrition monitoring in the United States: The directory of federal and state nutrition monitoring and related research activities.* Hyattsville, MD: National Center for Health Statistics.
14. Tippett KS, Enns CW, Moshfegh AJ. 1999. Food consumption surveys in the United States Department of Agriculture. *Nutrition Today* 34:33–46.
15. Hiza HAB, Bente L. 2011. Nutrient content of the U.S. food supply: Developments between 2000 and 2006. Home Economics Research Report No. 59. Washington, DC: U.S. Department of Agriculture, Center for Nutrition Policy and Promotion.
16. Muth MK, Karns SA, Nielsen SJ, Buzby JC, Wells HF. 2011. Consumer-level food loss estimates and their use in the ERS loss-adjusted food availability data. Technical Bulletin No. 1927. Washington, DC: U.S. Department of Agriculture, Economic Research Service.
17. Wells HF, Buzby JC. 2008. Dietary assessment of major trends in U.S. food consumption, 1970–2005. Economic Information Bulletin, No. 33. Washington, DC: U.S. Department of Agriculture, Economic Research Service.
18. McDowell M. 2003. U.S. Department of Health and Human Services–U.S. Department of Agriculture survey integration activities. *Journal of Food Composition and Analysis* 16:343–346.
19. Coleman-Jensen A, Nord M, Andrews M, Carlson S. 2011. Household food security in the United States in 2010. Economic Research Report No. 125. Washington, DC: U.S. Department of Agriculture, Economic Research Service.
20. Wunderlich GS, Norwood JL, (eds.). 2006. *Food insecurity and hunger in the United States: An assessment of the measure.* Committee on National Statistics, Division of Behavioral and Social Sciences and Education, National Research Council. Washington, DC: National Academies Press.
21. Yetley E, Johnson C. 1987. Nutritional applications of the health and nutrition examination surveys (HANES). *Annual Review of Nutrition* 7:441–463.
22. Citizens Board of Inquiry into Hunger and Malnutrition. 1968. *Hunger—USA.* Washington, DC: New Community Press.
23. Dwyer J, Picciano MF, Raiten DJ. 2003. Collection of food and dietary supplement intake data: What We Eat in America, NHANES. *Journal of Nutrition* 133:590S–600S.
24. National Center for Health Statistics. 1994. *Plan and operation of the Third National Health and Examination Survey, 1988–94.* Hyattsville, MD: U.S. Department of Health and Human Services, Public Health Service, Centers for Disease Control and Prevention.
25. Delgado JL, Johnson CL, Roy I, Treviño FM. 1990. Hispanic Health and Nutrition Examination Survey: Methodological considerations. *American Journal of Public Health* 80(suppl):65–105.
26. Woteki CE. 1990. The Hispanic Health and Nutrition Examination Survey (HHANES 1982–1984): Background and introduction. *American Journal of Clinical Nutrition* 51(suppl):897S–901S.
27. Chumlea WC, Guo S, Kuczmarski RJ, Johnson CL, Leahy CK. 1990. Reliability for anthropometric measurements in the Hispanic Health and Nutrition Examination Survey (HHANES 1982–1984). *American Journal of Clinical Nutrition* 51(suppl):902S–907S.
28. Roche AF, Guo S, Baumgartner RN, Chumlea WC, Ryan AS, Kuczmarski RJ. 1990. Reference data for weight, stature, and weight/stature in Mexican Americans from the Hispanic Health and Nutrition Examination Survey (HHANES 1982–1984). *American Journal of Clinical Nutrition* 51(suppl):917S–924S.
29. Woteki CE, Briefel R, Hitchcock D, Ezzati T, Maurer K. 1990. Selection of nutrition status indicators for field surveys: The NHANES III design. *Journal of Nutrition* 120:1440–1445.
30. Kuczmarski RJ, Ogden CL, Grummer-Strawn LM, Flegal KM, Guo SS, et al. 2000. *CDC growth charts: United States. Advance data from vital and health statistics; no. 314.* Hyattsville, MD: National Center for Health Statistics.
31. Woteki CE. 2003. Integrated NHANES: Uses in national policy. *Journal of Nutrition* 133:582S–584S.
32. http://www.fda.gov/Food/FoodSafety/FoodContaminantsAdulteration/TotalDietStudy/default.htm.
33. http://www.hc-sc.gc.ca/fn-an/surveill/total-diet/index-eng.php.
34. Byers T, Hubbard J. 1997. The Navajo Health and Nutrition Survey: Research that can make a difference. *Journal of Nutrition* 127:2075S–2077S.
35. Reinhold C, Dalenius K, Brindley P, Smith B, Grummer-Strawn L. 2011. *Pregnancy Nutrition Surveillance 2009 report.* Atlanta: U.S. Department of Health and Human Services, Centers for Disease Control and Prevention. www.cdc.gov/pednss.
36. Polhamus B, Dalenius K, Mackintosh H, Smith B, Grummer-Strawn L. 2011. *Pediatric Nutrition Surveillance 2009 report.* Atlanta: U.S. Department of Health and Human Services, Center for Disease Control and Prevention. www.cdc.gov/pednss.

37. Fact sheet: Key findings from 2002 and 2008 U.S. Food and Drug Administration's Health and Diet Survey. www.fda.gov/Food/LabelingNutrition/ucm202780.htm.
38. Behavioral Risk Factor Surveillance System, Centers for Disease Control and Prevention. www.cdc.gov/brfss/index.htm.
39. National Health Interview Survey, Centers for Disease Control and Prevention. www.cdc.gov/nchs/nhis.htm.
40. Morrison RM, Buzby JC, Wells HF. 2010. Guess who's turning 100? Tracking a century of American eating. *Amber Waves* 8(1):12–19. www.ers.usda.gov/amberwaves.
41. Hiza HAB, Bente L. 2007. Nutrient content of the U.S. food supply, 1909–2004: A summary report. Home Economics Research Report No. 57. Washington, DC: U.S. Department of Agriculture, Center for Nutrition Policy and Promotion.
42. Reedy J, Krebs-Smith SM. 2010. Dietary sources of energy, solid fats, and added sugars among children and adolescents in the United States. *Journal of the American Dietetic Association* 110:1477–1484.
43. Dietary Guidelines Advisory Committee. 2010. *Report of the Dietary Guidelines Advisory Committee on the Dietary Guidelines for Americans, 2010.* Washington, DC: U.S. Department of Agriculture, Agricultural Research Service.

Assessment Activity 4.1

Accessing Data from the Behavioral Risk Factor Surveillance System Website

As discussed earlier in this chapter, the Behavioral Risk Factor Surveillance System (BRFSS) is a state-based telephone survey of the U.S. noninstitutionalized civilian adult population established in 1984 by the U.S. Centers for Disease Control and Prevention (CDC). The BRFSS is intended to provide data on the prevalence of personal health practices identified as risk factors for one or more of the 10 leading causes of death. Data can be analyzed in several ways including by individual state or by smaller geographic areas within states known as metropolitan and micropolitan statistical areas (MMSAs). A metropolitan statistical area is a group of counties that contains at least one urbanized area of 50,000 or more inhabitants. A micropolitan statistical area is a group of counties that contains at least one urban cluster of at least 10,000 but less than 50,000 inhabitants. Data from the BRFSS are used by state and local health departments to plan, initiate, and guide health promotion and disease prevention programs as well as to monitor the success of such programs over time.

The CDC provides several different interactive databases for accessing data from the BRFSS, including prevalence and trend data on various health risks by individual states, all states, or selected metropolitan and micropolitan statistical areas. These and other data can be accessed by going to the Behavioral Risk Factor Surveillance System's website at http://www.cdc.gov/brfss/index.htm. In this Assessment Activity, students should familiarize themselves with the various interactive databases and then access information on various states or a particular metropolitan and micropolitan statistical area (MMSA). Some questions students might consider are:

- What are some of the risk factors that the BRFSS provides data about?
- How has the prevalence of these risk factors changed over time in a particular state?
- How does the prevalence of these risk factors differ from state to state?
- Why do you think the prevalence of certain risk factors differs among geographic regions?
- What are the different MMSAs, and does one include your home or the home of someone you know?
- How does the prevalence of some risk factors differ between two different MMSAs?

ASSESSMENT ACTIVITY 4.2

What's in the Foods You Eat?

The U.S. Department of Agriculture's Food Surveys Research Group has created a search tool it calls "What's in the Foods You Eat." This search tool provides easy online access to data on the nutrient content of about 13,000 foods that Americans typically eat every day; the search tool uses the data files in the Food and Nutrient Database for Dietary Studies, which is also used in processing *What We Eat in America,* the dietary intake interview component of NHANES. Users can easily search the database, view and select portions and weights for a food, and then view the nutrient composition of the food. The search tool is designed to provide nutrient composition data for foods as eaten, so it contains many food mixtures, common portion sizes, and some brand names. Each result can be printed by the user.

The search tool can be found at http://www.ars.usda.gov/foodsearch. In this Assessment Activity, students should go to the website of the Food Surveys Research Group and familiarize themselves with how the search tool works, how to search using the food name or descriptive words and food codes, how to select food amounts, how to view and understand the nutrient composition of the foods selected, and how to print results.

CHAPTER

5 Computerized Dietary Analysis Systems

Outline

Introduction: Using Computers in Nutritional Assessment

Factors to Consider in Selecting a Computerized Dietary Analysis System

Dietary Analysis on the Internet

Summary

References

Assessment Activity 5.1: Analysis of Your 24-Hour Recall on the Internet

Assessment Activity 5.2: Internet Sources for Sound Nutrition Information

Student Learning Outcomes

After reading this chapter, students will be able to:

1. Understand the role of computers in nutritional assessment.
2. List criteria for selecting a quality computerized dietary analysis system.
3. Use an Internet-based dietary analysis program.

Introduction: Using Computers in Nutritional Assessment

Prior to the development of computers and diet analysis software, the manual nutritional analysis of diets was difficult and time consuming. Consider, for example, the steps you would take to manually calculate intake of energy, protein, carbohydrate, total fat, calcium, iron, vitamin C, and other nutrients from a 24-hour recall using nutrient data from a published table. Your first step would be to find the appropriate food in the table and then compare the amount you actually ate with the portion size listed for the food. If these differed, you would have to mathematically adjust all of the nutrient values before listing them on a spreadsheet table. After doing this for each food in your 24-hour recall, you would have to add all of the values for each nutrient to calculate your final 24-hour intake. Next you would have to compare intake to a dietary standard, such as the RDA/DRI, and express this as a percentage. And you can imagine how much more difficult this process would be if you were analyzing a 7-day food record in which nutrient intake would have to be expressed as a daily average.

Clearly, computers are perfectly suited to this task of nutrient analysis, which is nothing more than number crunching, saving time, labor, and expense while reducing error (Figure 5.1).[1–5] Hundreds of software programs have been developed since the mid-1980s for all sorts of nutrition-related tasks, including analysis of food records and food frequency questionnaires, menu planning and forecasting, analysis of recipes, food service and food management tasks, nutrition education, patient interviews and counseling, and research.

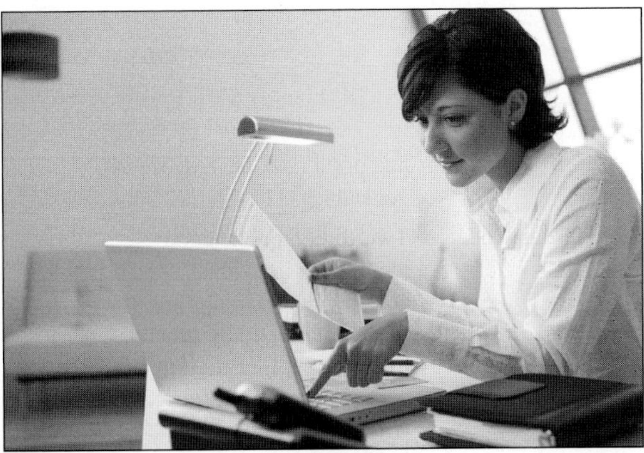

Figure 5.1
Computers are well suited to the task of nutrient analysis.
Source: Comstock Images/Getty Images.

The purpose of this chapter is to delineate important characteristics of computerized dietary analysis systems to aid you in selecting an appropriate software package for the analysis of food records, food frequency questionnaires, and recipes. Dietary analysis systems are now available on the Internet, and the strengths and weaknesses of these systems will be described.

Descriptions of computer applications in nutrition and dietetics first appeared in the literature in the late 1950s. Computer hardware cost is no longer the prohibitive factor it once used to be, and most hospitals, clinics, businesses, and educational facilities provide personal computer work stations for their employees. Computerized dietary intake analysis is an important skill for dietitians and nutritionists to master.

Factors to Consider in Selecting a Computerized Dietary Analysis System

Hundreds of dietary analysis software packages are available, ranging from simplified programs designed for elementary school students to comprehensive programs designed for researchers. In selecting a dietary analysis program, the first step is to establish the major needs for obtaining the software, with specific tasks defined. Once this has been accomplished, choose a dietary analysis system that is suitable to these needs and tasks. For example, a research professor in a university nutrition department will probably need a completely different type of computerized dietary analysis system than a public health nutritionist working with pregnant women at nutritional risk in a county health department.

In comparing software programs, dietitians and other health professionals should consider aspects of the database, program operation, and system output.[6–9]

Nutrient Database

The most important consideration to make when selecting a computerized diet analysis system is its nutrient database.[1,2,7] The database must be accurate, well documented, and large enough to meet all intended tasks. Software vendors begin development of their databases with data from the U.S. Department of Agriculture (USDA). The USDA began publishing food composition values in 1896 and has continually revised and expanded its food composition tables ever since.[10] The USDA has also contributed to the development of food composition tables for other countries for many years and has participated in the International Network of Food Data Systems (INFOODS), organized first in 1984. INFOODS is a comprehensive effort, under the United Nations University Food and Nutrition Program and cosponsored by the Food and Agriculture Organization (FAO) of the United Nations, to improve data on the nutrient composition of foods from all parts of the world. See http://www.fao.org/infoods/ for more information on INFOODS. A link to this and other websites related to computers in nutritional assessment are available on the *Nutritional Assessment* website at www.mhhe.com/lee-nieman6.

USDA Nutrient Data Laboratory

The Nutrient Data Laboratory (NDL) of the USDA is one of seven units in the Beltsville Human Nutrition Research Center (BHNRC) of the Agricultural Research Service (ARS). NDL has an interdisciplinary staff comprised of nutritionists, food technologists, and computer specialists. The mission of the NDL is to develop authoritative food composition databases and state-of-the-art methods to acquire, evaluate, compile, and disseminate composition data on foods available in the United States. As part of its mission, the NDL operates the National Nutrient Databank, a computerized information system for storing and summarizing data on the composition of foods. See Box 5.1 for a glossary of terms and acronyms used by the NDL.

The USDA NDL develops and maintains a number of databases, including the USDA Nutrient Database for Standard Reference (SR). SR nutrient data serve as the core for most commercial and many foreign databases and are the numerical foundation of essentially all public and private work in the field of human nutrition.

USDA Nutrient Databases

The Nutrient Databank System (NDBS) is a repository for information on up to 146 nutrients and food components found in more than 7900 foods. Until 1992, most of this information was published in the form of *Agriculture Handbook 8* (AH-8). However, AH-8 is no longer available in printed form. To facilitate dissemination, the information contained in AH-8 is provided in the SR at the website of the USDA NDL (http://www.ars.usda.gov/nutrientdata).

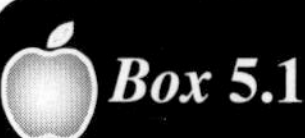

Box 5.1 Acronyms and Documentation Terms

The following is a list of definitions of acronyms and terms used in this chapter and in documentation for the USDA National Nutrient Database for Standard Reference.

Analytical	Data from laboratory analysis of one or more food samples
AOAC	Association of Official Analytical Chemists, independent scientific organization that published a reference of methods used in analyzing the composition of foods.
AMS	Agricultural Marketing Service, USDA
ARS	Agricultural Research Service, USDA
Atwater System	System developed by W. O. Atwater to calculate the energy contributed by protein, fat, and carbohydrates to foods.
BHNRC	Beltsville Human Nutrition Research Center
Calculated	Nutrient values computed or estimated by mathematical adjustment. Normalizing nutrients to an average moisture or fat value, use of retention factors, and substitution of similar ingredients in a formulation or recipe are examples of calculated values.
CFR	Code of Federal Regulations
CNPP	Center for Nutrition Policy and Promotion, USDA. Has information on the Dietary Guidelines, and MyPyramid.gov.
Derivation code	A 4-character, alphabetic code used to document Standard Reference nutrient data source and quality.
Discontinued item	Food product no longer sold or available commercially; item removed from Standard Reference Database.
FDA	Food and Drug Administration, U.S. Department of Health and Human Services
FNIC	Food and Nutrition Information Center. One of NAL's information centers.
Food Group	NDL categorizes foods into similar groups and assigns a Food Group Code, such as cereal grains and pasta (20), beverages (14), vegetables (11).
Food Group Code	Two-digit numeric code identifying individual Food Groups. Food Groups are further classified by subcodes, to produce a four-digit numeric code. For example, fresh pork is 1010, while cured pork is 1020. Food group codes are independent of NDB numbers.
Formulation	The estimated proportion by weight of ingredients in a multi-ingredient commercial food item when other characteristics of the food item are known or can be set. Characteristics that may be known or can be set include: order of predominance of ingredients, retention codes, target moisture level of individual ingredients and final product, and lower and upper bounds on the proportion of any individual ingredient. As a minimum, to derive a formulation, some nutrient values must be known and flagged for matching.
FSIS	Food Safety and Inspection Service, USDA
Handbook 8 (AH-8)	USDA Agriculture Handbook No. 8, *Composition of Foods*
HG-72	Home and Garden Bulletin No. 72, *Nutritive Value of Foods*
Household measure	Standard weight (sometimes with dimensions) or portion of individual food. Sometimes called serving size.
Imputed	Nutrient values developed when analytical values are unavailable. Nutrient values from another form of the same food, or another species of the same genus are examples of imputed values.
INFOODS	International Network of Food Data Systems
Item	Individual food or food product

Box 5.1 Continued

Key Foods	Identification of foods most highly consumed and also best sources of nutrients deemed important to national dietary health. Key Foods are identified as those foods contributing up to 75% of any one nutrient. Key Foods are used by NDL to set priorities for our nutrient analysis contracts.
Label	Data printed on a food label, as supplied by its manufacturer. The values are primarily company analytical or imputed; however, the values have been rounded and/or adjusted to provide uniform serving size weights.
NAL	National Agricultural Library, USDA located in Beltsville, Maryland
NCI	National Cancer Institute, NIH
NHANES	National Health and Nutrition Examination Survey. Conducted by the National Center for Health Statistics, U.S. Department of Health and Human Services
NHLBI	National Heart, Lung and Blood Institute, NIH
NNDB	USDA National Nutrient Databank
NDB No.	Identification number for food item in USDA Nutrient Database
NIH	National Institutes of Health
NIST	National Institute of Standards and Technology, U.S. Department of Commerce
NLEA	National Labeling and Education Act of 1990. Refers to food-labeling regulations promulgated by the FDA.
NTIS	National Technical Information Service, U.S. Department of Commerce
PDS	Primary Data Set for USDA Nationwide Food Surveys. No longer a separate database, but part of SR.
Recipe	The known weight or measure of ingredients in a multi-ingredient food item. Amounts of ingredients may be expressed in household volume measure units such as cups and tablespoons or may be expressed as gram weights. The term "recipe" is generally applied to a food item prepared from component ingredients in a household or institutional setting. The term may also apply to a commercial multi-ingredient food item for which the amounts of ingredients are set, rather than estimated (e.g., by Standards of Identity).
Refuse	Portion of food removed before consumption (meat bones, fruit pits, etc.).
RM	Reference Material used for evaluating the reliability of analytical methods
Source code	One-character numeric code to document source of nutrient data.
SRM	Standard Reference Material from NIST used for evaluating the reliability of analytical methods
Standard Reference (SR)	USDA National Nutrient Database for Standard Reference
Tagname	INFOODS Tag Names identify individual nutrients for international interchange of nutrient data.
UPC	Universal Product Code is a unique product identification number found on most product labels, represented by bar and number codes.
USDA	U.S. Department of Agriculture
USDA Commodity	Foods donated, or available for donation, by the Department under authorizing legislation, for use in any state in child nutrition programs, nonprofit summer camps for children, charitable institutions, nutrition programs for the elderly, the Commodity Supplemental Nutrition Program for Women, Infants, and Children (WIC), the Food Distribution Programs on Indian Reservations, and the assistance of needy people.
USDHHS	U.S. Department of Health and Human Services

Source: USDA Nutrient Data Laboratory, Agricultural Research Service. http://www.ars.usda.gov.

The SR includes the sections and supplements of AH-8 and has added new food group sections including "meals, entrees, and sidedishes," "snacks," "ethnic foods," and "restaurant foods."

As information is updated, new versions of the SR database are released. Release 24 (SR24) was published in September 2011 and contained data on 7900 food items and up to 146 nutrients and food components. Table 5.1 lists the 25 food groups included in SR24.

Data for SR24 were compiled from published and unpublished sources. Published sources included the scientific literature. Unpublished data were from the food industry, other government agencies, and research conducted under contracts initiated by the Agricultural Research Service (ARS). These analyses are currently conducted under the National Food and Nutrient Analysis Program (NFNAP), in cooperation with the National Cancer Institute and 16 other offices and institutes of the National Institutes of Health. Data from the food industry represent the nutrient content of a specific food or food product at the time the data are sent to NDL. Values in the database may be based on the results of laboratory analyses or calculated by using appropriate algorithms, factors, or recipes, as indicated by the source code in the Nutrient Data file.

Table 5.1 USDA Nutrient Database for Standard Reference, Release 24

	Food Group
01	Dairy and Egg Products
02	Spices and Herbs
03	Baby Foods
04	Fats and Oils
05	Poultry Products
06	Soups, Sauces, and Gravies
07	Sausages and Luncheon Meats
08	Breakfast Cereals
09	Fruits and Fruit Juices
10	Pork Products
11	Vegetables and Vegetable Products
12	Nut and Seed Products
13	Beef Products
14	Beverages
15	Finfish and Shellfish Products
16	Legumes and Legume Products
17	Lamb, Veal, and Game Products
18	Baked Products
19	Sweets
20	Cereal Grains and Pasta
21	Fast Foods
22	Meals, Entrees, and Sidedishes
25	Snacks
35	Ethnic Foods
36	Restaurant Foods

Source: U.S. Department of Agriculture, Agricultural Research Service. 2011. USDA Nutrient Database for Standard Reference, Release 24. http://www.ars.usda.gov/nutrientdata.

When nutrient data for prepared or cooked products are unavailable or incomplete, nutrient values are calculated from comparable raw items or by recipe. When values are calculated in a recipe or from the raw item, appropriate nutrient retention and food yield factors are applied. To obtain the content of nutrient per 100 g of cooked food, the nutrient content per 100 g of raw food is multiplied by the nutrient retention factor and, where appropriate, adjustments are made for fat and moisture gains and losses. Nutrient retention factors are based on data from USDA research contracts, research reported in the literature, and USDA publications.

Every food item may not contain a complete nutrient profile. Thus, blanks in the SR24 database are regarded as "missing data" or an indication of lack of reliable data. Table 5.2 summarizes the number of foods in the SR24 database containing selected nutrients.

Nutrient values per 100 grams and in edible portions of common measures (e.g., cup, tablespoon, or teaspoon) are contained in SR24. Other data are listed to further describe the mean value including the standard error, number of data points upon which the mean is based, the derivation code, and the source code. The derivation code documents the nutrient data source and quality. An "A," for example, means "analytical data." The source code field indicates how the data value was determined (for example, analytical, calculated, or assumed zero). Several support files that accompany SR24 provide more specific information on the source code, descriptive information about the food items, and descriptions of inedible material (for example, seeds, bone, skin).

Table 5.3 gives an example of the data that are available for each food in SR24. Analytical values represent the total amount of the nutrient present in the edible portion of the food, including any nutrients added in processing. The values do not necessarily represent the nutrient amounts available to the body.

The USDA Food and Nutrient Database for Dietary Studies (FNDDS) is a database of over 7000 foods, nutrient values, and weights for typical food portions (formerly called Survey Nutrient Database). The FNDDS is used to process data from the survey *What We Eat in America,* the dietary intake component of the National Health and Nutrition Examination Survey (NHANES). The FNDDS is available for use in other dietary research studies and can be downloaded free from the website of USDA's Food Surveys Research Group (FSRG), who develops and maintains the FNDDS. The FNDDS is designed for the coding and analysis of food consumption data. Many of the foods in FNDDS are mixtures that are not available in the SR. The SR is the source of the nutrient values for foods in FNDDS, including mixed foods whose nutrient

TABLE 5.2 Number of Foods in the Database (n = 7906) Containing a Value for the Specified Nutrient

Nutr. No.	Nutrient	Number of foods	Nutr. No.	Nutrient	Number of foods
255	Water* †	7901	573	Vitamin E, added*	4070
208	Energy* †	7906	341	β-tocopherol	1421
203	Protein* †	7906	342	γ-tocopherol	1416
204	Total lipid (fat)* †	7906	343	δ-tocopherol	1401
205	Carbohydrate, by difference* †	7906	328	Vitamin D ($D_2 + D_3$), μg * †	4635
207	Ash†	7899	325	Vitamin D_2 (ergocalciferol)	43
291	Total dietary fiber* †	7217	326	Vitamin D_3 (cholecalciferol)	1325
269	Total sugars* †	5765			
210	Sucrose	1250	324	Vitamin D, IU†	4636
211	Glucose	1252	428	Menaquinone-4	465
212	Fructose	1251	429	Dihydrophylloquinone	1284
213	Lactose	1232	606	Total saturated fatty acids* †	7574
214	Maltose	1220	607	4:0	4982
287	Galactose	1098	608	6:0	5027
209	Starch	837	609	8:0*	5286
301	Calcium* †	7771	610	10:0*	5752
303	Iron* †	7784	611	12:0	6021
304	Magnesium* †	7728	696	13:0	246
305	Phosphorus* †	7325	612	14:0	6397
306	Potassium* †	7486	652	15:0	1666
307	Sodium* †	7823	613	16:0*	6615
309	Zinc* †	7258	653	17:0	1881
312	Copper*	7050	614	18:0*	6603
315	Manganese†	6215	615	20:0	1980
317	Selenium* †	6488	624	22:0	1625
313	Fluoride	561	654	24:0	1353
401	Vitamin C, total ascorbic acid* †	7468	645	Total monounsaturated fatty acids* †	7209
404	Thiamin* †	7231	625	14:1	1885
405	Riboflavin* †	7253	697	15:1	1395
406	Niacin* †	7226	626	16:1 undifferentiated*	6361
410	Pantothenic acid†	6263	673	16:1 *cis*	573
415	Vitamin B_6* †	7062	662	16:1 *trans*	450
417	Folate, total* †	6839	687	17:1	1599
431	Folic acid* †	6489	617	18:1 undifferentiated*	6630
432	Food folate* †	6677	674	18:1 *cis*	1038
435	Folate (DFE)* †	6483	653	18:1 *trans*	1052
421	Choline, total* †	4157	859	18:1-1 *trans trans*	132
454	Betaine	1808	628	20:1*	5743
418	Vitamin B_{12}* †	6974	630	22:1 undifferentiated*	5201
578	Vitamin B_{12}, added*	4236	676	22:1 *cis*	476
320	Vitamin A (RAE)* †	6632	664	22:1 *trans*	369
319	Retinol* †	6409	671	24:1 *cis*	681
321	β-carotene* †	4757	646	Total polyunsaturated fatty acids* †	7216
322	α-carotene* †	4672			
334	β-cryptoxanthin* †	4663	618	18:2 undifferentiated*	6647
318	Vitamin A (IU)†	7476	675	18:2 n-6 *cis, cis*	996
337	Lycopene* †	4632	656	18:2 i (other isomers)	66
338	Lutein + zeaxanthin* †	4611	659	18:2 *trans, trans*	217
323	α-tocopherol (vitamin E)* †	4908	665	18:2 *trans*, not further defined	508

continued

TABLE 5.2 Number of Foods in the Database (n = 7906) Containing a Value for the Specified Nutrient—*continued*

Nutr. No.	Nutrient	Number of foods	Nutr. No.	Nutrient	Number of foods
619	18:3 undifferentiated*	6545	638	Stigmasterol	128
670	18:2 conjugated linoleic acid (CLAs)	665	639	Campesterol	127
			641	β-sitosterol	128
851	18:3 n-3 *cis, cis, cis* (ALA)	117	501	Tryptophan	4817
685	18:3 n-6 *cis, cis, cis*	1002	502	Threonine	4863
856	18:3 i (other isomers)	101	503	Isoleucine	4867
627	18:4*	5002	504	Leucine	4866
672	20:2 n-6 *cis, cis*	1663	505	Lysine	4880
689	20:3 undifferentiated	1484	506	Methionine	4877
852	20:3 n-3	369	507	Cystine	4805
853	30-3 n-6	451	508	Phenylalanine	4863
620	20:4 undifferentiated*	5756	509	Tyrosine	4832
855	20:4 n-6	9	510	Valine	4867
629	20:5 n-3* (EPA)	5170	511	Arginine	4852
857	21:5	104	512	Histidine	4860
858	22:4	516	513	Alanine	4806
631	22:5 n-3* (DPA)	5120	514	Aspartic acid	4809
621	22:6 n-3* (DHA)	5165	515	Glutamic acid	4809
605	Fatty acids, total *trans*	2149	516	Glycine	4806
693	Fatty acids, total *trans*-monoenoic	1020	517	Proline	4794
			518	Serine	4807
695	Fatty acids, total *trans*-polyenoic	769	521	Hydroxyproline	1114
			221	Alcohol*	4831
601	Cholesterol*†	7575	262	Caffeine*	4597
636	Phytosterols	516	263	Theobromine*	4573

*Indicates the 65 nutrients included in the USDA Food and Nutrient Database for Dietary Studies (FNDDS).

†Nutrients included in the Abbreviated file (p. 34).

Source: U.S. Department of Agriculture, Agricultural Research Service, USDA Nutrient Data Laboratory, 2011. USDA National Nutrient Database for Standard Reference, Release 24. USDA Nutrient Data Laboratory website: http://www.ars.usda.gov/nutrientdata

values are calculated using SR items as ingredients. The FNDDS portion weights are for the types of portion size that survey respondents report. For that reason, FNDDS includes additional weights for common food portion sizes that are not available in the SR. There are no missing values in the FNDDS, and each food has values for energy and 63 nutrients and food components. The FNDDS is updated every 2 years in conjunction with data released from *What We Eat in America, NHANES.*

Other data sets developed by NDL include retention tables and tables of special interest on nutrients such as choline, added sugars, flavonoids, fluoride, isoflavones, oxalic acid content of selected vegetables, oxygen radical absorbance capacity (ORAC), and proanthocyanidins. (See http://www.ars.usda.gov/ba/bhnrc/ndl) The USDA sponsors a yearly conference, the "National Nutrient Databank Conference," to facilitate cooperation among the USDA, university researchers, food companies, and others interested in nutrient data.

Criteria for Developing High-Quality Databases

Developers of commercial computerized dietary analysis systems are faced with several challenges in formulating high-quality databases.[6–9] Box 5.2 summarizes a checklist of criteria in choosing a good nutrient database.

The first challenge is to decide on how many foods and nutrients to include in the software program. Even though the USDA SR provides values on more than 140 nutrients and food components for more than 7900 foods, relatively few recipes and name brand foods are included. And, as emphasized in Table 5.2, a number of foods also have missing values for some nutrients, such as manganese, selenium, vitamin E, and newly introduced nutrients such as individual sugars and tocopherols.

Although the USDA releases substantial amounts of new or updated information each year, the typical supermarket contains 15,000 to 60,000 brand name food products. The best software vendors attempt to provide their customers with database updates at least once a year,

TABLE 5.3 An Example of the Nutrient Data Available for Each Food in SR24

NDB No. 09003
Apples, raw, with skin (1)
Malus domestica
Includes USDA commodity food A343

Refuse: 10% Core and stem

		Amount in 100 Grams of Edible Portion						Amount in Edible Portion of Common Measures of Food		
Nutrients and Units		**Mean**	**Std. Error**	**Number of Data Points**	**Deriv Code**	**Source Code**	**Confidence Code**	**Measure 1**	**Measure 2**	**Measure 3**
Proximates:										
Water	g	85.56	0.241	38	A	1		106.95	93.26	190.80
Energy	kcal	52		0	NC	4		65	57	116
Energy	kj	218		0	NC	4		272	237	486
Protein (N × 6.25)	g	0.26	0.019	29	A	1		0.33	0.29	0.59
Total lipid (fat)	g	0.17	0.011	35	A	1		0.22	0.19	0.39
Ash	g	0.19	0.018	29	A	1		0.24	0.21	0.43
Carbohydrate, by difference	g	13.81		0	NC	4		17.26	15.05	30.80
Fiber, total dietary	g	2.4	0.276	29	A	1		2.9	2.6	5.2
Sugars, total	g	10.39	0.112	25	A	1		12.99	11.32	23.17
Sucrose	g	2.07	0.049	25	A	1		2.58	2.25	4.61
Glucose (dextrose)	g	2.43	0.031	25	A	1		3.03	2.65	5.41
Fructose	g	5.90	0.059	25	A	1		7.37	6.43	13.15
Lactose	g	0.00	0.000	25	A	1		0.00	0.00	0.00
Maltose	g	0.00	0.000	25	A	1		0.00	0.00	0.00
Galactose	g	0.00	0.000	25	A	1		0.00	0.00	0.00
Starch	g	0.05	0.000	10	A	1		0.07	0.06	0.12
Minerals:										
Calcium, Ca	mg	6	0.340	26	A	1		7	6	13
Iron, Fe	mg	0.12	0.009	16	A	1		0.15	0.13	0.28
Magnesium, Mg	mg	5	0.073	26	A	1		6	6	12
Phosphorus, P	mg	11	0.337	23	A	1		14	12	25
Potassium, K	mg	107	2.211	26	A	1		134	117	239
Sodium, Na	mg	1	0.071	6	A	1		2	1	3
Zinc, Zn	mg	0.04	0.004	26	A	1		0.05	0.04	0.08
Copper, Cu	mg	0.027	0.001	13	A	1		0.034	0.030	0.060
Manganese, Mn	mg	0.035	0.002	26	A	1		0.044	0.038	0.079
Selenium, Se	mcg	0.0	0.000	7	A	1		0.0	0.0	0.0
Vitamins:										
Vitamin C, total ascorbic acid	mg	4.6	0.470	3	A	1		5.7	5.0	10.2
Thiamin	mg	0.017	0.002	23	A	1		0.022	0.019	0.039
Riboflavin	mg	0.026	0.004	20	A	1		0.032	0.028	0.058
Niacin	mg	0.091	0.006	13	A	1		0.114	0.099	0.203
Pantothenic acid	mg	0.061	0.012	23	A	1		0.076	0.066	0.135
Vitamin B_6	mg	0.041	0.001	23	A	1		0.051	0.045	0.092
Folate, total	mcg	3	0.611	23		1		4	3	6
Folic acid	mcg	0		0	Z	7		0	0	0
Folate, food	mcg	3	0.611	23		1		4	3	6

continued

TABLE 5.3 An Example of the Nutrient Data Available for Each Food in SR24—*continued*

NDB No. 09003
Apples, raw, with skin (1)
Malus domestica
Includes USDA commodity food A343

Refuse: 10% Core and stem

Nutrients and Units		Mean	Std. Error	Number of Data Points	Deriv Code	Source Code	Confidence Code	Measure 1	Measure 2	Measure 3
		Amount in 100 Grams of Edible Portion						**Amount in Edible Portion of Common Measures of Food**		
Folate, DFE	mcg_DFE	3		0	NC	4		4	3	6
Choline, total	mg	3.4		0	AS	1		4.3	3.8	7.7
Betaine	mg	0.1		1	A	1		0.1	0.1	0.2
Vitamin B_{12}	mcg	0.00		0	Z	7		0.00	0.00	0.00
Vitamin B_{12}, added	mcg	0.00		0	Z	7		0.00	0.00	0.00
Vitamin A, RAE	mcg_RAE	3	0.155	14	A	1		3	3	6
Retinol	mcg	0		0	Z	7		0	0	0
Carotene, beta	mcg	27	1.662	14	A	1		34	30	61
Carotene, alpha	mcg	0	0.000	14	A	1		0	0	0
Cryptoxanthin, beta	mcg	11	0.926	14	A	1		13	12	24
Vitamin A, IU	IU	54	3.108	14	A	1		68	59	121
Lycopene	mcg	0	0.000	14	A	1		0	0	0
Lutein + zeaxanthin	mcg	29	1.132	14	A	1		37	32	66
Vitamin E (alpha-tocopherol)	mg	0.18		10	A	1		0.23	0.20	0.41
Vitamin E, added	mg	0.00		0	Z	7		0.00	0.00	0.00
Tocopherol, beta	mg	0.00		10	A	1		0.00	0.00	0.00
Tocopherol, gamma	mg	0.00		10	A	1		0.00	0.00	0.00
Tocopherol, delta	mg	0.00		10	A	1		0.00	0.00	0.00
Vitamin D	IU									
Vitamin K (phylloquinone)	mcg	2.2	0.079	20	A	1		2.8	2.4	4.9
Lipids:										
Fatty acids, total saturated	g	0.028		0	NC	4		0.036	0.031	0.063
4:0	g	0.000		0		1		0.000	0.000	0.000
6:0	g	0.000		0		1		0.000	0.000	0.000
8:0	g	0.000		0		1		0.000	0.000	0.000
10:0	g	0.000		0		1		0.000	0.000	0.000
12:0	g	0.000		1		1		0.001	0.001	0.001
13:0	g									
14:0	g	0.001		1		1		0.001	0.001	0.002
15:0	g									
16:0	g	0.024		4		1		0.029	0.026	0.052
17:0	g									
18:0	g	0.003		4		1		0.004	0.004	0.008
20:0	g									
22:0	g									
24:0	g									

continued

TABLE 5.3 An Example of the Nutrient Data Available for Each Food in SR24—*continued*

NDB No. 09003
Apples, raw, with skin (1)
Malus domestica
Includes USDA commodity food A343

Refuse: 10% Core and stem

		Amount in 100 Grams of Edible Portion						Amount in Edible Portion of Common Measures of Food		
Nutrients and Units		**Mean**	**Std. Error**	**Number of Data Points**	**Deriv Code**	**Source Code**	**Confidence Code**	**Measure 1**	**Measure 2**	**Measure 3**
Fatty acids, total monounsaturated	g	0.007		0	NC	4		0.009	0.008	0.016
14:1	g									
15:1	g									
16:1 undifferentiated	g	0.000		1		1		0.001	0.001	0.001
17:1	g									
18:1 undifferentiated	g	0.007		4		1		0.009	0.007	0.015
20:1	g	0.000		0		1		0.000	0.000	0.000
22:1 undifferentiated	g	0.000		0		1		0.000	0.000	0.000
24:1 c	g									
Fatty acids, total polyunsaturated	g	0.051		0	NC	4		0.064	0.056	0.115
18:2 undifferentiated	g	0.043		4		1		0.053	0.046	0.095
18:3 undifferentiated	g	0.009		4		1		0.011	0.010	0.020
18:4	g	0.000		0		1		0.000	0.000	0.000
20:2 n-6 c,c	g									
20:3 undifferentiated	g									
20:4 undifferentiated	g	0.000		0		1		0.000	0.000	0.000
20:5 n-3	g	0.000		0		1		0.000	0.000	0.000
22:5 n-3	g	0.000		0		1		0.000	0.000	0.000
22:6 n-3	g	0.000		0		1		0.000	0.000	0.000
Fatty acids, total trans	g									
Cholesterol	mg	0		0	Z	7		0	0	0
Phytosterols	mg	12		0		1		15	13	27
Amino Acids:										
Tryptophan	g	0.001		0	A	1		0.001	0.001	0.002
Threonine	g	0.006		0	A	1		0.008	0.007	0.014
Isoleucine	g	0.006		0	A	1		0.007	0.006	0.013
Leucine	g	0.013		0	A	1		0.016	0.014	0.029
Lysine	g	0.012		0	A	1		0.015	0.013	0.027
Methionine	g	0.001		0	A	1		0.001	0.001	0.002
Cystine	g	0.001		0	A	1		0.001	0.001	0.002
Phenylalanine	g	0.006		0	A	1		0.008	0.007	0.014
Tyrosine	g	0.001		0	A	1		0.001	0.001	0.002
Valine	g	0.012		0	A	1		0.015	0.013	0.026
Arginine	g	0.006		0	A	1		0.007	0.006	0.012
Histidine	g	0.005		0	A	1		0.006	0.005	0.011
Alanine	g	0.011		0	A	1		0.014	0.012	0.025
Aspartic acid	g	0.070		0	A	1		0.087	0.076	0.156
Glutamic acid	g	0.025		0	A	1		0.031	0.027	0.055

continued

TABLE 5.3 An Example of the Nutrient Data Available for Each Food in SR24—*continued*

NDB No. 09003
Apples, raw, with skin (1)
Malus domestica
Includes USDA commodity food A343

Refuse: 10% Core and stem

Nutrients and Units		Amount in 100 Grams of Edible Portion: Mean	Std. Error	Number of Data Points	Deriv Code	Source Code	Confidence Code	Amount in Edible Portion of Common Measures of Food: Measure 1	Measure 2	Measure 3
Glycine	g	0.009		0	A	1		0.011	0.009	0.019
Proline	g	0.006		0	A	1		0.008	0.007	0.014
Serine	g	0.010		0	A	1		0.013	0.011	0.023
Hydroxyproline	g									
Others:										
Alcohol, ethyl	g	0.0		0		7		0.0	0.0	0.0
Caffeine	mg	0		0	Z	7		0	0	0
Theobromine	mg	0		0	Z	7		0	0	0

Blanks in the Mean column indicate lack of reliable data. The Number of Data Points column is the number of analyses upon which the mean is based. Number of Data Points of zero indicates the mean was either calculated (as for Energy) or estimated, usually from a recipe, another form of the same food, or similar food.

Common Measures:
Measure 1 = 125g: 1 cup, quartered or chopped
Measure 2 = 109g: 1 cup slices
Measure 3 = 223g: 1 large (3-1/4" dia)

Footnotes:
[1]Based on analytical data for red, delicious, golden delicious, gala, Granny Smith, and fuji varieties.
[2]3 and 5 pound bags of apples typically contain small and extra small sizes.

Calories Factors: Protein 3.36 **Fat** 8.37 **Carbohydrate** 3.6 **Food Group:** 09 Fruits and Fruit Juices

Source: USDA National Nutrient Database for Standard Reference, Release 24 (2011).

they use non-USDA sources to give information on brand name and ethnic foods, and they fill in missing data.

The total number of food items included in a database is important to ensure that substitution (choosing a similar food when the specific food is not in the database) is kept at a minimum.[11–13] For example, if a patient in a cardiac rehabilitation program provides a 3-day food record that includes several low-fat items not found in the database, some less than ideal substitutions with other similar foods will have to be made. However, more is not necessarily better. As the database size increases, the difficulty in finding the right food and the processing time can increase.

Some software packages report having more than 100 nutrients and food components in their databases, while others contain fewer than 30. Again, more is not necessarily better, because values for certain trace minerals (e.g., chromium, selenium, molybdenum, manganese), amino acids, some fatty acids, and some vitamins (e.g., alpha-tocopherol, total tocopherol, vitamin D, vitamin K, biotin) are unknown for many foods. Thus, with an increasing number of food components, the software package developer has to cope with an expanding bank of missing values. If missing data are entered as zero and not flagged (indicated by the software as missing), nutrient totals will appear lower than they actually are. During counseling sessions with patients or clients, some confusion can develop because, for many of these nutrients, low values represent a "database deficiency," not a deficiency in the diet of the patient. The best software packages will give information on how many missing values are present for each nutrient or will warn the dietitian or user about the issue.

One way to judge the quality of a computerized diet analysis system is to determine how the developer met the challenge of missing data in the management of its database.[7–9] Some developers go to unusual lengths to ensure that missing values are substituted with either non-USDA data or imputed values. Many food companies provide information on the nutrient content of their

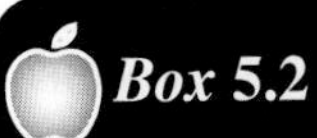

Box 5.2 Basic Checklist for Computerized Dietary Analysis Systems

1. **The Nutrient Database**
   - How many food items are in the database? Aim for more than 15,000 to minimize food substitution decisions during data entry.
   - Does the database contain a significant number of brand name items, fast foods, baby foods, and ethnic foods? If the database contains only the 7900 foods found in the USDA SR, few brand name foods will be available, and considerable food substitution decisions will have to be made.
   - How many nutrients and nutrient factors does the software program analyze for? It should at a minimum include the 12 basic components (energy sources, water, cholesterol, lipids, dietary fiber, and caffeine), 12 vitamins, and 9 minerals available from the USDA SR and FNDDS. Ensure that calculated nutrient factors such as percent of calories as fat, saturated fat, carbohydrate, protein, and alcohol are included. Decide if you need the large number of individual fatty acids and amino acids provided by the USDA SR and some software programs. Look for special features, such as *trans* fatty acids, animal and vegetable protein, carbohydrate components (fructose, sucrose, starch, etc.), soluble and insoluble dietary fiber, and unique nutrients, such as beta-carotene equivalents, vitamin K, tocopherol components, lycopene, and aspartame. Also review the software for its ability to provide nutrient ratios, such as the polyunsaturated to saturated fat ratio, cholesterol to saturated fatty acid index, calcium to phosphorus ratio, and potassium to sodium ratio.
   - How many missing values are in the database? The best software companies go well beyond the USDA SR to scientific journals, food composition tables from other countries, and food manufacturers to not only add additional foods but also ensure that blanks in the nutrient database are filled in with an appropriate value.
   - Can you add new food items to the database?
   - How often are database updates provided? Aim for one update every 1 to 2 years.

2. **Program Operation**
   - What is the cost of the software package? Most of the high-quality professional computerized dietary analysis systems cost more than $500.
   - What type of computer is needed to run the program? Make sure that you have the hardware to run the software.
   - How easy is it to search for foods in the database? The best programs allow you to type in any variation of the food name and still ensure that the food will be listed during the search.
   - Can the portion size or volume and weight measure be easily adapted to conform to those listed in your food record?
   - Can you view the nutrients for a food item during data entry? Access to this information makes food substitution decisions easier.
   - How easy is it to edit the food list during entry? You are bound to make mistakes during data entry, and the best programs make it easy to correct your errors.
   - Can you easily average multiple days of dietary input to derive a daily nutrient intake average?
   - Does the software package allow you to compare dietary intake with a wide variety of standards, such as the RDA/DRI, Canadian RNI, and USDA Dietary Guidelines for Americans?
   - How fast is the overall process of entering foods, analyzing and comparing with nutrient standards, and printing results? Some programs are slow and cumbersome to use.
   - Is the program so complex that it is difficult to learn and use? The best programs are user-friendly, with a small learning curve and a good help screen system.

3. **System Output**
   - Does the software provide nutrient information in the form of tables and graphs, and does it allow you to adapt the reports as desired? The best programs provide a diversity of attractive reports, which can be adapted and shared with a variety of clients and patients. Some programs allow you to add comments via a word processor.
   - Can you print out food exchanges or a MyPlate food guide that compares food group intake with USDA standards? MyPlate values are often among the most important data to provide clients and patients during counseling.
   - Can the nutrient report be printed out as a Nutrition Facts food label? This feature can enhance communication during counseling.
   - Can you rank or sort foods in a food record from high to low for any nutrient in the database? Nutrient sorting enhances your ability to personalize comments made to clients and patients during counseling.
   - Can you export nutrient output data to a spreadsheet for additional analyses? This is an important feature for investigators and administrators.
   - Does the program give an indication of the number of missing values when calculating nutrient intake? This feature can improve the decisions made during the preparation of reports to the client or patient.

products on request, but usually only for a small number of nutrients. Data on the composition of foods are frequently published in the scientific literature, with several journals (e.g., *Journal of Food Science* and *Journal of Food Composition*) specializing in reporting food composition data. Following established NDL criteria, the nutrient content of mixed dishes and recipes can be estimated. Calculations are also frequently used to impute values using data for another form of food or for a similar food. Replacing missing values with imputed values is not an easy process, and it is especially difficult when only limited information exists for a certain nutrient (e.g., trace minerals). The process requires nutritionists with expertise in data evaluation.

The computerized dietary analysis system should at a minimum include the basic nutrients and nutrient factors available from the USDA SR and FNDDS (review Box 5.2):

- Twelve basic components: energy, total fat, total carbohydrate, total protein, alcohol, water, cholesterol, total dietary fiber, caffeine, total saturated fatty acids, total monounsaturated fatty acids, and total polyunsaturated fatty acids
- Twelve vitamins (total vitamin A activity in retinol equivalents, total vitamin E activity in alpha-tocopherol equivalents, vitamin D, vitamin C, thiamin, riboflavin, niacin, vitamin B_6, folate, vitamin B_{12}, vitamin K, and choline)
- Nine minerals (calcium, iron, magnesium, phosphorus, potassium, sodium, zinc, copper, and selenium)

Ensure that calculated nutrient factors, such as percent of calories as fat, saturated fat, carbohydrate, protein, and alcohol, are included. Decide if you need the large number of individual fatty acids and amino acids provided by the USDA SR and FNDDS and some software programs. Look for special features, such as *trans* fatty acids, animal and vegetable protein, carbohydrate components (e.g., fructose, sucrose, starch), soluble and insoluble dietary fiber, and unique nutrients, such as beta-carotene equivalents, vitamin K, tocopherol components, lycopene, and aspartame. Also review the software for its ability to provide nutrient ratios, such as the polyunsaturated-to-saturated fat ratio, cholesterol-to-saturated fatty acid index, calcium-to-phosphorus ratio, and potassium-to-sodium ratio.

Other important measures for judging a vendor's ability to provide a high-quality database are the strength of its service policy, the number of years the vendor and the software have been in business, the frequency with which the nutrient database is updated, the credentials of the database developers, and the cost of upgrades and technical support.

In summary, the content quality of nutrient databases from different software vendors may vary widely, depending on the number of food items and nutrients included, whether the most recent USDA releases have been incorporated, and the degree to which non-USDA sources (e.g., food industry, scientific literature) or estimating calculations are used to fill in the missing values. Three questions to ask when evaluating a nutrient database for personal or professional use are

- Does the database contain all of the foods and nutrients of interest?
- Is the database complete for the nutrients of interest (i.e., few missing values)?
- Is the nutrient database kept up-to-date with the changing marketplace and the availability of new nutrient data?[2]

Program Operation

General operating features of the computerized diet analysis system are extremely important, determining whether a software package is easy to use while generating the desired information.[6–9] (Review Box 5.2 for a checklist of features to look for in the program operation of computerized dietary analysis systems.)

Important operating features include computer hardware requirements, cost of the software package, quality of help screens and user's manual, methods of searching for and entering foods to be analyzed (e.g., food codes, food names, and/or food groups), ability to preview single food nutrients while entering foods, ability to assign a variety of volume or weight measures for each food item, ease of editing the food list, food entry number limit, ease of averaging multiple days of dietary input, ability to compare results with a variety of dietary standards, and quality and variety of printed reports. The ability to modify the database (e.g., adding new foods, deleting old ones, or altering the nutrient values) is another important concern.

Most of the modern computerized diet analysis systems have been developed for personal computers, although several vendors also offer Macintosh versions. The amount of conventional RAM (random access memory), required hard disk space, type of central process unit (CPU), and Windows operating system version vary widely among software systems, and the user must carefully compare software requirements with hardware capabilities. Computer novices should seek the help of a local computer specialist before buying a diet analysis software program. Software package prices are typically more than $500 for high-quality programs used by nutrition professionals and researchers. However, some research-based systems can cost much more than this.

Several of the best computerized diet analysis systems come with help screens, which users can "pop up" during any segment of program operation (in other words, "context sensitive"). While many of the early computerized diet analysis systems were rather difficult to use, more recent versions tend to be user-friendly.

The method for searching and entering foods to be analyzed by the microcomputer is one of the most important program operation features. Most software programs allow users to search and enter foods by full name, partial name, or code numbers. However, diet analysis systems have different ways of accomplishing this task, with some requiring more effort and keystrokes than others. For example, some programs require the user to choose a food group prior to selecting the specific food, a step that can slow down the food entry process. Users tend to prefer searching for the appropriate foods using food names rather than code numbers (which requires use of a food code manual) or food groups. Most of the best programs have nearly instantaneous listing of foods after the user enters the food name. Some programs have a search capability, which allows the user to find the food quickly and directly using only a few appropriate keystrokes (e.g., the first few letters of each word of the food description in any order).

While searching the database for the appropriate food from a patient or client diet record, substitutions (using a food that is as similar as possible) often have to be made, even with databases containing more than 10,000 food items. Finding appropriate substitutes is much easier when the user is allowed to preview the nutrient breakdown of a certain food. Most of the top-quality programs provide a pop-up window during food search and entry, summarizing the nutrient components for the specific amount of the food chosen.

Once the appropriate food has been located in the database, the user must assign a volume or weight measure for each food item. In comparison with earlier software programs, many current diet analysis programs allow users to assign a wide variety of such measures in an easy and accurate manner.

Often there is the need to edit the food list either during or following food search and entry. Ease of editing the food list is an important feature to evaluate when deciding on a software program. The best programs allow users to easily delete or insert foods or allow the volume or weight measure to be changed with little additional effort.

Some of the earlier computerized diet analysis systems set low limits on the number of foods the user could enter prior to analysis. Although this wasn't a problem if only a 1-day food record was being analyzed, multiple-day food record analysis proved to be quite cumbersome, requiring multiple savings as separate meals and/or days prior to averaging. Many systems allow users to enter 200 or more food items, making it much easier to analyze multiple-day food records. For example, a typical 7-day food record may have 150 food items. All of these items can be entered into one list (without having to save each day separately), with nutrient values automatically divided by 7 after designating this number as the divisor.

Software packages often include a wide variety of dietary standards against which individual nutrient intake can be compared. These dietary standards typically include the Dietary Reference Intakes (DRIs), the Canadian Recommended Nutrient Intakes (RNIs), and the Food Guide Pyramid (see Chapter 2). Additionally, most programs compare basic food component intake (e.g., total fat, saturated fat, cholesterol, dietary fiber) with the USDA Dietary Guidelines for Americans. This comparison allows the tables and graphs to look complete and professional.

Food composition data are continually being updated. Users need to ensure that they are using the most current data available. There are times when a user may want to add foods, delete old ones, or add nutrients to the database. Nearly all dietary analysis systems allow users to modify the database in this fashion.

System Output

Once the data have been entered into the computerized dietary analysis system, two important features are the software program's ability to print out a variety of reports and its ability to export data to electronic files for further analysis. (Review Box 5.2.)

Most software packages allow users to preview the output in both tabular and graphic form on the monitor prior to storage on a disk and/or printing. A variety of output formats are desirable to present the nutrient analysis data, including graphic and tabular comparisons with the DRI, RNI, or other nutrient standards, and a spreadsheet table that outlines the nutrient values for each food in the analysis. While some software programs print a spreadsheet table with all of the nutrients for each food after one or two keystrokes, others will print only two to five nutrients for each food at a time, requiring the user to print out a series of repeated reports.

A few computerized dietary analysis systems have unique features that greatly improve the value of printed information. Few nutrient databases have no missing values. To aid in the interpretation of results, some software programs list missing nutrient values. For example, if a nutritionist is analyzing a 3-day food record with 70 foods, the number of missing values for zinc, vitamin E, copper, and so on are listed separately beside each nutrient. Some software packages allow users to sort and print the analyzed diet for nutrients that may be of concern. For example, if a patient's diet is low in iron, the iron values for each food within the diet can be printed in descending order, allowing the nutritionist to make individualized recommendations. A few software packages also allow personal messages from the nutritionist to the client or patient to be included with each printed report through use of a text editor. Another feature that is extremely useful is the automatic calculation of food exchanges or MyPlate food groups contained within the analyzed diet.

This allows the nutritionist to counsel the client or patient about potential deficiencies from a food group perspective. The scope, content, and presentation of the information generated vary greatly from one program to another, and users should ensure that printouts are appropriate, meaningful, and useful for specific needs.

Another system output feature that is useful to some nutritionists and most researchers is the ability of the software package to export the nutrient data to electronic files in a format that is useful for further statistical analysis. For example, if a researcher is analyzing the 7-day food records of 100 cancer patients, being able to electronically transport the nutrient summaries of each individual patient to a spreadsheet software program prior to statistical analysis can save a tremendous amount of effort.

Computerized Dietary Analysis Systems

Although several nutrition periodicals and journals regularly review general features of microcomputer dietary analysis systems (e.g., *Nutrition Today, Journal of Nutrition Education, Food and Nutrition News,* and *Journal of the American Dietetic Association*), very few comparative analyses have been published within the past 10 years.[6–8]

Box 5.3 lists general information on six computerized dietary analysis systems that meet most of the criteria listed in Box 5.2. ESHA Research (P.O. Box 13028, Salem, OR 97309) released the first version of Food Processor in 1984. Multiple versions have been released since then, and this program is the most popular and critically acclaimed computerized dietary analysis system among dietitians, nutritionists, nutrition professors, and allied health personnel. Another widely used dietary analysis system, Nutritionist Pro, was terminated by First DataBank in 2004, but then restarted and revised in 2005 by Axxya Systems (Stafford, Texas). The original Nutritionist Pro software was developed in 1982 and has remained popular despite sifting through three separate companies.

NutritionCalc Plus is available to students using this textbook and was jointly developed by The McGraw-Hill Companies and ESHA Research, Inc. NutritionCalc is a powerful dietary self-assessment tool that allows users to analyze and monitor personal diet goals. The program is easy to use and includes an abridged ESHA database with more than 27,000 foods and 27 nutrients. Dietary intake can be printed out using 11 different report options. Users can add unique foods and recipes to the database. In 1988, the Nutrition Coordinating Center (NCC) at the University of Minnesota released the Nutrition Data System, a microcomputer-based version of the mainframe computer system that had been developed beginning in 1974 in collaboration with the National Heart, Lung and Blood Institute (NHLBI) and outside experts in nutrition, statistics, computer science, and education. In 1998, NCC released the Nutrition Data System for Research (NDS-R), a Windows-based software package incorporating an up-to-date interface with its highly accurate database. The strength of the NDS-R is its extensive database, which contains more than 18,000 foods, 8000 brand name products, and many ethnic foods, with values for up to 162 nutrients and nutrient ratios, with virtually no missing nutrient values. There is a price, however, for this comprehensive database ($5500 and $3375/year support), and most users include medical and nutrition researchers, epidemiologists, and food and restaurant industries.

CyberSoft, Inc., entered the high-end dietary analysis software industry during the mid-1990s, with its Clinical NutriBase system (3851 E. Thunderhill Place, Phoenix, AZ 85044-6679). The NutriBase software package is an extremely sophisticated program, which contains a high number of food items and an amazing number of unique program operating features. Some may find this package too difficult to use, however, because it is complex,

Box 5.3 General Information for Selected Computerized Dietary Analysis Systems That Meet Most of the Criteria Listed in Box 5.2

Feature	Food Processor SQL	NutriBase Clinical	Nutrition Data System for Research	FoodWorks	Nutritionist Pro
Company name	ESHA Research	CyberSoft, Inc.	Nutrition Coordinating Center	The Nutrition Company	Axxya Systems
Telephone number	800-659-3742	877-223-5459	612-626-9450	888-659-6757	800-709-2799
Internet site http://www.	esha.com	nutribase.com	ncc.umn.edu	nutritionco.com	nutritionistpro.com
List price	$699	$795	$5500 and $3375/ year support	$200	$595
Number of foods database	>35,000	>37,000	>18,000	>39,000	>32,000
Number of nutrients/ food components	>160	>180	162	113	>90

with a high learning curve. CyberSoft, Inc., maintains an excellent Internet site (www.nutribase.com), which provides an involved comparison of its products with those from ESHA Research.

FoodWorks from The Nutrition Company features a large database and numerous attractive reports at a moderate price. Analysis results can be exported for use with word processors, and spreadsheet and presentation software. FoodWorks uses four dietary standards: RDA/DRI, Daily Values, Canadian RNI, and FAO/WHO. Users can estimate daily energy expenditure using an extensive list of physical activities. Foods can be searched by name, content of a selected nutrient, or by nutrient density.

Dietary Analysis on the Internet

Use of the Internet through work and home personal computers became widespread during the late 1990s and commonplace early in the twenty-first century. Thousands of websites provide nutrition-based information, and the quality of this information ranges from excellent to very poor. Box 5.4 lists several websites providing sound nutrition information.

Free dietary analysis on the Internet first became available during the mid-1990s. Box 5.5 summarizes three of the best Internet sites for dietary assessment. The top-rated online dietary assessment tool is the Choose My Plate Supertracker by the USDA's Center for Nutrition Policy and Promotion. Users at this site can enter food intake over several days and tabular reports on average nutrient intake and a comparison with MyPlate food group standards.

Online dietary assessment tools will become increasingly valuable to nutrition professionals and will more than likely supplant dietary analysis software programs for the PC as Internet access becomes more widespread, faster, and more sophisticated. The Food and Nutrition Information Center (FNIC) maintains an up-to-date listing of online dietary assessment tools (http://www.nal.usda.gov/fnic). ESHA Research provides online dietary assessment for students through publisher websites (e.g., NutritionCalc plus for users of this textbook).

Currently, online dietary assessment programs fall far short of dietary analysis software programs in several ways (although it is just a matter of time until these are resolved):

- Are slower and more cumbersome to use, and editing is more difficult

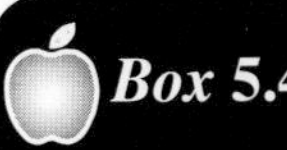

Box 5.4 Internet Sources for Sound Nutrition Information

- USDA Choose My Plate
  www.choosemyplate.gov and **www.usda.gov**
  Access point for learning how to build a healthy plate
- President's Council on Fitness, Sports & Nutrition
  www.fitness.gov
  Information on promoting health through fitness, sports, and nutrition
- Mayo Clinic
  www.mayoclinic.com
  Provides consumers with good nutrition information in a fun, user-friendly format
- Federal Citizen Information Center
  publications.USA.gov
  Provides access to hundreds of educational materials
- FDA Center for Food Safety and Applied Nutrition
  www.fda.gov/Food
  Provides government updates on food and nutrition issues and basic nutrition guidelines
- Meals for You (My Menus)
  www.MealsForYou.com
  Provides thousands of recipes with menu plans, shopping lists, and nutritional analysis
- USDA Food and Nutrition Information Center
  fnic.nal.usda.gov or **www.nutrition.gov** or **teamnutrition.usda.gov**
  Connects readers to the vast nutrition-related resources of the National Agricultural Library
- Healthfinder
  www.healthfinder.gov and **www.health.gov**
  Organizes the health and nutrition information from federal and state agencies
- Vegetarian Resource Group
  www.vrg.org
  Provides nutrition information and recipes for those interested in the vegetarian diet
- American Dietetic Association
  www.eatright.org
  Provides nutrition information for both consumers and dietitians
- International Food Information Council
  www.foodinsight.org
  Provides guidelines on nutrition and food safety for consumers and professionals
- Cyberdiet
  www.cyberdiet.com
  Gives information on foods, recipes, vitamins and minerals, and food planning

- Do not generally allow nutrient analysis of food intake from multiple days
- Have databases with fewer foods and nutrients
- Do not have as many special features (for example, nutrient sorting and database editing), and reports often limited to simple tables and graphs
- Often lack an adequate help function

As discussed in Chapter 3, there are both strengths and limitations in assessing dietary intake using 24-hour recalls, food records or food diaries, and food frequency questionnaires. The National Cancer Institute (NCI) has developed dietary analysis software for the analysis of food frequency questionnaires. The Block-NCI Health Habits and History Questionnaires (HHHQ) are food frequency questionnaires developed by Dr. Gladys Block and her colleagues at the NCI and have been repeatedly validated and used in epidemiologic studies.[14,15] Dr. Block is now associated with NutritionQuest (Berkeley, CA). Software was originally developed in the early 1980s as an analysis tool for the first Block-NCI HHHQ and then updated in 1987 and 1992 as the HHHQ was adapted. (See www.nutritionquest.com/ for more information.) This software program was cumbersome and difficult to use, and was primarily recommended for research purposes, especially the study of diet-disease relationships. The software program estimated intake of 33 nutrients and up to 20 user-defined food groups from the HHHQ. The NCI does not support the use of the 1992 HHHQ unless it is modified to keep up with recent changes in the food supply, particularly the increased number of low-fat and nonfat foods available in the marketplace and changes in the fat content of meat.

NCI investigators have developed a self-administered, scannable food frequency questionnaire, the Diet History Questionnaire (DHQ). Validity and calibration studies indicate that the DHQ performs better than the Block-NCI HHHQ in several ways, and it captures changes in the food supply since the 1990s. The DHQ and the Diet*Calc analysis software can be downloaded from the NCI Internet site: http://riskfactor.cancer.gov/DHQ/. The DHQ is recommended by the NCI for epidemiologic research and for nutrition professionals who prefer food frequency questionnaires over food records for estimation of nutrient intake. A Web-based DHQ is now available.

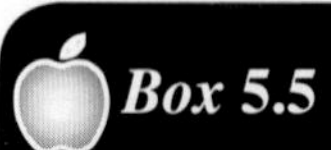

Dietary Assessment on the Internet

Choose My Plate SuperTracker
(www.choosemyplate.gov/SuperTracker)
The SuperTracker is a comprehensive diet and physical activity analysis resource available at ChooseMyPlate.gov. SuperTracker offers consumers the ability to (1) personalize recommendations for what and how much to eat and amount of physical activity; (2) track foods and physical activity from a database of foods and physical activities; (3) customize features such as goal setting, virtual coaching, weight tracking, and journaling; (4) measure progress with comprehensive reports ranging from a simple meal summary to in-depth analysis of food groups and nutrient intake over time; and (5) operationalize the 2008 Physical Activity Guidelines. The "Food-A-Pedia" option allows a nutrient comparison between two different foods. The "Food Tracker" option allows the user to enter food intake from multiple days and find the average intake of energy and 33 nutrients, and then compare to nutrition targets.

NutritionQuest Food Screeners for Adults
(www.nutritionquest.com)
NutritionQuest was founded by Dr. Gladys Block in 1993, initially to provide services to health researchers. NutritionQuest provides a full range of reliable, validated, up-to-date diet and physical activity assessment tools, in a variety of formats including food frequency questionnaires and short screening questionnaires.

Nutrition Analysis Tool (NAT)
(www.myfoodrecord.com)
NAT is provided as an Internet public service by the Food Science and Human Nutrition Department at the University of Illinois. The database used by NAT is composed of the *USDA Handbook #8* and information from food companies. The tabular report compares intake from a 1-day food record with the RDA for 19 nutrients. NAT provides a strong help function, and users can save food intake data.

Agricultural Research Service Nutrient Data Laboratory (www.nal.usda.gov/fnic/foodcomp/search)
This Internet page provides access to the *USDA Nutrient Database for Standard Reference.* You can either view the data or download the data files and documentation in several different formats for use later on your computer. A search tool is also provided, so you can look up the nutrient content (up to 146 food components with a complete breakdown of fatty acids and amino acids) of more than 7900 foods directly from this page. Users can view the nutrient content for one food at a time but cannot enter a 1-day food record for analysis.

NOTE: A link to these and other websites related to computers in nutritional assessment are available on the *Nutritional Assessment* website at www.mhhe.com/lee-nieman6.

SUMMARY

1. Computers are perfectly suited to the task of nutrient analysis, which is one of the most widespread applications of computer technology in dietetics. Computerized nutrient analysis tasks include clinical, educational, administrative, epidemiologic, and metabolic/experimental applications.
2. There are many factors to consider in selecting computerized dietary analysis systems. The first step is to establish the major needs for obtaining the software, with specific tasks defined. Once this has been accomplished, the next step is to choose a dietary analysis system that is suitable to these needs and tasks. There are three characteristics of software programs that dietitians and other health professionals can use to compare programs: (a) aspects of the database, (b) software program operation, and (c) system output.
3. The most important consideration to make when selecting a computerized diet analysis system is the nutrient database. The database must be accurate, verified, and large enough to meet all intended tasks.
4. The USDA Nutrient Data Laboratory develops and maintains a number of databases, including the USDA Nutrient Database for Standard Reference (SR) and the Food and Nutrient Database for Dietary Studies (FNDDS). SR and FNDDS nutrient data serve as the core for most commercial and many foreign databases and are the numerical foundation of essentially all public and private work on the field of human nutrition. These USDA nutrient databases can be downloaded from the Internet.
5. Developers of commercial computerized dietary analysis systems are faced with several challenges in formulating a high-quality database. These include deciding on how many foods and nutrients to include in the software program and use of non-USDA sources to give information on certain brand name foods and to fill in the missing data. The contents of nutrient databases from different software vendors may vary widely, depending on the number of food items and nutrients included, whether or not the most recent USDA releases have been incorporated, and the degree to which non-USDA sources (e.g., food industry, scientific literature) or estimating calculations are used to fill in the missing values.
6. The general operating features of the computerized diet analysis system are extremely important, determining whether a software package is easy to use while generating the desired information. These features include everything from search and entry of food items to the comparison of results with a variety of dietary standards.
7. Once the data have been entered into the computerized dietary analysis system, two important features are the software program's ability to print out a variety of printed reports, and export the data to a variety of electronic files for further analysis.
8. Use of the Internet through work and home personal computers became widespread during the late 1990s and commonplace early in the twenty-first century. Free dietary analysis on the Internet first became available during the mid-1990s. Online dietary assessment tools will become increasingly valuable to nutrition professionals and more than likely will supplant dietary analysis software programs for the PC as Internet access becomes more widespread, faster, and more sophisticated. Currently, online dietary assessment programs fall far short of dietary analysis software programs.

REFERENCES

1. Dwyer J, Picciano MF, Raiten DJ; National Health and Nutrition Examination Survey. 2003. Food and dietary supplement databases for What We Eat in America, NHANES. *Journal of Nutrition* 133:624S–634S.
2. Henríquez-Sánchez P, Sánchez-Villegas A, Doreste-Alonso J, Ortiz-Andrellucchi A, Pfrimer K, Serra-Majem L. 2009. Dietary assessment methods for micronutrient intake: A systematic review on vitamins. *British Journal of Nutrition* 102 Suppl 1:S10—37.
3. Illner AK, Nöthlings U, Wagner K, Ward H, Boeing H. 2010. The assessment of individual usual food intake in large-scale prospective studies. *Annals of Nutrition and Metabolism* 56:99–105.
4. Probst YC, Faraji S, Batterham M, Steel DG, Tapsell LC. 2008.

Computerized dietary assessments compare well with interviewer administered diet histories for patients with type 2 diabetes mellitus in the primary healthcare setting. *Patient Education and Counseling* 72:49–55.

5. Conway JM, Ingwersen LA, Moshfegh AJ. 2004. Accuracy of dietary recall using the USDA five-step multiple-pass method in men: An observational validation study. *Journal of the American Dietetic Association* 104:595–603.
6. Seaman C. 2008. Review of some computer software packages for dietary analysis. *Journal of Human Nutrition and Dietetics* 5:263–264.
7. Lee RD, Nieman DC, Rainwater M. 1995. Comparison of eight microcomputer dietary analysis programs with the USDA Nutrient Data Base for Standard Reference. *Journal of the American Dietetic Association* 95:858–867.
8. Nieman DC, Butterworth DE, Nieman CN, Lee KE, Lee RD. 1992. Comparison of six microcomputer dietary analysis systems with the USDA Nutrient Database for Standard Reference. *Journal of the American Dietetic Association* 92:48–56.
9. Nieman DC, Nieman CN. 1987. A comparative study of two microcomputer nutrient databases with the USDA Nutrient Database for Standard Reference. *Journal of the American Dietetic Association* 87:930–932.
10. Pao EM, Sykes KE, Cypel YS. 1990. Dietary intake—Large scale survey methods. *Nutrition Today* 25(6):11–17.
11. Lentjes MA, Bhaniani A, Mulligan AA, Khaw KT, Welch AA. 2010. Developing a database of vitamin and mineral supplements (ViMiS) for the Norfolk arm of the European Prospective Investigation into Cancer (EPIC-Norfolk). *Public Health Nutrition* 17:1—13.
12. Phillips KM, Patterson KY, Rasor AS, Exier J, Haytowitz DB, Holden JM, Pehrsson PR. 2006. Quality-control materials in the USDA National Food and Nutrient Analysis Program (NFNAP). *Analytical and Bioanalytical Chemistry* 384:1341–1355.
13. Yamini S, Juan W, Marcoe K, Britten P. 2006. Impact of using updated food consumption and composition data on selected MyPyramid Food Group nutrient profiles. *Journal of Nutrition Education and Behavior* 38(6 suppl):S136–S142.
14. Potischman N, Carroll RJ, Iturria SJ, Mittl B, Curtin J, Thompson FE, Brinton LA. 1999. Comparison of the 60- and 100-item NCI-Block questionnaires with validation data. *Nutrition and Cancer* 34:70–75.
15. Velie E, Kulldorff M, Schairer C, Block G, Albanes D, Schatzkin A. 2000. Dietary fat, fat subtypes, and breast cancer in postmenopausal women: A prospective cohort study. *Journal of the National Cancer Institute* 92:833–839.

Assessment Activity 5.1

Analysis of Your 24-Hour Recall on the Internet

Fill out a 24-hour recall (see Chapter 3) and analyze your nutrient intake using the SuperTracker as described in Box 5.5 (www.choosemyplate.gov/SuperTracker). Also, analyze your 24-hour recall using the NAT assessment tool (www.nat.uiuc.edu) listed in Box 5.5 and the ESHA NutritionCalc Plus program that can be found at the McGraw-Hill website for this textbook (www.mhhe.com/lee-nieman6). Print out results from each program and compare them in the following table. Then answer the questions that follow the table.

Nutrient	SuperTracker	NAT Program	NutritionCalc Plus
Energy (kcal)	______	______	______
Protein (gm)	______	______	______
Carbohydrate (gm)	______	______	______
Dietary fiber (gm)	______	______	______
Total fat (gm)	______	______	______
Cholesterol (mg)	______	______	______
Vitamin A (RE)	______	______	______
Vitamin C (mg)	______	______	______
Calcium (mg)	______	______	______
Iron (mg)	______	______	______
Zinc (mg)	______	______	______
Sodium (mg)	______	______	______

1. Did you find that some nutrient intake estimates from the three Internet programs varied more than 10%? List the nutrients that varied 10% or more.

2. What reasons can you list to explain the differences listed in question #1? Consider issues such as differences in databases, food substitution, program operation features, and program output.

ASSESSMENT ACTIVITY 5.2

Internet Sources for Sound Nutrition Information

Box 5.4 summarized Internet sites that provide sound nutrition information. Go to three of these sites and describe at least one topic that increased your understanding of nutrition.

Three Internet sites that contain some aspect of dietary analysis and are highly rated:

1. Name of Internet site: ______

New topic description: ______

2. Name of Internet site: ______

New topic description: ______

3. Name of Internet site: ______

New topic description: ______

CHAPTER

6 ANTHROPOMETRY

OUTLINE

Introduction
What Is Anthropometry?
Measuring Length, Stature, and Head Circumference
Measuring Weight
CDC Growth Charts
Weight Standards
Measuring Frame Size
Height-Weight Indices
Body Fat Distribution
Body Composition
Cadaveric Studies
Skinfold Measurements
Densitometry
Total Body Water
Total Body Potassium
Neutron Activation Analysis
Creatinine Excretion
3-Methylhistidine
Electrical Conductance
Infrared Interactance
Ultrasound
Computed Tomography
Magnetic Resonance Imaging
Dual-Energy X-Ray Absorptiometry
Summary
References
Assessment Activity 6.1: Assessment and Classification of Body Weight
Assessment Activity 6.2: Body Composition Evaluation Using Skinfold Measurements

STUDENT LEARNING OUTCOMES

After studying this chapter, the student will be able to:

1. Demonstrate the ability to accurately measure length, stature, and body weight.
2. Differentiate between the measurement of standing height or stature and the measurement of recumbent length.
3. Demonstrate the ability to calculate and interpret body mass index.
4. Demonstrate the ability to accurately measure waist circumference.
5. Discuss trends in the prevalence of overweight among American adults from the early 1960s to the present.
6. Discuss trends in the prevalence of obesity among American children and adolescents.
7. Distinguish between overweight and obesity.
8. Explain the difference between the two-compartment model and the four-compartment model of assessing body composition.
9. Discuss the value of measuring the triceps skinfold site.
10. Define residual volume and discuss how it can influence estimates of percent body fat based on underwater weighing.

INTRODUCTION

Anthropometry is of considerable interest to scientists and the public and is a valuable adjunct in assessing nutritional status. Concerns about the social and health implications of overweight and obesity have led many people to question the appropriateness of their weight, body composition, and body image. This has resulted in debate and confusion about which methods and standards should be used in assessing body weight and composition. Unfortunately, in some people it has led to such a preoccupation with body weight that their eating habits and body image have become disordered.

The effect of nutrition on human growth and development has made accurate measurement of the body's dimensions and weight indispensable to the practice of nutritional assessment. Properly assessing growth and development requires that standardized methods be followed for measuring the body. Assessment of the body's protein and muscle stores is fundamental to the diagnosis and treatment of malnutrition and to the evaluation of a patient's response to medical nutrition therapy. Nutritional research often depends on methods of accurately assessing changes in body growth and composition.

This chapter describes the available techniques for measuring the body's dimensions and composition. Some of these techniques are used daily by practitioners, and others are limited to nutritional research. This chapter establishes an essential foundation for applying the principles for assessing growth and development, nutritional status, and response to nutrition and other therapy.

Mastering and intelligently applying the techniques and information in this chapter will provide you with skills that will be invaluable to your work in the field of nutrition.

WHAT IS ANTHROPOMETRY?

Anthropometry is the measurement of body size, weight, and proportions.[1–3] Measures obtained from anthropometry can be sensitive indicators of health, development, and growth in infants and children.[2] Anthropometric measures can be used to evaluate nutritional status, whether it be obesity caused by overnutrition or emaciation resulting from protein-energy malnutrition. They are valuable in monitoring the effects of nutritional intervention for disease, trauma, surgery, or malnutrition.[1,4] Anthropometry also is considered the method of choice for estimating body composition in a clinical setting.[5]

MEASURING LENGTH, STATURE, AND HEAD CIRCUMFERENCE

Measurements of length, stature (or height), weight, and head circumference are among the most fundamental and easily obtained anthropometric measurements. Among infants and children, these measurements are the most sensitive and commonly used indicators of health. A child's growth and development can be assessed by comparing stature for age, weight for age, weight for stature, and BMI for age with standards obtained from studies of large numbers of healthy, normal children. The measurement of stature is important for calculating certain indices such as weight for stature, weight divided by stature, and the creatinine height index and for estimating basal energy expenditure.[6]

In measurements of length and stature, reference will be made to positioning the head in the **Frankfort horizontal plane.** As shown in Figure 6.1, this plane is represented by a line between the lowest point on the margin of the orbit (the bony socket of the eye) and the *tragion* (the notch above the tragus, the cartilaginous projection just anterior to the external opening of the ear). With the head in line with the spine, this plane should be horizontal.[7]

In all anthropometric measurements, consistency in technique and units of measurement (feet/inches, centimeter/millimeter, and so on) will help eliminate potential sources of error.[1,2]

Length

Length (also referred to as recumbent length) is obtained with the subject lying down, in a supine or face-up position, and generally is reserved for children up to 24 months of age or for children who cannot stand erectly without assistance.[2,7] The growth charts used for persons birth to 24 months of age are based on recumbent length, whereas the growth charts for those age 2 to 20 years are based on stature.[8,9] Measurement of recumbent length requires a special measuring device (Figure 6.2) with a

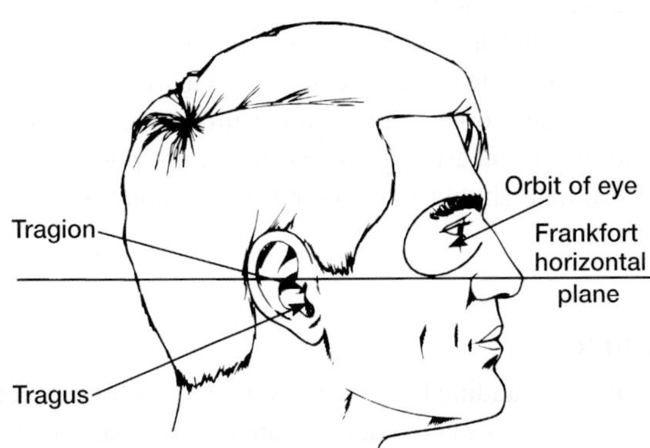

Figure 6.1
Length and stature are measured with the head in the Frankfort horizontal plane. This plane is represented by a line between the lowest point on the margin of the orbit (the bony socket of the eye) and the tragion (the notch above the tragus, the cartilaginous projection just anterior to the external opening of the ear).

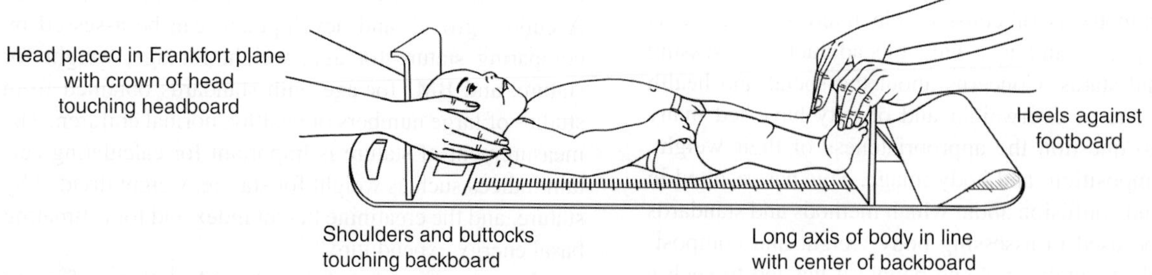

Figure 6.2 **Special device for measuring the length of children who cannot stand erectly without assistance; the device has a stationary headboard and a moveable footboard.**

stationary headboard and moveable footboard that are perpendicular to the backboard. The device's measuring scale (in millimeters or inches) should have its zero end at the edge of the headboard and allow the child's length to be read from the footboard.[2]

Two persons are required to measure recumbent length, as shown in Figure 6.2. With the child in the supine position (lying on his or her back), one person holds the child's head against the backboard, with the crown securely against the headboard and with the Frankfort plane perpendicular to the backboard. This person also keeps the long axis of the child's body aligned with the center line of the backboard, the child's shoulders and buttocks securely touching the backboard, and the shoulders and hips at right angles to the long axis of the body. The other person keeps the child's legs straight and against the backboard, slides the footboard against the bottom of the feet (without shoes or socks) with the toes pointing upward, and reads the measurement. The footboard should be pressed firmly enough to compress the soft tissues of the soles but without diminishing the vertebral column length. Length should be recorded to the nearest 0.1 cm or ⅛ in., using a consistent unit over repeated measurements.[2,7] Gentle restraint is often required to keep a squirming infant properly positioned during measuring. When this is not possible, the best estimate should be recorded with a notation of the circumstances.[2]

Stature

Stature, or standing height, can be measured for subjects 2 to 3 years of age and older who are cooperative and able to stand without assistance.[2,7] Stature can be measured in several ways. The simplest is to fasten a measuring stick or nonstretchable tape measure to a flat, vertical surface (for example, a wall) and use a right-angle headboard for reading the measurement. If a wall is used, it should not have a thick baseboard, and the subject should not stand on carpet, which could affect the accuracy of measurements.[7] Using the moveable rod on a platform scale is not recommended because it often lacks rigidity, the headboard is not always correctly aligned, there is no rigid surface against which to position the body, and the platform height will vary depending on the subject's weight.[9]

Another approach is to use a **stadiometer,** such as the Harpenden stadiometer or or a similar commercially available stadiometer. A list of suppliers of nutritional assessment equipment can be found in Appendix J or at the *Nutritional Assessment* website at www.mhhe.com/lee-nieman6. When being measured with the stadiometer, the subject should be barefoot and wear minimal clothing to facilitate correct positioning of the body. The subject should stand with heels together, arms to the side, legs straight, shoulders relaxed, and head in the Frankfort horizontal plane ("look straight ahead"). Heels, buttocks, scapulae (shoulder blades), and back of the head should, if possible, be against the vertical surface of the stadiometer, as shown in Figure 6.3. Some people may not be able to touch all four points against the stadiometer because of obesity, protruding buttocks, or curvature of the spine. Rather than creating an embarrassing situation by trying to force a subject into a physically impossible position, have the subject touch two or three of the four points to the vertical surface of the stadiometer or estimate height from knee height, as is discussed in Chapter 7.

Just before the measurement is taken, the subject should inhale deeply, hold the breath, and maintain an erect posture ("stand up tall") while the headboard is lowered on the highest point of the head with enough pressure to compress the hair.[1,2,7] The measurement should be read to the nearest 0.1 cm or ⅛ in. and with the eye level with the headboard to avoid errors caused by **parallax,** which is a difference in the apparent reading of a measurement scale (for example, a skinfold caliper's needle) when viewed from various points not in a straight line with the eye.[1,2,7] Hair ornamentation may have to be removed if this interferes with the measurement.

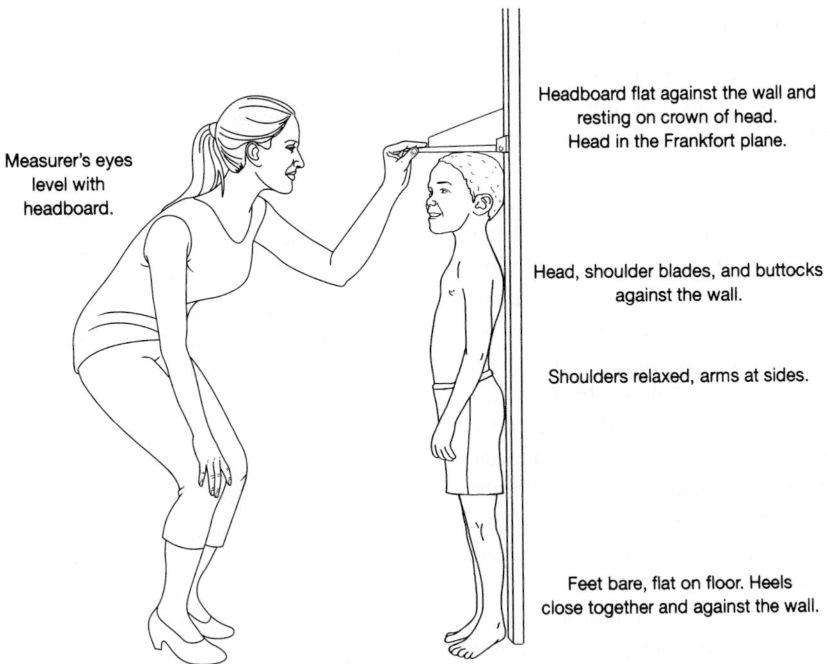

Figure 6.3 **Body position when measuring stature.**

Nonambulatory Persons

In nonambulatory persons (those unable to walk) or those who have such severe spinal curvature that measurement of height would be inaccurate, stature can be estimated from knee height.[1,6] This and other recumbent measures and their application in nutritional assessment of older persons are discussed in Chapter 7.

Head Circumference

Head circumference measurement is an important screening procedure to detect abnormalities of head and brain growth, especially in the first year of life. Although these conditions may or may not be related to nutritional factors, discussion of head circumference measurement is included here for convenience.[2] Head circumference increases rapidly during the first 12 months of life but, by 36 months, growth is much slower. Head circumference-for-age can be evaluated using a suitable pediatric growth chart, as discussed later in this chapter.[9]

Head circumference is most easily measured when the infant or child is sitting on the lap of the caregiver, although older children can be measured when they are standing.[2,7] A flexible, nonstretchable measuring tape is required. Objects such as pins should be removed from the hair. As shown in Figure 6.4, the lower edge of the tape should be positioned just above the eyebrows, above (not over) the ears, and around the back of the head, so that the maximum circumference is measured. The tape should be in the same plane on both sides of the head and pulled snug to compress the hair. The measurement is read to the nearest 0.1 cm or ⅛ in. and written in the infant's file. Reliability of the measurement should be verified with a second reading.[2,7]

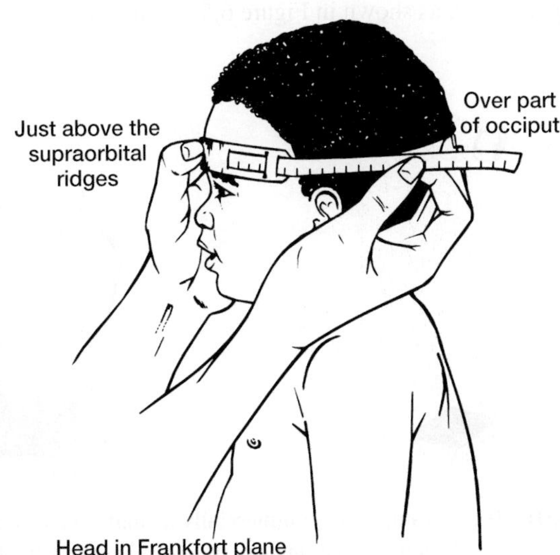

Figure 6.4
When measuring head circumference, the lower edge of the tape should be just above the eyebrows and ears, around the occipital prominence of the head, tight enough to compress the hair.

Measuring Weight

One of the most important measurements in nutritional assessment is body weight. Weight is an important variable in equations predicting caloric expenditure and in indices of body composition.[11]

Body weights should be obtained using an electronic scale, which is preferred over a balance-beam scale. Electronic scales tend to be lighter in weight, more portable, and faster and easier to use than balance-beam scales. They provide easy-to-read digital output in either metric or English units and, when properly calibrated, are highly accurate. Compared to most balance-beam scales, they have a much greater weight capacity, which can be as high as 1000 lb (450 kg). Most models can be connected to a computer network so that data on weight, height, and body mass index can be automatically entered into the patient's electronic medical record. They can record a subject's weight quickly, which is advantageous when weighing infants, who tend to resist lying still for very long. In addition to the types of electronic scales shown in Figure 6.5, there are models with a weight capacity of as much as 1000 lb (450 kg) that an extra-wide wheelchair can be easily rolled onto in order to weigh a patient seated in the wheelchair. When treated with care and operated according to the manufacturer's instructions, electronic scales are quite durable and long-lasting. Like any scale, they should be periodically checked for calibration by qualified instrument technicians and/or state inspectors.

Infants

Infants should be weighed on a pan-type pediatric electronic scale that is accurate to within at least 10 g (0.01 kg) or 0.5 oz, as shown in Figure 6.5.[2,7] Any cushion (for example, either a towel or diaper) used in the pan should be in place when the zero adjustments are made on the scale or its weight should be subtracted from the infant's weight. Whatever practice is used, it must be uniformly followed and noted in the infant's file. Infants can be weighed nude, or the weight of the infant's diaper can be subtracted from the infant's weight. The infant should be set lying down in the middle of the pan. The average of two or three weighings is recorded numerically in the infant's file to the nearest 10 g (0.01 kg) or 0.5 oz and then is plotted on the growth chart in the presence of the subject's caregiver. If, on comparison with previous data, the current values appear unusual, the measurements should be repeated.[2,7]

Excessive infant movement can make it difficult to obtain an accurate weight, in which case the weighing can be deferred until later in the examination. When too active to weigh on a baby scale, an infant can be weighed on a platform scale while being held by an adult with the weight derived by difference. Because this weight will be less accurate than desired (but still better than no weight), the method should be noted in the infant's chart.

Children and Adults

Children and adults who can stand without assistance are weighed on a platform electronic scale that is accurate to 100 g (0.1 kg) or 0.2 lb, as shown in Figure 6.5.[1,2,7] The subject should stand still in the middle of the scale's platform without touching anything and with the body weight equally distributed on both feet. The weight should be read to the nearest 100 g (0.1 kg) or 0.2 lb and recorded. Two measurements taken in immediate succession should agree to within 100 g (0.1 kg) or 0.2 lb.[1] The weight of

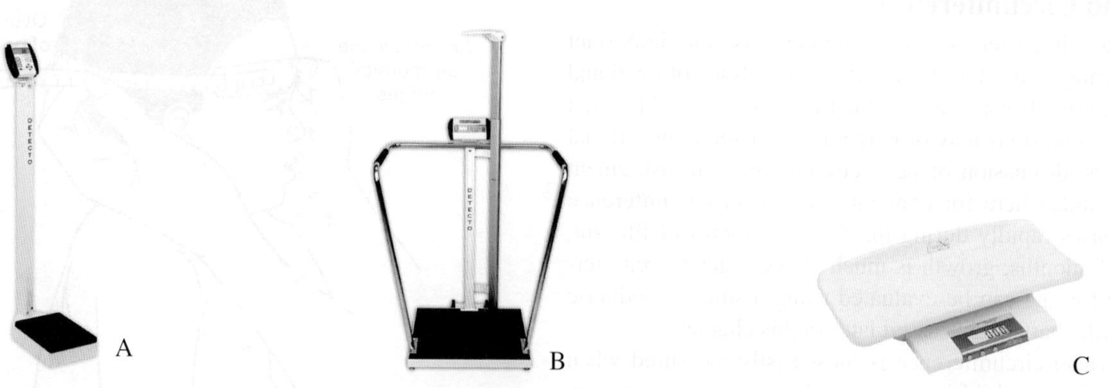

Figure 6.5 Examples of commercially available electronic scales.
The scale on the left (A) is a standard physician's scale with the digital display at eye level and a weight capacity of 500 lb (225 kg). The scale in the center (B) is a bariatric scale with the digital display at waist level, a hand rail attached to the platform on which the patient stands, an integrated digital height rod, and a weight capacity of 800 lb (360 kg). When height is measured along with weight, this unit is capable of calculating the patient's body mass index and displaying it on the digital read-out. The digital scale on the right (C) has a tray that is used for weighing infants and a weight capacity of 40 lb (20 kg). When the tray is removed, the scale can double as a floor scale for weighing toddlers who are capable of standing on their own without assistance.
Source: Images courtesy of DETECTO, a division of Cardinal Scale Manufacturing Company.

children then can be plotted on their growth charts. As with infants, if there seems to be any discrepancy between the current and past values, the measurement should be repeated for verification. Diurnal variations (cyclical changes occurring throughout the day) in weight of about 1 kg in children and 2 kg in adults are known to occur.[7,11] For this reason, it is a good practice to also record the time weight was measured.

Ideally, children and adults should be weighed after voiding and dressed in an examination gown of known weight or in light underclothing with the scales placed where adequate privacy is provided.[1,2,7] Should the weight of clothing be subtracted from the subject's weight? It depends on the purpose for which measurements are obtained and how accurate they need to be. In settings requiring a high degree of accuracy, subjects can be clothed in an examination gown of known weight for which consideration can be easily made. In situations having somewhat less stringent requirements, a reasonable estimate of clothing weight can be subtracted from a subject's weight.[1,7]

Nonambulatory Persons

Persons who cannot stand unassisted on a scale can be weighed in a bed scale or wheelchair scale.[1,7] The subject to be weighed in the bed scale (shown in Figure 6.6) is comfortably positioned in the weighing sling, which then is gently raised until the subject is suspended off the bed. In a chair scale, the subject sits upright in the center of the chair while leaning against the backrest. Using either method, once the subject is still, weight can be read and recorded to the nearest 100 g (0.1 kg) or 0.2 lb. Reliability of the measurement can be verified with a second reading, which should agree to within 100 g or 0.2 lb.[1]

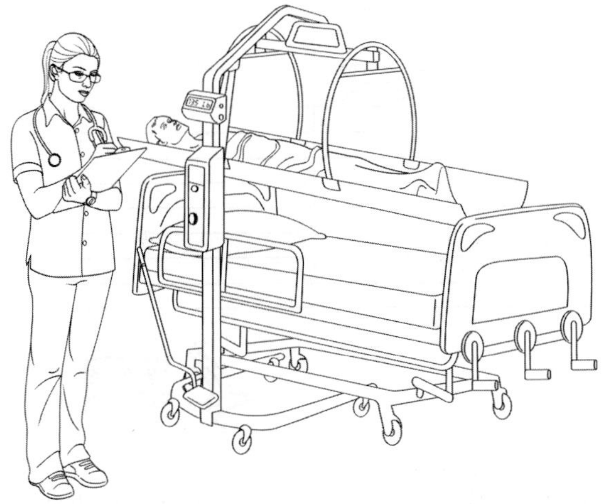

Figure 6.6
A bed scale can be used to weigh bedridden patients.

Body weight also can be computed from knee height, calf circumference, midarm circumference, and subscapular skinfold thickness.[1,10] Descriptions of these anthropometric measurements and computational formulas for computing body weight are given in Chapter 7.

CDC GROWTH CHARTS

The physical growth and development of infants and children are important indicators of the value a society places on the health and wellness of its most vulnerable members. Growth charts are a fundamental tool for evaluating physical growth and development and for assessing the nutritional status and general well-being of infants, children, and adolescents.[8–11] For at least a century they have been used to determine whether a child is adequately nourished and to screen for inadequate growth that might indicate some medical, nutritional, or developmental condition having an adverse effect on the child's health.[9] Growth charts also can be used for monitoring the growth of infants and children undergoing medical treatment so that dietary intake, including enteral or parenteral nutrition support, can be evaluated and adjusted to best meet the infant's or child's needs.[10] As valuable as they are, growth charts are intended to be used not as a sole diagnostic instrument but rather as tools contributing to the formation of an overall clinical impression for the child being measured. Traditionally, they have primarily been used for detecting malnutrition, but in the past few decades concerns about the rising prevalence of overweight and obesity among children and adolescents have led to the increased use of growth charts to screen for unhealthy weight gain, overweight, and obesity in the pediatric population.[9]

Figure 6.7 shows a CDC growth chart developed for assessing length-for-age and weight-for-age in females from birth to 24 months of age. The CDC has developed growth charts for females and males for two age intervals: birth to 24 months, and 2 to 20 years. The charts for the age interval birth to 24 months give **percentile** curves for length-for-age, weight-for-age, weight-for-length, and head circumference-for-age. For the age interval 2 to 20 years, the charts give percentile curves for stature-for-age, weight-for-age, body mass index-for-age, and weight-for-stature. Figure 6.8 shows the body mass index-for-age chart for females ages 2 to 20 years. All of the growth charts developed by the CDC and recommended for use in assessing the growth and development of children from birth up to 20 years of age are shown in Appendix K. When using the birth-to-24-months charts, length is measured in the recumbent position (lying down). When using the charts for persons 2 to 20 years old, stature (height) should be measured with the person standing. The median difference between length and stature at 2 years of age is 0.3 in. or

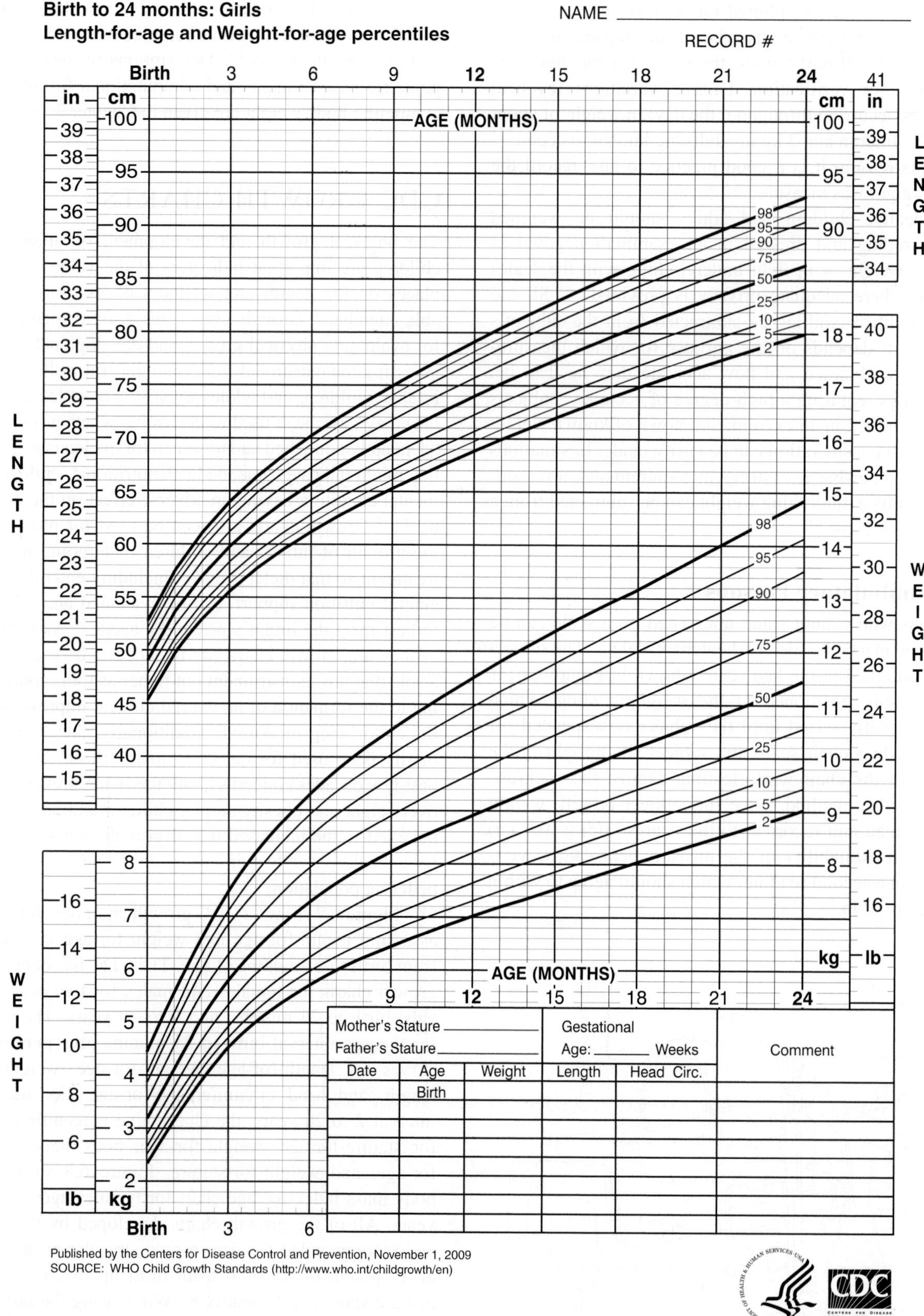

Figure 6.7
An example of a growth chart developed by the U.S. Centers for Disease Control and Prevention (CDC). This one assesses both length-for-age and weight-for-age in U.S. females from birth to 24 months. All of the growth charts recommended for use by the CDC are shown in Appendix K.

Source: U.S. Centers for Disease Control and Prevention. http://www.cdc.gov/growthcharts/

2 to 20 years: Girls
Body mass index-for-age percentiles

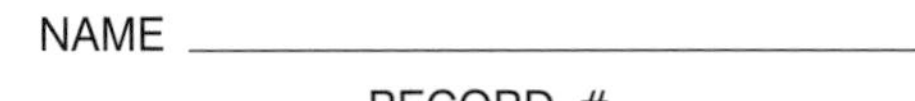

Date	Age	Weight	Stature	BMI*	Comments

***To Calculate BMI**: Weight (kg) ÷ Stature (cm) ÷ Stature (cm) x 10,000
or Weight (lb) ÷ Stature (in) ÷ Stature (in) x 703

BMI

35 34 33 32 31 30 29 28 27 26 25 24 23 22 21 20 19 18 17 16 15 14 13 12

95 90 85 75 50 25 10 5

kg/m² AGE (YEARS) kg/m²

2 3 4 5 6 7 8 9 10 11 12 13 14 15 16 17 18 19 20

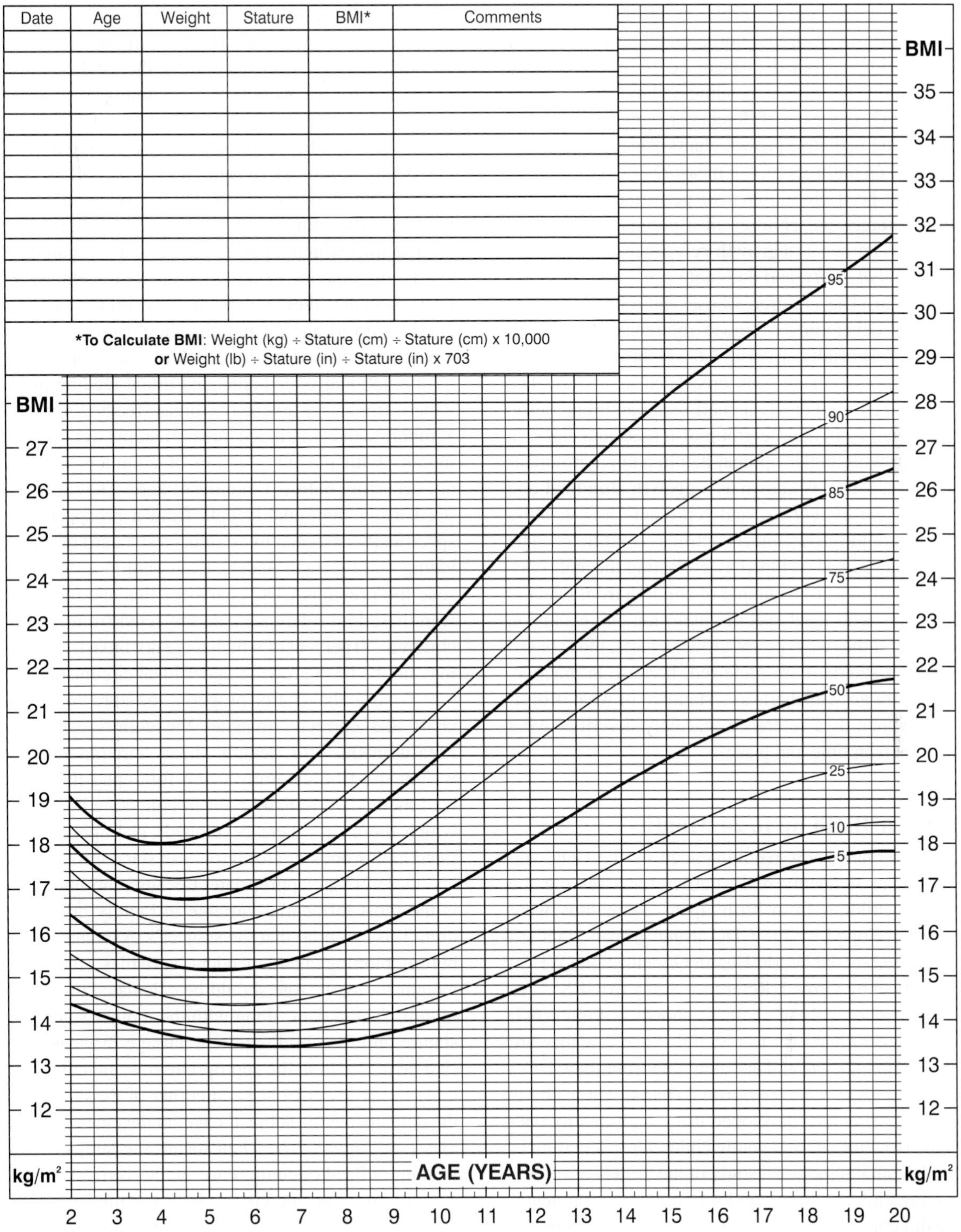

SOURCE: Developed by the National Center for Health Statistics in collaboration with the National Center for Chronic Disease Prevention and Health Promotion (2000).
http://www.cdc.gov/growthcharts

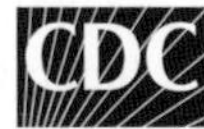

Figure 6.8
The body mass index-for-age growth charts developed by the CDC are an important advancement over the 1977 NCHS charts, which did not include BMI as an assessment variable. This chart is for females ages 2 to 20 years. The one for males is included in Appendix L.
Source: National Center for Health Statistics.

0.7–0.8 cm.[9] Head circumference, a variable included in the birth-to-24-months age charts, is omitted in the charts for those 2 to 20 years old.

Many users of growth charts assume that they represent an ideal or desirable norm, enabling clinicians to evaluate children for inadequate or excessive growth. But this may not be the case, depending on how the chart was developed. There are two different conceptual approaches to developing pediatric growth charts. One is to create a chart based on anthropometric measures (length, stature, weight, and head circumference) performed on a large group of infants and children in a particular place and time. This is known as a **growth reference** and describes *what is* or *what exists*, and does not necessarily represent what is ideal. The children whose anthropometric data are used in developing a growth reference may not all be healthy, especially in terms of weight or body mass index, or may not have been breast-fed as infants. The other approach is to create a chart using anthropometric data collected from a large group of infants and children who are growing under optimal health and environmental conditions. This is known as a **growth standard** and describes *what should be*, and represents how healthy children should grow under optimal conditions. The growth standard is developed by collecting the anthropometric data from a large number of children from selected communities who meet specific inclusion and exclusion criteria.[9,10] Of the two types of growth charts, those based on a growth standard are preferred, because in practice, clinicians use growth charts as a standard of what is optimal rather than as a reference that only describes what exists at a given time and place.

Charts for Birth up to 24 Months

The growth charts now recommended by the CDC and the American Academy of Pediatrics for assessing the growth of children from birth up to 24 months were recently developed by the CDC using growth standard data collected by the World Health Organization (WHO) in its Multicentre Growth Reference Study (MGRS).[9] An example of one of these charts is shown in Figure 6.7, while the other charts for use with this age category are shown in Appendix K and are available from the CDC's website (http://www.cdc.gov/growthcharts). These charts are a *growth standard* developed using high-quality data collected from infants and young children participating in the MGRS, an international study of the growth of infants and young children living under optimal environmental and health conditions. The study was conducted between 1997 and 2003 in six sites: Pelotas, Brazil; Accra, Ghana; Delhi, India; Oslo, Norway; Muscat, Oman; and Davis, California. Mothers, infants, and young children participating in the study had to meet strict inclusion and exclusion criteria. For example, mothers who smoked during pregnancy or lactation or who had a low socioeconomic status were excluded from the study. Infants born < 37 weeks of gestation or ≥ 42 weeks of gestation or who were part of a multiple delivery (when more than one fetus is carried to term in a single pregnancy) were excluded from the study.[9] The most important stipulation was that all infants participating in the MGRS were to be breast-fed for 12 months and predominantly breast-fed for at least 4 months (but preferably for 6 months) with complementary foods introduced by at least 6 months but not before 4 months of age. This is important because breast-feeding is the recommended standard for infant feeding and healthy breast-fed infants should be the standard against which all other infants are compared. These charts are superior to previous charts developed by the CDC because they represent how infants and young children up to age 24 months should grow under ideal environmental and health conditions and in accordance to internationally recommended infant feeding practices, which emphasize exclusive breast-feeding for at least 4 months and continued breast-feeding for at least 12 months with the introduction of complementary foods not occurring before 4 months of age.[9] They were developed using high-quality data from a prospective study specifically designed to establish a standard of infant and young child growth under ideal conditions. They supersede the previous CDC charts for this age range, which were based on reference data collected from infants and children, 50 percent of which were not breast-fed and who may not be been growing under ideal circumstances.[9–10]

To use the charts properly, be sure to select the chart that correctly matches the child's age and sex. Measurements for length, head circumference, and weight must be carefully taken following the standardized methods originally used in collecting the data from which the charts were developed. The approaches outlined in this book conform to those standardized methods and therefore are appropriate. Because chronological age is the most influential variable in rapidly growing children, it is essential that the subject's exact age be known before plotting age-dependent variables (for example, weight for age).[2] Age should be calculated to the nearest month.[2] These data, along with the mother's and father's stature and the child's gestational age in weeks, should first be recorded in the appropriate row and column in the table in the lower right-hand corner of the chart. To plot the data, locate the subject's age on the chart's horizontal axis (see Figure 6.7). Then locate the subject's length, weight, or head circumference on the vertical axis. Draw a small circle on the chart where the lines representing these two values intersect. Check to make sure that the circle you have drawn is at the correct point in reference to the two variables. A complete growth chart should include data that are both recorded numerically and plotted on the chart. If you plot the data while the subject is still present, you may repeat the measurements if unusual or changed values appear.[2] Variables on the chart, shown in Figure 6.7, are presented as nine percentile curves: 2, 5, 10, 25, 50, 75, 90, 95, and 98. A child's length for age, for example, would be considered average when, once it is plotted, it is on or near the 50th percentile curve. In other words, the 50th percentile is considered the average, or **median,** value for the specific population of interest. If the plotted length for age were on the 75th percentile curve, 75% of girls her age would be shorter than she is. If a child's height for age were at the 10th percentile, only 10% of children of the same age and sex would be shorter. Ranking persons this way is appropriate if they are part of the population from which the data were obtained. Values less than the 2nd percentile and greater than the 98th percentile warrant evaluation. If, over time, a subject's plotted values change markedly (i.e., cross two percentile lines), the reasons for that change should be investigated.

Charts for Ages 2 to 20 Years

The charts recommended for assessing growth in children and adolescents from age 2 up to 20 years were published in 2000 and developed by the CDC using *growth reference* data because high-quality growth standard data for this age range do not exist.[9] An example of one of these charts is shown in Figure 6.8, while the other charts for use with this age range are shown in Appendix K. These charts are based primarily on anthropometric measurements performed on nationally representative samples of infants, children, and adolescents during a series of national health examination surveys conducted by the CDC between 1963 and 1994. These include cycle II of the National Health Examination Survey (NHES) (1963–1965), cycle III of the NHES (1966–1970), the first National Health and Nutrition Examination Survey (NHANES I) (1971–1974), NHANES II (1976–1980), and NHANES III (1988–1994).[8]

There are some minor differences in how these charts are used, compared to the charts for children from birth up to 24 months of age. Stature (or standing height) is used instead of length, and head circumference is not used as a variable. The tables for recording this subject's anthropometric data and, when appropriate, the mother's and father's stature, are located in the upper left-hand corner of the charts. Another difference is in the number of percentile curves. In the stature-for-age and weight-for-age charts for both sexes, there are seven percentile curves: 5, 10, 25, 50, 75, 90, and 95. In the weight-for-stature charts for both sexes, there is an 85th percentile curve in addition to the other seven percentile curves. Values less than the 5th percentile and greater than the 95th percentile warrant evaluation, and if, over time, a subject's plotted values change markedly (i.e., cross two percentile lines), the reasons for that change should be investigated. The body mass index-for-age charts, an example of which is shown in Figure 6.8, also have an additional 85th percentile curve. As shown in Box 6.1, children and adolescents having a BMI-for-age

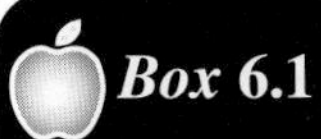

Box 6.1 Defining Overweight and Obesity in the Pediatric Population

The body mass index-for-age percentile charts developed by the CDC and published in 2000 should be used for classifying body mass index (BMI) in children and adolescents age 2 years of age and older, as shown below.[12–14] An example of the chart for females is shown in Figure 6.8 and the chart for males is in Appendix K. The charts are also available from the CDC's website (http://www.cdc.gov/growthcharts). Weight and stature should be carefully measured following the standardized methods outlined in this book, and recorded in the appropriate location in the table in the upper left-hand corner of the chart, along with the date and the subject's age to the nearest month. BMI should be accurately calculated to the nearest one-tenth (carried out one decimal point) and also recorded in the appropriate line of the table. Age should be plotted along the horizontal axis of the chart, and BMI should be plotted along the vertical axis. Draw a small circle on the chart where the lines representing these two values intersect. Check to make sure that the circle is at the correct point in reference to the two variables. A child or adolescent age 2 to 20 years having a BMI-for-age ≥ 85th percentile but <95th percentile is classified as "overweight," and a child or adolescent is classified as "obese" when the BMI-for-age is ≥ 95th percentile or the individual has a BMI ≥ 30 kg/m^2, whichever is smaller. Notice in Figure 6.8 that the 95th percentile curve exceeds a BMI of 30 kg/m^2 beginning at approximately 18 years of age. The BMI of an adolescent is classified as "obese" when it is ≥ 30 kg/m^2 even if it is less than the 95th percentile curve.[12–14]

Percentile Cut-Off Value	Classification of BMI
< 5th percentile	Underweight
≥ 5th and < 85th percentile	Healthy weight
≥ 85th and < 95th percentile	Overweight
≥ 95th percentile ***or*** ≥ 30 kg/m^2 (whichever is smaller)	Obese

≥ 85th percentile but < 95th percentile are classified as "overweight" and those having a BMI-for-age that is ≥ 95th percentile are classified as "obese."[12–14] In addition, an adolescent is considered obese when his or her BMI is ≥ 30 kg/m^2, even if the BMI-for-age percentile is less than the 95th percentile. For example, in adolescent females 18 to 20 years old (see Figure 6.8) and adolescent males 19 years old (see the BMI-for-age percentile chart in Appendix K), the 95th percentile exceeds a BMI of 30 kg/m^2.

Weight Standards

Technically speaking, **overweight** is defined as a body weight greater than some reference point of acceptable weight that usually is defined in relation to height. While it is possible for a highly muscular person to be overweight because of his or her muscle mass, in the vast majority of cases, particularly in developed countries such as the United States and Canada, people are overweight because their bodies contain an excess amount of body fat. **Obesity,** on the other hand, is technically defined as an excess amount of body fat in relation to lean body mass.[15] As will be discussed later in this chapter, determining the relative amounts of fat and lean tissue (i.e., body composition analysis) requires certain techniques. Body composition cannot be determined by simply measuring weight and height, for example, to calculate body mass index, or BMI (discussed later in this chapter), which is weight in kilograms divided by height in meters squared (BMI = kg ÷ m^2). However, because of the technical difficulties of body composition analysis and the ease by which weight and height can be measured and BMI can be calculated, clinicians often define overweight as a BMI ≥ 25 kg/m^2 but < 30 kg/m^2 and define obesity as a BMI ≥ 30 kg/m^2. Again, the assumption is that most people are overweight and obese because of excess body fat.

There is overwhelming scientific evidence that overweight and obese individuals, as a group, tend to die at a younger age compared to persons who are not overweight or obese.[16–20] Excess body fat is an important risk factor for type 2 diabetes, hypertension, coronary heart disease, certain types of cancer, osteoarthritis, and other health conditions. However, because excess body fat is only one of many factors influencing disease risk, it is difficult to estimate the extent to which excess body fat increases disease risk. Because disease risk is affected by factors other than excess body fat, such as cigarette smoking and physical inactivity, it is difficult to estimate the extent to which excess body fat increases disease risk. A recent study that pooled data from 57 different prospective studies with nearly 900,000 participants mostly from western Europe and North America showed that risk of death was lowest when BMI was approximately 22.5 kg/m^2 to 25.0 kg/m^2, which, according to this study, appears to be the optimal BMI range for adults.[16] Every additional 5 kg/m^2 of BMI greater than 25.0 kg/m^2 was associated with a 30% greater risk of death from all causes, a 40% greater risk of death from cardiovascular diseases, a 60% to 120% greater risk of death from diabetic, renal, and hepatic diseases, and a 10% increased risk of death from neoplastic diseases. Compared to those in the optimal BMI range, those whose BMI was in the 30.0 to 35.0 kg/m^2 range died two to four years earlier and those whose BMI was in the 40.0 to 45.0 kg/m^2 died eight to ten years earlier (which is comparable to the effects of cigarette smoking). Those having a BMI less than this optimal range of 22.5 to 25.0 kg/m^2 are also at increased risk of death compared to those whose BMI is in the optimal range, but much of the excess mortality seen in this group is primarily due to cigarette smoking.[16] This relationship between BMI and risk of death is illustrated in Figure 6.9.

A variety of approaches exist for determining a person's recommended (or "ideal") body weight range. Among these are the **Hamwi equations** which were first published in 1964 by George J. Hamwi, MD (1915–1967) who, at the time of his death, was Chief of the Division of Endocrinology and Metabolism, College of Medicine, The Ohio State University. For men, 106 lb are allowed

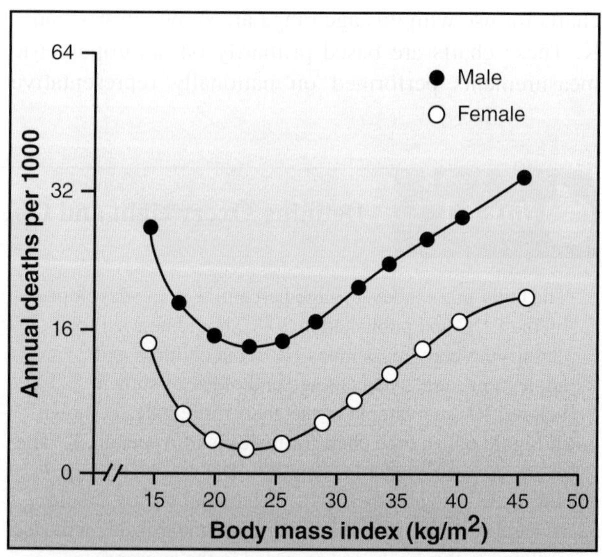

Figure 6.9 The relationship between body mass index (kg/m^2) and risk of death from all causes in males and females.

Risk of death is lowest when body mass index (BMI) is approximately 22.5 kg/m^2 to 25.0 kg/m^2 and for every 5 kg/m^2 greater BMI risk of death increases by 30%. Below 22.5 kg/m^2 risk of death increases, especially for smoking-related diseases such as respiratory diseases and lung cancer. The relationship between BMI and risk of death is referred to as "J-shaped" curve as illustrated in the figure.

Adapted from: Prospective Studies Collaboration. 2009. Body-mass index and cause-specific mortality in 900,000 adults: Collaborative analyses of 57 prospective studies. *Lancet* 373:1083-1096.

for the first 5 ft of stature and 6 lb are added for each additional inch over 5 ft. If the man is less than 5 ft tall, 6 lb are subtracted from the 106 lb for each inch under 5 ft. For women, 100 lb are allowed for the first 5 ft of stature and 5 lb are added for each additional inch over 5 ft. If the woman is less than 5 ft tall, 5 lb are subtracted from the 100 lb for each inch under 5 ft. This is then expressed as a range of plus or minus 10% to provide an allowance for the effects of frame size.

Men:

106 lb for the first 5 ft + 6 lb for each inch over 5 ft ± 10%

106 lb for the first 5 ft − 6 lb for each inch under 5 ft ± 10%

Women:

100 lb for the first 5 ft + 5 lb for each inch over 5 ft ± 10%

100 lb for the first 5 ft − 5 lb for each inch under 5 ft ± 10%

Consider, for example, a women who is 68 inches tall. Based on the Hamwi equation, her recommended body weight range would be 126 to 154 lb, which is 140 lb ± 10%.

Height-Weight Tables

Body weight can be assessed through the use of height-weight tables and the use of **relative weight** and **height-weight indices.** Height-weight tables are convenient, quick, easy to use, and understood by practically every adult. However, because of their limitations, they are obsolete and have been supplanted by better approaches, such as body mass index (kg/m^2).

The life insurance industry has been in the forefront of developing height-weight tables because of its access to the data necessary for generating them. The tables were developed by comparing the heights and weights of life insurance policyholders with statistical data (known as actuarial data) on mortality rates and/or longevity of policyholders. Actuarial data were compiled on literally millions of insured persons in the United States and Canada in an attempt to define weights associated with the greatest longevity and lowest mortality rates.[15,19,21] The insurance industry has used data from the tables to help screen applicants to avoid insuring persons who are poor risks. Good reviews of the topic have been published by Weigley,[21] Manson and coworkers.[22]

The Metropolitan Life Insurance Company published the Ideal Weight Tables in 1942 and 1943,[23,24] the Desirable Weight Tables in 1959,[25] and the Height-Weight Tables in 1983.[26] Table 6.1 is the 1983 Metropolitan Life table. Appendix L shows data for mean body weight, height, and body mass index for Americans as measured by national surveys conducted from 1960 to 2006.

Limitations of Height-Weight Tables

Height-weight tables have several limitations, which are summarized in Box 6.2.[19,22,27] Because tables are formulated from data drawn from specific groups or populations, they may not be applicable to other groups or populations. This is especially true of tables based on insurance industry data, which are derived from people who apply for life insurance—predominantly white, middle-class adults. African Americans, Asians, Native Americans, Hispanics, and low-income persons are not proportionally represented.[10]

The quality of the data on height and weight is variable. The same care in obtaining the NHANES data was not used in collecting data for the Metropolitan tables, where approximately 10% of the heights and weights were self-reported. Self-reporting of height and weight has been shown to be inaccurate, and the error is influenced by such factors as sex, actual height, and actual weight.[28–30] Rowland,[29] for example, showed that errors in self-reported weight were directly related to a person's

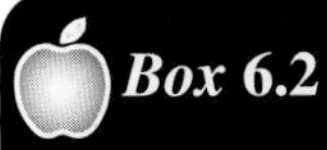

Box 6.2 Strengths and Limitations of Height-Weight Tables

STRENGTHS

Weight is an important distinguishing feature of identification

Weight and height can be accurately measured

Height-weight tables are easily understood by many

Height-weight tables are a part of our culture

LIMITATIONS

The data on which height-weight tables are based are not representative of the entire population

Quality of the data is variable

Some of the data are cross-sectional and do not allow associations between weight and mortality to be drawn

There is inadequate control of potentially confounding variables, especially smoking

It is not always clear how frame size was determined

Tables do not provide information on body composition

TABLE 6.1 Height-Weight Table for Persons Ages 25 to 59 Years (Height Without Shoes, Weight Without Clothing*)

Height		Small Frame		Medium Frame		Large Frame	
in.	cm	lb	kg	lb	kg	lb	kg
Men							
61	155	123–129	56–59	126–136	57–62	133–145	60–66
62	157	125–131	57–60	128–138	58–63	135–148	61–67
63	160	127–133	58–60	130–140	59–64	137–151	62–69
64	163	129–135	59–61	132–143	60–65	139–155	63–70
65	165	131–137	60–62	134–146	61–66	141–159	64–72
66	168	133–140	60–64	137–149	62–68	144–163	65–74
67	170	135–143	61–65	140–152	64–69	147–167	67–76
68	173	137–146	62–66	143–155	65–70	150–171	68–78
69	175	139–149	63–68	146–158	66–72	153–175	70–80
70	178	141–152	64–69	149–161	68–73	156–179	71–81
71	180	144–155	65–70	152–165	69–75	159–183	72–83
72	183	147–159	67–72	155–169	70–77	163–187	74–85
73	185	150–163	68–74	159–173	72–79	167–192	76–87
74	188	153–167	70–76	162–177	74–80	171–197	78–90
75	191	157–171	71–78	166–182	75–83	176–202	80–92
Women							
57	145	99–108	45–49	106–118	48–54	115–128	52–58
58	147	100–110	45–50	108–120	49–55	117–131	53–60
59	150	101–112	46–51	110–123	50–56	119–134	54–61
60	152	103–115	47–52	112–126	51–57	122–137	55–62
61	155	105–118	48–54	115–129	52–59	125–140	57–64
62	157	108–121	49–55	118–132	54–60	128–144	58–65
63	160	111–124	50–56	121–135	55–61	131–148	60–67
64	163	114–127	52–58	124–138	56–63	134–152	61–69
65	165	117–130	53–59	127–141	58–64	137–156	62–71
66	168	120–133	55–60	130–144	59–65	140–160	64–73
67	170	123–136	56–62	133–147	60–67	143–164	65–75
68	173	126–139	57–63	136–150	62–68	146–167	66–76
69	175	129–142	59–65	139–153	63–70	149–170	68–77
70	178	132–145	60–66	142–156	65–71	152–173	69–79
71	180	135–148	61–67	145–159	66–72	155–176	70–80

Adapted from 1983 Metropolitan Height and Weight Tables. 1983. *Statistical Bulletin of the Metropolitan Life Insurance Company* 64 (Jan.–June):3.

*Height without shoes obtained by subtracting 1 in. from heights with shoes for males and females. Weight without clothes obtained by subtracting 5 lb and 3 lb from weight with clothes for males and females, respectively.

overweight status and increased directly with the magnitude of overweight. The frequency of overreporting height increases with increasing height and is more common in males than females.[31]

There is often inadequate documentation and control of certain variables known to confound the relationships between weight and mortality.[22] Most important among these confounding variables is cigarette smoking. Smokers tend to weigh less than nonsmokers but have higher mortality rates because of smoking-related diseases. Including data on smokers in height-weight tables tends to make lower weights appear less healthy and higher weights appear more healthy.[32]

There have been problems associated with frame measurements.[27] The 1959 Metropolitan tables never defined how frame size was determined. The frame size measurements used in the 1983 Metropolitan tables are based on NHANES I and NHANES II data and are so devised that 25% of the population is classified as having a small frame, 50% as having a medium frame, and 25% as having a large frame. Within the range of body weights considered acceptable for a given height and sex, the lower end of the weight range was assumed to be for small-framed persons, the middle of the range for medium-framed persons, and the upper end of the range for large-framed persons. This practice may not be appropriate because data on height/weight and frame size were obtained from two distinct population groups.

The weight measurements used in compiling the data were only those taken when the subjects initially applied for life insurance.[27] If weight changed between issuance of the policy and death, this was not taken into account. Age also was not taken into account.

Finally, weight tables fail to provide information on actual body composition—the proportions of fat and lean tissue—or on the distribution of body fat. This is a critical weakness because the quantity of weight (a person's actual weight) is considerably less important than the quality of weight (how much of that weight is fat and how much is lean tissue). An unusually muscular person with a low body fat content (for example, a football player or weight lifter) may be overweight according to a height-weight table but not obese. Body composition can be estimated from measurements of skinfolds, densitometry (hydrostatic or underwater weighing), and other methods.

Strengths of Height-Weight Tables

Height-weight tables have some strengths. Body weight is an important concept, and next to age, sex, and race it is regarded as the most distinguishing feature of identification. Height and weight are easily measured, and most adults and many adolescents and children are able to understand and use height-weight tables.

Despite these strengths, height-weight tables are essentially obsolete. They have been replaced by body mass index (BMI), which is regarded as a better measure of adiposity.[19] A notable instance where BMI has replaced height-weight tables as the recommended approach for determining healthy weight is the *Dietary Guidelines for Americans,* as discussed in Chapter 2.

Measuring Frame Size

Several approaches to determining frame size have been proposed,[33,34] including biacromial breadth (distance between the tips of the biacromial processes at the top of the shoulders) and bitrochanteric breadth (distance between the most lateral projections of the greater trochanter of the two femurs),[33,35–37] the ratio of stature to wrist circumference;[38] breadth of the chest based on chest X rays,[39] knee and wrist breadth,[40] and elbow breadth.[41] The accessibility of the elbow and the ease by which elbow breadth can be measured makes it one of the most practical ways of determining frame size. The other methods are limited by such factors as lack of population norms, difficulty in obtaining measurements, and the influence of adiposity.[27,33]

When measuring elbow breadth, the subject stands erectly, with the right upper arm extended forward perpendicular to the body, as shown in Figure 6.10. The forearm is then flexed until the elbow forms a 90-degree angle, with fingers up, palm facing the subject. The measurer then should feel for the widest bony width of the elbow and place the heads of a flat-blade sliding caliper at those points. Pressure should be firm enough to compress soft tissues. The measurement should be read to the nearest 0.1 cm or 1/8 in.[35] Elbow breadth classifications for males and females of various stature are given in Table 6.2. Some data suggest that frame measurements do not materially improve the ability to predict body fat from body weight.[40,42] Other researchers suggest avoiding frame-adjusted tables because of the lack of data on the relationship of frame size to body weight.

The following formula can be used to determine frame size from the ratio of body height to wrist circumference,[38]

$$r = \frac{H}{C}$$

where r = the ratio of body height to wrist circumference; H = body height in centimeters; and C = circumference of the right wrist in centimeters. Compare the value for r with those in Table 6.3 to determine frame size.[38]

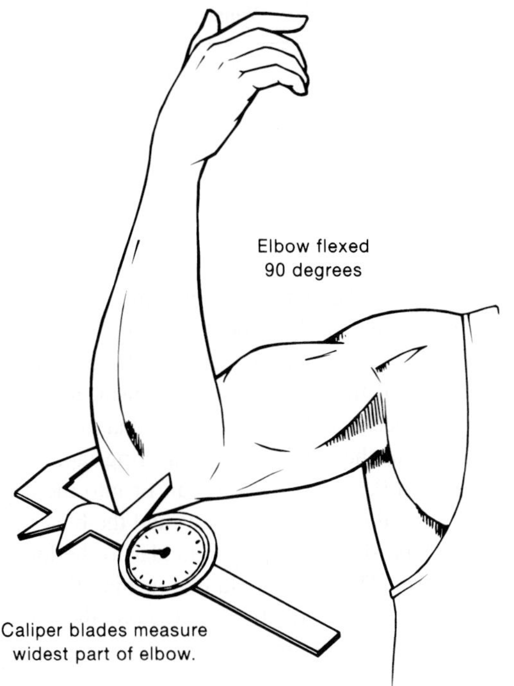

Figure 6.10
Elbow breadth is sometimes used for determining frame size. With the arm and hand in this position, a sliding caliper can be used to measure the widest point at the elbow.

TABLE 6.2 Elbow Breadth Classifications for Males and Females of Various Stature

Height*		Small Frame		Medium Frame		Large Frame	
in.	cm	in.	mm	in.	mm	in.	mm
Males							
61–62	155–158	< 2½	< 64	2½–2⅞	64–73	> 2⅞	> 73
63–66	159–168	< 2⅝	< 67	2⅝–2⅞	67–73	> 2⅞	> 73
67–70	169–178	< 2¾	< 70	2¾–3	70–76	> 3	> 76
71–74	179–188	2¾	< 70	2¾–3⅛	70–90	> 3⅛	> 79
≥ 75	≥ 189	< 2⅞	< 73	2⅞–3¼	73–83	> 3¼	> 83
Females							
57–58	145–148	< 2¼	< 57	2¼–2½	57–64	> 2½	> 64
59–62	149–158	< 2¼	< 57	2¼–2½	57–64	> 2½	> 64
63–66	159–168	< 2⅜	< 60	2⅜–2⅝	60–67	> 2⅝	> 67
67–70	169–178	< 2⅜	< 60	2⅜–2⅝	60–67	> 2⅝	> 67
≥ 71	≥ 79	< 2½	< 64	2½–2¾	64–70	> 2¾	> 70

Adapted from 1983 Metropolitan Height and Weight Tables. 1983. *Statistical Bulletin of the Metropolitan Life Insurance Company* 64 (Jan.–June):3.
*Table adapted to represent height without shoes.

TABLE 6.3 Determining Frame Size from the Ratio of Body Height to the Circumference of the Right Wrist

	r Value	
Frame Size	Women	Men
Small	> 10.9	> 10.4
Medium	10.9–9.9	10.4–9.6
Large	< 9.9	< 9.6

Adapted from Grant JP, Custer PB, Thurlow J. 1981. Current techniques of nutritional assessment. *Surgical Clinics of North America* 61:437–463.

To measure the right wrist circumference, the arm should be flexed at the elbow with the palm facing upward and the hand muscles relaxed. Place the measuring tape around the wrist crease just distal to (beyond) the styloid processes of the radius and ulna (the two bony prominences at the wrist). The measuring tape must be no wider than 0.7 cm, so that it can fit into the depressions between the styloid processes and the bones of the hand. The tape should be perpendicular to the long axis of the forearm. The tape should be touching the skin but not compressing the soft tissues. Record the measurement to the nearest 0.1 cm.[43]

HEIGHT-WEIGHT INDICES

In view of the shortcomings of height-weight tables, particularly their inability to provide information on actual body composition, investigators have sought better approaches to assessing body weight and fatness (or adiposity) that can be derived from easily obtainable anthropometric measures, such as weight and stature. This has led to the development of various height-weight indices or body mass indices which are shown in Table 6.4. An index is simply a ratio of one dimension (e.g., weight) to another dimension (e.g., height). The height-weight indices are of two types: relative weight and power-type indices.

Relative Weight

Relative weight is a person's *actual weight* divided by some *reference weight* for that person's height and multiplied by 100, so that it can be expressed as a percentage. Several approaches could be taken to arrive at a person's reference weight: the Hamwi equation, one of the height-weight tables discussed previously (e.g., the midpoint of the weight range for a person of medium frame from Table 6.1), the median weight for a given height and sex, the body weight for a given height and BMI, or the 50th percentile of weight-for-age or weight-for-stature using the CDC growth charts.

To calculate relative weight, take as an example a 19-year-old male who weighs 183 lb. Using the appropriate CDC growth chart in Appendix K (2 to 20 years: boys, stature-for-age and weight-for-age), the 50th percentile weight-for-age of a 19-year-old male would be 152 lb. The relative weight (RW) would be calculated as follows:

$$\frac{183 \text{ lb (actual weight)}}{152 \text{ lb (reference weight)}} \times 100 = 120\% \text{ RW}$$

Thus, this adolescent's relative weight (RW) is 120%, or his weight is 20% greater than the reference weight.

TABLE 6.4 Height-Weight Indices*

Relative weight:	$\frac{\text{Actual weight}}{\text{Reference weight}} \times 100$
Weight/height ratio:	$\frac{\text{Weight}}{\text{Height}}$
Quetelet's index:	$\frac{\text{Weight}}{\text{Height}^2}$
Khosla-Lowe index:	$\frac{\text{Weight}}{\text{Height}^3}$
Ponderal index:	$\frac{\text{Height}}{\text{Weight}^{1/3}}$
Benn's index:†	$\frac{\text{Weight}}{\text{Height}^p}$

Data from Lee J, Kolonel LN, Hinds MW. 1981. Relative merits of the weight-corrected-for-height indices. *American Journal of Clinical Nutrition* 34:2521–2529.

*The numerical values of the indices depend on the values used (for example, kilograms and meters or pounds and inches).

†"p" is a population-specific exponent derived from height-weight data of the population sample. Consequently, its value changes from sample to sample.

Depending as it does on some approach for determining reference weight, relative weight is subject to the same limitations as the approach used to determine reference weight. A relative weight within the range of 90% to 120% is generally considered acceptable.

Power-Type Indices

As shown in Table 6.4, several power-type indices are available for assessing body weight relative to height.[44–47] The preferred index should be maximally correlated with body mass (weight) and should be minimally correlated with stature. In other words, it should be equally good at indicating body mass, no matter how tall or short a person is. Of those indices shown in Table 6.4, there is general agreement among researchers and expert panels that Quetelet's index is preferred for assessing the body weight of children, adolescents, and adults.[19,48–50]

The most widely used height-weight index is the **Quetelet's index** (W/H^2), which is more commonly known as **body mass index (BMI).**[19,48–51] Because all the power-type indices are body mass indices, the more technically correct name for W/H^2 is Quetelet's index. Quetelet's index is obtained by dividing weight in kilograms by height in meters squared. Consider a male weighing 70 kg (154 lb) and standing 178 cm, or 1.78 m, (70 in.) tall. His body mass index would be

$$\frac{70 \text{ kg (weight in kilograms)}}{3.17 \text{ m}^2 \text{ (height in meters squared)}} = 22 \text{ kg/m}^2$$

Body mass index has a relatively high correlation with estimates of body fatness and a low correlation with stature.[48] Garrow and Webster,[47] for example, showed that Quetelet's index correlated well with estimates of body composition from three methods—body density, total body water, and total body potassium—and concluded that Quetelet's index "is both a convenient and reliable indicator of obesity." The National Institutes of Health[19] has recommended that physicians use Quetelet's index in evaluating patients. Many scientists consider Quetelet's index to be an appropriate way to assess body weight in children and adolescents.[52–55] Roche and coworkers[56] have found Quetelet's index to be the best single indicator of total body fat in girls and adults and the best single indicator of percent body fat in men. Of the other height-weight indices shown in Table 6.4, Quetelet's index has shown the closest correlation with estimates of body fatness by skinfold measurements and densitometry.[57,58]

Frisancho and Flegel[59] have shown Quetelet's index to correlate well with estimates of body fatness based on skinfold measurements, and they recommend combining Quetelet's index with skinfold measurements whenever possible. Investigators have suggested combining Quetelet's index with the rather easily obtained waist circumference as an improved means of assessing increased risk in adults for heart disease, stroke, type 2 diabetes, and premature death.[19,48,60,61]

A **nomogram** for determining Quetelet's index is shown in Figure 6.11. To use the nomogram, place

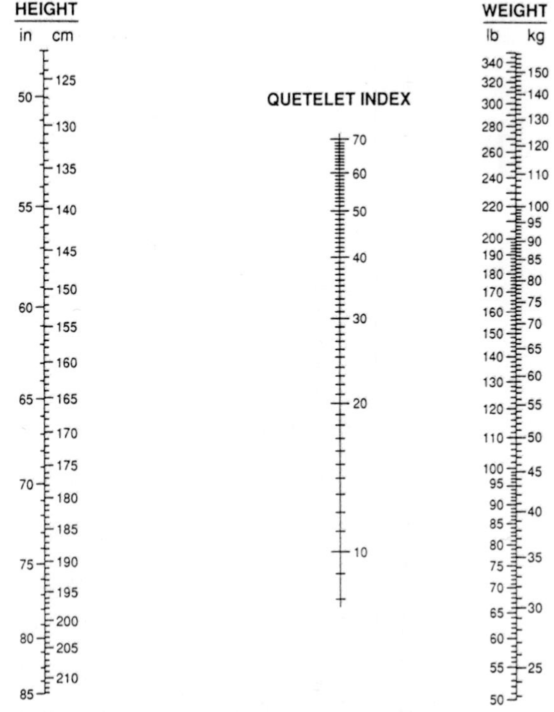

Figure 6.11

The Quetelet index (kg/m^2) is calculated from this nomogram by placing a straightedge on the measurements for height and body weight and reading the point at which the straightedge intersects the central scale.

Source: Adapted with permission from Nieman DC. 2003. *Exercise testing and prescription: A health-related approach,* 5th ed. Boston: McGraw-Hill Higher Education.

Table 6.5 Body Mass Index Table

To determine your BMI, first find your height (in inches without shoes) in the column at the far left of the table. Then, moving to the right along the row that represents your height, locate your weight in pounds. The number at the top of that column is the BMI for your height and weight.

	Healthy Weight						Overweight					Obese											Very Obese													
BMI	19	20	21	22	23	24	25	26	27	28	29	30	31	32	33	34	35	36	37	38	39	40	41	42	43	44	45	46	47	48	49	50	51	52	53	54
Height (in)	Body Weight (lb)																																			
58	91	96	100	105	110	115	119	124	129	134	138	143	148	153	158	162	167	172	177	181	186	191	196	201	205	210	215	220	224	229	234	239	244	248	253	258
59	94	99	104	109	114	119	124	128	133	138	143	148	153	158	163	168	173	178	183	188	193	198	203	208	212	217	222	227	232	237	242	247	252	257	262	267
60	97	102	107	112	118	123	128	133	138	143	148	153	158	163	168	174	179	184	189	194	199	204	209	215	220	225	230	235	240	245	250	255	261	266	271	276
61	100	106	111	116	122	127	132	137	143	148	153	158	164	169	174	180	185	190	195	201	206	211	217	222	227	232	238	243	248	254	259	264	269	275	280	285
62	104	109	115	120	126	131	136	142	147	153	158	164	169	175	180	186	191	196	202	207	213	218	224	229	235	240	246	251	256	262	267	273	278	284	289	295
63	107	113	118	124	130	135	141	146	152	158	163	169	175	180	186	191	197	203	208	214	220	225	231	237	242	248	254	259	265	270	278	282	287	293	299	304
64	110	116	122	128	134	140	145	151	157	163	169	174	180	186	192	197	204	209	215	221	227	232	238	244	250	256	262	267	273	279	285	291	296	302	308	314
65	114	120	126	132	138	144	150	156	162	168	174	180	186	192	198	204	210	216	222	228	234	240	246	252	258	264	270	276	282	288	294	300	306	312	318	324
66	118	124	130	136	142	148	155	161	167	173	179	186	192	198	204	210	216	223	229	235	241	247	253	260	266	272	278	284	291	297	303	309	315	322	328	334
67	121	127	134	140	146	153	159	166	172	178	185	191	198	204	211	217	223	230	236	242	249	255	261	268	274	280	287	293	299	306	312	319	325	331	338	344
68	125	131	138	144	151	158	164	171	177	184	190	197	203	210	216	223	230	236	243	249	256	262	269	276	282	289	295	302	308	315	322	328	335	341	348	354
69	128	135	142	149	155	162	169	176	182	189	196	203	209	216	223	230	236	243	250	257	263	270	277	284	291	297	304	311	318	324	331	338	345	351	358	365
70	132	139	146	153	160	167	174	181	188	195	202	209	216	222	229	236	243	250	257	264	271	278	285	292	299	306	313	320	327	334	341	348	355	362	369	376
71	136	143	150	157	165	172	179	186	193	200	208	215	222	229	236	243	250	257	265	272	279	286	293	301	308	315	322	329	338	343	351	358	365	372	379	386
72	140	147	154	162	169	177	184	191	199	206	213	221	228	235	242	250	258	265	272	279	287	294	302	309	316	324	331	338	346	353	361	368	375	383	390	397
73	144	151	159	166	174	182	189	197	204	212	219	227	235	242	250	257	265	272	280	288	295	302	310	318	325	333	340	348	355	363	371	378	386	393	401	408
74	148	155	163	171	179	186	194	202	210	218	225	233	241	249	256	264	272	280	287	295	303	311	319	326	334	342	350	358	365	373	381	389	396	404	412	420
75	152	160	168	176	184	192	200	208	216	224	232	240	248	256	264	272	279	287	295	303	311	319	327	335	343	351	359	367	375	383	391	399	407	415	423	431
76	156	164	172	180	189	197	205	213	221	230	238	246	254	263	271	279	287	295	304	312	320	328	336	344	353	361	369	377	385	394	402	410	418	426	435	443

a straightedge on the point of the height scale that corresponds to height in centimeters or inches and on the point of the weight scale that corresponds to weight in kilograms or pounds. Then read the Quetelet's index on the center scale. Use nomograms with caution. In some publications, nomograms may be inadvertently modified and thus rendered inaccurate.[62] This occurred in two highly respected reports: *The Surgeon General's Report on Nutrition and Health* and the National Research Council's *Diet and Health.* BMI can also be determined using Table 6.5.

Table 6.6 shows classifications of overweight and obesity and associated disease risk based on Quetelet's index (BMI) and waist circumference in adults. In Table 6.6, it should be noted that even in persons with a "normal" BMI, increased waist circumference can be a marker for increased risk of type 2 diabetes, hypertension, and cardiovascular disease.[60] There is no standard approach for using anthropometric measures to assess regional fat distribution in children. Consequently, use of waist circumference in conjunction with BMI is not recommended for children at this time.[49] The recommended approach for use of BMI for evaluating body weight in children and adolescents is use of the BMI-for-age growth charts developed by the CDC, discussed in the section "CDC Growth Charts" and in Box 6.1.

As BMI increases above approximately 25.0 kg/m^2, there is a gradual increase in risk of morbidity from such conditions as type 2 diabetes, hypertension, coronary heart disease, stroke, gallbladder disease, osteoarthritis, sleep apnea and other respiratory problems, and some types of cancer (prostate, colon, endometrial, and breast).[48,60] However, risk of morbidity and mortality from these conditions increases precipitously when BMI is greater than 30.0 kg/m^2. This observation resulted in *overweight* being defined as having a BMI of 25.0 to 29.9 kg/m^2 and in *obesity* being defined as a BMI of 30.0 kg/m^2 or greater.

Based on data from NHANES III, for example, the prevalence of hypertension in adults with a BMI < 25 kg/m^2 is 18.2% and 16.5% for males and females, respectively. At a BMI ≥ 30 kg/m^2, the prevalence of hypertension is 38.4% and 32.2% in males and females, respectively.[60] Data from the Nurses' Health Study show that risk for colon cancer is twice as high in women with a BMI > 29 kg/m^2 than in women with a BMI < 21 kg/m^2.[63] Data from the Women's Health Study showed that risk of type 2 diabetes in women increases as BMI increases.[18] This ongoing cohort study of nearly 40,000 female health professionals aged 45 years and older began in 1992 and relies on self-reported data on height, weight, sociodemographics, health habits, and medical history, all obtained using a questionnaire periodically completed by participants. Compared with women with a self-reported BMI of less than 25 kg/m^2, risk of type 2 diabetes is increased threefold in women having a BMI of 25 kg/m^2 to less than 30 kg/m^2 and is increased ninefold among women having a BMI of 30 kg/m^2 or greater.[18] This observed increase in morbidity and mortality with increased BMI is seen across all population groups. However, the specific degree of increased risk associated with any given level of overweight varies with race/ethnicity, age, gender, societal condition, physical activity, and family history of disease or presence of other disease risk factors. Consequently, the classifications of overweight and obesity and associated disease risks shown in Table 6.6 are approximations based on the best available data and are influenced by a variety of factors, which must be carefully considered by the clinician.[60]

How do the BMIs of American adults compare with these standards and how have they changed since the early 1960s? Figure 6.12 shows how the percent of American

Table 6.6 Classification of Overweight and Obesity by Body Mass Index (BMI), Waist Circumference, and Associated Disease Risk* in Adults

			Disease Risk* Relative to Normal Weight and Waist Circumference	
	BMI (kg/m^2)	Obesity Class	Men ≤ 40 in. (≤ 102 cm); Women ≤ 35 in. (≤ 88 cm)	Men > 40 in. (> 102 cm); Women > 35 in. (> 88 cm)
Underweight	< 18.5		—	—
Normal †	18.5–24.9		—	—
Overweight	25.0–29.9		Increased	High
Obesity	30.0–34.9	I	High	Very high
	35.0–39.9	II	Very high	Very high
Extreme obesity	≥ 40.0	III	Extremely high	Extremely high

Adapted from National Heart, Lung, and Blood Institute. 1998. *Clinical guidelines on the identification, evaluation, and treatment of overweight and obesity in adults.* Washington, DC: National Institutes of Health, U.S. Department of Health and Human Services.

* Disease risk for type 2 diabetes, hypertension, and cardiovascular disease.

† Increased waist circumference can also be a marker for increased risk even in persons of normal weight.

men and women with a BMI $\geq$ 25.0 kg/m^2 (includes both overweight and obese adults) and those with a BMI $\geq$ 30 kg/m^2 (obese adults) have changed between 1960 and 2010, based on measured weight and height collected by seven nationally representative surveys: the first National Health Examination Survey (NHES I), the first National Health and Nutrition Examination Survey (NHANES I), NHANES II, NHANES III, NHANES 1999–2002, NHANES 2003–2006, and NHANES 2007–2010. As shown in Figure 6.12, between 1960 and 1980 the percent of American men and women classified as obese (having a BMI $\geq$ 30.0 kg/m^2) remained relatively stable but then increased dramatically. For men the increase was nearly three-fold and for women it was two-fold. In recent years, the increase in the percent of American adults who are obese has slowed considerably, especially for women.

Figure 6.13 shows how the percent of obese American children and adolescents ages 2 to 5 years, 6 to 11 years, and 12 to 19 years changed between 1963 and 2010. These percentages are based on data from seven nationally representative surveys, NHES cycles II and III, NHANES I, NHANES II, NHANES III, NHANES 1999–2002, NHANES 2003–2006, and NHANES 2007–2010. During the first three surveys there were no obesity data for children 2 to 5 years of age. As outlined in Box 6.1, a BMI-for-age $\geq$ 95th percentile or a BMI $\geq$ 30 kg/m^2 (whichever is smaller) is used to define obesity in children and adolescents, which is associated with a significant likelihood of persistence of obesity into adulthood.[8,13,14,49] A BMI-for-age $\geq$ 95th percentile or a BMI $\geq$ 30 kg/m^2 is associated with elevated blood pressure and lipid and lipoprotein profiles that increase the risk for obesity-related disease and mortality. Pediatric obesity experts recommend that these children and adolescents have an in-depth medical assessment and possibly undergo treatment for weight loss.[14,49]

In most situations, people having a high BMI have a large amount of total body fat. However, BMI has limitations and in some instances is not a reliable indicator of total body fat.[60] For example, BMI overestimates total body fat in persons who are very muscular or who have clinically evident edema, and it underestimates body fat in persons who have lost muscle mass such as the frail and elderly. However, because of the ease of measuring weight and height and the ready availability of weight and height data, BMI is frequently used as a surrogate approach and is recommended as a practical approach for assessing body fat in the clinical setting.

Definitive measurement of body fat content requires using techniques that are expensive and/or often not readily available to most clinicians, such as skinfold measurements, underwater weighing, air displacement plethysmography, and bioelectrical impedance analysis. These measurement techniques and the concept of body composition are discussed in the next sections.

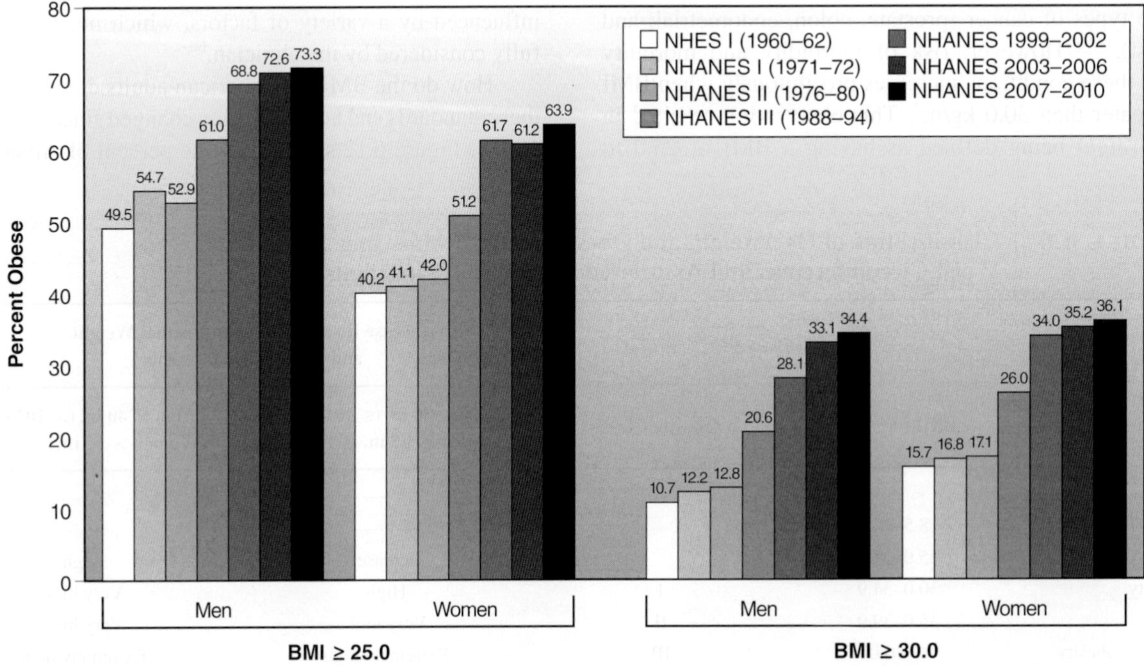

Figure 6.12 **Change in the percent of American men and women (20 to 74 years of age) with a BMI $\geq$ 25 kg/m^2 (includes both overweight and obese individuals) and those with BMI $\geq$ 30 kg/m^2 (obese individuals) between 1960 and 2010.**

Source: Data from the National Center for Health Statistics, http://www.cdc.gov/nchs/hus.htm.

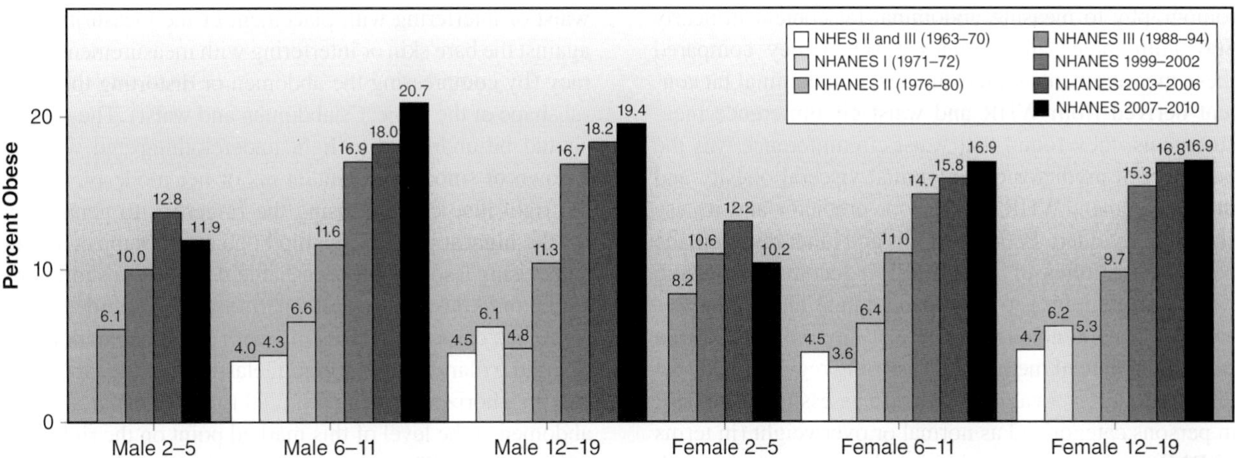

Figure 6.13 **Change in the percent of American children (2 to 5 years of age and 6 to 11 years of age) and adolescents (12 to 19 years of age) classified as obese between 1963 and 2010.**
Obese is defined as a BMI-for-age ≥ 95th percentile of BMI-for-age and sex using the CDC growth charts. Prior to NHANES III (1988–1994) there were no obesity data for children 2 to 5 years of age.
Source: Data from the National Center for Health Statistics, http://www.cdc.gov/nchs/hus.htm.

Body Fat Distribution

Body fat distribution is an important concept when considering the health implications of obesity.[15,19,60] Where fat is placed, or distributed, within the body may actually be more important than quantity of body fat. Body fat distribution can be classified into two types: (1) upper body, android, or male type, and (2) lower body, gynoid, or female type.[19] Obese persons having a greater proportion of fat within the upper body, especially within the abdomen, compared with that within the hips and thighs, have **android obesity.** Obese persons with most of their fat within the hips and thighs have **gynoid obesity.** Android obesity is generally (but not always) seen in obese males, whereas females generally carry a greater proportion of their body fat on the hips and thighs.[19]

Numerous studies have shown that risk for insulin resistance, hyperinsulinemia (elevated blood insulin levels), prediabetes (impaired glucose tolerance), type 2 diabetes mellitus, hypertension, hyperlipidemia (elevated blood cholesterol and triglyceride levels), and stroke, as well as risk for death are increased in persons with android obesity.[60,65,66] Although the approaches used to assess fat distribution varied somewhat among these studies, they consistently showed that disease risk is associated with upper-body placement of body fat.[19,60,65–67] They also showed that fat distribution is a more important risk factor for morbidity and mortality than is obesity per se.[19,68] In obese adolescent females, android obesity tends to be associated with elevated levels of triglyceride, serum cholesterol, and low-density lipoprotein (LDL) cholesterol. Android obesity in adolescent males tends to be associated with lower levels of high-density lipoprotein (HDL) cholesterol, a higher ratio of total cholesterol to HDL cholesterol, and higher levels of LDL cholesterol.[69]

Total abdominal fat has been described as the sum of the fat, or adipose tissue, present in three compartments of the body's abdominal region: subcutaneous (just under the skin), visceral (surrounding the organs within the peritoneal cavity), and retroperitoneal (outside of and posterior to the peritoneal cavity). Research suggests that excessive fat in the visceral compartment is most strongly correlated with increased risk for morbidity and mortality; however, this is a matter of debate and remains to be determined. What is certain is that the presence of increased total abdominal fat is an independent risk predictor, even when BMI is not markedly increased.[60,70] Total abdominal fat can be most accurately measured using magnetic resonance imaging or computed tomography. However, these approaches are expensive and not readily available in the clinical setting. Two other approaches for assessing total abdominal fat that are relatively easy to perform in the clinical setting are the waist-to-hip ratio and waist circumference. The waist-to-hip ratio (WHR) is calculated by dividing the waist circumference by the hip (or gluteal) circumference. Because of the increased risk for hypertension, prediabetes, type 2 diabetes, and hyperlipidemia associated with increased abdominal fat and the lower risks associated with fat placement in the hips and thighs, it is preferred that the waist circumference be less than the hip circumference, and consequently the WHR be somewhat less than 1. Some authorities recommend that the WHR be < 0.9 and < 0.8 for adult males and females, respectively, and that when WHR is greater than these cutpoints the risk for disease rises steeply.[15] In recent years, researchers have shown that waist circumference is actually a better predictor of total abdominal fat content than the WHR and a better predictor of disease risk.[60,65,71–73] For example, a team of Canadian researchers used computed tomography to measure abdominal fat content in nearly 800 adult males and females.[71] When they compared these measurements with estimates of abdominal fat content derived from WHR and waist circumference measurements, they found that waist circumference was the best overall predictor of abdominal visceral obesity and that, in women, WHR was a poor predictor and its use should be avoided. Because of this and other research, the National Institutes of Health (NIH) recommends using waist circumference to assess abdominal fat content.[60,70] The NIH has concluded that waist circumference is an easy and practical method for assessing regional body fat distribution. It is a valuable guide in assessing health risk in persons categorized as normal or overweight (in terms of BMI) and provides an independent prediction of risk over and above that of BMI.[60,70] Waist circumference has been shown to be positively correlated with the amount of fat within the abdomen and to serve as a good indicator of abdominal visceral obesity.[71]

Figure 6.14 illustrates how waist circumference is measured in adults.[60,70] Ask the subject to remove any outer clothing restricting easy access to the abdomen and waist or interfering with placement of the measuring tape against the bare skin or interfering with measurement accuracy (by compressing the abdomen or distorting the natural shape of the subject's abdomen and waist). The subject should be undressed to light underclothing and wearing a gown or smock to maintain his or her modesty. Locate the right iliac crest by using the fingertips to gently feel for the highest point of the hip bone on the subject's right side. Using a soft-tipped, washable pen, draw a short horizontal mark just above the uppermost lateral border of the right iliac crest. Then cross this with a vertical mark along the midaxillary line. Place an inelastic, flexible tape measure in a horizontal plane (parallel to the floor) around the abdomen at the level of this marked point on the right side of the subject. The subject should stand erectly, abdominal muscles relaxed, arms at the side, and feet together. The tape should be snug against the skin but not so tight as to compress the skin. Take the reading at the end of a normal expiration. Repeat the measurement once or twice to ensure that an accurate measurement has been obtained and record the measurement to the nearest 0.1 cm.

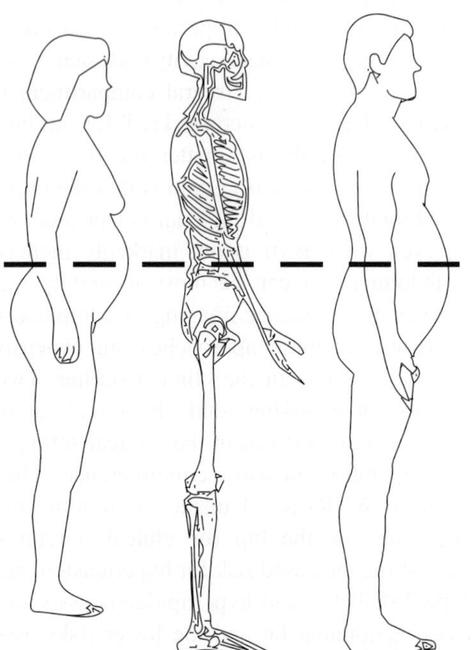

Figure 6.14
To measure waist circumference in adults, locate the top of the right iliac crest, the highest point of the hip bone on the right side. Place a measuring tape in a horizontal plane (parallel to the floor) around the abdomen at the level of the iliac crest. The tape should be snug but should not compress the skin. Take the reading at the end of a normal expiration. Repeat the measurement to ensure accuracy.

Source: National Heart, Lung, and Blood Institute. 1998. *The practical guide: Identification, evaluation, and treatment of overweight and obesity in adults.* Washington, DC: National Institutes of Health, U.S. Department of Health and Human Services.

As shown in Table 6.7, a "high-risk" waist circumference in adults is defined as > 40 in. (> 102 cm) in males and > 35 in. (> 88 cm) in females.[60,70] In addition to being used in the initial assessment of body weight and risk for disease, waist circumference is also useful for evaluating the success of weight loss treatment. Note that waist circumference has little predictive value in subjects having a BMI ≥ 35 kg/m^2 and that, in these persons, waist circumference does not need to be measured. Also, the cutpoints in Table 6.7 may not be applicable to persons whose height is < 60 in. (< 152 cm). The waist circumference cutpoints shown in Table 6.7 generally apply to all adult racial and ethnic groups in North America, although there are ethnic and age-related differences in regional body fat distribution that may influence the accuracy of waist circumference as a surrogate measure of abdominal fat content. For example, waist circumference is a better predictor of disease risk than is BMI for persons of Asian descent. In older persons, waist circumference is more valuable at estimating obesity-related disease risk.[60,70]

Body Composition

Interest in human body composition has increased over the past several decades, primarily because obesity has been associated with such diseases as diabetes

Table 6.7 **High-Risk Waist Circumferences for Adult Males and Females**

Males	> 40 in. (> 102 cm)
Females	> 35 in. (> 88 cm)

Source: National Institutes of Health.

mellitus, hypertension, and coronary heart disease.[16–18,74–76] Overweight is one of the most prevalent diet-related problems in the United States. As shown in Figures 6.12 and 6.13, the prevalence of obesity in the United States has markedly increased. Globally, the prevalence of obesity varies widely, from less than 5% in Japan and Korea to more than 33% in Chile and Mexico. Canada, the United Kingdom, Australia, and New Zealand have rates of approximately 25%.[77] Globally, the prevalence of obesity is increasing, as is the prevalence of obesity-linked diseases, such as type 2 diabetes, hypertension, and coronary heart disease.

Measurements of body fat are important in studying the nature of obesity and the obese person's response to treatment. As previously mentioned, the percent of body fat, as well as its placement, can have profound effects on health.

Estimating fat and protein reserves is a common practice in assessing a patient's nutritional status. During nutritional deprivation, these stores are depleted, leading to increased morbidity and mortality, caused at least in part by nutrition-related impairment of the body's immune system.[78,79] Simple techniques to screen fat and protein reserves of patients are critical in the light of reports that malnutrition is seen in as many as half of all hospitalized patients in the United States, Canada, and other industrialized countries.[80–82]

Body composition can be an important factor in certain athletic events. For example, carrying excess fat can be detrimental to the performance of runners and gymnasts. Body composition measurements can help these athletes maintain body fat at levels that are neither too high nor too low.[4] Too low a percent body fat can adversely affect metabolism and health. Female athletes will experience oligomenorrhea (abnormally infrequent menstruation) and amenorrhea (absence or abnormal cessation of menstruation) when their percent body fat is too low. This, in turn, can result in bone demineralization and increased risk of osteoporosis and bone fractures. Inadequate body fat may indicate disease, starvation, or an eating disorder, such as anorexia nervosa.

The perspective that the body consists of two chemically distinct compartments forms the model on which most body composition methods are based.[83,84] In the two-compartment model, the body can be divided into fat mass and fat-free mass, or, according to an alternative approach, into adipose tissue and lean body mass. In the former view, developed by Keys and Brozek,[85] the fat mass includes all the solvent-extractable lipids contained in both adipose tissue and other tissues, and the residual is the fat-free mass. The fat-free mass is composed of muscle, water, bone, and other tissues devoid of fat and lipid. For example, the solvent ether could be used to extract all the fat and lipid from a minced animal carcass. That remaining after all the fat and lipid were extracted would be the fat-free mass. The lean body mass of the latter approach is similar to the fat-free mass except that lean body mass includes a small amount of lipid that our bodies must have—for example, lipid that serves as a structural component of cell membranes or lipid contained in the nervous system.[86] This essential lipid constitutes about 1.5% to 3% of the weight of the lean body.

Body composition often is defined as the *ratio of fat to fat-free mass* and frequently is expressed as a percentage of body fat. Adipose tissue contains about 14% water, is nearly 100% free of the electrolyte potassium, and is assumed to have a density of 0.90 g/cm^3.[4,83] The less homogenous *fat-free compartment* is primarily composed of bone, muscle, other fat-free tissue, and body water. Its chemical composition is assumed to be relatively constant, with a water content of 72% to 74%, a potassium content of 60 to 70 mmol/kg in males and 50 to 60 mmol/kg in females, and a density of 1.10 g/cm^3 at normal body temperature.[83] However, several factors can affect the density of the fat-free compartment. Among these are age (the fat-free compartment in children is less dense than that of middle-aged persons, and bone density is decreased in elderly persons, especially those with osteoporosis), the degree of fitness (athletes have denser bone and muscle), and the body's state of hydration.[4] The use of anthropometry (measures of skinfold thicknesses, bone dimensions, and limb circumferences), determination of whole-body density (most commonly by underwater weighing), electrical conductance and impedance, and other methods to estimate body composition are based on the two-compartment model.[83]

An alternative approach to the two-compartment model is the four-compartment model, which views the human body as composed of four chemical groups: water, protein, mineral, and fat.[83] Methods for estimating body composition based on the four-compartment model include neutron activation analysis, isotope dilution techniques, bioelectrical impedance, total body electrical conductivity, and absorptiometry.[83]

A variety of methods exist for estimating body composition, and each has its strengths and limitations. Except for cadaveric studies, all of the following techniques are *indirect* measures.

CADAVERIC STUDIES

Only by analyzing cadavers can direct measurement of human body composition be made.[4] The most comprehensive direct study of body composition was the Brussels Cadaver Analysis Study (CAS), in which more than 30 cadavers were studied from 1979 to 1983.[87] The CAS helped validate various in vivo methods for estimating body composition and collected data for developing new anthropometric models for determining body composition.[87] Recumbent length, hydrostatic (underwater) weight, numerous girths and breadths, and skin surface area were measured. Skinfolds were measured at 14 standard sites. The skin and subcutaneous tissue then were cut open and carefully measured, so that skinfold measurements could be directly compared with measurements of skin and subcutaneous adipose tissue thickness. The skin, adipose tissue, skeletal muscle, bone, and viscera were dissected out and weighed in air and under water to determine density of the organs and tissues. The CAS allowed examination of several assumptions underlying the use of skinfold measurements and hydrostatic weighing to determine body composition. A major assumption of the CAS was that anthropometric measures and body composition in cadavers are similar to those of living subjects.[87,88]

Skinfold Measurements

The most widely used method of indirectly estimating percent body fat in clinical settings is to measure skinfolds—the thickness of a double fold of skin and compressed subcutaneous adipose tissue (Figure 6.15).[5,88] Although more accurate methods for assessing percent body fat exist, skinfold measurement has these advantages: the equipment needed is inexpensive and requires little space; measurements are easily and quickly obtained; and, when correctly done, skinfold measurement provides estimates of body composition that correlate well with those derived from hydrostatic weighing, the most widely used laboratory method for determining body composition.

Assumptions in Using Skinfold Measurements

Estimating body fat from skinfold thickness measurements involves several assumptions, outlined in Box 6.3,

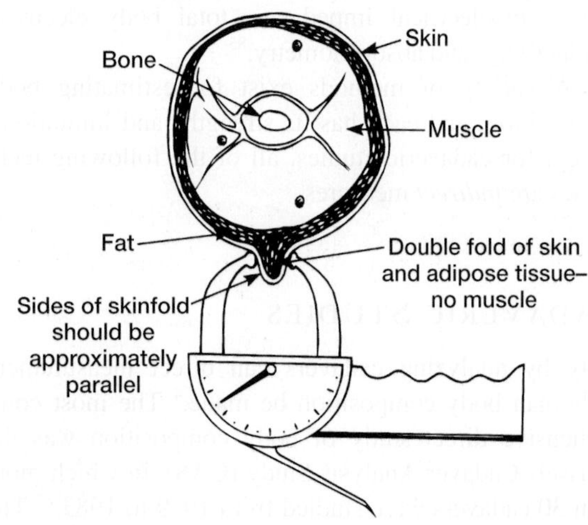

Figure 6.15
The double fold of skin and adipose tissue between the tips of the skinfold caliper should be large enough to form approximately parallel sides. Care should be taken to elevate only skin and adipose tissue, not muscle.

that may not always hold true.[88] When a caliper is initially applied to a skinfold, the caliper reading decreases as its tips compress the fold of skin and subcutaneous adipose tissue. Thus, it is recommended to read the caliper dial about 4 seconds after the caliper tips have been applied to the skinfold.[89] Research has shown significant differences in skinfold compressibility at a particular site among individuals (interindividual variation) and at different sites on one individual (intraindividual variation).[88,90] Even after the timing of caliper readings has been standardized, similar thicknesses of adipose tissue may yield different caliper readings because of differences in compressibility.[88] Alternatively, compressibility differences may result in skinfolds of different thicknesses yielding similar caliper readings.[33] Of all the assumptions considered in this section, this probably has the greatest potential for being a significant source of error in estimating body composition from skinfold measurements.[88]

The CAS showed that skin thickness as a percent of total caliper reading varies at different sites and that "while the contribution of skin to total skinfold thickness is generally not large, it may lead to significant error especially in lean subjects."[88]

Thickness of subcutaneous adipose tissue varies widely among different skinfold sites within individuals and for the same skinfold site between individuals.[87,88,91] Consequently, overall subcutaneous adipose tissue is best assessed by measuring multiple skinfold sites. A minimum of three is recommended. Proper site selection is critical because subcutaneous fat layer thickness can vary significantly within a 2- to 3-cm proximity of certain sites.[83,92] Research has shown that certain skinfold sites are highly correlated to total subcutaneous adipose tissue and that sites from the lower limbs should be included in body composition prediction formulas.[88,93]

Adipose tissue can be divided into external, or subcutaneous (what lies directly under the skin), and internal portions (that within and around muscles and surrounding organs).[92] The only direct data on the relationship of external-to-internal adipose tissue comes from the CAS. These data show that each kilogram of subcutaneous adipose tissue is associated with approximately 200 g of internal adipose tissue and that skinfolds are significantly correlated with total adiposity.[87]

Although estimating body composition by skinfold measurements fails to meet all the assumptions of Box 6.3, it is preferred over use of other anthropometric variables and is certainly better than height-weight indices.[94] Thus, skinfold measurement is the most widely used method of indirectly estimating percent body fat in clinical settings.

Measurement Technique

Proper measurement of skinfolds requires careful attention to site selection and strict adherence to the following protocol, which is standard among researchers who have

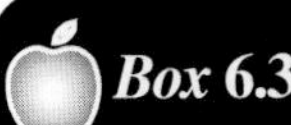

Box 6.3 **Assumptions Involved in Using Skinfold Thickness Measurements to Predict Body Fat**

1. The double thickness of skin and subcutaneous adipose tissue has a constant compressibility
2. Thickness of the skin is negligible or a constant fraction of the skinfold
3. The thickness of subcutaneous adipose tissue is constant or predictable within and between individuals
4. The fat content of adipose tissue is constant
5. The proportion of internal to external fat is constant
6. Body fat is normally distributed

Adapted from Martin AD, Ross WD, Drinkwater DT, Clarys JP. 1985. Prediction of body fat by skinfold caliper: Assumptions and cadaver evidence. *International Journal of Obesity* 9(suppl 1):31–39.

developed the prediction equations for determining body fatness from skinfold measurements.

1. Most North American investigators (including those conducting large national surveys from which reference data are derived) take skinfold measurements on the right side of the body. European investigators typically perform measurements on the left side.[95] From a practical standpoint, it matters little on which side measurements are taken. However, the authors of this textbook suggest that North American students be taught to take all measurements on the right side (except where indicated otherwise) to coincide with the efforts of most U.S. and Canadian researchers.
2. As a general rule, those with little experience in skinfold measurement should mark the site to be measured once it has been carefully identified. A flexible, nonstretchable tape measure can be used to locate midpoints on the body.[89]
3. The skinfold should be firmly grasped by the thumb and index finger of the left hand about 1 cm or ½ in. **proximal** to the skinfold site and pulled away from the body. This is usually easy with thin people, but it may be difficult with the obese and may be somewhat uncomfortable. The amount of tissue grasped must be enough to form a fold with approximately parallel sides. The thicker the fat layer under the skin, the wider the necessary fold.
4. The caliper is held in the right hand, perpendicular to the long axis of the skinfold and with the caliper's dial facing up and easily readable. The caliper tips should be placed on the site and should be about 1 cm or ½ in. **distal** to the fingers holding the skinfold, so that pressure from the fingers will not affect the measured value, as shown in Figure 6.16.
5. The caliper should not be placed too deeply into the skinfold or too close to the tip of the skinfold. The measurer should try to visualize where a true double fold of skin thickness is and place the caliper tips there. It is a good practice to position the caliper arms one at a time on the skinfold.
6. The dial is read approximately 4 seconds after the pressure from the measurer's hand has been released on the lever arm of the caliper. If caliper tips exert force for longer than 4 seconds, the reading will gradually become smaller as fluids are forced from the compressed tissues. The measurer's eyes and caliper dial should be positioned to avoid errors caused by parallax. Readings should be recorded to the nearest 1 mm.
7. A minimum of two measurements should be taken at each site. Measurements should be at least 15 seconds apart to allow the skinfold site to return to normal. If consecutive measurements vary by more than 1 mm, more should be taken until there is consistency.
8. The measurer should maintain pressure with the thumb and index finger throughout each measurement.
9. When measuring the obese, it may be impossible to elevate a skinfold with parallel sides, particularly over the abdomen. In this situation, the measurer should use both hands to pull the skinfold away while a partner attempts to measure the width. If the skinfold is too wide for the calipers, underwater weighing or another technique will have to be used.
10. Measurements should not be taken immediately after exercise or when the person being measured is overheated because the shift in body fluid to the skin will inflate normal skinfold size.
11. It takes practice to consistently grasp skinfolds at the same location every time. Accuracy can be tested by having several technicians take the same measurements and comparing results. It may take up to 50 practice sessions to become proficient in measuring skinfolds.

Several types of skinfold calipers are available (see Figure 6.17). The Lange skinfold caliper is most popular among U.S. researchers, whereas the Harpenden and

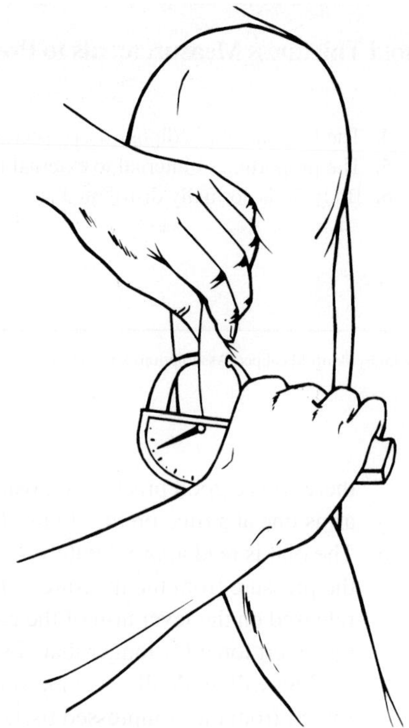

Figure 6.16
Accurate skinfold measurements require careful site selection and proper technique in placing and reading the caliper.

Holtain are commonly used in Great Britain and Europe. Several less expensive plastic calipers are available, such as the Slim Guide and the Fat-Control Caliper. Some of the plastic calipers have been shown to give results comparable to the more expensive calipers.[96,97] The Slim Guide, which is being used increasingly, may be an acceptable caliper for those who cannot afford a more expensive instrument. Currently, the Lange and Harpenden calipers are highly recommended because these were used in developing prediction equations and reference values. Whatever the caliper used, the jaw tips should exert a pressure of 10 g/mm^2 throughout the caliper's full measurement range. The calipers should be calibrated periodically (for example, before measuring skinfolds on groups of subjects) by checking the dial reading against a graduated calibration block. Caliper readings should be within at least ± 1 mm at each 5-mm interval from 5 to 50 mm.[98]

Site Selection

This section describes eight of the most commonly used skinfold sites following the Airlie Consensus Conference protocol as outlined in the *Anthropometric Standardization Reference Manual.*[93]

Chest

The chest, or pectoral skinfold site, is measured using a skinfold with its long axis running from the top of the anterior axillary fold to the nipple. The skinfold is grasped as high as possible on the anterior axillary fold, and the thickness of the fat fold is measured 1 cm or ½ in. below the fingers along the axis, as shown in Figures 6.18 and 6.19. The skinfold site is the same for males and females. Other than to help determine the long axis of the skinfold, the nipple is not used as a landmark for either males or females. This site can be measured on a female wearing a brassiere or two-piece bathing suit.

Triceps

Because of its accessibility, the triceps is the most commonly measured site. The triceps skinfold site is on the posterior aspect of the right arm, over the triceps muscle, midway between the lateral projection of the acromion process of the scapula and the inferior margin of the olecranon process of the ulna. These bony landmarks are shown in Figure 6.20. The midpoint between the acromion and olecranon processes should be marked along the *lateral* side of the arm with the elbow flexed 90 degrees, as shown in Figure 6.21. The subject's arm should now hang loosely at the side, with the palm of the hand facing *anteriorly* to

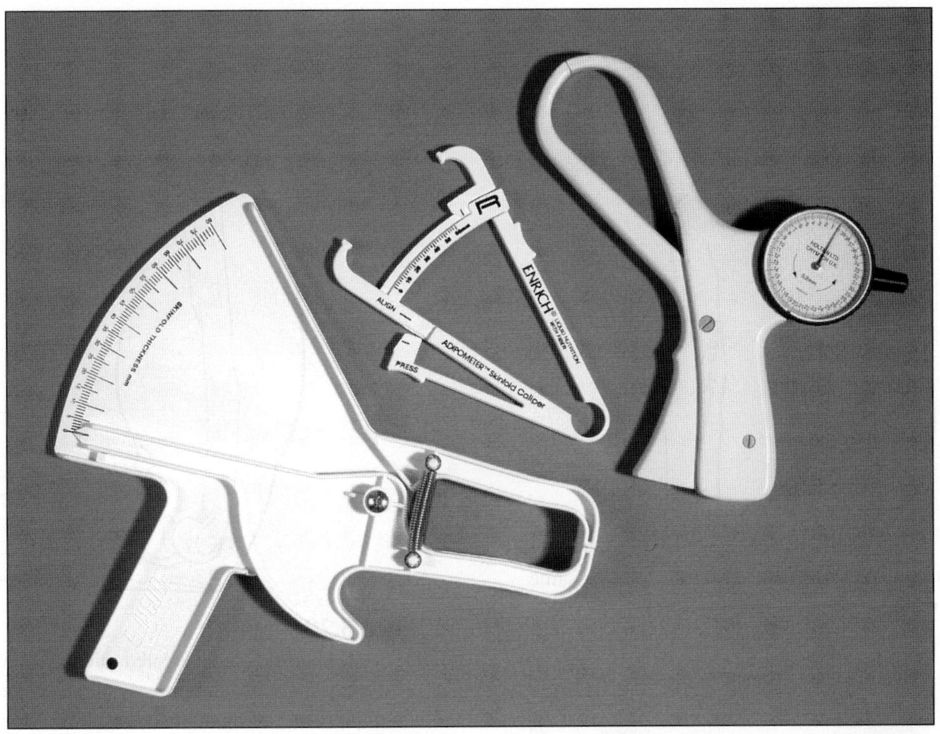

(a)

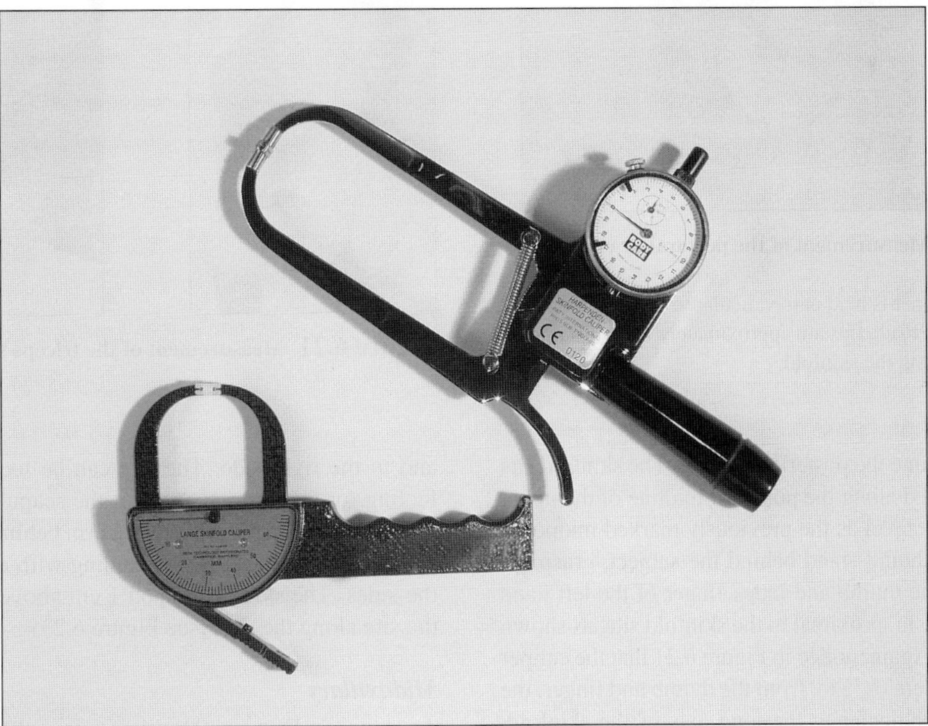

(b)

Figure 6.17 Examples of commercially available skinfold calipers. (a) Left to right: Slim Guide, Fat-Control, and Holtain. (b) Left to right: Lange and Harpenden.

Source: Photos by Mariah C. Doren.

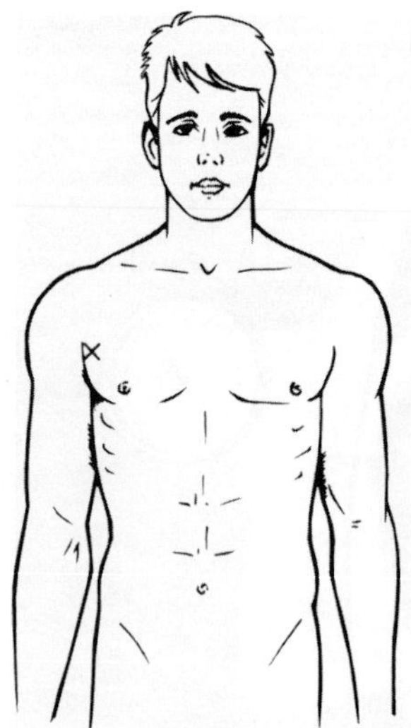

Figure 6.18
The location of the pectoral or chest skinfold site is the same for males and females.

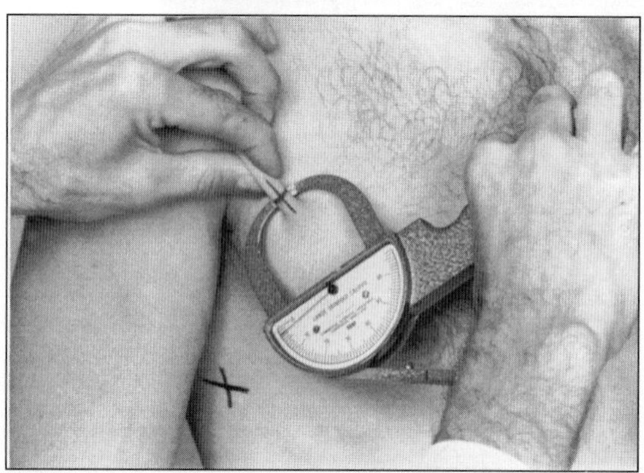

Figure 6.19 Measurement of the pectoral or chest skinfold.
Note that the caliper is held perpendicular to the long axis of the skinfold. The blade tips are approximately 1 cm distal to the fingers grasping the skinfold.

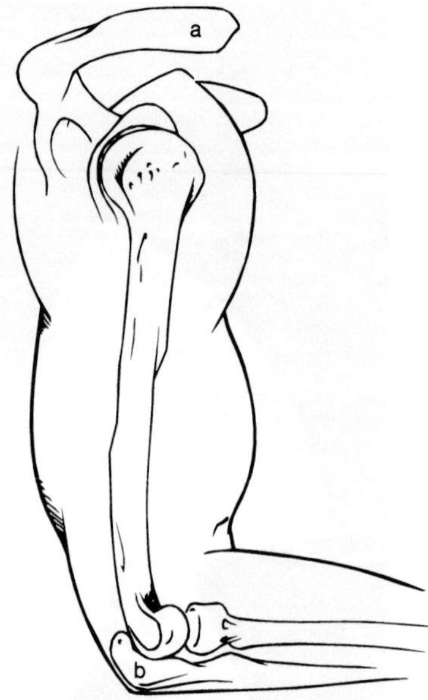

Figure 6.20
The triceps skinfold site is located midway between the lateral projection of the acromion process of the scapula, **a,** and the olecranon process of the ulna, **b,** with the elbow flexed 90 degrees.

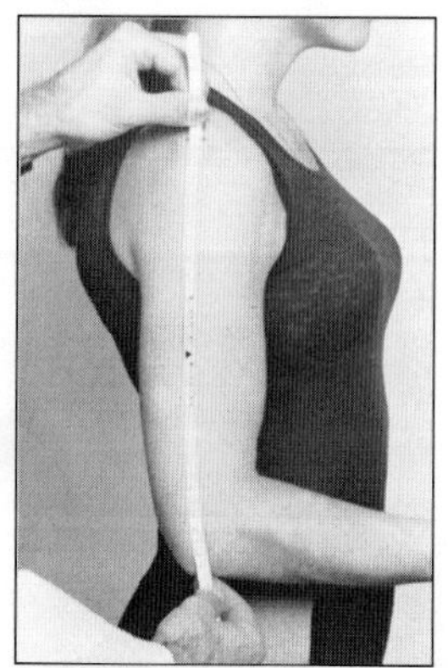

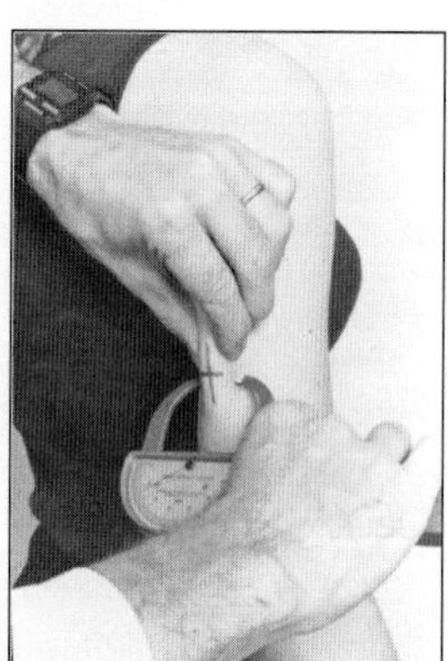

Figure 6.21 Measurement of the triceps skinfold.

properly determine the posterior midline. The skinfold site should be marked along the posterior midline of the upper arm at the same level as the previously marked midpoint. The measurer should stand behind the subject, grasp the skinfold with the thumb and index finger of the left hand about 1 cm or ½ in. proximal to the skinfold site, as shown in Figure 6.21. Again, notice in Figure 6.21 that the caliper tips are about 1 cm or ½ in. from the thumb and finger, the caliper is perpendicular to the long axis of the skinfold, and the dial can be easily read.

Subscapular

The subscapular site is 1 cm below the lowest, or inferior, angle of the scapula, as shown in Figure 6.22. The long axis of the skinfold is on a 45-degree angle directed down and to the right side. The site can be located by gently feeling for the inferior angle of the scapula or by having the subject place his or her right arm behind the back. It is measured with the subject standing with arms relaxed to the sides. The skin is grasped 1 cm above and medial to the site along the axis (see Figure 6.23).

Midaxillary

As shown in Figure 6.24, this site is at the right midaxillary line (a vertical line extending from the middle of the axilla) level with the xiphisternal junction (at the bottom of the sternum where the xiphoid process begins). It is measured with the subject standing erectly and with the right arm slightly abducted (moved away from center of the body) and flexed (bent posteriorly), as in Figure 6.25.

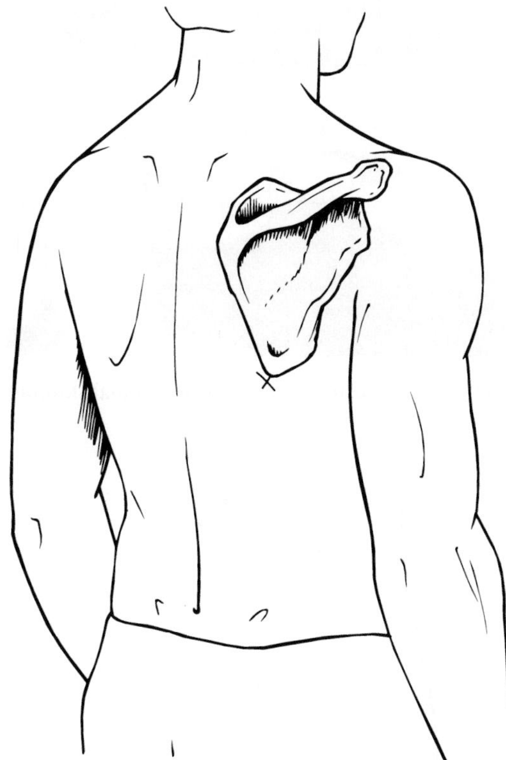

Figure 6.22
The subscapular skinfold site is just below the inferior border of the scapula. The long axis of the site runs at 45 degrees of horizontal.

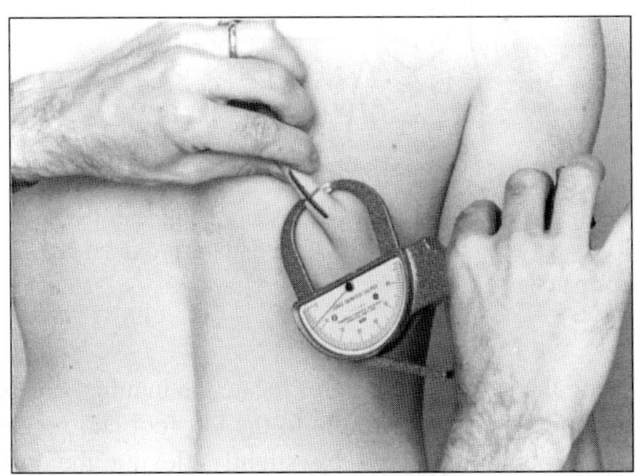

Figure 6.23 **Measurement of the subscapular skinfold site.**

Suprailiac

This skinfold is measured just above the iliac crest at the midaxillary line (see Figure 6.26 and Figure 6.27). The long axis follows the natural cleavage lines of the skin and runs diagonally. The subject should stand erectly with feet together and arms hanging at the sides, although the right arm can be abducted and flexed slightly to improve access to the site. The measurer should grasp the

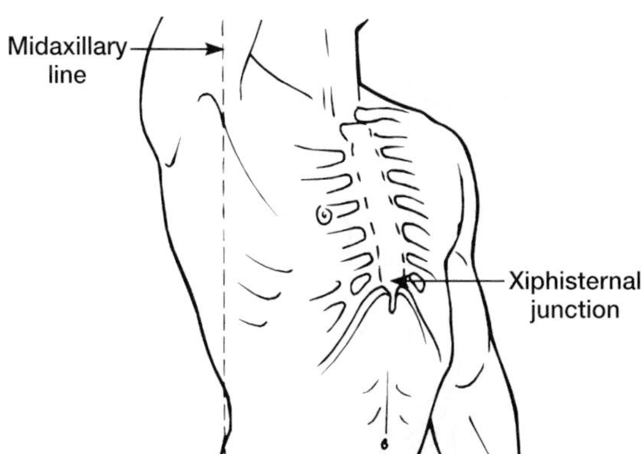

Figure 6.24
The midaxillary site is a horizontal skinfold along the midaxillary line at the level of the xiphisternal junction.

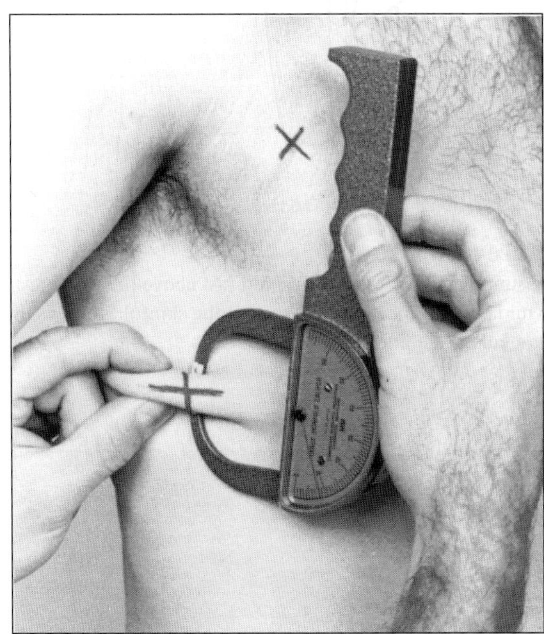

Figure 6.25 **Measurement of the midaxillary skinfold.**

skinfold about 1 cm posterior to the midaxillary line and measure the skinfold at the midaxillary line.

Abdomen

The subject stands erectly with the body weight evenly distributed on both feet, abdominal muscles relaxed, and breathing quietly. A horizontal skinfold 3 cm to the right of and 1 cm below the midpoint of the umbilicus is measured (Figure 6.28).

Thigh

This site is a vertical skinfold along the midline of the anterior aspect of the thigh midway between the junction of the midline and the inguinal crease and the proximal (upper) border of the patella, or knee cap (Figure 6.29).

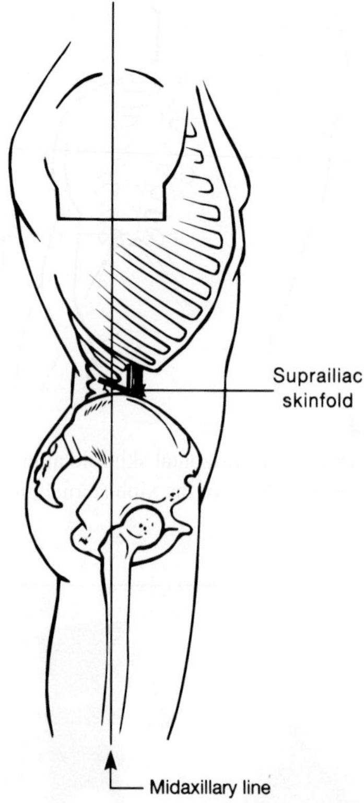

Figure 6.26
The suprailiac skinfold is measured just above the iliac crest at the midaxillary line. The long axis of the skinfold follows the natural cleavage lines of the skin.

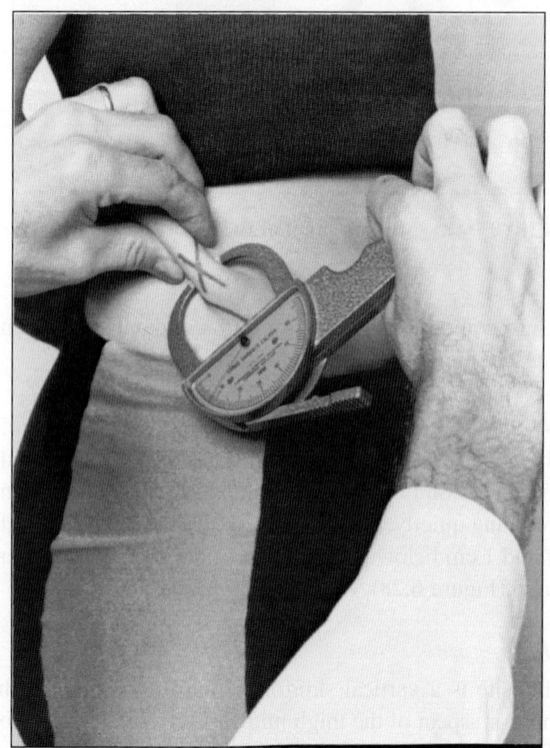

Figure 6.27 Measurement of the suprailiac skinfold.

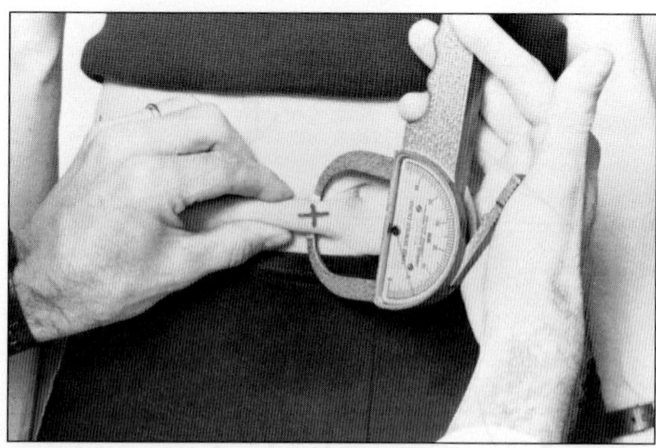

Figure 6.28 Measurement of the abdominal skinfold.

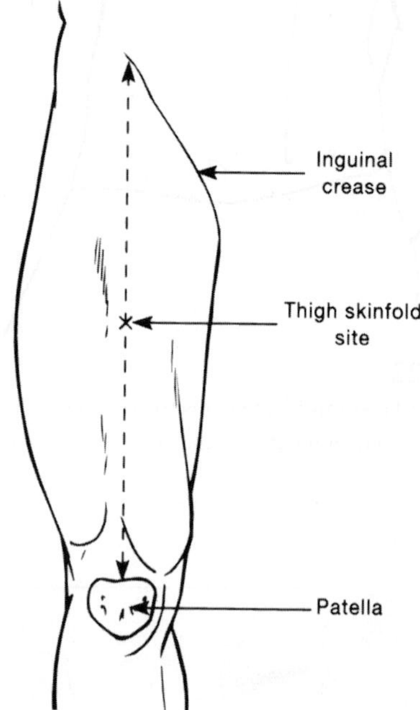

Figure 6.29
The thigh skinfold lies along the anterior midline of the thigh halfway between the inguinal crease and the proximal border of the patella.

Flexing the subject's hip helps locate the inguinal crease. The subject shifts the weight to the left foot and relaxes the leg being measured by slightly flexing the knee with the foot flat on the floor. The skinfold is measured as shown in Figure 6.30.

Medial Calf

With the subject sitting, the right leg is flexed about 90 degrees at the knee with the sole of the foot flat on the floor. The measurement also may be taken with the subject standing with the foot resting on a platform, so that the knee and hip are flexed about 90 degrees. The point of maximum calf circumference is marked at the medial (inner) aspect of the calf. A vertical skinfold is grasped about 1 cm proximal to the marked site and measured at the site (Figure 6.31).

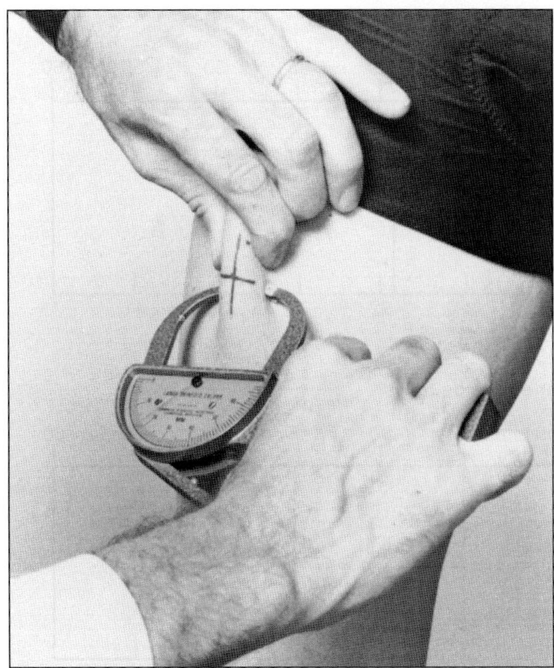

Figure 6.30 Measurement of the thigh skinfold.

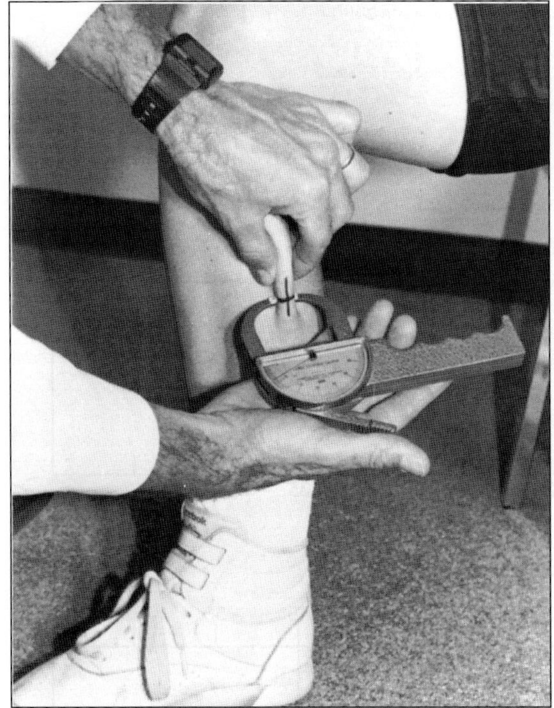

Figure 6.31 Measurement of the medial calf skinfold.

Single-Site Skinfold Measurements

The triceps is the most commonly used single site for assessing body composition. The ease by which it is accessed and measured has made it popular in large population studies, such as NHANES. Although single-site skinfold measurements cannot be used to estimate percent body fat, they are useful for making comparisons among subjects for which reference data are available. For example, the triceps skinfold measurements of a child can be compared with reference data on triceps skinfolds taken from a large group of children of a similar sex and age. Reference data derived from NHANES 2003–2006 are shown in Appendixes M and N. Using the tables, the 50th percentile represents the median value for each age/sex group. If a subject had a skinfold thickness at the 85th percentile for his or her age/sex group, 85% of the subjects studied in that group would have smaller measurements, and only 15% would have larger measurements.

Using single skinfold measurements has certain limitations: investigators disagree about what is the best single site to use as an index of body composition; no equations exist for estimating body fat using just the triceps skinfold measurement; and multiple anthropometric measures are required to achieve reasonably accurate body composition estimates because of variations in subcutaneous adipose tissue distribution. Therefore, single-site skinfold measurements must be interpreted with caution and should be used only as a rough approximation of total body fat percentage or to compare individuals for which reference data exist.

Two-Site Skinfold Measurements

The most commonly used approach to assessing body composition for young people age 6 years through the mid-20s uses the sum of the triceps and subscapular sites.[98,99] These sites have the following advantages: they are highly correlated with other measures of body fatness; they are more reliably and objectively measured than most other sites; and national norms are available for them. Figure 6.32 outlines skinfold and body fat standards developed for persons ages 6 to 17 years using the sum of the triceps and subscapular skinfolds.[99]

Because measurement of the subscapular skinfold may be embarrassing to some children and youth or may raise ethical questions about male teachers touching female students, norms using the sum of the triceps and medial calf skinfold measurements have been developed.[99,100] This sum has proved to be a reasonably valid and reliable indicator of body composition. The medial calf site is easily accessible and can be measured without raising concerns about modesty. In some persons, the skin at the site may be quite taut, making it difficult to measure the site. Figure 6.33 provides standards based on the sum of triceps and medial calf skinfold measurements for persons 6 to 17 years old.[99] Using Figures 6.32 and 6.33, obesity for 6- to 17-year-old males and females is greater than 25% body fat and greater than 32% body fat, respectively. An alternate approach for estimating percent body fat in children is to calculate the sum of biceps,

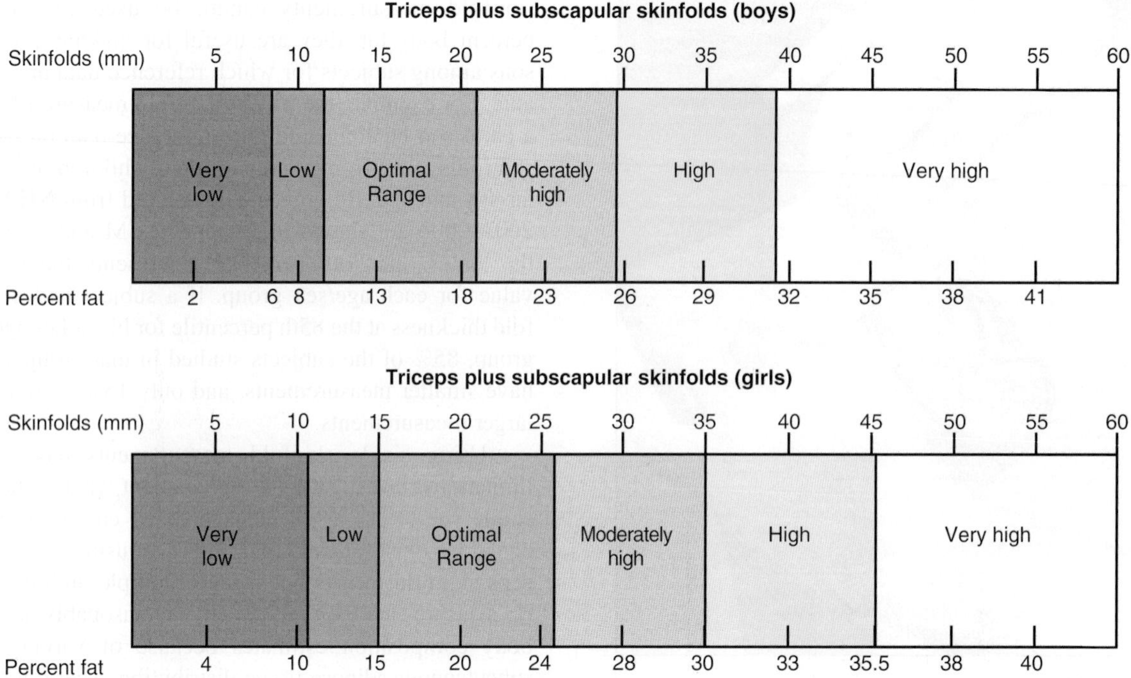

Figure 6.32 Body fat standards for persons 6 to 17 years old based on the sum of triceps and subscapular skinfold measurements.

Source: Reprinted with permission from the November/December 1987 *Journal of Physical Education, Recreation & Dance,* a publication of the American Alliance for Health, Physical Education, Recreation and Dance, 1900 Association Dr., Reston, VA 20191.

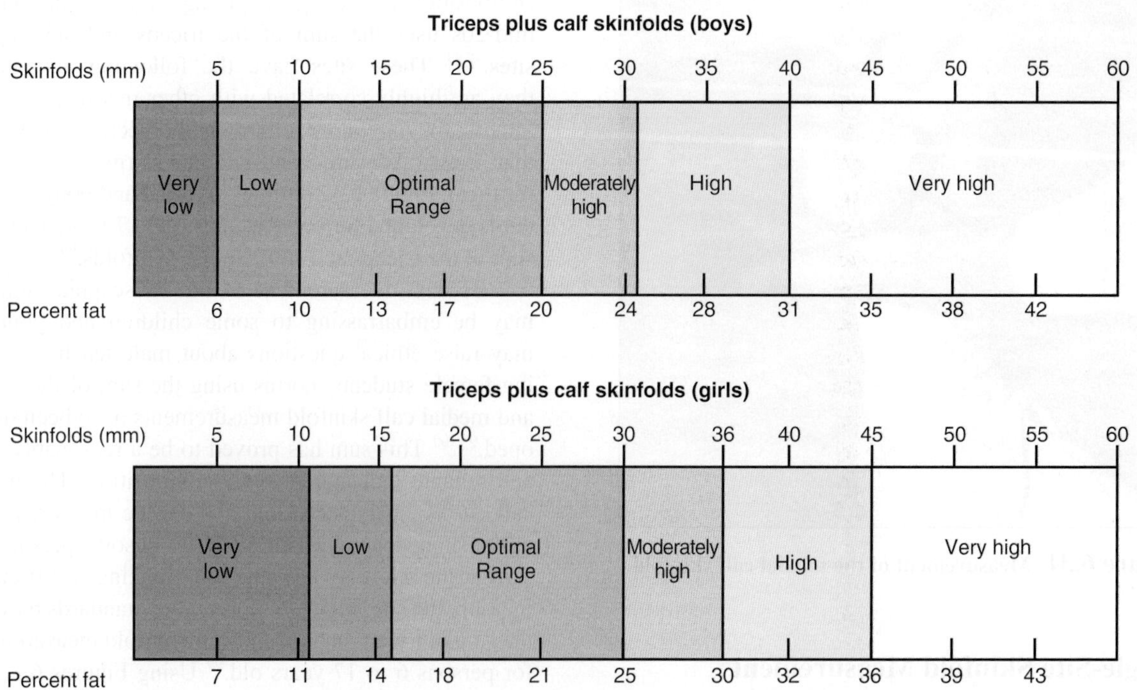

Figure 6.33 Body fat standards for persons 6 to 17 years old based on the sum of triceps and medial calf skinfold measurements.

Source: Reprinted with permission from the November/December 1987 *Journal of Physical Education, Recreation & Dance,* a publication of the American Alliance for Health, Physical Education, Recreation and Dance, 1900 Association Dr., Reston, VA 20191.

triceps, subscapular, and suprailiac skinfold measurements (discussed in the section "Multiple-Site Skinfold Measurements").

Multiple-Site Skinfold Measurements

Predicting body density and then percent of body fat from skinfold measurements requires regression equations. These formulas have been developed by comparing a variety of skinfold and other anthropometric measures with measurements of body density (usually by hydrostatic weighing) to see which anthropometric measures are best at predicting body density. A statistical process called multiple-regression analysis is used.[4,94,101–103] The measure or combinations of measures most highly correlated with body density as determined by a separate method are then used in the regression equation.

The more than 100 different regression equations that have been developed can be classified as either population-specific equations or generalized equations.[92,94] Population-specific equations are derived from data on groups of people sharing certain characteristics, such as age and gender. The first valid regression equations, for example, were developed in 1951 for young and middle-aged men.[104] Numerous other population-specific equations have been developed since then, but their use is limited. Equations developed from data on middle-aged females, for example, may not be valid for females of other ages.

More recently, generalized equations have been developed that are applicable to persons varying greatly in age and body fatness. The primary advantage of this approach is that one generalized equation can replace several population-specific equations with no loss in prediction accuracy.[5,94] Table 6.8 shows several generalized prediction equations for calculating body density or percent body fat. Because fat placement differs between males and females, separate equations are given for each sex.

Table 6.9 shows equations for estimating body density developed by Durnin and Womersley.[105] These have been used by many researchers and differ according to sex and age. The equations are based on the logarithm of the sum of four skinfolds—triceps, subscapular, suprailiac, and biceps. The biceps skinfold is a vertical fold on the anterior aspect of the arm, over the belly of the biceps muscle, directly opposite the triceps skinfold site.[89]

The equations in Table 6.8 and Table 6.9 predict either body fat percent or body density. Body density formulas require an additional calculation to estimate percent body fat. Two formulas are available for this step: the Brozek and the Siri equations:

Brozek: Percent body fat = (457 ÷ body density) − 414

Siri: Percent body fat = (495 ÷ body density) − 450

A programmable calculator will help in the use of these equations. The nomogram shown in Figure 6.34 greatly simplifies calculating percent body fat from the sum of three skinfold thicknesses.[106] For males, the sum of the chest, abdomen, and thigh skinfold measurements should be used. For females, the sum of the triceps, suprailiac, and thigh skinfold measurements should be used. The nomogram was developed from data on males from 18 to 61 years old and females 18 to 55 years old, with the sum of skinfold measurements ranging from 14 to 118 mm and 16 to 126 mm for males and females, respectively.[106] The nomogram should be used with caution for subjects outside these ranges.

Investigators in the Netherlands have proposed regression equations for estimating body density and percent body fat in persons from infancy to age 18 years.[107] Based on their equations, they have formulated a table

TABLE 6.8 Generalized Body Composition Equations for Male and Female Adults*

Males

Body density = $1.11200000 - 0.00043499(X_1) + 0.00000055\,(X_1)^2 - 0.00028826\,(X_8)$

Percent body fat = $0.29288\,(X_2) - 0.00050\,(X_2)^2 + 0.15845\,(X_8) - 5.76377$

Body density = $1.1093800 - 0.0008267\,(X_3) + 0.0000016\,(X_3)^2 - 0.0002574\,(X_8)$

Body density = $1.1125025 - 0.0013125\,(X_4) + 0.00000055\,(X_4)^2 - 0.0002440\,(X_8)$

Percent body fat = $0.39287\,(X_5) - 0.00105\,(X_5)^2 + 0.15772\,(X_8) - 5.18845$

Females

Body density = $1.0970 - 0.00046971\,(X_1) + 0.00000056\,(X_1)^2 - 0.00012828\,(X_8)$

Percent body fat = $0.29699\,(X_2) - 0.00043\,(X_2)^2 + 0.02963\,(X_8) + 1.4072$

Percent body fat = $0.41563\,(X_6) - 0.00112\,(X_6)^2 + 0.03661\,(X_8) + 4.03653$

Body density = $1.0994921 - 0.0009929\,(X_7) + 0.0000023\,(X_7)^2 - 0.0001392\,(X_8)$

Data from Jackson AS, Pollock ML. 1985. Practical assessment of body composition. *Physician and Sportsmedicine* 13(5):76–90; Golding LA, Myers CR, Sinning WE. 1989. *The Y's way to physical fitness,* 3rd ed. Champaign, IL: Human Kinetics Books.

*X_1 = sum of chest, midaxillary, triceps, subscapular, abdomen, suprailiac, and thigh skinfolds; X_2 = sum of abdomen, suprailiac, triceps, and thigh skinfolds; X_3 = sum of chest, abdomen, and subscapular skinfolds; X_4 = sum of chest, triceps, and subscapular skinfolds; X_5 = sum of abdomen, suprailiac, and triceps skinfolds; X_6 = sum of triceps, abdomen, and suprailiac skinfolds; X_7 = sum of triceps, suprailiac, and thigh skinfolds; X_8 = age in years.

TABLE 6.9 Age- and Sex-Specific Body Composition Equations Developed by Durnin and Womersley

Age Range (Years)	Equation
Males	
17–19	Body density = 1.1620 − 0.0630 × (log Σ)*
20–29	Body density = 1.1631 − 0.0632 × (log Σ)
30–39	Body density = 1.1422 − 0.0544 × (log Σ)
40–49	Body density = 1.1620 − 0.0700 × (log Σ)
50 +	Body density = 1.1715 − 0.0779 × (log Σ)
Females	
17–19	Body density = 1.1549 − 0.0678 × (log Σ)
20–29	Body density = 1.1599 − 0.0717 × (log Σ)
30–39	Body density = 1.1423 − 0.0632 × (log Σ)
40–49	Body density = 1.1333 − 0.0612 × (log Σ)
50 +	Body density = 1.1339 − 0.0645 × (log Σ)

Equations from Durnin JVGA, Womersley J. 1974. Body fat assessment from total body density and its estimation from skinfold thickness: Measurements on 481 men and women aged 16–72 years. *British Journal of Nutrition* 32:77–97.

*Σ = sum of the triceps, subscapular, suprailiac, and biceps skinfolds.

(Table 6.10) allowing the estimation of percent body fat of persons in this age range from the sum of biceps, triceps, subscapular, and suprailiac skinfold measurements.

What Is a Desirable Level of Fatness?

Determining with certainty just what constitutes a desirable level of body fatness is difficult. However, suggested percent body fat norms are given in Table 6.11. Note that the values are given in a range. This allows for error in measurement and for individual differences; what may be appropriate for one person may not be appropriate for another.[86,94]

Using the values in Table 6.11, the form shown in Figure 6.35, and the following formulas, a person can calculate a target weight necessary to achieve a certain percent body fat.[27]

Weight of fat = Total body weight × Percent body fat

Fat-free weight = Total body weight − Fat weight

Target weight = Present fat-free weight ÷ (100 − desired percent body fat)

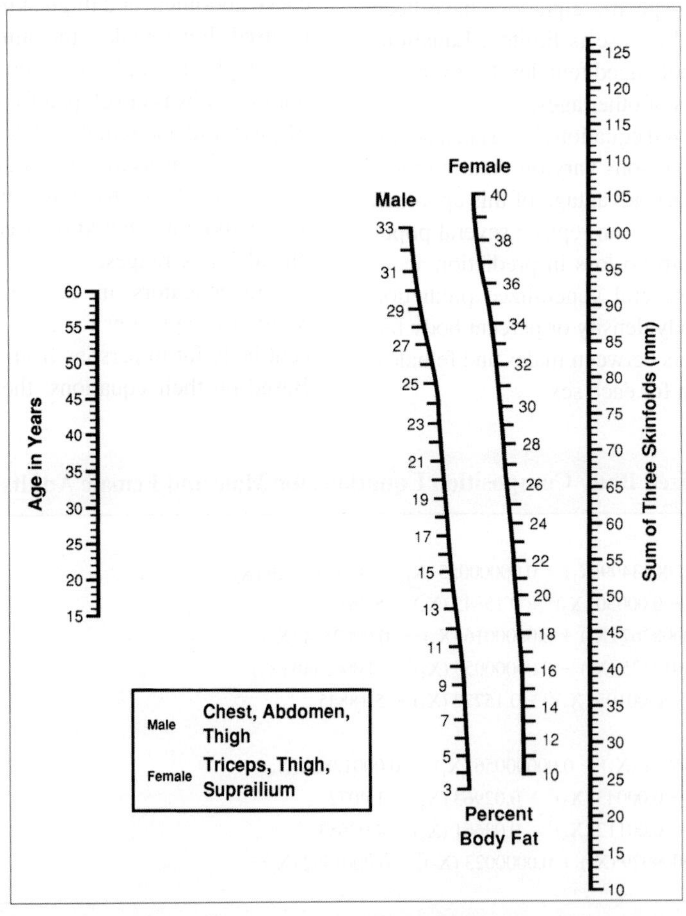

Figure 6.34 Nomogram for calculating percent of body fat from the sum of three skinfolds.
Use a straightedge to connect the subject's age (left axis) with the skinfold value (right axis). The percent body fat is read where the straightedge crosses the line representing the subject's sex.

Source: Reprinted with permission from the *Research Quarterly for Exercise and Sport* 52(3):1981. The *Research Quarterly for Exercise and Sport* is a publication of the American Alliance for Health, Physical Education, Recreation and Dance, 1900 Association Drive, Reston, VA 22091.

TABLE 6.10 Percent Body Fat Estimated from the Sum of Skinfold Thickness Measurements* in Persons from Infancy to Age 18 Years

	Percent Body Fat				
Age (Years)	15%	20%	25%	30%	35%
Male					
0†	17	22	30	40	52
1‡	18	24	32	43	58
2	18	25	34	45	60
4	20	27	37	51	68
6	22	30	41	57	78
8	32	33	46	64	88
10	25	36	51	72	101
12	27	40	57	81	115
14	27	44	63	92	132
16	32	48	71	104	152
18	34	52	79	117	175
Female					
0†	17	22	30	40	52
1‡	18	24	32	43	58
2	18	25	34	45	60
4	18	25	34	46	62
6	19	25	35	47	63
8	19	26	35	48	65
10	19	27	37	51	69
12	21	30	42	58	80
14	23	33	47	66	92
16	25	37	53	75	106
18	27	40	58	85	122

Adapted from Westrate JA, Deurenberg P. 1989. Body composition in children: Proposal for a method for calculating body fat percentage from total body density or skinfold-thickness measurements. *American Journal of Clinical Nutrition* 50:1104–1115.

*Sum of biceps, triceps, subscapular, and suprailiac skinfold measurements, given in millimeters.

†Mean age used was 6 months.

‡Mean age used was 18 months.

TABLE 6.11 Body Fat Ranges for Persons 18 Years of Age and Older

Classification	Males	Females
Unhealthy range (too low)	≤ 5%	≤ 8%
Acceptable range (lower end)	6–15%	9–23%
Acceptable range (upper end)	16–24%	24–31%
Unhealthy (too high)	≥ 25%	≥ 32%

Adapted from Nieman DC. 2003. *Exercise testing and prescription: A health-related approach,* 5th ed. Boston: McGraw-Hill Higher Education.

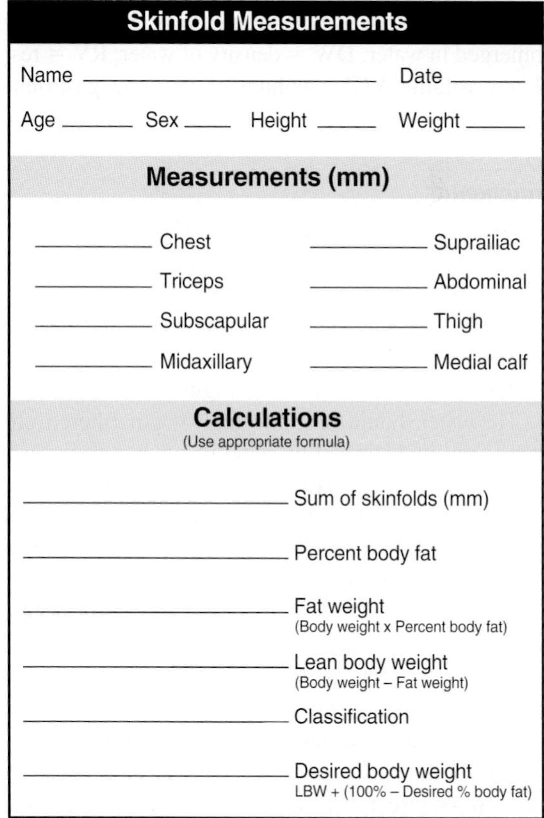

Figure 6.35 Skinfold recording and calculation form.

For example, take a subject who weighs 200 lb, has 25% body fat, and desires to have a 15% body fat:

$$\text{Weight of fat} = 200 \text{ lb} \times 0.25 = 50 \text{ lb}$$
$$\text{Fat-free weight} = 200 \text{ lb} - 50 \text{ lb} = 150 \text{ lb}$$
$$\text{Target weight} = 150 \text{ lb} \div 0.85 = 176 \text{ lb}$$

DENSITOMETRY

Densitometry is assessing body composition by measuring the density of the entire body.[83,84] Density is expressed as mass per unit volume and usually is obtained through **hydrostatic,** or underwater, weighing, although other methods have been developed as described in the section "Air Displacement Plethysmography."[108]

Underwater Weighing

The most widely used technique of determining whole-body density is hydrostatic, or underwater, weighing.[83,84] The technique is based on **Archimedes' principle,** which states that the volume of an object submerged in water equals the volume of water the object displaces. Thus, if the mass and the volume of a body are known, the density of that body can be calculated. Using another formula, percent body fat can be calculated from body density.

This approach is based on the two-compartment model of body composition: the fat and fat-free mass. The fat-free mass is assumed to have a constant level of hydration and a constant proportion of bone mineral to muscle. The approach also assumes a constant fat mass density of 0.90 g/cm^3 and a density of the fat-free mass of 1.10 g/cm^3.[83,84] The densities of bone and muscle tissue are greater than the density of water (density of distilled water = 1.00 g/cm^3), whereas fat is less dense than water. Thus, muscular subjects having a low percentage of body fat tend to weigh more submerged in water than do subjects having a higher percentage of body fat.

Body density can be calculated from the following formula,[4]

$$\text{Body density} = \frac{\text{WA}}{\frac{(\text{WA} - \text{WW})}{\text{DW}} - (\text{RV} + \text{VGI})}$$

where WA = body weight in air; WW = body weight submerged in water; DW = density of water; RV = residual lung volume; VGI = volume of gas in the gastrointestinal tract.

Equipment

The necessary equipment for underwater weighing includes a tank, tub, or pool of water of sufficient size for total body submersion; a scale or another method of determining the subject's underwater weight; and, attached to the scale, a chair or frame lowered into the water on which the subject sits (Figure 6.36).

The water should be comfortably warm, filtered, chlorinated, and undisturbed by wind or other activity in the water during testing.[27] A method of underwater weighing in a swimming pool using a wooden shell placed within the pool to reduce water movement, which can adversely affect weighing, has been described by Katch.[108]

The chair should be constructed so that the subject can sit under the water with legs slightly bent and the water at neck level, as shown in Figure 6.36. Weights should be attached to the chair, so that its empty or tare weight while under water is at least 3 kg for subjects of moderate body fatness and at least 4 to 6 kg for obese subjects.[10] Some researchers use a frame on which the subject lies submerged in the prone (face down) position while breathing through a snorkel.[4,108] They think that this position results in less up-and-down movement of the body in the water, thus resulting in fewer fluctuations of the scale.

Typically, an autopsy scale (such as the 9-kg capacity Chatillon autopsy scale shown in Figure 6.36) is used in underwater weighing. A strain gauge, or force cell, gives more precise measurements.[4,83,109] These instruments can be interfaced with a computer, which, with the appropriate software, can easily determine the midpoint of fluctuations and can use that as the basis for further calculations.[4]

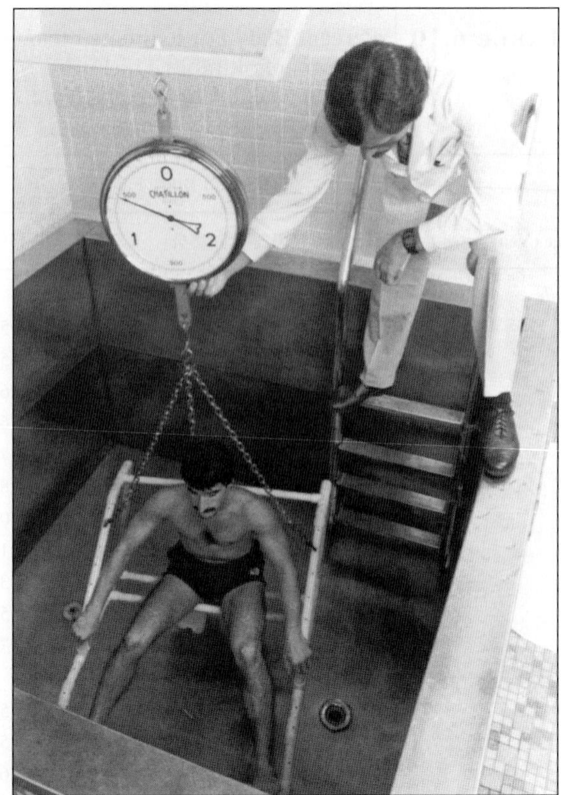

Figure 6.36
Equipment for underwater weighing includes a tank of sufficient size and shape for total human submersion, an accurate scale for measuring weight with 10-gram divisions, a method of measuring water temperature, and a chair that is weighted to prevent flotation.

Procedure[4,27]

1. Obtaining basic data: name, date, age, sex, stature, and weight (in kilograms) in air should be collected and recorded on a form such as the one shown in Figure 6.37. The tester should record the tare weight—the underwater weight of the chair (and any attached weights)—before the subject sits in it. The subject should be several hours **postprandial,** clean, wearing only a swimsuit. The subject should have urinated and defecated immediately before weighing. Carbonated beverages and flatus-causing foods should be avoided before the procedure because gastrointestinal tract gas will decrease the subject's underwater weight, resulting in erroneously low measurements of body density.
2. Measuring skinfolds: skinfold measurements can help verify results from underwater weighing. These can be recorded on the form shown in Figure 6.37.
3. Submerging: while comfortably seated in the chair, the subject exhales as fully as possible and slowly leans forward until the head is completely under the water, as shown in Figure 6.38. The subject continues to press as much air from the lungs as possible. After exhaling fully, the subject remains motionless and counts for 5 to 7 seconds before coming up for air. This allows the tester time to read

Body Composition Worksheet

Name ______________________ Date ______

Age ______ Sex _____ Height ____________

Skinfolds (mm)

_________ Chest _________ Suprailiac

_________ Triceps _________ Abdominal

_________ Subscapular _________ Thigh

_________ Midaxillary _________ Medial calf

Hydrostatic Measurements

_________ Weight in air (Wa)

_________ Tare weight

_________ Average gross weight (average of best two trials)

Underwater weighing trials

1 ____ 2 ____ 3 ____ 4 ____ 5 ____

6 ____ 7 ____ 8 ____ 9 ____ 10 ____

_________ Weight in water (Ww) (average gross weight—tare weight)

_________ Density of water (Dw)

_________ Residual volume (RV)

Calculations

$$\text{Density} = \frac{\text{Wa}}{\dfrac{(\text{Wa} - \text{Ww})}{\text{Dw}} - (\text{RV} + 100 \text{ ml})}$$

_______ Percent body fat = (495 ÷ density) – 450

_______ Fat weight (weight in the air x fat%)

_______ Lean body weight (weight in the air – fat weight)

_______ Classification

Figure 6.37 Body composition worksheet.

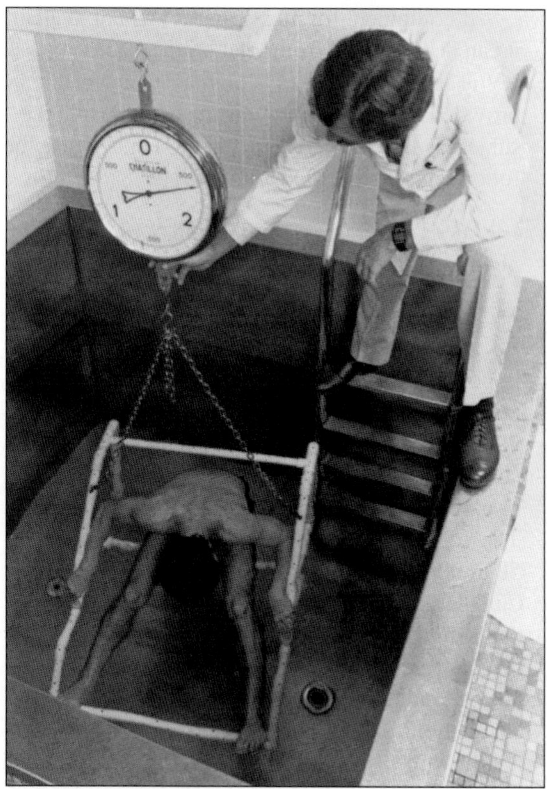

Figure 6.38 Subject's body position while submerged during underwater weighing.
The water should be kept as calm as possible to get a good reading on the scale. Note how the tester is steadying the scale with his hand. Once the scale is relatively steady, the tester should remove the hand and take the reading.

the scale. While in the water, the subject should move slowly and deliberately to prevent water turbulence, which can make the subject bob up and down and make scale reading difficult. When the subject submerges, the tester can keep one hand on the scale to steady it, as shown in Figure 6.38.

4. Recording underwater weight: several trials usually are necessary before the subject becomes accustomed to the procedure and consistent readings are obtained. Katch and coworkers[108] weighed subjects 9 or 10 times and took the average of the last 3 underwater readings as the "true" underwater weight. Underwater weight should be recorded on the Body Composition Worksheet (Figure 6.37) as the gross weight in water. The net body weight in water is the gross weight in water minus the tare weight. The temperature of the water should be measured, and water density should be determined from standard tables.
5. Determining residual volume: residual volume (RV) is the amount of air remaining in the lungs after a maximal exhalation. All other things being equal, a subject with a large RV will be more buoyant (have a lower underwater weight) than one with a smaller RV. Although RV often is estimated, whenever possible it should be measured directly. When RV is estimated, hydrostatically determined percent body fat is no more accurate than when derived from skinfold measurements.[27] Techniques for measuring RV include nitrogen washout, helium dilution, and oxygen dilution. The choice of technique is generally a matter of which is available to the investigator.[4] Whether RV should be measured at the same time as underwater weighing or immediately before or after is a point of contention among investigators.[4] Currently, there seems to be no clear advantage of one approach over the other.

If equipment for measuring RV is not available, it can be estimated from vital lung capacity.[110] RV is approximately 24% of vital lung capacity, provided the vital capacity is measured while the subject is in water.[4] Another approach is to use the following sex-specific formulas,[111]

$$\text{Male RV} = 0.017\text{ A} + 0.06858\text{ S} - 3.477$$
$$\text{Female RV} = 0.009\text{ A} + 0.08128\text{ S} - 3.900$$

where A = age in years and S = stature in inches. Because measuring gastrointestinal tract gas is impossible using conventional methods, it is nearly always estimated to be 100 mL in adults.[4,83] The value is likely smaller in children and larger in subjects who consumed flatus-producing foods or carbonated beverages before being measured.[4] The volume of gastrointestinal gas can range from 50 to 300 mL.[83]

6. Calculating density and percent body fat: using the formulas or the Body Composition Worksheet (Figure 6.37), you can calculate estimates of body density and percent body fat. The remainder of the calculations on the Body Composition Worksheet are the same as those discussed in the section "What Is a Desirable Level of Fatness?"

Weaknesses of Underwater Weighing

Underwater weighing has several weaknesses. It is not practical for testing large numbers of people. Subjects must be willing and able to remain submerged and motionless long enough for an accurate measurement of weight to be made. This requires considerable subject cooperation and training.[83,112,113] Consequently, about 10% to 20% of subjects find it difficult to be weighed under water. The technique requires some special equipment, experience, and financial investment. In many situations, skinfold measurements may be more practical.[27]

Densitometry is based on several assumptions. Perhaps the most tenuous of these is a constant density of the fat-free compartment.[4,83,87] A number of factors can affect the density of the fat-free mass, and these can influence the accuracy of body density measurement by 3% to 4%.[10] Athletes, for example, tend to have denser bone and muscle tissue, which may result in underestimation of body fat (possibly even *negative* body fat values), whereas the tendency of older persons to have less dense bones will likely result in overestimation of body fat.[4] Fat-free tissue density values for adults are probably not appropriate for use with children. Another concern is gas trapped in the gut, the amount of which can only be estimated. Other factors affecting the accuracy of body density measurements include the consumption of food and carbonated beverages shortly before underwater weighing, fluid loss during intensive training, fluid retention before menstruation, and the degree of forcible exhalation while submerged.[4] Despite these weaknesses, underwater weighing remains the standard laboratory technique for determining body density and percent body fat.[27,112,113]

Air Displacement Plethysmography

As an alternative to underwater weighing, body volume (and, consequently, body density and percent body fat) can be measured using a technique known as air displacement plethysmography. The fundamental principle behind air displacement plethysmography is that, when a subject enters a chamber of known volume, the subject's body volume is equal to the reduction in chamber volume.[114,115] An example of a commercially available air displacement plethysmograph (what the manufacturer calls the "Bod Pod®") is shown in Figure 6.39. Figure 6.40 illustrates the major components of the plethysmograph. The unit is constructed of fiberglass and consists of two chambers (front and rear), which are separated by a wall, which also serves as a molded seat on which the subject sits during testing. The subject enters and exits the front chamber of the unit through a hinged door containing a large acrylic window, giving the subject a comfortable sense of openness when the door is closed. The rear

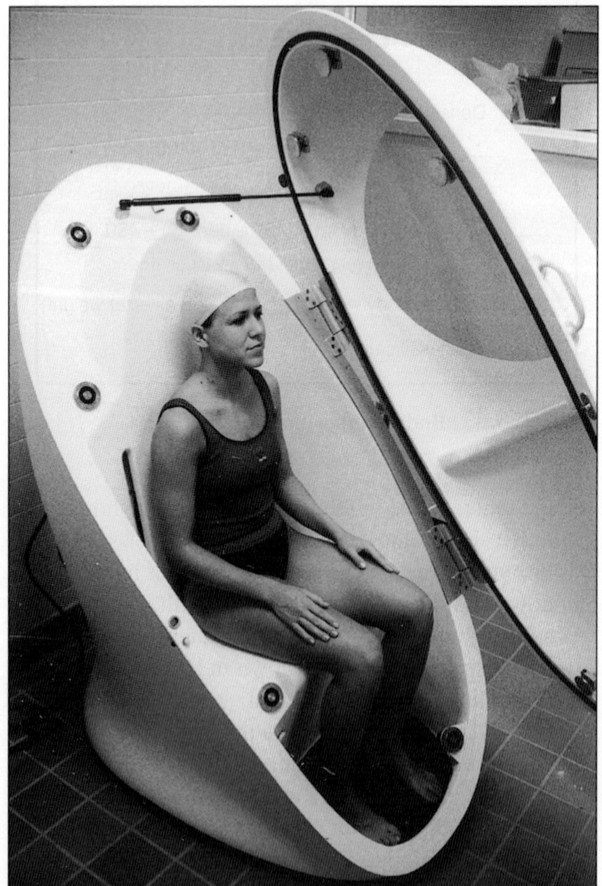

Figure 6.39 An air displacement plethysmograph.
Source: Photo by M. Ware.

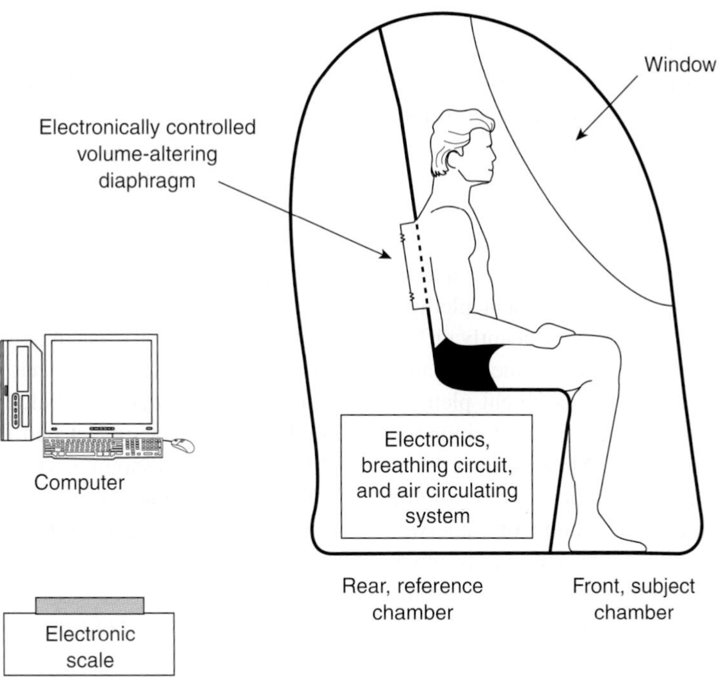

Figure 6.40 The major components of the air plethysmograph.

Source: Adapted from Dempster P, Aitkens S. 1995. *Medicine and Science in Sports and Exercise.* 27:1692–1697. Ellis KJ. 2000. *Physiological Reviews* 80:649–680.

chamber houses electronic instruments, an air circulation system, valves, pressure transducers, and a breathing circuit. Attached to the wall separating the two chambers is a diaphragm, which, when moved during calibration and subject measurement, slightly alters the volume of the two chambers. These volume alterations during calibration and subject measurement are used, along with other values, to calculate the subject's volume. Connected to but outside the unit are a scale for weighing the subject and a computer for controlling the system and for collecting, analyzing, and outputting data.[112,114] In order to accurately measure body volume, it is necessary to minimize or account for the effects of clothing, hair, body surface area, and thoracic (lung and airway) gas volume. The effects of clothing and hair are minimized by having the subject dress in a tight-fitting swimsuit and wear a swimcap to compress the hair. Body surface area is calculated using a formula and accurate measurement of height and weight. Thoracic gas volume is measured during the final step of the measurement process.[114,116]

After voiding, the subject is weighed on the system's scale, and height is measured using a stadiometer. A two-step calibration process is performed, first with the front chamber empty and the door closed and then with a 50-liter calibration cylinder in the front chamber with the door closed. During each step of the calibration process, the electronically controlled diaphragm oscillates back and forth to alter the volume in the two chambers.[114] The subject then enters the front chamber, the door is closed, and the subject relaxes and breathes normally while the diaphragm oscillates back and forth. At the end of this 20-second measurement, the door is momentarily opened and then closed and the measurement process is repeated. If these two volume measurements are within 150 mL of each other, the measurements are accepted and the mean value is used for calculations. If they are not within 150 mL, a third measurement is taken. Any two of the three measurements that are within 150 mL of each other are averaged, and that value is used in calculations of body volume. Pressure differences within the front chamber when it is empty and when the subject is present are used in calculating the subject's body volume.[114–116]

The final step is measurement of the subject's thoracic gas volume, which includes all air in the lungs and airways. The door is opened and the subject is given a single-use, disposable breathing tube, which is connected to a breathing circuit housed in the unit's rear chamber. The subject's nostrils are sealed with a nose clip and the subject is instructed to breathe quietly through the mouth. The door is then closed. After several normal breaths, a valve in the breathing circuit momentarily closes at the midpoint of an exhalation. As previously instructed, the subject compresses and then relaxes the diaphragm muscle. This produces small pressure fluctuations within the subject's airway and in the chamber, which are used to calculate thoracic gas volume. The final body volume is calculated based on the initial volume measurement, corrected for thoracic gas volume and the subject's body surface area. This is then used to calculate percent body fat mass and percent body lean mass.[115,116]

Measurements of body composition derived from air displacement plethysmography among different groups of subjects have been compared with those derived from other criterion methods, such as underwater weighing and dual-energy X-ray absorptiometry.[115–124] In general, these validation studies show good agreement between measurements of body composition based on air displacement plethysmography and these two other criterion methods when group means are compared. However, in some instances, air displacement plethysmography has been shown to provide significantly different estimates of body composition, and further research is needed.[116,121,122,124] Overall, air displacement plethysmography is a promising technique for body composition analysis in the clinical setting. Most noteworthy is the fact that plethysmography overcomes some of the methodological and technical constraints of underwater weighing. It is fairly quick and easy and is much more suitable for use with children, the elderly, and the disabled than is underwater weighing.[116–119,122,124] Like underwater weighing, calculations of body density from volume measurements derived from air displacement plethysmography are dependent on the assumption that fat-free tissue has a constant density.[112,117]

Total Body Water

Water is normally the largest component of the human body. It composes approximately 60% and 50% of the weight of the adult male and female body, respectively. As much as 90% of the weight of neonates is water.[4,112,113] Because fat is free of water, all the water in the body is found in the fat-free mass. It has been assumed that fat-free tissue has an average water content of approximately 73.2%. Based on this assumption, a measure of total body water (TBW) should allow calculation of total body fat from the following formula.[42,83]

$$\text{Total body fat} = (\text{Body weight}) - \frac{\text{TBW}}{0.732}$$

Total body water is measured indirectly using **dilution techniques** where a known concentration and volume of a certain substance (a tracer) is given orally or parenterally to a subject, time is allowed for the tracer to equilibrate with water in the subject's body, and the concentration of the tracer in a sample of the subject's blood, urine, or saliva is analyzed. From this data, TBW is measured using the following relationship:

$$C_1V_1 = C_2V_2$$

where C_1 and V_1 = the concentration and volume, respectively, of tracer given to the subject; C_2 = the concentration of tracer in the body fluid sample taken from the subject; and V_2 = the volume of water in the body, or TBW.[83]

Of the numerous tracers used throughout the years, three are currently in common use: water labeled with either **tritium** (^3H_2O), **deuterium** (^2H_2O), or the stable isotope of oxygen ($H_2{}^{18}O$). Of these three, the tritium and deuterium isotopes of water are the most frequently used.[4,42,83,112] A tracer at a specified concentration and volume is either ingested orally or injected intravenously. This is followed by an equilibration period and then a sampling period.[83]

Deuterium is a stable isotope of hydrogen (does not emit radiation) that has a mass twice that of ordinary hydrogen. Lukaski[125] has described TBW measurement using deuterium-labeled water (deuterium oxide, or D_2O). After a subject had fasted 10 hours overnight, blood and saliva samples were obtained. A 10-g oral dose of D_2O in fruit juice or deionized water was given to each subject. During the next 4 hours, the subjects remained in a quiet state. Blood and saliva samples were taken at 30, 60, 90, 120, 180, and 240 minutes following the dose. Concentrations of D_2O in samples were determined by infrared absorption.

The concentration of D_2O in blood or saliva also can be determined by gas chromatography and mass spectrometry.[83,112] The use of D_2O has been found to be simple, accurate, noninvasive (if saliva collections are used), and suitable for field studies.[4] In healthy subjects, the tracer equilibrates in the body's water within 2 hours after ingestion and remains at a constant concentration for the next 3 hours. In subjects experiencing edema, ascites, or some other form of water accumulation, 4 to 6 hours may be required for the D_2O to equilibrate.[82] Because deuterium is a stable isotope, its use is safe and ethical, even with children and females of childbearing age. Major drawbacks of the method are the cost of the equipment necessary to measure the D_2O in samples and the tedious work involved in preparing samples for analysis.[4,112,113]

Tritium (^3H) is a radioactive isotope of hydrogen with a mass three times that of ordinary hydrogen. Its use in measuring TBW is similar to that of deuterium oxide. Its radioactivity, however, makes it unsuitable in research involving children and females of childbearing age, or in studies requiring repeated administration of the tracer over a short period (for example, every 2 weeks or less).[83] The concentration of the isotope in body fluids is determined by a liquid scintillation counter, which measures the radioactive emission from the sample.[42,112,113]

The use of water labeled with the heavy isotope of oxygen (^{18}O) as a tracer in dilution studies is gaining popularity among researchers. It has the advantage of being a stable (nonradioactive) isotope, and exhaled carbon dioxide in the form of $C^{18}O_2$ is in isotopic equilibrium with body water and can be used as the sample for easy analysis by mass spectrometry.[42,112,113] These advantages are offset somewhat by the higher cost of $H_2{}^{18}O$ compared with that of the hydrogen isotopes.[42]

The three main sources of error in measuring total body water are failure to administer an accurately measured dose; consumption of beverages by subjects during the equilibration period, which may prevent equilibration from being reached; and contamination of the samples by atmospheric water before analysis. Calculation of the fat mass from TBW is based on the assumption that fat-free tissue has a constant water content that averages approximately 73%. This average value is based on analyses of a limited number of cadavers with actual values ranging from 67.4% to 77.5%. These variations can result in considerable error in calculating total body fat from TBW.[42] It also appears that fatter subjects tend to have a higher water content in their fat-free tissues. Failure to account for this will lead to an underestimation of fat mass based on TBW.

Total Body Potassium

Two factors make measurements of total body potassium of interest to those studying body composition. More than 90% of all the body's potassium is located within fat-free tissues (as an intracellular cation), and 0.012% of all potassium is the naturally occurring potassium-40 (^{40}K) isotope, which emits a very small yet detectable amount of high-energy gamma radiation.[4,42,83,112]

Measurement of total body potassium (TBK) requires a specially constructed counter fitted with multiple gamma-ray detectors, which are interfaced with a computer for data collection and processing. Because of the low levels of gamma radiation emitted from a subject, very sensitive detectors are required. The counter must be large enough to admit a subject and to be screened from external radiation (cosmic and local sources of ionizing radiation) by massive shields of lead or steel, thus making it very expensive.[42,112] The counting process requires about 30 minutes. Recently developed counters yield an estimate of TBK with a precision of about ± 3%.[42]

A major assumption of TBK measurement is that fat-free tissue has a known and constant potassium content. Researchers disagree on the concentration of potassium in fat-free tissue and whether there is a difference between the sexes.[4,42] The most widely published estimates are 66 and 60 mmol/kg of potassium in men and women, respectively.[42,112] It has been reported that the fat-free tissues of obese subjects tend to have a lower potassium content than the tissues of lean subjects. This may be due to actual differences in potassium content between obese and lean subjects. Another explanation may be that obese subjects have a thicker layer of potassium-poor fat surrounding a potassium-rich core of fat-free tissue, absorbing some of the radiation and thus leading to an underestimation of actual TBK and an overestimation of fat content in the obese.[42,112] It also has been reported that the potassium content of fat-free tissues decreases with increasing age.[42] Another factor affecting the performance of the counters is the presence of radioactive contamination on the subject's body and clothing from atmospheric radon gas.[4,83] Therefore, it is recommended that subjects shower, wash their hair, and wear clean clothes before undergoing TBK measurements.[83]

Despite the reported precision of ± 3%, the high cost and inherent limitations of the technique limit its use in estimating body composition. However, the technique does have value when used in conjunction with other measures. Combining the use of TBW measurements (which tend to underestimate body fat in obese subjects) with TBK measurements (which tend to overestimate body fat in the obese) may lead to more reliable estimates of body fat than either method alone.

Neutron Activation Analysis

Neutron activation analysis allows measurement of the body's content of calcium, iodine, hydrogen, sodium, chloride, phosphorus, carbon, and nitrogen.[4,83,112,126] Also known as in vivo neutron activation analysis, the method delivers a beam of neutrons to the subject, which interacts with the body's elements in several characteristic ways. In the most important of these (in terms of neutron activation analysis), atoms of target elements are activated, creating unstable isotopes, such as calcium-49 (^{49}Ca), nitrogen-15 (^{15}N), and sodium-24 (^{24}Na).[112,126,127] As these unstable isotopes revert back to their stable forms, gamma radiation of a characteristic energy is emitted from each. This is received by the system's detectors and analyzed by its computers. The unique energy level of the γ radiation identifies the element, and the radiation's level of activity represents its abundance. Gamma-ray emission can occur almost immediately (in which case, the technique is referred to as *prompt γ analysis*) or over a several-minute period (in which case, it is known as *delayed γ analysis*).[112,127]

Because a major component of muscle is nitrogen, the ability to measure nitrogen using neutron activation analysis allows the body's muscle and nonmuscle mass to be estimated.[83,112,126] The precision of repeated nitrogen determinations in healthy humans has been shown to be between 2% and 3%.[83]

Bone mineral content is of considerable interest to those studying osteoporosis, and neutron activation analysis is useful in measuring total body calcium, which is then used to quantitate total body bone mineral. The precision of repeated calcium measurements in healthy adults using neutron activation analysis has been 2.5%, making the method suitable for longitudinal studies of bone mass.[83] A more recent study of calcium content in phantoms (representations of the human body used for precision and accuracy testing) as measured by neutron activation analysis resulted in values within 3.6% of their known composition.[128]

Neutron activation analysis has been used successfully in clinical studies to assess the time required for body nitrogen to return to preoperative levels following aortic reconstruction surgery and to assess nutritional status in patients receiving continuous ambulatory peritoneal dialysis.[129,130] The accuracy and precision of the method are as good as, if not better than, those of other methods. It is preferable to isotope dilution techniques in patients requiring continuous intravenous fluid therapy and in those with large increases in body water. Newer, lighter-weight, portable units are making neutron activation analysis more available for body composition analysis in the clinical setting.[126] Neutron activation analysis is noninvasive and is not based on certain assumptions concerning ratios of major body compartments or their density, as are some of the methods used to assess body fat.[127]

The method has several drawbacks. It exposes subjects to ionizing radiation, is costly, and requires skilled operators.[79,112]

Creatinine Excretion

The amount of creatinine excreted in the urine over a 24-hour period can be used in estimating body muscle mass.[4,83] Creatinine is the only metabolite of creatine, a nitrogenous compound synthesized from amino acids in the liver and taken up by many tissues, but primarily by muscle. Ninety-eight percent of the body's creatine is found in muscle, primarily in the form of creatine phosphate (bound to adenosine triphosphate, where it serves as an immediate source of energy).[4,83] Creatine spontaneously dehydrates to form creatinine, which is then excreted unaltered in the urine. Therefore, measurement of creatinine in a 24-hour urine collection should reflect the level of total body creatinine and consequently total body muscle mass.[4]

Several problems are associated with this approach. The most notable of these are the influence of meat consumption on urinary creatinine levels and the large intraindividual variability in daily urinary creatinine excretion (about $\pm$ 11%) in persons consuming a meat-free diet.[83] Dietary creatine can influence urinary creatinine independently of muscle mass. Therefore, the diets of subjects undergoing urinary creatinine measurements should be meat free or be of a constant composition.[4] Urine collections must be complete because an error of 15 minutes in the timing of 24-hour urine collections can affect results of creatinine measurements by 1%.[4,83] Some researchers advise making three consecutive 24-hour urine collections to assure a representative creatinine excretion for an individual.[83] The precision of automated procedures for determining creatinine concentration in urine is approximately 1% to 2%, introducing further error.[83]

Despite these potential sources of error, estimates of fat-free mass based on 24-hour urinary excretion of creatinine have been shown to correlate reasonably well with those derived from measurements of body density, total body nitrogen, and total body potassium.[131,132] More accurate estimates of fat-free mass can be obtained from measurement of body density, total body nitrogen, and total body potassium. However, when the necessary facilities or resources are unavailable or when subjects are too ill to undergo such testing, urinary creatinine may be the most acceptable approach. Another urinary metabolite that appears better correlated with densitometrically determined fat-free mass is 3-methylhistidine.

3-Methylhistidine

3-Methylhistidine is an amino acid found in actin and myosin, the contractile proteins of muscle. 3-Methylhistidine is a *derived amino acid;* it is formed by the addition of methyl groups to histidine present in actin and myosin after these contractile proteins have been synthesized. When these proteins are catabolized, the 3-methylhistidine is released, not reutilized for protein synthesis, but excreted quantitatively in the urine. Assuming that muscle protein synthesis and degradation are balanced during steady-state periods, urinary 3-methylhistidine should be proportional to muscle mass.[4]

Lukaski and coworkers[131] have shown 24-hour urinary excretion of 3-methylhistidine to be well correlated to fat-free mass, determined by densitometry in healthy males age 23 to 52 years consuming a meat-free diet. In a later study, Lukaski and coworkers[132] assessed skeletal muscle mass in 14 healthy adult males on a meat-free diet using measurements of 3-methylhistidine, total body nitrogen, and total body potassium. Urinary excretion of 3-methylhistidine was significantly related to skeletal muscle mass and appeared to be a valid index of muscle and fat-free mass.

Measurement of urinary 3-methylhistidine excretion is subject to the same potential errors as are possible in measurement of urinary creatinine excretion.[4,83] Intraindividual variability is reported to range from 10% to 20%. Subjects should refrain from eating meat during the measurement period. Twenty-four-hour urine collections should be accurately timed and complete.[83] Before 3-methylhistidine can be used as a routine indicator of muscle mass, however, the effects of sex, age, maturity, fitness status, recent intense exercise, disease, and injury on 3-methylhistidine levels must be better understood.

Electrical Conductance

The use of electrical conductance to assess body composition is based on the marked difference in electrolyte content between fat and fat-free tissue.[112,133,134] Electrolytes such as sodium, chloride, potassium, and bicarbonate are found primarily in the fat-free tissues, whereas concentrations of these ions in adipose tissue are very low. Because electrolytes in body water are capable of conducting electricity, the body's fat-free mass has a greater electrical conductivity than its fat mass. This difference in conductivity is the basis of two body assessment methods: bioelectrical impedance and total body electrical conductivity.

Bioelectrical Impedance

When an electrical current is passed through the body, it is opposed by the nonconducting tissues (principally, fat and cell membranes) and is transmitted by electrolytes dissolved in water (largely found in the fat-free tissues, although adipose tissue contains about 14% water).[4,112,133,134] This opposition to an alternating current is called impedance, which is composed of two elements: resistance and reactance. In bioelectrical impedance analysis (BIA), an electronic instrument (Figure 6.41) generates an alternating current, which is passed through the body by means of four electrodes placed on the hand and foot. The current (50 kHz, 800 mA) is harmless and cannot be felt by the subject. The body's resistance to this current is measured by the instrument. Some BIA instruments simply provide the operator with a value for resistance, which is then used (along with the subject's stature, weight, and sex) to manually calculate total body water, fat-free mass, and percent of body fat. More sophisticated BIA instruments contain a computer and printer and are capable of automatically performing these calculations and providing a printed record.

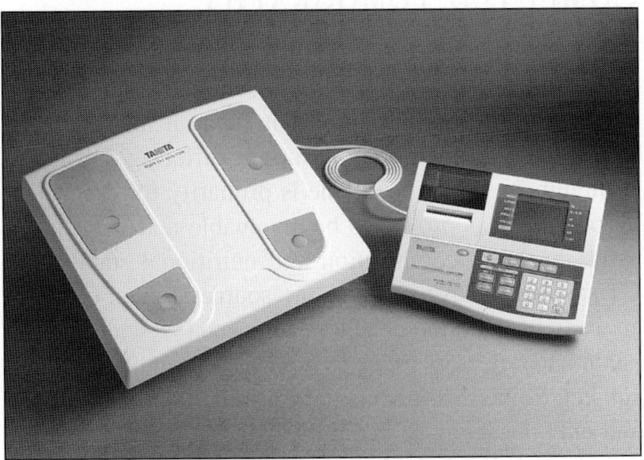

Figure 6.41
Bioelectrical impedance offers a convenient, rapid, noninvasive, and safe approach for assessing body composition. In this unit, four electrodes are built into the top of a digital scale (shown on the left). The subject stands on the scale, which simultaneously measures body weight and bioelectrical impedance. The microprocessor/printer (on the right) performs the calculations and provides visual and written output of body composition.
Source: Photo courtesy of Tanita Corporation of America.

Bioelectrical impedance analysis yields values for TBW that are very close to those obtained by dilution techniques.[112,113,133,134] One of the primary weaknesses of BIA, however, is estimating fat-free mass and percent of body fat from the value for TBW using regression equations. Because BIA relies on regression equations for calculating fat-free mass and percent of body fat, the method is only as good as the equation used.[112,135] Earlier equations tended to give inaccurate estimates of fat-free mass and percent of body fat; more recent equations are considerably better. Another weakness is that BIA assumes that subjects are normally hydrated. Dehydration caused by insufficient water intake, excessive perspiration, heavy exercise, or alcohol use (which stimulates urine production, possibly leading to dehydration) will result in overestimation of fat mass. To prevent this, subjects are advised to drink plenty of water, refrain from consuming alcohol the day before testing, and avoid heavy exercise 12 hours before testing.

When compared with estimates of percent body fat derived from underwater weighing, BIA has been shown to be as good as (if not slightly better than) skinfold measurements in predicting percent body fat.[133,134] The method has the advantage of being safe, convenient to use, portable, rapid, and noninvasive. Bioelectrical impedance is among the procedures used in NHANES. The only drawback is the instrument's cost, which can range from $2000 to $3000.

Total Body Electrical Conductivity

The degree to which an object placed in an electromagnetic field will tend to disrupt that field depends on the quantity of conducting material in the object. Because electrolytes within the fat-free mass are capable of conducting electricity, the degree to which a body placed in an electromagnetic field (EMF) disrupts that field is closely related to the amount of fat-free mass.[112,135] The instrument for measuring total body electrical conductivity (TOBEC) consists of a large solenoid coil driven by an oscillating radio-frequency current, which generates an EMF. The subject is placed on a table, which is slowly rolled into the coil. Changes in the EMF are measured between the conditions when the subject is inside the coil and when the coil is empty.[112] These changes are proportional to the total electrical conductivity of the subject's body. Using the statistical process of multiple-regression analysis, regression equations have been developed allowing TBW, TBK, fat-free mass, and percent body fat to be predicted from these changes.[112] Although TOBEC has been shown to compare favorably with other body composition assessment methods, the bulkiness and high cost of the units (approaching $100,000) seriously limit their use in nutritional assessment.

Infrared Interactance

When a material is exposed to infrared light, the light is absorbed, reflected, or transmitted, depending on the scattering and absorption properties of the material.[83] For example, water, protein, and fat have specific infrared absorption characteristics because of the stretching and bending of hydrogen bonds associated with the carbon, oxygen, and nitrogen they contain.[136] Information about the chemical composition (for example, water, protein, and fat content) of a material is contained in the infrared light reflected from the material.[83] Infrared instruments have been used successfully since about 1965 to determine the amount of moisture, protein, fat, and starch in grains and oil seeds.[83,136]

In human body composition analysis, a battery-powered, computerized infrared spectrophotometer has been developed. A probe, or "light wand," which acts as both an infrared transmitter and a detector, is attached to the unit by an electrical cord. The probe is placed on the subject's skin, and infrared light of two wavelengths is transmitted through the skin from the probe. Infrared light reflected from the skin and underlying tissues is detected by the probe. Estimates of body composition are made by analyzing certain characteristics of the reflected light (the shape of the interactance spectrum).[83,136,137] The instrument does not provide a measurement of fat thickness.

As an approach to estimating body composition, infrared interactance is marketed as safe, noninvasive, rapid, and convenient to use. These advantages have made infrared interactance a popular body composition technique at some hospitals, health clubs, and weight loss clinics.[138] Recent validation studies have raised questions about the accuracy of infrared interactance to estimate body composition.[138–141] When compared with other body composition methods (underwater weighing, skinfold measurements, and bioelectrical impedance analysis), infrared interactance overestimated percent body fat in lean subjects (< 8% body fat) and underestimated body fat in obese subjects (> 30% body fat).[138,141]

As a method for estimating body composition, most researchers report that infrared interactance is inferior to skinfold measurements and bioelectrical impedance.[138–142] At this time, it is not a recommended approach for determining body composition.

Ultrasound

Ultrasound is a widely used medical imaging method and has been studied as a possible tool in nutritional assessment. The heart of the technique is the transducer.[143] The transducer converts electrical energy into high-frequency sound and then converts that sound back into electrical energy; in other words, it acts as both a transmitter and a receiver. When the transducer is applied to the body surface, the ultrasound is transmitted into the body in the form of short pulses. As the ultrasound perpendicularly strikes the interface between two tissues differing in density (for example, adipose tissue and muscle), some of the sound is reflected and received by the transducer. The first reflection occurs at the transducer-skin interface. Each succeeding tissue interface results in a reflection, the intensity of which is reduced by the depth of the patient's tissues. This reflected sound is visually displayed on a video screen.[4,83,143]

In most published studies, ultrasonography has been compared with use of skinfold calipers. The results have been mixed and may be due to differences in instrumentation, technique, and interpretation.[144–146] Considerable skill is required in using the method and interpreting its results. The transducer must be applied to the skin surface with uniform and constant pressure to prevent differences in adipose and other soft tissue compression.[83,147] Differences in study populations could partly explain the conflicting results. For example, ultrasound may be preferable to skinfold calipers in measuring very obese individuals because of difficulty in accurately measuring skinfolds on them.[135,147]

Ultrasound has several advantages. It is noninvasive, nonradioactive, safe, and relatively portable, although less so than skinfold calipers. It may be a more appropriate technique for assessing persons whose skinfolds are thick and/or difficult to measure. Compared with the use of skinfold calipers, ultrasound is much more expensive and requires more training for its operation and interpretation.[83,135]

Computed Tomography

Computed tomography (CT) is an imaging technique producing highly detailed cross-sectional images of the body resulting from differences in the transmission of an X-ray beam through body tissues of differing density.[135] Although its role in medicine is primarily for diagnostic purposes, it has proved to be a valuable research tool in assessing body composition and nutritional status. The CT system consists of an X-ray source aligned opposite an array of radiation detectors. In some CT scanners, the beam and detectors rotate in a plane perpendicular to the subject. Some instruments have a full circle of detectors, and only the X-ray source moves.[112,143]

As the X-ray beam passes through the subject, it is weakened, or attenuated, by the body's tissues and eventually picked up by the detectors. The response of the detectors is then transmitted to a computer, which also considers the spatial arrangement of the subject and X-ray beam. From these data, the computer reconstructs the subject's cross-sectional anatomy, using mathematic equations adapted for computer processing.[112,143]

CT has been particularly useful in studying the relative deposition of subcutaneous and intraabdominal fat.[148–150] CT images can be used to differentiate among various types of lean tissue, such as skeletal muscle, visceral mass, or organ mass; to provide data on the amount and distribution of adipose tissue in skeletal muscle; and to discriminate between cortical and trabecular bone.[112,154] Estimates of subcutaneous and intraabdominal fat from CT have been shown to compare very closely with direct measurements in cadavers and laboratory animals.[151,152] CT scans at three sites—lower chest, abdomen, and midthigh—have been shown to be effective in estimating body fat mass in premenopausal obese women.[153]

The potential for using CT in assessing body composition and nutritional status has been limited by problems of radiation exposure and the high cost and limited availability of the instrument.[83,112] Multiple scans of the same individual, whole-body scans, and use of CT with children and women of childbearing age are not encouraged because of the exposure to ionizing radiation. The use of the technology in nutritional assessment is restricted, for the most part, to special research applications. Recently, however, techniques have been used to reduce radiation exposure without compromising the accuracy of measurements of abdominal fat volume and distribution.[112,150,155]

Magnetic Resonance Imaging

Magnetic resonance imaging (MRI) is a technology that allows both imaging of the body and in vivo chemical analysis without hazard to the subject.[112,156] Originally referred to as nuclear magnetic resonance, this approach is based on the fact that the nucleus of an atom acts as a magnet; it has north and south poles and is said to be a *magnetic dipole.* Ordinarily, nuclei or magnetic dipoles are oriented randomly. However, if a subject is placed in a large bore magnet generating a very strong magnetic field, the magnetic dipoles become aligned in relation to the magnetic field. If a radio-frequency wave is then directed into the subject's body, some of the nuclei will absorb energy from the radio wave and change their orientation with respect to the magnetic field. When the radio wave is discontinued, the nuclei gradually return to their equilibrium state (relaxation) and emit a signal that can be received by the system. These data are then processed by computer to generate an image much the same way as in CT.[83,112,135]

The hydrogen nucleus is particularly well suited for analysis because of its high concentration and abundance in the body and its easy detection by MRI. Tissue levels of phosphorus also can be detected in tissues using MRI. This allows investigators to quantify the relative amounts of ATP, phosphocreatine, and inorganic phosphorus in the body's tissues.[112] MRI allows researchers to monitor the metabolic functions of certain tissues and organs in response to certain treatments, including various nutritional regimens.[112,156]

MRI is a valuable tool for assessing muscle mass and regional fat distribution, giving accurate and precise measurements of muscle and adipose tissue content, when compared with direct measures in cadavers. For example, MRI was used to measure the intraabdominal, retroperitoneal, and subcutaneous adipose tissue content in three unembalmed cadavers, which were subsequently dissected so that the adipose tissue in these three compartments could be accurately weighed.[157] MRI was shown to be an accurate technique to evaluate the content of the adipose tissue in these compartments. In a similar study, MRI was used to measure adipose tissue–free skeletal muscle cross-sectional area, adipose tissue embedded in muscle (interstitial adipose tissue), and adipose tissue surrounding muscle (subcutaneous adipose tissue) in nearly 120 arms and legs of cadavers.[158] The limbs were then carefully dissected and the corresponding tissues weighed. Values obtained from MRI compared favorably with those obtained from direct analysis of the tissues involved. The accuracy and precision with which MRI can make these measurements has made MRI the "method of choice for calibration of field methods designed to measure body fat and skeletal muscle *in vivo.*"[156]

The advantages of MRI are several. It is totally noninvasive, uses no ionizing radiation (thus, it is safe for children, females of childbearing age, and multiple studies on the same subject), produces high-quality images of the body, allows the amount and distribution of body fat to be studied, and can be used to study the metabolic activity of tissues or organs. MRI can image hydrogen, phosphorus, carbon, fluoride, sodium, and potassium.[112] The low-contrast resolution of MRI is much better than that of CT. Drawbacks of the method are its restricted availability and high cost.[83]

Dual-Energy X-Ray Absorptiometry

Dual-energy X-ray absorptiometry (DXA) was originally developed as a means of assessing bone mineral density for the diagnosis of osteoporosis, an area in which it is particularly well suited because of its high precision in measuring bone mineral density, as discussed in Chapter 8. However, in recent years it has become one of the most widely used approaches for determining fat mass and fat-free mass.[159–161] As a body composition assessment method, DXA has the advantage of being fast and safe. A whole-body scan takes about 3 minutes, and the radiation exposure is 0.01 to 0.04 millirem, an extremely low dose compared to the exposure from a conventional chest X ray, which is approximately 40 millirem. The fact that the procedure requires little cooperation from patients makes it an attractive body composition assessment method for the very young, the very old, and the sick. The use of effective and user-friendly software allows personnel with minimal training to operate the instrument and produce high-quality output.[159] Body composition estimates from DXA have been shown to be highly correlated with those from underwater weighing and measurement of total body water.[160,161] DXA is used by NHANES for determining bone mineral density and analysis of body composition.

As with any technology, DXA has some limitations. Marked differences in the hydration of lean tissue from that seen in healthy adults may adversely affect the accuracy of body composition measures. Consequently, concerns have been raised about the appropriateness of using DXA for assessing body composition in infants (who tend to have a higher degree of lean tissue hydration than adults) and in persons with acute or chronic alterations in body water. Body composition measurements may be affected by the thickness of the body part being scanned, possibly resulting in systematic differences between thin and obese persons or affecting the accuracy of serial measurements in persons losing or gaining weight. The accuracy of regional soft tissue measurements can be adversely affected by the presence of bone (especially by ribs in the thorax) and the calcification of soft tissues (as is seen in the aortas of older people).[160–162] Differences in instruments between various manufacturers as well as between different models produced by the same manufacturer have been reported.[160] However, ongoing improvements in scanner technology and the software used by the scanners has led to DXA becoming an increasingly common technique for body composition analysis in the clinical setting.[117,159,162]

Summary

1. Anthropometry is the measurement of body size, weight, and proportions. Adherence to proper technique is critical to obtaining accurate and precise measurements. Among children, length, stature, weight, and head circumference are the most sensitive and commonly used anthropometric indicators of health.
2. Body weight, one of the most important measurements in nutritional assessment, should be obtained using an electronic or balance-beam scale with nondetachable weights that is appropriate for the subject. Attention must be given to regular calibration of balance-beam scales, especially after they have been moved.
3. Standards for assessing physical growth of persons from birth to age 20 years have been developed by the Centers for Disease Control and Prevention. These growth charts allow a child's development to be easily categorized relative to the development of other children of similar age and sex.
4. Overweight is a body weight above some reference weight, which usually is defined in relation to stature. Obesity is an excess of body fat in relation to lean body mass. Overweight persons tend to die sooner than average-weight persons, especially those who are overweight at younger ages. The lowest mortality in the United States is associated with body weights that are somewhat below average for a given group based on sex and stature.
5. Approaches to assessing body weight include height-weight tables, relative weight, and height-weight indices. The life insurance industry, a leader in the development of height-weight tables, has attempted to define body weights for a given sex and stature that are associated with the lowest mortality.
6. Height-weight tables fail to provide information on body composition. Their data are not drawn from representative population samples and are sometimes self-reported. They inadequately control for confounding variables, such as cigarette smoking, which tend to make lower body weights appear less healthy.
7. Relative weight is a person's actual weight divided by some reference weight for that person's height, multiplied by 100, and expressed as a percentage of reference weight. Relative weights between 90% and 120% are considered within normal limits.
8. Of the various body mass indices available, the most common is Quetelet's index—weight in kilograms divided by height in meters squared. Although body mass indices tend to be better predictors of obesity than height-weight tables or relative weight, they still do not distinguish between overweight resulting from obesity and that resulting from unusual muscular development.
9. The distribution of body fat may be as important a consideration as total quantity of fat. Body fat distribution can be classified into two types:

upper body (android, or male, type) and lower body (gynoid, or female, type). Android obesity is associated with increased risk of insulin resistance, hyperinsulinemia, impaired glucose tolerance (prediabetes), type 2 diabetes mellitus, hypertension, hyperlipidemia, stroke, and death. The waist-to-hip ratio and waist circumference are valuable indices of regional body fat distribution.

10. Body composition analysis can provide estimates of the body's reserves of fat, protein, water, and several minerals. The two-compartment model divides the body into fat and fat-free masses. The four-compartment model views the human body as composed of four chemical groups: water, protein, mineral, and fat. Most approaches to determining body composition are indirect measures.

11. Measurement of skinfolds is the most widely used method of indirectly estimating percent body fat. What is actually measured is the thickness of a double fold of skin and compressed subcutaneous adipose tissue.

12. Skinfold measures have several advantages. The equipment is inexpensive and portable. Measurements can be easily and quickly obtained, and they correlate well with body density measurements. Proper measurement of skinfolds requires careful site selection and strict adherence to the standardized techniques outlined in this chapter.

13. The triceps is the most commonly used single skinfold site. Single-site skinfold measurements must be interpreted with caution and should be used only as a rough approximation of total body fat percentage. Results should be compared with reference data derived from large population surveys, such as NHANES.

14. For assessing body composition of young people, the sum of two sites (triceps and subscapular or triceps and medial calf) often is used. These sites correlate with other measures of body fatness and are more reliably and objectively measured than most other sites, and reference data are available.

15. Regression equations allow body density and percent body fat to be estimated from multiple skinfold measures. These equations were developed by seeing which combination of anthropometric measures best predict body density. Generalized equations can be applied to groups varying greatly in age and body fatness and can replace several population-specific equations with little loss in prediction accuracy.

16. Densitometry involves measuring the density of the entire body, usually by hydrostatic (underwater) weighing. If mass and volume of the body are known, its density can be calculated. However, hydrostatic weighing is not practical for testing large groups. It requires considerable subject cooperation, special equipment, experience, and financial investment.

17. Despite its weaknesses, underwater weighing remains the standard laboratory technique for determining body density and percent body fat. Compared with other body density methods and more sophisticated body composition techniques, the costs are low.

18. Air displacement plethysmography involves using a specially designed two-chambered unit for measuring the body's volume, which is then used to calculate body density and composition. Subjects better tolerate this method than underwater weighing. It requires less subject cooperation, and residual lung volume measurements are not needed. It appears as accurate and precise as underwater weighing, but the equipment is considerably more complex and costly.

19. Total body water is measured indirectly using dilution techniques where a tracer of known concentration and volume is given to a subject, time is allowed for the tracer to equilibrate with the subject's body water, and the concentration of the tracer in a sample of the subject's blood, urine, or saliva is analyzed. Commonly used tracers include deuterium oxide and water labeled with the heavy isotope of oxygen.

20. Measurement of total body potassium can also be used to evaluate body composition. More than 90% of body potassium is located within fat-free tissues, and 0.012% of potassium is potassium-40 isotope, which emits gamma radiation.

21. Neutron activation analysis is based on the response of elements (e.g., nitrogen, calcium, and carbon) to neutron beam irradiation and is particularly useful in estimating total body muscle. The method's drawbacks include ionizing radiation exposure, high cost, and limited availability.

22. Measurement of creatinine in a 24-hour urine collection reflects total body muscle mass. Despite limitations by such factors as dietary creatine, intraindividual variation, and timing of urine collections, estimates of fat-free mass based on urinary creatinine correlate reasonably well with estimates derived from measurements of body density, total body nitrogen, and total body potassium.

23. 3-Methylhistidine is an amino acid found in the contractile proteins actin and myosin. When these proteins are catabolized, 3-methylhistidine is released and excreted in the urine. Urinary excretion has been shown to be a valid index of muscle

and fat-free mass. However, its measurement is subject to the same potential errors as those in measurements of urinary creatinine excretion.

24. The marked difference in electrolyte content between fat and fat-free tissues is a basic principle behind body composition estimates from bioelectrical impedance analysis (BIA) and total body electrical conductivity (TOBEC). In BIA, the body's resistance to a minute electrical current is used to calculate total body water, from which the percentages of body fat and fat-free mass are calculated using various formulas.

25. In TOBEC, the degree to which a body placed in an electromagnetic field (EMF) disrupts that field is closely related to the amount of fat-free mass. TOBEC uses an instrument consisting of a large solenoid coil driven by an oscillating radio-frequency current, which generates an EMF. Like BIA, the accuracy of total body water estimates can be affected by dehydration. It appears to be an acceptable technique for body composition assessment, but its use is limited by high cost.

26. When infrared light is projected through the skin, some of the energy is reflected from the skin and underlying tissues. Estimates of body composition are made by analyzing certain characteristics of this reflected energy. The approach tends to overestimate percent body fat in lean subjects and underestimate percent body fat in obese subjects. This method is inferior to skinfold measurements and is not recommended for determining body composition.

27. In ultrasound, high-frequency sound waves are transmitted into the body from a transducer applied to the skin surface. As ultrasound strikes the interface between two tissues differing in density (for example, adipose tissue and muscle), some of it is reflected and received by the transducer. The time lag between reflections allows tissue layer depth to be calculated. Ultrasound compares favorably with skinfold measurements but may be preferable to skinfold measurements when evaluating very obese people.

28. Computed tomography is an imaging technique producing highly detailed cross-sectional images of the body caused by differences in the transmission of an X-ray beam through body tissues of differing density.

29. Magnetic resonance imaging is a technology allowing both imaging of the body and in vivo chemical analysis without radiation hazard to the subject.

30. Body composition estimates derived from dual-energy X-ray absorptiometry (DXA) compare favorably with those from underwater weighing. DXA has the advantage of requiring little subject cooperation, being relatively quick, and having a low radiation dose. Differences in hydration and the presence of bone or calcified soft tissues may affect the accuracy of body composition measurements.

References

1. Chumlea WC, Roche AF, Mukherjee D. 1987. *Nutritional assessment of the elderly through anthropometry.* Columbus, OH: Ross Laboratories.
2. Moore WM, Roche AF. 1983. *Pediatric anthropometry,* 2nd ed. Columbus, OH: Ross Laboratories.
3. Heymsfield SB, Casper K. 1987. Anthropometric assessment of the adult hospitalized patient. *Journal of Parenteral and Enteral Nutrition* 11(suppl):36S–41S.
4. Brodie DA. 1988. Techniques of measurement of body composition. Part I. *Sports Medicine* 5:11–40.
5. Pollock ML, Jackson AS. 1984. Research progress in validation of clinical methods of assessing body composition. *Medicine and Science in Sports and Exercise* 16:606–613.
6. Chumlea WC, Roche AF, Steinbaugh ML. 1985. Estimating stature from knee height for persons 60 to 90 years of age. *Journal of the American Geriatrics Society* 33:116–120.
7. Gordon CC, Chumlea WC, Roche AF. 1988. Stature, recumbent length, and weight. In Lohman TG, Roche AF, Martorell R (eds.), *Anthropometric standardization reference manual.* Champaign, IL: Human Kinetics Books.
8. Kuczmarski RJ, Ogden CL, Guo SS, et al. 2002. *2000 CDC growth charts for the United States: Methods and development.* National Center for Health Statistics. Vital and Health Statistics, Series 11, Number 246.
9. Centers for Disease Control and Prevention. 2010. Use of World Health Organization and CDC Growth Charts for children aged 0–59 months in the United States. *Morbidity and Mortality Weekly Report* 59(No. RR-9):1–15.
10. Parsons HG, George MA, Innis SM. 2011. Growth assessment in clinical practice: Whose growth curve? *Current Gastroenterology Reports* 13:286–292.
11. Mei Z, Grummer-Strawn LM. 2011. Comparison of changes in

growth percentiles of US children on CDC 2000 growth charts with corresponding changes on WHO 2006 growth charts. *Clinical Pediatrics* 50:402–407.

12. Ogden CL, Flegel KM. 2010. Changes in terminology for childhood overweight and obesity. National Health Statistics Reports No. 25, National Center for Health Statistics, U.S. Centers for Disease Control and Prevention, U.S. Department of Health and Human Services.
13. Krebs NS, Himes JH, Jacobson D, Nicklas TA, Guilday P. 2007. Assessment of child and adolsescent overweight and obesity. *Pediatrics* 120(suppl 4):S193–S228.
14. Barlow SE. 2007. Expert committee recommendations regarding the prevention, assessment, and treatment of child and adolescent overweight and obesity: Summary report. *Pediatrics* 120(suppl 4):S164–S192.
15. Food and Nutrition Board, National Research Council. 1989. *Diet and health: Implications for reducing chronic disease risk.* Washington, DC: National Academy Press.
16. Prospective Studies Collaboration. 2009. Body-mass index and cause-specific mortality in 900,000 adults: Collaborative analyses of 57 prospective studies. *Lancet* 373:1083–1096.
17. Manson JE, Skerrett PJ, Greenland P, VanItallie TB. 2004. The escalating pandemics of obesity and sedentary lifestyle: A call to action for clinicians. *Archives of Internal Medicine* 164:249–258.
18. Weinstein AR, Sesso HD, Lee IM, Cook NR, Manson JE, Buring JE, Gaziano JM. 2004. Relationship of physical activity vs. body mass index with type 2 diabetes in women. *Journal of the American Medical Association* 292:1188–1194.
19. National Task Force on the Prevention and Treatment of Obesity. 2000. Overweight, obesity, and health risk. *Archives of Internal Medicine* 160:898–904.
20. May AL, Kuklina EV, Yoon PW. 2012. Prevalence of cardiovascular disease risk factors among US adolescents, 1999–2008. *Pediatrics* 129:1035–1041.
21. Weigley ES. 1984. Average? Ideal? Desirable? A brief overview of height-weight tables in the United States. *Journal of the American Dietetic Association* 84:417–423.
22. Manson JE, Stampfer MJ, Hennekens CH, Willett WC. 1987. Body weight and longevity: A reassessment. *Journal of the American Medical Association* 257:353–358.
23. Ideal weights for women. 1942. *Statistical bulletin of the Metropolitan Life Insurance Company* 23(October):6–8.
24. Ideal weights for men. 1943. *Statistical bulletin of the Metropolitan Life Insurance Company* 24(June):6–8.
25. New weight standards for men and women. 1959. *Statistical bulletin of the Metropolitan Life Insurance Company* 40(November– December):1–3.
26. Metropolitan height and weight tables. 1983. *Statistical bulletin of the Metropolitan Life Insurance Company* 64(January–June):2.
27. Nieman DC. 2003. *Exercise testing and prescription: A health-related approach,* 5th ed. Boston: McGraw-Hill.
28. Pirie P, Jacobs D, Jeffery R, Hannan P. 1981. Distortion in self-reported height and weight data. *Journal of the American Dietetic Association* 78:601–606.
29. Rowland ML. 1991. Self-reported weight and height. *American Journal of Clinical Nutrition* 52:1125–1133.
30. Schlichting PF, Hoilund-Carlsen PF, Quaade F, Lauritzen SL. 1981. Comparison of self-reported height and weight with controlled height and weight in women and men. *International Journal of Obesity* 5:67–76.
31. DelPrete LR, Caldwell M, English C, Banspach SW, Lefebvre C. 1992. Self-reported and measured weights and heights of participants in community-based weight loss programs. *Journal of the American Dietetic Association* 92:1483–1486.
32. Willett WC, Stampfer M, Manson J, VanItallie T. 1991. New weight guidelines for Americans: Justified or injudicious? *American Journal of Clinical Nutrition* 53:1102–1103.
33. Frisancho AR. 1990. *Anthropometric standards for the assessment of growth and nutritional status.* Ann Arbor: University of Michigan Press.
34. Novascone MA, Smith EP. 1989. Frame size estimation: A comparative analysis of methods based on height, wrist circumference, and elbow breadth. *Journal of the American Dietetic Association* 89:964–966.
35. Wilmore JH, Frisancho RA, Gordon CC, Himes JH, Martin AD, Martorell R, Seefeldt VD. 1988. Body breadth equipment and measurement techniques. In Lohman TG, Roche AF, Martorell R, eds. *Anthropometric standardization reference manual.* Champaign, IL: Human Kinetics Books.
36. Katch VL, Freedson PS. 1982. Body size and shape: Derivation of the HAT frame size model. *American Journal of Clinical Nutrition* 36:669–675.
37. Katch VL, Freedson PS, Katch FI, Smith L. 1982. Body frame size: Validity of self-appraisal. *American Journal of Clinical Nutrition* 36:676–679.
38. Grant JP, Custer PB, Thurlow J. 1981. Current techniques of nutritional assessment. *Surgical Clinics of North America* 61:437–463.
39. Garn SM, Pesick SD, Hawthorne VM. 1983. The bony chest breadth as a frame size standard in nutritional assessment. *American Journal of Clinical Nutrition* 37:315–318.
40. Baecke JAH, Burema J, Deurenberg P. 1982. Body fatness, relative weight and frame size in young adults. *British Journal of Nutrition* 48:1–6.
41. Frisancho AR, Flegel PN. 1983. Elbow breadth as a measure of

frame size for U.S. males and females. *American Journal of Clinical Nutrition* 37:311–314.

42. Garrow JS. 1983. Indices of adiposity. *Nutrition Abstracts and Reviews* 53:697–708.
43. Callaway CW, Chumlea WC, Bouchard C, Himes JH, Lohman GT, Martin AD, Mitchell CD, Mueller WH, Roche AF, Seefeldt VD. 1988. Circumferences. In Lohman TG, Roche AF, Martorell R, eds. *Anthropometric standardization reference manual.* Champaign, IL: Human Kinetics Books.
44. Lee J, Kolonel LN, Hinds MW. 1981. Relative merits of the weight-corrected-for-height indices. *American Journal of Clinical Nutrition* 34:2521–2529.
45. Lee J, Kolonel LN, Hinds MW. 1982. Relative merits of old and new indices of body mass: A commentary. *American Journal of Clinical Nutrition* 36:727–728.
46. Lee J, Kolonel LN. 1983. Body mass indices: A further commentary. *American Journal of Clinical Nutrition* 38:660–661.
47. Garrow JS, Webster J. 1985. Quetelet's index (W/H^2) as a measure of fatness. *International Journal of Obesity* 9:147–153.
48. Willett WC, Dietz WH, Colditz GA. 1999. Guidelines for healthy weight. *New England Journal of Medicine* 341:427–434.
49. Barlow SE, Dietz WH. 1998. Obesity evaluation and treatment: Expert committee recommendations. *Pediatrics* 102(3). http://www.pediatrics.org/cgi/content/full/102/3/e29.
50. Flegal KM. 1999. The obesity epidemic in children and adults: Current evidence and research issues. *Medicine and Science in Sports and Exercise* 31(suppl):S509–S514.
51. Smalley KJ, Knerr AN, Kendrick ZV, Colliver JA, Owen OE. 1990. Reassessment of body mass indices. *American Journal of Clinical Nutrition* 52:405–408.
52. Dietz WH, Robinson TN. 1998. Uses of the body mass index as a measure of overweight in children and adolescents. *Journal of Pediatrics* 132:191–193.
53. Killeen J, Vanderburg D, Harlan W. 1978. Application of weight-height ratios and body mass indices to juvenile populations—the National Health Examination Survey data. *Journal of Chronic Diseases* 31:529–537.
54. Dietz WH, Bellizzi MC. 1999. Introduction: The use of body mass index to assess obesity in children. *American Journal of Clinical Nutrition* 70(suppl):S123–S125.
55. Bellizzi MC, Dietz WC. 1999. Workshop on childhood obesity: Summary of the discussion. *American Journal of Clinical Nutrition* 70(suppl):S173–S175.
56. Roche AF, Siervogel RM, Chumlea WC, Webb P. 1981. Grading body fatness from limited anthropometric data. *American Journal of Clinical Nutrition* 34:2831–2838.
57. Keys A, Fidanza F, Karvonen MJ, Kimura N, Taylor HL. 1972. Indices of relative weight and obesity. *Journal of Chronic Diseases* 25:329–343.
58. Norgan NG, Ferro-Luzzi A. 1982. Weight-height indices as estimators of fatness in men. *Human Nutrition: Clinical Nutrition* 36C:363–372.
59. Frisancho AR, Flegel PN. 1982. Relative merits of old and new indices of body mass with reference to skinfold thickness. *American Journal of Clinical Nutrition* 36:697–699.
60. National Institutes of Health. 1998. *Clinical guidelines on the identification, evaluation, and treatment of overweight and obesity in adults.* National Heart, Lung, and Blood Institute. NIH publication number 98-4083.
61. U.S. Department of Health and Human Services and U.S. Department of Agriculture. 2010. *Dietary Guidelines for Americans, 2010.* Washington, DC: U.S. Government Printing Office. www.dietaryguidelines.gov.
62. Kahn HS. 1991. A major error in nomograms for estimating body mass index. *American Journal of Clinical Nutrition* 54:435–437.
63. Giovannucci E, Colditz GA, Stampfer MJ, Willett WC. 1996. Physical activity, obesity, and risk of colorectal adenoma in women (United States). *Cancer Causes and Control* 7:253–263.
64. Troiano RP, Flegal KM. 1999. Overweight prevalence among youth in the United States: Why so many different numbers? *International Journal of Obesity* 23(suppl 2):S22–S27.
65. Wang Y, Rimm EB, Stampfer MJ, Willett WC, Hu FB. 2005. Comparison of abdominal adiposity and overall obesity in predicting risk of type 2 diabetes among men. *American Journal of Clinical Nutrition* 81:555–563.
66. Bray GA, Champagne CM. 2004. Obesity and the metabolic syndrome: Implications for dietetics practitioners. *Journal of the American Dietetic Association* 104:86–89.
67. Kaye SA, Folsom AR, Prineas RJ, Potter JD, Gapstur SM. 1990. The association of body fat distribution with lifestyle and reproductive factors in a population study of postmenopausal women. *International Journal of Obesity* 14:583–591.
68. Troisi RJ, Weiss ST, Segal MR, Cassano PA, Vokonas PS, Landsberg L. 1990. The relationship of body fat distribution to blood pressure in normotensive men: The normative aging study. *International Journal of Obesity* 14:515–525.
69. Zwiauer K, Widhalm K, Kerbl B. 1990. Relationship between body fat distribution and blood lipids in obese adolescents. *International Journal of Obesity* 14:271–277.
70. National Institutes of Health. 2000. *The practical guide; identification, evaluation, and treatment of overweight and obesity in adults.* National Heart, Lung, and Blood Institute. NIH publication number 00-4084.
71. Rankinen T, Kim SY, Perusse L, Despres JP, Bouchard C. 1999. The prediction of abdominal visceral fat level from body composition and anthropometry: ROC analysis. *International*

Journal of Obesity and Related Metabolic Research 23:801–809.

72. Turcato E, Bosello O, Francesco VD, Harris TB, Zoico E, et al. 2000. Waist circumference and abdominal sagittal diameter as surrogates of body fat distribution in the elderly: Their relation with cardiovascular risk factors. *International Journal of Obesity and Related Metabolic Research* 24:1005–1010.
73. Clasey JL, Bouchard C, Teates CD, Riblett JE, Thorner MO, et al. 1999. The use of anthropometric and dual-energy x-ray absorptiometry (DXA) measures to estimate total abdominal and abdominal visceral fat in men and women. *Obesity Research* 7:256–264.
74. Must A, Strauss RS. 1999. Risk and consequences of childhood and adolescent obesity. *International Journal of Obesity and Related Metabolic Disorders* 23(suppl 2): S2–S11.
75. Flegal KM. 1999. The obesity epidemic in children and adults: Current evidence and research issues. *Medicine and Science in Sports and Exercise* 31(suppl):S509–S514.
76. Colditz GA. 1999. Economic costs of obesity and overweight. *Medicine and Science in Sports and Exercise* 31(suppl):S663–S667.
77. Sassi F. 2010. *Obesity and the economics of prevention.* Paris: Organisation for Economic Cooperation and Development.
78. Chandra RK. 1981. Immunodeficiency in undernutrition and overnutrition. *Nutrition Reviews* 39:225–231.
79. Chandra RK. 1991. 1990 McCollum Award lecture. Nutrition and immunity: Lessons from the past and new insights into the future. *American Journal of Clinical Nutrition* 53:1087–1101.
80. Bistrian BR, Blackburn GL, Hallowel E, Heddle R. 1974. Protein status of general surgical patients. *Journal of the American Medical Association* 230:858–860.
81. Bistrian BR, Blackburn GL, Vitale J, Cochran D, Naylor J. 1976. Prevalence of malnutrition in general medical patients. *Journal of the American Medical Association* 235:1567–1570.
82. Coats KG, Morgan SL, Bartolucci AA, Weinsier RL. 1993. Hospital-associated malnutrition: A reevaluation 12 years later. *Journal of the American Dietetic Association* 93:27–33.
83. Lukaski HC. 1987. Methods for the assessment of human body composition: Traditional and new. *American Journal of Clinical Nutrition* 46:537–556.
84. Wang J, Thornton JC, Kolesnik S, Pierson RN. 2000. Anthropometry in body composition. An overview. *Annals of the New York Academy of Sciences* 904:317–326.
85. Keys A, Brozek J. 1953. Body fat in adult man. *Physiological Reviews* 33:245–325.
86. Wilmore JH, Buskirk ER, DiGirolamo M, Lohman TG. 1986. Body composition: A round table. *Physician and Sportsmedicine* 14:144–162.
87. Clarys JP, Martin AD, Drinkwater DT, Marfell-Jones MJ. 1987. The skinfold: Myth and reality. *Journal of Sports Sciences* 5:3–33.
88. Martin AD, Ross WD, Drinkwater DT, Clarys JP. 1985. Prediction of body fat by skinfold caliper: Assumptions and cadaver evidence. *International Journal of Obesity* 9:31–39.
89. Harrison GG, Buskirk EB, Carter JEL, Johnston JE, Lohman TG, Pollock ML, Roche AF, Wilmore J. 1988. Skinfold thicknesses and measurement technique. In Lohman TG, Roche AF, Martorell R (eds.), *Anthropometric standardization reference manual.* Champaign, IL: Human Kinetics Books.
90. Himes JH, Roche AF, Siervogel RM. 1979. Compressibility of skinfolds and the measurement of subcutaneous fatness. *American Journal of Clinical Nutrition* 32:1734–1740.
91. Siervogel RM, Roche AF, Himes JH, Chumlea WC, McCammon R. 1982. Subcutaneous fat distribution in males and females from 1 to 39 years of age. *American Journal of Clinical Nutrition* 36:162–171.
92. Lohman TG. 1981. Skinfolds and body density and their relation of body fatness: A review. *Human Biology* 53:181–225.
93. Lohman TG. 1988. Anthropometry and body composition. In Lohman TG, Roche AF, Martorell R (eds.), *Anthropometric standardization reference manual.* Champaign, IL: Human Kinetics Books.
94. Jackson AS, Pollock ML. 1985. Practical assessment of body composition. *Physician and Sportsmedicine* 13(5):76–90.
95. Martorell R, Mendoza F, Mueller WH, Pawson IG. 1988. Which side to measure: Right or left? In Lohman TG, Roche AF, Martorell R (eds.), *Anthropometric standardization reference manual.* Champaign, IL: Human Kinetics Books.
96. Leger LA, Lambert J, Martin P. 1982. Validity of plastic skinfold caliper measurements. *Human Biology* 54:667–675.
97. Burgert SL, Anderson CF. 1979. A comparison of triceps skinfold values as measured by the plastic McGaw caliper and Lange caliper. *American Journal of Clinical Nutrition* 32:1531–1533.
98. Ross JG, Pate RR, Delpy LA, Gold RS, Svilar M. 1987. New health-related fitness norms. *Journal of Physical Education, Recreation, and Dance* 58:(9)66–70.
99. Lohman TG. 1987. The use of skinfolds to estimate body fatness on children and youth. *Journal of Physical Education, Recreation, and Dance* 58(9):98–102.
100. American Alliance for Health, Physical Education, Recreation, and Dance. 1985. *Norms for college students: Health-related physical fitness test.* Reston, VA: American Alliance for Health, Physical Education, Recreation, and Dance.
101. Jackson AS, Pollock ML, Ward A. 1980. Generalized equations for predicting body density of women. *Medicine and Science in Sports and Exercise* 12:175–182.
102. Pollock ML, Laughridge EE, Coleman B, Linnerud AC, Jackson A. 1975. Prediction

of body density in young and middle-aged women. *Journal of Applied Physiology* 38:745–749.

103. Jackson AS, Pollock ML. 1978. Generalized equations for predicting body density in men. *British Journal of Nutrition* 40:497–504.
104. Brozek J, Keys A. 1951. The evaluation of leanness-fatness in man: Norms and intercorrelations. *British Journal of Nutrition* 5:194–205.
105. Durnin JVGA, Womersley J. 1974. Body fat assessment from total body density and its estimation from skinfold thickness: Measurements on 481 men and women aged 16–72 years. *British Journal of Nutrition* 32:77–97.
106. Baun WB, Baun MR, Raven PB. 1981. A nomogram for the estimate of percent body fat from generalized equations. *Research Quarterly for Exercise and Sport* 52:380–384.
107. Westrate JA, Deurenberg P. 1989. Body composition in children: Proposal for a method for calculating body fat percentage from total body density or skinfold-thickness measurements. *American Journal of Clinical Nutrition* 50:1104–1115.
108. Katch F, Michael ED, Horvath SM. 1967. Estimation of body volume by underwater weighing: Description of a simple method. *Journal of Applied Physiology* 23:811–813.
109. Akers R, Buskirk ER. 1969. An underwater weighing system utilizing "force cube" transducers. *Journal of Applied Physiology* 26:649–652.
110. Wilmore JH. 1969. A simplified method for determination of residual volumes. *Journal of Applied Physiology* 27:96–100.
111. Goldman HI, Becklake MR. 1959. Respiratory function tests: Normal values at median altitudes and the prediction of normal results. *American Review of Tuberculosis and Pulmonary Diseases* 79:457–467.
112. Ellis KJ. 2000. Human body composition: In vivo methods. *Physiological Reviews* 80:649–680.
113. Wagner DR, Heyward VH. 1999. Techniques of body composition assessment: A review of laboratory and field methods. *Research Quarterly for Exercise and Sport* 70:135–149.
114. Dempster P, Aitkens S. 1995. A new air displacement method for the determination of human body composition. *Medicine and Science in Sports and Exercise* 27:1692–1697.
115. McCrory MA, Gomez TD, Bernauer EM, Molé PA. 1995. Evaluation of a new air displacement plethysmograph for measuring human body composition. *Medicine and Science in Sports and Exercise* 27:1686–1691.
116. Sardinha LB, Lohman TG, Teixeira PJ, Guedes DP, Going SB. 1998. Comparison of air displacement plethysmography with dual-energy x-ray absorptiometry and 3 field methods for estimating body composition in middle-aged men. *American Journal of Clinical Nutrition* 68:786–793.
117. Fields DA, Goran MJ, McCrory MA. 2002. Body-composition assessment via air-displacement plethysmography in adults and children: A review. *American Journal of Clinical Nutrition* 75:453–467.
118. Radley D, Gately PJ, Cooke CB, Carroll S, Oldroyd B, Truscott JG. 2005. Percentage fat in overweight and obese children: Comparison of DXA and air displacement plethysmography. *Obesity Research* 13:75–85.
119. Demerath EW, Guo SS, Chumlea WC, Towne B, Roche AF, Siervogel RM. 2002. Comparison of percent body fat estimates using air displacement plethysmography and hydrodensitometry in adults and children. *International Journal of Obesity and Related Metabolic Disorders* 26:389–397.
120. Fields DA, Hunter GR, Goran MI. 2000. Validation of the Bod Pod with hydrostatic weighing: Influence of body clothing. *International Journal of Obesity* 24:200–205.
121. Collins MA, Millard-Stafford ML, Sparling PB, Snow TK, Rosskopf LB, Webb SA, Omar J. 1999. Evaluation of the Bod Pod for assessing body fat in collegiate football players. *Medicine and Science in Sports and Exercise* 31:1350–1356.
122. Dewit O, Fuller NJ, Fewtrell MS, Wells JCK. 2000. Whole body air displacement plethysmography compared with hydrodensitometry for body composition analysis. *Archives of Disease in Childhood* 82:159–164.
123. Biaggi RR, Vollman MW, Nies MA, Brener CE, Flakoll PJ, et al. 1999. Comparison of air-displacement plethysmography with hydrostatic weighing and bioelectrical impedance analysis for the assessment of body composition in healthy adults. *American Journal of Clinical Nutrition* 69:898–903.
124. Nunez C, Kovera AJ, Pietrobelli A, Heshka S, Horlick M, Kehayias JJ, et al. 1999. Body composition in children and adults by air displacement plethysmography. *European Journal of Clinical Nutrition* 53:382–387.
125. Lukaski HC, Johnson PE. 1985. A simple, inexpensive method of determining total body water using a tracer dose of D2O and infrared absorption of biological fluids. *American Journal of Clinical Nutrition* 41:363–370.
126. Kehayias JJ, Valtuena S. 1999. Neutron activation analysis determination of body composition. *Current Opinion in Clinical Nutrition and Metabolic Care* 2:453–463.
127. Beddoe AH, Hill GL. 1985. Clinical measurement of body composition using in vivo neutron activation analysis. *Journal of Parenteral and Enteral Nutrition* 9:504–520.
128. Ryde SJ, Morgan WD, Compston J, Evans CJ. 1990. Measurements of total body calcium by prompt-gamma neutron activation analysis using a 252Cf source. *Biological Trace Element Research* 26-27:429–437.

129. Fletcher JP, Allen BJ, Blagojevic N. 1990. Changes in body protein composition following aortic reconstruction. *Australian and New Zealand Journal of Surgery* 60:209–211.

130. Pollock CA, Allen BJ, Warden RA, Caterson RJ, Blagojevic N, Cocksedge B, Mahoney JF, Waugh DA, Ibels LS. 1990. Total body nitrogen by neutron activation in maintenance dialysis. *American Journal of Kidney Diseases* 16:38–45.

131. Lukaski HC, Mendez J. 1980. Relationship between fat free weight and urinary 3-methylhistidine excretion in man. *Metabolism* 29:758–761.

132. Lukaski HC, Mendez J, Buskirk ER, Cohn SH. 1981. Relationship between endogenous 3-methylhistidine excretion and body composition. *American Journal of Physiology* 240:E302–307.

133. Segal KR, Gutin B, Presta E, Wang J, VanItallie TB. 1985. Estimation of human body composition by electrical impedance methods: A comparative study. *Journal of Applied Physiology* 58:1565–1571.

134. Lukaski HC, Bolonchuk WW, Hall CB, Siders WA. 1986. Validation of tetrapolar bioelectrical impedance method to assess human body composition. *Journal of Applied Physiology* 60:1327–1332.

135. Brodie DA. 1988. Techniques of measurement of body composition. Part II. *Sports Medicine* 5:74–98.

136. Conway JM, Norris KH. 1987. Noninvasive body composition in humans by near infrared interactance. In Ellis KJ, Yasumura S, Morgan WD (eds.), *In vivo body composition studies.* London, England: Institute of Physical Sciences in Medicine.

137. Conway JM, Norris KH, Bodwell CE. 1984. A new approach for the estimation of body composition: Infrared interactance. *American Journal of Clinical Nutrition* 40:1123–1130.

138. Mclean KP, Skinner JS. 1992. Validity of Futrex-5000 for body composition determination. *Medicine and Science in Sports and Exercise* 24:253–258.

139. Williams DP, Going SB, Milliken LA, Hall MC, Lohman TG. 1995. Practical techniques for assessing body composition in middle-aged and older adults. *Medicine and Science in Sports and Exercise* 27:776–783.

140. Thomas DW, Ryde SJ, Ali PA, Birks JL, Evans CJ, Saunders NH, et al. 1997. The performance of an infra-red interactance instrument for assessing total body fat. *Physiological Measurement* 18:305–315.

141. Brooke-Wavell K, Jones PR, Norgan NG, Hardman AE. 1995. Evaluation of near infra-red interactance for assessment of subcutaneous and total body fat. *European Journal of Clinical Nutrition* 49:57–65.

142. Wilmore KM, McBride PJ, Wilmore JH. 1994. Comparison of bioelectrical impedance and near-infrared interactance for body composition assessment in a population of self-perceived overweight adults. *International Journal of Obesity* 18:375–381.

143. Bushong SC. 1993. *Radiologic science for technologists: Physics, biology, and protection,* 5th ed. St. Louis, MO: Mosby.

144. Borkan GA, Hults DE, Cardarelli JC, Burrows BA. 1982. Comparison of ultrasound and skinfold measurements in assessment of subcutaneous and total fatness. *American Journal of Physical Anthropology* 58:307–313.

145. Fanelli MT, Kuczmarski RJ. 1984. Ultrasound as an approach to assessing body composition. *American Journal of Clinical Nutrition* 39:703–709.

146. Chiba T, Lloyd DA, Bowen A, Condon-Meyers A. 1989. Ultrasonography as a method of nutritional assessment. *Journal of Parenteral and Enteral Nutrition* 13:529–534.

147. Booth RAD, Goddard A, Paton A. 1966. Measurement of fat thickness in man: A comparison of ultrasound, Harpenden calipers and electrical conductivity. *British Journal of Nutrition* 20:719–725.

148. Weits T, van der Beek EJ, Wedel M, Hubben MW, Koppeschaar HP. 1989. Fat patterning during weight reduction: A multimodal investigation. *Netherlands Journal of Medicine* 35:174–184.

149. Seidell JC, Bakker CJG, van der Kooy K. 1990. Imaging techniques for measuring adipose-tissue distribution—A comparison between computed tomography and 1.5-T magnetic resonance. *American Journal of Clinical Nutrition* 51:953–957.

150. Rogalla P, Meiri N, Hoksch B, Boeing H, Hamm B. 1998. Low-dose spiral computed tomography for measuring abdominal fat volume and distribution in a clinical setting. *European Journal of Clinical Nutrition* 52:597–602.

151. Rössner S, Bo WJ, Hiltbrandt E, Hinson W, Karstaedt N, Santago P, Sobol WT, Crouse JR. 1990. Adipose tissue determinations in cadavers—A comparison between cross-sectional planimetry and computed tomography. *International Journal of Obesity* 14:893–902.

152. Weingand KW, Hartke GT, Noordsy TW, Ledeboer DA. 1988. A minipig model of body adipose tissue distribution. *International Journal of Obesity* 13:347–355.

153. Ferland M, Despres JP, Tremblay A, Pinault S, Nadeau A, Moorjani S, Lupien PJ, Theriault G, Bouchard C. 1989. Assessment of adipose tissue distribution by computed axial tomography in obese women: Association with body density and anthropometric measurements. *British Journal of Nutrition* 61:139–148.

154. Goodpaster BH, Thaete FL, Kelley DE. 2000. Composition of skeletal muscle evaluated with computed tomography. *Annals of the New York Academy of Sciences* 904:18–24.

155. Starck G, Lonn L, Cederblad A, Alpsten M, Sjostrom L, Ekholm

S. 1998. Dose reduction for body composition measurements with CT. *Applied Radiation and Isotopes* 49:561–563.

156. Ross R, Goodpaster B, Kelley D, Boada F. 2000. Magnetic resonance imaging in human body composition research. *Annals of the New York Academy of Sciences* 904:12–17.

157. Abate N, Burns D, Peshock RM, Garg A, Grundy SM. 1994. Estimation of adipose tissue mass by magnetic resonance imaging: Validation against dissection in human cadavers. *Journal of Lipid Research* 35:1490–1496.

158. Mitsiopoulos N, Baumgartner RN, Heymsfield SB, Lyons W, Gallagher D, Ross R. 1998. Cadaver validation of skeletal muscle measurement by magnetic resonance imaging and computerized tomography. *Journal of Applied Physiology* 85:115–122.

159. Albanese CV, Diessel E, Genant HK. 2003. Clinical applications of body composition measurements using DXA. *Journal of Clinical Densitometry* 6:75–85.

160. Schoeller DA, Tylavsky FA, Baer DJ, Chumlea WC, Earthman CP, Fuerst T, et al. 2005. QDR 4500A dual-energy X-ray absorptiometer underestimates fat mass in comparison to criterion methods in adults. *American Journal of Clinical Nutrition* 81:1018–1025.

161. Bolanowski M, Nilsson BE. 2001. Assessment of human body composition using dual-energy X-ray absorptiometry and bioelectrical impedance analysis. *Medical Science Monitor* 7:1029–1033.

162. Foster BJ, Leonard MB. 2004. Measuring nutritional status in children with chronic kidney disease. *American Journal of Clinical Nutrition* 80:801–814.

Assessment Activity 6.1

Assessment and Classification of Body Weight

Successful treatment of overweight begins with the assessment and classification of body weight. This assessment activity explains how to assess and classify body weight, waist circumference, and risk status using the approaches recommended by the U.S. National Institutes of Health in its publication *The Practical Guide; Identification, Evaluation, and Treatment of Overweight and Obesity in Adults.*[70] Although several accurate methods exist for measuring body fat, most of these methods are not readily available in the clinical setting. Body mass index (BMI) is recommended as the most practical approach for assessing body weight in the clinical setting and can be used as a surrogate method for assessing body fat content. Table 6.6 gave classifications of overweight and obesity, based on BMI. It should be noted that BMI overestimates body fat in very muscular persons and in patients with edema. It can underestimate body fat in persons who have lost muscle mass (such as the elderly). Waist circumference is recommended as the most practical tool for assessing a person's abdominal fat content. The cutpoints for high-risk waist circumference were given in Table 6.7. BMI and waist circumference also can be used to monitor response to weight management treatment in persons whose BMI is < 35 kg/m^2.

Begin this assessment activity by accurately measuring your stature, body weight, and waist circumference and then calculating your body mass index (BMI), following the instructions in this chapter. Classify your BMI and waist circumference (high-risk or low-risk) using Tables 6.6 and 6.7 and Figure 6.42; if applicable, classify your disease risk ("increased," "high," "very high," or "extremely high") using Table 6.6. Record your results in the following spaces:

Body weight:

_____ lb _____ kg (pounds ÷ 2.2 = kg)

Body stature:

_____ in. _____ m (inches × 0.0254 = m)

Waist circumference:

_____ in. _____ cm (inches × 2.54 = cm)

Body mass index:

_____ kg/m^2

BMI classification:

____

Waist circumference classification:

____

Disease risk classification:

____

Elevated BMI, high-risk waist circumference, or both suggest the need for weight loss but do not indicate the required intensity of intervention. Patients who have certain obesity-related diseases (*comorbidities*) or who have cardiovascular disease risk factors (Table 6.12) are at a higher risk for mortality than those who do not have these diseases or risk factors. Consequently, patients need to be screened for these diseases and risk factors and, when present, placed on a program of intense risk-factor modification and weight management intervention.

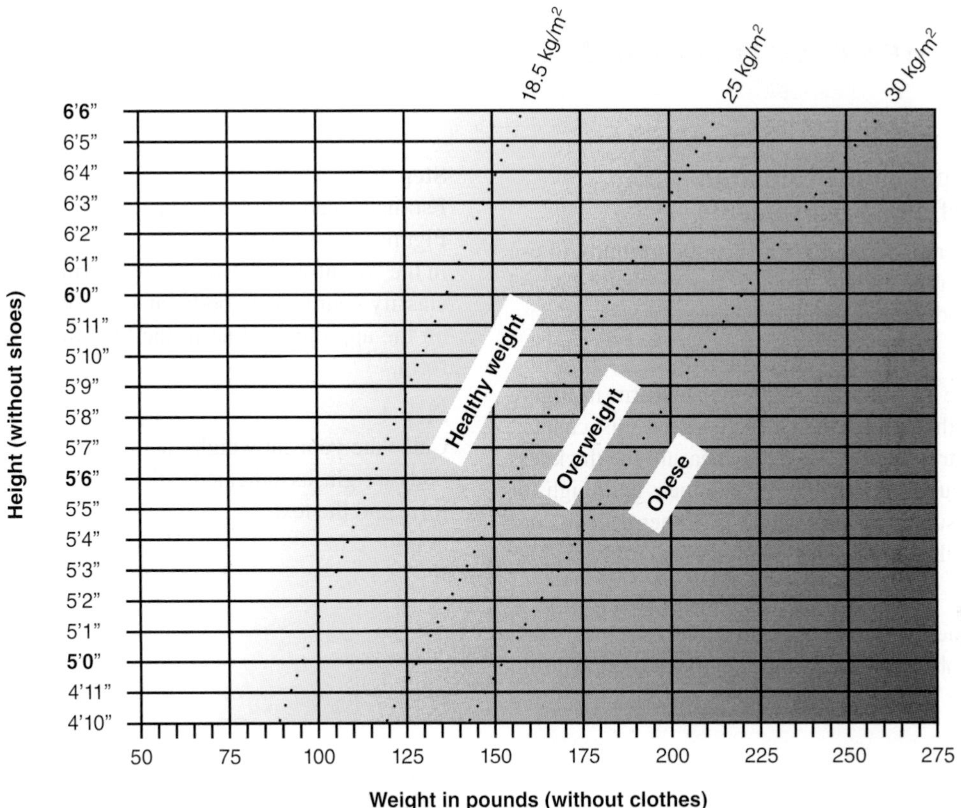

Figure 6.42

Using body mass index (BMI), body weight can be grouped into three categories. Healthy weight is defined as a BMI of 18.5 kg/m^2 up to 25 kg/m^2, overweight is a BMI of 25 kg/m^2 up to 30 kg/m^2, and obese is a BMI of 30 kg/m^2 or greater.

TABLE 6.12 Diseases and Risk Factors That Place Patients at Increased Risk for Mortality

Diseases Placing Patients at Very High Risk for Mortality

- Established coronary heart disease
- Atherosclerotic diseases other than coronary heart disease (e.g., peripheral arterial disease, abdominal aortic aneurysm, symptomatic carotid artery disease)
- Type 2 diabetes (fasting plasma glucose ≥ 126 mg/dL or 2-hour postprandial plasma glucose ≥ 200 mg/dL)
- Sleep apnea

Cardiovascular Disease Risk Factors

- Cigarette smoking
- Hypertension (systolic blood pressure ≥ 140 mm Hg or diastolic blood pressure ≥ 90 mm Hg) or current use of antihypertensive medication
- High-risk low-density lipoprotein cholesterol (≥ 160 mg/dL) or borderline high-risk (130 to 159 mg/dL), along with two or more other risk factors
- Low high-density lipoprotein cholesterol (< 35 mg/dL)
- Impaired fasting glucose (between 110 and 125 mg/dL)
- Family history of premature coronary heart disease
- Age (if male, ≥ 45 years; if female, ≥ 55 years or postmenopausal)
- Physical inactivity

Assessment Activity 6.2

Body Composition Evaluation Using Skinfold Measurements

This assessment activity gives you an opportunity to use skinfold measurements to estimate percent body fat and to evaluate body composition.

Step 1
Photocopy the "Skinfold Measurements" form in Figure 6.35. Using the information described in this chapter, have your instructor or a classmate measure the thickness of three of your skinfolds (chest, abdomen, and thigh for men; triceps, suprailiac, and thigh for women), and record the values on the "Skinfold Measurements" form.

Step 2
Total the values of the three skinfold measurements and enter this number on the appropriate line in the "Skinfold Measurements" form.

Step 3
Estimate percent body fat using the nomogram in Figure 6.34. Enter this percentage on the appropriate line in the "Skinfold Measurements" form. Using Table 6.11, classify your percent body fat and write that classification on the appropriate line in the "Skinfold Measurements" form.

Step 4
Calculate your fat weight, lean body weight, and desired body weight, as indicated in the "Skinfold Measurements" form and the text.

CHAPTER 7

Assessment of the Hospitalized Patient

Outline

Introduction
Assessing Nutritional Status
Determining Energy Requirements
Determining Protein Requirements
Mini Nutritional Assessment
Malnutrition Universal Screening Tool
Summary
References
Assessment Activity 7.1: Estimating Stature and Body Weight
Assessment Activity 7.2: Arm Muscle Area

Student Learning Outcomes

After studying this chapter, the student will be able to:

1. Differentiate between nutritional assessment and nutritional screening.
2. Discuss the characteristics of the nutritional screening process.
3. Identify some of the diagnoses and problems that can increase risk of malnutrition in hospitalized patients.
4. Given the appropriate data, correctly calculate the following: percent desirable body weight, percent usual weight, and percent weight change.
5. Compare and contrast the Harris-Benedict equations, the World Health Organization equations, and the equations used to calculate EER in terms of the variables they require, how they were developed, how they are applied, and their accuracy.
6. Differentiate between resting energy expenditure and basal metabolic rate.
7. Describe how various stresses (diseases or traumatic events) affect resting energy expenditure and energy requirement in humans.
8. Describe how various stresses (diseases or traumatic events) affect nitrogen excretion and protein requirement in humans.
9. Demonstrate the ability to correctly screen the nutritional status of a patient using the Mini Nutritional Assessment and the Malnutrition Universal Screening Tool.

Introduction

In today's cost-conscious health care environment, the demand to control health care costs supports the assessment of the nutritional status of hospitalized patients. Estimates of the prevalence of protein-energy malnutrition (PEM) among hospitalized patients typically range from 20% to 50%.[1] These estimates vary, depending on the measures used to define PEM and the population studied (elderly and more acutely ill patients are more likely to have PEM than younger and less acutely ill patients). Compared with their well-nourished counterparts, patients with PEM have a greater risk of postoperative infection, with an increased length of hospital stay, a higher risk for mortality, and a greater likelihood of readmission to the hospital following discharge.[1] Appropriate nutritional support of these patients can result in faster recovery and shorter hospital stays, which translate into reduced health care expenditures. Another reason that nutritional assessment of hospitalized patients is important is our increasing capability to provide nutritional support to these patients through enteral and parenteral routes.

This chapter discusses approaches to assessing the nutritional status of hospitalized patients. It brings together many of the various assessment techniques discussed in previous chapters (e.g., anthropometric and dietary) and shows how they are used to evaluate nutritional status in hospitalized patients. It also builds on Chapter 6 by introducing several new anthropometric techniques that are unique to the acute-care setting.

Assessing Nutritional Status

Assessing the nutritional status of the hospitalized patient involves four steps:[2,3] First, all patients must receive a *nutritional screening* to determine whether they are at risk of impaired nutritional status. Second, patients who are nutritionally at risk should receive a more in-depth *nutritional assessment* to determine the severity and causes of their nutritional impairment. Although both undernutrition and overnutrition can negatively affect health, most frequently it is undernutrition (particularly, protein-energy malnutrition) that is of greatest concern in hospitalized patients. Third, if the patient is nutritionally impaired, the dietitian should develop a nutritional support plan for improving the patient's nutritional status. Finally, the patient should be monitored to ensure an appropriate response to nutritional support.

Nutritional Screening

Nutritional screening "is the process of identifying characteristics known to be associated with nutrition problems. Its purpose is to pinpoint individuals who are malnourished or at nutritional risk."[4] The standards for nutrition care established by the Joint Commission on the Accreditation of Health Care Organizations (JCAHO) do not require that nutritional screening be done within a specific time following admission but, rather, indicate that it be carried out "in a timely, effective, and efficient manner." Considering the emphasis given to short hospitalizations in order to contain health care costs, it is reasonable to expect that a nutritional screen be done on all patients within the first 24 to 48 hours following admission, although, the earlier the screen is performed and acted on, the sooner the patient will, if necessary, receive and benefit from nutritional support. Nutritional screening can be done by any member of the health care team. Because it does not require the high degree of nutrition knowledge and expertise of a registered dietitian, it is best done by a dietetic technician. Box 7.1 outlines the characteristics of the nutritional screening process.[4]

Screening can be greatly facilitated by using a checklist or form on which pertinent patient information can be entered. Once completed, this form can be placed in the patient's medical record for other members of the health care team to refer to. An example of a nutritional screening form is shown in Figure 7.1.[5] Information required to complete the form includes anthropometric, biochemical, clinical, and dietary data. Much of this information can be obtained from the patient's medical record. To use the

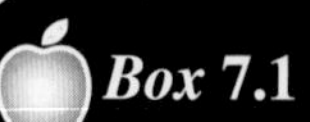

Box 7.1 Characteristics of the Nutritional Screening Process

- It can be completed in any setting, either through personal contact with the patient or by collecting data from the patient's chart
- It facilitates completion of early intervention
- It includes the collection of relevant data on risk factors and the interpretation of data for intervention and treatment
- It determines the need for a more in-depth nutritional assessment
- It is cost-effective

Adapted from Posthauer ME, Dorse B, Foiles RA, et al. 1994. ADA's definitions for nutrition screening and nutrition assessment. *Journal of the American Dietetic Association* 94:838–839.

Nutritional Screening Form

Laboratory Values

1. ☐ Albumin ≤ 2.9 mg/dl ________ 6. ☐ Albumin < 3.5 mg/dl ________

Anthropometrics

Ht ______ Admit Wt ______ Usual Wt ______ DBW ______

BMI ______ % DBW ______ % Wt Lost ______

2. ☐ <80% DBW 7. ☐ 80%-90% of Usual Wt

3. ☐ >10% Wt Lost 8. ☐ 5%-10% Wt Lost

Feeding

4. ☐ Parenteral/Enteral Feeding 9. ☐ Loss of appetite (<1/2 trays)

10. ☐ Chewing or swallowing difficulty

11. ☐ >3 days of NPO, dextrose, and/or clear liquids only

Nutrition-Related Problems/Diagnoses

5. ☐ Malnutrition ☐ Sepsis 12. ☐ Nutrition-related diagnosis/problems ____________

☐ Pressure ulcers ☐ AIDS

☐ Dysphagia/renal/hepatic diet restrictions

13. ☐ Serum cholesterol ≥ 200 mg/dL

14. ☐ Random glucose ≥ 200 mg/dL

15. ☐ BMI ≥ 27 kg/m^2 women; ≥ 28 kg/m^2 men

☐ No further nutrition evaluation recommended at this time

☐ Patient may benefit from further nutritional evaluation and will be seen by a Registered Dietitian or Dietetic Technician

☐ Care Level I ☐ Care Level II ☐ Care Level III

☐ Diet counseling/education/classes recommended (1 risk in criteria 13-15), which requires a physician order

Patient Information

Current diet order: ____________

Screened by: ____________

Date: ____________

Figure 7.1 **An example of a form that can be used to screen patients for nutritional risk.**

Source: Adapted from Hedberg AM, Garcia N, Trejus IJ, Weinmann-Winkler S, Gabriel ML, Lutz AL. 1988. Nutritional risk screening: Development of a standardized protocol using dietetic technicians. *Journal of the American Dietetic Association* 88:1553–1556.

screening form in Figure 7.1, place a check in every box that applies to the patient and, when appropriate, enter pertinent patient data on the line next to certain items.

Suppose your patient's serum albumin were 2.5 mg/dL. Check the box following number 1 to indicate that the serum albumin level is ≤ 2.9 mg/dL. Then enter the patient's serum albumin level on the line following that item. Enter the patient's anthropometric data next (Ht = height; Admit Wt = body weight on admission; DBW = desirable body weight). A patient's usual weight is his or her stable weight in the past 6 to 12 months. It can be determined by asking the patient or a significant other or looking in the nurses' notes or in the medical records of previous hospitalizations, if these are available.

Desirable (or reference) body weight can be obtained from a height-weight chart or calculated using the BMI equation with a given BMI of 22 kg/m^2 (the approximate mid-point of the healthy BMI range for adults) and given the patient's height and solving for weight. The particular height-weight chart used varies among health care facilities. Calculate the percent of desirable weight (or relative weight) and percent of weight lost (these are discussed in the section on Physical Examination. Enter the values in the appropriate lines and place checks in the appropriate boxes. Check on the form whether the patient is receiving parenteral feedings (administered directly into a central or peripheral vein) or enteral feedings (administered into the stomach or small intestine), has experienced loss of appetite (eating less than one-half of the food on the meal trays), has been NPO ("non per os," meaning "nothing by mouth"), or has received only intravenous fluids (e.g., 5% dextrose in water) or clear liquids for more than 3 days. Certain diagnoses, such as pressure ulcers, sepsis, HIV/AIDS, diet restrictions because of dysphagia, renal or hepatic disease, and, of course, a diagnosis of malnutrition, place a patient at nutritional risk. Nutritional risk is increased when serum cholesterol, random (or nonfasting) serum glucose, and body mass index are above certain cutpoints. Nutritional risk can also be elevated in certain nutrition-related diagnoses and problems, as listed in Box 7.2.

A patient receiving one check for items 6 through 12 (found along the right side of the form) falls in Care Level I. Follow-up for these patients can be done by a registered dietitian or a dietetic technician. A patient having one or more checks for items 1 through 5 (found on the left side of the form) or two or more checks for items 6 through 12 falls within Care Level II and should receive further evaluation by a registered dietitian. Patients receiving enteral or parenteral nutritional support are placed in Care Level III and are further evaluated by a registered dietitian. A patient not meeting these criteria requires no further nutritional evaluation unless a change in his or her condition warrants it. If a patient receives a check for items 13 through 15, he or she would likely benefit from diet counseling or education. A check is placed in the appropriate box (diet counseling/education/classes and so on) to signal the patient's physician, who can then order any necessary intervention.

Nutritional Assessment

Once nutritional screening has identified a patient to be at nutritional risk, a nutritional assessment should be done to determine the severity and causes of the patient's nutritional impairment, to evaluate whether the nutritional impairment is a factor contributing to the worsening of the patient's medical condition, and to monitor the patient's response to nutritional support. If the nutritional impairment is identified and documented as a factor appreciably worsening the patient's health (what is called a comorbidity and complicating condition), it could increase the reimbursement the health care facility receives for that patient's care.[4,6,7] This is an important consideration for dietitians who want to document the revenue-generating ability and cost-effectiveness of nutrition services rather than being a nonreimbursable service and easy target of draconian budget cuts.

Because no single measurement or test by itself is capable of providing information sufficient to evaluate a patient's nutritional status, a variety of available measurements and tests must be used. Much of the basic information needed to assess a patient's nutritional status is fairly easy to obtain by simply asking the patient (or a close friend or relative of the patient) or by using relatively

Box 7.2 Diagnoses and Problems That Can Increase Risk of Malnutrition

Trauma: fracture, burn, closed head injury, gunshot wound, spinal cord injury, motor vehicle accident
Dysphagia
Bowel resection
Short bowel syndrome
Small bowel obstruction
Hypoglycemia
Failure to thrive
Congenital heart disease
Chronic obstructive pulmonary disease
Anorexia
Cancer
HIV/AIDS
Vomiting or diarrhea
Anemia
Stroke or hemiparesis
Gastrointestinal bleeding
Crohn's disease
Dumping syndrome
Pressure ulcers
Organ transplant
Diabetes mellitus
Coronary artery disease
Pancreatitis

inexpensive tests or measurements. It is important to note that some of this information is routinely collected by the medical and nursing staff and is recorded in the patient's medical record. This basic information includes the patient's stature, usual and present weight, and past and current dietary practices; any significant changes in eating habits; and the presence of any nutrition-related problems. The medical record can provide much relevant information from the physician's history and physical exam, relevant information about previous hospitalizations, reports from consulting physicians, and results of various X-ray, imaging, and diagnostic tests, including routine laboratory tests, such as a complete blood count and chemistry profile (see Chapter 9 for additional information about laboratory tests). Important information can be obtained from the notes recorded by nurses and allied health professionals. In many instances, this information is sufficient to assess the nutritional status of less critically ill patients or those with more obvious nutritional deficits.

For more critically ill patients or those with less obvious nutritional deficits, more detailed anthropometric, laboratory, and dietary information may need to be collected. Included among anthropometric measures are skinfold measurements (usually only triceps and subscapular), and measurements of midarm and midcalf circumferences. Additional biochemical measurements include 24-hour urinary creatinine (for calculating the creatinine-height index), 24-hour urine urea nitrogen (for estimating nitrogen balance), serum proteins (which are more sensitive indicators of protein nutriture and repletion than serum albumin), and tests of delayed cutaneous hypersensitivity. Indirect calorimetry may be used to measure energy expenditure and energy needs. Dietary assessment may include calorie counts, more extensive patient interviewing, and questioning of surrogates having knowledge of the patient's dietary intake.

In addition, more sophisticated and specialized nutritional assessment techniques are available. These include neutron activation analysis, isotope dilution, whole-body potassium measurement, computed tomography, and magnetic resonance imaging to determine body composition and response to nutritional therapy. Because of high cost, restricted availability, and other drawbacks, these methods are infrequently used in assessing the critically ill. Instead, their use is limited to research applications.

History

Obtaining a patient's history is the first step in clinical assessment of nutritional status.[8] Data on the patient's history can be obtained from the medical record and from interviews with the patient or others knowledgeable about the patient's habits. Parts of the medical record that are particularly helpful include the medical history; entries made by physicians, nurses, social workers, and other members of the health care team; and medical records from previous admissions.[9] Other essential components of a patient's history include pertinent facts about past and current health, use of medications, and personal and household information. Components of the medical history and psychosocial factors to consider in nutritional assessment are discussed in Chapter 10.

Dietary Information

Dietary information includes the patient's food preferences, allergies and intolerances, and usual eating pattern (timing and location of meals and snacks). Data should also be collected about the amount of money available for purchasing food, ability to obtain and prepare food, eligibility for and access to food assistance programs, and use of vitamin, mineral, and other supplements (if not obtained in the history).

A 24-hour recall or simple food frequency questionnaire can provide important data on usual eating patterns and can help generate additional questions on dietary intake. Patients sent home to return for later follow-up visits can be asked to complete a food frequency questionnaire or a multiple-day (usually a 3-day) diet record. Hospitalized patients' food intake can be evaluated by a calorie count, in which the caloric and nutrient value of foods eaten from the patient's tray for 1 or more days are calculated and recorded.

Physical Examination

Two of the most important measurements to obtain are body weight and stature (or length, in the case of infants and young children unable to stand without assistance). Weight is a gross measure of the body's fluid and tissue mass, and serial weighings indicate changes in those body constituents. Marked, unintentional weight loss is generally viewed as a manifestation of serious disease.[1] Weight is an important variable in equations predicting energy expenditure and in Quetelet's index (BMI).[10] Stature is necessary for determining weight for stature and for calculating Quetelet's index, the creatinine height index, body surface area, and energy expenditure.[11]

Body weight gain can indicate repletion of lean and fat tissues, development of obesity, or abnormal accumulation of body fluids, as in edema, ascites, pleural effusion, or fluid overload in a patient receiving excessive intravenous fluid. Loss of body weight can represent the presence, severity, or progress of a disease or nutritional impairment. It can also be seen in patients receiving diuretics, which increase renal excretion of water. Depletion of lean body mass can be masked by the simultaneous retention of fluid. For these reasons, body weight measurements need to be carefully scrutinized.

One way to evaluate body weight is to compare it to some reference, or "desirable," weight. This can be expressed as a percent of desirable body weight. This is the same as relative weight, which was discussed in

Chapter 6. The following equation is used for calculating percent of desirable weight (relative weight):

$$\text{Percent desirable body weight} = \frac{\text{Current weight}}{\text{“Desirable,” or reference, weight}} \times 100$$

The value for desirable or reference weight depends on what a particular health care facility has chosen for its standard. Usually, this is a height-weight table similar to the ones shown in Chapter 6. If the patient's percent of desirable body weight (%DBW) is 80%, he or she is 20% below desirable body weight. Many authors regard a %DBW of < 80% as substandard.[8]

Recent changes in body weight are a better indicator of nutritional status than are static weight measurements.[1] One way to assess change in body weight is to calculate percent of usual weight. This can be done using the following equation:

$$\%\text{ usual weight} = \frac{\text{Current or admit weight}}{\text{Usual weight}} \times 100$$

Information about usual weight can be obtained from the patient, a person close to the patient, nurses' notes, or medical records of previous admissions. An alternate approach to assessing recent changes in body weight is to calculate percent of weight change using the following equation:

$$\%\text{ weight change} = \frac{\text{Usual weight} - \text{Current weight}}{\text{Usual weight}} \times 100$$

A weight loss < 5% is considered small. A 5% to 10% weight loss is considered potentially significant. A weight loss > 10% is considered definitely significant.[1,12] Rapid changes in body weight should be interpreted with caution. A change in body weight > 1 lb/d (0.5 kg/d) indicates an accumulation or loss of water in the body and not a gain or loss of lean or fat tissue. Considering the fact that one pint (16 fluid ounces) of water weighs 1 pound, rapid changes in body weight can occur from relatively modest changes in fluid levels in the body.

The rate of weight loss is as important to consider as the amount lost. A 12% weight loss during the past 6 months is more significant than a similar weight loss during the past 12 months. The pattern of weight loss is also important to consider. Imagine two patients, Patient A and Patient B. Patient A lost 12% of her usual weight over a period 6 months to 1 month prior to admission but regained half that weight in the month just before admission and is continuing to regain. Consequently, she has a net loss of 6% of her body weight. Patient B lost 6% of his usual weight during the 6 months prior to admission and is continuing to lose weight. Some health care professionals would consider the nutritional status of Patient A to be better than that of Patient B.[12]

Because important clinical decisions are based on the patient's weight and stature, it is important to obtain measurements that are as accurate and precise as possible. This can be done by following the techniques outlined in Chapter 6. Although the patient should be asked about his or her weight history, actual weight and stature should be measured or estimated using the appropriate equation, rather than relying on the patient's stated weight and stature. If stated weight and stature are recorded in the patient's chart, they should be labeled as such.

Weighing can be complicated by the patient's condition and the presence of casts, traction devices, and life-support equipment. Nonambulatory patients, for example, can be weighed using bed or wheelchair scales (see Chapter 6), or weight can be estimated from various anthropometric measures, including subscapular skinfold, calf circumference, knee height, and midarm circumference (explained later in this chapter).[13] When patients cannot stand for stature measurements or when stature is likely to be inaccurate because of skeletal deformity, it can be estimated from knee height, as explained in the section "Knee Height."[11,13] As discussed in Chapter 6, body weight for stature can be compared with height-weight charts, and relative weight and Quetelet's index can be calculated and compared with various standards.

Another valuable indicator of nutritional status is arm muscle area. Arm muscle area is calculated from measures of the triceps skinfold and the midarm circumference.[14] Arm muscle area has been shown to be a useful index of total body muscle in young children[8] and in adults.[14]

Besides weight, stature, and other anthropometric measures, the physical examination involves numerous measurements and observations, including measurement of heart and respiratory rate and body temperature; observation of heart, respiratory, and bowel sounds; examination of the head, neck, thorax, abdomen, extremities, and integument (skin, hair, and nails); and examination of the nervous and circulatory systems. This information is gathered during the physical examination and initial work-up on admission and is available in the patient's chart.

Knee Height

Knee height is measured with the subject in the supine position (lying facing up), using one of several commercially available large, broadblade sliding calipers (see Appendix J for sources).[11,13,15,16]

Measurements are made on the *left leg* because this side was used by researchers in developing the equations given in Table 7.1.[11] The knee and ankle of the left leg are positioned at a 90-degree angle, as shown in Figure 7.2. These angles should be verified by a right triangle, square, or other appropriate device. The fixed blade of the caliper is placed under the heel of the left

TABLE 7.1 Equations for Estimating Stature from Knee Height for Various Groups

Age*	Equation†	Error‡
Black Females		
> 60	S = 58.72 + (1.96 KH)	8.26 cm
19–60	S = 68.10 + (1.86 KH) − (0.06 A)	7.60 cm
6–18	S = 46.59 + (2.02 KH)	8.78 cm
White Females		
> 60	S = 75.00 + (1.91 KH) − (0.17 A)	8.82 cm
19–60	S = 70.25 + (1.87 KH) − (0.06 A)	7.20 cm
6–18	S = 43.21 + (2.14 KH)	7.80 cm
Black Males		
> 60	S = 95.79 + (1.37 KH)	8.44 cm
19–60	S = 73.42 + (1.79 KH)	7.20 cm
6–18	S = 39.60 + (2.18 KH)	9.16 cm
White Males		
> 60	S = 59.01 + (2.08 KH)	7.84 cm
19–60	S = 71.85 + (1.88 KH)	7.94 cm
6–18	S = 40.54 + (2.22 KH)	8.42 cm

Adapted from Chumlea WC, Guo SS, Steinbaugh ML. 1994. Prediction of stature from knee height for black and white adults and children with application to mobility-impaired or handicapped persons. *Journal of the American Dietetic Association* 94:1385–1388.

*Age in years rounded to the nearest year.

†S = stature; KH = knee height; A = age in years.

‡Estimated stature will be within this value for 95% of persons within each age, sex, race group.

foot, and the moveable blade is placed on the anterior surface of the left thigh. The caliper shaft is positioned parallel to the fibula (the outside bone of the lower leg), over the lateral malleolus (the most prominent bony projection on the outer side of the left ankle), and just posterior to the head of the fibula (Figures 7.3 and 7.4). Pressure is applied to the two blades to compress the soft tissues.[13,15,16] The measurement is recorded to the nearest 0.1 cm. Two measurements made in quick succession should agree to within 0.5 cm.

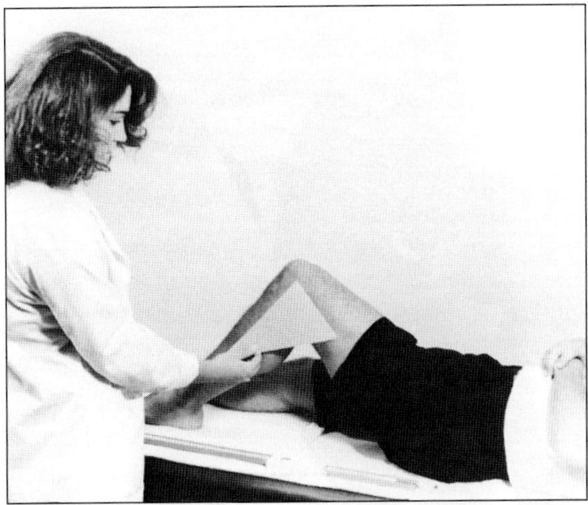

Figure 7.2
When knee height is being measured, the knee and ankle of the left leg should be bent at 90-degree angles.

Estimating Stature

For most patients, stature can be easily obtained. However, for persons who are nonambulatory or who have contractures, severe arthritis, paralysis, amputations, or other conditions limiting their ability to stand erectly, stature may have to be estimated. The most common approach is to estimate stature from knee height because knee height has been shown to correlate highly with stature.[11,17,18] An alternate approach is estimating stature from either upper-arm or lower-arm length as described by Jarzem.[19]

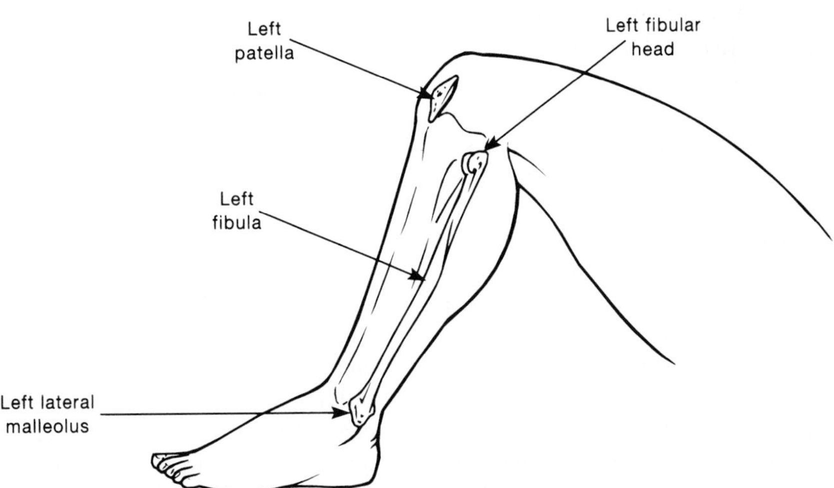

Figure 7.3 Anatomical landmarks for proper placement of the knee height caliper.

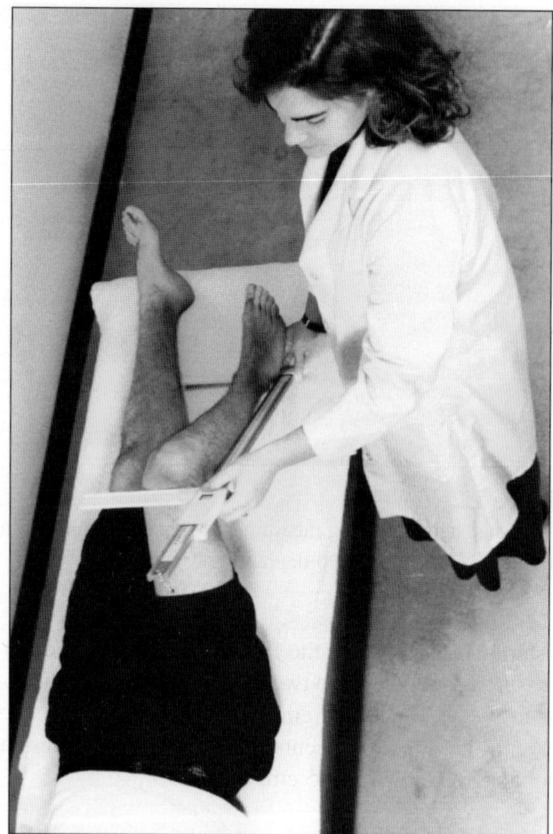

Figure 7.4
The fixed blade of the caliper is placed under the heel, and the moveable shaft is positioned parallel to the fibula, over the lateral malleolus, and just behind the head of the fibula.

The sex-, age-, and race-specific equations in Table 7.1 can be used for estimating stature in children, adults, and older persons. Data from national surveys of healthy, able-bodied persons were used to develop these equations, and they reflect normal patterns of growth and development. The nomogram in Figure 7.5 can be used for estimating stature from age and knee height in persons 60 to 90 years old.

An alternative approach to measuring the stature of a bedridden patient who has no skeletal abnormalities or contractures is to align his or her body so that the lower extremities, trunk, shoulders, and head are in a straight line and mark on the bedsheet the position of the base of the heels and top of the crown, as shown in Figure 7.6. The distance between these two lines can then be measured using a suitable tape measure.

When done carefully, this approach is somewhat more accurate than estimates derived from knee height in patients without skeletal abnormalities or contractures. However, it is always preferable to obtain standing measurements of stature when patients are able to stand and when these measurements are not contraindicated by the patient's condition.

Midarm Circumference

Midarm circumference (MAC), also known as upper midarm circumference, can be used in equations for calculating arm muscle area and estimated body weight.[2,13,16] As an indicator of muscle and subcutaneous adipose tissue, it is an accepted measure of nutritional status. It and related upper-arm anthropometric measurements can be obtained quickly and noninvasively.[20] MAC is the circumference of the upper arm at the triceps skinfold site. In the ambulatory patient, the triceps skinfold site is measured and marked as described in Chapter 6. The arm is relaxed to the side with the palm of the hand facing the thigh. A nonstretchable measuring tape is placed around the arm, perpendicular to the long axis of the arm, and at the level of the triceps skinfold site (see Figure 7.7). The tape should be placed in contact with the arm but without compressing the soft tissues. The measurement should be recorded to the nearest 0.1 cm.[15]

In the nonambulatory patient, MAC is measured while the patient is in the supine position.[11,21] Either the right or left side can be used for this and subsequent recumbent measurements.[15] With the upper arm approximately parallel to the body, the forearm is placed palm down across the middle of the body with the elbow bent 90 degrees. Using a nonstretchable tape measure, the midpoint of the upper arm is located between the tip of the acromion process and the olecranon process and marked, as shown in Figure 7.8.[13,21] (These are the same anatomical landmarks used for determining the triceps skinfold site described in Chapter 6.)

Once the midpoint of the upper arm is properly marked, the arm is returned to the patient's side with the palm facing upward. The arm is then raised slightly off the surface of the examination table by placing a folded pillow or towel under the patient's elbow. A nonstretchable tape measure is placed around the upper arm at the level of the marked midpoint and perpendicular to the long axis of the arm (Figure 7.9). The tape should come in contact with the skin of the arm but should not be pulled so tight that it indents or compresses the soft tissues. The measurement should be recorded to the nearest 0.1 cm.[13,21]

Calf Circumference

Calf circumference is used in some equations for estimating body weight and is a measure of muscle and subcutaneous adipose tissue. In elderly men, it is significantly correlated with lean body mass.[22] Calf circumference can be measured with the subject standing, sitting, or lying in the supine position. If ambulatory, the subject can either sit on an examination table with the right or left leg hanging freely or stand with the feet about 20 cm (8 in.) apart, with the body weight equally distributed on both feet.[21] A nonstretchable measuring tape should be looped horizontally around the calf and moved up

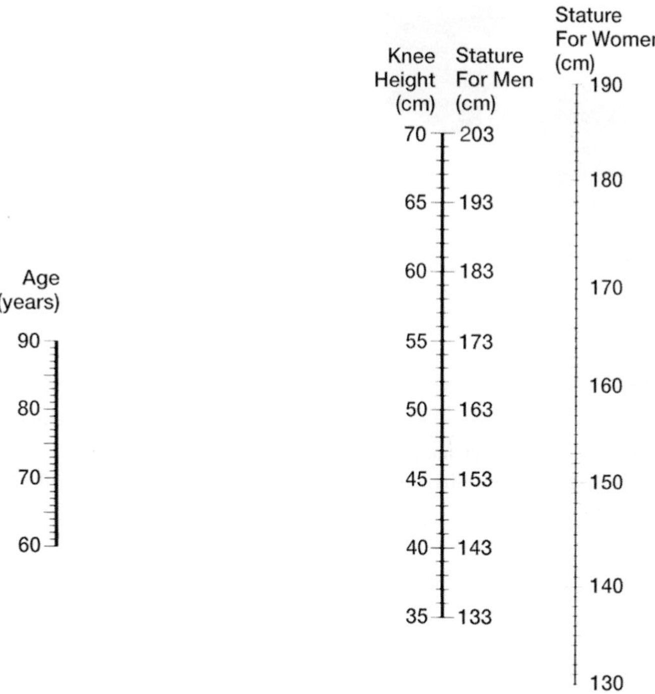

Figure 7.5 Nomogram for estimating stature from knee height in persons ages 60 to 90 years.
To use, locate the patient's age and knee height on the appropriate columns and connect these points with a straightedge. The estimated stature can be read where the straightedge crosses the appropriate sex-specific column.

Source: Adapted from Chumlea WC, Roche AF, Mukherjee D. 1987. *Nutritional assessment of the elderly through anthropometry*. Columbus, OH: Ross Laboratories.

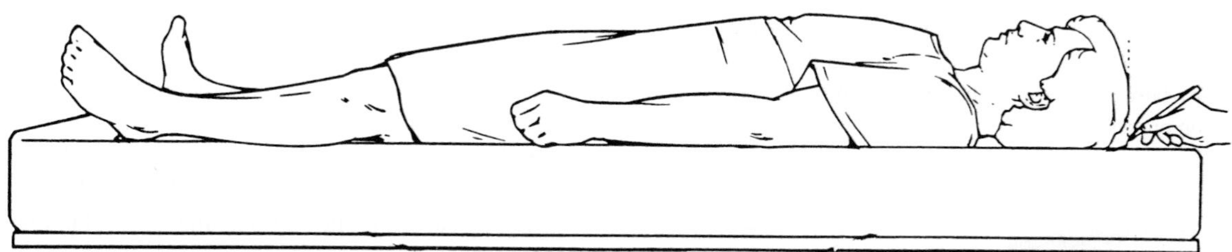

Figure 7.6
An alternative approach to measuring recumbent length in the bedridden patient is simply to place a mark on the bed sheet at the top of the patient's head and at the bottom of the heel. With the patient out of bed or rolled to one side, measure the distance.

and down until the greatest calf circumference is found. The tape should be tightened around the calf so that it contacts the skin without indenting or compressing the soft tissues. The circumference should be recorded to the nearest 0.1 cm.[21]

If nonambulatory, the subject should be in the supine position with the knee bent at a 90-degree angle. The tape measure should be looped around the calf in a plane perpendicular to the long axis of the lower leg (Figure 7.10) and moved up and down. When the greatest circumference of the lower leg is found, the tape should be tightened around the calf so that it contacts the skin without indenting or compressing the soft tissues. The circumference should be recorded to the nearest 0.1 cm.[13,15]

Recumbent Skinfold Measurements

In the recumbent patient, the triceps and subscapular skinfolds can be measured with the patient lying on the right or left side.[15] Apart from differences in body positioning, the techniques for measuring skinfolds in

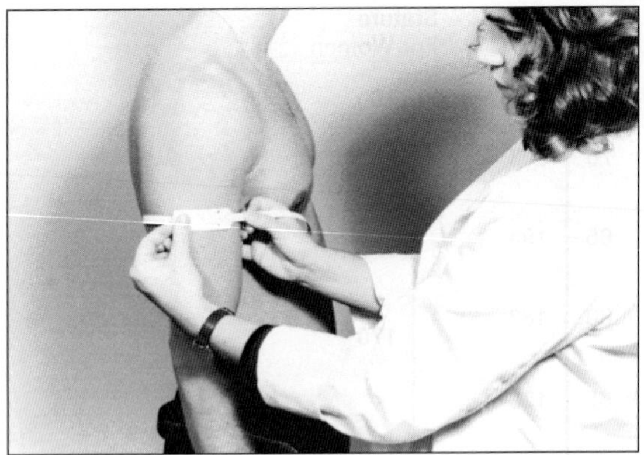

Figure 7.7
Midarm circumference is measured with the subject standing. The tape is placed around the arm, perpendicular to the long axis, and at the level of the triceps skinfold site.

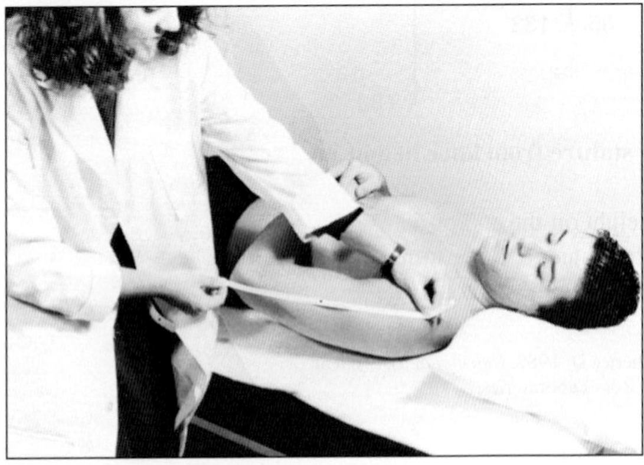

Figure 7.8
When the subject cannot stand, midarm circumference is measured by first locating and marking the midpoint of the upper arm between the tip of the acromion process and the olecranon process.

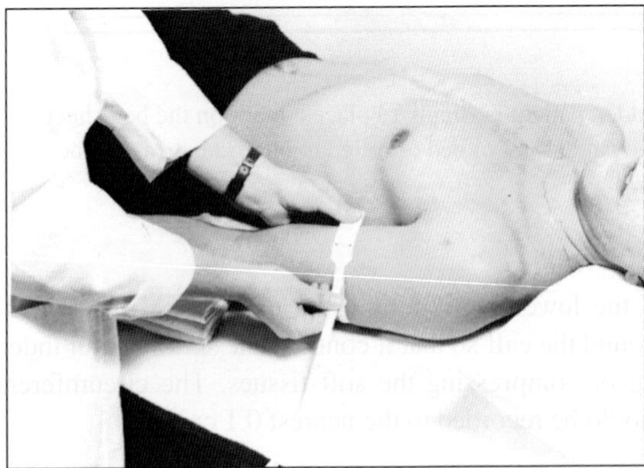

Figure 7.9 Measurement of the midarm circumference of the recumbent subject.
A folded towel under the elbow raises the arm off the surface of the table. The tape is perpendicular to the long axis of the arm and touches the arm without compressing soft tissues.

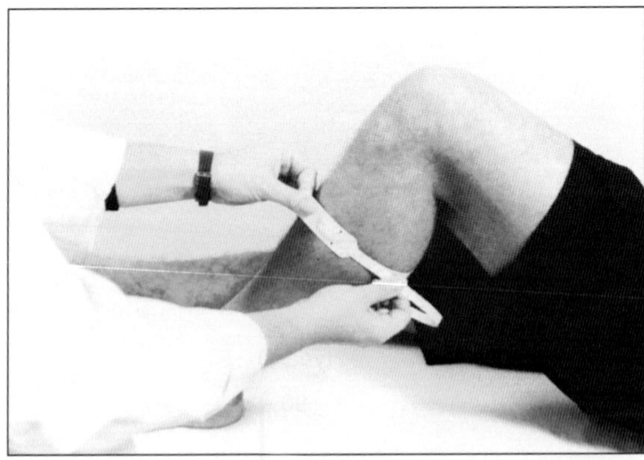

Figure 7.10 Measurement of calf circumference of the recumbent subject.
The tape measure is kept in a plane perpendicular to the long axis of the lower leg.

the recumbent patient are essentially the same as those described in Chapter 6.

The subject is positioned as shown in Figure 7.11. The right arm is in front of the body at a 45-degree angle, the trunk is in a straight line, the shoulders are perpendicular to the spine and examination table, and the arm to be measured is lying on the trunk with the palm down. The legs are slightly flexed at the hips and knees.[13,15]

As in the standing ambulatory patient, the triceps skinfold is measured at the back of the upper arm at the level of the marked midpoint. With the thumb and index finger of the left hand, the measurer grasps a double fold of skin and adipose tissue about 1 cm (½ in.) above the marked midpoint of the upper arm. The long axes of the skinfold and arm must be parallel. Holding the skinfold, the measurer places the caliper tips on the skinfold and reads the dial after about 4 seconds (Figure 7.12). The measurer's eyes should be in line with the needle and dial of the caliper to avoid errors caused by parallax.[13,15]

For measuring the subscapular skinfold, the body is positioned as shown in Figure 7.11. The same site is used as when the subject is standing, and the skinfold is grasped and measured along the same axis (see Chapter 6). Because the subject is lying on the right side, however, the measurement technique is somewhat different. The subscapular skinfold site is just distal to the inferior angle of the left scapula. As shown in Figure 7.13, the measurer grasps the double layer of skin and adipose tissue along the axis of the skinfold, so that the thumb and index finger of the left hand are about 1 cm (½ in.) from the actual measurement site. Note that the left hand is distal and lateral to the skinfold site. Holding the skinfold, the measurer places the caliper tips at the site and reads the dial after about 4 seconds. The measurer should look directly at the dial of the caliper to avoid errors caused by parallax.[13,15] A minimum of two measurements should be taken at each site. Successive measurements should be

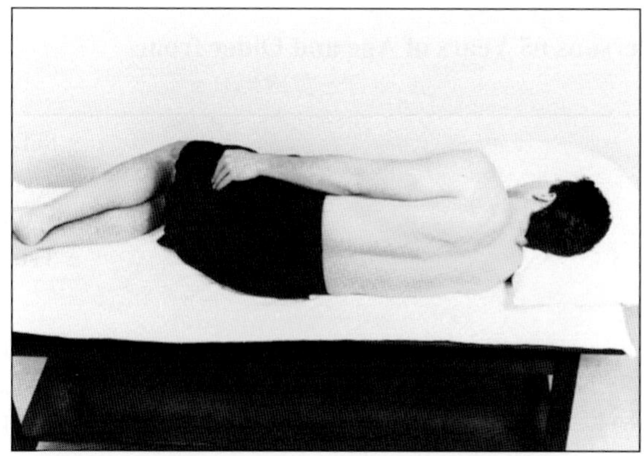

Figure 7.11 Body position for measurement of triceps and subscapular skinfolds of the recumbent subject.

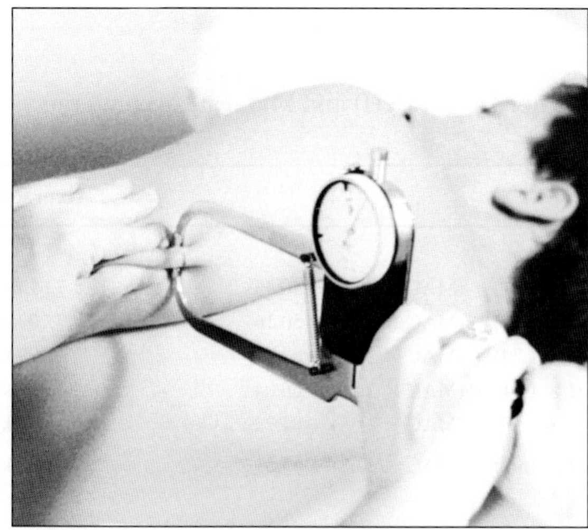

Figure 7.12 Measurement of triceps skinfold of the recumbent subject.

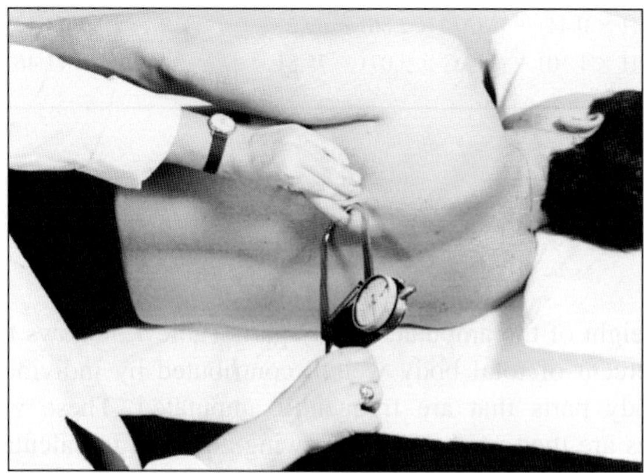

Figure 7.13 Measurement of subscapular skinfold of the recumbent subject.

at least 15 seconds apart from each other to allow the skinfold site to return to normal. If consecutive measurements vary by more than 1 mm, additional measurements should be taken until the readings are consistent.

The sum of the triceps and subscapular skinfold thicknesses can be used as an indicator of the body's energy reserves. Appendix O provides percentiles for the sum of triceps and subscapular skinfold thicknesses for males and females ages 2 to 90 years. Although researchers disagree about which standards are the most appropriate, the guidelines in Table 7.2 can be used for interpreting these age-, sex-, and race-specific percentile values.[1] The cutoff point for excess fat was chosen as greater than the 85th percentile because it has been observed that persons above this point are at significantly greater risk of hypertension and hypercholesterolemia than persons at or below the 85th percentile.[23]

Estimating Body Weight

Most patients can be weighed on scales, but sometimes it is difficult or impossible to obtain a patient's weight. This may be because of the patient's medical condition, equipment attached to the patient (for example, life support devices, traction equipment, casts, or braces), or lack of a suitable bed or wheelchair scale. Despite the critical importance of body weight in delivering nutritional therapy, it is estimated that about 22% of hospitalized adults receiving nutritional support have no record of body weight.[24]

When it is difficult or impossible to obtain a patient's body weight directly, it can be estimated from various anthropometric measures (that is, knee height, midarm circumference, calf circumference, and subscapular skinfold thickness) using the equations given in Tables 7.3 and 7.4. The decision of which equation to use will depend on the patient's age and the anthropometric measures that can be obtained or are available.

From Tables 7.3 and 7.4, it can be noted that a certain amount of error is inherent in the process of estimating body weight from anthropometric measures. This error can be minimized by using an equation requiring

TABLE 7.2 Guidelines for Interpreting the Age-, Sex-, and Race-Specific Percentile Values for the Sum of Triceps and Subscapular Skinfold Thicknesses for Males and Females Given in Appendix P

Percentile	Category
≤ 5th	Lean
> 5th but ≤ 15th	Below average
> 15th but ≤ 75th	Average
> 75th but ≤ 85th	Above average
> 85th	Excess fat

Adapted from Frisancho AR. 1990. *Anthropometric standards for the assessment of growth and nutritional status.* Ann Arbor: University of Michigan Press.

Table 7.3 Equations for Estimating Body Weight in Persons 65 Years of Age and Older from Anthropometric Measures

	SEE†
Females*	
Weight = (MAC × 1.63) + (CC × 1.43) − 37.46	± 4.96 kg
Weight = (MAC × 0.92) + (CC × 1.50) + (SSF × 0.42) − 26.19	± 4.21 kg
Weight = (MAC × 0.98) + (CC × 1.27) + (SSF × 0.40) + (KH × 0.87) − 62.35	± 3.80 kg
Males*	
Weight = (MAC × 2.31) + (CC × 1.50) − 50.10	± 5.37 kg
Weight = (MAC × 1.92) + (CC × 1.44) + (SSF × 0.26) − 39.97	± 5.34 kg
Weight = (MAC × 1.73) + (CC × 0.98) + (SSF × 0.37) + (KH × 1.16) − 81.69	± 4.48 kg

Adapted from Chumlea WC, Guo S, Roche AF, Steinbaugh ML. 1988. Prediction of body weight for the nonambulatory elderly from anthropometry. *Journal of the American Dietetic Association* 88:564–568.

*Weight is in kg; MAC = midarm circumference, in cm; CC = calf circumference, in cm; SSF = subscapular skinfold thickness, in mm; KH = knee height, in cm.

†SEE = standard error of the estimate.

Table 7.4 Equations for Estimating Body Weight from Knee Height (KH) and Midarm Circumference (MAC) for Various Groups

Age*	Race	Equation†	Accuracy‡
Females			
6–18	Black	Weight = (KH × 0.71) + (MAC × 2.59) − 50.43	± 7.65 kg
6–18	White	Weight = (KH × 0.77) + (MAC × 2.47) − 50.16	± 7.20 kg
19–59	Black	Weight = (KH × 1.24) + (MAC × 2.97) − 82.48	± 11.98 kg
19–59	White	Weight = (KH × 1.01) + (MAC × 2.81) − 66.04	± 10.60 kg
60–80	Black	Weight = (KH × 1.50) + (MAC × 2.58) − 84.22	± 14.52 kg
60–80	White	Weight = (KH × 1.09) + (MAC × 2.68) − 65.51	± 11.42 kg
Males			
6–18	Black	Weight = (KH × 0.59) + (MAC × 2.73) − 48.32	± 7.50 kg
6–18	White	Weight = (KH × 0.68) + (MAC × 2.64) − 50.08	± 7.82 kg
19–59	Black	Weight = (KH × 1.09) + (MAC × 3.14) − 83.72	± 11.30 kg
19–59	White	Weight = (KH × 1.19) + (MAC × 3.21) − 86.82	± 11.42 kg
60–80	Black	Weight = (KH × 0.44) + (MAC × 2.86) − 39.21	± 7.04 kg
60–80	White	Weight = (KH × 1.10) + (MAC × 3.07) − 75.81	± 11.46 kg

* Age (in years) is rounded to the nearest year.

†Weight is in kg: lb ÷ 2.2 = kg; kg × 2.2 = lb. Knee height is in cm; in. × 2.54 = cm; cm ÷ 2.54 = in.

‡For persons within each group, estimated body weight should be within the stated value for 95% of the subjects.

a larger number of variables (four as opposed to two) and by paying strict attention to measurement technique. Although estimates of body weight may be as much as 14 kg greater than or less than actual body weight, an estimate of body weight recorded on a patient's chart is better than no weight recorded. The use of estimated weights should be reserved for patients who cannot be weighed or for whom weights would be inaccurate, and every reasonable effort should be made to obtain direct measurements of body weights on patients.

If a patient has had an amputation, the patient's current body weight can be adjusted to account for the weight of the amputated body part. Table 7.5 shows the percent of total body weight contributed by individual body parts that are frequently amputated. These values are then used in the following equation to calculate adjusted body weight.[8,25]

$$\text{Adjusted wt} = \frac{\text{Current weight}}{100 - \%\text{ of amputation}} \times 100$$

Suppose you have a patient whose current weight is 157 lb and whose leg has been amputated at the right knee (right lower leg and foot removed). From Table 7.5, it can be seen that the lower leg and foot contribute approximately

TABLE 7.5 Percent of Total Body Weight Contributed by Individual Body Parts

Body Part	Contribution to Body Weight (%)
Entire arm	6.5
Upper arm	3.5
Forearm	2.3
Hand	0.8
Entire leg	18.5
Upper leg	11.6
Lower leg	5.3
Foot	1.8

Adapted from Brunnstrom S. 1983. *Clinical kinesiology*, 4th ed. Philadelphia: Davis.

7.1% of total body weight. Given this information and the equation, adjusted body weight can be calculated:

$$\text{Adjusted wt} = \frac{157 \text{ lb}}{100 - 7.1} \times 100$$

$$\text{Adjusted wt} = 169 \text{ lb}$$

Thus, this patient's adjusted body weight (approximately what it would be without the amputation) is 169 lb.

Arm Muscle Area

Arm muscle area (AMA) is used as an index of lean tissue or muscle in the body.[13,26] This is based on the observation that an organism facing nutritional deprivation draws on its nutritional reserves in the form of adipose tissue, visceral protein, and skeletal protein. In the case of upper-arm anthropometry, thickness of the triceps skinfold is used as an index of fat stores, and arm muscle size is used to represent muscle protein reserves.[26]

As the size of arm muscle changes in response to growth, development, and nutritional status, the resulting change in arm muscle area is greater than the change in midarm circumference. Consequently, changes in upper-arm musculature are not as easily detected by measurement of midarm circumference as by measurement of AMA. Therefore, AMA is the preferred nutritional index.[26]

AMA is correlated with creatinine excretion in children[9] and is related to total body muscle mass in adults.[14] It is particularly valuable in assessing persons with edema, whose body weights would be augmented by increased intracellular water, and in assessing persons who have undergone amputation.

AMA is estimated from the triceps skinfold measurement and midarm circumference.[13,14,26] The standard equation for calculating arm muscle area is[26]

$$\text{AMA} = \frac{[\text{MAC} - (\pi \times \text{TSF})]^2}{4\pi}$$

where AMA = arm muscle area in mm^2; MAC = midarm circumference in mm; and TSF = triceps skinfold thickness in mm. Use of this formula is based on the following assumptions. In cross section, both the midarm and midarm muscle compartment are circular; the triceps skinfold thickness is twice the average thickness of the subcutaneous fat layer; bone atrophies in proportion to muscle wasting in protein-energy malnutrition; and the cross-sectional area of bone and the sheath containing the nervous and vascular tissues of the upper arm are small and insignificant.[14] In reality, however, several of these factors are significant sources of error in estimating AMA. When estimates of AMA derived from this equation were compared with AMA measured by computed tomography (see Chapter 6), the equation overestimated AMA by 20% to 25%.[14]

Heymsfield and coworkers[14] developed the following revised equations, which partially correct for the overestimation of AMA by subtracting a constant that accounts for the presence of bone, nervous tissue, and vascular tissue in the upper arm:

$$\text{cAMA for females} = \frac{[\text{MAC} - (\pi \times \text{TSF})]^2}{4\pi} - 6.5$$

$$\text{cAMA for males} = \frac{[\text{MAC} - (\pi \times \text{TSF})]^2}{4\pi} - 10$$

where cAMA = corrected arm muscle area in cm^2; MAC = midarm circumference in cm; and TSF = triceps skinfold thickness in cm. Note that these equations call for all measurements to be made in *centimeters*. The nomogram in Figure 7.14 facilitates calculation of cAMA. Estimates of cAMA have been shown to be within ± 8% of actual AMA, based on computed tomography. It should be noted that measurements must be carefully taken by trained observers and that the equations and nomogram for cAMA have not been validated for use with elderly persons.[14] In the obese, all of the equations tend to overestimate AMA when compared with values derived from computed tomography, and the magnitude of overestimation is proportional to the degree of adiposity. Heymsfield[14] recommends that AMA prediction equations not be used for persons having a relative weight of ≥ 125 percent, but Frisancho[23] suggests they not be used for persons whose triceps skinfold thickness exceeds the 85th age and sex percentile. Despite these limitations, estimates of muscle mass derived from anthropometry can be collected inexpensively and easily and are helpful in assessing nutritional status and response to nutritional support.

Appendix P provides means and percentiles of AMA for males and females ages 2 to 90 years. For persons ages 18 years and older, the values are for corrected AMA. The guidelines in Table 7.6 can be used for interpreting these age/sex percentile values. No single index (for example, AMA) can be used as a reliable indicator

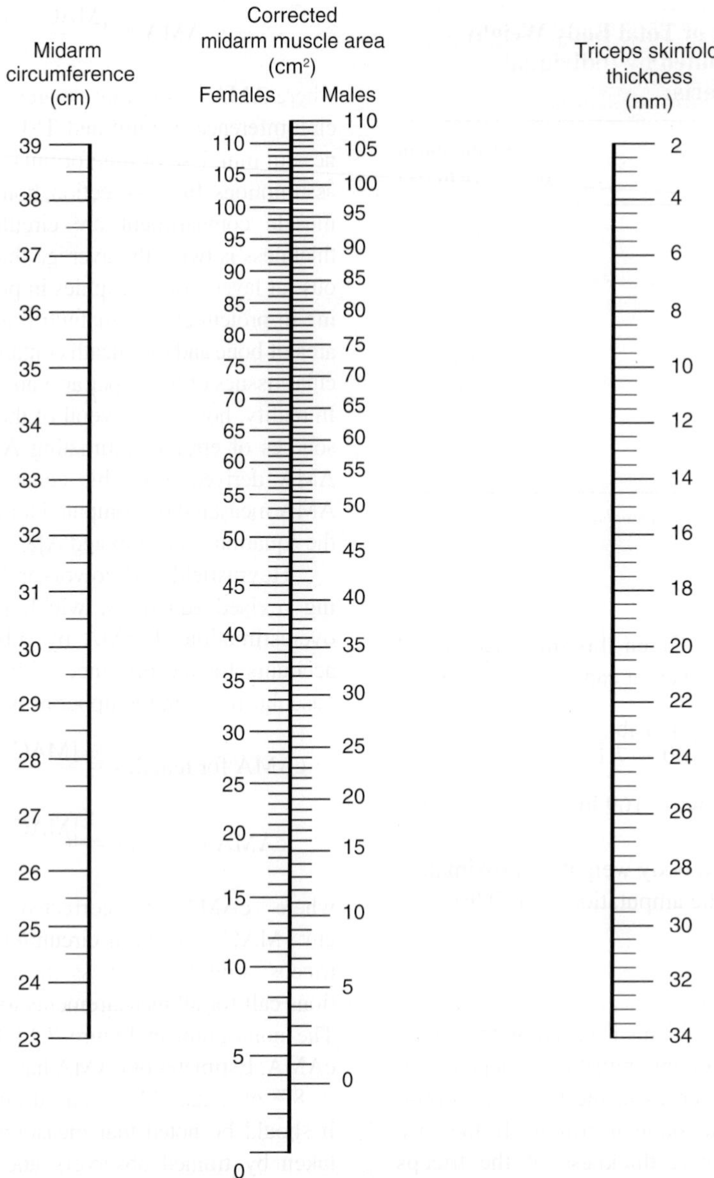

Figure 7.14 **Nomogram for estimating corrected arm muscle area.** To use, locate the patient's midarm circumference and triceps skinfold in the appropriate columns. Connect these points with a straightedge. The corrected arm muscle area is read where the straightedge crosses the arm muscle area column. Note that there are values for females and males.

Source: Adapted from Chumlea WC, Roche AF, Mukherjee D. 1987. *Nutritional assessment of the elderly through anthropometry.* Columbus, OH: Ross Laboratories.

of nutritional status. Basic assumptions inferred from anthropometry should be corroborated by data derived from dietary, biochemical, and clinical observations.[23]

Determining Energy Requirements

Twenty-four-hour energy expenditure is primarily determined by resting energy expenditure, the thermic effect of food, the thermic effect of exercise, and whether disease or injury is present.[27] As Sims and Danforth[27] pointed out, these "components of energy expenditure are not entirely discrete but are useful divisions when attempting to investigate factors that might regulate or control them."

Twenty-four-hour energy expenditure can be represented by the following equation:

$$\text{24-EE} = \text{REE} + \text{TEF} + \text{TEE} + \text{TED}$$

where 24-EE = 24-hour energy expenditure; REE = resting energy expenditure; TEF = thermic effect of food;

TABLE 7.6 Guidelines for Interpreting the Age/Sex Percentile Values for Arm Muscle Area Given in Appendix P

Percentile	Category
≤ 5th	Wasted
> 5th but ≤ 15th	Below average
> 15th but ≤ 85th	Average
> 85th but ≤ 95th	Above average
> 95th	High muscle

Adapted from Frisancho AR. 1990. *Anthropometric standards for the assessment of growth and nutritional status.* Ann Arbor: University of Michigan Press.

TEE = thermic effect of exercise; and TED = thermic effect of disease and injury.

Basal metabolic rate (BMR) is defined as the lowest rate of energy expenditure of an individual. It is calculated from oxygen consumption measured over a 6- to 12-minute period when the subject is in a postabsorptive state (no food consumed during the previous 12 hours) and has rested quietly during the previous 30 minutes in a thermally neutral environment (room temperature is perceived as neither hot nor cold). To be precise, however, the point of lowest energy expenditure—the true BMR—occurs in the early morning hours of deep sleep. Obtaining a truly basal metabolic measurement is impractical in most instances. Therefore, a more appropriate term for metabolic rate or energy expenditure in the awake, resting, postabsorptive subject is *resting energy expenditure (REE).*

In the clinical setting, achieving optimal conditions for determining REE can be difficult sometimes because of the continuous care patients undergo. In these situations, the term *REE* is used in the scientific literature to represent energy expenditure measured by indirect calorimetry under conditions that are as controlled as the clinical situation allows.[28,29] As shown in Figure 7.15, REE is the largest component of 24-hour energy expenditure, accounting for roughly 65% to 75% of 24-hour energy expenditure in healthy persons.

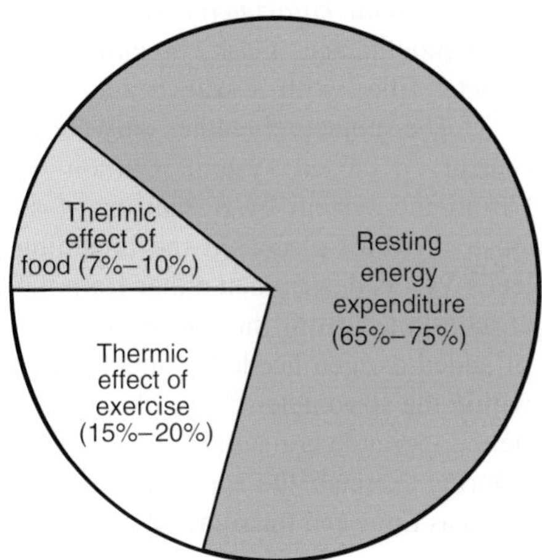

Figure 7.15 The components of 24-hour energy expenditure in healthy persons.

The second largest contributor to 24-hour energy expenditure is the energy expended for muscular work, or the thermic effect of exercise (TEE).[27] Of all the components of a healthy person's 24-hour energy expenditure, it is the most variable. For most North Americans, it accounts for about 15% to 20% of 24-hour energy expenditure but can increase by a factor of two or more with regular, high-intensity, long-duration physical activity.[27] Energy expended in exercise generally exceeds the REE in athletes who train several hours daily.

The thermic effect of food (TEF), also known as diet-induced thermogenesis or the specific dynamic action of food, is the increased energy expenditure following food consumption or administration of parenteral or enteral nutrition. The TEF is the energy cost of nutrient absorption, transport, storage, and metabolism. It accounts for about 7% to 10% of 24-hour energy expenditure.[27]

The energy needs of patients can be determined in two ways: measuring energy expenditure or estimating these needs using a variety of guidelines.[2,28]

Measuring Energy Expenditure

Calorimetry is the measurement of the body's energy expenditure. Direct calorimetry measures the body's heat output, whereas indirect calorimetry determines energy expenditure by measuring the body's oxygen consumption and carbon dioxide production. Because energy expenditure measurements using direct and indirect calorimetry are performed in a laboratory, they may not accurately represent energy expenditure of free-living subjects (i.e., persons living at home and engaged in typical work and leisure-time activities). To more accurately measure the energy expenditure of free-living subjects, researchers can use two other methods: doubly labeled water and the bicarbonate-urea method.

Direct Calorimetry

Direct calorimetry uses a specially designed chamber to measure the amount of heat given off by the body through radiation, convection, and evaporation.[30] Direct calorimeters range in size from just large enough to comfortably accommodate an adult human lying in the recumbent position to those the size of a small room, such as the one located at the USDA Human Nutrition Research Center at Beltsville, Maryland, and shown in Figure 7.16.[28,31] The walls of the USDA direct calorimeter contain a layer of water that is warmed by the subject's body heat. Changes in the water temperature are recorded, and the amount of energy expended by the subject is calculated.

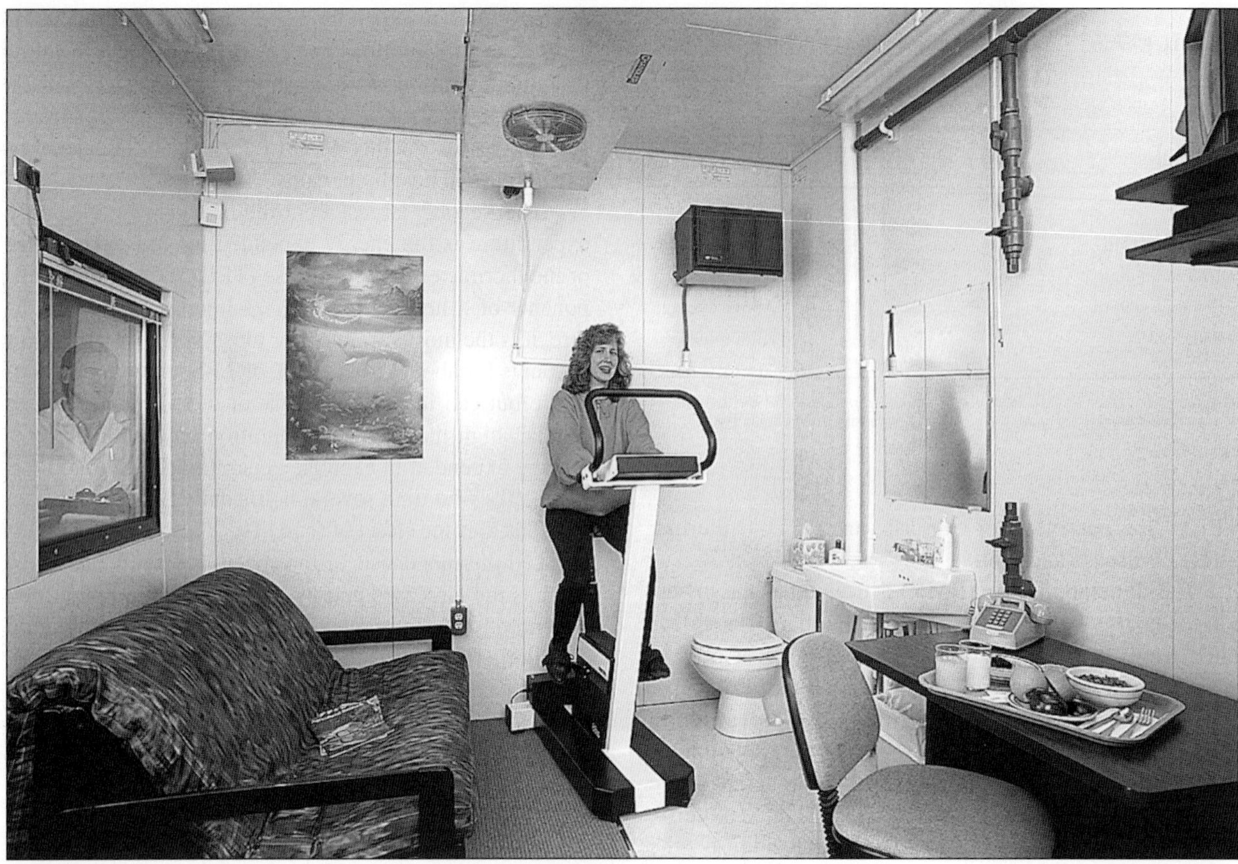

Figure 7.16
The interior of the USDA Human Nutrition Research Center's direct calorimeter provides a small but comfortable living space to subjects undergoing energy expenditure measurements lasting as long as 24 hours.
Source: Photo courtesy of U.S. Department of Agriculture, Agriculture Research Service, Beltsville Human Nutrition Research Center.

The composition of air entering and exiting the chamber is analyzed to determine the subject's production of carbon dioxide and methane and consumption of oxygen. Temperature, pressure, and humidity within the chamber and the subject's motion are measured. A total of 30 different measurements are monitored, recorded, and analyzed using electronic instrumentation. The interior of the chamber measures 8 ft by 9 ft by 10 ft and is comfortably furnished with a bed, table, toilet, sink, video monitor, telephone, and exercise equipment, as shown in Figure 7.16. The calorimeter provides highly accurate measurements of human energy expenditure for periods as long as 24 hours. However, the expense of building and maintaining the chamber and instrumentation is prohibitive, and thus, this approach is rarely used.[28,30–32]

Indirect Calorimetry

Indirect calorimetry is based on the fact that energy metabolism ultimately depends on oxygen utilization (VO_2) and carbon dioxide production (VCO_2).[30,32] Thus, expired air contains less oxygen and more carbon dioxide than inspired air. When the volume of expired air is known and the differences in oxygen and carbon dioxide concentrations in inspired and expired air are known, the body's energy expenditure can be calculated. Estimations of energy expenditure by indirect calorimetry have been shown to be practically identical to those derived from direct calorimetry.

Several techniques can be used in indirect calorimetry. In *closed circuit calorimetry,* the subject is connected via a mouthpiece, mask, or endotracheal tube to a spirometer filled with a known amount of 100% oxygen.[29,30,32] The subject rebreathes only the gas within the spirometer—a closed system. Carbon dioxide is removed from the system by a canister of soda lime (potassium hydroxide) placed in the breathing circuit. The subject's VO_2 is determined either from the amount of oxygen consumed from the spirometer or from the amount of added oxygen needed to maintain a constant volume within the spirometer.[29] The closed circuit technique is neither portable nor suitable to use on exercising subjects. During exercise, the apparatus offers excessive resistance to gas flow, and the removal of carbon dioxide is inadequate.

In *open circuit calorimetry,* the subject breathes through a two-way valve in which room air is inspired from one side of the valve, and expired air passes through the opposite side to where it is either analyzed immediately or collected for later analysis. In the *Douglas bag method* of open circuit calorimetry, the expired air is collected in large vinyl bags or latex rubber meteorologic balloons for later analysis. A lightweight, portable apparatus strapped to the subject's back also can be used to measure ventilation and can periodically collect samples of expired air for later analysis.[28]

A more common approach to open circuit indirect calorimetry in clinical settings is use of a *computerized metabolic monitor,* which can be taken to the bedside for measuring energy expenditure of patients who are either spontaneously breathing or breathing with the assistance of a mechanical ventilator.[28,31] The portable computerized metabolic monitor shown in Figure 7.17 has a ventilated hood, which can be placed over the face of a patient while in bed and can be made air-tight with a snugly fitting collar. The volume of inspired and expired air (known as minute ventilation) is typically measured using a pneumotachograph. Gas analyzers in the unit determine the oxygen and carbon dioxide content of both inspired and expired air, and they determine the caloric requirements and substrate utilization. Data can be displayed on the unit's video screen, recorded on an optional printer, or downloaded to a computer for storage and/or further analysis. Use of a mouthpiece or face mask often results in discomfort and stress to the patient, which can affect test results. The hood on the monitor in Figure 7.17 avoids this problem and can result in an accurate and representative measurement of metabolic rate in the critically ill patient.[28,30,32]

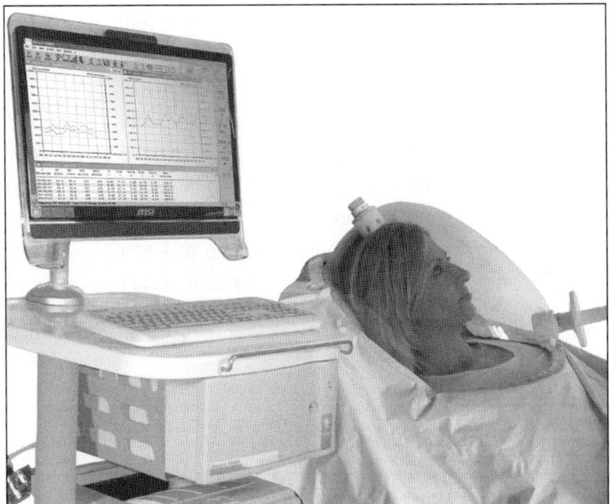

Figure 7.17 An example of a computerized metabolic monitor in operation.
This unit uses indirect calorimetry to determine a patient's resting energy expenditure. The plastic hood allows expired air to be collected without the annoyance of a mask or mouthpiece.
Source: Photo courtesy of COSMED USA, Inc.

Another approach to indirect calorimetry is the use of small, handheld calorimeters for measuring resting metabolic rate and oxygen consumption, designed to allow dietitians and other allied health professionals to quickly assess the REE of their clients.[33–35] The user holds the unit while breathing through an attached mouthpiece or face mask for 5 to 12 minutes. While breathing through the unit, the user wears a nose clip to ensure that all air entering and exiting the user's lungs pass through the unit. Sensors in the handheld calorimeter measure oxygen consumption, minute ventilation, temperature, humidity, and barometric pressure to provide a digital readout of REE in kilocalories per day. Caution should be exercised when using handheld calorimeters, because units from some manufacturers might be inaccurate.[33–35]

Doubly Labeled Water

Another approach to measuring energy expenditure is the doubly labeled water (DLW) method. Using this approach, a subject drinks a known amount of two different stable isotopic forms of water: $H_2{}^{18}O$ and ^2H_2O. Ordinary water is a molecule composed of two atoms of hydrogen, each having an atomic mass of one (^1H), and one atom of oxygen having an atomic mass of 16 (^{16}O). Although hydrogen atoms with an atomic mass of two (^2H, or deuterium) and oxygen atoms with an atomic mass of 18 (^{18}O) are naturally present in nature, they are found only in extremely minute quantities. Consequently, it is reasonable to assume that essentially all the ^2H and ^{18}O present in the body came from the doubly labeled water. After the subject drinks the two different isotopic forms of water, they mix with the body's water and are gradually eliminated from the body. The ^2H_2O is lost from the body only as water and reflects water flux, whereas the $H_2{}^{18}O$ is lost from the body in water and as $C^{18}O_2$ and reflects both water flux and CO_2 produced by the body.[31,32,36,37] Over the next 1 to 3 weeks the subject provides a series of urine samples that are used to measure the rate at which the two isotopes disappear from the body. The rate of disappearance is then used to calculate energy expenditure. The method is noninvasive and provides an accurate measurement of energy expenditure over a period of 1 to 3 weeks, and because the two isotopes are stable (nonradioactive), the procedure is considered safe to use even on infants and females who are pregnant or lactating.

The method has been validated in humans by use of carefully performed energy balance studies and by direct and indirect calorimetry.[37,38] In laboratory testing, DLW has demonstrated an accuracy of 1% and a coefficient of variation of 3% to 6%.[36] The DLW technique is considered the best available method for providing average estimates of the 24-hour energy expenditure of free-living subjects (those outside a controlled setting) over an extended period of time of 1 to 3 weeks. Although it does not provide a direct measurement of energy expended in physical activity (thermic effect of exercise), this can be calculated by subtracting estimates of resting metabolic rate and the thermic effect of food from measured 24-hour energy expenditure. Use of DLW is limited by the expense of the isotopes and its dependence on isotope ratio mass spectrometry for analysis of urine samples, and consequently it is not ideally suited for use in large, epidemiologic studies.[31,37–39] As mentioned in Chapter 3, comparisons of energy expenditure determined by DLW with reported energy intake from 24-hour recalls and food records have raised serious questions about the accuracy of reported energy intakes in dietary studies.[32,36,40–42]

Bicarbonate-Urea Method

Another approach for measuring total energy expenditure in free-living subjects over relatively short periods of time (several hours to several days) is the bicarbonate-urea method.[31,37,43] Like doubly labeled water, the bicarbonate-urea method relies on an estimate of carbon dioxide production to calculate energy expenditure in free-living subjects. However, in this approach, the isotope used is ^{14}C administered intravenously or subcutaneously in the form of bicarbonate ($H^{14}CO_3-$). The labeled bicarbonate mixes freely with and becomes diluted by the endogenous CO_2 produced by the body. Most of the labeled carbon is eliminated from the body through expired CO_2, while some is eliminated as urea in urine. The amount of labeled carbon in the urea is used to estimate CO_2 production from which energy expenditure is estimated.[37,44]

British researchers have shown that energy expenditure estimates based on the bicarbonate-urea method compare favorably with those derived from whole-body calorimetry in apparently healthy subjects and those with HIV infection and lung cancer.[44–46] The researchers used an insulin pump to continuously administer the labeled bicarbonate via subcutaneous injection to each free-living subject over a several-day study period. Compared with doubly labeled water, the bicarbonate-urea method has the advantage of being less costly and providing estimates of total energy expenditure over shorter periods of time (several hours to several days), allowing the day-to-day variations in energy expenditure to be studied.[37]

Estimating Energy Needs

In most clinical settings, energy expenditure is not usually measured. Instead, it is estimated using one of numerous available formulas such as the Harris-Benedict equations, those recently developed by the Institute of Medicine for calculating Estimated Energy Requirement, or the World Health Organization equations.

Commonly Used Equations

There are approximately 200 published guidelines for estimating the nonprotein energy requirements of hospitalized patients.[30,47–53] Commonly used equations for predicting REE are those published in 1919 by Harris and Benedict[47] and those developed by an expert panel of the World Health Organization, which are shown in Table 7.7. Harris and Benedict used indirect calorimetry to determine the REE of 239 healthy young adults (136 males and 103 females with a mean age of 27 and 31 years, respectively). From these data, they derived regression equations (Table 7.7) that best predicted REE using the variables weight, stature, age, and sex.[47,48] Research has shown the Harris-Benedict equations' accuracy of prediction among healthy, adequately nourished persons to be within ± 14% of REE measured by indirect calorimetry.[48,49] In malnourished, ill patients, however, the Harris-Benedict equations tend to underestimate REE

TABLE 7.7 Examples of Equations for Estimating Resting Energy Expenditure in Healthy Persons

Harris-Benedict			
Females	REE = 655.096 + 9.563 W + 1.850 S − 4.676 A		
Males	REE = 66.473 + 13.752 W + 5.003 S − 6.755 A		
Harris-Benedict (Values Rounded for Simplicity)			
Females	REE = 655.1 + 9.6 W + 1.9 S − 4.7 A		
Males	REE = 66.5 + 13.8 W + 5.0 S − 6.8 A		
World Health Organization (WHO)			***SD****
Females	3–9 years old	22.5 W + 499	± 63
	10–17 years old	12.2 W + 746	± 117
	18–29 years old	14.7 W + 496	± 121
	30–60 years old	8.7 W + 829	± 108
	>60 years old	10.5 W + 596	± 108
Males	3–9 years old	22.7 W + 495	± 62
	10–17 years old	17.5 W + 651	± 100
	18–29 years old	15.3 W + 679	± 151
	30–60 years old	11.6 W + 879	± 164
	>60 years old	13.5 W + 487	± 148
National Institutes of Health			
REE = 638 + (15.9 × FFM)			
University of Vermont			
REE = 418 + (20.3 × FFM)			

Abbreviations: W = weight in kilograms; A = age in years; S = stature in cm; FFM = fat-free mass in kilograms.

*SD = standard deviation of the differences between actual and computed values—68% of the time the actual REE will be within ± 1 standard deviation of the predicted REE.

Adapted from Harris JA, Benedict FG. 1919. *A biometric study of basal metabolism in man.* Publication 279. Washington, DC: Carnegie Institution of Washington; World Health Organization. 1985. *Energy and protein requirements. Report of a joint FAO/WHO/UNU expert consultation.* Technical Report Series 724. Geneva, Switzerland: World Health Organization; Nieman DC. 2003. *Exercise testing and prescription: A health-related approach,* 5th ed. Boston: McGraw-Hill.

by as much as 22%.[48] Despite these shortcomings, the Harris-Benedict equations are often widely used in estimating the energy needs of patients in clinical settings.

A major decision in developing prediction equations is which variables to include. The major determinant of REE is fat-free mass—what some researchers call the active protoplasmic tissue, or the body cell mass.[48–51] These cells are the body's metabolically active, energy-consuming cells, and they determine about 70% to 80% of the variance in REE. The remaining 20% to 30% of variance in REE is primarily determined by genetics.[50] As discussed in Chapter 6, fat-free mass can be determined using a variety of approaches such as skinfold measurement, underwater weighing, air displacement plethysmography, or dual-energy X-ray absorptiometry. If known, an individual's fat-free mass in kilograms can be used to estimate resting energy expenditure using equations shown in Table 7.7.

Numerous other equations for predicting REE in healthy populations are available.[49,51] Some are derived from original research, and others are based on a reanalysis of data published by Harris and Benedict between 1919 and 1935.[48,52] The WHO equations (shown in Table 7.7) were developed by a group of experts.[53] Because stature was not found to significantly improve the predictive ability of the equations, it was omitted from those developed by the WHO. Using measured energy expenditure based on the doubly labeled water technique, the National Academy of Sciences developed a set of equations for estimating REE in healthy people. These are shown in Table 7.8.

The equations in Table 7.7 and Table 7.8 predict REE in kilocalories, and to arrive at estimates of 24-hour energy expenditure, the REE must be increased to account for TEE. This is done by multiplying REE by one of the activity factors shown in Box 7.3 to arrive at TEE. Theoretically, REE includes TEF as well as TEE. In most clinical settings, however, no additional allowance is made for TEF. Use of an additional factor to account for increased metabolism caused by disease, injury, and surgery is often necessary to estimate the 24-hour energy expenditure of patients.

Statistical analysis of the data (stepwise multiple-regression analysis) has shown that stature and body weight are reasonably well correlated with REE, and because these measures can be easily and accurately performed, one or both are included in most equations. Some of the earlier REE equations used body surface area as a variable.

When using these equations, keep in mind that there is a large interindividual variability in energy requirements. Even though a particular equation may be able to predict the mean REE for a given group of people with a rather high degree of accuracy, the accuracy of that same equation in predicting one individual's value

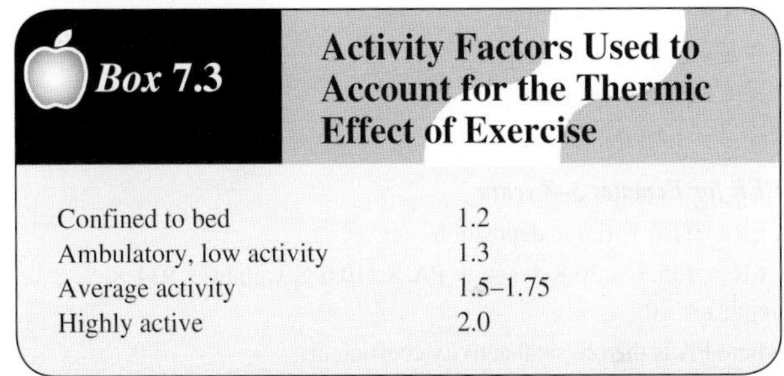

Box 7.3 Activity Factors Used to Account for the Thermic Effect of Exercise

Confined to bed	1.2
Ambulatory, low activity	1.3
Average activity	1.5–1.75
Highly active	2.0

Source: Adapted from Zeman FJ. 1991. *Clinical nutrition and dietetics.* New York: Macmillian; Long CL. 1984. The energy and protein requirements of the critically ill patient. In Wright RA, Heymsfield SB (eds.), *Nutritional assessment.* Boston: Blackwell Scientific Publications.

TABLE 7.8 Equations for Calculating Resting Energy Expenditure (REE) in Kilocalories per Day

REE for males ages 3–18 years, healthy weight (BMI < 85th percentile for age and sex)

REE = 68 − (43.3 × age) + (712 × height) + (19.2 × weight)

REE for males ages 3–18, at risk of overweight or overweight (BMI ≥ 85th percentile for age and sex)

REE = 419.9 − (33.5 × age) + (418.9 × height) + (16.7 × weight)

REE for females ages 3–18 years, healthy weight (BMI < 85th percentile for age and sex)

REE = 189 − (17.6 × age) + (625 × height) + (7.9 × weight)

REE for females ages 3–18, at risk of overweight or overweight (BMI ≥ 85th percentile for age and sex)

REE = 515.8 − (26.8 × age) + (347 × height) + (12.4 × weight)

REE for males ages 19 and older

REE = 293 − (3.8 × age) + (456.4 × height) + (10.12 × weight)

REE for females ages 19 and older

REE = 247 − (2.67 × age) + (401.5 × height) + (8.6 × weight)

Abbreviations: REE = resting energy expenditure; age is in years; height is in meters; weight is in kilograms.

Source: Adapted from Panel on Macronutrients, Panel on the Definition of Dietary Fiber, Subcommittee on Upper Reference Levels of Nutrients, Subcommittee on Interpretation and Uses of Dietary Reference Intakes, Standing Committee on the Scientific Evaluation of Dietary Reference Intakes. 2002. *Dietary reference intakes for energy, carbohydrate, fiber, fat, fatty acids, cholesterol, protein, and amino acids.* Washington, DC: National Academy Press.

may be quite low. Thus, remember that even the best prediction equation provides only an approximation of an individual's energy requirement.

Estimated Energy Requirement Equations

The National Academy of Sciences, as part of its ongoing work in developing the Dietary Reference Intakes (DRIs) (discussed in Chapter 2), has developed a set of prediction equations to calculate the Estimated Energy Requirement (EER).[50] These equations are shown in Table 7.9. The EER is defined as the average dietary energy intake that is predicted to maintain energy balance in a healthy person of a defined age, gender, weight, height, and level of physical activity consistent with good health.[50] For

TABLE 7.9 Equations for Calculating Estimated Energy Requirement (EER) in Kilocalories per Day

EER for Infants and Young Children

EER = TEE + tissue deposition[a]

0–3 months	(89 × weight − 100) + 175
4–6 months	(89 × weight − 100) + 56
7–12 months	(89 × weight − 100) + 22
13–35 months	(89 × weight − 100) + 20

EER for Males 3–8 years

EER = TEE + tissue deposition

EER = 88.5 − 61.9 × age + PA × (26.7 × weight + 903 × height) + 20

where PA is the physical activity coefficient:

- PA = 1.00 for sedentary
- PA = 1.13 for low active
- PA = 1.26 for active
- PA = 1.42 for very active

EER for Females 3–8 years

EER = TEE + tissue deposition

EER = 135.3 − 30.8 × age + PA × (10.0 × weight + 934 × height) + 20

where PA is the physical activity coefficient:

- PA = 1.00 for sedentary
- PA = 1.16 for low active
- PA = 1.31 for active
- PA = 1.56 for very active

EER for Males 9–18 years

EER = TEE + tissue deposition

EER = 88.5 − 61.9 × age + PA × (26.7 × weight + 903 × height) + 25

where PA is the physical activity coefficient:

- PA = 1.00 for sedentary
- PA = 1.13 for low active
- PA = 1.26 for active
- PA = 1.42 for very active

EER for Females 9–18 years

EER = TEE + tissue deposition

EER = 135.3 − 30.8 × age + PA × (10.0 × weight + 934 × height) + 25

where PA is the physical activity coefficient:

- PA = 1.00 for sedentary
- PA = 1.16 for low active
- PA = 1.31 for active
- PA = 1.56 for very active

EER for Males 19 years of age and older

EER = TEE

EER = 662 − 9.53 × age + PA × (15.91 × weight + 539.6 × height)

where PA is the physical activity coefficient:

- PA = 1.00 for sedentary
- PA = 1.11 for low active
- PA = 1.25 for active
- PA = 1.48 for very active

EER for Females 19 years of age and older

EER = TEE

EER = 354 − 6.91 × age + PA × (9.36 × weight + 726 × height)

where PA is the physical activity coefficient:

- PA = 1.00 for sedentary
- PA = 1.12 for low active
- PA = 1.27 for active
- PA = 1.45 for very active

EER for Pregnancy

EER = EER for age + pregnancy energy needs[b] + tissue deposition

1st trimester = EER for age + 0

2nd trimester = EER for age + 160 + 180

3rd trimester = EER for age + 272 + 180

EER for Lactation

EER = EER for age + milk energy output[c] − weight loss[d]

1st 6 months = EER for age + 500 − 170

2nd 6 months = EER for age + 400 − 0

Abbreviations: EER = Estimated Energy Requirement; TEE = Total Energy Expenditure; PA = physical activity coefficient; age is in years; height is in meters; weight is in kilograms.

[a]Tissue deposition represents the energy cost of growth during infancy, childhood, adolescence, and pregnancy as measured in kilocalories.

[b]Pregnancy energy needs represents the additional energy required to support the metabolic demands of pregnancy.

[c]Milk energy output represents the energy needed to produce the milk during lactation. Milk output is somewhat greater in the first 6 months than in the second 6 months of breastfeeding.

[d]Weight loss represents an average decline in EER of 170 kcal/day that well-nourished lactating women experience during the first 6 months postpartum, resulting in an average weight loss of 0.8 kg/month.

Source: Adapted from Panel on Macronutrients, Panel on the Definition of Dietary Fiber, Subcommittee on Upper Reference Levels of Nutrients, Subcommittee on Interpretation and Uses of Dietary Reference Intakes, Standing Committee on the Scientific Evaluation of Dietary Reference Intakes. 2002. *Dietary reference intakes for energy, carbohydrate, fiber, fat, fatty acids, cholesterol, protein, and amino acids.* Washington, DC: National Academy Press.

infants, children, and adolescents the EER includes the energy needed for a desirable level of physical activity and optimal growth, maturation, and development at an age- and gender-appropriate rate that is consistent with good health, including maintenance of a healthy body weight and appropriate body composition. For females who are pregnant or lactating, the EER includes the energy needed for physical activity, maternal and fetal development, and lactation at a rate consistent with good health.[50]

The EER is calculated using a series of prediction equations developed by the DRI Committee for healthy-weight individuals age 0 to 100 years based on the 24-hour total energy expenditures of more than 1200 subjects measured using the doubly labeled water technique.[50] Using measured 24-hour total energy expenditure data obtained from these healthy-weight subjects, the DRI Committee developed a series of regression equations that best predict the energy requirement of healthy-weight individuals using such variables as age, gender, life stage (pregnant or lactating), body weight, height, and physical activity level. As shown in Table 7.9, EER equations have been developed for infants and young children of both sexes age 0 to 35 months, males and females age 3 to 8 years, males and females age 9 to 18 years, males and females age 19 years and older, and females who are pregnant or lactating. Except for those for infants and young children age 0 to 35 months, the equations contain a physical activity coefficient (PA) that represents one of four different categories of physical activity level: sedentary, low active, active, and very active. Energy expenditure at the sedentary level includes basal energy expenditure, the thermic effect of food, and physical activities required for independent living. A low active lifestyle would be roughly equivalent to the energy expended by a 70 kg (154 lb) adult walking 2.2 miles per day at a rate of 3 to 4 miles per hour (or an equivalent amount of energy expended in other activities) in addition to the activities necessary for independent living. An active lifestyle would be roughly equivalent to the energy expended by a 70 kg (154 lb) adult walking 7 miles per day at a rate of 3 to 4 miles per hour in addition to the activities related to independent living. Energy expenditure by a very active lifestyle would be equivalent to walking 17 miles per day in addition to the activities of independent living. The extra energy needed for growth during infancy, childhood, adolescence, and pregnancy is included in an allowance referred to as tissue deposition. During pregnancy, metabolic rate is also increased because of the energy requirements of the uterus and fetus and the increased work of the heart and lungs. During lactation, extra energy is needed to support milk production, which is somewhat greater in the first 6 months of breastfeeding than in the second 6 months. Because most women lose an average of 0.8 kg per month in the first 6 months postpartum (i.e., after delivery), EER is, on average, 170 kcal per day less.[50]

EER equations apply only to persons having a healthy weight, and EER values have not been established for persons who are overweight or obese.[50] Instead, the DRI Committee has developed a separate set of equations for calculating total energy expenditure (TEE) for the maintenance of weight for adults age 19 years and older who are overweight (BMI between 25.0 kg/m^2 and 29.9 kg/m^2) and or obese (BMI $\geq$ 30.0 kg/m^2), and an additional set were developed for children and adolescents age 3 to 18 years who are overweight (a BMI for age and sex $\geq$ 95th percentile).[50] These equations are shown in Table 7.10. The DRI Committee adopted the definition of healthy weight for adults (age 19 years and older) used by the Dietary Guidelines for Americans, which is a BMI $\geq$ 18.5 kg/m^2 but $\leq$ 24.9 kg/m^2. Healthy weight for persons age 2 to 18 years is defined as a BMI that is > 5th percentile but < 85th percentile of BMI for age and sex, a concept discussed at length in Chapter 6. The equations developed for overweight or obese persons shown in Table 7.10 allow calculation of the TEE necessary for weight maintenance using the variables of gender, age, weight, height, and physical activity level. If weight loss is desired, a recommended approach is to reduce energy intake by 500 to 1000 kilocalories less than that needed for maintenance and to increase energy expenditure by engaging in moderate physical activity for approximately 60 minutes per day on most days of the week.

Energy Expenditure in Disease and Injury

Surgery, trauma, infection, burns, and various diseases can cause 24-hour energy expenditure and urinary nitrogen excretion to increase markedly.[28,29] The effect of various stresses on REE in hospitalized patients is shown in Figure 7.18.[28] The normal range of resting

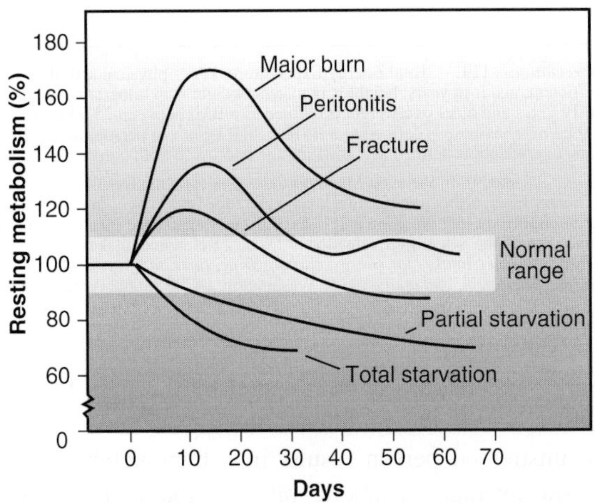

Figure 7.18 Effect of various stresses on resting energy expenditure in hospitalized patients.

Source: Adapted from Long CL, Schaffel N, et al. 1979. Metabolic response to injury and illness: Estimation of energy and protein needs from indirect calorimetry and nitrogen balance. *Journal of Parenteral and Enteral Nutrition* 3:452–456.

TABLE 7.10	Equations for Calculating Total Energy Expenditure (TEE) for Weight Maintenance in Kilocalories per Day for Overweight and Obese Adults and for Overweight Children and Adolescents

TEE for Overweight and Obese Males Age 19 Years and Older

TEE = 1086 − 10.1 × age + PA × (13.7 × weight + 416 × height)

where PA is the physical activity coefficient:

PA = 1.00 for sedentary

PA = 1.12 for low active

PA = 1.29 for active

PA = 1.59 for very active

TEE for Overweight and Obese Females Age 19 Years and Older

TEE = 448 − 7.95 × age + PA × (11.4 × weight + 619 × height)

where PA is the physical activity coefficient:

PA = 1.00 for sedentary

PA = 1.16 for low active

PA = 1.27 for active

PA = 1.44 for very active

TEE for Overweight Males Age 3–18 Years

TEE = 114 − 50.9 × age + PA × (19.5 × weight + 1161.4 × height)

where PA is the physical activity coefficient:

PA = 1.00 for sedentary

PA = 1.12 for low active

PA = 1.24 for active

PA = 1.45 for very active

TEE for Overweight Females Age 3–18 Years

TEE = 389 − 41.2 × age + PA × (15.0 × weight + 701.6 × height)

where PA is the physical activity coefficient:

PA = 1.00 for sedentary

PA = 1.18 for low active

PA = 1.35 for active

PA = 1.60 for very active

Abbreviations: TEE = Total Energy Expenditure; PA = physical activity coefficient; age is in years; height is in meters; weight is in kilograms. In persons age 19 years and older overweight is defined as a BMI between 25.0 kg/m^2 and 29.9 kg/m^2 and obese is defined as a BMI ≥ 30.0 kg/m^2. In persons age 3–18 years, overweight is defined as a BMI for age and sex ≥ 95th percentile.[54]

Source: Adapted from Panel on Macronutrients, Panel on the Definition of Dietary Fiber, Subcommittee on Upper Reference Levels of Nutrients, Subcommittee on Interpretation and Uses of Dietary Reference Intakes, Standing Committee on the Scientific Evaluation of Dietary Reference Intakes. 2002. *Dietary reference intakes for energy, carbohydrate, fiber, fat, fatty acids, cholesterol, protein, and amino acids.* Washington, DC: National Academy Press.

energy expenditure is represented by the light horizontal bar across the middle of the figure. Starvation in the unstressed person results in a hypometabolic state (below average metabolic rate) as the body attempts to conserve its energy reserves. The time when peak energy expenditure occurs in response to stress varies, depending on the severity of the illness or injury, and energy needs gradually return to normal during recovery. Figure 7.18 represents average values for both males and females of varying ages and body sizes and assumes no secondary complications, which can prolong periods of increased energy needs. The clinical course of individual patients can be expected to vary somewhat from these average values.

A common approach to estimating a patient's energy needs is to calculate the 24-hour energy expenditure, as outlined in Box 7.4, and then to increase this value by the appropriate injury factors shown in Table 7.11. This second step is necessary because the equations developed by Harris-Benedict, the DRI equations for calculating EER, and the World Health Organization equations are all based on data collected from healthy subjects.

Of all the conditions in Table 7.11, burns have the greatest potential for increasing energy expenditure.[54–59] When caloric intake fails to adequately meet energy expenditure in burn patients, weight loss, delayed wound healing, and poor clinical outcome will result. A number of equations or approaches have been proposed for estimating the energy and protein needs of burn patients.[56–58,60–63] Several of these are shown in Table 7.12. An approach to estimating the energy requirements of a burn patient is to simply calculate his or her REE using the Harris-Benedict equation and then increase this value by an injury factor (1.6 to 2.2) and possibly an activity factor to account for energy the patient expends while in therapy.[63] A very simple approach, shown in Table 7.12, is merely to double the REE derived from the Harris-Benedict equation.[60]

The equations developed by Curreri and coworkers, shown in Table 7.12, have been frequently used

TABLE 7.11	Injury Factors Used to Account for the Thermic Effect of Disease and Injury

Condition	Injury Factor*
Minor surgery	1.0–1.1
Major surgery	1.1–1.3
Mild infection	1.0–1.2
Moderate infection	1.2–1.4
Severe infection	1.4–1.8
Skeletal or blunt trauma	1.2–1.4
Skeletal or head trauma (steroid treated)	1.6–1.8
Burns involving ≤ 20% BSA†	1.2–1.5
Burns involving 20% to 40% BSA	1.5–1.8
Burns involving > 40% BSA	1.8–2.0

Adapted from Long CL. 1984. The energy and protein requirements of the critically ill patient. In Wright RA, Heymsfield SB, eds. *Nutritional assessment.* Boston: Blackwell Scientific Publications.

*Multiply the predicted resting energy expenditure adjusted for the thermic effect of food and the thermic effect of exercise by the appropriate injury factor to arrive at an estimate of the patient's 24-hour energy expenditure. The range in values allows adjustment depending on the severity of the disease or injury.

†BSA = body surface area.

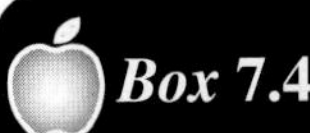

Box 7.4 Estimating Resting Energy Expenditure (REE) and 24-Hour Energy Expenditure Using the World Health Organization (WHO) Equations

Using the WHO equations in Table 7.7, the Harris-Benedict equations in Table 7.7, or the DRI equations for calculating REE in Table 7.8 is quite easy. As an example, take a 23-year-old female with a body weight of 64 kg (141 lb). Begin by selecting the proper equation for the subject's sex and age. Then calculate the predicted REE using the appropriate WHO equation.

$$\text{REE} = 14.7\text{ W} + 496$$

$$\text{REE} = (14.7 \times 64) + 496$$

$$\text{REE} = 941 + 496$$

$$\text{REE} = 1437 \text{ kcal}$$

To arrive at an estimate of 24-hour energy expenditure, the value for REE (1437 kcal) is then multiplied by an activity factor (Box 7.3) that accounts for the thermic effect of exercise—the calories expended during physical activity. Assuming this person has an activity level at the low end of the average activity category, the activity factor of 1.5 will be used.

$$1437 \text{ kcal} \times 1.5 = 2156 \text{ kcal}$$

This gives an estimated 24-hour energy expenditure of 2156 kcal. Assuming that the subject is 168 cm (66 in) tall, how do these values compare with those obtained by using the DRI equations for calculating EER?

for calculating the energy needs of burned patients.[56,64] In these equations, energy requirements for patients of different ages are estimated by adding resting energy expenditure (REE) as predicted by the Harris-Benedict equation to the product of the percent of body surface area burned (%BSAB) and an age-dependent constant. In the originally published equation for adults, resting or basal energy requirement was estimated by multiplying the patient's body weight in kilograms by 25.[64] This is based on the observation that REE is approximately 25 kcal/kg of body weight. The Curreri equations have the advantage of linking energy estimates with percent of body surface area burned. However, studies comparing the energy needs of severely burned patients as measured by indirect calorimetry and as estimated by the Curreri equations show that the equations tend to overestimate energy needs, resulting in overfeeding.[58,65,66] One explanation for this may be that recent advances in the management of severe burns result in less of a hypermetabolic response to the thermal injury as when the Curreri formula[58] was originally developed in the early 1970s.[58]

TABLE 7.12 Equations for Estimating the Energy Requirements of Patients with Burns*

Age	Equation
Allard[67]	
Adults	kcal = −4343 + (10.5 × %BSAB) + (0.23 CI) + (0.84 REE) + (114 T) − (4.5 PBD)
Cunningham[60]	
0–3 yr	kcal = 2 × REE
Curreri[64]	
0–1 yr	kcal = REE + (15 × %BSAB)
1–3 yr	kcal = REE + (25 × %BSAB)
4–15 yr	kcal = REE + (40 × %BSAB)
16–59 yr	kcal = REE + (40 × %BSAB)
≥ 60 yr	kcal = REE + (65 × %BSAB)
Hildreth[62]	
Child	kcal = (1800 × m^2 BSA) + (2200 × m^2 BSAB)
Adolescent	kcal = (1500 × m^2 BSA) + (1500 × m^2 BSAB)
Long	
Any age	kcal = REE × injury factor × activity factor

*kcal = estimated daily energy requirement in kilocalories; REE = resting energy expenditure as predicted by the Harris-Benedict equation; BSA = body surface area in m^2; BSAB = body surface area burned in m^2; %BSAB = percent of body surface area burned; CI = the number of kilocalories the patient received in the previous 24 hours; T = average rectal temperature of the previous 24 hours in degrees Celsius; PBD = the number of postburn days prior to the day the energy requirements are calculated; see Box 7.3 for activity factors and Table 7.8 for injury factors.

The equation in Table 7.12 developed by Allard and coworkers[61] has been shown to fairly accurately predict the energy requirements of burned patients, compared with energy expenditure measured by indirect calorimetry. Referred to as the "Toronto formula," it was derived by multiple-regression analysis of data collected from 23 patients with a mean burned body surface area of 39%.[67] Energy requirement is estimated by beginning with a negative value of 4343 kcal and adding or subtracting to this value various products. The equation requires information on the percent body surface area burned (estimated on admission and corrected where amputation was performed); the number of kilocalories the patient received in the previous 24 hours, including all dextrose infusions, parenteral and enteral feedings; REE calculated from the Harris-Benedict equation; the average of the hourly rectal temperatures from the previous 24 hours expressed in degrees Celsius; and the number of postburn days as of the previous day. The Toronto formula has been shown to more closely predict the energy requirements of severely burned patients than the modified Curreri or the practice of doubling REE derived from the Harris-Benedict equation, both of which tend to overestimate energy requirements.[61] Energy expenditure predictions derived from the Toronto formula have also been shown to compare favorably with measured resting energy expenditure of clinically stable, mechanically ventilated burn patients.[68] The Toronto formula is unique in that it considers the thermic effect of food (which tends to be elevated in critically ill patients), the increased metabolic rate caused by elevations in body temperature, and the gradual fall in metabolic rate with time.

Energy Needs: Estimated or Measured?

Estimates of energy expenditure obtained from equations are just that—estimates. They are approximate and should be used only as rough guidelines.[58,69] However, for most hospital patients, estimates of energy expenditure are acceptable in providing the care their conditions demand. For these patients, the time and financial costs of measuring energy needs are not warranted. However, in some instances, it may be cost-effective to determine energy expenditure rather than to rely solely on estimates.[35] The use of total parenteral nutrition (TPN) is quite expensive; not only are the solutions themselves costly but their administration requires a considerable time investment by nurses, pharmacists, physicians, and registered dietitians. Basing the administration of TPN solutions on measured energy expenditure may help prevent excessive use of TPN.[30,35] Not only is undernutrition associated with increased morbidity and mortality, but overnutrition can have negative clinical outcomes as well.[30,35] Measuring energy expenditure allows administration of TPN solutions to be based on physiologic need and promotes patient recovery. Thus, the cost of indirect calorimetry may be justified by both improved patient care and savings resulting from more judicious use of costly resources, such as TPN solutions and staff time and savings to the hospital because of shorter hospital stays.[30,35] In the case of burn patients, routine use of indirect calorimetry allows tailoring of nutritional support and is valuable in the early detection of significant undernutrition or overnutrition.[65] Considering the seriousness of thermal injury and the importance of nutritional support in its management, measuring the energy expenditure of severely burned patients should be standard practice.[69]

Determining Protein Requirements

Protein serves as a functional component of body tissues and enzymes and as a fuel source. The protein needs of healthy, nonpregnant, nonlactating adults generally can be met with an intake of 0.8 g/kg body weight per day. In trauma or burn patients, protein catabolism increases markedly, as does protein loss, as indicated by urinary nitrogen excretion. Nitrogen makes up about 16% of protein and serves as a convenient way of measuring protein intake and losses.

Protein Losses in Disease and Injury

Figure 7.19 shows how urinary nitrogen losses vary over time among different conditions.[28] The normal range of urinary nitrogen loss is represented by the figure's light horizontal bar. Partial or total starvation in the unstressed person often results in *reduced* nitrogen losses as the body attempts to spare protein. The opposite is true in trauma or burn patients, even though their energy and protein intake often are reduced substantially. Trauma and burns are usually associated with increased protein catabolism and urinary nitrogen losses, although the patient's nutritional status before injury can affect the extent of loss. All other factors being equal, nitrogen losses after trauma and thermal injury are less in depleted persons and the elderly. Under these conditions, the protein reserves may be so depleted that the response is blunted or may not even be observed.

As with changes in REE seen in response to injury and illness (Figure 7.18), urinary nitrogen losses vary in degree and duration with the severity of the injury, may take several days after onset of the disease or trauma to reach their peak, and gradually return to the normal range.

Estimating Protein Needs

In practice, there is no single best method for conclusively determining the amount of protein that should be

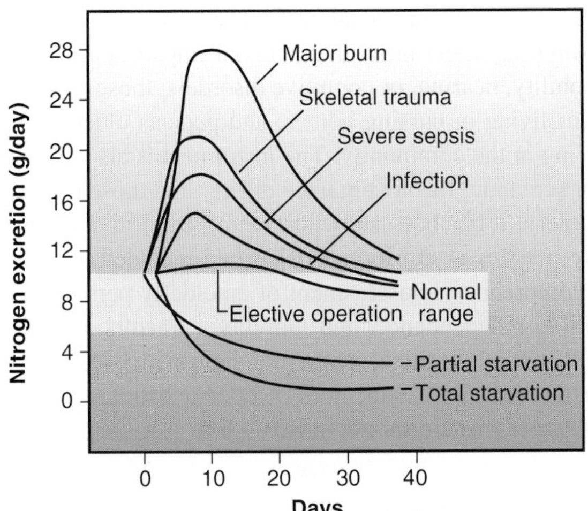

Figure 7.19 Effect of various stresses on urinary nitrogen excretion in hospitalized patients.

Source: Adapted from Long CL, Schaffel N, et al. 1979. Metabolic response to injury and illness: Estimation of energy and protein needs from indirect calorimetry and nitrogen balance. *Journal of Parenteral and Enteral Nutrition* 3:452–456.

TABLE 7.13 Suggested Ranges of Protein Intake per Kilogram of Body Weight During Peak Catabolic Response for Various Injuries and Conditions in Adults

Stress Level	Condition	Protein (g/kg/d)
Normal	Healthy	0.8
Mild	Minor surgery, mild infection	0.8–1.2
Moderate	Major surgery, moderate infection, moderate skeletal trauma	1.2–1.8
Severe	Severe infection, multiple injuries, severe trauma, major burns	1.6–2.2

Adapted from Ireton-Jones CS, Hasse JM. 1992. Comprehensive nutritional assessment: The dietitian's contribution to the team effort. *Nutrition* 8:75–81; Long CL. 1984. The energy and protein requirements of the critically ill patient. In Wright RA, Heymsfield SB, eds. *Nutritional assessment.* Boston: Blackwell Scientific Publications; Waymack JP, Herndon DN. 1992. Nutritional support of the burned patient. *World Journal of Surgery* 16:80–86; Mentegut WJ, Lowry SF. 1993. Nutrition in burn patients. *Seminars in Nephrology* 13:400–408.

in the diet of patients suffering from trauma, burns, and other injuries. The protein requirements of these patients can only be estimated. Three approaches are commonly used—basing protein intake on body weight, caloric intake, or nitrogen balance.[28] Table 7.13 provides some suggested ranges of protein intake per kilogram of body weight for various injuries and situations. If the energy needs of a patient are reasonably well defined, these can be used to estimate protein requirements. Some authorities consider 1 g of nitrogen (or 6.25 g of protein) for every 150 nonprotein kilocalories to be an adequate daily protein intake for critically ill adults and adults with burns when the percent body surface area burned is ≤ 10.[28] When injuries are very severe or the burn involves more than 10% body surface area, 1 g of nitrogen is recommended for every 100 nonprotein kilocalories.

Nitrogen balance (discussed in Chapter 9) involves 24-hour measurement of protein intake and an estimate of nitrogen losses where N Bal = nitrogen balance; protein intake = protein intake in g/24 hours; and UUN = urine urea nitrogen in g/24 hours.

$$\text{N Bal} = \frac{\text{Protein intake}}{6.25} - \text{UUN} - 4$$

Protein intake is divided by 6.25 to arrive at an estimate of nitrogen intake. Because protein is 16% nitrogen, dividing grams of protein by 6.25 gives you grams of nitrogen. Nitrogen loss is *estimated* by measuring urine urea nitrogen (which accounts for 85% to 90% of total urinary nitrogen) and subtracting a constant (4 g in the equation, although this value can vary from 2 to 4 g) to account for dermal, fecal, and nonurea nitrogen losses, which cannot be easily measured.[70,71]

Measuring total urinary nitrogen (TUN) is more difficult, expensive, and time consuming than measuring urinary urea nitrogen (UUN). Consequently, estimating TUN from measurements of UUN is standard practice. However, some researchers question the appropriateness of this practice, suggesting that in trauma and burn patients UUN represents only about 65% of TUN, as opposed to 80% to 90% in healthy persons.[72,73] They suggest that TUN should be measured directly rather than estimated from UUN. Other researchers report that estimates of TUN based on UUN are significantly different from direct measures of TUN but that the differences are small and clinically insignificant to justify the added expense and trouble of directly measuring TUN.[74]

Despite the problems associated with measuring protein intake and nitrogen excretion, nitrogen balance is generally accepted as an appropriate and cost-effective way of monitoring the protein status of burn and other critically ill patients.[28,58,72,74] Although not an exact indicator of nutritional adequacy, nitrogen balance studies serve as an excellent guide to nutritional support when used in conjunction with changes in body weight and energy expenditure measured by indirect calorimetry.[74] However, even if more protein is provided a patient than is calculated from losses in the urine, nitrogen balance is difficult to achieve in the early stage of severe trauma and thermal injury. The catabolism associated with the stress of trauma and thermal injury, as well as the atrophy of muscle caused by immobilization and disuse, result in considerable urinary nitrogen losses. Given time and the provision of adequate energy and protein, the patient gradually will begin to retain more protein than is excreted and will replace lost body protein.[28,58]

Mini Nutritional Assessment

The Mini Nutritional Assessment (MNA) is a validated nutritional screening instrument designed to identify elderly persons who are malnourished or at risk of malnutrition. Developed by Nestlé, it uses data that are relatively easy to obtain, and it can be administered in clinical settings such as hospitals or physicians' offices or in community settings.[76–81] The MNA, shown in Figure 7.20, is designed to provide primary care health professionals with a single tool to efficiently identify elderly patients at nutritional risk who may subsequently need a more extensive nutritional assessment.[76] It is primarily intended for evaluating the so-called frail elderly—older persons exhibiting some kind of functional impairment, such as mobility, hearing, or cognitive disorders; those older persons living in nursing homes; and persons older than 85 living in the community. The instrument is also effective for screening the hospitalized elderly and those requiring surgery. It has been shown to be most useful at identifying persons at nutritional risk when included as part of a comprehensive assessment of an elderly person's cognition, independence, and mobility.[76] Factors associated with poor nutritional status are shown in Box 7.5, and major and minor indicators of poor nutritional status in older persons are shown in Box 7.6.[75]

Mini Nutritional Assessment
MNA®

Nestlé
NutritionInstitute

Last name: First name:
Sex: Age: Weight, kg: Height, cm: Date:

Complete the screen by filling in the boxes with the appropriate numbers.
Add the numbers for the screen. If score is 11 or less, continue with the assessment to gain a Malnutrition Indicator Score.

Screening

A Has food intake declined over the past 3 months due to loss of appetite, digestive problems, chewing or swallowing difficulties?
0 = severe decrease in food intake
1 = moderate decrease in food intake
2 = no decrease in food intake ☐

B Weight loss during the last 3 months
0 = weight loss greater than 3kg (6.6lbs)
1 = does not know
2 = weight loss between 1 and 3kg (2.2 and 6.6 lbs)
3 = no weight loss ☐

C Mobility
0 = bed or chair bound
1 = able to get out of bed / chair but does not go out
2 = goes out ☐

D Has suffered psychological stress or acute disease in the past 3 months?
0 = yes 2 = no ☐

E Neuropsychological problems
0 = severe dementia or depression
1 = mild dementia
2 = no psychological problems ☐

F Body Mass Index (BMI) (weight in kg) / (height in m²)
0 = BMI less than 19
1 = BMI 19 to less than 21
2 = BMI 21 to less than 23
3 = BMI 23 or greater ☐

Screening score (subtotal max. 14 points) ☐☐
12-14 points: Normal nutritional status
8-11 points: At risk of malnutrition
0-7 points: Malnourished
For a more in-depth assessment, continue with questions G-R

Assessment

G Lives independently (not in nursing home or hospital)
1 = yes 0 = no ☐

H Takes more than 3 prescription drugs per day
0 = yes 1 = no ☐

I Pressure sores or skin ulcers
0 = yes 1 = no ☐

J How many full meals does the patient eat daily?
0 = 1 meal
1 = 2 meals
2 = 3 meals ☐

K Selected consumption markers for protein intake
- At least one serving of dairy products (milk, cheese, yoghurt) per day yes ☐ no ☐
- Two or more servings of legumes or eggs per week yes ☐ no ☐
- Meat, fish or poultry every day yes ☐ no ☐

0.0 = if 0 or 1 yes
0.5 = if 2 yes
1.0 = if 3 yes ☐.☐

L Consumes two or more servings of fruit or vegetables per day?
0 = no 1 = yes ☐

M How much fluid (water, juice, coffee, tea, milk...) is consumed per day?
0.0 = less than 3 cups
0.5 = 3 to 5 cups
1.0 = more than 5 cups ☐.☐

N Mode of feeding
0 = unable to eat without assistance
1 = self-fed with some difficulty
2 = self-fed without any problem ☐

O Self view of nutritional status
0 = views self as being malnourished
1 = is uncertain of nutritional state
2 = views self as having no nutritional problem ☐

P In comparison with other people of the same age, how does the patient consider his / her health status?
0.0 = not as good
0.5 = does not know
1.0 = as good
2.0 = better ☐.☐

Q Mid-arm circumference (MAC) in cm
0.0 = MAC less than 21
0.5 = MAC 21 to 22
1.0 = MAC 22 or greater ☐.☐

R Calf circumference (CC) in cm
0 = CC less than 31
1 = CC 31 or greater ☐

Assessment (max. 16 points) ☐☐.☐
Screening score ☐☐.☐
Total Assessment (max. 30 points) ☐☐.☐

Malnutrition Indicator Score

24 to 30 points	☐	Normal nutritional status
17 to 23.5 points	☐	At risk of malnutrition
Less than 17 points	☐	Malnourished

References
1. Vellas B, Villars H, Abellan G, *et al.* Overview of the MNA® - Its History and Challenges. *J Nutr Health Aging*. 2006; **10:456**-465.
2. Rubenstein LZ, Harker JO, Salva A, Guigoz Y, Vellas B. Screening for Undernutrition in Geriatric Practice: Developing the Short-Form Mini Nutritional Assessment (MNA-SF). *J. Geront*. 2001; **56A**: M366-377
3. Guigoz Y. The Mini-Nutritional Assessment (MNA®) Review of the Literature - What does it tell us? *J Nutr Health Aging*. 2006; **10**:466-487.

For more information: www.mna-elderly.com

Figure 7.20 The Mini Nutritional Assessment.
The full Mini Nutritional Assessment (full MNA) comprises questions A through R and takes 10 to 15 minutes to complete. The short form of the MNA (the MNA-SF) comprises questions A through F and takes less than 5 minutes to complete.
Source: Reprinted courtesy of Société des Produits Nestlé S.A., Vevey, Switzerland, Trademark Owners.

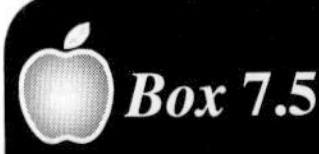

Box 7.5 Risk Factors for Poor Nutritional Status in Older Adults

- Inappropriate food intake
- Poverty
- Social isolation
- Dependency/disability
- Acute/chronic diseases or conditions
- Chronic medication use
- Advanced age (≥ 80 years)

Adapted from: White JV, Ham RJ, Lipschitz DA, Dwyer JT, Wellman NS. 1991. Consensus of the Nutrition Screening Initiative:Risk factors and indicators of poor nutritional status in older Americans. *Journal of the American Dietetic Association* 91:783–787.

Approximately 10 to 15 minutes are needed to complete the full MNA questionnaire (questions A through R in the instrument shown in Figure 7.20). An abbreviated version of the instrument, the Mini Nutrition Assessment–Short Form (MNA-SF), comprises questions A through F in the instrument shown in Figure 7.20, and can be completed in less than 5 minutes. The MNA-SF retains the validity of the full MNA but is practical for use in clinical and community settings because it can be more quickly administered than the full version. There is also a self-administered version of the instrument, the Self MNA (shown in Figure 7.21) composed of six questions. Individuals whose scores suggest they are malnourished or at risk of malnutrition are advised to consult with a health care professional. There are also "apps" for smart phones and tablets, such as the iPhone and iPad.

Most of the information required to complete the full MNA can be obtained from a physical examination and from a brief interview with the patient or someone knowledgeable about the patient's condition and dietary habits. In addition, some anthropometric data are necessary, including height and weight (for calculating body mass index), mid-arm circumference, and calf circumference.[76–81]

The full MNA was developed and thoroughly evaluated by researchers at Toulouse University Hospital, Toulouse, France; the University of New Mexico, Albuquerque; and the Nestlé Research Center in Lausanne, Switzerland.[76] The full MNA is completed by assigning points for each of the 18 items in the instrument, which are then summed to provide a "malnutrition indicator score." When the malnutrition indicator score is ≥ 24, the patient's nutritional status can be considered normal, and these patients should be given general dietary and lifestyle information about how to remain in good health. A patient whose malnutrition indicator score is < 17 is likely to be at high risk for protein-energy malnutrition and should be followed up with a comprehensive nutritional assessment. Those whose malnutrition indicator score is between 17 and 23.5 are at increased risk for malnutrition and should also receive further evaluation of their nutritional status. Research shows the full MNA and MNA-SF to be practical, noninvasive, and cost-effective instruments for identifying elderly persons at risk for malnutrition.[77–81]

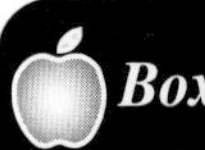

Box 7.6 Major and Minor Indicators of Poor Nutritional Status in Older Adults

MAJOR INDICATORS

- Weight loss ≤ 10 lb
- Underweight or overweight
- Serum albumin < 3.5 g/dL
- Change in functional status
- Inappropriate food intake
- Midarm muscle circumference < 10th percentile
- Triceps skinfold < 10th percentile or > 95th percentile
- Obesity
- Nutrition-related disorders
- Osteoporosis
- Osteomalacia
- Folate deficiency
- Vitamin B_{12} deficiency

MINOR INDICATORS

- Alcoholism
- Cognitive impairment
- Chronic renal insufficiency
- Multiple concurrent medications
- Malabsorption syndromes
- Anorexia, nausea, dysphagia
- Change in bowel habits
- Fatigue, apathy, memory loss
- Poor oral/dental status
- Dehydration
- Poorly healing wounds
- Loss of subcutaneous fat or muscle mass
- Fluid retention
- Reduced iron, ascorbic acid, zinc

Adapted from White JV, Ham RJ, Lipschitz DA, Dwyer JT, Wellman NS. 1991. Consensus of the Nutrition Screening Initiative:Risk factors and indicators of poor nutritional status in older Americans. *Journal of the American Dietetic Association* 91:783–787.

Malnutrition Universal Screening Tool

The Malnutrition Universal Screening Tool (MUST) is a validated, evidence-based nutrition screening instrument designed to identify adults who are malnourished, at risk of malnutrition, underweight, as well as obese.[80,82,83] It is easy to use and takes 3 to 5 minutes to complete.[82] The MUST uses a five-step process to evaluate three different components: BMI, history of unintentional weight loss during the previous three to six months, and the presence of decreased food intake due to acute illness the patient is experiencing (acute disease effects). In the first step, height and weight are measured and BMI is calculated and scored. A BMI > 20.0 kg/m^2 receives a score of 0, a BMI of 18.5 to 20.0 kg/m^2 receives a score of 1, and a BMI < 18.5 kg/m^2 receives a score of 2. In the second step, a score is assigned based on any recent unintentional weight loss (within the past three to six months). If the patient has unintentionally lost < 5% of his or her usual weight in the past three to six months, a score of 0 is assigned. If the unintentional weight loss has been 5% to 10%, a score of 1 is given. If the weight loss has been > 10%, a score of 2 is given. The third step evaluates the effects of any acute illness the patient has on nutritional intake. If the patient has been acutely ill and there has been, or there is likely to be, no nutritional intake for more than five days, a score of 2 is assigned. In the

Nestlé
NutritionInstitute

Self MNA®

Mini Nutritional Assessment

For Adults 65 years of Age and Older

Last name: ____________________ First name: ____________________

Date: ____________________ Age: ____________________

Complete the screen by filling in the boxes with the appropriate numbers. Total the numbers for the final screening score.

Screening		
A Has your food intake declined over the past 3 months? [ENTER ONE NUMBER] *Please enter the most appropriate number (0, 1, or 2) in the box to the right.*	0 = severe decrease in food intake 1 = moderate decrease in food intake 2 = no decrease in food intake	☐
B How much weight have you lost in the past 3 months? [ENTER ONE NUMBER] *Please enter the most appropriate number (0, 1, 2, or 3) in the box to the right.*	0 = weight loss greater than 7 pounds 1 = do not know the amount of weight lost 2 = weight loss between 2 and 7 pounds 3 = no weight loss or weight loss less than 2 pounds	☐
C How would you describe your current mobility? [ENTER ONE NUMBER] *Please enter the most appropriate number (0, 1, or 2) in the box to the right.*	0 = unable to get out of a bed, a chair, or a wheelchair without the assistance of another person 1 = able to get out of a bed or a chair, but unable to go out of my home 2 = able to leave my home	☐
D Have you been stressed or severely ill in the past 3 months? [ENTER ONE NUMBER] *Please enter the most appropriate number (0 or 2) in the box to the right.*	0 = yes 2 = no	☐
E Are you currently experiencing dementia and/or prolonged severe sadness? [ENTER ONE NUMBER] *Please enter the most appropriate number (0, 1, or 2) in the box to the right.*	0 = yes, severe dementia and/or prolonged severe sadness 1 = yes, mild dementia, but no prolonged severe sadness 2 = neither dementia nor prolonged severe sadness	☐
Please total all of the numbers you entered in the boxes for questions A-E and write that number here:		☐

continued

Figure 7.21 The Self MNA is a self-administered version of the Mini Nutritional Assessment. Individuals whose scores suggest they are malnourished or at risk of malnutrition (≤ 11) are advised to consult with a health care professional.

Source: Reprinted courtesy of Société des Produits Nestlé S.A., Vevey, Switzerland, Trademark Owners.

Now, please CHOOSE ONE of the following two questions – F1 or F2 – to answer.

Question F1

Height (feet & inches)	Body Weight (pounds)			
4'10"	Less than 91	91-99	100-109	110 or more
4'11"	Less than 94	94-103	104-113	114 or more
5'0"	Less than 97	97-106	107-117	118 or more
5'1"	Less than 100	100-110	111-121	122 or more
5'2"	Less than 104	104-114	115-125	126 or more
5'3"	Less than 107	107-117	118-129	130 or more
5'4"	Less than 110	110-121	122-133	134 or more
5'5"	Less than 114	114-125	126-137	138 or more
5'6"	Less than 118	118-129	130-141	142 or more
5'7"	Less than 121	121-133	134-145	146 or more
5'8"	Less than 125	125-137	138-150	151 or more
5'9"	Less than 128	128-141	142-154	155 or more
5'10"	Less than 132	132-145	146-159	160 or more
5'11"	Less than 136	136-149	150-164	165 or more
6'0"	Less than 140	140-153	154-168	169 or more
6'1"	Less than 144	144-158	159-173	174 or more
6'2"	Less than 148	148-162	163-178	179 or more
6'3"	Less than 152	152-167	168-183	184 or more
6'4"	Less than 156	156-171	172-188	189 or more
Group	0	1	2	3

Please refer to the chart on the left and follow these instructions:

1. Find your height on the left-hand column of the chart.
2. Go across that row and circle the range that your weight falls into.
3. Look to the bottom of the chart to find what group number (0, 1, 2, or 3) your circled weight range falls into.

Write the Group Number (0, 1, 2, or 3) here: ☐

Write sum of questions A-E (from page 1) here: ☐

Lastly, calculate the sum of these 2 numbers: ☐

Question F2 DO NOT ANSWER QUESTION F2 IF QUESTION F1 IS ALREADY COMPLETED.

Measure the circumference of your LEFT calf by following the instructions below:

Loop a tape measure all the way around your calf to measure its size.

Record the measurement in inches: ___________

If Less than 12 inches, enter "0" in box to the right.

If 12 inches or Greater, enter "3" in box to the right. ☐

© SIGVARIS

Write the sum of questions A-E (from page 1) here: ☐

Lastly, calculate the sum of these 2 numbers: ☐

Screening Score 14 points maximum

12 – 14 points:	Normal nutritional status
8 – 11 points:	At risk of malnutrition
0 – 7 points:	Malnourished

☐

If you score between 0 - 11, please take this form to a healthcare professional for consultation.

Figure 7.21 ***Continued***

fourth step, the overall risk of malnutrition is determined by adding together the scores from the first three steps, and in the fifth step, an appropriate patient care plan is developed and implemented. If the total score is 0, the patient is considered at low risk of malnutrition and is given routine clinical care. If the total score is 1, the patient is considered at medium risk of malnutrition and is observed or treated, as is appropriate. If the total score is 2 or more, the patient is considered at high risk of malnutrition and is treated, as is appropriate.[84]

The MUST has been shown very effective in predicting clinical outcomes such as length of hospitalization and mortality in older persons, and for providing guidance in the discharge destination of orthopedic and other patients.[82,83] The MUST was developed in 2003 by the Malnutrition Advisory Group of the British Association for Parenteral and Enteral Nutrition and has been independently reviewed by a number of independent clinicians and health care practitioners as well as several prestigious health care groups in the United Kingdom, including the Royal College of Physicians, Royal College of Obstetricians and Gynaecologists, Royal College of Nursing, and British Dietetic Association. It is reviewed annually and updated as needed. It is the most widely used nutritional screening tool in the UK and is commonly used in other countries worldwide.[82–84] The questionnaire and a variety of print and online support materials, including an "app" for the iPhone and iPad, are available from the website of the British Association for Parenteral and Enteral Nutrition (www.bapen.org.uk).

Summary

1. Assessing the nutritional status of hospitalized patients involves at least four goals: identifying those at nutritional risk, determining the severity and causes of nutritional impairment, determining the patient's risk of dying from the undernutrition or developing a related disease condition, and monitoring to evaluate response to nutrition therapy.
2. The purpose of nutritional screening is to identify potentially malnourished individuals at nutritional risk. Screening should be done on all patients within the first 24 to 48 hours following admission. It is best done by a dietetic technician.
3. Because no single measurement or test is capable of evaluating a patient's nutritional status, a variety of data must be used. The most fundamental include the patient's stature, usual and present weight, and past and current dietary practices; significant changes in eating habits; and the presence of any nutrition-related problems. Some of this information is routinely collected by the nursing and medical staff and can be found in the patient's medical record. For critically ill patients or those with less obvious nutritional deficits, detailed anthropometric, laboratory, and dietary information may need to be collected.
4. The history includes facts about past and current health, use of medications, and personal and household information as it pertains to nutritional status. Dietary information relates to food intake, food preferences, intolerances and allergies, usual eating pattern, use of supplements, and resources for purchasing and preparing food. Physical examination includes anthropometric data as well as findings from the physical examination available from the patient's chart.
5. Stature and body weight are important measures to be obtained from hospitalized patients. Under certain conditions they may have to be calculated from such variables as the patient's knee height, calf circumference, age, and sex, or they may be obtained by measuring body length while the patient is lying in bed. When calculations are performed, care should be exercised in selecting the proper equation.
6. Midarm circumference is the circumference of the upper arm at the triceps skinfold site. It is an indicator of muscle and subcutaneous adipose tissue and can be obtained quickly and noninvasively in both ambulatory and nonambulatory patients. Arm muscle area, calculated from the triceps skinfold measurement and midarm circumference, is used as an index of lean tissue or muscle in the body.
7. Calf circumference is used in estimating body weight and as an indicator of muscle and subcutaneous adipose tissue. Obtaining calf circumference and measures of skinfold thickness in bedridden patients is somewhat different than in ambulatory persons, and the standardized protocol outlined in this chapter should be strictly followed.
8. Energy needs are based on an individual's 24-hour energy expenditure, which is determined by resting energy expenditure, the thermic effect of food, energy expended in physical activity, and whether disease or injury is present. Resting energy expenditure is the largest component of 24-hour energy expenditure.
9. Twenty-four-hour energy expenditure can be determined through indirect calorimetry or roughly approximated from a variety of equations. Indirect calorimetry involves measurement of the body's oxygen consumption and carbon dioxide production and often uses a computerized metabolic monitor.

The energy expenditure of patients usually is estimated. In critically ill persons or those receiving parenteral or enteral feedings, indirect calorimetry may be preferable to estimating energy expenditure.

10. Surgery, trauma, infection, burns, and various diseases can cause 24-hour energy expenditure and urinary excretion of nitrogen to increase markedly. Energy expenditure in patients can be obtained through indirect calorimetry or estimates using a variety of equations.

11. The degree and duration of increased protein catabolism following injury vary with the trauma's severity. Protein catabolism may take several days to peak before gradually returning to normal. Recommended protein intake can be based on nitrogen balance, body weight, or energy intake.

12. The full Mini Nutritional Assessment (MNA) is an 18-item questionnaire designed to identify elderly patients at nutritional risk who may subsequently need a more extensive nutritional assessment. A short form of the questionnaire, the MNA-SF, comprises the first six items of the full version and takes less than 5 minutes to complete. A self-administered version is also available.

13. The Malnutrition Universal Screening Tool (MUST) is a validated, evidence-based five-step screening tool for identifying adults who are malnourished or at risk of malnutrition. It uses BMI, history of recent unintentional weight loss, and the effects of any acute illness on nutritional intake to arrive at an overall malnutrition risk score.

REFERENCES

1. Corish CA, Kennedy NP. 2000. Protein-energy undernutrition in hospital in-patients. *British Journal of Nutrition* 83:575–591.
2. Klein S, Kinney J, Jeejeebhoy K, Alpers D, Hellerstein M, Murray M, Twomey P. 1997. Nutrition support in clinical practice: Review of published data and recommendations for future research directions. *American Journal of Clinical Nutrition* 66:683–706.
3. McMahon K, Brown JK. 2000. Nutritional screening and assessment. *Seminars in Oncology Nursing* 16:106–112.
4. Posthauer ME, Dorse B, Foiles RA, et al. 1994. ADA's definitions for nutrition screening and nutrition assessment. *Journal of the American Dietetic Association* 94:838–839.
5. Green SM, Watson R. 2005. Nutritional screening and assessment tools for use by nurses: Literature review. *Journal of Advanced Nursing* 50:69–83.
6. Trimble JM. 1992. Reimbursement enhancement in a New Jersey hospital: Coding for malnutrition in prospective payment systems. *Journal of the American Dietetic Association* 92:737–738.
7. Sayarath VG. 1993. Nutrition screening for malnutrition: Potential economic impact at a community hospital. *Journal of the American Dietetic Association* 93:1440–1442.
8. Ireton-Jones CS, Hasse JM. 1992. Comprehensive nutritional assessment: The dietitian's contribution to the team effort. *Nutrition* 8:75–81.
9. Hopkins B. 1993. Assessment of nutritional status. In Gottschlich MM, Matarese LE, Shronts EP, eds. *Nutrition support dietetics core curriculum,* 2nd ed. Silver Spring, MD: American Society for Parenteral and Enteral Nutrition.
10. Chumlea WC, Guo S, Roche AF, Steinbaugh ML. 1988. Prediction of body weight for the nonambulatory elderly from anthropometry. *Journal of the American Dietetic Association* 88:564–568.
11. Chumlea WC, Guo SS, Steinbaugh ML. 1994. Prediction of stature from knee height for black and white adults and children with application to mobility-impaired or handicapped persons. *Journal of the American Dietetic Association* 94:1385–1388.
12. Detsky AS, Smalley PS, Change J. 1994. Is this patient malnourished? *Journal of the American Medical Association* 271:54–58.
13. Chumlea WC, Roche AF, Mukherjee D. 1987. *Nutritional assessment of the elderly through anthropometry.* Columbus, OH: Ross Laboratories.
14. Heymsfield SB, McManus C, Smith J, Stevens V, Nixon DW. 1982. Anthropometric measurement of muscle mass: Revised equations for calculating bone-free arm muscle area. *American Journal of Clinical Nutrition* 36:680–690.
15. Chumlea WC. 1988. Methods of nutritional anthropometric assessment for special groups. In Lohman TG, Roche AF, Martorell R (eds.), *Anthropometric standardization reference manual.* Champaign, IL: Human Kinetics Books.
16. Chumlea WC, Roche AF. 1988. Assessment of the nutritional status of healthy and handicapped adults. In Lohman TG, Roche AF, Martorell R (eds.), *Anthropometric standardization reference manual.* Champaign, IL: Human Kinetics Books.

17. Cockram DB, Baumgartner RN. 1990. Evaluation of accuracy and reliability of calipers for measuring recumbent knee height in elderly people. *American Journal of Clinical Nutrition* 52:397–400.
18. Muncie HL, Sobal J, Hoopes JM, Tenney JH, Warren JW. 1987. A practical method of estimating stature of bedridden female nursing home patients. *Journal of the American Geriatrics Society* 35:285–289.
19. Jarzem PF, Gledhill RB. 1993. Predicting height from arm measurements. *Journal of Pediatric Orthopaedics* 13:761–765.
20. Falciglia G, O'Conner J, Gedling E. 1988. Upper arm anthropometric norms in elderly white subjects. *Journal of the American Dietetic Association* 88:569–574.
21. Callaway CW, Chumlea WC, Bouchard C, Himes JH, Lohman TG, Martin AD, Mitchell CD, Mueller WH, Roche AF, Seefeldt VD. 1988. Circumferences. In Lohman TG, Roche AF, Martorell R (eds.), *Anthropometric standardization reference manual.* Champaign, IL: Human Kinetics Books.
22. Chumlea WC, Roche AF, Webb P. 1984. Body size, subcutaneous fatness and total body fat in older adults. *International Journal of Obesity* 8:311–317.
23. Frisancho AR. 2008. *Anthropometric standards: An interactive nutritional reference of body size and body composition for children and adults.* Ann Arbor: University of Michigan Press.
24. Guenter PA, Moore K, Crosby LO, Buzby GP, Mullen JL. 1982. Body weight measurement of patients receiving nutritional support. *Journal of Parenteral and Enteral Nutrition* 6:441–443.
25. Brunnstrom S. 1983. *Clinical kinesiology,* 4th ed. Philadelphia: Davis.
26. Frisancho AR. 1981. New norms of upper limb fat and muscle areas for assessment of nutritional status. *American Journal of Clinical Nutrition* 34:2540–2545.
27. Sims AH, Danforth E. 1987. Expenditure and storage of energy in man. *Journal of Clinical Investigation* 79:1019–1025.
28. Long CL. 1984. The energy and protein requirements of the critically ill patient. In Wright RA, Heymsfield SB (eds.), *Nutritional assessment.* Boston: Blackwell Scientific Publications.
29. Damask MC, Schwarz Y, Weissman C. 1987. Energy measurements and requirements of critically ill patients. *Critical Care Clinics* 3:71–96.
30. Committee on Metabolic Monitoring for Military Field Applications, Standing Committee on Military Nutrition Research, Food and Nutrition Board. 2004. *Monitoring metabolic status: Predicting decrements in physiological and cognitive performance.* Washington, DC: National Academy Press.
31. Seale JL, Rumpler WV, Moe PW. 1991. Description of a direct-indirect room-sized calorimeter. *American Journal of Physiology* 260:E306–E320.
32. Ainslie PN, Reilly T, Westerterp KR. 2003. Estimating human energy expenditure: a review of techniques with particular reference to doubly labelled water. *Sports Medicine* 33:683–698.
33. Hipskind P, Glass C, Charlton D, Nowak D, Dasarathy S. 2011. Do handheld calorimeters have a role in assessment of nutrition needs in hospitalized patients? A systematic review of literature. *Nutrition in Clinical Practice* 26:426–433.
34. Nieman DC, Austin MD, Chilcote SM, Benezra L. 2005. Validation of a new handheld device for measuring resting metabolic rate and oxygen consumption in children. *International Journal of Sport Nutrition and Exercise Metabolism* 15:186–194.
35. McDoniel SO. 2007. A systematic review on use of a handheld indirect calorimeter to assess energy needs in adults and children. *International Journal of Sport Nutrition and Exercise Metabolism* 17:491–500.
36. Schoeller DA. 1990. How accurate is self-reported dietary energy intake? *Nutrition Reviews* 48:373–379.
37. Gibney ER. 2000. Energy expenditure in disease: Time to revisit? *Proceedings of the Nutrition Society* 59:199–207.
38. Levine JA. 2005. Measurement of energy expenditure. *Public Health Nutrition* 8:1123–1132.
39. Livingstone MBE, Prentice AM, Coward AW, Ceesay SM, Strain JJ, McKenna PG, Nevin GB, Barker ME, Hickey RJ. 1990. Simultaneous measurement of free-living energy expenditure by the doubly labeled water method and heart-rate monitoring. *American Journal of Clinical Nutrition* 52:59–65.
40. Bandini LG, Schoeller DA, Dietz WH. 1990. Energy expenditure in obese and nonobese adolescents. *Pediatric Research* 27:198–202.
41. Prentice AM, Black AE, Coward WA, Davies HL, Goldberg GR, Murgatroyd PR, Ashford J, Sawyer M, Whitehead RG. 1986. High levels of energy expenditure in obese women. *British Medical Journal* 292:983–987.
42. Johnson RK, Goran MI, Poehlman ET. 1994. Correlates of over- and underreporting of energy intake in healthy older men and women. *American Journal of Clinical Nutrition* 59:1286–1290.
43. Elia M, Fuller N, Murgatroyd P. 1988. The potential use of the labelled bicarbonate method for estimating energy expenditure in man. *Proceedings from the Nutrition Society* 47:247–258.
44. Elia M, Jones MG, Jennings G, Poppitt SD, Fuller NJ, Murgatroyd PR, Jebb SA. 1995. Estimating energy expenditure from specific activity of urine urea during lengthy subcutaneous $NaH^{14}CO_3$ infusion. *American Journal of Physiology* 269:E172–E182.
45. Gibney E, Elia M, Jebb SA, Murgatroyd P, Jennings G. 1997. Total energy expenditure in patients with small-cell lung cancer: Results of a validated study using the bicarbonate-urea method. *Metabolism* 46:1412–1417.

46. Paton NI, Elia M, Jebb SA, Jennings G, Macallan DC, Griffin GE. 1996. Total energy expenditure and physical activity measured with the bicarbonate-urea method in patients with human immunodeficiency virus infection. *Clinical Science* 91:241–245.

47. Harris JA, Benedict FG. 1919. *A biometric study of basal metabolism in man.* Publication 279. Washington, DC: Carnegie Institution of Washington.

48. Roza AM, Shizgal HM. 1984. The Harris Benedict equation reevaluated: Resting energy requirements and the body cell mass. *American Journal of Clinical Nutrition* 40:168–182.

49. Owen OE, Holup JL, D'Alessio DA, Craig ES, Polansky M, Smalley KJ, Karle EC, Bushman MC, Owen LR, Mozzoli MA, Kedrick ZV, Boden GH. 1987. A reappraisal of the caloric requirement of men. *American Journal of Clinical Nutrition* 46:875–885.

50. Panel on Macronutrients, Panel on the Definition of Dietary Fiber, Subcommittee on Upper Reference Levels of Nutrients, Subcommittee on Interpretation and Uses of Dietary Reference Intakes, Standing Committee on the Scientific Evaluation of Dietary Reference Intakes. 2002. *Dietary reference intakes for energy, carbohydrate, fiber, fat, fatty acids, cholesterol, protein, and amino acids.* Washington, DC: National Academy Press.

51. Mifflin MD, St Jeor ST, Hill LA, Scott BJ, Daugherty SA, Koh YO. 1990. A new predictive equation for resting energy expenditure in healthy individuals. *American Journal of Clinical Nutrition* 51:241–247.

52. Cunningham JJ. 1980. A reanalysis of the factors influencing basal metabolic rate in normal adults. *American Journal of Clinical Nutrition* 33:2372–2374.

53. World Health Organization. 1985. *Energy and protein requirements. Report of a joint FAO/WHO/UNU expert consultation.* Technical Report Series 724. Geneva, Switzerland: World Health Organization.

54. Mayes T. 1997. Enteral support for the burn patient. *Nutrition in Clinical Practice* 12:S43–S45.

55. Flynn MB. 2004. Nutritional support for the burn-injured patient. *Critical Care Nursing Clinics of North America* 16:139–144.

56. Curreri PW. 1990. Assessing nutritional needs for the burned patient. *Journal of Trauma* 30(12 suppl):S20–S23.

57. Bell SJ, Wyatt J. 1986. Nutrition guidelines for burned patients. *Journal of the American Dietetic Association* 86:648–653.

58. Waymack JP, Herndon DN. 1992. Nutritional support of the burned patient. *World Journal of Surgery* 16:80–86.

59. Montegut WJ, Lowry SF. 1993. Nutrition in burn patients. *Seminars in Nephrology* 13:400–408.

60. Cunningham JJ, Lydon MK, Russell WE. 1990. Calorie and protein provision for recovery from severe burns in infants and young children. *American Journal of Clinical Nutrition* 51:533–537.

61. Allard JP, Pichard C, Hoshino E, Stechison S, Fareholm L, Peters WJ, Jeejeebhoy KN. 1990. Validation of a new formula for calculating the energy requirements of burn patients. *Journal of Parenteral and Enteral Nutrition* 14:115–118.

62. Hildreth MA, Herndon DN, Parks KH. 1987. Evaluation of a caloric requirement formula in burned children treated with early excision. *Journal of Trauma* 27:188–189.

63. Hansbrough JF. 1998. Enteral nutritional support in burn patients. *Gastrointestinal Endoscopy Clinics of North America* 8:645–667.

64. Curreri PW, Richmond D, Marvin J, Baxter CR. 1974. Dietary requirements of patients with major burns. *Journal of the American Dietetic Association* 65:415–417.

65. Saffle JR, Medina E, Raymond J, Westenskow D. 1985. Use of indirect calorimetry in the nutritional management of burned patients. *Journal of Trauma* 25:32–39.

66. Turner WW, Ireton CS, Hunt JL, Baster CR. 1985. Predicting energy expenditure in burned patients. *Journal of Trauma* 25:11–16.

67. Allard JP, Jeejeebhoy KN, Whitwell J, Pashutinski L, Peters WJ. 1988. Factors influencing energy expenditure in patients with burns. *Journal of Trauma* 28:199–202.

68. Royall D, Fairholm L, Peters WJ, Jeejeebhoy KJ, Allard JP. 1994. Continuous measurement of energy expenditure in ventilated burn patients: An analysis. *Critical Care Medicine* 22:399–406.

69. Mancusi-Ungaro HR, Van Way CW, McCool C. 1992. Caloric and nitrogen balance as predictors of nutritional outcome in patients with burns. *Journal of Burn Care and Rehabilitation* 13:695–702.

70. Benjamin DR. 1989. Laboratory tests and nutritional assessment: Protein-energy status. *Pediatric Clinics of North America* 36:139–161.

71. Alcock NW. Laboratory tests for assessing nutritional status. In Shils ME, Olson JA, Shike M, Ross AC (eds.), *Modern nutrition in health and disease,* 9th ed. Baltimore, MD: Williams & Wilkins.

72. Konstantinides FN, Radmer WJ, Becker WK, Herman VK, Warren WE, Solem LD, Williams JB, Cerra FB. 1992. Inaccuracy of nitrogen balance determinations in thermal injury with calculated total urinary nitrogen. *Journal of Burn Care and Rehabilitation* 13:254–260.

73. Loder PB, Kee AJ, Horsburgh R, Jones M, Smith RC. 1989. Validity of urinary urea nitrogen as a measure of total urinary nitrogen in adult patients requiring parenteral nutrition. *Critical Care Medicine* 17:309–312.

74. Milner EA, Cioffi WG, Mason AD, McManus WF, Pruitt BA. 1993. Accuracy of urinary urea nitrogen for predicting total urinary nitrogen in thermally injured patients. *Journal of Parenteral and Enteral Nutrition* 17:414–416.

75. White JV, Ham RJ, Lipschitz DA, Dwyer JT, Wellman NS. 1991. Consensus of the Nutrition Screening Initiative: Risk factors and indicators of poor nutritional status in older Americans. *Journal of the American Dietetic Association* 91:783–787.

76. Vellas B, Guigoz Y, Garry PJ, Nourhashemi F, Bennahum D, Lauque S, Albarede JL. 1999. The Mini Nutritional Assessment (MNA) and its use in grading the nutritional state of elderly patients. *Nutrition* 15:116–122.

77. Guigoz Y, Vellas B, Garry PJ. 1996. Assessing the nutritional status of the elderly: The Mini Nutritional Assessment as part of the geriatric evaluation. *Nutrition Reviews* 54(Suppl):S59–S65.

78. Vellas B, Guigoz Y, Baumgartner M, Garry PJ, Lauque S, Albarede JL. 2000. Relationships between nutritional markers and the Mini Nutritional Assessment in 155 older persons. *Journal of the American Geriatrics Society* 48:1300–1309.

79. Rubenstein LZ, Harker JO, Salva A, Guigoz Y, Vellas B. 2001. Screening for undernutrition in geriatric practice: Developing the short-form Mini Nutritional Assessment (MNA-SF). *Journals of Gerontology: Series A, Biological Sciences and Medical Sciences* 56:M366–M372.

80. Phillips MB, Foley AL, Barnard R, Isenring EA, Miller MD. 2010. Nutritional screening in community-dwelling older adults: A systematic literature review. *Asia Pacific Journal of Clinical Nutrition* 19:440–449.

81. Kaiser MJ, Bauer JM, Ramsch C, Uter W, Guigoz Y, Dederholm T, et al. 2009. Validation of the Mini Nutritional Assessment Short Form (MNA-SF): A practical tool for identification of nutritional status. *Journal of Nutrition, Health & Aging* 13:782–788.

82. Ahmed T, Haboubi N. 2010. Assessment and management of nutrition in older people and its importance to health. *Clinical Interventions in Aging* 5:207–216.

83. Anthony PS. 2008. Nutrition screening tools for hospitalized patients. *Nutrition in Clinical Practice* 23:373–382.

84. Todorovic V, Russell C, Elia M, eds. 2011. *The "MUST" explanatory booklet: A guide to the Malnutrition Universal Screening Tool for adults.* British Association for Parenteral and Enteral Nutrition (www.bapen.org.uk).

Assessment Activity 7.1

Estimating Stature and Body Weight

Although stature and body weight usually can be easily obtained by direct measurement, there are times when they have to be estimated. Stature can be estimated from knee height, age, sex, and race using the equations in Table 7.1. Body weight can be estimated from knee height, age, sex, race, and midarm circumference using the equations in Tables 7.3 and 7.4. In this assessment activity, you will have an opportunity to practice measuring knee height, midarm circumference, stature, and body weight. You will use the appropriate formulas in Tables 7.1, 7.3, and 7.4 for calculating estimates of stature and body weight and then will compare these estimates with values obtained by direct measurement.

Your class can divide into groups of two or three students and measure each other's knee height and midarm circumference as outlined in this chapter. Two consecutive measurements of knee height should agree with each other to within 0.5 cm and be recorded. Measurements of midarm circumference should be recorded to within 0.1 cm. Be sure to mark the triceps skinfold site (where the midarm circumference is measured) if you plan to measure the triceps skinfold site in Assessment Activity 7.2. These values then can be substituted into the appropriate equations to obtain estimates of stature and body weight. Stature and body weight then can be measured directly following the guidelines in Chapter 6.

Once all students have completed their measurements and calculations, these can be listed on the board or on a sheet of paper distributed to all students. The means and standard deviations of all estimates and measures can be quickly calculated using a pocket calculator with statistical functions. In addition, the differences between estimated and measured values for stature and body weight can be calculated, and the mean and standard deviations of these can be calculated as well.

What was the difference between the estimated and measured values? Although it is clearly better to directly measure stature and body weight, estimates are generally better than no values at all.

ASSESSMENT ACTIVITY 7.2

Arm Muscle Area

Arm muscle area is used as an index of lean tissue or muscle in the body and represents muscle protein reserves. This assessment activity will help familiarize you with the anthropometric measurements and calculations required in arriving at estimates of arm muscle area.

In addition to midarm circumference (already obtained in Assessment Activity 7.1), the formula for arm muscle area requires measurement of the triceps skinfold. If you marked the triceps skinfold site in Assessment Activity 7.1, it will be easy to make this measurement. Review the section on triceps skinfold measurement in Chapter 6 if necessary. A pocket calculator and the following equations can be used for calculating corrected arm muscle area:

$$\text{cAMA for females} = \frac{[\text{MAC} - (\pi \times \text{TSF})]^2}{4\pi} - 6.5$$

$$\text{cAMA for males} = \frac{[\text{MAC} - (\pi \times \text{TSF})]^2}{4\pi} - 10$$

where cAMA = corrected arm muscle area in cm^2; MAC = midarm circumference in cm; and TSF = triceps skinfold thickness in cm. Note that these equations call for all measurements to be made in *centimeters.* The nomogram in Figure 7.14 also can be used to calculate corrected arm muscle area.

Appendix Q provides means, standard deviations, and percentiles of arm muscle area for males and females ages 1 to 74 years. For persons ages 18 years and older, the values are for corrected arm muscle area. Table 7.6 can be used for interpreting these age/sex percentile values. No single index (for example, arm muscle area) is a reliable indicator of nutritional status. Basic assumptions inferred from anthropometry should be corroborated by data derived from dietary, biochemical, and clinical observations.

CHAPTER

8 Nutritional Assessment in Disease Prevention

Chapter Outline

Introduction

Coronary Heart Disease

Cardiovascular Disease in Youth

Dietary Treatment in Coronary Heart Disease

Issues in Measuring Lipid and Lipoprotein Levels

Hypertension

Osteoporosis

Diabetes Mellitus

Summary

References

Assessment Activity 8.1: Lipid and Lipoprotein Levels and Coronary Heart Disease Risk

Assessment Activity 8.2: Calculating 10-Year Coronary Heart Disease Risk

Assessment Activity 8.3: Categorizing Blood Pressure in Children and Adolescents

Assessment Activity 8.4: Estimating Your Calcium Intake

Student Learning Outcomes

After studying this chapter, the student will be able to:

1. Identify the positive and negative risk factors for coronary heart disease.
2. Discuss the dietary and other lifestyle factors influencing serum levels of total cholesterol, low-density-lipoprotein cholesterol, and high-density-lipoprotein cholesterol.
3. Explain the rationale for primordial and primary prevention of CVD in children and adolescents.
4. Describe the Cardiovascular Health Integrated Lifestyle Diet (CHILD 1) recommended by the NHLBI's Expert Panel on Integrated Guidelines for Cardiovascular Health and Risk Reduction in Children and Adolescents.
5. Given the necessary information about a hypothetical patient, estimate that patient's risk of CHD in the next ten years.
6. Discuss the various preanalytical factors that influence a person's usual serum cholesterol level.
7. Given a certain blood pressure reading, evaluate it using the most recent classifications as published by the National Heart, Lung, and Blood Institute.
8. Discuss the various modifiable risk factors for hypertension mentioned in the textbook.
9. Identify the most recent diagnostic criteria for diabetes as established by the American Diabetes Association.
10. Define glycosylated hemoglobin and discuss how it is used to assess and manage glycemic control.

INTRODUCTION

The prominent role of diet and nutritional status in several leading causes of death for North Americans gives nutritional assessment an important role to play in disease prevention. This chapter addresses nutritional assessment as it relates to three major causes of death and disability: coronary heart disease, osteoporosis, and diabetes.

Several risk factors of coronary heart disease, the leading cause of death for North Americans, are related to diet. Among these are elevated serum total and low-density-lipoprotein cholesterol (LDL-C), low levels of high-density-lipoprotein cholesterol (HDL-C), obesity, hypertension, and diabetes. This chapter also discusses issues in measuring lipid and lipoprotein levels, which apply to practically all measurements in nutritional assessment.

Osteoporosis, a reduction in bone mineral density that leaves bones weakened and more likely to fracture, is a major cause of disability and death among older persons. Available methods for assessing bone mineral content are discussed. The chapter concludes with a discussion of criteria for diagnosing diabetes.

Reducing the individual and societal burden imposed by these and other diseases lies in our ability to prevent their premature onset through risk factor modification, early diagnosis, and research into more effective preventive measures. Nutritional assessment plays a prominent role in each of these.

CORONARY HEART DISEASE

Coronary heart disease, also referred to as coronary artery disease, is one of more than 50 different diseases affecting the heart and blood vessels, which collectively are known as cardiovascular diseases. Coronary heart disease occurs when the coronary arteries supplying the heart with oxygen and nutrients become narrowed and inelastic because of atherosclerosis. There is substantial scientific evidence that atherosclerosis begins in childhood with the formation of fatty streaks as lipids (primarily cholesterol and its esters) become deposited in macrophages (large phagocytic cells located within connective tissue) and smooth muscle cells within the inner lining of large elastic and muscular arteries. These early lesions do not disturb blood flow in the affected artery. As more lipid collects within the artery wall during adolescence and early adulthood, a fibrous plaque develops that projects into the channel, or lumen, of the artery, resulting in ischemia, or impaired blood flow. Ischemia within the heart muscle or myocardium can result in angina pectoris, which is chest pain caused by insufficient blood flow to the heart. If the impaired blood flow is severe enough, the tissues fed by the obstructed artery may die. This is known as an **infarction.** When this process affects the coronary arteries, a heart attack, or **myocardial infarction,** occurs. When the cerebral arteries are affected (known as cerebrovascular disease), a **stroke** results. Atherosclerotic changes within the aorta and iliac and femoral arteries can result in **peripheral vascular disease.**

Coronary heart disease (CHD) is the leading cause of death of American males and females.[1] Nearly 16.5 million American adults alive today have CHD, and nearly 9 million Americans have survived a heart attack. According to American Heart Association estimates, every year about 800,000 Americans experience a heart attack, and of these, about 400,000 die from their heart attack. In Canada, cardiovascular disease is the second leading cause of death, accounting for 22% of all male deaths and 20% of all female deaths.[2] In Europe, CHD is the leading cause of death, accounting for 21% of deaths among males and 22% of deaths among females.[3] In North America, nearly half of these deaths occur before the victims reach the hospital. This is due in part to the unfortunate fact that about half of all heart attack victims wait more than 2 hours before seeking help. Everyone should be familiar with the warning signs of heart attack (outlined in Box 8.1) and promptly seek medical care if these symptoms occur. Despite a more than 26% decline in the death rate from CHD since 1995, it remains the leading cause of death in the United States.[1] Over the

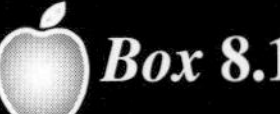

Box 8.1 Heart Attack Warning Signs

- **Chest discomfort or pain:** Most heart attacks involve discomfort or pain in the center of the chest that lasts more than a few minutes or that goes away and comes back. It can feel like uncomfortable pressure, tightness, squeezing, burning, heaviness, or pain.
- **Pain or discomfort in other regions of the upper body:** Symptoms can include pain or discomfort in one or both arms, the back, neck, jaw, or stomach.
- **Shortness of breath:** This feeling often comes along with chest discomfort. But it can occur before the chest discomfort.
- **Other signs:** Symptoms may include sweating, nausea, or dizziness. If you or someone you're with has chest discomfort, especially with one or more of the other signs, don't wait longer than a few minutes (no more than 5) before calling for help or going to a hospital.

Source: Adapted from American Heart Association Statistics Committee and Stroke Statistics Subcommittee. 2012. Heart Disease and Stroke Statistics—2012 Update. *Circulation* 125:e2–e220. http://circ.ahajournals.org/content/125/1/e2.

past 30 years death rates from CHD have been falling rapidly in most Northern and Western European countries but are rising rapidly in most Central and Eastern European countries. Between 1994 and 2004, CHD death rates for males less than 65 years of age living in Finland and the United Kingdom fell by 37% and 42%, respectively. During the same period of time, death rates rose by 57% for males living in Albania and by 19% for males living in Ukraine. For females less than 65 years of age living in Finland and the United Kingdom, CHD death rates fell by 35% and 49%, respectively, but rose by 46% for females living in Albania and by 19% for females living in Ukraine.[3]

Coronary Heart Disease Risk Factors

As discussed in Chapter 1, several factors or traits influence a person's risk of developing CHD and how rapidly atherosclerosis progresses.[1,4] The risk factors other than LDL-C levels are shown in Box 8.2. The "positive" risk factors are those that increase CHD risk. An HDL-C level ≥ 60 mg/dL is considered a "negative" risk factor because it decreases risk of CHD. Some of these risk factors are modifiable (e.g., cigarette smoking and, to a somewhat lesser degree, hypertension) while others are obviously not modifiable (e.g., age, male sex, and family history of premature CHD).

Serum Lipids and Lipoproteins

Cholesterol is a lipid, or fatlike, substance present only in foods of animal origin and synthesized by the body. It serves as a structural component of cell membranes and a precursor for steroid hormones and vitamin D, and it is used by the liver to form bile acids, which facilitate fat digestion and absorption. About 93% of the body's cholesterol is present in cell membranes, whereas only about 7% circulates in the blood. Triglyceride, a compound consisting of three fatty acids esterified to a molecule of glycerol, is the usual storage form of lipid in humans and animals.

There is a strong causal relationship between elevated low-density-lipoprotein cholesterol (LDL-C) and incidence of and mortality from CHD.[4–7] As serum LDL-C concentration increases, risk of CHD rises proportionally. CHD is rare in groups having a low serum LDL-C concentration, even when other CHD risk factors, such as cigarette smoking, hypertension, and diabetes mellitus, are relatively common.[5,6] The National Cholesterol Education Program has concluded that elevated LDL cholesterol is a major cause of CHD and, in its *Third Report of the National Cholesterol Education Program Expert Panel on Detection, Evaluation, and Treatment of High Blood Cholesterol in Adults* (referred to as the *Adult Treatment Panel III* or *ATP III*), the primary goals for the prevention and treatment of CHD are stated in terms of serum concentration of LDL-C.[4]

Because lipids such as cholesterol and triglycerides are fat soluble, they must be transported within the bloodstream from sites of absorption or synthesis to sites of storage or metabolism by lipoproteins. The major lipid-transporting lipoproteins are chylomicrons, very low-density lipoprotein (VLDL), low-density lipoproteins (LDL), and high-density lipoprotein (HDL).[5,8] Lipoproteins are spherical macromolecular complexes of lipids (triglycerides, cholesterol, cholesterol esters, and phospholipids) and proteins known as apoproteins.

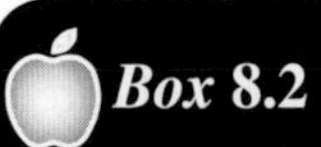

Box 8.2 Major Coronary Heart Disease Risk Factors Other Than LDL Cholesterol*

Positive Risk Factors

- Current cigarette smoking
- Hypertension (blood pressure ≥ 140/90 mm Hg or on antihypertensive medication)
- Low HDL cholesterol (< 40 mg/dL)
- Family history of premature CHD (CHD in a male first-degree relative < 55 years old or CHD in a female first-degree relative < 65 years old)**
- Presence of CHD risk equivalents†
- Age (men ≥ 45 years old; women ≥ 55 years old)

**A first-degree relative is one's parent, sibling, or offspring.
† CHD risk equivalents include diabetes mellitus; clinical forms of atherosclerotic disease (other than CHD), such as peripheral arterial disease, abdominal aortic aneurysm, and symptomatic carotid artery disease; and the presence of multiple risk factors, which together confer a 10-year risk for CHD that is greater than 20%.

Negative Risk Factor‡

- HDL cholesterol ≥ 60 mg/dL

*The presence of one or more risk factors influences low-density lipoprotein treatment goals. Age (defined differently for men and women) is treated as a risk factor because rates of CHD are higher in the elderly than in the young, and higher in men than in women of the same age. Obesity is not listed as a risk factor because it operates through other risk factors that are included (hypertension, hyperlipidemia, decreased HDL-C), but it should be considered a target for intervention. Physical inactivity is similarly not listed as a risk factor, but it, too, should be considered a target for intervention, and physical activity is recommended as desirable for everyone.
‡ If HDL-C is ≥ 60 mg/dL, subtract one risk factor because high HDL-C decreases CHD risk.

Adapted from National Cholesterol Education Program. 2001. *Third report of the expert panel on detection, evaluation, and treatment of high blood cholesterol in adults.* Bethesda, MD: U.S. Department of Health and Human Services, Public Health Service; National Institutes of Health; National Heart, Lung, and Blood Institute.

Apoproteins control the interaction and metabolic fate of lipoproteins. They activate enzymes that modify the composition and structure of lipoproteins, they are involved in the binding and ingestion of lipoproteins by cells, and they participate in the exchange of lipids among lipoproteins of different classes.[8] Figure 8.1 shows the relative size and the lipid composition of the three major lipoprotein particles.

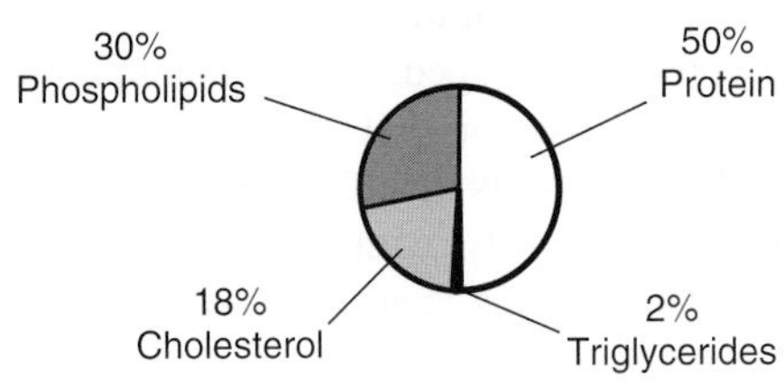

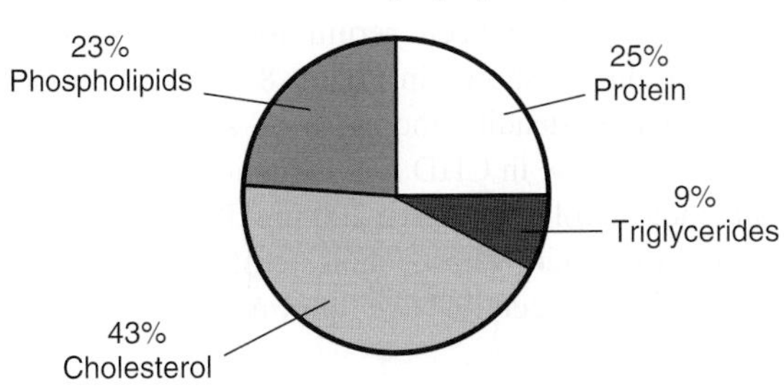

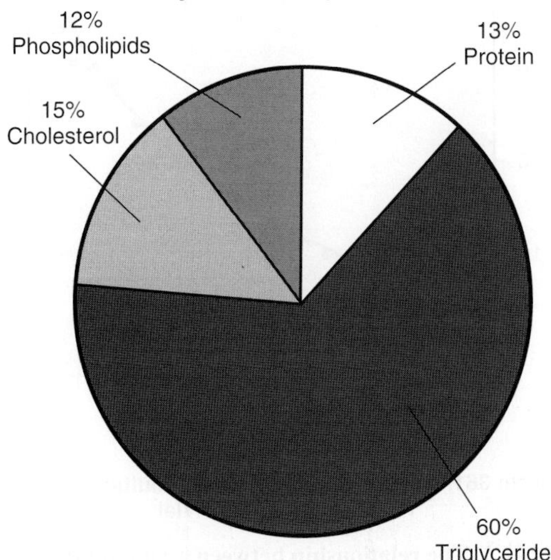

Figure 8.1 The relative size and the lipid composition of the three major lipoprotein particles found in fasting serum.

Source: Adapted from Haskell WL. 1994. The influence of exercise on the concentrations of triglyceride and cholesterol in human plasma. *Exercise and Sports Science Review* 12:205–244.

Chylomicrons are the largest lipoproteins, containing about 90% triglycerides by weight. They are synthesized in the intestine and transport dietary triglycerides from the small intestine to adipose tissue, muscle, and the liver. The dietary cholesterol they carry is taken up by the liver for production of bile acids or later incorporation into VLDL. Chylomicrons are not found in fasting serum, except in certain disease states.[8]

VLDL is 60% triglyceride by weight and contains 10% to 15% of the serum's total cholesterol. It is synthesized in the liver and primarily carries triglyceride to the cells for storage and metabolism. Removal of triglyceride from VLDL results in smaller, denser particles known as intermediate-density lipoprotein (IDL). The density of IDL falls between that of VLDL and LDL. About half the IDL is catabolized by the liver, and the remaining IDL undergoes additional changes (for example, uptake of cholesterol) that transforms it into LDL. Thus, LDL levels are linked to hepatic VLDL production and IDL catabolism.

The primary role of LDL is to transport cholesterol to the various cells of the body. LDL contains approximately 70% of the serum's total cholesterol, is considered the most atherogenic (atherosclerosis-producing) lipoprotein, and *is the prime target of attempts to lower serum cholesterol.* Clinical trials have shown, for example, that, for every 1% decrease in serum total cholesterol (most of which is found in the LDL particle), CHD risk falls roughly 2%. About 70% to 80% of LDL is removed from the serum by LDL receptors located on the plasma membranes of hepatic and peripheral cells. The remaining 20% to 30% is degraded by macrophages.

Most clinical laboratories do not measure LDL-C directly. Instead, they calculate it based on measurements of total cholesterol, HDL-C, and triglyceride. In this procedure, VLDL cholesterol (VLDL-C) is estimated by dividing **triglyceride** by 5. The following equation, known as the Friedewald equation, is recommended by the National Cholesterol Education Program:[4]

$$\text{LDL-C} = \text{TC} - \text{HDL-C} - (\text{TG} \div 5)$$

where TC = total cholesterol and TG = triglyceride. This formula cannot be used when the triglyceride level is $\geqslant$ 400 mg/dL.

HDL is the smallest and densest of the lipoproteins. Secreted by the liver and small intestine in a disc-shaped form, HDL eventually assumes a spherical shape as it takes up phospholipids and cholesterol from other lipoproteins and body cells. There is an *inverse* relationship between risk of CHD and serum HDL-cholesterol (the cholesterol carried by the HDL particle, referred to as HDL-C). Compared to those with a lower level of serum HDL-C, those with a higher serum HDL-C level are at a lower risk of CHD.[4,7,9] Data from several studies have shown that a 1% greater serum HDL-C translates into a 1.5% to 2% reduction in CHD risk. However, what is uncertain is whether higher serum levels of HDL-C *cause* this reduction or are merely *associated* with this reduction. Recent research suggests that the relationship between higher serum levels of HDL-C and lower CHD risk may only be an association and that perhaps a higher serum level of HDL-C is a marker for other factors that reduce CHD risk, such as having a healthier body weight, being more physically active, being a nonsmoker, and not being insulin resistant.[9]

In recent years there has been growing interest in several emerging substances found in the plasma that have potential value in predicting the risk of CHD or in guiding treatment of established CHD. Known as plasma-based markers or biomarkers, they include high-sensitivity C-reactive protein, homocysteine, and lipoprotein(a).[10,11] Interest in biomarkers is driven by the fact that more than half of all instances of CHD occur in persons who do not have overt hyperlipidemia and that measurement of certain biomarkers may improve the ability of clinicians to identify persons at high risk of CHD. High-sensitivity C-reactive protein (hs-CRP) is a marker of inflammation, which is an important process in the development of atherosclerosis and in thrombosis, the formation of blood clots.[10,11] Numerous prospective studies have shown that elevated hs-CRP is an independent predictor of risk of myocardial infarction, stroke, peripheral vascular disease, and sudden cardiac death, even in apparently healthy individuals.[10,11] The American Heart Association and the Centers for Disease Control and Prevention suggest that clinicians consider evaluating CRP levels in patients who are at intermediate risk of CHD.[12] A plasma level of hs-CRP < 1.0 mg/L is associated with a low risk of CHD, whereas levels 1.0 to 3.0 mg/L and > 3.0 mg/L are associated with moderate and higher CHD risk, respectively.[13] Currently, no evidence shows that lowering plasma hs-CRP reduces risk of CHD, although weight loss, physical activity, smoking cessation, and lipid-lowering drugs all reduce plasma hs-CRP levels.[10]

Elevated plasma levels of the amino acid homocysteine are associated with platelet aggregation, dysfunction of the endothelial cells lining the blood vessels, inflammation, and accelerated oxidation of LDL-C, all of which have the potential to increase risk of CHD.[10,11] Measurement of plasma homocysteine is not recommended for the general adult population, but may be considered in persons with CHD having few of the traditional risk factors shown in Box 8.2 and for patients with renal failure.[10] Mild elevations of homocysteine are common among people with a low dietary intake of folic acid and vitamin B_{12}. Folic acid supplementation has been shown to reduce plasma homocysteine by approximately 25%, and vitamin B_{12} supplementation can result in a further reduction of about 7%. No evidence shows that lowering plasma homocysteine levels reduces CHD risk, although several ongoing clinical trials are evaluating the efficacy of folic acid supplementation for the primary and secondary prevention of CHD.[10,11]

Another biomarker of interest is lipoprotein(a) [Lp(a)] or "lipoprotein small a." Lp(a) is a low-density lipoprotein-like particle that shares many characteristics with plasminogen.[10,11] Research shows that elevated plasma Lp(a) is associated with increased risk of myocardial infarction and angina pectoris, particularly in men who also had elevated plasma LDL-C.[11] However, no evidence shows that lowering Lp(a) reduces CHD risk.[10,11] Simple and accurate methods for measuring Lp(a) have yet to be developed, and its potential use as a marker of increased risk for CHD is still in the research stage.[10] In addition, there is no effective therapy for lowering elevated Lp(a) levels, with the exception of very high doses of niacin, which is not well tolerated by most patients.[11]

Lipoproteins, Cholesterol, and Coronary Heart Disease

The relationship between serum total cholesterol and CHD mortality is shown in Figure 8.2.[4] It can be noted that CHD risk steadily increases as serum cholesterol rises. The increase in CHD risk is particularly steep after serum cholesterol rises above 200 mg/dL (5.17 mmol/L). For example, men whose cholesterol levels are at or above the 90th percentile have four times the risk of CHD

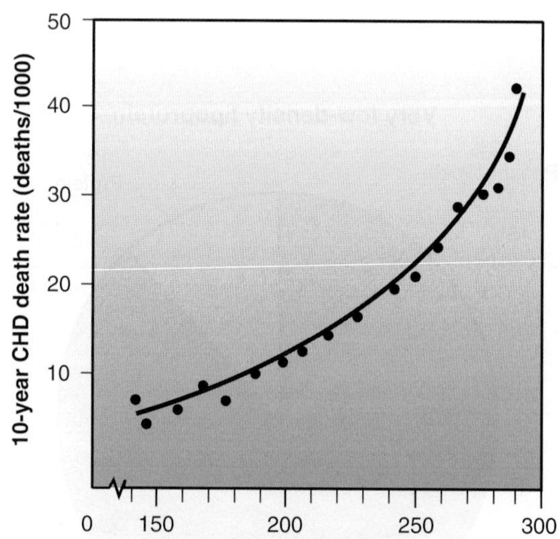

Figure 8.2 **The relationship between serum total cholesterol and coronary heart disease (CHD) mortality in men.**

Source: From National Cholesterol Education Program. 1993. *Second report of the expert panel on detection, evaluation, and treatment of high blood cholesterol in adults.* Bethesda, MD: U.S. Department of Health and Human Services, Public Health Service; National Institutes of Health; National Heart, Lung, and Blood Institute.

compared with men whose cholesterol levels are at or below the 10th percentile.[4]

Guidelines developed by the National Cholesterol Education Program (NCEP) for classifying total cholesterol and HDL-C levels in adults are shown in Table 8.1. The cutoff point that defines "high blood cholesterol" (total cholesterol of 240 mg/dL) is the value above which risk of CHD rises steeply and corresponds to approximately the 80th percentile for the adult U.S. population based on data from the third National Health and Nutrition Examination Survey (NHANES III). Reference values for serum levels of total cholesterol, LDL cholesterol, and HDL cholesterol and the ratio of total cholesterol to HDL cholesterol (TC/HDL-C) are given in Appendix R. As explained in Box 8.3, to change a cholesterol value from mg/dL to mmol/L, simply multiply the value in mg/dL by 0.0259. This operation is appropriate for total cholesterol, HDL cholesterol, and LDL cholesterol.

The atherosclerotic process begins in childhood and progresses slowly into adulthood.[4,14] There is also evidence that children and adolescents with elevated serum cholesterol frequently come from families whose adult members have a high incidence of CHD or elevated serum cholesterol levels.[14] For these reasons, the NCEP has established guidelines for classifying total cholesterol and LDL-C levels in children and adolescents from families with elevated serum cholesterol levels or premature CHD. These are shown in Table 8.2. The average total cholesterol and LDL-C levels in persons ages 1 to 19 years are approximately 160 mg/dL (4.14 mmol/L) and 100 mg/dL (2.59 mmol/L), respectively. The cutoff points for the "borderline" (170 mg/dL) and "high" (200 mg/dL) values in this age group correspond to the 75th and 95th percentiles, respectively.

TABLE 8.1 Classification of LDL, Total, and HDL Cholesterol*

	mg/dL	mmol/L
LDL Cholesterol		
Optimal	< 100	< 2.59
Near optimal/above optimal	100–129	2.59–3.35
Borderline high	130–159	3.36–4.13
High	160–189	4.14–4.90
Very high	≥ 190	≥ 4.91
Total Cholesterol		
Desirable	< 200	< 5.17
Borderline high	200–239	5.17–6.19
High	≥ 240	≥ 6.20
HDL Cholesterol		
Low (undesirable)	< 40	< 1.03
High (desirable)	≥ 60	≥ 1.55

From National Cholesterol Education Program. 2001. *Third report of the expert panel on detection, evaluation, and treatment of high blood cholesterol in adults.* Bethesda, MD: U.S. Department of Health and Human Services, Public Health Service; National Institutes of Health; National Heart, Lung, and Blood Institute.

*LDL = low-density lipoprotein; HDL = high-density lipoprotein.

Cholesterol in mg/dL × 0.0259 = cholesterol in mmol/L.

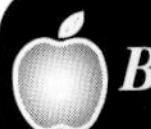

Box 8.3 Using the SI Units

The International System of Units (abbreviated SI from the French *Le Système International d'Unités*) is the world's most widely used system of measurement, both for everyday commerce and for science. It was established in 1960 as an updated, modern form of the older metric system, and is periodically modified and updated through international agreement as the technology of measurement progresses, and as the precision of measurements improves. The SI units are nearly universally employed with the notable exception of the United States, which continues to use customary units in addition to SI.

Throughout Chapter 8, both conventional units and SI units are used to express the amounts of such laboratory components as serum lipids and lipoproteins, and plasma glucose. Below is a list of these components, the abbreviations of the conventional and SI units, and a factor for converting the values from the conventional unit to the SI unit. To convert values from conventional units to SI units, multiply the value in conventional units by the conversion factor. To convert values from SI units to conventional units, divide the SI value by the conversion factor.

Component	Conventional Unit	Conversion Factor	SI Unit
Cholesterol	mg/dL	0.0259	mmol/L
Glucose	mg/dL	0.0555	mmol/L
High-density-lipoprotein cholesterol	mg/dL	0.0259	mmol/L
Low-density-lipoprotein cholesterol	mg/dL	0.0259	mmol/L
Triglyceride	mg/dL	0.0113	mmol/L

Source: National Institute of Standards and Technology. 2008. *Guide for the use of the International System of Units (SI).* NIST Special Publication 811. Gaithersburg, MD: National Institute of Standards and Technology.

TABLE 8.2 The National Cholesterol Education Program's Classification of Total Cholesterol and LDL-C Levels in Children and Adolescents from Families with Hypercholesterolemia or Premature Coronary Heart Disease

	Total Cholesterol		Low-Density-Lipoprotein Cholesterol	
	mg/dL	mmol/L	mg/dL	mmol/L
Acceptable	< 170	< 4.40	< 110	< 2.84
Borderline high	170–199	4.40–5.16	110–129	2.84–3.35
High	≥ 200	≥ 5.17	≥ 130	≥ 3.36

From National Cholesterol Education Program. 1991. *Report of the expert panel on blood cholesterol levels in children and adolescents.* Bethesda, MD: U.S. Department of Health and Human Services, Public Health Service; National Institutes of Health; National Heart, Lung, and Blood Institute.

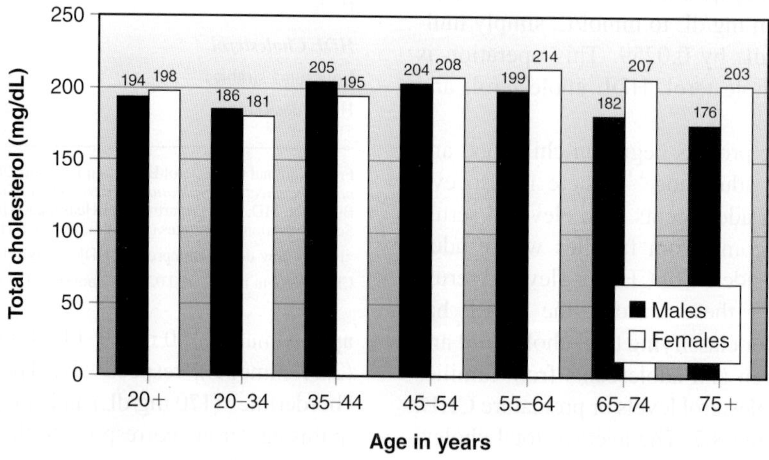

Figure 8.3 Mean total cholesterol levels of adult Americans, 2007–2010. Throughout adulthood, the mean serum total cholesterol levels of Americans change. Beginning at about age 35 years in males and 45 years in females, they rise above the levels recommended by the National Cholesterol Education Program. In the later decades of life, they tend to decline especially for males.
Source: Data from the National Center for Health Statistics.

How do mean (average) cholesterol levels for adult Americans compare with these standards? According to data from NHANES, shown in Figure 8.3, the mean total cholesterol levels for U.S. males and females 20 years of age and older are 194 mg/dL and 198 mg/dL, respectively. Mean total cholesterol levels for males ages 20 to 34 years and for females ages 20 to 44 years are within the range considered "desirable" by the NCEP. Beginning at about age 35 years in males and 45 years in females, they rise above the levels recommended by the National Cholesterol Education Program. In the later decades of life, they tend to decline, especially for males.

In contrast to total cholesterol and LDL-C levels, higher serum levels of HDL-C are associated with a lower risk of CHD. According to data from the Framingham Heart Study, in the presence of high serum HDL-C levels, the risk of CHD is relatively low, even in subjects with increased serum total cholesterol or LDL-C. In contrast, persons with low HDL-C levels are at increased CHD risk, even if their total cholesterol and LDL-C levels are within the "desirable" range. Exactly why greater levels of serum HDL-C are associated with a reduction in CHD risk remains unclear.[9]

According to the NCEP, an HDL-C level below 40 mg/dL (1.03 mmol/L) is defined as a "low" serum level and is considered a major risk factor. An HDL-C level ≥ 60 mg/dL (≥ 1.55 mmol/L) is considered a "negative risk factor," which decreases CHD risk.[4]

Lipoprotein Ratios

Another approach to evaluating HDL-C levels that is suggested by some investigators is to calculate the ratio of two lipid values—for example, the LDL-C/HDL-C ratio (LDL-C level divided by HDL-C level) and the TC/HDL-C ratio (total cholesterol level divided by HDL-C level).[15–17] Data from the Framingham Heart Study show that, the higher a person's TC/HDL-C ratio, the greater is his or her risk of having symptomatic CHD. In other words, as total cholesterol increases in proportion to HDL-C, CHD risk increases as well. According to Framingham data, 50- to 70-year-old men having a TC/HDL-C ratio of 4.4 have an average risk for CHD, compared with men their age. This cutoff point roughly corresponds to a total cholesterol of 200 mg/dL (5.17 mmol/L) and an HDL-C of 45 mg/dL (1.16 mmol/L). Those having a TC/HDL-C ratio of 3.0 have half the risk, and those with a ratio of 6.2, 7.7, or 9.5 have two, three, or four times the average risk, respectively.[16] Although not a substitute for measurements of individual lipid and lipoprotein levels, the TC/HDL-C ratio appears, in many instances, to be a valuable adjunct to evaluating CHD risk.[15–17]

Figure 8.4 illustrates the relationship between the total cholesterol/HDL-C ratio and risk of myocardial infarction. The figure is based on data collected by Harvard University researchers as part of the Health Professionals Follow-Up Study.[18] The researchers considered a ratio of less than 3.0 to be optimal. As a subject's ratio increased above 3.0, relative risk of myocardial infarction increased. The average American male has a ratio of 4.6, while the average American female's ratio is 4.0.

Triglyceride and Coronary Heart Disease

The connection between serum triglyceride levels and CHD risk is controversial.[4,19,20] Most population studies show serum plasma triglyceride levels to be positively associated with increased CHD risk. However, in most of these studies, triglyceride was not shown to act independently to increase CHD risk after statistical adjustments were made for closely associated factors, such as total cholesterol, HDL-C, high blood pressure, cigarette smoking, and obesity.[19] Some researchers argue that elevated triglyceride levels reflect certain lipoprotein alterations (elevated VLDL-C and LDL-C and decreased HDL-C) or accompany other disease states known to increase CHD risk, such as diabetes mellitus, nephrotic syndrome, and chronic renal disease.[4,19,20] More recent meta-analyses of prospective studies, however, suggest that elevated serum triglyceride is an independent risk factor for CHD, particularly in persons with low HDL-C.[19,20] Consequently, the NCEP, in its *Adult Treatment Panel III,* now recognizes elevated triglyceride as an independent risk factor for CHD and has identified VLDL cholesterol as a target for cholesterol-lowering therapy. Table 8.3 provides NCEP guidelines for classifying serum triglyceride. To change a triglyceride value from mg/dL to mmol/L, simply multiply the triglyceride value in mg/dL by 0.0113.

TABLE 8.3 Classification of Serum Triglyceride

	mg/dL	mmol/L
Normal	< 150	< 1.69
Borderline high	150–199	1.69–2.25
High	200–499	2.26–5.64
Very high	≥ 500	≥ 5.65

From National Cholesterol Education Program. 2001. *Third report of the expert panel on detection, evaluation, and treatment of high blood cholesterol in adults.* Bethesda, MD: U.S. Department of Health and Human Services, Public Health Service; National Institutes of Health; National Heart, Lung, and Blood Institute.

Triglyceride in mg/dL × 0.0113 = triglyceride in mmol/L.

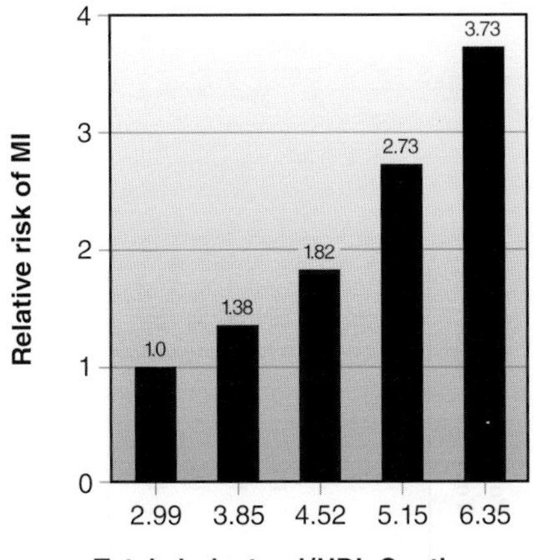

Figure 8.4 Total cholesterol/HDL-C ratio and risk for myocardial infarction.

As the total cholesterol/HDL cholesterol ratio increases, the risk of myocardial infarction (MI) increases.

Source: Data from Stampfer MJ, Sacks FM, Salvini S, Willett WC, Hennekens CH. 1991. A prospective study of cholesterol, apolipoproteins, and the risk of myocardial infarction. *New England Journal of Medicine* 325:373–381.

Estimating CHD Risk

The National Cholesterol Education Program has developed charts for estimating the actual likelihood (or "absolute risk") that one will develop CHD within the next 10 years.[4,21] Table 8.4 shows the chart for adult males, and Table 8.5 shows the chart for adult females. The charts are based on data collected from the Framingham Study and use the following variables: age, total serum cholesterol, serum HDL cholesterol, systolic blood pressure, whether one is being treated for hypertension, and cigarette smoking. Total and HDL cholesterol measurements should be the average of at least two measurements obtained from lipoprotein analysis. Although the charts use total and HDL cholesterol as variables, LDL cholesterol remains the primary target of cholesterol-lowering therapy. Systolic blood pressure should be based on the average of several blood pressure measurements. Note that the number of points assigned for systolic blood pressure depends on whether one is taking medication to treat hypertension ("treated") or not receiving any antihypertensive treatment ("untreated"). The term *smoker* applies to any cigarette smoking in the past month.

TABLE 8.4 Estimating Risk of CHD in the Next 10 Years, Men

Ages	Points
20–34	−9
35–39	−4
40–44	0
45–49	3
50–54	6
55–59	8
60–64	10
65–69	11
70–74	12
75–79	13

Total Cholesterol*	Points at Ages 20–39	Points at Ages 40–49	Points at Ages 50–59	Points at Ages 60–69	Points at Ages 70–79
< 160	0	0	0	0	0
160–199	4	3	2	1	0
200–239	7	5	3	1	0
240–279	9	6	4	2	1
≥ 280	11	8	5	3	1

HDL*	Points
≥ 60	−1
50–59	0
40–49	1
< 40	2

	Points at Ages 20–39	Points at Ages 40–49	Points at Ages 50–59	Points at Ages 60–69	Points at Ages 70–79
Nonsmoker	0	0	0	0	0
Smoker	8	5	3	1	1

Systolic BP[†]	Untreated	Treated
< 120	0	0
120–129	0	1
130–139	1	2
140–159	1	2
≥ 160	2	3

Point Total	10-Year Risk (%)	Point Total	10-Year Risk (%)
< 0	< 1	11	8
0–4	1	12	10
5–6	2	13	12
7	3	14	16
8	4	15	20
9	5	16	25
10	6	≥ 17	≥ 30

How to Use This Risk-Prediction Chart

1. Determine the points for each variable and then total the points in the spaces below:

____ Age + ____ Total Cholesterol + ____ HDL + ____ Smoking + ____ Systolic BP = ____ Point Total

2. Compare point total with the chart to the left to determine one's risk of developing CHD in the next 10 years.

Adapted from National Cholesterol Education Program. 2001. *Third report of the expert panel on detection, evaluation, and treatment of high blood cholesterol in adults.* Bethesda, MD: U.S. Department of Health and Human Services, Public Health Service; National Institutes of Health; National Heart, Lung, and Blood Institute.

*Measured in mg/dL

[†]Measured in mm Hg

TABLE 8.5 Estimating Risk of CHD in the Next 10 Years, Women

Ages	Points
20–34	−7
35–39	−3
40–44	0
45–49	3
50–54	6
55–59	8
60–64	10
65–69	12
70–74	14
75–79	16

Total Cholesterol*	Points at Ages 20–39	Points at Ages 40–49	Points at Ages 50–59	Points at Ages 60–69	Points at Ages 70–79
< 160	0	0	0	0	0
160–199	4	3	2	1	1
200–239	8	6	4	2	1
240–279	11	8	5	3	2
≥ 280	13	10	7	4	2

HDL*	Points
≥ 60	−1
50–59	0
40–49	1
< 40	2

	Points at Ages 20–39	Points at Ages 40–49	Points at Ages 50–59	Points at Ages 60–69	Points at Ages 70–79
Nonsmoker	0	0	0	0	0
Smoker	9	7	4	2	1

Systolic BP[†]	Untreated	Treated
< 120	0	0
120–129	1	3
130–139	2	4
140–159	3	5
≥ 160	4	6

Point Total	10-Year Risk (%)	Point Total	10-Year Risk (%)
< 9	< 1	19	8
9–12	1	20	11
13–14	2	21	14
15	3	22	17
16	4	23	22
17	5	24	27
18	6	≥ 25	≥ 30

How to Use This Risk-Prediction Chart

1. Determine the points for each variable and then total the points in the spaces below:

____		____		____		____		____		____
Age	+	**Total Cholesterol**	+	**HDL**	+	**Smoking**	+	**Systolic BP**	=	**Point Total**

2. Compare point total with the chart to the left to determine one's risk of developing CHD in the next 10 years.

Adapted from National Cholesterol Education Program. 2001. *Third report of the expert panel on detection, evaluation, and treatment of high blood cholesterol in adults.* Bethesda, MD: U.S. Department of Health and Human Services, Public Health Service; National Institutes of Health; National Heart, Lung, and Blood Institute.

*Measured in mg/dL

[†]Measured in mm Hg

To estimate the likelihood that one will develop CHD in the next 10 years, select the appropriate chart (male or female), determine the points for each variable, enter these in the appropriate spaces, and then determine the point total. By comparing the point total with the values in the table at the bottom left corner of each chart, it is possible to determine one's "absolute" 10-year risk for CHD—in other words, the person's actual likelihood of developing coronary heart disease. For example, if one's absolute 10-year risk is ⩾ 20%, then there is a greater than 1 in 5 chance of developing CHD in the next 10 years. The *ATP III* guidelines recommend that this assessment of absolute 10-year risk be used in determining the intensity of therapy for reducing CHD risk for persons with two or more CHD risk factors.[4,21] In persons with 0 to 1 risk factor, short-term and long-term CHD is so low that use of the charts is not considered necessary.

National Cholesterol Education Program's Guidelines

The NCEP was created by the National Heart, Lung, and Blood Institute in November 1985 with the overall goal of reducing the prevalence of high blood cholesterol in the United States. It has issued reports, written by different panels of experts, that address elevated cholesterol levels in several populations.[4,22–24] These reports recommend the *patient-based approach* and/or the *population-based, or public health, approach.* The former establishes guidelines for the identification and treatment by physicians of individuals with elevated cholesterol levels. The latter approach emphasizes dietary and lifestyle changes that can be made by all people to lower average cholesterol levels and modify risk factors in the entire population. The two approaches are complementary, and together they represent a coordinated strategy for reducing coronary risk.

Two somewhat related concepts are primary prevention and secondary prevention. *Primary prevention* involves risk factor reduction (smoking cessation, lowering of elevated total and LDL cholesterol levels, control of high blood pressure, and so on) in patients with no evidence or diagnosis of CHD. *Secondary prevention* involves risk factor reduction in patients who have evidence of CHD and in whom CHD or some other atherosclerotic disease has been diagnosed. The National Cholesterol Education Program considers primary prevention to be the most effective approach for reducing the prevalence of CHD in the United States.[4]

In 1988, the NCEP published the *Report of the Expert Panel on Detection, Evaluation, and Treatment of High Blood Cholesterol in Adults.*[22] This report was revised in 1993, when the NCEP published its *Second Report of the Expert Panel on Detection, Evaluation, and Treatment of High Blood Cholesterol in Adults.*[23] Another revision, the *Third Report of the Expert Panel on Detection, Evaluation, and Treatment of High Blood Cholesterol in Adults* (the *ATP III*), was published in 2001.[4] In 1990, the *Report of the Expert Panel on Population Strategies for Blood Cholesterol Reduction* was published.[24] As the title indicates, this report took a population-based, or public health, approach to the problem of elevated blood cholesterol levels among Americans. The *Report of the Expert Panel on Blood Cholesterol Levels in Children and Adolescents,* published by the NCEP in 1991, made recommendations that were both patient-based and population-based.[14] All of these reports make similar dietary and other lifestyle recommendations.

Assessing Risk for Coronary Heart Disease

The *Third Report of the Expert Panel on Detection, Evaluation, and Treatment of High Blood Cholesterol in Adults* (also known as the *Adult Treatment Panel III* or *ATP III*), identifies risk assessment as the first step to be taken in reducing one's risk for CHD. Risk assessment is the basis for establishing the goal for serum LDL cholesterol and other targets for CHD risk reduction, such as dietary change, blood pressure control, smoking cessation, weight reduction, and increased physical activity. Risk assessment involves three components: (1) a complete lipoprotein profile (measurement of serum total cholesterol, LDL cholesterol, HDL cholesterol, and triglycerides); (2) identification of the presence of clinical CHD as well as what the *ATP III* calls "CHD risk equivalents"; and (3) identification of the major, independent CHD risk factors other than elevated LDL-C (review Box 8.2).

The *ATP III* recommends that all adults ages 20 years or more have a fasting lipoprotein profile performed at least once every 5 years. Because of potential analytical errors, the profile should be done twice within a period of 1 to 8 weeks and the values averaged. If the values for LDL-C from the two profiles differ by more than 30 mg/dL, a third profile should be performed and the three values averaged. Fasting is necessary for the accurate measurement of triglyceride, which is required for the calculation of LDL-C. However, total cholesterol and HDL-C can be accurately measured in the nonfasting state. If the nonfasting total cholesterol is ≥ 200 mg/dL or HDL-C is < 40 mg/dL, then measurement of LDL-C is warranted, and a fasting lipoprotein profile is recommended for proper management of serum lipids and lipoprotein values based on LDL-C. The *ATP III* classifications of total cholesterol, LDL-C, and HDL-C were shown in Table 8.1. Results of the lipoprotein profile must be interpreted with caution in persons recovering from a recent heart attack or unstable angina. When LDL-C is > 100 mg/dL, a clinical evaluation should be done to rule out a genetic disorder or secondary causes.

A prior diagnosis of CHD (the presence of preexisting CHD) markedly increases one's risk of recurrent CHD. The presence of CHD risk equivalents also markedly increases one's risk for coronary heart disease. CHD risk equivalents are conditions or combinations of CHD risk factors that increase the risk of CHD to a level equivalent to that of diagnosed CHD. CHD risk equivalents include clinical forms of atherosclerotic disease other than CHD (e.g., peripheral arterial disease, abdominal aortic aneurysm, and symptomatic carotid artery disease), diabetes, and CHD risk factors that together result in an absolute 10-year CHD risk of greater than 20%.[4] It is important to note that diabetes is considered a CHD risk equivalent due to the markedly elevated risk of CHD in persons with diabetes.

The presence of other CHD risk factors that were shown in Box 8.2 should then be assessed. Persons with two or more of these risk factors should have their absolute 10-year (short-term) CHD risk evaluated, using the charts in Tables 8.4 and 8.5. A 10-year CHD risk greater than 20% is considered a CHD risk equivalent. Those with zero to one CHD risk factor do not need to have their absolute CHD risk assessed because their CHD risk is likely to be so low as to make this additional step unnecessary.

Results of the assessment are then used to determine the goal for serum LDL-C, as shown in Table 8.6. Persons having zero to one of the major, independent risk factors listed in Box 8.2 have an LDL-C goal of < 160 mg/dL. Those with two or more of these risk factors have an LDL-C goal of < 130 mg/dL. Persons at the greatest risk for CHD, those already diagnosed with CHD or having a CHD risk equivalent, have an LDL-C goal of < 100 mg/dL.

Besides the major, independent risk factors listed in Box 8.2, the *ATP III* recognizes two additional categories of factors that potentially increase one's risk for CHD: life-habit risk factors and emerging risk factors.[4] The life-habit risk factors include obesity, physical inactivity, and an atherogenic diet. Although the LDL-C goals shown in Table 8.6 are not necessarily lowered when a person is found to have one or more of these life-habit risk factors, they are regarded as "direct targets for clinical intervention." The emerging risk factors include elevated serum levels of lipoprotein(a), homocysteine, and C-reactive protein and the presence of other factors that increase the formation of blood clots (prothrombotic factors) or that may inflame the arterial wall (proinflammatory factors). The emerging risk factors do not categorically alter the LDL-C treatment goals but may be considered when determining the intensity of risk reduction therapy.[4]

Many persons at higher risk for CHD likely have various combinations of major risk factors, life-habit risk factors, and emerging risk factors, which together constitute what is known as the "metabolic syndrome." The metabolic syndrome is characterized by abdominal obesity (discussed in Chapter 6), atherogenic dyslipidemia (elevated triglyceride, small LDL particles, low HDL-C), elevated blood pressure, insulin resistance (with or without glucose intolerance), and prothrombotic and proinflammatory factors. The *ATP III* considers the metabolic syndrome to be a "secondary target" of risk reduction therapy after serum LDL-C, the primary risk reduction target. Table 8.7 lists the clinical determinants of the metabolic syndrome as identified by the *ATP III*. A diagnosis of metabolic syndrome can be made when three or more of these risk factors are present.[4]

Therapeutic Lifestyle Changes

The term *therapeutic lifestyle changes* is used by the *ATP III* to identify multifaceted lifestyle approaches to reduce risk for CHD. Included among the therapeutic lifestyle changes (TLC) are various dietary recommendations, as shown in

TABLE 8.6 Three Categories of Risk that Modify LDL Cholesterol Goals

Risk Category	LDL Goal (mg/dL)
Zero to one risk factor	< 160
Multiple (two or more) risk factors*	< 130
Presence of CHD or CHD risk equivalents	< 100

Adapted from National Cholesterol Education Program. 2001. *Third report of the expert panel on detection, evaluation, and treatment of high blood cholesterol in adults*. Bethesda, MD: U.S. Department of Health and Human Services, Public Health Service; National Institutes of Health; National Heart, Lung, and Blood Institute.

*Risk factors that modify the LDL goal were shown in Box 8.2.

TABLE 8.7 Clinical Determinants of the Metabolic Syndrome

Risk Factor	Defining Level
Abdominal obesity*	Waist circumference:† males > 40 in females > 35 in
Triglycerides	≥ 150 mg/dL
HDL cholesterol	Males < 40 mg/dL Females < 50 mg/dL
Blood pressure	Systolic ≥ 130 mm Hg Diastolic ≥ 85 mm Hg
Fasting plasma glucose	≥ 110 mg/dL

Adapted from National Cholesterol Education Program. 2001. *Third report of the expert panel on detection, evaluation, and treatment of high blood cholesterol in adults*. Bethesda, MD: U.S. Department of Health and Human Services, Public Health Service; National Institutes of Health; National Heart, Lung, and Blood Institute.

*Overweight and obesity are associated with insulin resistance and the metabolic syndrome. However, the presence of abdominal obesity is more highly correlated with risk for the metabolic syndrome than is an elevated body mass index (BMI). Therefore, the simple measure of waist circumference is recommended to identify the presence of abdominal obesity.

†Some male patients can develop multiple metabolic risk factors when the waist circumference is only marginally increased (e.g., 37–39 in. or 94–102 cm). Such patients may have a strong genetic contribution to insulin resistance. They should benefit from changes in life habits, similarly to men with categorical increases in waist circumference.

TABLE 8.8 Nutrient Composition of the Therapeutic Lifestyle Change Diet

Nutrient	Recommended Intake
Saturated fat*	Less than 7% of total calories
Polyunsaturated fat	Up to 10% of total calories
Monounsaturated fat	Up to 20% of total calories
Total fat	25% to 35% of total calories
Carbohydrate†	50% to 60% of total calories
Fiber	20 to 30 g/d
Protein	Approximately 15% of total calories
Cholesterol	Less than 200 mg/day
Total calories (energy)‡	Balance energy intake and expenditure to maintain healthy body weight or to prevent weight gain.

From National Cholesterol Education Program. 2001. *Third report of the expert panel on detection, evaluation, and treatment of high blood cholesterol in adults.* Bethesda, MD: U.S. Department of Health and Human Services, Public Health Service; National Institutes of Health; National Heart, Lung, and Blood Institute.

**Trans* fatty acids are another LDL-raising fat that should be kept at a low intake.

†Carbohydrate should be derived predominantly from foods rich in complex carbohydrates, including grains, especially whole grains, fruits, and vegetables.

‡Daily energy expenditure should include at least moderate physical activity (contributing approximately 200 kcal per day).

Table 8.8, increased consumption of plant stanols/sterols (2 g/d) and viscous (soluble) dietary fiber (10–25g/d), weight reduction when indicated, and increased physical activity. The TLC dietary recommendations shown in Table 8.8 are, for the most part, consistent with the *Dietary Guidelines for Americans* (discussed in Chapter 2). The *Dietary Guidelines for Americans* recommend that most persons ages 2 years and older limit their intake of saturated fat to no more than about 10% of calories. Because the TLC diet is targeted to persons with increased risk of CHD, especially elevated LDL-C, it makes the more conservative recommendation of no more than 7% of calories from saturated fat and that intake of *trans* fatty acids should be kept low. This reflects the fact that saturated fat and *trans* fatty acids are the most important determinants of serum total and LDL cholesterol levels. The second most important factor influencing serum total and LDL cholesterol levels is dietary cholesterol. The *Dietary Guidelines for Americans* recommend < 300 mg/d, compared with the TLC's recommendation of < 200 mg/d. In contrast to previous recommendations to limit fat intake to < 30% of energy, both the *Dietary Guidelines for Americans* and the TLC diet now recommend that up to 35% of total calories come from fat but that a majority of energy from fat come from oils that are monounsaturated. This modest increase in the proportion of energy from fat (primarily from monounsaturated fats) with a commensurate decrease in energy from carbohydrate may help reduce elevated triglycerides in some persons. Despite this more liberal fat recommendation, total energy intake should be balanced with energy expenditure to maintain a healthy weight or to prevent unhealthful weight gain.

Once CHD risk has been assessed and found to be elevated, application of lifestyle therapy should begin. A model of steps to follow in applying the various therapeutic lifestyle changes is shown in Figure 8.5. At the first visit with the health care provider following risk assessment,

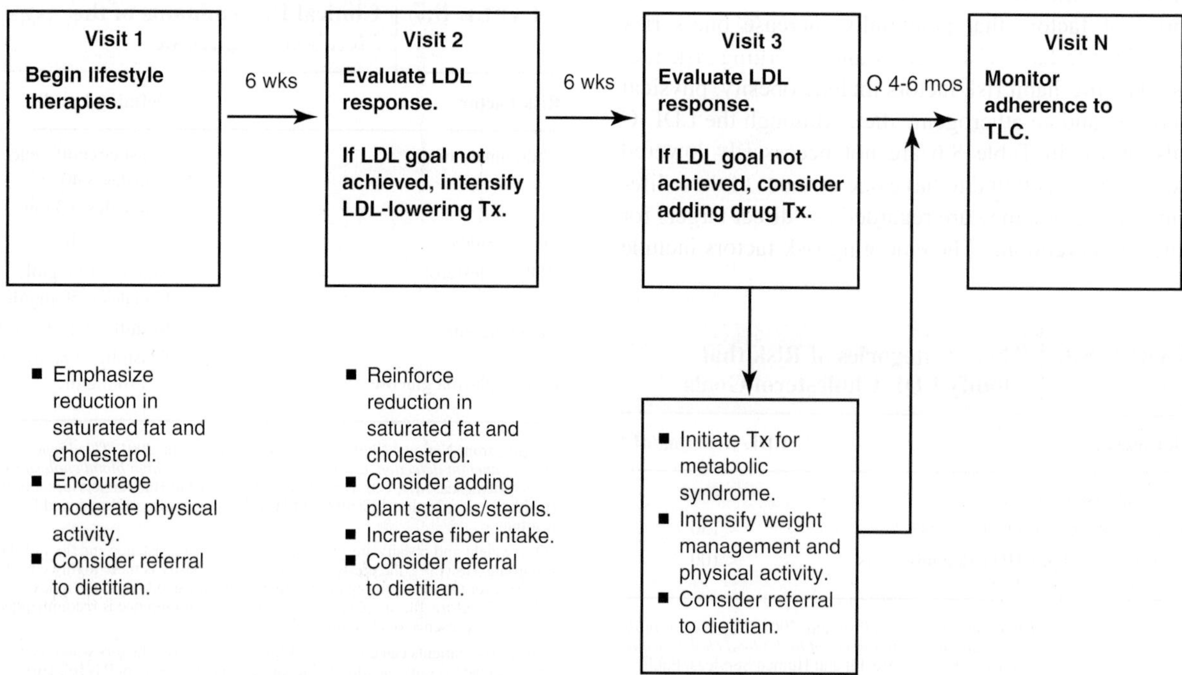

Figure 8.5 A model for applying therapeutic lifestyle changes.

Source: From National Cholesterol Education Program. 2001. *Third report of the expert panel on detection, evaluation, and treatment of high blood cholesterol in adults.* Bethesda, MD: U.S. Department of Health and Human Services, Public Health Service; National Institutes of Health; National Heart, Lung, and Blood Institute.

the therapeutic lifestyle changes are initiated, with an emphasis on reducing intake of saturated fat and dietary cholesterol to levels indicated in Table 8.8. Referral to a registered dietitian competent in medical nutrition therapy of CHD and related risk factors should be considered. Physical activity level should be assessed, and, if necessary, moderate physical activity should be encouraged. After 6 weeks, the lipoprotein profile should be repeated to evaluate any changes in serum LDL-C in response to therapeutic lifestyle changes. If the LDL-C goal is not achieved at this point, application of the therapeutic lifestyle changes should be intensified, reduction of saturated fat and dietary cholesterol intake should be reinforced (preferably with the help of a dietitian), and consideration should be given to other options for further lowering LDL-C, such as increasing intake of viscous (soluble) dietary fibers and including plant stanols/sterols in the diet.

Another 6 weeks are given for determining the maximum effect of dietary therapy on reducing LDL-C. If dietary therapies alone are not effective at achieving the LDL-C goal, increased attention should be given to managing body weight, maintaining adequate physical activity, and, if necessary, addressing any of the clinical determinants of the metabolic syndrome (shown in Table 8.7). Administration of cholesterol-lowering drugs should also be considered at this point. However, in the presence of markedly increased levels of LDL-C and multiple CHD risk factors or CHD equivalents, it may be necessary to begin drug treatment simultaneously with therapeutic lifestyle changes. Table 8.9 outlines the LDL-C goals and cutpoints at which therapeutic lifestyle changes and drug therapy are initiated. For example, consider a person previously diagnosed with CHD or who had CHD risk equivalents and an LDL-C level of greater than 130 mg/dL. Therapeutic lifestyle changes and cholesterol-lowering drug therapy would begin simultaneously. If this person had an LDL-C level between 100 and 129 mg/dL, cholesterol lowering drug therapy would be considered optional.

Therapeutic lifestyle change is considered the cornerstone of therapy to reduce blood cholesterol levels. The general aim of dietary therapy is to reduce serum total and LDL cholesterol while providing a nutritionally adequate diet. The rationale for the TLC dietary recommendations given in Table 8.8 is thoroughly discussed in the *ATP III* report and in the American Heart Association's dietary guidelines, and they are briefly reviewed later in this chapter in Dietary Treatment in Coronary Heart Disease.[25] It is important to assess the patient's current eating habits before initiating medical nutrition therapy for CHD risk reduction. This can be done using the MEDFICTS dietary assessment questionnaire, discussed in Chapter 3 and shown in Appendix F. With adequate training, physicians or members of their staffs can assist patients in nutritional education and behavioral change. However, some patients may need counseling from a registered dietitian from the outset. It should be emphasized to patients that the goal is not a temporary "diet" but, rather, a permanent change in eating behavior.[4]

Inadequate lowering of cholesterol levels can result from several factors.[4] Inherited metabolic disorders of lipid metabolism (for example, absent or dysfunctional LDL receptors or hepatic lipoprotein overproduction) can result in severe elevations of serum cholesterol that are resistant to lowering, no matter how strict the diet. Some patients are biologically resistant to LDL lowering by dietary modification and will not achieve the cholesterol-lowering goal despite good adherence to diet.

Some patients refuse to change their eating habits despite the intensive efforts of the physician and counselors. However, a concerted effort by health professionals to promote behavioral change should minimize the size of this patient group. It may take up to a year, or

TABLE 8.9 LDL-C Goals and Cutpoints for Therapeutic Lifestyle Changes and Drug Therapy in Different Risk Categories

Risk Category	LDL Goal	LDL Level at Which to Initiate Therapeutic Lifestyle Changes (TLC)	LDL Level at Which to Consider Drug Therapy
CHD or CHD risk equivalents 10-year risk < 20%	< 100 mg/dL	≥ 100 mg/dL	≥ 130 mg/dL (100–129 mg/dL: drug optional)*
Two or more risk factors 10-year risk 10–20%	< 130 mg/dL	≥ 130 mg/dL	≥ 130 mg/dL
Two or more risk factors 10-year risk < 10%	< 130 mg/dL	≥ 130 mg/dL	≥ 160 mg/dL
Zero to one risk factor†	< 160 mg/dL	≥ 160 mg/dL	≥ 190 mg/dL (160–189 mg/dL: drug optional)

From National Cholesterol Education Program. 2001. *Third report of the expert panel on detection, evaluation, and treatment of high blood cholesterol in adults.* Bethesda, MD: U.S. Department of Health and Human Services, Public Health Service; National Institutes of Health; National Heart, Lung, and Blood Institute.

*Some authorities recommend use of LDL-lowering drugs in this category if an LDL cholesterol < 100 mg/dL cannot be achieved by therapeutic lifestyle changes. Others prefer use of drugs that primarily modify triglycerides and HDL, such as nicotinic acid or fibrate. Clinical judgment also may call for deferring drug therapy in this subcategory.

†Almost all people with zero to one risk factor have a 10-year risk < 10%; thus, 10-year risk assessment in people with zero to one risk factor is not necessary.

even longer, for some patients to adopt the recommended dietary changes. Thus, adequate time should be allowed for patients to attempt to modify their diets to achieve the desired therapeutic goals.[4]

Lowering Cholesterol in the Population

In the *Report of the Expert Panel on Population Strategies for Blood Cholesterol Reduction,* similar CHD risk factors are identified as in the *ATP III* report and similar total cholesterol and LDL-C cutoff points are used in classifying persons.[24] The Expert Panel has recommended that all healthy Americans about age 2 years and older adopt a diet similar to the one outlined in Table 8.8. The rationale for this diet is outlined in the section "Dietary Treatment in Coronary Heart Disease."

Will population strategies be successful in lowering the average serum cholesterol levels of Americans? Even before government agencies made a concerted effort to promote a heart-healthy diet, the average cholesterol level of Americans was declining, as shown in Figure 8.6. A comparison of data from the first National Health Examination Survey (1960–1962) with data collected from NHANES 2007–2010 shows that mean serum total cholesterol levels of U.S. adult males and females have declined 26 mg/dL, or approximately 12%. This fact, along with a decrease in cigarette smoking and a possible increase in leisure-time physical activity, have no doubt contributed to the nearly 70% decline in heart disease mortality between 1950 and 2010, as shown in Figure 8.7. During the same period, there was a nearly 80% reduction in age-adjusted stroke mortality, as shown in Figure 8.8. Despite these reductions,

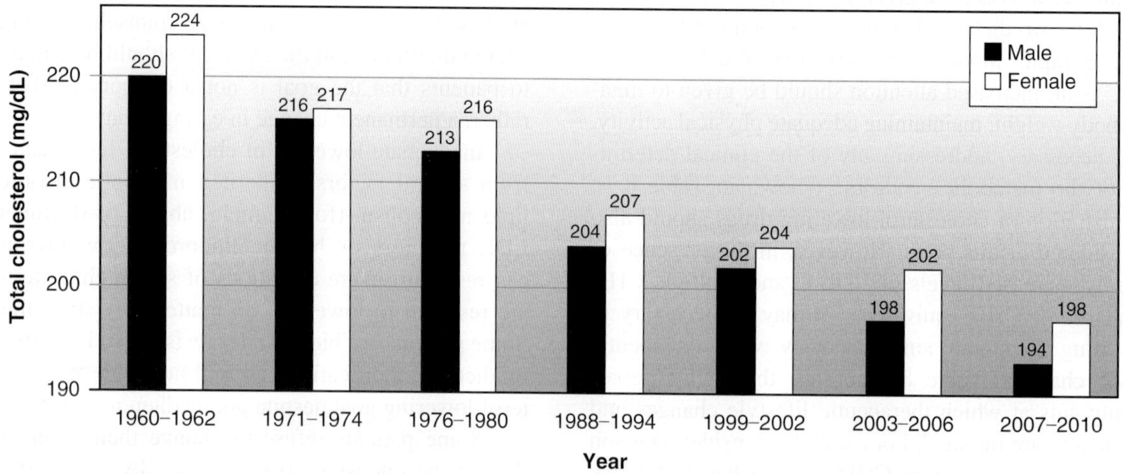

Figure 8.6 Mean total serum cholesterol in U.S. adults, 1960–2010.
Since the early 1960s, the mean serum cholesterol levels of U.S. adults have declined 26 mg/dL, or approximately 12%.
Source: Data from the National Center for Health Statistics.

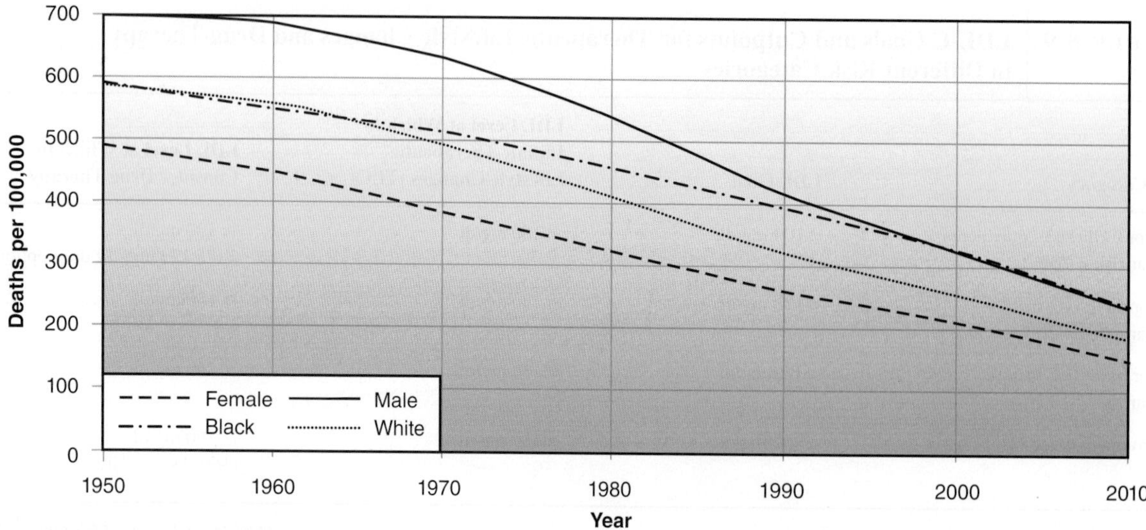

Figure 8.7 Age-adjusted death rate (per 100,000 resident population) for diseases of the heart by sex and race, United States, 1950–2010.
Source: Data from the National Center for Health Statistics.

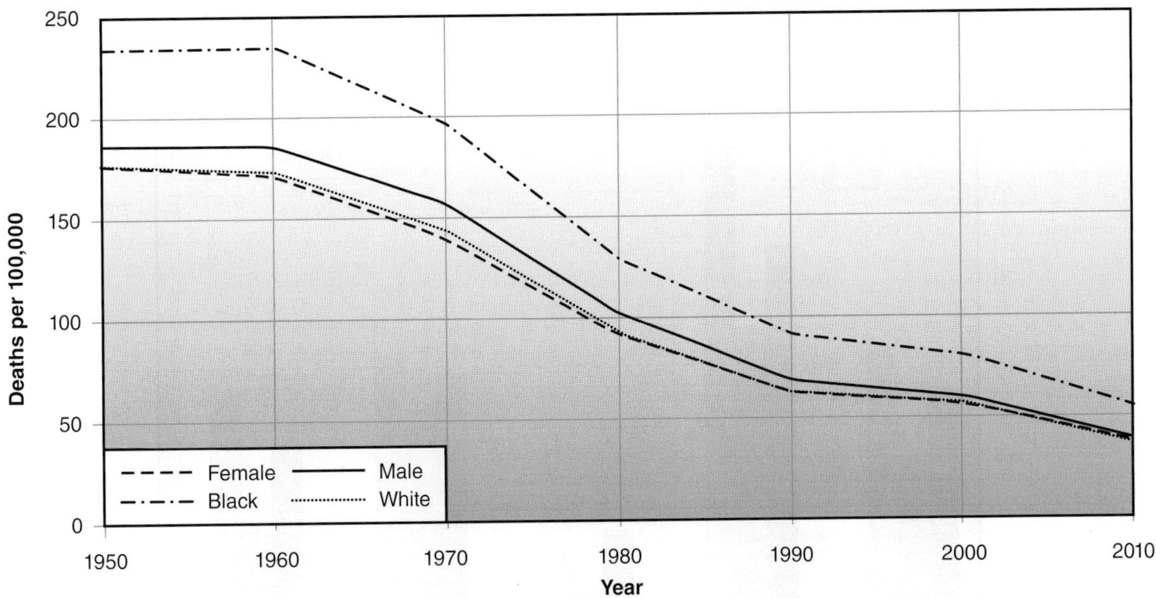

Figure 8.8 Age-adjusted death rate (per 100,000 resident population) for stroke by sex and race, United States, 1950–2010.

Source: Data from the National Center for Health Statistics.

heart disease mortality is 50% greater for blacks than it is for whites. Stroke mortality is nearly twice as high for blacks as for whites.

Not only is there good evidence that lowering serum cholesterol levels reduces CHD risk, but several studies have shown that cholesterol lowering can slow the progression of and even reverse atherosclerotic narrowing.[26–32] According to the NCEP, "the conclusion now seems inescapable that definite regression can be expected in 16% to 47% of patients, provided that large decreases in LDL-cholesterol (of the order of 34% to 48%) are induced for a period of 2 to 5 years."[14]

Cardiovascular Disease in Youth

Although symptomatic or clinically manifest cardiovascular disease (CVD) is rare in children and adolescents, there is strong evidence that risk factors and risk behaviors adopted in childhood initiate and accelerate the development of CVD, which is then manifest during adulthood. There is also increasing evidence that risk reduction in childhood and adolescence delays the progression of CVD. For example, there are good data indicating that atherosclerosis was present in the coronary arteries of U.S. soldiers killed in the Korean and Vietnam wars.[33,34] In these studies, postmortem examination of the coronary arteries revealed lesions and narrowing consistent with coronary heart disease in 77% of the soldiers, whose average age was 22 years. Data from a number of researchers studying the development and progression of coronary artery lesions in infants and children support the view that atherosclerosis begins in childhood and progresses slowly into adulthood.[35–38]

Evidence from two ongoing, prospective cohort studies, the Pathobiological Determinants of Atherosclerosis in Youth (PDAY) study and the Bogalusa Heart Study, indicate that the presence and severity of atherosclerotic lesions in the coronary arteries of adolescents and young adults as determined by postmortem examination are associated with smoking, high serum total cholesterol, LDL-C and VLDL-C levels, low HDL-C levels, and diabetes. Both studies show that the presence and intensity of these CHD risk factors in children and young adults are associated with the extent and severity of atherosclerotic lesions as determined by autopsy of subjects who died from unintentional causes.[39–45]

Recent technological advances in computed tomography imaging and ultrasonography now allow clinicians to noninvasively assess subclinical atherosclerosis in children and adolescents without having to resort to postmortem analysis.[35] These noninvasive techniques reveal that evidence of subclinical atherosclerosis is more likely seen in children with obesity, hypertension, type 1 diabetes, and marked elevations in LDL-C, and in children exposed to cigarette smoke, either actively or passively. There is now a substantial body of scientific evidence indicating that hypertension, dyslipidemia, diabetes, obesity, and cigarette smoking contribute to the early development of atherosclerosis in children and adolescents. Furthermore, normalization of blood pressure, dyslipidemia, glucose metabolism, and body weight has been associated with a reversal of subclinical atherosclerosis.[39–45] Research also shows that risk factors present during childhood, especially obesity, are often carried or "track" into adulthood.[46]

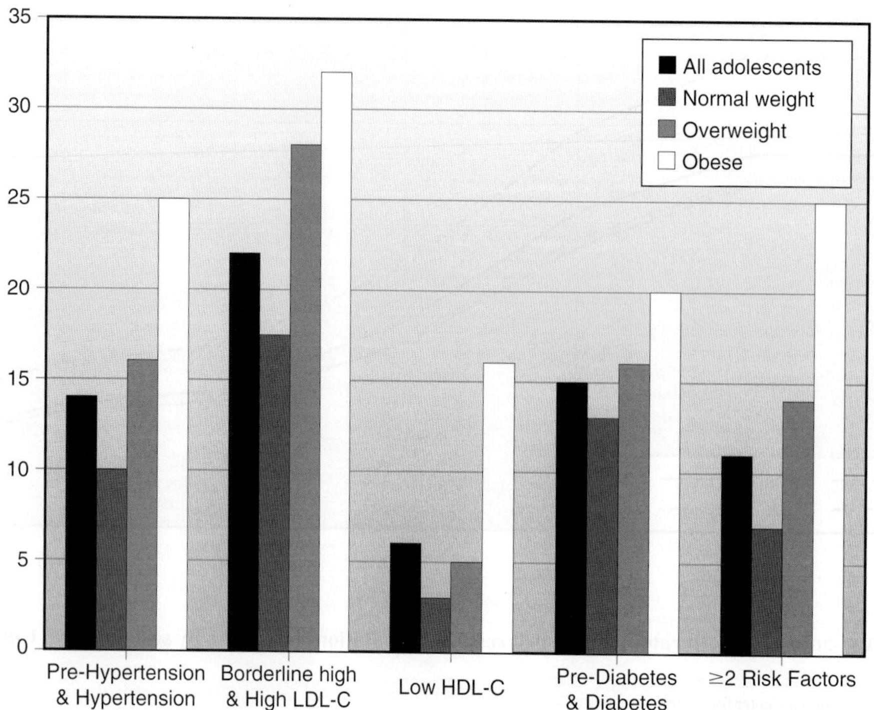

Figure 8.9 Prevalence of selected CVD risk factors among U.S. adolescents, 12 to 19 years of age, by BMI classification, NHANES 1999–2008.
Compared to adolescents whose BMI is in the normal weight category, the prevalence of these risk factors is increased among those in the overweight category, and even more so among adolescents in the obese category. BMI is classified using the 2000 CDC sex-specific growth charts as explained in Chapter 6. Risk factor definitions are given in the text.
Source: Adapted from: May AL, Kuklina EV, Yoon PW. 2012. Prevalence of cardiovascular disease risk factors among US adolescents, 1999–2008. *Pediatrics* 129:1035–1041.

CVD risk factors are commonly seen in young people in the United States, as shown in Figure 8.9.[47] According to data from NHANES collected between 1999 to 2008, 14% of U.S. adolescents 12 to 19 years of age had either prehypertension or hypertension, which are defined following the methodology explained later in this chapter. The same data show that 22% of 12- to 19-year-olds in the United States had borderline high LDL-C (defined as ≥ 110 mg/dL to < 129 mg/dL) or high LDL-C (defined as ≥ 130 mg/dL), 6% had a low HDL-C (defined as < 35 mg/dL), 15% had either prediabetes (a fasting plasma glucose level > 99 mg/dL to < 126 mg/dL) or diabetes (a fasting plasma glucose level ≥ 126 mg/dL), and that 11% of all adolescents had two or more of these risk factors at the same time.[47–49] Figure 8.9 also shows that compared to adolescents whose BMI was in the normal weight category, the prevalence of these risk factors was increased among those in the overweight category, and even more so among adolescents in the obese category. Prevalence of normal weight, overweight, and obesity in adolescents having at least one risk factor was 37%, 49%, and 61%, respectively.[47] Thus, U.S. adolescents carry a significant burden of cardiovascular disease risk factors, especially those whose BMI classifies them as overweight or obese.

Cardiovascular Disease Risk Reduction in Children and Adolescents

The National Heart, Lung, and Blood Institute (NHLBI) recently updated its clinical practice guidelines for CVD risk reduction in children in a report entitled *Expert Panel on Integrated Guidelines for Cardiovascular Health and Risk Reduction in Children and Adolescents* (www.nhlbi.nih.gov/guidelines/cvd_ped/index.htm). This is the first major update in recommendations addressing atherosclerotic cardiovascular disease in children and adolescents since 1992. The Expert Panel's report reflects not only a much larger knowledge base surrounding the link between dyslipidemia and increased CVD risk, but also the fact that a much greater number of children and adolescents have dyslipidemia, in part due to the increased prevalence of pediatric overweight and obesity that has occurred over the past two decades. The Expert Panel recommends that preventing cardiovascular disease must begin in childhood and address two fundamental goals:

preventing the development of CVD risk factors in children (referred to as *primordial prevention*) and preventing future CVD by effectively managing any identified risk factors (referred to as *primary prevention*).[51] The Expert Panel's recommendations address all of the recognized cardiovascular disease risk factors that are relevant in childhood, such as family history, physical activity, tobacco exposure, high blood pressure, dyslipidemia, overweight and obesity, and abnormal glucose metabolism. The dietary and nutrition recommendations affirm the 2010 *Dietary Guidelines for Americans* as the basis for promoting optimal growth and development and preventing chronic disease in persons beginning at the age of 2 years. But because the Expert Panel's recommendations are intended to be used by pediatric care providers to reduce CVD risk in youth, they also provide guidance on specific dietary fatty acids and energy components to prevent dyslipidemia and obesity, as well as advice on dietary composition and micronutrient intake to promote a healthy blood pressure.[51]

Accompanying the Expert Panel's report is a set of evidence-based dietary recommendations for patients of pediatric care providers called the Cardiovascular Health Integrated Lifestyle Diet (CHILD 1), which is shown in Table 8.10. The Expert Panel stresses that good nutrition beginning at birth can have profound health benefits and potentially decrease future CVD risk, and emphasizes the importance of exclusive breast-feeding for the first six months of life and continued breast-feeding for at least 12 months of age with the addition of appropriate complementary foods. Infants who cannot be fed directly from the breast should be fed expressed human milk from a bottle. Infants for whom expressed milk is not available should be fed an iron-fortified infant formula. Research has shown that individuals who were breast-fed during infancy have long-term cardiovascular health benefits such as lower risk of obesity, lower total cholesterol levels and carotid intima-media thickness in adulthood, and lower risk of type 2 diabetes mellitus.[52,53] The recommendations in Table 8.10 are consistent with the 2010 *Dietary Guidelines for Americans*

TABLE 8.10 Evidence-Based Dietary Recommendations for Patients of Pediatric Care Providers: Cardiovascular Health Integrated Lifestyle Diet (CHILD 1)

CHILD 1 is the recommended first step diet for all children and adolescents at elevated cardiovascular risk.

Birth–6 months	Infants should be exclusively breast-fed (no supplemental formula or other foods) until age 6 months. Infants who cannot be fed directly at the breast should be fed expressed milk. Infants for whom expressed milk is not available should be fed iron-fortified infant formula.
6–12 months	Continue breast-feeding until at least age 12 months while gradually adding solids. Transition to an iron-fortified formula until 12 months if reducing breast-feeding. Infants who cannot be fed directly at the breast should be fed expressed milk. Infants for whom expressed milk is not available should be fed iron-fortified infant formula. Fat intake in infants younger than 12 months of age should not be restricted without medical indication. Limit other drinks to 100% fruit juice ≤ 4 oz/d. No sweetened beverages. Encourage water.
12–24 months	Transition to reduced-fat (2% to fat-free) unflavored cow's milk. Toddlers 12–24 months of age with a family history of obesity, heart disease, or high cholesterol should discuss transition to reduced-fat milk with pediatric care provider after 12 months of age. Continued breast-feeding is still appropriate and nutritionally superior to cows milk. Milk reduced in fat should be used only in the context of an overall diet that supplies 30% of calories from fat. Limit/avoid sugar-sweetened beverage intake. Encourage water. Transition to table food with: • Total fat 30% of daily kcal* • Saturated fat 8–10% of daily kcal* • Avoid *trans* fat as much as possible • Monounsaturated and polyunsaturated fat up to 20% of daily kcal* • Cholesterol < 300 mg/d Supportive actions: • The fat content of cow's milk to introduce at ages 12–24 months should be decided together by parents and health care providers based on the child's growth, appetite, intake of other nutrient-dense foods, intake of other sources of fat, and potential risk for obesity and CVD. • Limit 100% fruit juice (from a cup) to no more than 4 oz/d. • Limit sodium intake. • Consider DASH-type diet rich in fruits, vegetables, whole grains, low-fat/fat-free milk and milk products; lower in sugar.
2–10 years	Primary beverage: Fat-free unflavored milk. Limit/avoid sugar-sweetened beverages. Encourage water.

continued

Table 8.10 Evidence-Based Dietary Recommendations for Patients of Pediatric Care Providers: Cardiovascular Health Integrated Lifestyle Diet (CHILD 1)—*continued*

	Fat content: • Total fat 25–30% of daily kcal* • Saturated fat 8–10% of daily kcal* • Avoid *trans* fats as much as possible • Monounsaturated and polyunsaturated fat up to 20% of daily kcal* • Cholesterol < 300 mg/d Encourage high dietary fiber intake from foods. Naturally fiber-rich foods are recommended (fruits, vegetables, whole grains); fiber supplements are not advised. Limit refined carbohydrates (sugars, white rice, white bread). Supportive actions: • Teach portions based on EER for age/gender/activity. • Encourage moderately increased energy intake during periods of rapid growth and/or regular moderate-to-vigorous physical activity. • Encourage dietary fiber from foods: Age + 5 g/d. • Limit naturally sweetened juice (no added sugar) to 4 oz/d. • Limit sodium intake. • Support DASH-style eating plan.
11–21 years	Primary beverage: Fat-free unflavored milk. Limit/avoid sugar-sweetened beverages. Encourage water. Fat content: • Total fat 25–30% of daily kcal* • Saturated fat 8–10% of daily kcal* • Avoid *trans* fat as much as possible • Monounsaturated and polyunsaturated fat up to 20% of daily kcal* • Cholesterol < 300 mg/d Encourage high dietary fiber intake from foods. Naturally fiber-rich foods are recommended (fruits, vegetables, whole grains); fiber supplements are not advised. Limit refined carbohydrates (sugars, white rice, white bread). Supportive actions: • Teach portions based on EER for age/gender/activity. • Encourage moderately increased energy intake during periods of rapid growth and/or regular moderate-to-vigorous physical activity. • Advocate dietary fiber: Goal of 14 g/1000 kcal. • Limit naturally sweetened juice (no added sugar) to 4–6 oz/d. • Limit sodium intake. • Encourage healthy eating habits: Breakfast every day, eating meals as a family, limiting fast-food meals. • Support DASH-style eating plan.

*Kcal intake should be based on the Estimated Energy Requirement (EER) per day according to age and gender.

Source: Adapted from Expert Panel on Integrated Guidelines for Cardiovascular Health and Risk Reduction in Children and Adolescents. 2011. *Expert Panel on Integrated Guidelines for Cardiovascular Health and Risk Reduction in Children and Adolescents: Full report.* National Heart, Lung, Blood Institute, National Institutes of Health, U.S. Department of Health and Human Services. www.nhlbi.nih.gov/guidelines/cvd_ped/index.htm.

and those of professional groups such as the American Academy of Pediatrics and the American Academy of Family Physicians, while providing additional guidance specifically targeting children and adolescents at increased risk of CVD.

Given the high prevalence of pediatric overweight and obesity and the increased CVD risk associated with overweight and obesity, age-appropriate energy intake matched with energy expenditure is critical. Table 8.11 lists the Estimated Energy Requirements (EER) per day by age, gender, and physical activity level using the EER formulas included in the Dietary Reference Intakes, as previously discussed in Chapter 7. The Expert Panel's report also addresses the important role that regular physical activity and avoidance of tobacco smoke play in promoting cardiovascular health. The report's recommendations for blood pressure measurement and diagnosis of hypertension in children and adolescents are consistent with earlier clinical practice guidelines issued by the National High Blood Pressure Education Program in 2004 and discussed later in this chapter. The DASH eating plan is emphasized along with a reduction in dietary sodium intake.

The most controversial aspect of the Expert Panel's report are its guidelines for lipid assessment, which recommend universal screening for lipid levels in all children at 9 to 11 years of age and then again for all adolescents at 17 to 21 years of age.[51] The report does not recommend lipid screening in the first 2 years of life. Between the ages of 2 to 8 years and between 12 and 16 years, routine lipid screening is not recommended but

TABLE 8.11 Estimated Energy Requirements per Day by Age, Gender, and Physical Activity Level[a]

Estimated amounts of calories needed to maintain caloric balance for various gender and age groups at three different levels of physical activity. The estimates are rounded to the nearest 200 calories. An individual's calorie needs may be higher or lower than these average estimates

		Calorie Requirements (kcals) by Activity Level[b]		
Gender	**Age (Years)**	**Sedentary**	**Moderately Active**	**Active**
Child	2–3	1,000–1,200	1,000–1,400[c]	1,000–1,400[c]
Female[d]	4–8	1,200–1,400	1,400–1,600	1,400–1,800
	9–13	1,400–1,600	1,600–2,000	1,800–2,200
	14–18	1,800	2,000	2,400
	19–30	1,800–2,000	2,000–2,200	2,400
Male	4–8	1,200–1,400	1,400–1,600	1,600–2,000
	9–13	1,600–2,000	1,800–2,200	2,000–2,600
	14–18	2,000–2,400	2,400–2,800	2,800–3,200
	19–30	2,400–2,600	2,600–2,800	3,000

a. Based on Estimated Energy Requirements (EER) equations, using reference heights (average) and reference weights (health) for each age/gender group. For children and adolescents, reference height and weight vary. For adults, the reference man is 5 feet 10 inches tall and weighs 154 pounds. The reference woman is 5 feet 4 inches tall and weighs 126 pounds. EER equations are from the Institute of Medicine. *Dietary Reference Intakes for Energy, Carbohydrate, Fiber, Fat, Fatty Acids, Cholesterol, Protein, and Amino Acids.* Washington, DC: The National Academies Press; 2002.

b. Sedentary means a lifestyle that includes only the light physical activity associated with typical day-to-day life. Moderately active means a lifestyle that includes physical activity equivalent to walking about 1.5 to 3 miles per day at 3 to 4 miles per hour, in addition to the light physical activity associated with typical day-to-day life. Active means a lifestyle that includes physical activity equivalent to walking more than 3 miles per day at 3 to 4 miles per hour, in addition to the light physical activity associated with typical day-to-day life.

c. The calorie ranges shown are to accommodate needs of different ages within the group. For children and adolescents, more calories are needed at older ages. For adults, fewer calories are needed at older ages.

d. Estimates for females do not include women who are pregnant or breastfeeding.

Source: U.S. Department of Health and Human Services and U.S. Department Agriculture. 2010. *Dietary Guidelines for Americans, 2010.* Washington, DC: U.S. Government Printing Office. www.dietaryguidelines.gov.

should occur if there is a family history of early CVD, a parent has a high total cholesterol level, or the child has a major CVD risk factor such as diabetes, hypertension, obesity, cigarette smoking, or a medical condition placing the child at increased CVD risk.[51] The cut points for classifying lipid and lipoprotein levels in children and adolescents and in young adults are shown in Table 8.12 and Table 8.13, respectively. The tables include values for non-high-density-lipoprotein cholesterol (non-HDL-C), which can be calculated from total cholesterol and HDL-C values using the following equation:

$$\text{non-HDL-C} = \text{total cholesterol} - \text{HDL-C}$$

Non-HDL-C has been shown to be a significant predictor of the presence of atherosclerosis in children and adolescents, as powerful as any other lipoprotein cholesterol measurement. Compared to total cholesterol, LDL-C, and HDL-C alone, non-HDL-C appears to be a better indicator of persistent dyslipidemia, atherosclerosis, and future CHD. An important advantage of non-HDL-C is that it can be determined in the nonfasting state because it is calculated using values for total cholesterol and HDL-C, both of which can be measured in the nonfasting state. The Expert Panel suggests that non-HDL-C be used as a screening test for the identification of dyslipidemia in children and adolescents.[51]

TABLE 8.12 Acceptable, Borderline High, and High Plasma Lipid and Lipoprotein Levels (mg/dL) for Children and Adolescents, Birth to 19 Years of Age

Category	Acceptable	Borderline High	High
Total cholesterol	< 170	170–199	≥ 200
Low-density-lipoprotein cholesterol	< 110	110–129	≥ 130
Non-high-density-lipoprotein cholesterol	< 120	120–144	≥ 145
Triglyceride			
0–9 years of age	< 75	75–99	≥ 100
10–19 years of age	< 90	90–129	≥ 130
Category	**Acceptable**	**Borderline Low**	**Low**
High-density-lipoprotein cholesterol	> 45	40–45	< 40

Source: Adapted from Expert Panel on Integrated Guidelines for Cardiovascular Health and Risk Reduction in Children and Adolescents. 2011. *Expert Panel on Integrated Guidelines for Cardiovascular Health and Risk Reduction in Children and Adolescents: Full report.* National Heart, Lung, Blood Institute, National Institutes of Health, U.S. Department of Health and Human Services. www.nhlbi.nih.gov/guidelines/cvd_ped/index.htm.

TABLE 8.13 Recommended Cut Points for Lipid and Lipoprotein Levels (mg/dL) in Young Adults, 20 to 24 Years of Age

Category	Acceptable	Borderline High	High
Total cholesterol	< 190	190–224	≥ 225
Low-density-lipoprotein cholesterol	< 120	120–159	≥ 160
Non-high-density-lipoprotein cholesterol	< 150	150–189	≥ 190
Triglyceride	< 115	115–149	≥ 150
Category	**Acceptable**	**Borderline Low**	**Low**
High-density-lipoprotein cholesterol	> 45	40–45	< 40

Source: Adapted from Expert Panel on Integrated Guidelines for Cardiovascular Health and Risk Reduction in Children and Adolescents. 2011. *Expert Panel on Integrated Guidelines for Cardiovascular Health and Risk Reduction in Children and Adolescents: Full report.* National Heart, Lung, Blood Institute, National Institutes of Health, U.S. Department of Health and Human Services. www.nhlbi.nih.gov/guidelines/cvd_ped/index.htm.

Dietary Treatment in Coronary Heart Disease

In the past 5 decades, government agencies and private organizations have developed a variety of dietary and lifestyle recommendations for promoting healthy levels of serum lipids and lipoproteins and for reducing overall coronary heart disease risk. Several of these are discussed at length in Chapter 2. Consistent features among these various recommendations have been limiting consumption of foods rich in total fats, saturated fatty acids, and dietary cholesterol; maintaining a healthy body weight by balancing energy intake with energy expenditure; and keeping sodium intake moderate.

Among the most authoritative and comprehensive sets of dietary recommendations for reducing the risk of cardiovascular disease are the *ATP III*'s "therapeutic lifestyle changes," which were outlined in Table 8.8, and the American Heart Association's diet and lifestyle goals and recommendations for reducing risk of cardiovascular disease, which are outlined in Box 8.4. The American Heart Association's recommendations are appropriate for the general public, including adults and children over the age of 2 years, and are intentionally flexible to meet the unique requirements of growth, development, and aging.[25] These recommendations may have to be modified to accommodate medical nutrition therapy for individuals presenting with such conditions as preexisting cardiovascular disease, specific lipid disorders (e.g., elevated serum triglyceride, low serum HDL-C, or the presence of chylomicrons in fasting serum), diabetes mellitus, insulin resistance, congestive heart failure, and kidney disease.[25]

Saturated Fatty Acids

Saturated fatty acids (SFA) are the most important dietary determinant of serum total cholesterol and LDL-C levels.[4,25] One exception to this rule is stearic acid (18:0), an SFA that appears to have a neutral effect on serum cholesterol and lipoprotein levels. Moderation should still be practiced in the consumption of fats high in stearic acid, such as beef

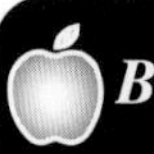

Box 8.4 The American Heart Association's Diet and Lifestyle Goals and Recommendations for Cardiovascular Disease Risk Reduction, Revised in 2006

Diet and Lifestyle Goals for Cardiovascular Disease Risk Reduction

- Consume an overall healthy diet
- Aim for a healthy body weight
- Aim for recommended levels of low-density lipoprotein (LDL) cholesterol, high-density lipoprotein (HDL) cholesterol, and triglycerides
- Aim for a normal blood pressure
- Aim for a normal blood glucose level
- Be physically active
- Avoid use of and exposure to tobacco products

Diet and Lifestyle Recommendations for Cardiovascular Disease Risk Reduction

- Balance calorie intake and physical activity to achieve or maintain a healthy body weight
- Consume a diet rich in vegetables and fruits
- Choose whole-grain, high-fiber foods
- Consume fish, especially oily fish, at least twice a week
- Limit intake of saturated fat to < 7% of energy, *trans* fat to < 1% of energy, and cholesterol to < 300 mg per day by
    - choosing lean meats and vegetable alternatives
    - selecting fat-free (skim), 1%-fat, and low-fat dairy products
    - minimizing intake of partially hydrogenated fats
- Minimize your intake of beverages and foods with added sugars
- Choose and prepare foods with little or no salt
- If you consume alcohol, do so in moderation
- When eating food prepared outside of the home, follow the AHA Diet and Lifestyle Recommendations

Source: Adapted from Lichtenstein AH, Appel LJ, Brands M, Carnethon M, Daniels S, Franch HA, et al. 2006. Diet and lifestyle recommendations: Revision 2006. *Circulation* 114:82–96.

fat and cocoa butter, because these fats contain a substantial amount of the other SFAs that raise serum cholesterol.

The American Heart Association recommends that members of the general population (ages > 2 years) limit their intake of SFA to < 7% of energy. This is consistent with the recommendation of the Expert Panel on Integrated Guidelines for Cardiovascular Health and Risk Reduction in Children and Adolescents.[51] According to data from NHANES 2008–2010, SFAs provide, on average, 11.0% of energy.

During the past several decades, average SFA intake among Americans has declined from a high of nearly 20% of energy to the current level of 11.0%. This is recognized as a major factor in the decline of mean total serum cholesterol levels. However, more progress is needed in further reducing SFA intake to meet the American Heart Association's goals. This can be done by identifying foods rich in saturated fat and substituting foods containing less saturated fat. Major food sources of saturated fat in the diets of U.S. adults include full-fat dairy products, beef, poultry, stick margarine, pastries, cookies, and quick breads made with meat fats and hydrogenated vegetable fats. Particular attention should be given to monitoring the intake of these foods when evaluating the diets of persons with elevated serum levels of total cholesterol and LDL-C.

Trans *Fatty Acids*

Consumption of dietary *trans* unsaturated fatty acids increases LDL-C and reduces HDL-C.[54,55] Although saturated fatty acids appear to increase LDL-C to a somewhat greater extent than an equal amount of dietary *trans* unsaturated fatty acids, the detrimental effects of dietary *trans* unsaturated fatty acids on serum lipid and lipoprotein levels has led to recommendations to limit intake of foods rich in *trans* unsaturated fatty acids.[4,25,56] It is estimated that average intake of *trans* fatty acids in the U.S. diet is approximately 2.7% of energy. As shown in Box 8.4, the American Heart Association recommends that *trans* fat be restricted to < 1% of energy.[25] The *ATP III*'s therapeutic lifestyle change diet recommends that intake of *trans* unsaturated fatty acids be kept as low as possible, which is consistent with the recommendation of the Expert Panel on Integrated Guidelines for Cardiovascular Health and Risk Reduction in Children and Adolescents.[51]

Trans fatty acids are unsaturated fatty acids containing at least one double bond in the *trans* configuration. In most naturally occurring unsaturated fatty acids (particularly those found in vegetable oils), double bonds are typically in the *cis* configuration. However, unsaturated *trans* fatty acids naturally occur at relatively low levels in meat and dairy foods as by-products of fermentation in ruminant animals.[57] The richest sources of *trans* fatty acids are partially hydrogenated vegetable fats, such as vegetable shortening and some margarines. Foods prepared with partially hydrogenated vegetable fats include cookies, crackers, doughnuts, and other baked goods, as well as commercially prepared fried foods.[58] With the introduction of mandatory *trans* fat labeling on January 1, 2006, it has been much easier for consumers to identify and limit their consumption of *trans* fatty acids. However, the presence of small amounts of naturally occurring *trans* fatty acids in meat and dairy products will make it difficult to entirely eliminate *trans* fatty acids from the diet.[25,57,58]

Dietary Cholesterol

Dietary cholesterol (cholesterol in food) also raises serum total cholesterol and LDL-C levels (especially the latter), although the elevations are not as great as those seen in diets high in SFA.[4,25,59–61] As is the case with intake of saturated fatty acids, the response of serum total cholesterol and LDL-C to dietary intake of cholesterol varies widely among individuals.[4,25,62] Epidemiologic studies suggest that dietary cholesterol intake is also associated with increased risk for coronary heart disease.[63–66] In several studies, researchers have found dietary cholesterol to be an independent predictor of CHD, *apart from its effects on serum cholesterol.*[63,67]

According to data from NHANES 2008–2010, mean dietary cholesterol intake for American males and females is 362 mg and 230 mg per day, respectively. However, mean dietary cholesterol intake for males and females ages 20 to 29 years is approximately 355 mg and 216 mg per day, respectively. The American Heart Association recommends that members of the general population (age > 2 years) limit their intake of dietary cholesterol to < 300 mg per day, which is consistent with the recommendation of the Expert Panel on Integrated Guidelines for Cardiovascular Health and Risk Reduction in Children and Adolescents.[51] Persons following the *ATP III*'s therapeutic lifestyle change diet are advised to limit their dietary cholesterol intake to < 200 mg per day.[4] Identification of foods containing dietary cholesterol is relatively easy, given the fact that dietary cholesterol is found only in foods of animal origin. Particularly rich sources include egg yolk, full-fat dairy products, and organ meats (e.g., liver, kidney, and brain). Most foods high in saturated fat are also sources of dietary cholesterol. Consequently, reducing consumption of these foods results in a double benefit of reduced intake of saturated fat and dietary cholesterol.

Confusion about dietary cholesterol's influence on serum cholesterol is primarily due to the high variability of response of serum total cholesterol and LDL-C to consumption of dietary cholesterol.[4] A report of an 88-year-old man having a plasma total cholesterol level of 200 mg/dL (5.17 mmol/L) despite eating about 25 eggs per day for more than 15 years is a case in point.[68] Amazingly, he was almost completely free of any clinically important atherosclerosis. He absorbed only 18% of the cholesterol he ate (people normally absorb 45% to 55%), he had twice the normal rate of bile acid synthesis, and his body synthesized less than average amounts of cholesterol. Despite this *one* individual's highly unusual cholesterol metabolism, it remains prudent for the rest of us with more normal cholesterol metabolism to follow a low-cholesterol diet.

Total Calories

Another significant dietary factor is total caloric intake, with its implications for obesity. Because obesity is associated with elevated serum LDL-C, increased risk for hypertension and type 2 diabetes mellitus, and is an independent risk factor for CHD, the *ATP III* and American Heart Association recommend balancing energy intake with energy expenditure to prevent weight gain once an adult has attained his or her healthy weight or to maintain a healthy body weight.[4,25] For many adults, this can be accomplished by modestly reducing energy intake (consuming 500 to 1000 fewer kilocalories per day) and increasing energy expenditure through moderate physical activity on most days of the week. Emphasizing foods with a low energy density (e.g., fruits, vegetables, legumes, whole-grain products, fat-free dairy products, and lean meats) is recommended.[25] Dietary approaches to weight management for children and adolescents must be consistent with appropriate growth and development. The American Heart Association does not recommend the use of very low-fat diets or high-protein diets for weight management in the general population.[25] In overweight persons, weight reduction has been shown to lower serum LDL-C and triglycerides, to raise HDL-C, to assist in the control of hypertension, and to improve glycemic control in persons with type 2 diabetes.[4,25]

Total and Unsaturated Fat

Most people in the general population older than 2 years will benefit from a diet providing a moderate intake of total fat while saturated and *trans* fatty acids and dietary cholesterol are kept low and polyunsaturated fatty acids do not exceed 10% of energy.[4,25] A diet providing no more than 30% of energy from fat and moderately restricted in total energy (a daily deficit of 500 to 1000 kilocalories) can be particularly beneficial for overweight and obese individuals when combined with regular physical activity of moderate intensity and duration. However, in persons with the metabolic syndrome and type 2 diabetes, the amount of carbohydrate (50% to 60% of energy) in a moderately fat-restricted diet (≤ 30% of energy) may elevate serum triglyceride and depress serum HDL-C.[4,25] Consequently, a dietary treatment strategy for patients presenting with elevated triglycerides and low HDL-C is to moderately restrict percent of energy from carbohydrate and increase the proportion of energy from monounsaturated fats, while keeping intake of dietary cholesterol and polyunsaturated, saturated, and *trans* fatty acids low.[4,25] Weight reduction is also recommended by keeping total energy intake moderate while increasing physical activity. Individuals with severe hypertriglyceridemia (≥ 1000 mg/dL) may benefit from a very low-fat diet (< 10% of energy from all forms of fat) and pharmacologic treatment.[25]

Protein and Carbohydrate

The *ATP III* recommends that protein compose about 15% of total calories and that emphasis be given to plant-based sources of protein.[4] Although some studies have suggested that soy protein had particularly beneficial effects on LDL cholesterol levels and other CHD risk factors, more recent research has not confirmed these results.[69–73,25] Still, plant foods have unique advantages over animal products. Plant foods contain no cholesterol (unless prepared with some type of animal product) and tend to be low in both total and saturated fat. Mortality from CHD is higher in nonvegetarians than in vegetarians, who generally rely heavily on plant foods for protein, energy, and other nutrient needs.[74,75] Most of the decreased CHD mortality rate in vegetarians is likely due to the differences in the types and amounts of fat found in plants compared with foods of animal origin; however, several nondietary factors no doubt play a role as well. Plants also contain phytochemicals, some of which have antioxidant and other beneficial properties that confer protection against heart disease, stroke, and cancer.

An intake of carbohydrates at 55% or more of total calories is generally recommended. This includes simple sugars (monosaccharides and disaccharides), complex digestible carbohydrates (starches), and complex indigestible carbohydrates (fiber). To ensure that adequate vitamins, minerals, and fiber are consumed, intake of complex digestible carbohydrates should be kept high and that of simple sugars relatively low. In most people, when digestible carbohydrates are substituted for saturated fatty acids, serum LDL-C generally falls to about the same extent as when oleic and linoleic acids are substituted in this manner.[4]

Fiber can be defined as plant materials in the diet that are resistant to digestion by enzymes produced by the human intestinal tract.[76] Fiber can be divided into the soluble and insoluble fractions. The soluble fibers (gums, pectins, mucilages, and some hemicelluloses) are effective in lowering serum total cholesterol and LDL-C levels, although these effects are not as pronounced in persons with lower serum total cholesterol as it is in those having higher levels.[76–78]

Probable mechanisms for this effect include soluble fiber's ability to bind bile acids and promote their excretion in the feces and the reduction of cholesterol absorption by fiber's interference with micelle formation.[79,80] The release of short-chain fatty acids (especially propionate) from the bacterial fermentation of dietary fiber may decrease hepatic cholesterol synthesis, thus lowering serum cholesterol levels and providing several other beneficial effects.[81,82]

General Principles

The goals of the *ATP III*'s therapeutic lifestyle change diet for the treatment of elevated cholesterol levels and the American Heart Association's recommendations are not a temporary "diet" but, rather, a permanent change in eating behavior that is consistent with good overall nutrition. Consumption of a variety of foods is important because no single food item provides all the essential nutrients in the amounts needed. One of the best ways to ensure an adequate diet is to include in one's meals a variety of foods from all food groups.

Although preventing obesity by controlling energy consumption is a major concern of many people, supplying the nutrient and energy needs of growing and developing children and adolescents must not be overlooked. For example, the energy needs of 2- to 3-year-old children per unit of body weight are particularly high. In addition, the capacity of a child's gastrointestinal tract for food at any one time is limited. Consequently, children's diets should include foods that are good sources of energy and nutrients and yet low in SFA and cholesterol. Some young children may need snacks to help them meet their energy and nutrient needs, and suitable selections are available that will keep children's diets within the recommended guidelines.

Issues in Measuring Lipid and Lipoprotein Levels

The public health impact of cardiovascular disease and the causal relationships between cardiovascular disease and serum lipid and lipoprotein levels make measurement of total cholesterol, low-density-lipoprotein cholesterol, and high-density-lipoprotein cholesterol among the most important in the clinical laboratory.[83] The presence of specific and detailed guidelines for detecting, evaluating, and treating elevated blood cholesterol levels in adults (e.g., the *Adult Treatment Panel III*) require that serum lipid and lipoprotein measurement meet certain standards for *precision, accuracy,* and *total analytical error.* Although these three particularly important aspects apply to any measurement, whether a clinical laboratory test (such as serum total cholesterol) or measurement of weight or stature, they are discussed in this section as they relate to measurement of lipid and lipoprotein levels.

Precision (or reproducibility) relates to the difference in results when the same measurement is repeatedly performed. The difference, or variability, in results from repeated, or replicate, measurements should be within acceptable limits. *Accuracy* relates to the difference between the measured value as reported by a clinical laboratory and the "true," or "real," measurement value obtained by using the definitive analytical process known as the "reference method" of measurement. Accuracy is often expressed in terms of *bias,* which is defined as the average deviation of the measured value from the true, or real, value. *Total analytical error* is the National Cholesterol Education's primary criterion for evaluating the performance of an analytical test (e.g., measuring serum cholesterol), and it accounts for both accuracy and precision.[83,84]

Precision

Precision and its relationship to bias are illustrated in Figure 8.10. Precision is high when multiple analyses of the same sample result in values that are reasonably close. In Figure 8.10, high precision can be thought of as multiple shots at the target being in close proximity of each other, as seen in Figure 8.10a and 8.10b. Precision is low when multiple analyses performed on one sample result in values differing considerably, as illustrated in Figure 8.10c and 8.10d. Ideally, replicate analyses of a single sample would yield the same measurement result, but the reality is that these replicate measurements vary somewhat because of potential variation in sample preparation (some analyses require precipitation and ultracentrifugation of the serum or plasma) and analytical variation inherent in the automatic analyzers used in clinical laboratories. Automatic analyzers are subject to slight variation in function over time. In addition, the reagents used in the analyzers can vary slightly from lot to lot. Obviously, the challenge to the clinical laboratory and the reagent manufacturer is to minimize such fluctuations.[84]

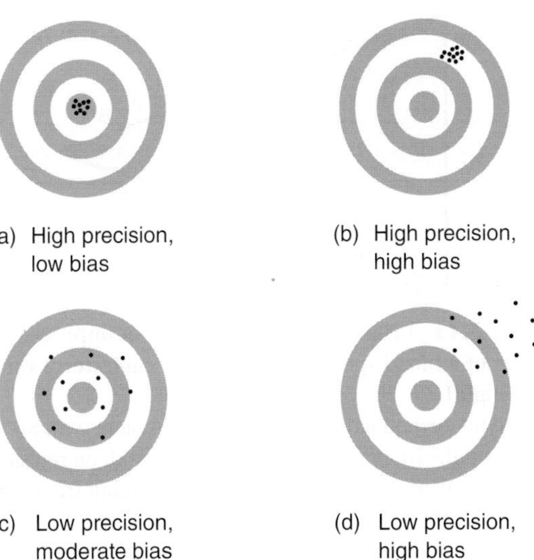

Figure 8.10
Multiple shots at a target can be used to illustrate precision and bias. Note that high precision is necessary for low bias to exist.

The importance of precision in diagnosing and monitoring persons with high cholesterol levels is illustrated in Figure 8.11. The figure shows the effect of differing degrees of imprecision (sometimes referred to as "random error" or "analytical noise") in cholesterol measurement. If a person's serum sample has a true cholesterol value of 240 mg/dL (6.21 mmol/L), values from replicate analyses of that sample could be scattered over a wide range, depending on the precision of the analytical method. Replicate analyses of a single specimen allow calculation of the measurement as represented by the coefficient of variation (CV). CV is a measure of imprecision and is calculated by dividing the standard deviation (SD) of replicate analyses by the mean of those replicate analyses and then multiplying them by 100 (CV = SD ÷ mean × 100).[83]

Figure 8.11 shows, for example, that, if the precision of an analytical method for serum total cholesterol were such that the CV were 10%, replicate cholesterol analyses of a single specimen having a true value of 240 mg/dL would yield values ranging from 192 to 288 mg/dL. Obviously, with this degree of imprecision, it would be very difficult to properly identify persons with elevated serum cholesterol. Surveys indicate that the analytical CV of clinical laboratories is in the range of 3% to 7%, with an average of 4%.[84] The National Cholesterol Education Program believes that a modern, well-controlled clinical laboratory should be able to maintain analytical CVs of less than 4%.[84] Analytical performance goals established by the National Cholesterol Education Program are shown in Table 8.14.

Accuracy

Accuracy and bias (also referred to as systematic error or overall inaccuracy) and their relationship to precision

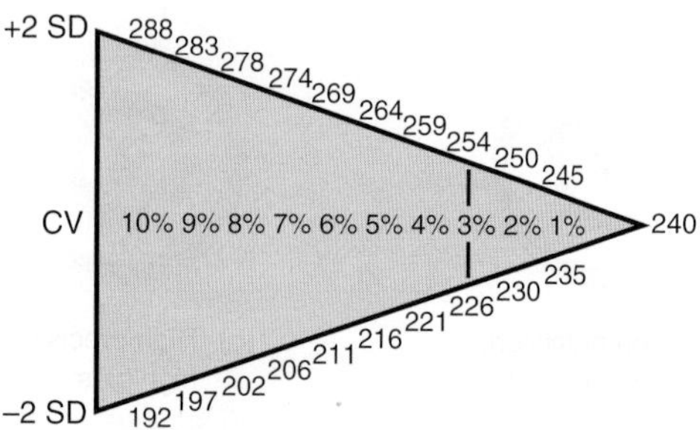

Figure 8.11 Effect of differing degrees of imprecision in analysis of a blood specimen with a true cholesterol value of 240 mg/dL.

An analytic method having a precision consistent with a coefficient of variation (CV) of 3% would yield, on repeat measurements of the same sample, values ranging from 226 to 254 mg/dL. SD = standard deviation.

Source: From National Cholesterol Education Program. 1988. *Current status of blood cholesterol measurement in clinical laboratories in the United States: A report from the Laboratory Standardization Panel of the National Cholesterol Education Program.* Bethesda, MD: U.S. Department of Health and Human Services, Public Health Service; National Institutes of Health; National Heart, Lung, and Blood Institute.

TABLE 8.14 Analytical Performance Goals for Lipid and Lipoprotein Measurements Established by the National Cholesterol Education Program

	Imprecision*	Bias†	Total Analytical Error‡
Total cholesterol	CV ≤ 3%	≤ ± 3%	≤ 8.9%
Triglyceride	CV ≤ 5%	≤ ± 5%	≤ 15.0%
HDL cholesterol	CV ≤ 6%	≤ ± 10%	≤ 22.0%
LDL cholesterol	CV ≤ 4%	≤ ± 4%	≤ 12.0%

Adapted from National Cholesterol Education Program. 1995. *Recommendations on lipoprotein measurement from the working group on lipoprotein measurement.* Bethesda, MD: U.S. Department of Health and Human Services, Public Health Service; National Institutes of Health; National Heart, Lung, and Blood Institute.

*CV = coefficient of variation.

†Percent difference between the measured value and the true value when analyzed using the reference method.

‡Total analytical error = percent bias + (1.96 × CV). Total analytical error is the National Cholesterol Education Program's primary criterion for analytical performance.

were illustrated in Figure 8.10. Bias is low when multiple shots at the target repeatedly hit the "bull's eye," as shown in Figure 8.10a. When bias is low, precision is simultaneously high. However, it is impossible for bias to be low when precision is low; thus, precision is a prerequisite for accuracy. Note, also, that high precision does not ensure accuracy, as illustrated in Figure 8.10b. Accuracy is necessary to correctly identify patients with elevated lipid and lipoprotein levels and to monitor their response to treatment. Clinical misdiagnosis can occur from inaccurate measurements, resulting in the reporting of false positive values (measurement results falsely classifying a person as having a condition) or false negative values (measurement results falsely classifying a person as not having a condition).

The true value of a measurement is determined using the reference method, which can be thought of as the "gold standard" measurement process. The U.S. Centers for Disease Control and Prevention (CDC) has established reference methods for measuring each of the lipids and lipoproteins. The CDC-sponsored Cholesterol Reference Method Laboratory Network has established a formal certification program for clinical laboratories, manufacturers of automated analyzers, and organizations providing laboratory standardization and proficiency testing. Laboratory standardization and proficiency testing programs provide clinical laboratories with an opportunity to determine the precision and accuracy of their instruments. The bias of a particular analytical method or automated analyzer can be determined by comparing the mean value of replicate analyses performed on the particular analyzer with the mean value of replicate analyses of the same sample performed using the reference method. The percentage difference between the mean results of the clinical laboratory undergoing evaluation and that of the reference method is known as the relative bias.[83]

If a laboratory's particular analytical method of measuring serum total cholesterol has a *positive bias* of 10% and a subject's true cholesterol value is 200 mg/dL (5.17 mmol/L), the laboratory's reported value is 220 mg/dL (5.69 mmol/L), or 10% greater than the true value. If a person's true value is 240 mg/dL (6.21 mmol/L), a 10% negative bias results in a reported value of 216 mg/dL (5.59 mmol/L), or 10% less than the true value. If the true value is 240 mg/dL (6.21 mmol/L), a 10% positive bias yields a reported value of 264 mg/dL (6.83 mmol/L). Thus, at a given bias, the higher the true cholesterol value, the greater the magnitude of the error. The National Cholesterol Education Program's goals for bias were shown in Table 8.14.

Total Analytical Error

The National Cholesterol Education Program's primary criterion for analytical performance is expressed in terms of *total analytical error*, which takes into account both accuracy (represented as bias) and precision (represented as the coefficient of variation).[84] Total analytical error is calculated using the following equation: total analytical error = percent bias + (1.96 × coefficient of variation).[84] Because calculation of total analytical error includes both bias and the coefficient of variation, a greater inaccuracy (larger bias) can be tolerated if the measurements are very precise.[84] On the other hand, if the measurements are more accurate (bias is low), then a greater degree of imprecision (larger coefficient of variation) can be tolerated. The National Cholesterol Education Program's goals for total analytical error were shown in Table 8.14.

Sources of Error in Cholesterol Measurement

Approximately one-third of within-individual variability in cholesterol analyses is due to laboratory errors. These factors are beyond the scope of this text and will not be addressed.

The remaining two-thirds of within-individual variability is due to a variety of factors occurring before the sample is actually analyzed. These can be referred to as *preanalytical factors*.[83–85] Preanalytical factors operate before or during blood sampling or during sample storage or shipment to the laboratory. They can be divided into biological factors contributing to the patient's usual cholesterol level and those factors altering the patient's usual cholesterol level (Table 8.15).

As can be seen in Table 8.15, numerous factors have the potential for altering usual cholesterol level. Some of these can be controlled by those persons involved in the drawing, preparation, storage, and shipment of blood specimens. In addition, certain conditions call for postponing measurement of serum lipid and lipoprotein levels. Among those identified by the National Cholesterol Education Program are recent myocardial infarction, stroke, trauma, acute infections, and pregnancy.

TABLE 8.15 Preanalytical Factors Affecting Within-Individual Variability in Cholesterol Levels

Biological	Behavioral	Clinical (Disease-Induced)	Clinical (Drug-Induced)	Sample Collecting and Handling
Age Individual biology Race	Usual diet Alcohol Caffeine	Acute and transient: burns, infections, recent myocardial infarction, recent stroke, trauma	Antihypertensives: beta-blockers, chlorothalidone, thiazides Immunosupressives: cyclosporine, prednisolone, tacrolimus	Anticoagulants/preservatives Fasting status Diurnal variation/time of day
Sex	Exercise Smoking Stress	Endocrine: diabetes mellitus, hypothyroidism, hypopituitarism, pregnancy	Steroids: estrogen, progestin	Hemoconcentration Posture Specimen storage
		Hepatic: congenital biliary atresia		
		Renal: chronic renal failure, nephrotic syndrome		Venous vs. capillary blood Venous occlusion
		Storage diseases: Gaucher disease, glycogen storage disease, Tay-Sachs disease		
		Other: anorexia nervosa, systemic lupus erythematosus		

Adapted from Rifai N, Dufour R, Cooper GR. 1997. Preanalytical variation in lipid, lipoprotein, and apolipoprotein testing. In Rifai N, Warnick GR, Dominiczak MH, eds. *Handbook of lipoprotein testing*. Washington, DC: American Association of Clinical Chemistry, pp. 75–97; Warnick GR. 2000. Measurement of cholesterol and other lipoprotein constituents in the clinical laboratory. *Clinical Chemistry and Laboratory Medicine* 38:287–300.

Fasting

Total cholesterol and HDL-C levels can be measured in nonfasting persons. Recent food intake affects plasma total cholesterol levels by only about 1.5% or less.[86] The NCEP recommended that plasma triglyceride concentrations be measured only after a fast of at least 12 hours because absorption of fat after a meal elevates blood triglyceride levels. When a patient's LDL-C value is desired, a fast of at least 12 hours also is necessary because LDL-C typically is calculated from measurements of triglyceride, cholesterol, and HDL-C. If the triglyceride concentration is > 400 mg/dL (> 4.52 mmol/L), the LDL-C should be measured directly instead of being calculated.[86]

Posture

When a person sits or lies down after standing for several minutes, his or her plasma volume increases, and the concentration of cholesterol (and other non-diffusible plasma components) decreases. Compared with values in blood drawn while a person is standing, cholesterol levels can be significantly lower in blood drawn from the same person after he or she has been lying down for 5 minutes and may be as much as 10% to 15% lower in blood drawn after the person has been lying down for 20 minutes. Cholesterol levels in blood drawn after a person has been sitting for 10 to 15 minutes have been shown to be 6% lower than those in blood drawn from the same person while standing. It is recommended that blood sampling conditions be standardized to the sitting position. The patient should sit quietly for about 5 minutes before the sample is drawn.[86]

Venous Occlusion

If a tourniquet is applied to a vein for a prolonged period, the concentration of cholesterol (and other nondiffusible plasma components) will increase. The cholesterol concentration of blood drawn from a vein following a 2-minute tourniquet application can be 2% to 5% higher than that of venous blood drawn after a 30- to 60-second tourniquet application. A 10% to 15% average increase can result from a 5-minute tourniquet application. Venipuncture should be completed as rapidly as possible, preferably within 1 minute.[86]

Anticoagulants

Plasma is derived from whole blood, which is treated with an anticoagulant. The anticoagulants heparin and ethylenediamine tetraacetic acid are preferred. Fluoride, citrate, and oxalate anticoagulants should not be used because they cause plasma components to be diluted (cholesterol concentration is lower when these are used).[86,87]

Recent Heart Attack and Stroke

When a person has suffered a heart attack or stroke, his or her total cholesterol and LDL-C should not be measured for 8 weeks following the attack. These levels fall considerably in a heart attack or stroke victim and remain low for several weeks.

Trauma and Acute Infections

Cholesterol levels can fall by as much as 40% in a person who has suffered severe trauma and can fall temporarily in response to severe pain, surgery, and short-term physical strain. Cholesterol measurements should be performed no sooner than 8 weeks after such conditions have occurred.

Pregnancy

Increases in LDL and VLDL during pregnancy can lead to increases in cholesterol levels by as much as 35%. It is recommended that lipid measurements not be made until 3 to 4 months after delivery.

Hypertension

Hypertension (high blood pressure) is one of the most common risk factors for cardiovascular and renal diseases. It is associated with increased risk of developing CHD, stroke, congestive heart failure, renal insufficiency, and peripheral vascular disease.[88,89] Figure 8.12 shows that, as systolic blood pressure (SBP) or diastolic blood pressure (DBP) increase, there is an increased risk of death from cardiovascular disease.

Arterial blood pressure is measured using a device called a sphygmomanometer ("blood pressure cuff") and is expressed in millimeters of mercury (mm Hg). Systolic blood pressure is the blood pressure following systole, the phase of cardiac contraction. Diastolic blood pressure is that following diastole, the phase of cardiac relaxation. Blood pressure is expressed as two numbers, as in 120/80. The first number (120 mm Hg) is systolic blood pressure, and the second is diastolic blood pressure (80 mm Hg). From the standpoint of cardiovascular disease, a normal blood pressure is one that is less than 120/80, although unusually low blood pressure readings should be evaluated for clinical significance.

There are three types of sphygmomanometers: mercury, aneroid, and electronic. Mercury sphygmomanometers are simple in design, accurate, reliable, and easy to calibrate; however, concerns about the potential of mercury spillage contaminating the environment have resulted in increased use of aneroid and electronic units, which do not contain mercury. Aneroid and electronic sphygmomanometers must be appropriately validated and regularly checked for accuracy.[88] The subject of a blood pressure measurement should be seated quietly in a chair (rather than on an examination table) for at least 5 minutes with both feet on the floor and the arms supported at heart level. To ensure accuracy, an appropriately sized cuff should be used; the bladder cuff should circle at least 80% of the arm. At least two measurements should be made and the average

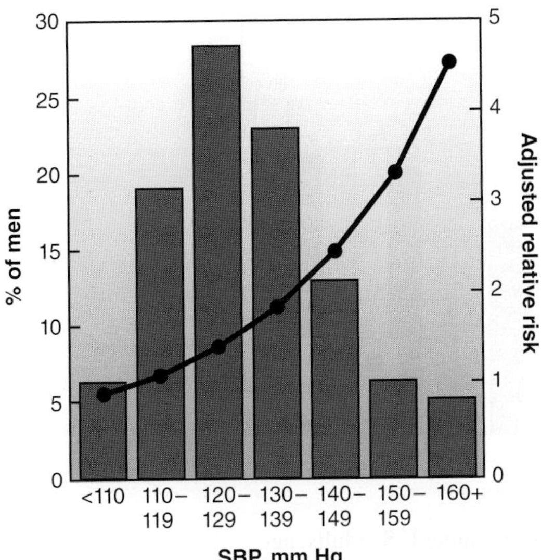

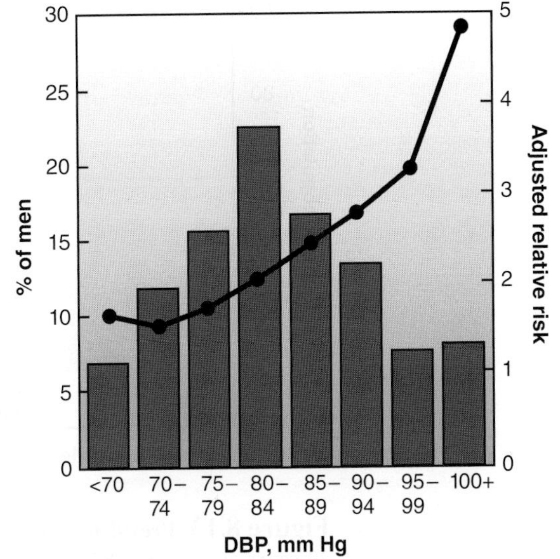

Figure 8.12

The bars in this figure represent the distribution of systolic blood pressure (chart on the left) and diastolic blood pressure (chart on the right) for males ages 35 to 57 years participating in the Multiple Risk Factor Intervention Trial (N = 347,978). The curved lines represent the 12-year rate of cardiovascular mortality for each level of systolic blood pressure (SBP) and diastolic blood pressure (DBP). As either SBP or DBP increases, risk of death from cardiovascular disease increases.

Source: Adapted from National High Blood Pressure Education Program Working Group. 1993. National High Blood Pressure Education Program Working Group report on primary prevention of hypertension. *Archives of Internal Medicine* 153:186–208.

value recorded.[88] In ambulatory blood pressure monitoring (ABPM), the subject wears a device that periodically measures and records blood pressure over a period of 24 hours or longer. For some patients, ABPM is a better indicator of average blood pressure, particularly for patients who experience "white-coat hypertension," a temporary increase in blood pressure when it is measured in the medical care environment. Values obtained from ABPM are generally lower than those obtained when blood pressure is measured in a clinic setting. Self-monitoring of blood pressure is also a recommended approach, as long as the sphygmomanometer is reliable and properly calibrated and the subject is instructed in the correct operation of the unit.[88]

Table 8.16 shows the guidelines developed by the National High Blood Pressure Education Program for classifying blood pressure.[88] To be considered within the normal range, systolic blood pressure must be < 120 mm Hg and diastolic pressure must be < 80 mm Hg. The recently introduced classification of *prehypertension* is defined as a systolic blood pressure ranging from 120 to 139 mm Hg and/or a diastolic blood pressure of 80 to 89 mm Hg. Introduction of the prehypertension category reflects the fact that the risk of cardiovascular and kidney disease is increased at levels of blood pressure previously thought to be normal. While prehypertension is not a disease category, it identifies high-risk persons who should modify their lifestyle practices to reduce their blood pressure, to decrease the risk that their blood pressure will progress to hypertensive levels with increasing age, or to prevent hypertension entirely.[88] Lifestyle modifications are generally sufficient to normalize the blood pressure in persons with prehypertension. However, persons with prehypertension who also have diabetes or kidney disease should be considered candidates for appropriate drug therapy if lifestyle modifications fail to normalize their blood pressure.[88] Approximately 30% of U.S. adults (more than 75 million people) have hypertension and another 30% have prehypertension.[1] Risk of hypertension increases with age, as shown in Figure 8.13. Not

TABLE 8.16 Classification of Blood Pressure for Persons Age 18 Years and Older*

	Systolic BP (mm Hg)		Diastolic BP (mm Hg)
Normal†	< 120	and	< 80
Prehypertension	120–139	or	80–89
Stage 1 hypertension	140–159	or	90–99
Stage 2 hypertension	≥ 160	or	≥ 100

Adapted from National High Blood Pressure Education Program. 2004. *The seventh report of the Joint National Committee on Prevention, Detection, Evaluation, and Treatment of High Blood Pressure.* U.S. Department of Health and Human Services, National Institutes of Health, National Heart, Lung, and Blood Institute.

*Not taking antihypertensive drugs and not acutely ill.

†Based on the average of two or more properly measured, seated, blood pressure readings taken at each of two or more visits after an initial screening.

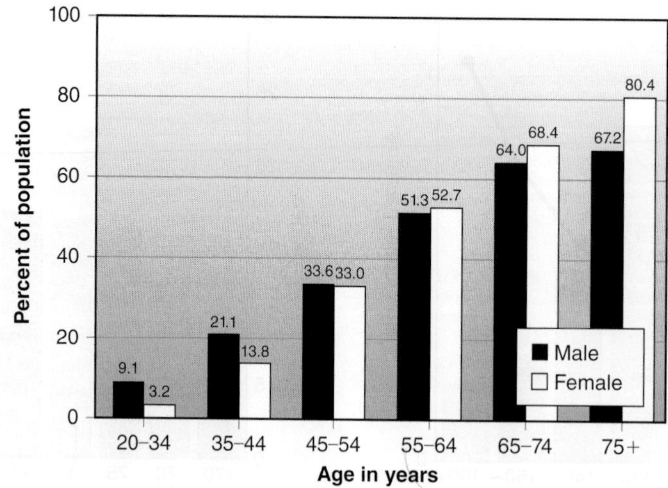

Figure 8.13 Prevalence of hypertension among U.S. adults, age 20 years and older, 2007–2010.
A person with hypertension is defined as someone taking antihypertensive medication or having a systolic blood pressure ≥ 140 mm Hg or a diastolic blood pressure ≥ 90 mm Hg.
Source: Data from the National Center for Health Statistics.

only are black males and females more likely to have hypertension than are white males and females (as shown in Figure 8.14), but hypertension among blacks is more severe, develops at an earlier age, and leads to more health problems such as coronary heart disease, stroke, and kidney failure.[88]

Efforts to reduce morbidity and mortality related to hypertension can be grouped into two broad categories: the patient-based, or clinical, approach and the population-based, or public health, approach. Early efforts to reduce hypertension-related morbidity and mortality centered on the patient-based approach, which involves clinicians detecting and treating individual cases of hypertension. More recently, greater attention has been given to the population-based approach, which stresses increased public awareness of hypertension and encourages every adult to know his or her blood pressure and to avoid those behaviors identified as risk factors for hyper tension. These efforts have been quite successful, as demonstrated by the dramatic decline in deaths from coronary heart disease and stroke, as was shown in Figures 8.7 and 8.8.

Another indicator of success is shown in Figure 8.15. Using data from NHANES II (1976–80), NHANES III Phase 1 (1988–91), NHANES III Phase 2 (1991–94), NHANES 1999–2000, and NHANES 2005–2008, Figure 8.15 shows general improvement during those years in the percentage of persons with hypertension who are aware of their condition, who are being treated, and whose hypertension is under control. According to the latest data shown in Figure 8.15, 80% of persons with hypertension are aware of their condition, 71% are treated, and 48% have adequate control of their blood pressure. This lack of awareness and inadequate control can result in significant vascular damage to the eyes, heart, kidneys, and brain. Although pharmacologic therapy for hypertension markedly reduces mortality and

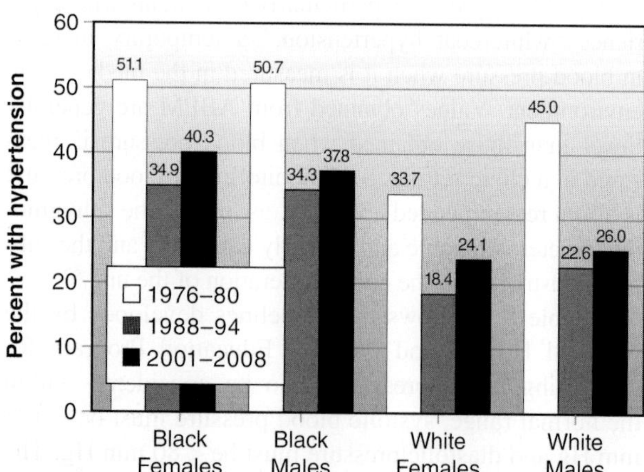

Figure 8.14 The age-adjusted prevalence of hypertension among U.S. adults, 20 to 74 years of age, by sex and race, 1976–80, 1988–94, 2001–2008.
Between the survey periods of 1976–80 and 1988–94 the prevalence of hypertension decreased in all four of the groups shown, but it increased in the most recent survey period. Blacks have a higher prevalence of hypertension than whites. Hypertension is defined as a systolic blood pressure ≥ 140 mm Hg or a diastolic blood pressure ≥ 90 mm Hg or the need to take antihypertensive medication.
Source: Data from the National Center for Health Statistics.

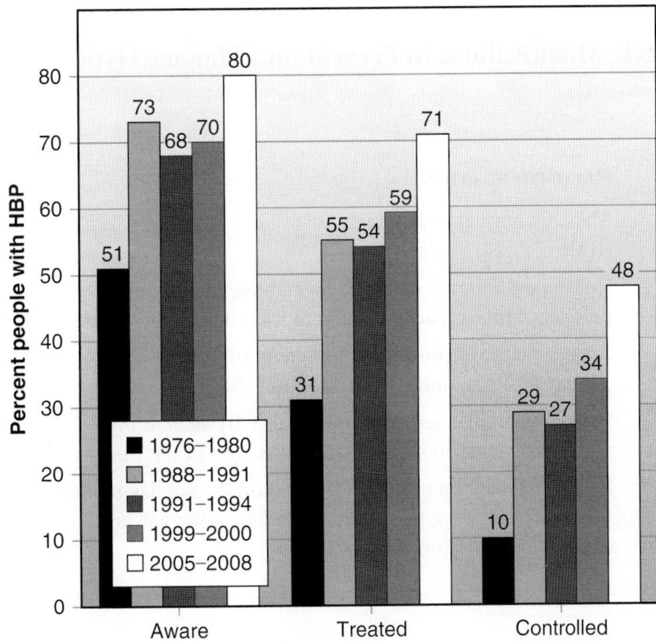

Figure 8.15 Trends in the awareness, treatment, and control of hypertension among U.S. adults, 18 to 74 years of age, 1976–1980, 1988–1991, 1991–1994, 1999–2000, and 2005–2008.
Since the survey period of 1976–1980, the percentage of Americans with hypertension who are aware of their condition, who are being treated, and whose hypertension is controlled has increased considerably.
Source: Data from the National Center for Health Statistics.

morbidity from cardiovascular disease and stroke, long-term pharmacologic therapy involves the expense of ongoing medical supervision and carries with it undesirable side effects. Even with optimal blood pressure control, persons with hypertension still have a higher morbidity and mortality than persons with normal or optimal blood pressure.[88] Thus, there remains a need to increase efforts to promote hypertension awareness and to identify and modify risk factors leading to high blood pressure.

Increasing attention is being given to primary prevention of hypertension using the population-based approach by modifying risk factors associated with hypertension. The most important of these risk factors are a high sodium intake, excessive consumption of energy, physical inactivity, excessive alcohol consumption, and inadequate potassium intake. Box 8.5 lists lifestyle modifications having proven efficacy in preventing and managing hypertension and approximate reduction in systolic blood pressure expected from the modification. Clinical trials have shown that lifestyle modifications involving these lifestyle factors can lower elevated blood pressure at little cost, with minimal risk, and to an extent equal to or greater than single-drug therapy.[88–91] Even when these modifications fail to control hypertension, they can reduce the number and dosage of antihypertensive medications needed to manage the condition—what is referred to as a "step-down" in therapy. Primary prevention is particularly helpful in lowering the elevated blood pressures of persons in groups at higher risk of hypertension, such as African Americans, older persons, and persons with hypertension or diabetes.[88]

Body Weight

The evidence linking body weight to blood pressure and overweight to hypertension is strong and consistent. A body mass index $\geq$ 27 kg/m^2 is closely correlated with increased blood pressure. Excess adipose tissue within the abdomen (abdominal fat) has been associated with increased risk of hypertension, dyslipidemia, type 2 diabetes, and coronary heart disease.[88] As discussed in Chapter 6, the best clinical approach to assessing abdominal adiposity is measuring waist circumference. A high-risk waist circumference in adult males and females as > 40 in. and > 35 in., respectively. Several studies have shown that loss of excess body weight reduces both SBP and DBP and that the degree of blood pressure reduction is related to the extent of weight loss. A weight reduction of as little as 10 pounds is effective at reducing elevated blood pressure in overweight persons with hypertension, while enhancing the effectiveness of antihypertensive drugs and reducing

Box 8.5 Lifestyle Modifications to Prevent and Manage Hypertension

Modification	Recommendation	Approximate Systolic BP Reduction (Range)[1]
Weight reduction	Maintain normal body weight (BMI 18.5–24.9 kg/m^2)	5–20 mm Hg per 10 kg weight loss
Adopt DASH eating plan[2]	Consume a diet rich in fruits, vegetables, and lowfat dairy products with a reduced content of saturated and total fat	8–14 mm Hg
Dietary sodium reduction	Reduce dietary sodium intake to no more than 100 mmol per day (2.4 g sodium or 6.0 g sodium chloride)	2–8 mm Hg
Physical activity	Engage in regular aerobic physical activity such as brisk walking (at least 30 min per day, most days of the week)	4–9 mm Hg
Moderation of alcohol consumption	Limit consumption to no more than 2 drinks per day in most men and to no more than 1 drink per day in women and lighter weight persons	2–4 mm Hg

[1]The effects of implementing these modifications are dose and time dependent and could be greater for some individuals.
[2]DASH = Dietary Approaches to Stop Hypertension.
For overall cardiovascular risk reduction, stop smoking.

Source: National High Blood Pressure Education Program. 2004. *The seventh report of the Joint National Committee on Prevention, Detection, Evaluation, and Treatment of High Blood Pressure.* U.S. Department of Health and Human Services, National Institutes of Health, National Heart, Lung, and Blood Institute.

cardiovascular disease risk by enhancing the management of type 2 diabetes and dyslipidemia.[88]

The largest randomized controlled trial to evaluate the impact of weight loss in persons with high-normal blood pressure, the Trials of Hypertension Prevention, showed that an average weight loss of 8.4 lb (3.8 kg) resulted in a 2.9 mm Hg and 2.3 mm Hg reduction in SBP and DBP, respectively.[89,92] Although this may seem like an insignificant decline in blood pressure, it has been estimated that a 2 mm Hg decline in the population mean SBP might reduce the annual mortality from stroke, CHD, and all causes by 6%, 4%, and 3%, respectively.[88] Not only is weight loss an effective means of lowering blood pressure, but it also tends to improve the lipid and lipoprotein profile and reduce the risk of developing noninsulin-dependent diabetes mellitus and possibly breast cancer.

Sodium

Research on the association between sodium intake and blood pressure has been hampered by several methodologic challenges. These include difficulty in measuring sodium intake, variable adherence to the prescribed reduction in sodium, the large day-to-day intraindividual (within-person) variation in sodium intake, the wide range of blood pressure values at any level of sodium intake, the small interindividual (between-person) variation in sodium intakes within a given population group, inadequate trial design, small numbers of subjects, and limitations in analysis and presentation of research findings. Despite these challenges, there is unequivocal evidence that a causal relationship exists between sodium intake and risk of hypertension, particularly from those studies that determine sodium intake by measuring 24-hour urinary sodium excretion, which is the definitive method for determining sodium intake.[92–94]

Based on data from NHANES 2008–2010, the estimated mean sodium intake of American males age 20 years of age and older is approximately 4043 mg per day, and for American females of the same age it is approximately 2900 mg per day. This intake is far in excess of human physiologic need and is much greater than the typical intakes of people in less industrialized societies, who do not experience North America's age-related increase in blood pressure. The Adequate Intake (AI) (discussed in Chapter 2) for sodium for males and females ages 14 to 50 years in 1500 mg per day.[93] The AI for persons 51 to 70 years of age is 1300 mg per day, and for persons older than 70 years it is 1200 mg per day. The Tolerable Upper Intake Level (UL) (discussed in Chapter 2) for sodium for all age groups is 2300 mg per day.[93] The *Dietary Guidelines for Americans* recommend limiting sodium intake to less than 2300 mg per day. However, persons 51 years of age and older and those of any age who are African American or have hypertension, diabetes, or chronic kidney disease should limit their sodium intake to 1500 mg per day. The 1500 mg recommendations applies to about 50% of the U.S. population, including children and the majority of adults. Research shows that for most people, a reduction in sodium intake to the current AI of 1500 mg per day is safe and is an effective way to reduce risk for hypertension.[88,90,93,94] Furthermore, the blood pressures of blacks, middle-aged and older persons, and those with hypertension are more responsive to changes in dietary sodium. A modest reduction in sodium intake to less than 2300 mg per day and adoption of some of the other lifestyle changes shown in Box 8.5 are sufficient to control mild hypertension in many patients. For those still needing antihypertensive medication, these steps will reduce their requirement for medication (result in a step-down in therapy).[88,90,94]

Data from the Dietary Approaches to Stop Hypertension (DASH) trial show that a further reduction in sodium intake to 1.5 g per day provides a safe and effective way to further reduce risk for hypertension. The DASH trial was a multicenter, randomized feeding trial testing the effects of certain dietary patterns on blood pressure. These and other data provide a scientific basis for a lower goal for dietary sodium than the level currently recommended.[90,94]

Maintaining a sodium intake of < 2300 mg per day is difficult, considering the high-salt food environment in the United States and the fact that approximately 77% of sodium in the U.S. diet comes from processed foods. Between the early 1970s and 2000, sodium intake in the United States rose 55%, primarily because of increased consumption of fast foods and convenience foods during that interval.[95] A sodium intake of < 2300 mg per day has been a "cornerstone" of the recommendations from the National Heart, Lung, and Blood Institute's National High Blood Pressure Education Program and other groups working to decrease the prevalence of hypertension in the United States. One of the *Healthy People 2020* objectives is for Americans 2 years of age and older to reduce their sodium intake to no more than 2300 mg per day.[95] In 2003, the American Public Health Association adopted a resolution calling for a 50% reduction in the amount of sodium in processed and restaurant foods over a 10-year period. In 2006, the American Medical Association issued a report that urged the U.S. Food and Drug Administration to revoke the "generally recognized as safe" (GRAS) status of salt and to develop regulatory measures to limit sodium in processed and restaurant foods. The report also called for at least a 50% reduction in the amount of sodium in processed and restaurant foods over a 10-year period, new labeling initiatives to assist consumers in understanding the amount of sodium in processed foods, and a public health campaign to educate consumers about the long-term benefits of reducing sodium intake.[95] In 2007, the World Health Organization issued a report that said there is conclusive evidence that excess sodium causes hypertension and that called for the global reformulation of processed and prepared foods to achieve the lowest possible sodium content along with consumer education and the creation of a food environment that facilitates the selection of low-sodium foods.[95]

Alcohol

Despite the difficulty of measuring the alcohol intake of study participants, there is consistent evidence of a strong positive relationship between alcohol consumption and blood pressure. It is estimated that as much as 5% to 7% of the overall prevalence of hypertension in the United States can be attributed to an alcohol intake of three drinks or more per day.[88] One drink of alcohol (0.5 fluid ounce of ethanol) is equivalent to 12 fluid ounces of beer, 4 fluid ounces of wine, or 1 ounce of 100-proof spirits. Furthermore, when alcohol intake is reduced, there is a subsequent reduction in blood pressure. A reduction in alcohol intake has been shown to be effective in lowering blood pressure in both hypertensive and normotensive individuals, and it may help prevent hypertension. Persons with hypertension should be advised to limit their alcohol intake to no more than two drinks per day.[88]

Physical Activity

Numerous studies have shown an inverse relationship between leisure-time and work-related physical activity and blood pressure. Other studies have shown that blood pressure tends to be lower in physically fit individuals. Although these studies have certain design limitations, they provide consistent evidence that increased physical activity results in an average reduction of approximately 6 to 7 mm Hg for both SBP and DBP. This reduction is not dependent on weight loss. A low to moderate exercise intensity (40% to 60% of maximum oxygen consumption) is as effective at lowering blood pressure in patients with mild to moderate hypertension as higher-intensity exercise. This can be achieved by brisk walking for 30 to 45 minutes most days of the week.[88]

Dietary Pattern

A number of studies have identified an inverse relationship between blood pressure and consumption of foods providing potassium, calcium, and magnesium. Persons consuming vegetarian diets, for example, tend to have a lower blood pressure than nonvegetarians. Aspects of the vegetarian diet believed to reduce blood pressure include minerals (potassium, calcium, and magnesium), reduced fat content, and possibly dietary fiber.[96,97] In studies investigating individual nutrients, often when provided in supplemental form, the reduction in blood pressure is typically small and inconsistent, probably because the blood pressure–lowering effect of a single nutrient is too small to detect in clinical trials. However, when these nutrients are consumed together, the cumulative effect is sufficient to bring about a statistically and clinically significant lowering of blood pressure. Food is incredibly complex and contains countless nutrients and components other than those few being examined in trials or measured in observational studies. When evaluating the blood pressure–lowering effects of foods, these nutrients and food components and the complex interactions among them must be considered.[96,97]

Consequently, increased attention is being given to the overall dietary pattern, rather than to a few individual nutrients. This is in large part due to results from the Dietary Approaches to Stop Hypertension (DASH) trial.[90,97] The DASH trial showed that a diet rich in fruits, vegetables, and fat-free or low-fat dairy products lowers elevated blood pressure, particularly when sodium intake is kept moderate.[90,97] The DASH diet, combined with a moderate sodium restriction and sustained efforts to modify the other factors associated with hypertension, which were listed in Box 8.5, is a safe, effective, and low-cost nonpharmacologic approach for promoting optimal to normal blood pressure.

Evaluating Blood Pressure in Children and Adolescents

As shown in Box 8.6, hypertension in children and adolescents age 1 to 17 years is defined as an average systolic blood pressure (SBP) and/or diastolic blood pressure (DBP) that is greater than or equal to the 95th percentile of blood pressure for a young person of a given sex, age, and height.[98] Prehypertension in children and adolescents age 1 to 17 years is defined as average SBP or DBP levels that are ≥ 90th percentile but < 95th percentile. This somewhat arbitrary definition of hypertension is based on the normative distribution of blood pressure in apparently healthy children and adolescents in which those in the top 5% for a given sex, age, and height are categorized as hypertensive. In adults, blood pressure is categorized on the basis of clinical outcomes, with a normal blood pressure being one associated with a low-risk of disease and with hypertension associated with increasing risk of disease such as CHD, stroke, or kidney failure. Because these diseases are rarely *clinically evident* in young people, even those with hypertension, a different strategy must be used to establish categories of normal blood pressure, prehypertension, and hypertension.[98] It is important to identify and effectively treat children with hypertension because target-organ damage can occur at a young age in children and adolescents with hypertension.[98,99]

To evaluate the blood pressure of a child or adolescent, it is necessary to determine his or her percentile of height for sex and age. This is done using the sex- and age-appropriate CDC growth charts that provide the length-for-age percentiles (for children ≤ 3 years of age who are unable to stand on their own without assistance) or the stature-for-age percentiles (for those ≥ 2 years of age who are able to stand on their own without assistance). The CDC growth charts are discussed in Chapter 6 and shown in Appendix K. Once the subject's percentile of height is determined, Table 8.17 or 8.18 is used to determine the blood pressure percentile. Consider, for example, a 9-year-old male who is 53 inches tall and whose blood pressure, averaged from multiple measurements taken during three different visits to a physician's office, is shown to be 116/76 mm Hg. Using the appropriate CDC growth chart (2 to 20 years: boys, stature-for-age and weight-for-age percentiles) shown in Appendix K, it is determined that this youngster is at the 50th percentile of height (i.e., stature) for age. Table 8.17 is then used to categorize the systolic and diastolic blood pressure. For this youngster, an SBP of 116 mm Hg lies between the values of 114 and 118 mm Hg, which is between the 90th and 95th percentiles of SBP. The DBP of 76 mm Hg lies between the values of 75 and 79 mm Hg, which is between the 90th and 95th percentiles of DBP. Based on the information given in Box 8.6, this youngster's blood pressure would be categorized as prehypertension.[98]

The National High Blood Pressure Education Program recommends that after 3 years of age, all children and adolescents have their blood pressure measured every time they are seen in a health care setting.[98] Measuring blood pressure in children less than 3 years of age is not recommended unless special circumstances exist, such

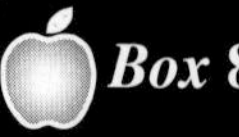

Box 8.6 Evaluating Blood Pressure in Children and Adolescents

- Hypertension is defined as an average SBP and/or DBP that is greater than or equal to the 95th percentile for sex, age, and height on three or more occasions.
- Prehypertension in children is defined as average SBP or DBP levels that are greater than or equal to the 90th percentile but less than the 95th percentile.
- As with adults, adolescents with BP levels greater than or equal to 120/80 mm Hg but less than the 95th percentile should be considered prehypertensive.
- A patient with BP levels above the 95th percentile in a physician's office or clinic but who is normotensive outside a clinical setting has white-coat hypertension. Ambulatory BP monitoring (ABPM) is usually required to make this diagnosis.

Source: National High Blood Pressure Education Program. 2005. *The fourth report on the diagnosis, evaluation, and treatment of high blood pressure in children and adolescents.* U.S. Department of Health and Human Services, National Institutes of Health, National Heart, Lung, and Blood Institute.

TABLE 8.17 Blood Pressure Levels for Males by Age and Height Percentiles

Age, y	BP percentile	SBP, mm Hg							DBP, mm Hg						
		Percentile of height							Percentile of height						
		5th	10th	25th	50th	75th	90th	95th	5th	10th	25th	50th	75th	90th	95th
1	50th	80	81	83	85	87	88	89	34	35	36	37	38	39	39
	90th	94	95	97	99	100	102	103	49	50	51	52	53	53	54
	95th	98	99	101	103	104	106	106	54	54	55	56	57	58	58
	99th	105	106	108	110	112	113	114	61	62	63	64	65	66	66
2	50th	84	85	87	88	90	92	92	39	40	41	42	43	44	44
	90th	97	99	100	102	104	105	106	54	55	56	57	58	58	59
	95th	101	102	104	106	108	109	110	59	59	60	61	62	63	63
	99th	109	110	111	113	115	117	117	66	67	68	69	70	71	71
3	50th	86	87	89	91	93	94	95	44	44	45	46	47	48	48
	90th	100	101	103	105	107	108	109	59	59	60	61	62	63	63
	95th	104	105	107	109	110	112	113	63	63	64	65	66	67	67
	99th	111	112	114	116	118	119	120	71	71	72	73	74	75	75
4	50th	88	89	91	93	95	96	97	47	48	49	50	51	51	52
	90th	102	103	105	107	109	110	111	62	63	64	65	66	66	67
	95th	106	107	109	111	112	114	115	66	67	68	69	70	71	71
	99th	113	114	116	118	120	121	122	74	75	76	77	78	78	79
5	50th	90	91	93	95	96	98	98	50	51	52	53	54	55	55
	90th	104	105	106	108	110	111	112	65	66	67	68	69	69	70
	95th	108	109	110	112	114	115	116	69	70	71	72	73	74	74
	99th	115	116	118	120	121	123	123	77	78	79	80	81	81	82
6	50th	91	92	94	96	98	99	100	53	53	54	55	56	57	57
	90th	105	106	108	110	111	113	113	68	68	69	70	71	72	72
	95th	109	110	112	114	115	117	117	72	72	73	74	75	76	76
	99th	116	117	119	121	123	124	125	80	80	81	82	83	84	84
7	50th	92	94	95	97	99	100	101	55	55	56	57	58	59	59
	90th	106	107	109	111	113	114	115	70	70	71	72	73	74	74
	95th	110	111	113	115	117	118	119	74	74	75	76	77	78	78
	99th	117	118	120	122	124	125	126	82	82	83	84	85	86	86
8	50th	94	95	97	99	100	102	102	56	57	58	59	60	60	61
	90th	107	109	110	112	114	115	116	71	72	72	73	74	75	76
	95th	111	112	114	116	118	119	120	75	76	77	78	79	79	80
	99th	119	120	122	123	125	127	127	83	84	85	86	87	87	88
9	50th	95	96	98	100	102	103	104	57	58	59	60	61	61	62
	90th	109	110	112	114	115	117	118	72	73	74	75	76	76	77
	95th	113	114	116	118	119	121	121	76	77	78	79	80	81	81
	99th	120	121	123	125	127	128	129	84	85	86	87	88	88	89

(continued)

Table 8.17 Blood Pressure Levels for Males by Age and Height Percentiles—*continued*

		SBP, mm Hg							DBP, mm Hg						
		Percentile of height							Percentile of height						
Age, y	BP percentile	5th	10th	25th	50th	75th	90th	95th	5th	10th	25th	50th	75th	90th	95th
10	50th	97	98	100	102	103	105	106	58	59	60	61	61	62	63
	90th	111	112	114	115	117	119	119	73	73	74	75	76	77	78
	95th	115	116	117	119	121	122	123	77	78	79	80	81	81	82
	99th	122	123	125	127	128	130	130	85	86	86	88	88	89	90
11	50th	99	100	102	104	105	107	107	59	59	60	61	62	63	63
	90th	113	114	115	117	119	120	121	74	74	75	76	77	78	78
	95th	117	118	119	121	123	124	125	78	78	79	80	81	82	82
	99th	124	125	127	129	130	132	132	86	86	87	88	89	90	90
12	50th	101	102	104	106	108	109	110	59	60	61	62	63	63	64
	90th	115	116	118	120	121	123	123	74	75	75	76	77	78	79
	95th	119	120	122	123	125	127	127	78	79	80	81	82	82	83
	99th	126	127	129	131	133	134	135	86	87	88	89	90	90	91
13	50th	104	105	106	108	110	111	112	60	60	61	62	63	64	64
	90th	117	118	120	122	124	125	126	75	75	76	77	78	79	79
	95th	121	122	124	126	128	129	130	79	79	80	81	82	83	83
	99th	128	130	131	133	135	136	137	87	87	88	89	90	91	91
14	50th	106	107	109	111	113	114	115	60	61	62	63	64	65	65
	90th	120	121	123	125	126	128	128	75	76	77	78	79	79	80
	95th	124	125	127	128	130	132	132	80	80	81	82	83	84	84
	99th	131	132	134	136	138	139	140	87	88	89	90	91	92	92
15	50th	109	110	112	113	115	117	117	61	62	63	64	65	66	66
	90th	122	124	125	127	129	130	131	76	77	78	79	80	80	81
	95th	126	127	129	131	133	134	135	81	81	82	83	84	85	85
	99th	134	135	136	138	140	142	142	88	89	90	91	92	93	93
16	50th	111	112	114	116	118	119	120	63	63	64	65	66	67	67
	90th	125	126	128	130	131	133	134	78	78	79	80	81	82	82
	95th	129	130	132	134	135	137	137	82	83	83	84	85	86	87
	99th	136	137	139	141	143	144	145	90	90	91	92	93	94	94
17	50th	114	115	116	118	120	121	122	65	66	66	67	68	69	70
	90th	127	128	130	132	134	135	136	80	80	81	82	83	84	84
	95th	131	132	134	136	138	139	140	84	85	86	87	87	88	89
	99th	139	140	141	143	145	146	147	92	93	93	94	95	96	97

SBP = systolic blood pressure; DBP = diastolic blood pressure; Age is in years.

National High Blood Pressure Education Program. 2005. *The fourth report on the diagnosis, evaluation, and treatment of high blood pressure in children and adolescents.* Bethesda, MD: U.S. Department of Health and Human Services, National Institutes of Health, National Heart, Lung, and Blood Institute.

Table 8.18 Blood Pressure Levels for Females by Age and Height Percentiles

Age, y	BP percentile	SBP, mm Hg							DBP, mm Hg						
		Percentile of height							Percentile of height						
		5th	10th	25th	50th	75th	90th	95th	5th	10th	25th	50th	75th	90th	95th
1	50th	83	84	85	86	88	89	90	38	39	39	40	41	41	42
	90th	97	97	98	100	101	102	103	52	53	53	54	55	55	56
	95th	100	101	102	104	105	106	107	56	57	57	58	59	59	60
	99th	108	108	109	111	112	113	114	64	64	65	65	66	67	67
2	50th	85	85	87	88	89	91	91	43	44	44	45	46	46	47
	90th	98	99	100	101	103	104	105	57	58	58	59	60	61	61
	95th	102	103	104	105	107	108	109	61	62	62	63	64	65	65
	99th	109	110	111	112	114	115	116	69	69	70	70	71	72	72
3	50th	86	87	88	89	91	92	93	47	48	48	49	50	50	51
	90th	100	100	102	103	104	106	106	61	62	62	63	64	64	65
	95th	104	104	105	107	108	109	110	65	66	66	67	68	68	69
	99th	111	111	113	114	115	116	117	73	73	74	74	75	76	76
4	50th	88	88	90	91	92	94	94	50	50	51	52	52	53	54
	90th	101	102	103	104	106	107	108	64	64	65	66	67	67	68
	95th	105	106	107	108	110	111	112	68	68	69	70	71	71	72
	99th	112	113	114	115	117	118	119	76	76	76	77	78	79	79
5	50th	89	90	91	93	94	95	96	52	53	53	54	55	55	56
	90th	103	103	105	106	107	109	109	66	67	67	68	69	69	70
	95th	107	107	108	110	111	112	113	70	71	71	72	73	73	74
	99th	114	114	116	117	118	120	120	78	78	79	79	80	81	81
6	50th	91	92	93	94	96	97	98	54	54	55	56	56	57	58
	90th	104	105	106	108	109	110	111	68	68	69	70	70	71	72
	95th	108	109	110	111	113	114	115	72	72	73	74	74	75	76
	99th	115	116	117	119	120	121	122	80	80	80	81	82	83	83
7	50th	93	93	95	96	97	99	99	55	56	56	57	58	58	59
	90th	106	107	108	109	111	112	113	69	70	70	71	72	72	73
	95th	110	111	112	113	115	116	116	73	74	74	75	76	76	77
	99th	117	118	119	120	122	123	124	81	81	82	82	83	84	84
8	50th	95	95	96	98	99	100	101	57	57	57	58	59	60	60
	90th	108	109	110	111	113	114	114	71	71	71	72	73	74	74
	95th	112	112	114	115	116	118	118	75	75	75	76	77	78	78
	99th	119	120	121	122	123	125	125	82	82	83	83	84	85	86
9	50th	96	97	98	100	101	102	103	58	58	58	59	60	61	61
	90th	110	110	112	113	114	116	116	72	72	72	73	74	75	75
	95th	114	114	115	117	118	119	120	76	76	76	77	78	79	79
	99th	121	121	123	124	125	127	127	83	83	84	84	85	86	87

(continued)

TABLE 8.18 Blood Pressure Levels for Females by Age and Height Percentiles—*continued*

		SBP, mm Hg							DBP, mm Hg						
		Percentile of height							Percentile of height						
Age, y	BP percentile	5th	10th	25th	50th	75th	90th	95th	5th	10th	25th	50th	75th	90th	95th
10	50th	98	99	100	102	103	104	105	59	59	59	60	61	62	62
	90th	112	112	114	115	116	118	118	73	73	73	74	75	76	76
	95th	116	116	117	119	120	121	122	77	77	77	78	79	80	80
	99th	123	123	125	126	127	129	129	84	84	85	86	86	87	88
11	50th	100	101	102	103	105	106	107	60	60	60	61	62	63	63
	90th	114	114	116	117	118	119	120	74	74	74	75	76	77	77
	95th	118	118	119	121	122	123	124	78	78	78	79	80	81	81
	99th	125	125	126	128	129	130	131	85	85	86	87	87	88	89
12	50th	102	103	104	105	107	108	109	61	61	61	62	63	64	64
	90th	116	116	117	119	120	121	122	75	75	75	76	77	78	78
	95th	119	120	121	123	124	125	126	79	79	79	80	81	82	82
	99th	127	127	128	130	131	132	133	86	86	87	88	88	89	90
13	50th	104	105	106	107	109	110	110	62	62	62	63	64	65	65
	90th	117	118	119	121	122	123	124	76	76	76	77	78	79	79
	95th	121	122	123	124	126	127	128	80	80	80	81	82	83	83
	99th	128	129	130	132	133	134	135	87	87	88	89	89	90	91
14	50th	106	106	107	109	110	111	112	63	63	63	64	65	66	66
	90th	119	120	121	122	124	125	125	77	77	77	78	79	80	80
	95th	123	123	125	126	127	129	129	81	81	81	82	83	84	84
	99th	130	131	132	133	135	136	136	88	88	89	90	90	91	92
15	50th	107	108	109	110	111	113	113	64	64	64	65	66	67	67
	90th	120	121	122	123	125	126	127	78	78	78	79	80	81	81
	95th	124	125	126	127	129	130	131	82	82	82	83	84	85	85
	99th	131	132	133	134	136	137	138	89	89	90	91	91	92	93
16	50th	108	108	110	111	112	114	114	64	64	65	66	66	67	68
	90th	121	122	123	124	126	127	128	78	78	79	80	81	81	82
	95th	125	126	127	128	130	131	132	82	82	83	84	85	85	86
	99th	132	133	134	135	137	138	139	90	90	90	91	92	93	93
17	50th	108	109	110	111	113	114	115	64	65	65	66	67	67	68
	90th	122	122	123	125	126	127	128	78	79	79	80	81	81	82
	95th	125	126	127	129	130	131	132	82	83	83	84	85	85	86
	99th	133	133	134	136	137	138	139	90	90	91	91	92	93	93

SBP = systolic blood pressure; DBP = diastolic blood pressure; Age is in years.

National High Blood Pressure Education Program. 2005. *The fourth report on the diagnosis, evaluation, and treatment of high blood pressure in children and adolescents.* Bethesda, MD: U.S. Department of Health and Human Services, National Institutes of Health, National Heart, Lung, and Blood Institute.

as a previous neonatal complication that required intensive care, congenital heart disease, recurrent urinary tract problems, treatment with drugs known to raise blood pressure, or the presence of some other disease associated with hypertension.[98] Blood pressure should be measured after the subject has been quietly and comfortably seated for 5 minutes with both feet on the floor and the back supported. Subjects should avoid consuming stimulant drugs or foods prior to the visit with the health care provider. Using the appropriate size cuff is important, and specific recommendations on cuff size have been published.[98] If the cuff size is too small, the blood pressure measurement will be erroneously high. A cuff that is too large will cause blood pressure to be underestimated, but not to the extent that an inappropriately small cuff will cause blood pressure to be overestimated.[98] An instance of elevated systolic and/or diastolic blood pressure must be confirmed by repeat measurement on at least two additional occasions in order to confirm a diagnosis of prehypertension or hypertension. Blood pressure should be measured two or more times per health care visit, and values obtained over the course of at least three different visits should be averaged.

OSTEOPOROSIS

Osteoporosis, the most common bone disorder in humans, is characterized by the loss of bone mass and deterioration of bone microarchitecture, compromised bone strength, and an increased susceptibility to fracture and painful morbidity.[100,101] Bone strength is a function of two factors: bone mineral density and bone quality. Bone mineral density accounts for approximately 70% of bone strength and is expressed as grams of mineral per area or volume of bone. Bone density is determined by peak bone mass and the amount of bone loss. Bone quality relates to bone architecture, bone turnover, mineralization, and the accumulation of damage to the bone (e.g., microfractures). Figure 8.16 illustrates how bone architecture and density can differ between normal bone and that from an individual with osteoporosis. When sufficient force is applied to osteoporotic bone, a fracture occurs, making osteoporosis a significant risk factor for fracture. A fracture can occur not only from a traumatic event, such as a fall, but also from the stress placed on bone during normal lifting and bending.[100,101]

Osteoporosis is a major public health problem. In the United States and Canada, approximately 25% of postmenopausal white women have osteoporosis and an additional 50% of postmenopausal white women have low BMD and thus are at increased risk of fracture and future development of osteoporosis.[102,103] One out of every two white women in North America will experience an osteoporotic fracture at some time in her life.[102] Although osteoporosis is often considered a disease of women, it is a major health care problem in men. According to World Health Organization (WHO) estimates, the risk of suffering an osteoporotic fracture over the course of life is about 40% for women and about 13% for men.[103] Hip fractures have the greatest morbidity, mortality, and socioeconomic impact. Of those persons having a hip fracture, 20% die within 1 year, 28% require long-term care, and 50% never recover the ability to walk without assistance.[101,103] Hip and vertebral fractures often result in serious depression as patients grapple with pain, physical limitations, and lifestyle changes. Vertebral fractures result in back pain, height loss, and kyphosis, an abnormal backward curvature of the spine. Postural and height changes associated with kyphosis can limit activity (e.g., bending and reaching), cause restrictive lung disease, and alter abdominal anatomy, leading to constipation,

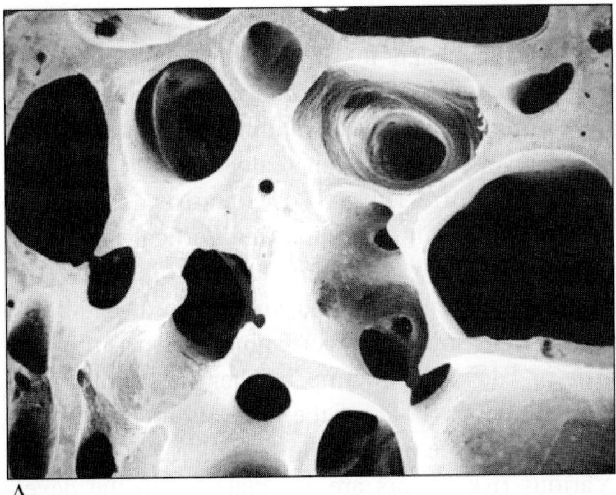

A

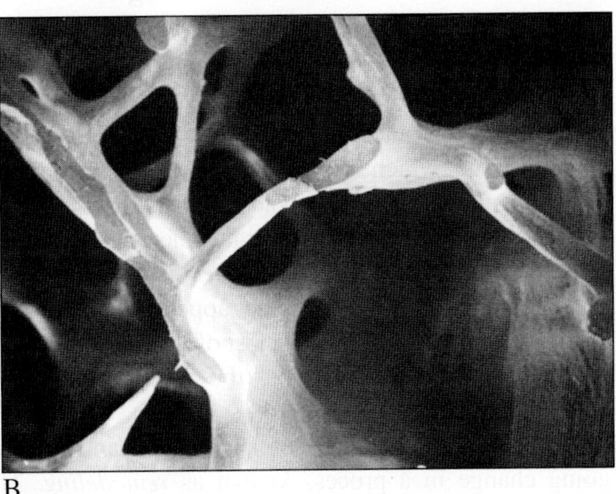

B

Figure 8.16 Scanning electron micrographs of bone biopsy specimens from the iliac crest: A is normal, and B is from a person with osteoporosis.

Source: Dempster DW, Shone E, Horbert W, Lindsay R. 1986. A simple method for correlative light and scanning electron microscopy of human iliac crest bone biopsies: Qualitative observations in normal and osteoporotic subjects. *Journal of Bone and Mineral Research* 1:15–21. Copyright © American Society for Bone and Mineral Research.

abdominal pain, reduced appetite, and premature satiety.[101–103] The annual economic burden of health care costs is estimated to be as high as $18 billion. Along with heart disease and breast cancer, it is one of the three most serious diseases affecting women.[101] Among Americans ages 50 years and older, 50% of females and 12% of males will have a osteoporosis-related fracture in their lifetime. For any given age, osteoporotic fractures are twice as common in females than in males, and, because they live longer than males, females experience an even higher absolute incidence during their lifetime.[101]

At about age 20 or 25 years, the bones of the human skeleton reach 90% to 95% of their *peak bone mass* (the point of maximum bone mineralization). Over the next 10 years, the final 5% to 10% of bone mineral is added, in a process known as *consolidation.* There is considerable interindividual variation in peak bone mass because of such factors as heredity, sex, race, and environmental factors. On average, males have 10% to 15% greater peak bone mass than females, and the bones of black persons are about 10% denser than those of white persons. Black males have the most dense bones, followed by white males, black females, and white females.[101,104]

Once peak mass is reached, bone mineral content begins to decline in both sexes at an annual rate of 0.3% to 0.5%.[101] In males, this gradual decline remains fairly constant, resulting in a lifetime bone mineral loss of 20% to 30%. In females, around the time of menopause (generally occurring at age 45 to 55 years) or following surgical removal of both ovaries, the rate of bone mineral loss temporarily accelerates to as high as 4% to 8% annually. Lifetime losses in females may be 40% to 50% or more of peak bone mass. The major factor in the higher rate of bone demineralization in the years immediately following menopause is apparently due to estrogen deficiency.[101]

Bones: Structure and Remodeling

Bones can be classified as being composed of two types of structural tissue: *cortical,* or *compact,* tissue and *trabecular,* or *cancellous,* tissue. The very dense cortical tissue forms the outer shells of bones, encasing the trabecular tissue, which is composed of a fine, spongelike mesh with numerous small voids. The marrow elements occupy these voids.[105,106] The total skeleton is composed of 80% cortical bone and 20% trabecular bone. Cortical bone is found primarily in the appendicular skeleton (bones of the limbs), whereas most of the trabecular bone is found in the axial skeleton (the skull and vertebral bones).[105,106]

Bone is a dynamic tissue and is constantly undergoing change in a process known as *remodeling.* The bone resorption cells, or osteoclasts, are active at numerous points within bone. They secrete enzymes that dissolve bone before it is reformed and provide a source of blood calcium when dietary intake is inadequate. The bone-forming cells, or osteoblasts, secrete an organic matrix composed largely of collagen. This matrix then becomes hardened by deposits of calcium and phosphate crystals known as *hydroxyapatite.* The rate of remodeling, or turnover rate, is approximately eight times faster in trabecular bone than in cortical bone, leading to a faster decline in bone mineral content in trabecular bone.[105] Consequently, symptoms of osteoporosis appear earlier in trabecular bone—in for example the spine (vertebral bodies) and wrist (distal radius).[105]

Osteoporosis: Classification and Risk Factors

Osteoporosis can be classified as either primary (not related to other disease) or secondary (when an identifiable cause other than age or menopause is present). Osteoporosis can be secondary to such conditions as Cushing's syndrome, malignancies of the bone (myeloma), hyperthyroidism, hyperparathyroidism, male hypogonadism, and amenorrhea. Certain inherited diseases, such as osteogenesis imperfecta, can also result in osteoporosis, as can long-term use of such medications as thiazide diuretics and heparin.[100,105] The most common form is primary osteoporosis, in which no other disease is apparent. This is most frequently seen in middle-aged and older females and older males. In these age groups, Type I and Type II primary osteoporosis are most commonly seen.[100,105]

Type I is seen in postmenopausal females between 51 and 75 years of age and primarily involves loss of trabecular bone. Low estrogen levels accompanying menopause lead to increased bone remodeling and accelerated bone loss. Production of vitamin D_3 and intestinal absorption of calcium often are decreased in postmenopausal women, exacerbating bone loss. This leads to fractures at sites where trabecular bone predominates (for example, vertebral bodies and the distal radius).[100,105]

Type II osteoporosis is seen in both sexes after age 70 years. It is related to several age-related changes, such as decreased osteoblast function, decreased calcium absorption, decreased vitamin D_3 synthesis, and decreased levels of calcitonin (calcitonin inhibits bone resorption).[100,105] In Type II osteoporosis, bone mineral is lost from both trabecular and cortical bone. The most common sites of fractures are the hip and vertebrae. Multiple fractures of the vertebrae can lead to a marked curvature of the thoracic spine known as *thoracic kyphosis* or "dowager's hump." Other sites include the proximal humerus (bone of the upper arm), pelvis, and proximal tibia (large bone of the lower leg).

Various risk factors are associated with the development of osteoporosis. These are shown in Table 8.19. Early menopause, either natural or surgically induced by removal of both ovaries (bilateral oophorectomy), shortens the time that a woman experiences estrogen's

TABLE 8.19 Risk Factors for Osteoporosis Fracture

Major Risk Factors
- Low bone mineral density
- Personal history of fracture as an adult
- History of fracture in a parent or sibling
- Female sex
- Age 65 years or older
- Caucasian race
- Menopause before age 45 years
- Premenopausal amenorrhea for 1 year or more
- Glucocorticoid therapy for ≥ 3 months
- Recurrent falls

Minor Risk Factors
- Impaired vision
- Dementia
- Alcoholism
- Low lifelong calcium and vitamin D intake
- Physical inactivity
- Poor health/frailty
- Current cigarette smoking
- Body weight < 127 lb (< 58 kg)

Adapted from National Osteoporosis Foundation. 2008. *Clinician's guide to prevention and treatment of osteoporosis.* Washington, DC: National Osteoporosis Foundation; Lindsay R, Cosman F. 2005. Osteoporosis. In Kasper DL, Braunwald E, Fauci AS, Hauser SL, Longo DL, Jameson JL (eds.), *Harrison's principles of internal medicine,* 16th ed. New York: McGraw-Hill, 2268–2278; Brown JP, Josse RG. 2002. 2002 clinical practice guidelines for the diagnosis and management of osteoporosis in Canada. *CMAJ* 167 (10 suppl):S1–S34.

protective effects and thus increases risk. Risk is also increased by menstrual irregularities (oligomenorrhea or amenorrhea) resulting from an unhealthfully low percent body fat. This may be due to excessive physical activity coupled with caloric restriction (as seen in some long-distance runners, gymnasts, and ballet dancers) or from eating disorders, such as anorexia nervosa or bulimia.

Peak bone mass is a major factor determining risk of developing osteoporosis. At any given age, risk for fracture is less in people who have achieved a greater peak bone mass during the period of bone development than in those with a lower peak bone mass. Because they have the greatest average peak bone mass, black males tend to develop osteoporosis least often of any sex/race group. Compared with white females, black females have a higher peak bone mass and, consequently, less incidence of osteoporosis.[100,101]

Diagnosing Osteoporosis

The most widely used method for diagnosing osteoporosis is bone densitometry, which is the measurement of bone mineral density (BMD).[100,101] At this time, there is no accurate way of measuring overall bone strength. However, because BMD accounts for approximately 60% to 80% of the variation in bone strength, it is generally used as a proxy measure of bone strength.[107–110] BMD measurements correlate strongly with the load-bearing capacity of the hip and spine and with fracture risk.[100–102] Over the past several decades, a variety of methods have been used to quantify bone mineral density. These included radiogrammetry (use of conventional X rays of the bones), single-photon absorptiometry, dual-photon absorptiometry, dual-energy X-ray absorptiometry, quantitative computed tomography, and quantitative ultrasound.[108–110] Other techniques, such as neutron activation analysis, Compton scattering, ultrasonic transmission velocity or attenuation, and magnetic resonance, are either not widely available or are in the early stages of development.[108–111] Of all these methods, the best and most widely used is dual-energy X-ray absorptiometry (DXA).[108,111] Another method used for screening individuals at high risk of low BMD is quantitative ultrasound.[111]

Dual-Energy X-Ray Absorptiometry

DXA is the preferred approach for measuring BMD because of its capacity to measure bone mineral content at axial and appendicular sites, its superior capabilities for monitoring changes in the skeleton over time and in response to osteoporosis treatment, its rapid scan time and low radiation exposure, and its superior quality-control procedures.[101–104,108–111] Figure 8.17 shows an example of a commercially available DXA unit, and Figure 8.18 gives an example of a DXA scan of the hip. In DXA, X-ray beams of two different energy levels are projected through the body and received by a detector opposite the X-ray source. As the X-ray beam passes through tissues that have different densities, the tissues attenuate or absorb X-ray energy differently; the difference in attenuation between soft tissues and bone at the two different energy levels is used to calculate BMD. A DXA scan of the spine or hip can be accomplished in approximately 10 seconds with negligible radiation exposure. A whole-body scan takes about 3 minutes and the radiation exposure is 0.01 to 0.04 millirem, an extremely low dose compared to the exposure from a conventional chest X ray, which is approximately 40 millirem.

Osteoporosis is generally diagnosed by comparing a patient's BMD (determined by DXA) with the mean normal BMD in a population of healthy young adults of the same sex and assigning what is referred to as a **T-score**.[100,101,109,110] The comparison group serves as the reference population and is considered the standard for peak bone mass. The T-score is the number of standard deviations above or below the mean BMD of the reference population. The most widely accepted diagnostic criterion for osteoporosis is that developed by the World Health Organization (WHO), which defines osteoporosis as a T-score at or below −2.5, as shown in Table 8.20. When the T-score is between −1.0 and −2.5 standard deviations, a condition known as **osteopenia** is present. Osteopenia is not considered a diagnosis but, rather, is a term used to describe a bone mineral density that is

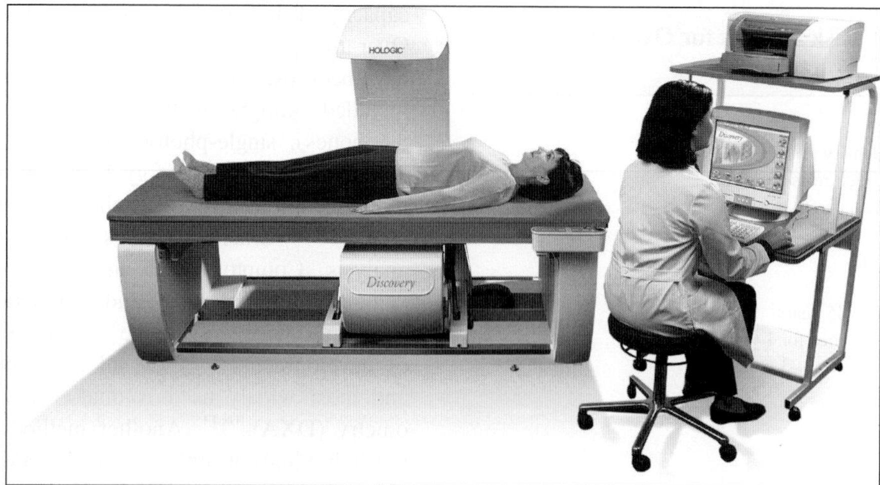

Figure 8.17 An example of a commercially available dual-energy X-ray absorptiometry (DXA) unit in operation.
Source: Photo courtesy of Hologic Incorporated.

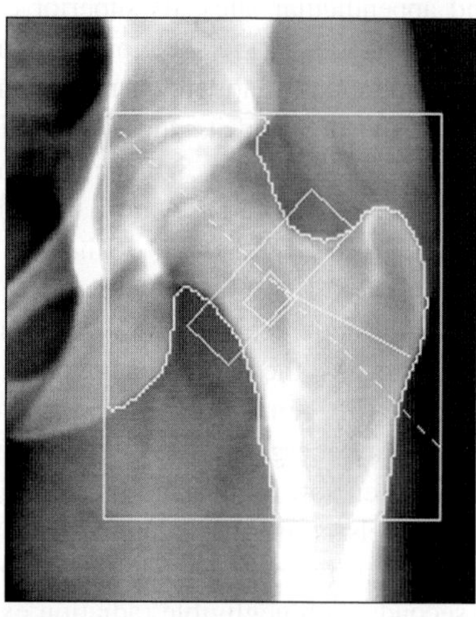

Figure 8.18 An example of a dual-energy X-ray absorptiometry scan of the hip.
Source: Photo courtesy of Hologic Incorporated.

Table 8.20 World Health Organization T-Score Criteria for Classifying Normal Bone Mineral Density (BMD), Osteopenia, and Osteoporosis

Classification	T-score
Normal BMD	−1.0 or greater
Osteopenia	Between −1.0 and −2.5
Osteoporosis	−2.5 or less
Severe osteoporosis	−2.5 or less and fragility fracture

Adapted from the World Health Organization and the International Society for Clinical Densitometry.

somewhat low but not so low as to warrant a diagnosis of osteoporosis. Risk of fracture is increased in osteopenia, but not to the extent seen in osteoporosis.[101,102] A normal T-score is −1.0 or greater.

Figure 8.19 shows the distribution of bone mineral density in the reference population used for establishing the T-score. In this large group of apparently healthy women aged 30 to 40 years, the average BMD (represented by the peak height of the curve) is assigned a T-score of 0. Individuals having a BMD that is greater than the mean have a T-score greater than 0, and those whose BMD is less than average have a T-score less than 0. Consider the case of a 75-year-old female whose DXA scan of the skeleton revealed that her bone mineral density was 2.6 standard deviations or more below the mean BMD of the reference population. This patient's T-score would be −2.6, and according to the WHO criteria in Table 8.17, she would be diagnosed as having osteoporosis. Measurements of BMD at any skeletal site have value in predicting fracture risk, and the lower the BMD, the greater the fracture risk.[102] It is estimated that fracture risk increases 1.5 to 3.0 times for each standard deviation decrease in bone density.[112,113] Clinical determinations of BMD are usually made at the lumbar spine and hip, but hip BMD is the best predictor of risk of hip fracture and is useful for predicting fractures at other sites.[100–102] Once a patient's T-score is known, it can be used to help guide clinicians in their treatment of patients. Figure 8.20 provides clinical guidelines for preventing and treating osteoporosis based on various patient characteristics and the results of bone density testing.[101]

Quantitative Ultrasound

For years, ultrasound has been successfully used for nondestructive material testing. Characteristic changes in the

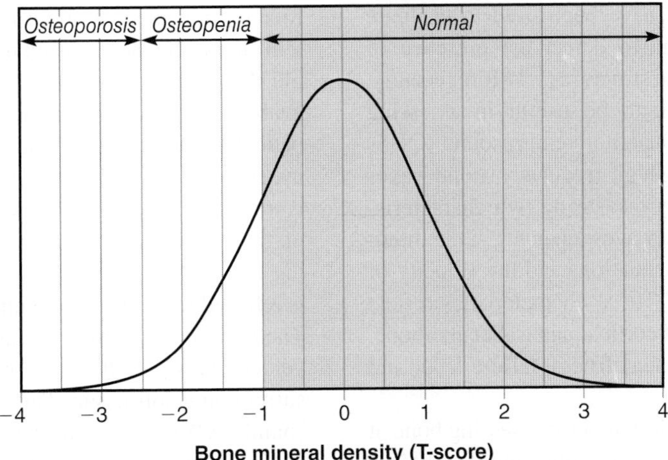

Figure 8.19 The distribution of bone mineral density (BMD) in healthy females, 30 to 40 years of age, the group that serves as the reference population for establishing the T-score for females. Females who have an average BMD are assigned a T-score of 0. According to the World Health Organization, osteopenia exists when a female's T-score is between −1.0 and −2.5. A T-score of −2.5 is diagnostic for osteoporosis.

Source: Adapted from Kanis JA. 2002. Diagnosis of osteoporosis and assessment of fracture risk. *Lancet* 359:1929–1936.

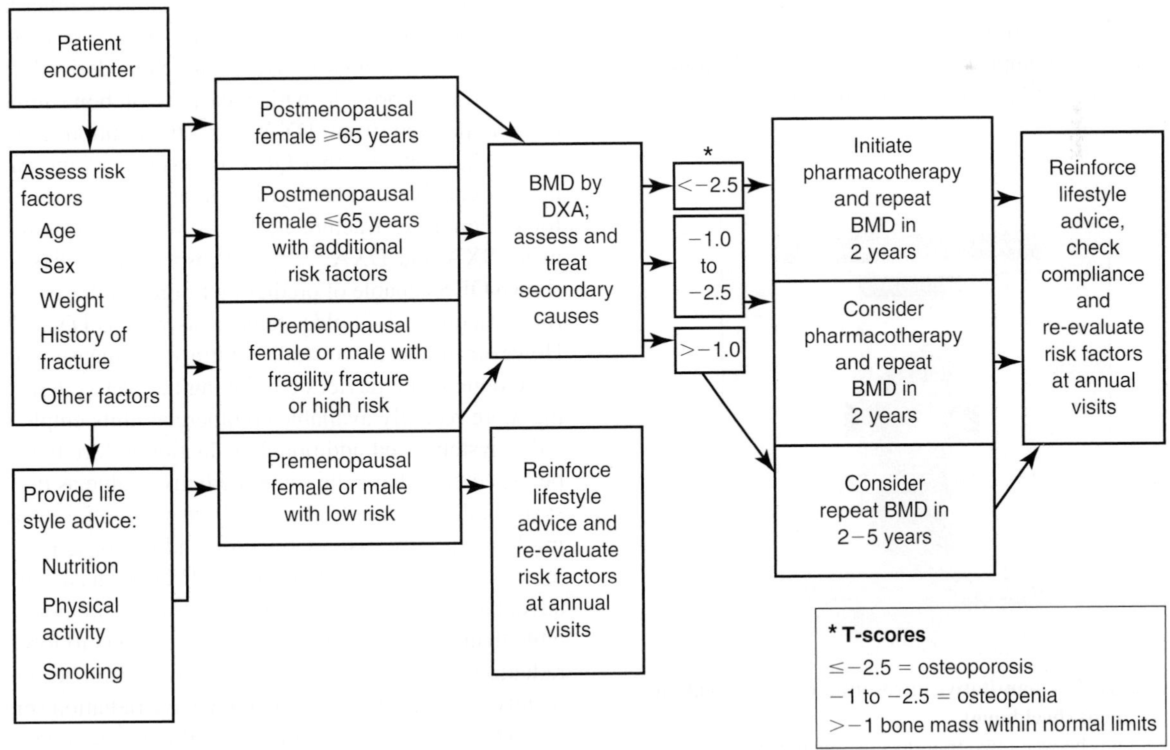

Figure 8.20 This flow chart outlines a broad approach to assessing bone health and preventing bone disease, recommending who should have bone density measurements and when pharmacologic treatment for osteoporosis should be initiated.

Source: Adapted from U.S. Department of Health and Human Services. 2004. *Bone Health and Osteoporosis: A Report of the Surgeon General.* Rockville, MD: U.S. Department of Health and Human Services, Office of the Surgeon General.

transmission of ultrasound have been used to evaluate mechanical competence and to detect the presence of damage in both materials and structures.[114] More recently, ultrasound has been shown to be useful in assessing osteoporotic fracture risk. Quantitative ultrasound (QUS) assesses skeletal status using high-frequency sound waves transmitted through bone by measuring two characteristics of the transmitted sound waves: changes in the intensity of the sound waves (attenuation) and the velocity of the transmitted sound.[114,115] These characteristics reflect the mechanical properties of cortical and trabecular bone, which in turn determine bone stiffness, failure load, and fracture risk.[114–116]

Sonometers have been designed for assessing bone at different anatomic sites, such as the tibia and the phalanges (bones of the fingers), but the most common measurement site is the calcaneus (heel bone). The calcaneus is easily accessible, has a high percentage of trabecular bone, is weight bearing, and has a pattern of osteoporotic loss similar to that of the spine.[115,116] When using a sonometer, the heel of the foot is positioned between two transducers, which transmit and receive the ultrasound signals (typically in the frequency range of 0.1 to 1.0 MHz) as illustrated in Figure 8.21. The ultrasonic wave is transmitted from one transducer, through the heel, and is received by the other transducer. Maintaining good acoustic contact between the transducers and the skin of the heel is essential to allow high transmission of the ultrasound between the transducers and the tissues of the foot. Two methods are used to accomplish this. A "wet system" utilizes a temperature-stabilized water bath in which the patient's foot is immersed. A more recently developed "dry system" uses silicone pads and ultrasound gel to directly couple the transducers to the heel.[115–117] The commercially available dry systems have the advantage of processing patients at a faster rate, and they are more convenient to use (no water bath is necessary). When the ultrasonic wave is transmitted through the tissues of the heel, the intensity of the sound wave is dampened, or weakened, depending on various physical characteristics of the bone. This is referred to as broadband ultrasound attenuation (BUA). The other characteristic of ultrasound transmission is the velocity at which the sound waves pass through bone and surrounding soft tissue. This is referred to as the speed of sound (SOS) and is considered an index of bone strength. A high SOS suggests that the bone is strong and less susceptible to fracture. In some commercial QUS units, BUA and SOS are used to calculate a third parameter shown to be related to fracture risk. Depending on the manufacturer of the unit, this third parameter is referred to as "stiffness" or a "quantitative ultrasound index."[114–117]

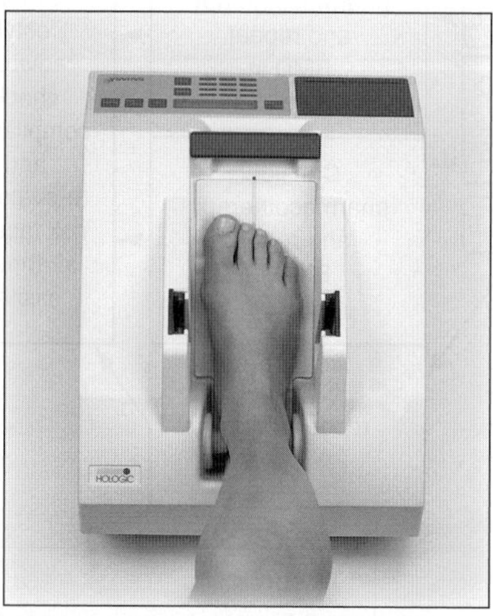

Figure 8.21 Quantitative ultrasound measurement on the calcaneus (heel bone).
The heel lies between two transducers: one transmits the ultrasonic wave through the calcaneus while the other receives the wave. A foot-positioning aide (not shown in this illustration) ensures precise placement of the foot and heel within the unit.
Source: Photo courtesy of Hologic Incorporated.

Exactly what QUS measures is still under investigation.[115] QUS does not actually measure bone mineral content. Rather, it assesses bone mass and several aspects of bone microarchitecture, such as the connectivity, spacing, thickness, and number of trabeculae in bone, all of which appear to be important determinants of fracture risk. It has been suggested that QUS assesses factors important to osteoporotic fracture risk other than bone mineral density, which cannot be assessed using DXA.[115–117] Measures of BUA and SOS derived from QUS closely correlate with measures of bone mineral content derived from DXA.[116,117] In addition, several studies have shown that QUS assessment of the calcaneus is capable of identifying persons at increased risk for osteoporotic fracture nearly as well as assessments using SXA and DXA.[114,116,117] Prospective studies have shown QUS capable of predicting future risk for osteoporotic fracture risk in older females as well as DXA.[116,117] However, in these two studies, ultrasound measurements were done using devices employing the wet system, and the more recently available commercial units employing a dry system need additional evaluation before they can be expected to have the same predictive value as the wet systems. DXA remains the definitive method for evaluating bone density, risk of fracture, and response to treatment for osteoporosis. However, QUS does have several advantages over DXA. It is less expensive and more portable than DXA and does not expose patients to ionizing radiation. Consequently, QUS instruments can be conveniently located in rooms that do not have radiation shielding. The regulations for training and licensing operators of QUS instruments are considerably less stringent than those required for DXA. QUS is a promising new technique for bone assessment, but because of limited experience in applying this new technology it cannot yet be recommended as the sole means of assessing fracture risk and monitoring skeletal changes in response to treatment. At this time, it appears that QUS is better suited as a screening method and that abnormal QUS values should be followed up by a regular DXA measurement to confirm the presence of osteoporosis.[114–117]

Preventing Osteoporosis

Preventing osteoporosis involves attaining the greatest genetically possible bone mineral density and then minimizing its loss. The three major interacting factors influencing bone health are diet, exercise, and estrogen. Primary prevention of osteoporosis begins in childhood and continues throughout adolescence and into the mid-30s, when the skeleton is acquiring its genetically programmed peak mineral mass. Secondary prevention is also critical to reducing morbidity and mortality. It is estimated that adequate nutrition can reduce the impact of osteoporosis by one-half or more. Researchers have identified a number of risk factors for osteoporosis as well as basic steps people can take to reduce their risk of osteoporosis. These are outlined in Table 8.21.

TABLE 8.21 Risk Factors for Osteoporosis and Steps to Reduce Risk of Osteoporosis

Risk Factors for Osteoporosis

- Personal history of fracture after age 45
- Current low bone mass
- Being female
- Being thin or having a small frame (weight < 127 lb)
- Advanced age
- Family history of osteoporosis
- Estrogen deficiency as a result of early menopause (before age 45 years) or surgically induced
- Amenorrhea
- Anorexia nervosa
- Low lifetime calcium intake
- Low testosterone levels in men
- Inactive lifestyle and minimal weight-bearing exercise
- Current cigarette smoking
- Excessive use of alcohol
- Being Caucasian or Asian

Steps to Reduce Risk of Osteoporosis

- Maintain a balanced diet rich in calcium and vitamin D.
- Participate in regular weight-bearing exercise.
- Practice a healthy lifestyle with no smoking or excessive alcohol intake.
- Talk to a health care professional about bone health.
- If indicated, obtain bone mineral density testing and take medication, if appropriate.

Sources: National Osteoporosis Foundation, http://www.nof.org; U.S. Department of Health and Human Services. 2004. *Bone Health and Osteoporosis: A report of the Surgeon General.* Rockville, MD: U.S. Department of Health and Human Services, Office of the Surgeon General.

There is compelling evidence that in North America and Europe, where risk of osteoporosis is high, calcium intakes less than 400 mg/day have an adverse impact on BMD and are associated with increased risk of osteoporosis and fracture.[100,112] However, when North Americans and Europeans have calcium intakes in the range of 600 to 800 mg/day, there is much less certainty about calcium intake and risk of osteoporosis and fracture. Calcium requirements vary among humans depending on each individual's biology, diet, lifestyle, and environment. Furthermore, risk of osteoporosis is influenced by factors other than calcium intake. Paradoxically, in many developing countries where calcium intake tends to be low, hip fracture incidence also tends to be low, whereas in highly developed Western nations that have the highest rates of hip fracture, calcium intake tends to be greater. A plausible explanation for this paradox is that people living in the less-industrialized developing countries tend to have lower intakes of animal proteins, sodium, and caffeine, increased consumption of fruits, vegetables, legumes, and whole grain products, and higher levels of physical activity and sun exposure, all of which have the potential to reduce calcium losses (and thus calcium requirements) and to enhance bone mineral density.[112] Nevertheless, North Americans are advised to maintain the recommended calcium intake, preferably by consuming a variety of calcium-rich foods. These include milk (liquid and powdered), milk products (e.g., cheese, yogurt, and kefir), dark green vegetables (mustard and turnip greens, kale, and broccoli), some nuts (e.g., almonds), some seeds (e.g., sesame), tofu (manufactured using calcium sulfate as opposed to magnesium chloride), corn tortillas, and a variety of calcium-fortified foods such as citrus juice and soy beverages.[100–102,111] Table 8.22 lists calcium-containing foods, organized by their calcium content per serving. Persons with lactose intolerance, a condition more commonly seen in persons who are of African, Hispanic, Asian, and Native North American descent, should be advised to consume a variety of calcium-rich, lactose-free foods.[101,111]

Vitamin D acts to increase blood concentrations of calcium and phosphorus by promoting their absorption by the GI tract and promoting their reabsorption by the kidney. Research has shown that adequate intake of calcium and vitamin D slows bone loss in elderly males and females and reduces fracture risk, including fractures of the hip, by as much as 20% to 30%.[100,112,113] Adequate intake of vitamin D and calcium is a safe, effective, and inexpensive way to reduce risk of fracture.[102] Vitamin D and calcium supplementation is now advocated as the basic minimum for treating osteoporosis and reducing risk of fracture in older females and males.[112] Recommendations for calcium, vitamin D, physical activity, and bone density testing for promoting good bone health are shown in Figure 8.22.

Bone mineral density increases and risk of hip fracture decreases in response to the stress bones receive from

TABLE 8.22 Calcium-Containing Foods Organized by Calcium Content per Serving

Food	Serving size	Calcium, mg
> 400 mg		
Tofu, regular with calcium sulfate	½ cup	434
Tofu, firm with calcium sulfate	½ cup	860
Fortified cereal	¾ cup	varies by brand
300–400 mg		
Whole milk	1 cup	291
Milkshake	8 oz.	300
Lowfat yogurt	8 oz.	300
Fortified orange juice	1 cup	300
Fortified soy milk	1 cup	300
Fortified rice milk	1 cup	300
Skim, 1%, or 2% milk	1 cup	321
Fortified cereal	¾ cup	varies by brand
Fortified oatmeal	1 pkt	350
200–300 mg		
Cheddar, monterey or provolone cheese	1 oz.	206
Soybeans, roasted	1 cup	237
Spinach (cooked)	1 cup	245
Mixed cheese dish	1 cup	250
Fortified energy bar	1	250
Soybeans (cooked)	1 cup	261
Swiss cheese	1 oz.	272
Plain yogurt	8 oz	274
100–200 mg		
Pizza	1 slice	100
Fortified waffles	2	100
Fortified butter or margarine	1 Tbsp.	100
Sherbet	1 cup	103
Mustard greens (cooked), bok choy	1 cup	104
Spaghetti, lasagna	1 cup	125
Cottage cheese	1 cup	138
Baked beans	1 cup	142
Dandelion greens or turnip greens (cooked)	1 cup	147
Ice cream	1 cup	151
Frozen yogurt or pudding	½ cup	152
American, feta, or mozzarella cheese	1 oz.	174
Soybeans, boiled	1 cup	175

Source: U.S. Department of Health and Human Services. 2004. *Bone Health and Osteoporosis: A report of the Surgeon General.* Rockville, MD: U.S. Department of Health and Human Services, Office of the Surgeon General.

weight-bearing or impact-type physical activities such as physically demanding occupations, walking, jogging, jumping rope, climbing stairs, high-impact aerobics, and a variety of sports such as tennis, soccer, basketball, and gymnastics. Persons living in rural communities and in countries in which physical activity is maintained into adult life have a lower fracture risk compared to those living in more urban, sedentary societies.[100,103,113] Although the benefits of nonimpact activities on BMD in postmenopausal females are inconsistent, activities leading to improvements in flexibility, balance, agility, and muscle strength are associated with fewer falls and a significant reduction in fracture risk. This finding is particularly true when such activities are coupled with an assessment and modification of fall hazards in the home, a review of prescription medications for side effects that may affect stability and balance, and a correction of hearing and vision.[102,103]

While there is no consistent evidence that moderate alcohol consumption has an adverse impact on bone health and fracture risk, heavy alcohol use is associated with decreased BMD, reduced bone formation, and increased risk of fracture, and chronic alcoholism is considered a major risk factor for osteoporosis. Heavy alcohol use increases calcium and magnesium losses from the body and adversely impacts vitamin D and overall nutritional status.[100–102,112,113] Even moderate alcohol consumption can increase the risk of falling and other types of skeletal trauma, thus increasing the risk of fracture.[101] Cigarette smoking has been shown to be causally related to lower bone density, increased bone mineral loss, and increased risk of fracture in males and females.[100,101,113]

The role of several other nutrients, foods, and food components in the prevention of osteoporosis has been studied, including fruit and vegetable intake, sodium, caffeine, fluoride, and trace minerals. Higher BMD is associated with diets rich in fruits, vegetables, and vegetable proteins that provide ample potassium and magnesium.[112] As dietary sodium intake increases, so does urinary calcium excretion. High-sodium diets are associated with increased excretion of calcium in the urine.[101,113] Although there is convincing evidence that reducing sodium intake results in a lowering of urinary calcium excretion, research has not yet demonstrated whether a low-sodium diet is an effective approach for preventing osteoporosis and reducing risk of fracture. However, considering the beneficial effects on blood pressure of diets providing ample amounts of vegetables and fruits, adequate intakes of nonfat dairy products, and moderate amounts of lean meats, there is strong rationale for patients to follow such a dietary pattern.[112]

DIABETES MELLITUS

Diabetes mellitus is a group of diseases characterized by a defect in insulin secretion and/or increased cellular resistance to insulin, resulting in elevated plasma (or serum) glucose levels, abnormalities of carbohydrate and lipid metabolism, characteristic pathologic changes in the nerves and small blood vessels, and aggravation of atherosclerosis.[118] Since 1932, diabetes mellitus has been

	Calcium (mg/day)	Vitamin D (IU/day)	Physical Activity	Bone Density Testing	Patients at Increased Risk
Infants					
0–6 Months	210	200	Interactive play.	As clinically indicated in high risk patients.	Frequent fractures, anorexia, amenorrhea, chronic hepatic, renal, gastrointestinal, autoimmune disease.
6–12 Months	270				
Children and Adolescents					
1–3 years	500	200	Moderate to vigorous activity at least 60 minutes per day. Emphasize weight bearing activity.	As clinically indicated in high risk patients.	
4–8 years	800				
9–18 years	1300				
Adults					
18–50 years	1000	200	Moderate activity at least 30 minutes per day, on most, preferably all, days of the week. Emphasize weight bearing activity. Fall prevention programs, modified for the frail elderly and spine fracture patients.	As clinically indicated in high risk patients.	
51–70 years	1200	400		Bone density testing by DXA in all women over age 65; consider in women under age 65 with risk factors. No consensus on men.	Individuals with risk factors.
>70 years	1200	600			

Figure 8.22 Recommendations for calcium, vitamin D, physical activity, and bone density testing for promoting good bone health.

Source: Adapted from U.S. Department of Health and Human Services. 2004. *Bone health and osteoporosis: A report of the Surgeon General.* Rockville, MD: U.S. Department of Health and Human Services, Office of the Surgeon General.

among the top 10 leading causes of death in America. It is a major cause of blindness, renal failure, congenital malformation, and lower extremity amputation. The prevalence of coronary artery disease and peripheral vascular disease is twice as common among persons with diabetes, compared with those without diabetes. Nearly 26 million Americans, or 8.3% of the population, have diabetes.

Types of Diabetes

There are five categories of patients with diabetes, or impaired glucose metabolism: type 1 diabetes, type 2 diabetes, gestational diabetes mellitus, impaired fasting glucose, and impaired glucose tolerance, also known as prediabetes. The vast majority of diabetes cases fall into two broad categories, type 1 diabetes and type 2 diabetes.[118] Type 1 diabetes is that form resulting from the destruction of the insulin-secreting beta cells of the pancreas. The beta cells are typically destroyed by an autoimmune process in which antibodies produced by the patient's own immune system destroy these insulin-secreting cells.[118] Although the rate and extent of beta cell destruction can vary considerably among persons with type 1 diabetes, most patients eventually become dependent on insulin injections for survival and to prevent life-threatening ketoacidosis.[118] Although onset of type 1 diabetes can occur at any age, it is generally diagnosed in children and young adults and accounts for 5% to 10% of diabetes cases.

Type 2 diabetes is that form resulting from insulin resistance and a "relative" insulin deficiency. *Insulin resistance* refers to abnormalities in the binding of insulin to the insulin receptor located within the cell's plasma membrane, to defects in glucose transport into the cell, and to abnormalities in other intracellular processes involved in glucose metabolism, including insulin-stimulated glycogen synthesis.[118] Although blood insulin levels in patients with type 2 diabetes may appear normal or even elevated, they are inadequate to compensate for insulin resistance, and a relative insulin deficiency is said to exist. Type 2 is the most common form of diabetes, seen in 90% to 95% of persons with diabetes. Historically, type 2 was generally diagnosed in persons older than 30 years of age but is now seen in all age groups, and its incidence is rising fastest in children and young adults, in large part due to the high prevalence of obesity and physical inactivity among youth. Most patients with type 2 diabetes are obese or have increased amounts of adipose tissue in the abdominal region. The risk factors for type 2 diabetes are shown in Box 8.7. Type 2 frequently

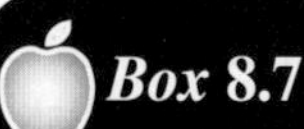

Box 8.7 **Risk Factors for Type 2 Diabetes**

- Overweight (BMI ≥ 25 kg/m^2*)
- Age ≥ 45 years
- Parent, sibling, or offspring with diabetes
- Physical inactivity
- High-risk race/ethnicity (e.g., African, Asian, Latino, Native American, Pacific Islander)
- Previously identified impaired fasting glucose (IFG) or impaired glucose tolerance (IGT)
- HbA_{1c} ≥ 5.7%
- History of gestational diabetes mellitus (GDM) or delivery of a baby weighing > 9 lb
- Hypertension (≥ 140/90 mm Hg in adults) or on therapy for hypertension
- HDL cholesterol < 35 mg/dL (0.90 mmol/L) and/or a triglyceride level > 250 mg/dL (2.82 mmol/L)
- Polycystic ovary syndrome
- History of cardiovascular disease

*At-risk BMI may be lower in some ethnic groups.

Source: Adapted from American Diabetes Association. 2012. Standards of medical care in diabetes–2012. *Diabetes Care* 35(Supplement 1):S11–S63.

goes undiagnosed for years because hyperglycemia develops gradually. Ketoacidosis seldom occurs spontaneously and generally arises only in response to the stress of another illness, such as an acute infection.[118,119] The American Diabetes Association recommends that testing for diabetes begin at age 45 years and that adults who are overweight and have one or more additional risk factor for type 2 diabetes (as indicated in Box 8.7) should be tested for diabetes. If the test results are normal, testing should be repeated at least every 3 years and more frequently if risk factor status changes. Persons with prediabetes should be tested annually.[119]

Gestational diabetes mellitus (GDM) is a class of diabetes defined by any degree of glucose intolerance with onset or first recognition during pregnancy unless a woman is diagnosed with diabetes as a result of testing at her initial prenatal visit, in which case she received a diagnosis of overt diabetes, not gestational diabetes.[118,119] The classification of GDM is assigned regardless of whether insulin or diet modification is used for treatment or whether the condition persists after delivery. In the United States more than 200,000 cases of GDM are diagnosed each year. About 7% of all pregnancies are complicated by GDM, but the prevalence ranges from 1% to 14%, depending on the diagnostic tests used and the population studied, because some groups are at higher risk of GDM than others.[118] Of all pregnancies complicated by diabetes, 90% involve GDM, making it the most common medical disorder affecting pregnancy. Early diagnosis and effective management of GDM is important to reduce the risk of perinatal morbidity and mortality and to reduce the risk for cesarean delivery.[118,120]

Impaired fasting glucose (IFG) and *impaired glucose tolerance* (IGT) refer to a metabolic stage between normal glucose homeostasis and diabetes.[118] Impaired fasting glucose occurs when fasting plasma glucose levels are greater than the upper limit of normal but are not sufficiently elevated to be diagnostic for diabetes (i.e., fasting plasma glucose is ≥ 100 mg/dL but < 126 mg/dL). Individuals with impaired glucose tolerance often have normal blood glucose levels (are euglycemic) in their daily lives and may exhibit hyperglycemia only when tested for diabetes using an oral glucose tolerance test.[118] IGT is diagnosed when the plasma glucose level is ≥ 140 mg/dL but < 200 mg/dL when tested two hours after consuming a drink containing 75 grams of glucose.[118] IFG and IGT are sometimes referred to as *prediabetes* based on the observation that most people have either IFG or IGT before they are diagnosed with type 2 diabetes.[119] In addition, individuals having a hemoglobin A_{1C} (HbA_{1C}) value in the range of 5.7 to 6.4% are at increased risk of diabetes and, therefore, could be considered to have prediabetes. The American Diabetes Association estimates that 79 million people in the United States have prediabetes. Research shows that a plasma glucose level greater than normal but less than the diagnostic threshold for diabetes can, over time, cause long-term damage to the body, especially the heart and circulatory system, substantially increase the risk for cardiovascular disease and death, is a risk factor for future diabetes, and is associated with the metabolic syndrome.[118,119] Medical nutrition therapy resulting in a modest weight loss of 5% to 10% and moderate regular physical activity can prevent or delay the progression of prediabetes to type 2 diabetes.[118,119]

Diagnosis of Diabetes

Despite the public health significance of diabetes, data from NHANES show that about 30% of people with diabetes are not diagnosed. Four testing criteria are recognized for diagnosing diabetes, as shown in Box 8.8.[118] In the absence of unequivocal hyperglycemia, criteria 1–3 in Box 8.8 should be confirmed by repeat testing. Beginning in 2010, the American Diabetes Association

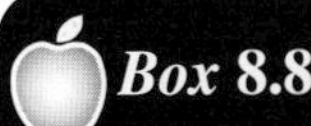

Box 8.8 Diagnostic Criteria for Diabetes

1. **A hemoglobin A_{1C} (HbA_{1C}) value ≥ 6.5%.** The test should be performed by a laboratory using a method that is certified by the National Glycohemoglobin Standardization Program (NGSP) and standardized or traceable to the Diabetes Control and Complication Trial reference assay.*
2. **Fasting plasma glucose (FPG) ≥ 126 mg/dL (7.0 mmol/L).** Fasting is defined as no caloric intake for at least 8 hours.*
3. **An oral glucose tolerance test (OGTT) with a 2-hour plasma glucose ≥ 200 mg/dL (11.1 mmol/L).** The test should adhere to World Health Organization protocol with a glucose load containing the equivalent of 75 g of anhydrous glucose dissolved in water.*
4. **Presence of the classic symptoms of hyperglycemia or hyperglycemic crisis plus a random (nonfasting) plasma glucose ≥ 200 mg/dL (11.1 mmol/L).** Classic symptoms of diabetes include polyuria (excessive urination), polydipsia (excessive thirst), polyphagia (excessive consumption of food), unexplained weight loss, blurred vision, and recurrent infections.

** In the absence of unequivocal hyperglycemia, criteria 1–3 should be confirmed by repeat testing.*

Source: Adapted from American Diabetes Association. 2012. Diagnosis and classification of diabetes mellitus. *Diabetes Care* 35(Supplement 1):S64–S71.

added to this set of diagnostic criteria a hemoglobin A1C (HbAIC) value ≥ 6.5%.

A normal fasting plasma glucose level is considered < 100 mg/dL. For the purpose of some glucose measurements, fasting can be defined as no consumption of food or beverage other than water for at least 8 hours before testing.[118]

Oral Glucose Tolerance Test

The oral glucose tolerance test (OGTT) involves having the patient who is fasting drink a beverage containing a known amount of glucose, usually 75 grams for adults or 1.75 g/kg for children. A fasting venous blood sample is drawn immediately before the glucose beverage is consumed and then at set intervals following consumption to monitor changes in blood sugar level. In preparing for the OGTT, it is best for the patient to consume more than 150 g of carbohydrate per day, abstain from alcohol, and have unrestricted activity for 3 days before the test.[118,119] On the morning of the test, the fasting subject consumes the glucose beverage within a 5- to 10-minute period. Plasma glucose is measured while fasting and usually at 1-hour intervals for 2 or 3 hours.

A plasma glucose level ≥ 200 mg/dL (≥ 11.1 mmol/L) at 2 hours is diagnostic of diabetes. Figure 8.23 shows examples of how plasma glucose might respond to an OGTT in a person with diabetes, a person with impaired glucose tolerance, and a person without diabetes. In the curve representing the person with diabetes, the plasma glucose exceeds 200 mg/dL at 2 hours after consuming the glucose load. Impaired glucose tolerance is diagnosed when plasma glucose level is 140 mg/dL but is < 200 mg/dL.

The 2-hour, 75-g OGTT is also used as a one-step test for GDM. However, different cutpoints are used in diagnosing GDM than are used to diagnose persons with diabetes or impaired glucose tolerance. At the first prenatal visit, all pregnant women should be screened for risk factors for diabetes (see Box 8.7). Those who are at high risk for diabetes should be tested. If, at this time, a pregnant woman is found to have diabetes, she should receive a diagnosis of overt diabetes, not gestational diabetes mellitus. If, at this initial prenatal visit, she is not diagnosed with overt diabetes, she should be tested for GDM at 24 to 28 weeks of gestation with a 75-g OGTT. The American Diabetes Association now recommends that all pregnant women not known to have diabetes should be tested for GDM at 24 to 28 weeks of gestation with a 75-g OGTT.[118–120] The OGTT should be performed in the morning after an overnight fast of at least 8 hours. A diagnosis of GDM is made if any one of the following plasma glucose values are obtained: fasting plasma glucose ≥ 92 mg/dL (5.1 mmol/L), 1-hour plasma glucose ≥ 180 mg/dL (10.0 mmol/L), or 2-hour plasma glucose ≥ 153 mg/dL (8.5 mmol/L).[118,119]

Self-Monitoring of Blood Glucose

In self-monitoring of blood glucose (SMBG), persons with diabetes periodically measure the amount of glucose in a small sample of their blood. It allows patients to evaluate their response to therapy and to assess whether their treatment goals are being met. It is valuable in preventing hypoglycemia and adjusting medical nutrition therapy, physical activity, and medications, especially insulin doses given immediately before meals.[119] Self-monitoring of blood glucose can be accurately and precisely done using a commercially available blood glucose

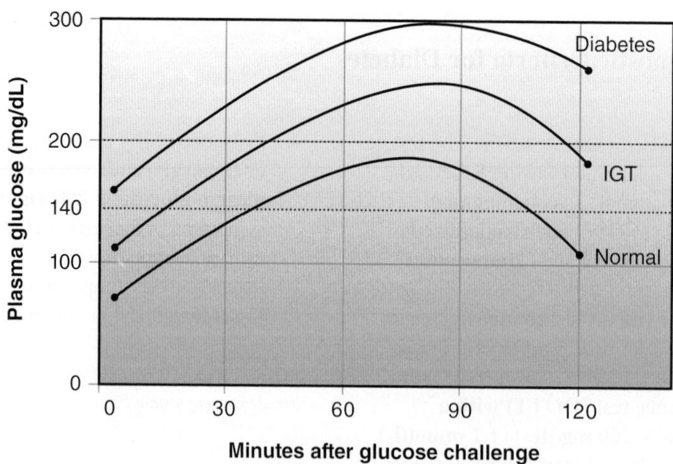

Figure 8.23 Diagnosis of diabetes using the oral glucose tolerance test (OGTT).
Normally, plasma glucose should be < 140 mg/dL 2 hours after ingesting 75 g of glucose (the so-called glucose challenge). A diagnostic criterion for impaired glucose tolerance (IGT) is a 2-hour plasma glucose ≥ 140 mg/dL and < 200 mg/dL. A 2-hour plasma glucose ≥ 200 mg/dL is a diagnostic criterion for diabetes.

meter such as the one shown in Figure 8.24. A test strip is inserted into the meter, the side of a fingertip is pricked using a lancet to draw a drop of blood for testing, and the tip of the test strip is touched to the drop of blood. Capillary action draws the blood into the strip for analysis by the meter, which provides a digital readout of the blood glucose level. Before testing, patients should be instructed to wash their hands using soap and warm water. Gently massaging the tip of the finger that will be lanced improves blood flow to that area and makes the lancing more successful.

The frequency of SMBG depends primarily on the type of diabetes and a person's overall therapy. It is especially important for preventing hypoglycemia and hyperglycemia in patients treated with insulin. For most patients with type 1 diabetes and pregnant women taking insulin, monitoring as often as three or more times a day is appropriate. More frequent testing may be required in order to reach targets for HbA_{1C} without experiencing hypoglycemia. In patients attempting tight glycemic control, testing might be recommended before performing critical tasks such as driving. In a large study of children and adolescents with type 1 diabetes, each additional test per day up to a maximum of 5 tests per day was associated with a reduction in HbA_{1C} of 0.2%. Testing should be more frequent when there are changes in a person's schedule, exercise habits, medications, diet, and body weight and during illness. There is uncertainty about the optimal frequency of SMBG in patients with type 2 diabetes who are not treated with insulin. Some research suggests that in patients not treated with insulin, SMBG may not be cost-effective. Because many of the studies investigating the benefits of SMBG on improved glycemic control also included patient education on diet and physical activity, separating the effect of SMBG from these other efforts is difficult.

The accuracy and precision of blood glucose measurements using a commercially available meter are dependent on the instrument and the user. Patients need to be instructed on the correct use of the instrument and monitored initially and periodically to ensure that they are using proper technique. Patients also need to be instructed on how to use the SMBG data to adjust their diet and physical activity and any medications they are taking.[119]

Glycated Hemoglobin

During the average life span of a red blood cell (approximately 120 days), glucose in the blood binds to the major form of hemoglobin (Hb) in the red blood cell, hemoglobin A (HbA). When this occurs, the hemoglobin is said to be glycated. There are several forms of HbA in the red blood cell. The form of glycated HbA that most closely correlates with mean blood glucose levels is referred to as hemoglobin $A1_C$ (HbA_{1C}), or what is sometimes simply called an $A1_C$ test.[118,119] The binding of glucose to HbA is almost irreversible during the life span of the red blood cell. Consequently, HbA_{1C} reflects average blood glucose levels during the past 8 to 12 weeks or 2 to 3 months. The proportion of HbA_{1C} does not decline with a temporary fall in blood glucose. It decreases only when glycemic control has been consistent over a period of several weeks, and older red blood cells with a high proportion of HbA_{1C} are replaced by new red blood cells with a lower proportion of HbA_{1C}. Consequently, the test is a good

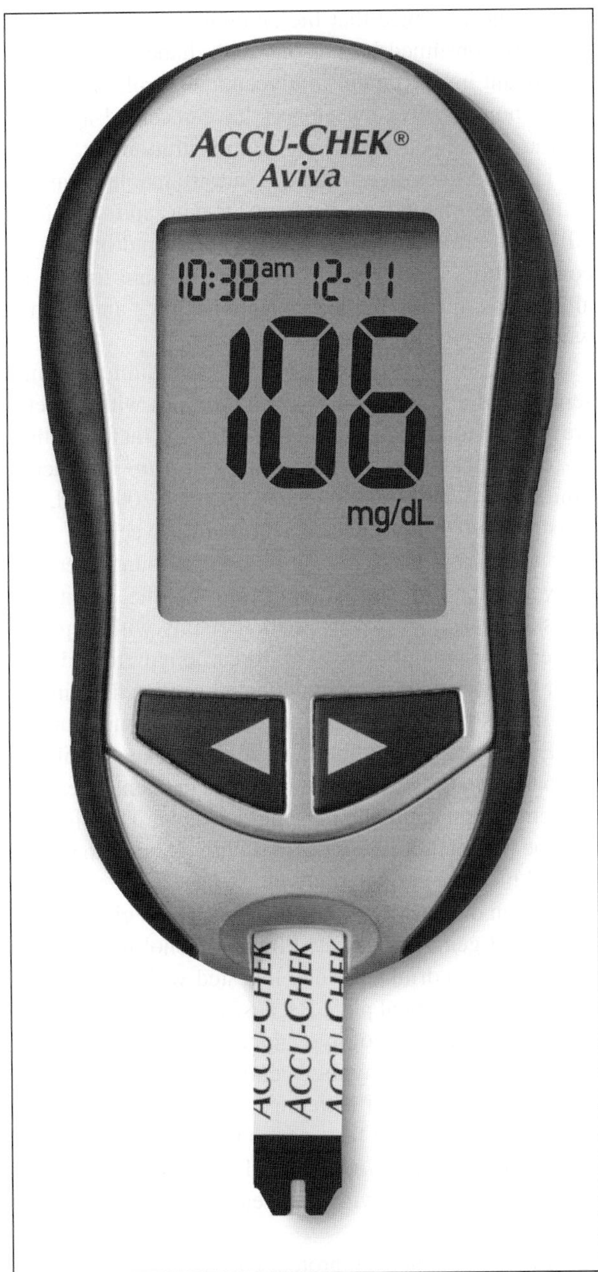

Figure 8.24 **Example of a portable, battery-operated glucose meter for performing self-monitoring of blood glucose. This unit is approximately 4 inches high and 2 inches wide and weighs approximately 2 ounces.**

Source: Photo courtesy of Roche Diabetes Care, makers of ACCU-CHEK® products and services.

way to assess a patient's adherence to his or her program of blood glucose control. It can also serve as a check on the accuracy of the patient's glucose meter and how accurately the patient is reported results from SMBG.[119]

The American Diabetes Association recommends that HbA_{1C} testing be done routinely in all patients with diabetes during their initial assessment and then periodically, depending on the patient's clinical situation, the treatment regimen used, and the judgment of the clinician.[119] Testing approximately every three months is useful in determining whether a patient's glycemic targets have been reached and are maintained. For patients meeting treatment goals and maintaining stable glycemic control, testing twice a year is considered sufficient. For patients whose therapy has changed or who are not meeting glycemic goals, quarterly testing may be warranted.[119] There are limitations to HbA_{1C} testing. It does not serve as a measure of glycemic variability or hypoglycemia. In conditions that accelerate red blood cell turnover such as anemia from hemolysis, blood loss, and iron deficiency, plasma glucose levels must be used in diagnosing and monitoring patients. Some HbA_{1C} tests may give inaccurately high or low readings in patients with hemoglobin variants such as sickle-cell trait, in which case a testing method that yields accurate results should be specifically selected.[118,119]

Medical Nutrition Therapy

In 1994, the American Diabetes Association published a major revision of its nutrition recommendations and principles for people with diabetes.[121] These recommendations presented two major philosophical changes in the nutritional management of diabetes. One was that the focus of therapy for persons with diabetes should include reasonable goals for the control of blood glucose and lipid levels, in addition to weight loss, if necessary. The other philosophical change was that a patient's diet should be individually tailored according to his or her lifestyle and nutritional and metabolic needs. Rather than patients merely receiving and following a generic set of instructions from health professionals through the process of "diabetes patient education," they are encouraged to become more fully informed of and involved in the management of their condition through the process of "self-management training." Instead of "diet therapy" for persons with diabetes, the new recommendations use "medical nutrition therapy."[121,122]

Medical nutrition therapy is a four-part approach that involves assessing an individual's nutritional, metabolic, and lifestyle needs; identifying nutritional and lifestyle goals; designing an intervention to achieve these goals; and evaluating therapeutic outcomes. Medical nutrition therapy is assessment-based; goal setting, intervention, and evaluation depend in large part on data collected through nutritional assessment. Assessment begins with establishing rapport with the client and then proceeds with collecting pertinent clinical data, obtaining a diet history, and assessing current nutrient intake. Nutritional assessment shows what the patient is currently doing, suggests what he or she is able and willing to do, and determines how likely he or she will be to adhere to nutritional recommendations. Once data from the assessment are discussed with the patient, the process of goal setting can begin. Goal setting allows the patient to set his or her own goals that are reasonable, specific, and measurable. Although goal setting is the responsibility of the patient, the dietitian can negotiate with the patient so that goals promote positive changes in eating and other lifestyle habits, resulting in improvements in blood glucose and lipid levels and nutrient intake. Remember that, as a patient's metabolic control changes over time (e.g., glucose and lipid levels improve), goals will also change.

Rather than prescribing a set energy level and percentage of energy from carbohydrates, protein, and fat, the nutrition intervention should be individually tailored to address any metabolic abnormality. Through self-management training, the intervention should help the patient acquire the knowledge and meal planning skills necessary to adapt diet and lifestyle to achieve his or her goals, despite the various situations demanded by modern life.

Over the course of the twentieth century, nutrition recommendations for diabetes have changed. Overall, the recommended proportion of energy from carbohydrate has increased while the recommended proportion of energy from fat, particularly saturated fat, has decreased. Because carbohydrate has a much greater impact on blood glucose level than protein or fat, considerable attention has been given to the amounts and types of carbohydrate in the diets of persons with diabetes. Scientific evidence supports the concept that the total amount of carbohydrate in meals and snacks is more important than the source or type of carbohydrate.[122] Sucrose (e.g., table sugar) does not increase blood glucose level to a greater extent than does an isocaloric amount of starch. Consequently, sucrose and sucrose-containing foods do not necessarily need to be restricted by people with diabetes, as long as they are substituted, gram for gram, for other carbohydrate sources. If sucrose and sucrose-containing foods are added to the meal plan, the administration of insulin or other glucose-lowering medication may need adjustment to cover the increased carbohydrate intake. When selecting carbohydrate sources, emphasis should be given to whole grains, fruits, vegetables, and nonfat dairy products because these foods have a high nutrient density, are relatively low in kilocalories, and provide vitamins, minerals, dietary fiber, and numerous other dietary components necessary for good health.[122] Dietary fiber is a beneficial food component and useful in preventing and treating constipation, and soluble fiber has the potential to lower elevated serum lipid levels. However, the American Diabetes Association's dietary fiber recommendation for people with diabetes is the same as for the general population: 20 to 35 g of dietary fiber per day from a wide variety of food sources.[122] Although fructose produces a lower postprandial glycemic response when used in place of sucrose or starch, its use may increase blood lipid levels. Consequently, the American Diabetes Association does not recommend the use of added fructose as a sweetening agent. Sugar alcohols (polyols) also produce a lower postprandial glycemic response than do sucrose, fructose, or glucose, but there is no evidence that the amounts of sugar alcohols typically consumed by persons with diabetes result in a significant improvement in glycemic control. Seven different non-nutritive sweeteners have received approval by the U.S. Food and Drug Administration for use in the United States: acesulfame K, aspartame, luo han guo fruit extract, neotame, saccharin, stevia, and sucralose. All seven provide a sweet taste to foods and beverages, contain little, if any, energy, and appear safe for use by all persons, including persons with diabetes and women who are pregnant or lactating.[123]

Because of the importance of maintaining optimal serum lipid and lipoprotein levels, persons with diabetes are advised to limit their intake of saturated fat to less than 7% of total calories, minimize intake of *trans* fatty acids, limit dietary cholesterol intake to less than 200 mg/d, and consume two or more servings of fish per week.

Apart from these restrictions, the amount of energy derived from fat should be based on the nutritional assessment and treatment goals. Persons with hypertriglyceridemia may be sensitive to carbohydrate and may want to lower their carbohydrate and saturated fat intake and modestly increase their intake of monounsaturated fat. Evidence is mounting that a high-fat diet contributes to obesity and that a low-fat diet, independent of energy reduction, is beneficial in weight loss.[122] Therefore, it may be prudent for obese persons with diabetes to reduce fat and increase carbohydrate intake.

When diabetes is well controlled, blood glucose levels are not generally affected by an alcohol intake of no more than two drinks per day ingested with and in addition to the usual meal plan. Because alcohol consumption may increase the risk of hypoglycemia in persons treated with insulin and oral hypoglycemic agents, if consumed, it should be consumed with meals. Abstention is advised during pregnancy and for persons with a history of alcohol abuse. Abstention or reduced intake may be advisable for individuals with pancreatitis, dyslipidemia, or nephropathy.

Energy supplied by protein can range between 15% and 20%, although with the onset of nephropathy, a protein intake approaching the RDA (0.8 g/kg of body weight per day, or about 10% of energy) should be considered. Reducing sodium intake lowers blood pressure in both normotensive and hypertensive persons. However, the blood pressure response to sodium reduction is generally greater in those with diabetes and hypertension. The goal is to reduce sodium intake to less than 2300 mg per day and to consume a diet high in vegetables, fruits, and low-fat dairy products as recommended by the DASH eating plan. Potassium supplementation may be required in some persons taking diuretics. Vitamin and mineral supplementation is not necessary for most people with diabetes when dietary intake is adequate. There appears to be no benefit in taking chromium and magnesium supplements unless a documented deficiency of these nutrients exists.[122]

SUMMARY

1. Coronary heart disease (CHD) remains the leading cause of death in the United States and is causally associated with several risk factors, especially elevated blood cholesterol levels, high blood pressure, and cigarette smoking.
2. Because cholesterol, triglycerides, and other lipids are fat soluble, they are transported in the blood by lipoproteins. CHD risk is directly related to serum levels of total cholesterol and low-density-lipoprotein cholesterol (LDL-C) and inversely related to levels of high-density-lipoprotein cholesterol (HDL-C). The National Cholesterol Education Program (NCEP) has set desirable levels of total cholesterol in adults at < 200 mg/dL.
3. Although clinically manifest CVD is rare in children and adolescents, risk factors during childhood initiate and accelerate the development of CVD, which is then manifest in adulthood. According to the Expert Panel on Integrated Guidelines for Cardiovascular Health and Risk Reduction in Children and Adolescents, preventing CVD must begin in childhood and address two fundamental goals: preventing development of CVD risk factors (*primordial prevention*) and preventing future CVD by managing any identified risk factors (*primary prevention*).
4. The Expert Panel developed dietary recommendations for children and adolescents called the Cardiovascular Health Integrated Lifestyle Diet (CHILD 1). These are consistent with the 2010 *Dietary Guidelines for Americans* and provide additional guidance specifically targeting children and adolescents at increased risk of CVD. The Expert Panel also recommends universal lipid screening in all children at 9 to 11 years of age and then again for all adolescents at 17 to 21 years of age.
5. Two ways of addressing the problem of high serum cholesterol levels are the population-based and the patient-based approaches. The former emphasizes dietary and lifestyle changes for all people to lower average cholesterol levels in the entire population. The latter promotes identification and treatment of individuals with elevated cholesterol levels by physicians.
6. The *Third Report of the National Cholesterol Education Program Expert Panel on Detection, Evaluation, and Treatment of High Blood Cholesterol in Adults* uses a multifaceted lifestyle approach called *therapeutic lifestyle changes* as a component of CHD risk reduction. The therapeutic lifestyle changes diet recommends that saturated fat intake be limited to < 7% of total calories, that dietary cholesterol intake be less than 200 mg/day, and that polyunsaturated and monounsaturated fat provide no more than 10% and 20% of calories, respectively. The recommendation for total fat is liberalized somewhat to 25% to 35% of calories, recognizing that a slight decrease in calories from carbohydrate and a slight increase in calories from monounsaturated fat will lower serum triglycerides in some patients.
7. A number of dietary factors can influence serum cholesterol and lipoprotein levels. Saturated fatty acids tend to raise total cholesterol and LDL-C levels, whereas substitution of saturated fats with polyunsaturated and monounsaturated fats tends to lower total cholesterol and LDL-C. Dietary cholesterol tends to raise serum cholesterol, but it is not as potent an elevator as saturated fats. Obesity elevates total cholesterol and LDL-C levels and depresses HDL-C levels. Consumption of soluble dietary fiber tends to lower elevated total cholesterol and LDL-C levels.
8. Precision, or reproducibility, relates to the difference in results when the same blood sample is measured repeatedly. The coefficient of variation (CV) is a measure of precision and is calculated by dividing the standard deviation (SD) by the mean and multiplying by 100 (CV = SD ÷ mean × 100). The NCEP recommends that laboratories achieve a CV ≤ 3%.
9. Accuracy relates to the difference between the measured value reported by the clinical laboratory and the true, or real, value that has been previously established by comparison with a known standard (reference material) and/or a definitive measurement method. Bias is a measure of inaccuracy, or departure from accuracy. Inaccurate measurement leads to clinical misdiagnosis caused by reporting of false positive or false negative values.
10. Hypertension is one of the most common risk factors for cardiovascular and renal diseases. One of every four Americans has hypertension or is taking antihypertensive medication. As systolic blood pressure increases above 120 mm Hg and diastolic blood pressure increases above 80 mm Hg, risk for death from cardiovascular disease increases.
11. The most important risk factors for hypertension are high sodium intake, excessive energy consumption

and physical inactivity (both promoting obesity), excessive alcohol consumption, and inadequate potassium intake.

12. Osteoporosis is a condition in which bone mineral content is decreased, resulting in greater susceptibility to fracture. Common fracture sites include the pelvis, vertebrae, hip, distal forearm, and humerus. Osteoporotic fractures are twice as common in females than in males, and, because they live longer than males, females experience an even higher absolute incidence during their lifetime.

13. Peak bone mass, a major factor determining risk of osteoporosis development, varies considerably among individuals because of heredity, sex, race, and environmental factors. On average, males have 20% to 30% greater peak bone mass than females, and the bones of black males and females are about 10% denser than those of white males and females.

14. Bone densitometry, the measurement of bone mineral content, is important in early detection and treatment of osteoporosis and in monitoring its progression and response to treatment. Dual-energy X-ray absorptiometry (DXA) is the most widely used technology for determining bone mineral density and is the method of choice for diagnosing osteoporosis. Quantitative ultrasonography (QUS) is commonly used to identify persons at high risk of osteoporosis who are likely to benefit from more definitive DXA testing.

15. In children and adolescents, optimal calcium intake increases bone mineral density. In postmenopausal women, calcium and vitamin D supplementation and estrogen replacement therapy decrease the rate of bone demineralization and reduce fracture risk.

16. Diabetes is a group of diseases characterized by lack of insulin secretion and/or increased insulin resistance, elevated plasma glucose levels, abnormal carbohydrate and lipid metabolism, pathologic changes in the nerves and small blood vessels, and aggravation of atherosclerosis. Among the diseases classified as diabetes are type 1 diabetes, type 2 diabetes, gestational diabetes mellitus, impaired fasting glucose, and impaired glucose tolerance.

17. Despite its public health significance, diabetes is undiagnosed in about 30% of people who have the disease. Diagnostic criteria for diabetes include the presence of symptoms of diabetes and fasting glucose measurements of ≥ 126 mg/dL (≥ 7.0 mmol/L) on two occasions. The oral glucose tolerance test also can be used to diagnose diabetes, especially gestational diabetes.

18. Glycated hemoglobin (HbA_{1C}), or simply called an A1C test is useful for assessing a person's mean glucose levels during the past 8 to 12 weeks. Self-monitoring blood glucose is helpful in evaluating how changes in diet, exercise, and medications affect glycemic control. Glycemic control has been shown to be effective in reducing the risk of microvascular complications in persons with type 1 diabetes.

19. The American Diabetes Association's nutrition recommendations encourage people with diabetes to become better informed about diabetes and its nutritional management, rather than simply follow a standard "diabetic diet."

20. Medical nutrition therapy is an approach involving nutritional assessment, goal setting, intervention, and evaluation. Its goals are to control blood glucose, blood lipids, and blood pressure; to provide adequate calories for normal growth and development, pregnancy, and lactation; to prevent, delay, or treat nutrition-related complications of diabetes; and to improve health through optimal nutrition.

References

1. American Heart Association Statistics Committee and Stroke Statistics Subcommittee. 2012. Heart disease and stroke statistics—2012 update. *Circulation*125:e2–e220. doi: 0.1161/CIR.0b013e31823ac046. http://circ.ahajournals.org/content/125/1/e2.
2. Statistics Canada. 2011. *Leading Cause of Death in Canada, 2004–2008.* Ottawa, Ontario: Statistics Canada.
3. Allender S, Scarborough P, Peto V, Rayner M. 2008. *European Cardiovascular Disease Statistics.* London: British Heart Foundation.
4. National Cholesterol Education Program. 2001. *Third report of*

the expert panel on detection, evaluation, and treatment of high blood cholesterol in adults. Bethesda, MD: U.S. Department of Health and Human Services, Public Health Service; National Institutes of Health; National Heart, Lung, and Blood Institute.

5. Grundy SM. 2006. Nutrition in the management of disorders of serum lipids and lipoproteins. In Shils ME, Shike M, Ross AC, Caballero B, Cousins RJ, eds. *Modern nutrition in health and disease,* 10th ed. Philadelphia: Lippincott Williams & Wilkins.
6. Stamler J, Daviglus ML, Garside DB, Dyer AR, Greenland P, Neaton JD. 2000. Relationship of baseline serum cholesterol levels in 3 large cohorts of younger men to long-term coronary, cardiovascular, and all-cause mortality and to longevity. *Journal of the American Medical Association* 284:365–367.
7. Jeppesen J, Hein HO, Suadicani P, Gyntelberg F. 2001. Low triglycerides-high high-density lipoprotein cholesterol and risk of ischemic heart disease. *Archives of Internal Medicine* 161:361–366.
8. Denke MA. 2006. Nutrient and genetic regulation of lipoprotein metabolism. In Shils ME, Shike M, Ross AC, Caballero B, Cousins RJ, eds. *Modern nutrition in health and disease,* 10th ed. Philadelphia: Lippincott Williams & Wilkins.
9. Voight BF, Peloso GM, et al. 2012. Plasma HDL cholesterol and risk of myocardial infarction: A Mendelian randomisation study. *The Lancet.* May 17. doi:10.1016/S0140-6736(12)60312-2.
10. Ridker PM, Brown NJ, Vaughan DE, Harrison DG, Mehta JL. 2004. Established and emerging plasma biomarkers in the prediction of first atherosclerotic events. *Circulation* 109(Supplement IV):IV-6–IV-19.
11. Fruchart JC, Nierman MC, Stroes ESG, Kastelein JJP, Duriez P. 2004. New risk factors for atherosclerosis and patient risk assessment. *Circulation* 109(Supplement III):III-15–III-19.
12. Pearson TA, Mensah GA, Alexander RW, Anderson JL, et al. 2003. Markers of inflammation and cardiovascular disease: Application to clinical and public health practice. A statement for healthcare professionals from the Centers for Disease Control and Prevention and the American Heart Association. *Circulation* 107:499–511.
13. Ridker, PM, Rifai N, Rose L, Buring JE, Cook NR. 2002. Comparison of C-reactive protein and low-density lipoprotein cholesterol levels in the prediction of first cardiovascular events. *New England Journal of Medicine* 347:1557–1565.
14. National Cholesterol Education Program. 1991. *Report of the expert panel on blood cholesterol levels in children and adolescents.* Bethesda, MD: U.S. Department of Health and Human Services, Public Health Service; National Institutes of Health; National Heart, Lung, and Blood Institute.
15. Linn S, Fulwood R, Carroll M, Brook JG, Johnson C, Kalsbeek WD, Rifkind BM. 1991. Serum total cholesterol: HDL cholesterol ratios in U.S. white and black adults by selected demographic and socioeconomic variables (HANES II). *American Journal of Public Health* 81:1038–1043.
16. Kinosian B, Glick H, Garland G. 1994. Cholesterol and coronary heart disease: Predicting risk by levels and ratios. *Annals of Internal Medicine* 121:641–647.
17. Assmann G, Cullen P, Fruchart C, Lewis B, Mancini M, Carmena R. 1999. Coronary heart disease prevention task force. *European Heart Journal* 20:841–844.
18. Stampfer MJ, Sacks FM, Salvini S, Willett WC, Hennekens CH. 1991. A prospective study of cholesterol, apolipoproteins, and the risk of myocardial infarction. *New England Journal of Medicine* 325:373–381.
19. Gotto AM. 2002. High-density lipoprotein cholesterol and triglycerides as therapeutic targets for preventing and treating coronary artery disease. *American Heart Journal* 144:S33–S42.
20. Miller M, Cosgrove B, Havas S. 2002. Update on the role of triglycerides as a risk factor for coronary heart disease. *Current Atherosclerosis Reports* 4:414–418.
21. Lauer MS, Fontanarosa PB. 2001. Updated guidelines for cholesterol management. *Journal of the American Medical Association* 285:2508–2509.
22. National Cholesterol Education Program. 1988. *Report of the expert panel on detection, evaluation, and treatment of high blood cholesterol in adults.* Bethesda, MD: U.S. Department of Health and Human Services, Public Health Service; National Institutes of Health; National Heart, Lung, and Blood Institute.
23. National Cholesterol Education Program. 1993. *Second report of the expert panel on detection, evaluation, and treatment of high blood cholesterol in adults.* Bethesda, MD: U.S. Department of Health and Human Services, Public Health Service; National Institutes of Health; National Heart, Lung, and Blood Institute.
24. National Cholesterol Education Program. 1990. *Report of the expert panel on population strategies for blood cholesterol reduction.* Bethesda, MD: U.S. Department of Health and Human Services, Public Health Service; National Institutes of Health; National Heart, Lung, and Blood Institute.
25. Lichtenstein AH, Appel LJ, Brands M, Carnethon M, Daniels S, Franch HA, et al. 2006. Diet and lifestyle recommendations: Revision 2006. *Circulation* 114:82–96.
26. Blankenhorn DH, Johnson RL, Mack WJ, El Zein HA, Vailas LI. 1990. The influence of diet on the appearance of new lesions in human coronary arteries. *Journal of the American Medical Association* 263:1646–1652.
27. Buchwald H, Varco RL, Matts JP, Long JM, Fitch LL, Campbell GS, POSCH Group. 1990. Effect of partial ileal bypass surgery on mortality and morbidity from coronary heart disease on patients with hypercholesterolemia: Report

of the Program on the Surgical Control of Hyperlipidemias (POSCH). *New England Journal of Medicine* 323:946–955.

28. Kane JP, Mallory MJ, Ports TA, Phillips R, Diehl JC, Havel RJ. 1990. Regression of coronary atherosclerosis during treatment of familial hypercholesterolemia with combined drug regimens. *Journal of the American Medical Association* 264:3007–3012.
29. Ornish D, Brown SE, Scherwitz LW, Billings JH, Armstrong WT, Ports TA, McLanahan SM, Kirkeeide RL, Brand RJ, Gould KL. 1990. Can lifestyle changes reverse coronary heart disease? *Lancet* 336:129–133.
30. Ornish D, Scherwitz LW, Billings JH, Gould KL, Merritt TA, Sparler S, et al. 1998. Intensive lifestyle change for reversal of coronary heart disease. *Journal of the American Medical Association* 280:2001–2007.
31. Stampfer MJ, Hu FB, Manson JE, Rimm EB, Willett WC. 2000. Primary prevention of coronary heart disease in women through diet and lifestyle. *New England Journal of Medicine* 343:16–22.
32. Haskell WL, Alderman EL, Fair JM, Maron DJ, Mackey SF, Superko HR, et al. 1994. Effects of intensive multiple risk factor reduction on coronary atherosclerosis and clinical events in men and women with coronary artery disease. The Stanford Coronary Risk Intervention Project (SCRIP). *Circulation* 89:975–990.
33. Enos WF, Beyer JC, Holmes RH. 1955. Pathogenesis of coronary disease in American soldiers killed in Korea. *Journal of the American Medical Association* 158:912–914.
34. McNamara JJ, Molot MA, Stremple JF, Cutting RT. 1971. Coronary artery disease in combat casualties in Vietnam. *Journal of the American Medical Association* 216:1185–1187.
35. Expert Panel on Integrated Guidelines for Cardiovascular Health and Risk Reduction in Children and Adolescents. 2011. Expert Panel on Integrated Guidelines for Cardiovascular Health and Risk Reduction in Children and Adolescents: Summary report. *Pediatrics* 128(Suppl 5):S213–S256. doi:10.1542/peds.2009–2107C.
36. Stary HC. 1990. The sequence of cell and matrix changes in atherosclerotic lesions of coronary arteries in the first forty years of life. *European Heart Journal* 11(suppl):E3–E19.
37. McGill HC, McMahan CA. 1998. Determinants of atherosclerosis in the young. Pathobiological Determinants of Atherosclerosis in Youth (PDAY) Research Group. *American Journal of Cardiology* 82(suppl):30T–36T.
38. Wissler RW, Strong JP, and the PDAY Research Group. 1998. Risk factors and progression of atherosclerosis in youth. *American Journal of Pathology* 153:1023–1033.
39. Parikh NI, Hwang SJ, Larson MG, Cupples LA, Fox CS, Manders ES, Murabito JM, Massaro JM, Hoffmann U, O'Donnell CJ. 2007. Parental occurrence of premature cardiovascular disease predicts increased coronary artery and abdominal aortic calcification in the Framingham Offspring and Third Generation cohorts. *Circulation* 116:1473–1481.
40. Zieske AW, Malcolm GT, Strong JP. 2002. Natural history and risk factors of atherosclerosis in children and youth: PDAY study. *Pediatric Pathology and Molecular Medicine* 21:213–237.
41. Davis PH, Dawson JD, Riley WA, Lauer RM. 2001. Carotid intimal-medial thickness is related to cardiovascular risk factors measured from childhood through middle age: The Muscatine Study. *Circulation* 104:2815–2819.
42. Berenson GS, Srinivasan SR, Bao W, Newman WP III, Tracey RE, Wattigney WA. 1998. Association between multiple cardiovascular risk factors and atherosclerosis in children and young adults: The Bogalusa Heart Study. *New England Journal of Medicine* 338:1650–1656.
43. McGill HC, McMahan CA, Zieske AW, Malcom GT, Tracy RE, Strong JP. 2001. Effects of nonlipid factors on atherosclerosis in youth with a favorable lipoprotein profile. *Circulation* 103:1546–1550.
44. Raitakari OT, Juonala M, Kahbnen M, Taittonen L, Laitinen T, Maki-Torkko N, Jarvisalo MJ, Uhari M, Jokinen E, Rb'nnemaa T, Akerblom HK, Viikari JS. 2003. Cardiovascular risk factors in childhood and carotid artery intima-media thickness in adulthood: The Cardiovascular Risk in Young Finns Study. *Journal of the American Medical Association* 290:2277–2283.
45. Loria CM, Liu K, Lewis CE, Hulley SB, Sidney S, Schreiner PJ, Williams OD, Bild DE, Detrano R. 2007. Early adult risk factor levels and subsequent coronary artery calcification: The CARDIA Study. *Journal of the American College of Cardiology* 49:2013–2020.
46. Freedman DS, Mei Z, Srinivasan SR, Berenson GS, Dietz WH. 2007. Cardiovascular risk factors and excess adiposity among overweight children and adolescents: The Bogalusa Heart Study. *Journal of Pediatrics* 150:12–17.
47. May AL, Kuklina EV, Yoon PW. 2012. Prevalence of cardiovascular disease risk factors among US adolescents, 1999–2008. *Pediatrics* 129:10351041.
48. Daniels SR, Greer FR. 2008. Lipid screening and cardiovascular health in childhood. *Pediatrics* 122:198–208.
49. American Diabetes Association. 2000. Type 2 diabetes in children and adolescents. *Pediatrics* 105:671–680.
50. Reinehr T, Wunsch R. 2011. Intima media thickness-related risk factors in childhood obesity. *International Journal of Pediatric Obesity* 6 (Supplement 1):46–52.
51. Expert Panel on Integrated Guidelines for Cardiovascular Health and Risk Reduction in Children and Adolescents. 2011. *Expert Panel on Integrated Guidelines for Cardiovascular Health and Risk Reduction in*

Children and Adolescents: Full report. National Heart, Lung, Blood Institute, National Institutes of Health, U.S. Department of Health and Human Services. http://www.nhlbi.nih.gov/guidelines/cvd_ped/index.htm.

52. Arenz S, Ruckerl R, Koletzko B, von Kries R. 2004. Breast-feeding and childhood obesity—A systematic review. *International Journal of Obesity and Related Metabolic Disorders* 28:1247–1256.
53. Schack-Nielsen L, Michaelsen KF. 2006. Breast feeding and future health. *Current Opinion in Clinical Nutrition and Metabolic Care* 9:289–296.
54. Judd JT, Clevidence BA, Muesing RA, Wittes J, Sunkin ME, Podczasy JJ. 1994. Dietary trans fatty acids: Effects on plasma lipids and lipoproteins of healthy men and women. *American Journal of Clinical Nutrition* 59:861–868.
55. Lichtenstein AH, Ausman LM, Jalbert SM, Schaefer EJ. 1999. Effects of different forms of dietary hydrogenated fats on serum lipoprotein cholesterol levels. *New England Journal of Medicine* 340:1933–1940.
56. U.S. Department of Health and Human Services and U.S. Department of Agriculture. 2010. *Dietary Guidelines for Americans, 2010.* Washington, DC: U.S. Government Printing Office. http://www.dietaryguidelines.gov.
57. Lichtenstein AH. 2000. Dietary trans fatty acid. *Journal of Cardiopulmonary Rehabilitation* 20:143–146.
58. Katan MB. 2000. *Trans* fatty acids and plasma lipoproteins. *Nutrition Reviews* 58:188–191.
59. Hegsted DM, Ausman LM, Johnson JA, Dallal GE. 1993. Dietary fat and serum lipids: An evaluation of the experimental data. *American Journal of Clinical Nutrition* 57:875–883.
60. Beynen AC, Katan MB. 1985. Effect of egg yolk feeding on the concentration and composition of serum lipoprotein in man. *Atherosclerosis* 54:157–166.
61. Schonfeld G, Patsch W, Rudel LL, Nelson C, Epstein M, Olson RE. 1982. Effects of dietary cholesterol and fatty acids on plasma lipoproteins. *Journal of Clinical Investigation* 69:1072–1080.
62. Beynen AC, Katan MB. 1985. Reproducibility of the variations between humans in the response of serum cholesterol to cessation of egg consumption. *Atherosclerosis* 57:19–31.
63. Shekelle RB, Stamler J. 1989. Dietary cholesterol and ischaemic heart disease. *Lancet* 1:1177–1179.
64. McGee DL, Reed DM, Yano K, Kagan A, Tillotson J. 1984. Ten-year incidence of coronary heart disease in the Honolulu Heart Program. Relationship to nutrient intake. *American Journal of Epidemiology* 119:667–676.
65. Kromhout D, de Lezenne Coulander C. 1984. Diet, prevalence and 10-year mortality from coronary heart disease in 871 middle-aged men. The Zutphen Study. *American Journal of Epidemiology* 119:733–741.
66. Kushi LH, Lew RA, Stare FJ, Ellison CR, Lozy M, Bourke G, Daly L, Graham I, Hickey N, Mulcahy R, Kevaney J. 1985. Diet and 20-year mortality from coronary heart disease. The Ireland-Boston Diet-Heart Study. *New England Journal of Medicine* 312:811–818.
67. Gotto AM. 1991. Cholesterol intake and serum cholesterol level. *New England Journal of Medicine* 324:912–913.
68. Kern F. 1991. Normal plasma cholesterol in an 88-year-old man who eats 25 eggs a day. *New England Journal of Medicine* 312:896–899.
69. Carroll KK. 1991. Review of clinical studies on cholesterol-lowering response to soy protein. *Journal of the American Dietetic Association* 91:820–827.
70. Anderson JW, Johnstone BM, Cook-Newell ME. 1995. Meta-analysis of the effects of soy protein intake on serum lipids. *New England Journal of Medicine* 333:276–282.
71. Teixeira SR, Potter SM, Weigel R, Hannum S, Erdman JW, Hasler CM. 2000. Effects of feeding 4 levels of soy protein for 3 and 6 wk on blood lipids and apolipoproteins in moderately hypercholesterolemic men. *American Journal of Clinical Nutrition* 71:1077–1084.
72. Crouse JR, Morgan T, Terry JG, Ellis J, Vitolins M, Burke GL. 1999. A randomized trial comparing the effect of casein with that of soy protein containing varying amounts of isoflavones on plasma concentrations of lipids and lipoproteins. *Archives of Internal Medicine* 159:2070–2076.
73. Potter SM, Baum JA, Teng H, Stillman RJ, Shay NF, Erdman JW. 1998. Soy protein and isoflavones: Their effects on blood lipids and bone density in postmenopausal women. *American Journal of Clinical Nutrition* 68(suppl):1375S–1379S.
74. Burr ML, Sweetnam PM. 1982. Vegetarianism, dietary fiber, and mortality. *American Journal of Clinical Nutrition* 36:873–877.
75. Phillips RL, Kuzma JW, Beeson WL, Lotz T. 1980. Influence of selection versus lifestyle on risk of fatal cancer and cardiovascular disease among Seventh-day Adventists. *American Journal of Epidemiology* 112:296–314.
76. Life Sciences Research Office. 1987. *Physiological effects and health consequences of dietary fiber.* Bethesda, MD: Life Sciences Research Office, Federation of American Societies for Experimental Biology.
77. Ludwig DS, Pereira MA, Kroenke CH, Hilner JE, Van Horn L, Slattery ML, Jacobs DR. 1999. Dietary fiber, weight gain, and cardiovascular disease risk factors in young adults. *Journal of the American Medical Association* 282:1539–1546.
78. Van Horn L. 1997. Fiber, lipids, and coronary heart disease. A statement for healthcare professionals from the Nutrition Committee, American Heart Association. *Circulation* 95:2701–2704.

79. Story JA, Kritchevsky D. 1976. Comparison of the binding of various bile acids and bile salts in vitro by several types of fiber. *Journal of Nutrition* 106:1292–1294.

80. Story JA. 1985. Dietary fiber and lipid metabolism. *Proceedings of the Society for Experimental Biology and Medicine* 180:447–452.

81. Chen WJL, Anderson JW, Jennings D. 1984. Propionate may mediate the hypocholesterolemic effects of certain soluble plant fibers in cholesterol-fed rats. *Proceedings of the Society for Experimental Biology and Medicine* 175:215–218.

82. Cummings JH, Englyst HN. 1987. Fermentation in the human large intestine and the available substrates. *American Journal of Clinical Nutrition* 45:1243–1255.

83. Warnick GR. 2000. Measurement of cholesterol and other lipoprotein constituents in the clinical laboratory. *Clinical Chemistry and Laboratory Medicine* 38:287–300.

84. National Cholesterol Education Program. 1995. *Recommendations on lipoprotein measurement from the Working Group on Lipoprotein Measurement.* Bethesda, MD: U.S. Department of Health and Human Services, Public Health Service; National Institutes of Health; National Heart, Lung, and Blood Institute.

85. Rifai N, Dufour R, Cooper GR. 1997. Preanalytical variation in lipid, lipoprotein, and apolipoprotein testing. In Rifai N, Warnick GR, Dominiczak MH, eds. *Handbook of lipoprotein testing.* Washington, DC: American Association of Clinical Chemistry, pp. 75–97.

86. National Cholesterol Education Program. 1990. *Recommendations for improving cholesterol measurement: A report from the Laboratory Standardization Panel of the National Cholesterol Education Program.* Bethesda, MD: U.S. Department of Health and Human Services, Public Health Service; National Institutes of Health; National Heart, Lung, and Blood Institute.

87. Cooper GR, Myers GL, Smith SJ, Schlant RC. 1992. Blood lipid measurements: Variations and practical utility. *Journal of the American Medical Association* 267:1652–1660.

88. National High Blood Pressure Education Program. 2004. *The seventh report of the Joint National Committee on Prevention, Detection, Evaluation, and Treatment of High Blood Pressure.* U.S. Department of Health and Human Services, National Institutes of Health; National Heart, Lung, and Blood Institute.

89. Stevens VJ, Obarzanek E, Cook NR, Lee IM, Appel LJ, et al. 2001. Long-term weight loss and changes in blood pressure: Results of the Trials of Hypertension Prevention, phase II. *Annals of Internal Medicine* 134:1–11.

90. Sacks FM, Svetkey LP, Vollmer WM, Appel LJ, et al. 2001. Effects on blood pressure of reduced sodium and the Dietary Approaches to Stop Hypertension (DASH) diet. *New England Journal of Medicine* 344:3–10.

91. Appel LJ, Espeland MA, Easter L, Wilson AC, Folmar S, Lacy CR. 2001. Effect of reduced sodium intake on hypertension control in older individuals. *Archive of Internal Medicine* 161:685–693.

92. The Trials of Hypertension Prevention Collaborative Research Group. 1992. The effects of nonpharmacologic interventions on blood pressure of persons with high normal levels: Results of the Trials of Hypertension Prevention. Phase I. *Journal of the American Medical Association* 267:1213–1220.

93. Panel on Dietary Reference Intakes for Electrolytes and Water, Standing Committee on the Scientific Evaluation of Dietary Reference Intakes, Food and Nutrition Board. 2004. *Dietary reference intakes for water, potassium, sodium, chloride, and sulfate.* Washington, DC: National Academy Press.

94. Greenland P. 2001. Beating high blood pressure with low-sodium DASH. *New England Journal of Medicine* 344:53–55.

95. Havas S, Dickinson BD, Wilson M. 2007. The urgent need to reduce sodium consumption. *Journal of the American Medical Association* 298:1439–1441.

96. Kotchen TA, McCarron DA. 1998. Dietary electrolytes and blood pressure. A statement for healthcare professionals from the American Heart Association Nutrition Committee. *Circulation* 98:613–617.

97. Appel LJ, Moore TJ, Obarzanek E, Vollmer WM, Svetkey LP, Sacks FM, et al. 1997. A clinical trial of the effects of dietary patterns on blood pressure. *New England Journal of Medicine* 336:1117–1124.

98. National High Blood Pressure Education Program. 2005. *The fourth report on the diagnosis, evaluation, and treatment of high blood pressure in children and adolescents.* U.S. Department of Health and Human Services, National Institutes of Health; National Heart, Lung, and Blood Institute.

99. Sorof JM, Lai D, Turner J, Poffenbarger T, Portman RJ. 2004. Overweight, ethnicity, and the prevalence of hypertension in school-aged children. *Pediatrics* 113:475–482.

100. Lindsay R, Cosman F. 2005. Osteoporosis. In Kasper DL, Braunwald E, Fauci AS, Hauser SL, Longo DL, Jameson JL (eds.), *Harrison's principles of internal medicine,* 16th ed. New York: McGraw-Hill, 2268–2278.

101. U.S. Department of Health and Human Services. 2004. *Bone health and osteoporosis: A report of the Surgeon General.* Rockville, MD: U.S. Department of Health and Human Services, Office of the Surgeon General.

102. National Osteoporosis Foundation. 2003. *Physician's guide to prevention and treatment of osteoporosis.* Washington, DC: National Osteoporosis Foundation.

103. Brown JP, Josse RG. 2002. 2002 clinical practice guidelines for the diagnosis and management of osteoporosis in Canada. *Canadian Medical Association Journal* 167(10 suppl):S1–S34.

104. National Institutes of Health. 2000. Osteoporosis prevention, diagnosis, and therapy. *NIH Consensus Statements* 17(1):1–52. http://consensus.nih.gov/cons/111/111_statement.pdf.

105. Porth CM. 2005. Structure and function of the musculoskeletal system. In Porth CM (ed.), *Pathophysiology: Concepts of altered health status,* 7th ed. Philadelphia: Lippincott Williams & Wilkins, 1357–1366.

106. Saladin KS. 2004. *Anatomy and physiology: The unity of form and function,* 3rd ed. Boston: McGraw-Hill.

107. Hightower MK, Gunta KE. 2005. Disorders of skeletal function: Developmental and metabolic disorders. In Porth CM (ed.), *Pathophysiology: Concepts of altered health status,* 7th ed. Philadelphia: Lippincott Williams & Wilkins, 1393–1415.

108. Theodorou SJ, Theodorou DJ, Sartoris DJ. 2003. Evaluation of osteoporosis in orthopedic practice: A review of current diagnostic modalities. *American Journal of Orthopedics* 32:178–188.

109. Richmond B. 2003. DXA scanning to diagnose osteoporosis: Do you know what the results mean? *Cleveland Clinic Journal of Medicine* 70:353–360.

110. Brown SA, Rosen CJ. 2003. Osteoporosis. *Medical Clinics of North America* 87:1039–1063.

111. Sartoris DJ, Resnick D. 1990. Current and innovative methods for noninvasive bone densitometry. *Orthopedics* 28:257–278.

112. Prentice A. 2004. Diet, nutrition and the prevention of osteoporosis. *Public Health Nutrition* 7:227–243.

113. Krall EA, Dawson-Hughes B. 1999. Osteoporosis. In Shils ME, Olson JA, Shike M, Ross AC (eds.), *Modern nutrition in health and disease,* 9th ed. Baltimore: Williams & Wilkins, 1353–1364.

114. Gluer CC. 1997. Quantitative ultrasound techniques for the assessment of osteoporosis: Expert agreement on current status. The International Quantitative Ultrasound Consensus Group. *Journal of Bone and Mineral Research* 12:1280–1288.

115. Maurice M, Chen Z. 2000. Bone densitometry. *Clinics in Laboratory Medicine* 20:469–488.

116. Stewart A, Reid DM. 2002. Quantitative ultrasound in osteoporosis. *Seminars in Musculoskeletal Radiology* 6:229–232.

117. Gonnelli S, Cepollaro C. 2002. The use of ultrasound in the assessment of bone status. *Journal of Endocrinological Investigation* 25:389–397.

118. American Diabetes Association. 2012. Diagnosis and classification of diabetes mellitus. *Diabetes Care* 35(Supplement 1):S64–S71.

119. American Diabetes Association. 2008. Nutrition recommendations and interventions for diabetes. *Diabetes Care* 31(Suppl 1):S61–S78.

120. International Association of Diabetes and Pregnancy Study Groups Consensus Panel. 2010. International Association of Diabetes and Pregnancy Study Groups recommendations on the diagnosis and classification of hyperglycemia in pregnancy. *Diabetes Care* 33:676–882.

121. American Diabetes Association. 1994. Nutrition recommendations and principles for people with diabetes mellitus. *Diabetes Care* 17:519–522.

122. American Diabetes Association. 2008. Nutrition recommendations and interventions for diabetes. *Diabetes Care* 31(Suppl 1):S61–S78.

123. Academy of Nutrition and Dietetics. 2012. Position of the Academy of Nutrition and Dietetics: Use of nutritive and nonnutritive sweeteners. *Journal of the American Academy of Nutrition and Dietetics* 112:739–758.

ASSESSMENT ACTIVITY 8.1

Lipid and Lipoprotein Levels and Coronary Heart Disease Risk

The National Cholesterol Education Program recommends that all adults 20 years of age or older know their serum total cholesterol. Values < 200 mg/dL (5.17 mmol/L) can be repeated at least every 5 years. Values of 200 mg/dL (5.17 mmol/L) or greater should be verified by a repeat measurement within 1 to 8 weeks. If the second value is within 30 mg/dL (0.8 mmol/L) of the first, the average of the two can be used as a guide for subsequent decisions. Otherwise, a third test should be obtained in another 1 to 8 weeks and the average of the three values used.

You are encouraged to have your blood lipid and lipoprotein levels measured and to know these values. There are several ways you can do this. Your professor may be able to arrange with student health services or a local hospital or clinical laboratory to have cholesterol and lipoprotein measurements performed on all interested students in your class. If measurements are done on several members of your class, they may be done at a reduced price; for example, triglycerides, total cholesterol, low-density-lipoprotein cholesterol, and high-density-lipoprotein cholesterol may be measured for $30 or less, or you may want to have your cholesterol or lipid and lipoprotein levels measured on your own. Some hospitals offer low-priced testing as a community service.

When you receive your results, answer the following questions:

1. What are the highest, lowest, mean, and median values for each of the lipids and lipoproteins measured?

2. How do these compare with the population norms given in Appendix Q?
3. What are the highest, lowest, mean, and median values for the ratio of total cholesterol to high-density-lipoprotein cholesterol?
4. How do these compare with the values shown in Appendix Q?
5. Is there anyone in your class needing follow-up testing, according to the National Cholesterol Education Program's guidelines given in this chapter?

Assessment Activity 8.2

Calculating 10-Year Coronary Heart Disease Risk

Using data obtained from the Framingham Heart Study, the National Cholesterol Education Program has developed tables for calculating the likelihood of a person's having a myocardial infarction or dying from coronary heart disease (CHD) within the next 10 years (review Tables 8.4 and 8.5). The values for total cholesterol and high-density-lipoprotein cholesterol (HDL-C) used to score risk should be the average of at least two measurements obtained from lipoprotein analysis. The average of several blood pressure measurements is needed for an accurate assessment of baseline systolic blood pressure. A person taking medication for hypertension is considered treated and at increased risk for CHD, as reflected in a higher risk score. The designation "smoker" means any cigarette smoking in the past month.

Consider, for example, a nonsmoking, 45-year-old male who has a total cholesterol of 223 mg/dL, a high-density-lipoprotein cholesterol (HDL-C) level of 43 mg/dL, and a systolic blood pressure of 127 mm Hg. Also assume that this individual is not being treated for hypertension. In Table 8.4, this male would receive 0 points for being a nonsmoker, 3 points for age, 5 points for total cholesterol at age 45 years, 1 point for HDL-C, and 0 points for systolic blood pressure. The total of all points would be 9, giving this individual a 10-year risk for myocardial infarction or death from CHD of 5%. You are encouraged to estimate your own 10-year risk and that of several hypothetical patients.

In Tables 8.4 and 8.5, the points assigned for total cholesterol and cigarette smoking decline with advancing age, suggesting that the risk for CHD from these two variables decreases with advancing age. However, this decline is more apparent than real because of the exponential rise in risk with mounting Framingham points. For example, for males, a change in total points from 9 to 10 increases the 10-year risk a mere 1%, but a change from 15 to 16 points increases risk by 5%. Thus, in older persons who have several points due to age alone, the addition of fewer points for high total cholesterol or smoking increases absolute risk as much as or more than do more points at a younger age. Thus, Tables 8.4 and 8.5 should not be misconstrued to mean that risk contributed by total cholesterol and smoking declines in importance with advancing age.

Assessment Activity 8.3

Categorizing Blood Pressure in Children and Adolescents

As discussed in this chapter, an entirely different approach is used to categorize blood pressure (BP) in children and adolescents than that used to categorize blood pressure in adults. As shown in Box 8.6, in children and adolescents 1 to 17 years of age, hypertension is defined as an average systolic blood pressure (SBP) and/or diastolic blood pressure (DBP) that is ≥ 95th percentile of BP for a young person of a given sex, age, and stature or height. Prehypertension is defined as average SBP or DBP levels that are ≥ 90th percentile but < 95th percentile. To categorize the BP of a person in this age group, it is necessary to determine his or her percentile of stature for sex and age using the sex- and age-appropriate CDC growth chart that provides the length-for-age percentiles or stature-for-age percentiles. The CDC growth charts are discussed in Chapter 6 and shown in Appendix K. Once the subject's percentile of length or stature is determined, Table 8.17 or 8.18 is used to determine the BP percentile that is then used to categorize BP.

Keep in mind that following proper technique is critical to measuring BP in any age group. Categorization of BP in children and adolescents is based on the average of multiple BP measurements. At each visit with a health care provider, BP should be measured two or three times following the protocol discussed in this chapter. Furthermore, categorization of BP is done on an average of multiple BP measurements taken during at least three different visits with the health care provider. A diagnosis of hypertension cannot be made on the basis of a single BP measurement or on values taken during a single visit with a health care provider.

Working through the following three cases will help you understand how to categorize blood pressure in children and adolescents.

1. A 7-year-old female is 4 feet tall. Using multiple measurements of BP taken during three different visits with a health care provider, it was determined that this child's average BP is 110/72 mm Hg. What is this child's percentile of stature for sex and age?

   ____

   This child's BP would be categorized as:

   A. normal

   B. prehypertension

   C. hypertension

2. A 14-year-old female is 156 cm tall and has an average BP of 127/83 Hg. What is this adolescent's percentile of stature for sex and age?

   ____

   This adolescent's BP would be categorized as:

   A. normal

   B. prehypertension

   C. hypertension

3. What would be the 50th to 90th percentile range of BP for 10-year-old males who are at the 50th percentile of stature-for-age?

   _____ to _____ / _____ to _____

ASSESSMENT ACTIVITY 8.4

Estimating Your Calcium Intake

You can use the list below to calculate your calcium points based on your average diet. Begin by thinking about your average daily food intake. When you see a food in the list below that's in your diet, circle the points that correspond to that food. If your typical serving is larger or smaller than what is given in the list, adjust the points accordingly. Total your calcium points and then compare that total to the number of points you need based on your age. How do you rate?

Food	Calcium (mg)	Points
Fortified oatmeal, 1 packet	350	3
Sardines, canned in oil, with edible bones, 3 oz.	324	3
Cheddar cheese, 1½ oz. shredded	306	3
Milk, nonfat, 1 cup	302	3
Milkshake, 1 cup	300	3
Yogurt, plain, low-fat, 1 cup	300	3
Soybeans, cooked, 1 cup	261	3
Tofu, firm, with calcium, ½ cup	204	2
Orange juice, fortified with calcium, 6 oz.	200–260 (varies)	2–3
Salmon, canned, with edible bones, 3 oz.	181	2
Pudding, instant, (chocolate, banana, etc.) made with 2% milk, ½ cup	153	2
Baked beans, 1 cup	142	1
Cottage cheese, 1% milk fat, 1 cup	138	1
Spaghetti, lasagna, 1 cup	125	1
Frozen yogurt, vanilla, soft-serve, ½ cup	103	1

continued

continued

Food	Calcium (mg)	Points
Ready-to-eat cereal, fortified with calcium, 1 cup	100–1000 (varies)	1–10
Cheese pizza, 1 slice	100	1
Fortified waffles, 2	100	1
Turnip greens, boiled, ½ cup	99	1
Broccoli, raw, 1 cup	90	1
Ice cream, vanilla, ½ cup	85	1
Soy or rice milk, fortified with calcium, 1 cup	80–500 (varies)	1–5
How do you rate?	Total calcium points ___________	

Points Needed:

Infants/toddlers (ages 0–3 years)	2–5
Children (ages 4–8 years)	8
Teens	23
Adults (< 50 years of age)	10
Adults (≥ 50 years of age)	12

Source: Adapted from U.S. Department of Health and Human Services. 2004. *Bone health and osteoporosis: A report of the Surgeon General.* Rockville, MD: U.S. Department of Health and Human Services, Office of the Surgeon General.

CHAPTER 9

Biochemical Assessment of Nutritional Status

Outline

Introduction
Use of Biochemical Measures
Protein Status
Iron Status
Calcium Status
Zinc Status
Iodine Status
Vitamin A Status
Vitamin D Status
Vitamin C Status
Vitamin B_6 Status
Folate Status
Vitamin B_{12} Status
Blood Chemistry Tests
Summary
References
Assessment Activity 9.1: Visiting a Clinical Laboratory
Assessment Activity 9.2: Chemistry Profile, Complete Blood Count, and Coronary Risk Profile

Student Learning Outcomes

After studying this chapter, the student will be able to:

1. Discuss the biochemical tests for assessing visceral and somatic protein status.
2. Recall the formula for determining nitrogen balance and calculate nitrogen balance given a patient's protein intake and urine urea nitrogen value.
3. Discuss the advantages and disadvantages of using serum proteins for assessing nutritional status.
4. Discuss the strengths and weaknesses of the models used for assessing iron status.
5. Describe the state of iron nutriture in the United States using data from NHANES.
6. Describe the state of iodine nutriture in the United States using data from NHANES.
7. Explain how vitamin D status is assessed.
8. Describe how indicators of folate status have changed since the FDA required the addition of folate to refined cereal products.

Introduction

Compared with the other methods of nutritional assessment (anthropometric, clinical methods, and dietary), biochemical tests can potentially provide more objective and quantitative data on nutritional status. Biochemical tests, also known as biomarkers, often can detect nutrient deficits long before anthropometric measures are altered and clinical signs and symptoms appear. Some of these tests are useful indicators of recent nutrient intake and can be used in conjunction with dietary methods to assess food and nutrient consumption.

This chapter discusses the topic of biochemical methods in nutritional assessment, reviews the more commonly encountered tests for those nutrients of public health importance, and provides examples of various biochemical techniques in nutritional assessment.

Nutritional science is a relatively young discipline, and use of biochemical methods as indicators of nutritional status is still in its early development. This, along with all that yet remains unknown about the human body, makes the use of these measures in nutritional assessment a rapidly developing field and one with many research opportunities.

Use of Biochemical Measures

Biochemical tests available for assessing nutritional status can be grouped into two general and somewhat arbitrary categories: *static tests* and *functional tests.* These are sometimes referred to as *direct* and *indirect tests,* respectively. Static tests are also referred to as qualitative and quantitative biochemical indicators. Functional tests are also referred to as biological, functional, and histologic indicators.[1]

Static tests are based on measurement of a nutrient or its metabolite in the blood, urine, or body tissue—for example, serum measurements of folate, retinol, vitamin B_{12}, vitamin D. These are among the most readily available tests, but they have certain limitations. Although they may indicate nutrient levels in the particular tissue or fluid sampled, they often fail to reflect the overall nutrient status of an individual or whether the body as a whole is in a state of nutrient excess or depletion.[2] For example, the amount of calcium in serum can be easily determined, but that single static measurement is a poor indicator of the body's overall calcium status or of bone mineral content.

Functional tests of nutritional status are based on the ultimate outcome of a nutrient deficiency which is the failure of the physiologic processes that rely on that nutrient for optimal performance. Included among these functional tests are measurement of dark adaptation (assesses vitamin A status) and urinary excretion of xanthurenic acid in response to consumption of tryptophan (assesses vitamin B_6 status). Although many functional tests remain in the experimental stage, this is an area of active research and one that is likely to be fruitful. One drawback of some functional tests, however, is a tendency to be nonspecific; they may indicate general nutritional status but not allow identification of specific nutrient deficiencies.

Biochemical tests can also be used to examine the validity of various methods of measuring dietary intake or to determine if respondents are underreporting or overreporting what they eat. The ability of a food frequency questionnaire to accurately measure protein intake, for example, can be assessed by comparing reported protein intake with 24-hour urine nitrogen excretion. When properly used, this method is sufficiently accurate to use as a validation method in dietary surveys. As with any test requiring a 24-hour urine sample, however, each collection must be complete (i.e., respondents must collect all urine during an exact 24-hour period). Urinary nitrogen is best estimated using multiple 24-hour urine samples, and any extrarenal nitrogen losses must be accounted for.[3] The doubly labeled water technique, as mentioned in Chapters 3 and 7, is another biochemical test useful for determining validity and accuracy of reporting. It can be an accurate way of measuring energy expenditure without interfering with a respondent's everyday life.[4] If reported energy and protein consumption fail to match estimates of energy and protein intake derived from these properly performed biochemical tests, then the dietary assessment method may be faulty or the respondent did not accurately report food intake.

Biochemical tests are a valuable adjunct in assessing and managing nutritional status; however, their use is not without problems. Most notable among these is the influence that nonnutritional factors can have on test results. A variety of pathologic conditions, use of certain medications, and technical problems in a sample collection or assay can affect test results in ways that make them unusable. Another problem with some biochemical tests is their nonspecificity. A certain test may indicate that a patient's general nutritional status is impaired yet lack the specificity to indicate which nutrient is deficient. Additionally, no single test, index, or group of tests by itself is sufficient for monitoring nutritional status. Biochemical tests must be used in conjunction with measures of dietary intake, anthropometric measures, and clinical methods.

Protein Status

Assessing protein status can be approached by use of anthropometric (Chapters 6 and 7), biochemical, clinical (Chapter 10), and dietary data (Chapters 3 and 4).

Biochemical assessment of protein status has typically been approached from the perspective of the two-compartment model: evaluation of somatic protein and visceral protein status. The body's somatic protein is found within skeletal muscle. Visceral protein can be regarded as consisting of protein within the organs or viscera of the body (liver, kidneys, pancreas, heart, and so on), the erythrocytes (red blood cells), and the granulocytes and lymphocytes (white blood cells), as well as the serum proteins.[5,6] The somatic and visceral pools contain the metabolically available protein (known as body cell mass), which can be drawn on, when necessary, to meet various bodily needs. The somatic and visceral protein pools comprise about 75% and 25% of the body cell mass, respectively. Together, they comprise about 30% to 50% of total body protein.[5] The remaining body protein is found primarily in the skin and connective tissue (bone matrix, cartilage, tendons, and ligaments) and is not readily exchangeable with the somatic and visceral protein pools. Division of the body's protein into these two compartments is somewhat arbitrary and artificial.

Although the somatic compartment is homogeneous, the visceral protein pool is composed of hundreds of different proteins serving many structural and functional roles.

Although protein is not considered a public health issue among the general population of developed nations, protein-energy malnutrition (PEM), also known as protein-calorie malnutrition, can be a result of certain diseases and is clearly a pressing concern in many developing nations. Protein-energy malnutrition can be seen in persons with cancer and acquired immune deficiency syndrome (AIDS), children who fail to thrive, and homeless persons.

Because of its high prevalence and relationship to infant mortality and impaired physical growth, PEM is considered the most important nutritional disease in developing countries.[7] It is also of concern in developed nations. According to some reports, PEM has been observed in nearly half of the patients hospitalized in medical and surgical wards in the United States. In more recent studies, the prevalence of PEM ranged from 30% to 40% among patients with hip fractures, patients undergoing thoracic surgery for lung cancer, patients receiving ambulatory peritoneal dialysis, and children and adolescents with juvenile rheumatoid arthritis.[2,7–9]

Assessment of protein status is central to the prevention, diagnosis, and treatment of PEM. The causes of PEM can be either primary (inadequate food intake) or secondary (other diseases leading to insufficient food intake, inadequate nutrient absorption or utilization, increased nutritional requirement, and increased nutrient losses).[7–9] The protein and energy needs of hospitalized patients can be two or more times those of healthy persons as a result of hypermetabolism accompanying trauma, infection, burns, and surgical recovery. PEM can result in kwashiorkor (principally a protein deficiency), marasmus (predominantly an energy deficiency), or marasmic kwashiorkor (a combination of chronic energy deficit and chronic or acute protein deficiency).[7] Clinical findings pertinent to kwashiorkor and marasmus are discussed in Chapter 10.

Body weight is a readily obtained indicator of energy and protein reserves. However, it must be carefully interpreted because it fails to distinguish between fat mass and fat-free mass, and losses of skeletal muscle and adipose tissue can be masked by water retention resulting from edema and ascites. The creatinine-height index is also well suited to the clinical setting but has limited precision and accuracy. Use of midarm muscle circumference and midarm muscle area are two other approaches to assessing somatic protein status.[7] These are discussed in Chapter 7.

Rather than relying on any single indicator, a combination of measures can produce a more complete picture of protein status. The choice of approaches depends on methods available to the particular facility. Biochemical data on nutritional status constitute only part of the necessary information to evaluate the severity of nutritional depletion and PEM. Data relating to dietary intake, pertinent anthropometric measures, and clinical findings are necessary as well.

Creatinine Excretion and Creatinine-Height Index

A biochemical test sometimes used for estimating body muscle mass is 24-hour urinary creatinine excretion. Creatinine, a product of skeletal muscle, is excreted in a relatively constant proportion to the mass of muscle in the body. It is readily measured by any clinical laboratory. Lean body mass can be estimated by comparing 24-hour urine creatinine excretion with a standard based on stature (Table 9.1) or from reference values of 23 and 18 mg/kg of recommended body weight for males and females, respectively. Another approach is using the creatinine-height index (CHI), a ratio of a patient's measured 24-hour urinary creatinine excretion and the expected excretion of a reference adult of the same sex and stature. The CHI is expressed by the following formula:

$$\text{CHI} = \frac{\text{24-hr urine creatinine (mg)} \times 100}{\text{Expected 24-hr urine creatinine (mg)}}$$

Expected 24-hour urine creatinine values are shown in Table 9.1. These should be matched to the subject's sex and height.

The CHI is expressed as a percent of expected value. A CHI of 60% to 80% is considered indicative of mild protein depletion; 40% to 60% reflects moderate protein depletion; and a value under 40% represents severe depletion.[5–7]

TABLE 9.1 Expected 24-Hour Urinary Creatinine Values for Height for Adult Males and Females

Adult Males*		Adult Females†	
Height (cm)	Creatinine (mg)	Height (cm)	Creatinine (mg)
157.5	1288	147.3	830
160.0	1325	149.9	851
162.6	1359	152.4	875
165.1	1386	154.9	900
167.6	1426	157.5	925
170.2	1467	160.0	949
172.7	1513	162.6	977
175.3	1555	165.1	1006
177.8	1596	167.6	1044
180.3	1642	170.2	1076
182.9	1691	172.7	1109
185.4	1739	175.3	1141
188.0	1785	177.8	1174
190.5	1831	180.3	1206
193.0	1891	182.9	1240

Adapted from Blackburn GL, Bistrian BR, Maini BS, Schlamm HT, Smith MR. 1977. Nutritional and metabolic assessment of the hospitalized patient. *Journal of Parenteral and Enteral Nutrition* 1:11–12.

*Creatinine coefficient for males = 23 mg/kg of "ideal" body weight.

†Creatinine coefficient for females = 18 mg/kg of "ideal" body weight.

As mentioned in the section "Use of Biochemical Measures," a major concern when using any test requiring a 24-hour urine sample is obtaining a complete urine sample collected during an exact 24-hour period. The value of protein status measurements based on urinary creatinine measurements can also be compromised by the effect of diet on urine creatinine levels, variability in creatinine excretion, and the use of height-weight tables for determining expected creatinine excretion based on sex and stature.[5] These limitations are discussed in Chapter 6.

Nitrogen Balance

A person is said to be in nitrogen balance when the amount of nitrogen (consumed as protein) equals the amount excreted by the body. It is the difference between nitrogen intake and the amount excreted from the body in urine and feces or lost in miscellaneous ways such as the sloughing of skin cells and blood loss.[10] Nitrogen balance is the expected state of the healthy adult. It occurs when the rate of protein synthesis, or anabolism, equals the rate of protein degradation or catabolism. Positive nitrogen balance occurs when nitrogen intake exceeds nitrogen loss and is seen in periods of anabolism, such as childhood or recovery from trauma, surgery, or illness. Negative nitrogen balance occurs when nitrogen losses exceed nitrogen intake and can result from insufficient protein intake, catabolic states (for example, sepsis, trauma, surgery, and cancer), or during periods of excessive protein loss (as a result of burns or certain gastrointestinal and renal diseases characterized by unusual protein loss). Nutritional support can help return a patient to positive nitrogen balance or at least prevent severe losses of energy stores and body protein.[5–7]

Nitrogen balance studies involve 24-hour measurement of protein intake and an estimate of nitrogen losses from the body. The following formula is used:

$$N_2\,\text{Balance} = \frac{\text{PRO}}{6.25} - \text{UUN} - 4$$

where N_2 Balance = nitrogen balance; PRO = protein intake (g/24 h); and UUN = urine urea nitrogen (g/24 h).

Protein intake, measured by dietary assessment methods, is divided by 6.25 to arrive at an estimate of nitrogen intake. Nitrogen loss is generally estimated by measuring urine urea nitrogen (which accounts for 85% to 90% of nitrogen in the urine) and adding a constant (for example, 4 g) to account for nitrogen losses from the skin, stool, wound drainage, nonurea nitrogen, and so on, which cannot be easily measured.[5–7,10]

Problems associated with measuring protein intake and nitrogen excretion limit the usefulness of this approach. For example, it is difficult to account for the unusually high nonurine nitrogen losses seen in some patients with burns, diarrhea, vomiting, or fistula drainage. In such cases, this approach to calculating nitrogen balance may not yield accurate results.

Serum Proteins

Serum protein concentrations can be useful in assessing protein status, in determining whether a patient is at risk of experiencing medical complications, and for evaluating a patient's response to nutritional support. The serum proteins of primary interest in nutritional assessment are shown in Table 9.2.[2] In most instances, their measurement is simple and accurate. Use of serum protein measurements is based on the assumption that decreases in serum concentrations are due to decreased liver production (the primary site of synthesis). This is considered a consequence of a limited supply of amino acids from which the serum proteins are synthesized or a decrease in the liver's capacity to synthesize serum proteins. The extent to which nutritional status or liver function affects serum protein concentrations cannot always be determined. A number of factors other than inadequate protein intake affect serum protein concentrations. These are noted in Table 9.2.

Albumin

The most familiar and abundant of the serum proteins, as well as the most readily available clinically, is albumin. Serum albumin level has been shown to be an indicator of depleted protein status and decreased dietary protein intake. Measured over the course of several weeks, it has been shown to correlate with other measures of protein status and to respond to protein repletion. Low concentrations of serum albumin are associated with increased morbidity and mortality in hospitalized patients.[2,5–7,11] Despite these correlations, the value of albumin as a protein status indicator is severely limited by several factors. Its relatively long half-life (14 to 20 days) and large body pool (4 to 5 g/kg of body weight) cause serum levels to respond very slowly to nutritional change.[2,5–7,11] Because it is neither sensitive to, nor specific for, acute PEM or a patient's response to nutritional support, it is not a useful indicator of protein depletion or repletion.[2,11]

Serum albumin level is determined by several factors: the rate of synthesis, its distribution in the body, the rate at which it is catabolized, abnormal losses from the body, and altered fluid status.[2,11] About 60% of the body's albumin is found outside the bloodstream. When serum concentrations begin falling during early PEM, this extravascular albumin moves into the bloodstream, helping maintain normal serum concentrations despite protein and energy deficit. During the acute catabolic phase of an injury, an infection, or surgery, there is increased synthesis of substances known as acute-phase reactants. Included among these are C-reactive protein, fibrinogen, haptoglobin, and $Á_1$-glycoprotein. Acute-phase reactants decrease synthesis of albumin, prealbumin, and transferrin. Consequently, levels of these serum proteins may remain low during this catabolic phase

TABLE 9.2 Serum Proteins Used in Nutritional Assessment

Serum Protein		Half-Life	Function	Comments*
Albumin		18–20 days	Maintains plasma oncotic pressure; carrier for small molecules	In addition to protein status, other factors affect serum concentrations.
Normal:	3.5–5.0 g/L			
Mild depletion:	3.0–3.4 g/L			
Moderate depletion:	2.4–2.9 g/L			
Severe depletion:	< 2.4 g/L			
Transferrin		8–9 days	Binds iron in plasma and transports to bone marrow	Iron deficiency increases hepatic synthesis and plasma levels; increases during pregnancy, during estrogen therapy, and in acute hepatitis; reduced in protein-losing enteropathy and nephropathy, chronic infections, uremia, and acute catabolic states; often measured indirectly by total iron-binding capacity; equations for indirect prediction should be developed locally.
Normal:	200–400 mg/dL			
Mild depletion:	150–200 mg/dL			
Moderate depletion:	100–149 mg/dL			
Severe depletion:	< 100 mg/dL			
Prealbumin (Transthyretin)		2–3 days	Binds T_3 and, to a lesser extent, T_4; carrier for retinol-binding protein	Level is increased in patients with chronic renal failure on dialysis due to decreased renal catabolism; reduced in acute catabolic states, after surgery, in hyperthyroidism, in protein-losing enteropathy; increased in some cases of nephrotic syndrome; serum level determined by overall energy balance as well as nitrogen balance.
Normal:	16–40 mg/dL			
Mild depletion:	10–15 mg/dL			
Moderate depletion:	5–9 mg/dL			
Severe depletion:	< 5 mg/dL			
Retinol-binding protein (RBP)		12 hours	Transports vitamin A in plasma; binds noncovalently to prealbumin	It is catabolized in renal proximal tubular cell; with renal disease, RBP increases and half-life is prolonged; low in vitamin A deficiency, acute catabolic states, after surgery, and in hyperthyroidism.
Normal:	2.1–6.4 mg/dL			

Adapted from Heimburger DC. 2012. Malnutrition and nutritional assessment. In Longo DL, Fauci AS, Kasper DL, Hauser SL, Jameson JL, Loscalzo J (eds.), *Harrison's principles of internal medicine,* 18th ed. New York: McGraw-Hill, 605–612; and Charney P, Malone AM. 2009. *ADA pocket guide to nutrition assessment,* 2nd ed. Chicago: American Dietetic Association.

* All the listed proteins are influenced by hydration and the presence of hepatocellular dysfunction.

despite the provision of adequate nutritional support.[14] The practice of administering albumin to severely ill patients also can interfere with its use as an indicator of protein status.

Transferrin

Serum transferrin is a β-globulin synthesized in the liver that binds and transports iron in the plasma. Because of its smaller body pool and shorter half-life, it has been considered a better index of changes in protein status compared with albumin.[2,11] Although serum transferrin has been shown to be associated with clinical outcome in children with kwashiorkor and marasmus, its use to predict morbidity and mortality outcomes in hospitalized patients has produced conflicting results.[5]

Serum transferrin can be measured directly (by radial immunodiffusion and nephelometry), but it is frequently estimated indirectly from total iron-binding capacity (TIBC) using a prediction formula suited to the particular facility's method for measuring TIBC.[5]

The use of transferrin as an index of nutritional status and repletion is limited by several factors other than protein status that affect its serum concentration. As was outlined in Table 9.2, transferrin levels decrease in chronic infections, protein-losing enteropathy, chronically draining wounds, nephropathy, acute catabolic states (e.g., surgery and trauma), and uremia. Serum levels can be increased during pregnancy, estrogen therapy, and acute hepatitis.[14,18]

Prealbumin

Prealbumin, also known as transthyretin and thyroxine-binding prealbumin, is synthesized in the liver and serves as a transport protein for thyroxine (T_4) and as a carrier protein for retinol-binding protein. Because of its short half-life (2 to 3 days) and small body pool (0.01 g/kg body weight), it is considered a more sensitive indicator of protein nutriture and one that responds more rapidly to changes in protein status than albumin or transferrin.

Prealbumin decreases rapidly in response to deficits of either protein or energy and is sensitive to the early stages of malnutrition. Because serum concentration quickly returns to expected levels once adequate nutritional therapy begins, it is not recommended as an end-point for terminating nutritional support. It may prove to be better suited as an indicator of recent dietary intake than as a means of assessing nutritional status.[2] Serum concentration also will return to expected levels in response to adequate energy in the absence of sufficient protein intake. Its use as an indicator of protein status appears to be preferable to the use of albumin or transferrin. However, like the other serum proteins outlined in Table 9.2, several factors other than protein status affect its concentration in serum. Levels are reduced in liver disease, sepsis, protein-losing enteropathies, hyperthyroidism, and acute catabolic states (e.g., following surgery or trauma). Serum prealbumin can be increased in patients with chronic renal failure who are on dialysis due to decreased renal catabolism.[2,11]

Retinol-Binding Protein

Retinol-binding protein, a liver protein, acts as a carrier for retinol (vitamin A alcohol) when complexed with prealbumin. It circulates in the blood as a 1:1:1 trimolecular complex with retinol and prealbumin.[13] Retinol-binding protein shares several features with prealbumin. It responds quickly to protein-energy deprivation and adequate nutritional therapy, as well as to ample energy in the absence of sufficient protein. Like prealbumin, it may be a better indicator of recent dietary intake than of overall nutritional status. It has a much shorter half-life (about 12 hours) than prealbumin. Its smaller body pool (0.002 g/kg body weight), however, complicates its precise measurement. There is no convincing evidence that its use in nutritional assessment is preferred over prealbumin. Because it is catabolized in the renal proximal tubule cell, serum levels are increased in renal disease and its half-life is prolonged. Serum levels can be decreased in vitamin A deficiency, acute catabolic states, and hyperthyroidism.[2,13]

Iron Status

Iron deficiency is the most common single nutrient deficiency in the United States and the most common cause of anemia. Preschool children and women of childbearing age are at highest risk of iron deficiency.[14]

Iron deficiency results when ingestion or absorption of dietary iron is inadequate to meet iron losses or iron requirements imposed by growth or pregnancy. Considerable iron can be lost from heavy menstruation, frequent blood donations, early feeding of cow's milk to infants, frequent aspirin use, or disorders characterized by gastrointestinal bleeding. Risk of iron deficiency increases during periods of rapid growth—notably, in infancy (especially in premature infants), adolescence, and pregnancy. The consequences of iron deficiency include reduced work capacity, impaired body temperature regulation, impairments in behavior and intellectual performance, increased susceptibility to lead poisoning, and decreased resistance to infections. During pregnancy, iron deficiency increases risk of maternal death, prematurity, low birth weight, and neonatal mortality. During early childhood it can have adverse effects on cognitive, motor, and emotional development that may be only partially reversible.[15,16] The public health significance of iron deficiency is underscored by the fact that two of the objectives for *Healthy People 2020* relate to reducing iron deficiency among young children and females of childbearing age and among pregnant females.[14]

Anemia is a hemoglobin level below the normal reference range for individuals of the same sex and age. Descriptive terms such as *microcytic, macrocytic,* and *hypochromic* are sometimes used to describe anemias. *Microcytic* refers to abnormally small red blood cells defined by a mean corpuscular volume (MCV) < 80 femtoliters (fL), whereas *macrocytic* describes unusually large red blood cells defined as an MCV > 100 fL. Hypochromic cells are those with abnormally low levels of hemoglobin as defined by a mean corpuscular hemoglobin concentration < 320 g of hemoglobin/L or by a mean corpuscular hemoglobin < 27 picograms (pg, 10^{-12} grams).

Although the most common cause of anemia is iron deficiency, other common causes include inflammation, infection, tissue injury, and cancer, which are collectively referred to as anemia of inflammation. Anemia can also result from deficiencies of folate and vitamin B_{12}. Of particular concern to physicians working with individual patients and nutritional epidemiologists attempting to estimate the prevalence of iron deficiency in populations is differentiating iron-deficiency anemia from anemia caused by inflammatory disease, infection, chronic diseases, and thalassemia traits.[17,18]

Stages of Iron Depletion

The risk of iron deficiency increases as the body's iron stores are depleted. Iron depletion can be divided into three stages. These stages and the biochemical tests used in identifying them are shown in Table 9.3. Figure 9.1 illustrates how values for these tests change throughout the stages of iron deficiency.

The first stage of iron depletion, depleted iron stores, is not associated with any adverse physiologic effects, but it does represent a state of vulnerability.[16,18] Low stores occur in healthy persons and appear to be the usual physiologic condition for growing children and menstruating women.[18,19] As shown in Figure 9.1, during this first stage, low iron stores are reflected by decreased serum ferritin levels, but values for the other biochemical tests remain within normal limits.

The second stage of iron depletion, early functional iron deficiency without anemia, can be considered representative of early or mild iron deficiency because, at this point, adverse physiologic consequences can begin to occur. This stage is characterized by changes indicating insufficient iron for normal production of hemoglobin and other essential iron compounds (for example, myoglobin and iron-containing enzymes).[16,18,19] As shown in Figure 9.1, this stage is characterized by decreased transferrin saturation and increased erythrocyte protoporphyrin levels. A precursor of hemoglobin, erythrocyte protoporphyrin increases when too little iron is available for optimal hemoglobin

TABLE 9.3 The Three Stages of Iron Deficiency and the Indicators Used to Identify Them

Stage of Iron Deficiency	Indicator	Diagnostic Range
1. Depleted stores	Serum ferritin concentration	< 12 μg/L
	Total iron binding capacity	> 400 μg/dL
2. Early functional iron deficiency (without anemia)	Transferrin saturation	< 16%
	Free erythrocyte protoporphyrin	> 70 μg/dL erythrocyte
	Serum transferrin receptor	> 8.5 mg/L
3. Iron deficiency anemia	Hemoglobin concentration	< 130 g/L in males < 120 g/L in females
	Mean corpuscular volume	< 80 fL

Source: Adapted from Panel on Micronutrients, Subcommittee on Upper Reference Levels of Nutrients and of Interpretation and Uses of Dietary Reference Intakes, Standing Committee on the Scientific Evaluation of Dietary Reference Intakes. 2001. *Dietary Reference Intakes for Vitamin A, Vitamin K, Arsenic, Boron, Chromium, Copper, Iodine, Iron, Manganese, Molybdenum, Nickel, Silicon, Vanadium, and Zinc.* Washington, DC: National Academy Press.

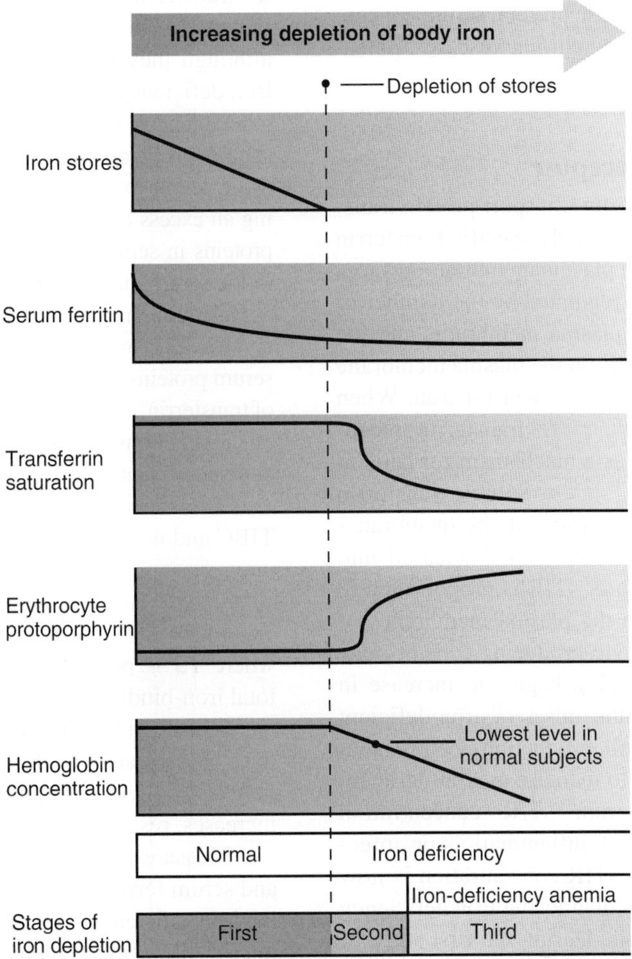

Figure 9.1 Changes in body iron compartments and laboratory assessments of iron status during the stages of iron depletion.

synthesis. Although hemoglobin may be decreased at this stage, it may not fall below the lowest levels seen in normal subjects. Consequently, hemoglobin is not a useful indicator of either stage 1 or stage 2 iron depletion.[16]

The third stage of iron depletion, iron-deficiency anemia, is characterized by decreased serum ferritin, transferrin saturation, hemoglobin, and MCV and increased erythrocyte protoporphyrin.[18,19]

No single biochemical test is diagnostic of impaired iron status. Several different static tests used together provide a much better measure of iron status.[16,18,19]

Serum Ferritin

When the protein apoferritin combines with iron, ferritin is formed. Ferritin, the primary storage form for iron in the body, is found primarily in the liver, spleen, and bone marrow. In healthy persons, approximately 30% of all iron in the body is in the storage form, most of this as ferritin but some as hemosiderin. As iron stores become depleted, tissue ferritin levels decrease. This is accompanied by a fall in serum ferritin concentration.[18–20] Although low serum ferritin concentration is a sensitive indicator of early iron deficiency, it does not necessarily reflect the severity of the depletion as it progresses. Because ferritin is an acute-phase protein, serum concentration is increased in acute and chronic diseases, potentially masking iron deficiency.[20]

Soluble Transferrin Receptor

Cells acquire iron when the iron transport protein transferrin forms a complex with a highly specific transferrin receptor (TfR) located on the plasma membrane surfaces of cells. Intracellular iron is regulated by the number of transferrin receptors on the plasma membrane, and the number of transferrin receptors on the plasma membrane is proportional to the cell's requirement for iron. When cellular iron content is low, more transferrin receptors appear on cell surfaces as a mechanism for cells to sequester the iron they need.[16,17,20–22] Soluble transferrin receptor (sTfR) is a shortened form of the membrane-bound TfR that is cleaved from TfR and released into the serum. The concentration of sTfR is proportional to the concentration of TfR on the plasma membranes of cells, especially the erythrocyte-producing cells of bone marrow. The sTfR concentration begins to increase in early iron deficiency with the onset of iron-deficient erythropoiesis (red blood cell production) before anemia develops and continues to increase as iron-deficient erythropoiesis worsens. Serum sTfR concentration is not affected by concurrent inflammation or infection. Measurement of serum sTfR concentration is now regarded as a valuable tool in diagnosing iron deficiency and monitoring erythropoiesis. During the first stage of iron depletion, when there are residual iron stores in the body, serum ferritin is the most sensitive index of iron status. However, sTfR concentration is a more sensitive index of iron status when iron stores are depleted and before anemia develops.[20–22] NHANES began measuring serum sTfR concentration beginning in 2003, and it is one of the key variables in the model now used by NHANES to assess iron status in children 1 to 5 years of age and in women of childbearing age.[14,20]

Transferrin, Serum Iron, and Total Iron-Binding Capacity

Iron is transported in the blood bound to transferrin, a β-globulin protein molecule synthesized in the liver. Transferrin accepts iron from sites of hemoglobin destruction (the primary source for iron bound to transferrin), from storage sites, and from iron absorbed through the intestinal tract. It then delivers the iron to sites where it is used—primarily the bone marrow for hemoglobin synthesis, as well as to storage sites, to the placenta for fetal needs, and to all cells for incorporation into iron-containing enzymes. Each molecule of transferrin has the capacity to transport two atoms of iron, but under most circumstances only about 30% of the available iron-binding sites are occupied or saturated.[34]

Because iron is carried in the blood by transferrin, serum iron level is a measure of the amount of iron bound to transferrin. Levels fall sometime between depletion of tissue iron stores and development of anemia, although they may actually be normal in persons with iron deficiency.[18,19]

Total iron-binding capacity measures the amount of iron capable of being bound to serum proteins and provides an estimate of serum transferrin. It is usually measured by adding an excess of iron to serum (thus saturating iron-binding proteins in serum), removing all iron not bound to protein in the serum, and then measuring serum iron. Because it is assumed that most serum iron is bound to transferrin, TIBC is an indirect measure of serum transferrin. Because other serum proteins can bind iron, TIBC is not an exact measure of transferrin, especially in cases of iron overload and certain other conditions. In about 30% to 40% of persons with iron-deficiency anemia, TIBC is not elevated.[18,19]

Transferrin saturation is the ratio of serum iron to TIBC and is calculated using the following formula:

$$TS = \frac{\text{Serum iron } (\mu \text{ mol/L})}{\text{TIBC } (\mu \text{ mol/L})} \times 100$$

where TS = percent transferrin saturation and TIBC = total iron-binding capacity.

Transferrin saturation is the percent of transferrin that is saturated with iron. In uncomplicated iron-deficiency anemia, serum iron levels decrease and TIBC increases, resulting in a decreased transferrin saturation.

Measures of serum iron, TIBC, transferrin saturation, and serum ferritin concentration are useful in distinguishing iron deficiency from other disorders capable of causing microcytic anemias (anemias in which the erythrocytes are smaller than normal).[18,19] Transferrin saturation, however, is considered to be a more sensitive indicator of iron deficiency than either serum iron or TIBC.[35]

Erythrocyte Protoporphyrin

Protoporphyrin is a precursor of heme and accumulates in red blood cells (erythrocytes) when the amount of heme that can be produced is limited by iron deficiency.

Protoporphyrin concentration is generally reported in the range of 0.622 ± 0.27 μmol/L of red blood cells, although the value can vary depending on the analytic method. Iron deficiency can lead to a more than twofold increase over normal values. Erythrocyte protoporphyrin increases as iron depletion worsens, as can be seen in Figure 9.1. Lead poisoning also can result in increased erythrocyte protoporphyrin levels.

Hemoglobin

Hemoglobin is an iron-containing molecule found in red blood cells that is capable of carrying oxygen and carbon dioxide. It also acts as an important acid-base buffer system. It is used as an index of the blood's oxygen-carrying capacity. The amount of hemoglobin in blood depends primarily on the number of red blood cells and to a lesser extent on the amount of hemoglobin in each red blood cell.[12,18,19] Despite its use as a screening test for iron deficiency anemia, isolated measurements of hemoglobin concentration or hematocrit level are not suitable as the sole indicator of iron status.[17] They tend not to become abnormal until the late stages of iron deficiency and are not good indicators of early iron deficiency. In addition, hemoglobin fails to distinguish between iron deficiency anemia and anemia of inflammation.[17] Normal ranges for hemoglobin and hematocrit are shown in Table 9.4.

The use of cutoff points (as in Table 9.4) to evaluate laboratory values inevitably results in some degree of misclassification. For example, no matter where the cutoff value is placed in Figure 9.2, there will be some individuals with adequate iron status whose hemoglobin levels fall below the cutoff value. These are the false positives. There will be some, on the other hand, with an inadequate iron status whose hemoglobin levels fall above the cutoff value. These are the false negatives.

TABLE 9.4 Normal Ranges for Hemoglobin and Hematocrit

Age Group	Hemoglobin (g/dL)	Hematocrit (%)
Newborn	14–24	44–64
2–8 weeks	12–20	39–59
2–6 months	10–17	35–50
6–12 months	9.5–14	29–43
1–6 years	9.5–14	30–40
6–18 years	10–15.5	32–44
Adult male	14–18	42–52
Adult female	12–16	37–47
Pregnant female	> 11	> 33

Source: Adapted from Pagana KD, Pagana TJ. 2010. *Mosby's Manual of Diagnostic and Laboratory Tests,* 4th ed. St. Louis: Mosby Elsevier.

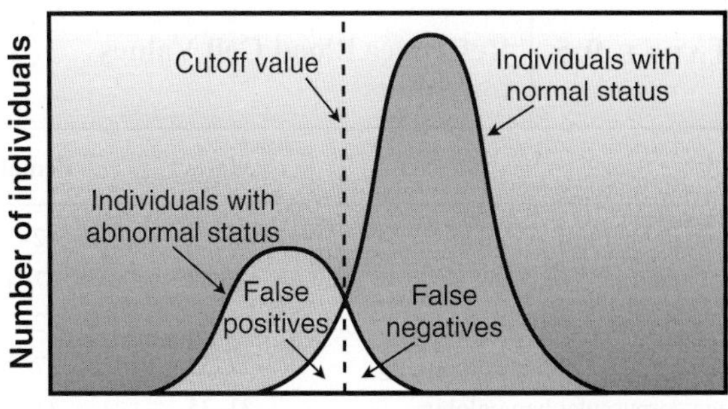

Figure 9.2 Effect of applying a cutoff value for an indicator of nutritional status to the distributions of values for individuals with adequate status and individuals with inadequate status.

Hematocrit

Hematocrit (also known as *packed cell volume*) is defined as the percentage of red blood cells making up the entire volume of whole blood. It can be measured manually by comparing the height of whole blood in a capillary tube with the height of the RBC column after the tube is centrifuged. In automated counters, it is calculated from the RBC count (number of RBCs per liter of blood) and the mean corpuscular volume. Hematocrit depends largely on the number of red blood cells and to a lesser extent on their average size. Normal ranges for hematocrit are shown in Table 9.4. As is the case with hemoglobin, isolated measurement of hematocrit are not suitable as a sole indicator of iron status.[17]

Mean Corpuscular Hemoglobin

The mean corpuscular hemoglobin (MCH) is the amount of hemoglobin in red blood cells. It is calculated by dividing hemoglobin level by the red blood cell count. Reference values are approximately 26 to 34 pg. MCH is influenced by the size of the red blood cell and the amount of hemoglobin in relation to the size of the cell.[18,19]

A similar measure, mean corpuscular hemoglobin concentration (MCHC) is the average concentration of hemoglobin in the average red blood cell. It is calculated by dividing the hemoglobin value by the value for hematocrit. Normal values lie in the range of 320 to 360 g/L (32 to 36 g/dL).[18,19]

Mean Corpuscular Volume

Mean corpuscular volume (MCV) is the average volume of red blood cells. It is calculated by dividing the hematocrit value by the RBC count. Values for MCV are normally in the range of 80 to 100 fL for both males and females.

Factors increasing MCV (resulting in macrocytosis) include deficiencies of folate or vitamin B_{12}, chronic liver disease, alcoholism, and cytotoxic chemotherapy. Among factors decreasing MCV (resulting in microcytosis) are

Table 9.5 Reference Blood Cell Values for Adults

	Males	Females
Hemoglobin (g/dL of blood)	14–18	12–16
Hematocrit (%)	40–54	37–47
Red cell count (× 10^{12}/L blood)	4.7–6.1	4.2–5.4
Mean corpuscular hemoglobin (pg)	27–33	27–33
Mean corpuscular hemoglobin concentration (g/dL of blood)	31–35	31–35
Mean corpuscular volume (fL)	82–98	82–98

Adapted from Ravel R. 1994. *Clinical laboratory medicine: Clinical application of laboratory data,* 6th ed. St. Louis: Mosby.

chronic iron deficiency, thalassemia, anemia of chronic diseases, and lead poisoning.[18,19] Reference blood cell values for adults are shown in Table 9.5.

Assessing Iron Status

One of the challenges of addressing iron deficiency has been uncertainty about the best approach for assessing iron status.[17] Because no single biochemical test exists for reliably assessing iron status, models using two or more different indicators of iron status have been developed. Three of these models are shown in Table 9.6. The two most commonly used are the ferritin model and the more recently introduced body iron model. The ferritin model (also known as the three-indicator model) uses three indicators: serum ferritin, transferrin saturation, and erythrocyte protoporphyrin.[14,16,23,24] The body iron model uses two indicators: serum ferritin and soluble transferrin receptor (sTfR).[14,15,17,20–23] Another model, the mean corpuscular volume (MCV) model uses MCV, transferrin saturation, and erythrocyte protoporphyrin as indicators.[25] Both the ferritin model and the MCV model require that at least two of the three indicators be abnormal.[23–25] The ferritin model tends to overestimate the presence of iron deficiency because it includes ferritin, which reflects stores in the first stage of iron depletion. The MCV model, on the other hand, includes three biochemical tests, all of which reflect altered red blood cell formation.[26] Both models are capable of identifying persons in the second and third stages of iron depletion, but they may fail to distinguish iron-deficiency anemia from the other common causes of anemia, such as inflammation, acute and chronic disease, and lead poisoning, because they include erythrocyte protoporphyrin as a variable.[24–26]

Table 9.6 Models for Assessing Iron Status

Model	Measurements Used
Body iron model*	Soluble transferrin receptor (sTfR) Serum ferritin
Ferritin model†	Serum ferritin Transferrin saturation Erythrocyte protoporphyrin
Mean corpuscular volume (MCV) model†	MCV Transferrin saturation Erythrocyte protoporphyrin

*Measurements used to calculate the sTfR to serum ferritin ratio.

†Two of three values must be abnormal.

The MCV model was employed to assess iron status using data from NHANES II (1976–1980).[25] The ferritin model was used in NHANES III as well as the first few years of the continuous NHANES survey that began in 1999.[20] Beginning in 2003, NHANES limited its interest in assessing iron status to children 1–5 years of age and to women of childbearing age (12–49 years of age) and introduced the measurement of sTfR. Since 2003, NHANES has used the body iron model to assess body iron in the two groups of interest (children 1–5 years and women 12–49 years).[20] Of the three models, the body iron model is considered superior because it is less affected by inflammation than are the ferritin and MCV models. In addition, only two measures are used in the body model, whereas three measures are used in the other models. The greater simplicity of the body iron model makes it more suitable for use in areas where resources are limited and where anemia due to inflammation, chronic disease, and nutrient deficiencies other than iron are relatively common.[14,15,20–22] Using the body iron model, body iron can be estimated from the ratio of sTfR to serum ferritin. Body iron is in positive balance (≥ 0 mg of iron per kg of body weight or ≥ 0 mg/kg) when there is residual storage iron or in a negative balance (< 0 mg of iron per kg of body weight or < 0 mg/kg) during functional iron deficiency when there is a lack of iron required to maintain a normal hemoglobin concentration.[20] Both sTfR and serum ferritin can be measured using a small capillary blood specimen. Body iron is expressed in mg of iron per kg of body weight, controlling for the effect of body weight when estimating body iron and increasing the utility of this model for assessing the iron status of younger persons. Figure 9.3 shows the age-adjusted prevalence estimates of low body iron stores (< 0 mg/kg) in U.S. children and women by race/ethnicity using data from NHANES 2003–2006. The highest prevalence of low body iron assessed using the body iron model was seen in Mexican American children 1–5 years of age and in non-Hispanic black women 12–49 years of age.[20]

Iron Overload

A second disorder of iron metabolism is iron overload, which is the accumulation of excess iron in body tissues. Iron overload is most often the result of hemochromatosis, a group of genetic diseases characterized by excessive

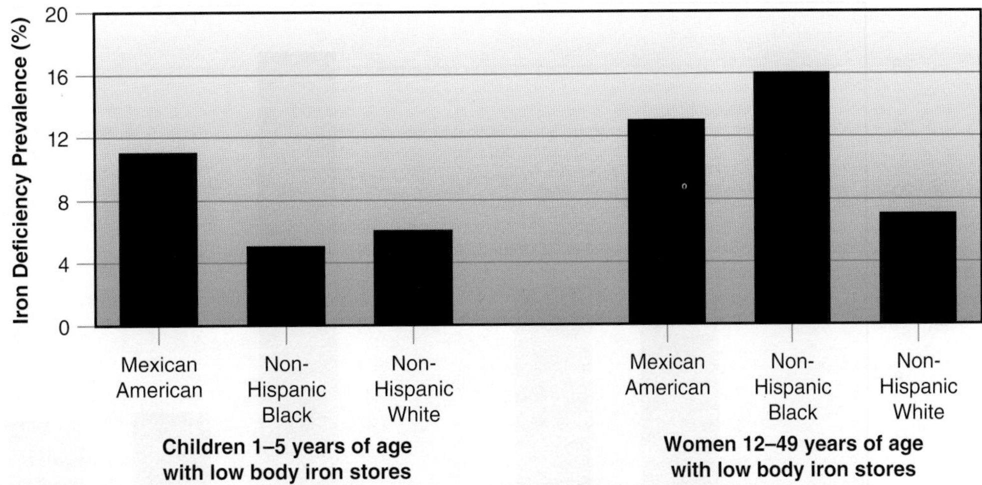

Figure 9.3 Age-adjusted prevalence estimates of low body iron stores (< 0 mg/kg) in U.S. children and women by race/ethnicity, NHANES 2003–2006.

The highest prevalence of low body iron assessed using the body iron model was seen in Mexican American children 1–5 years of age and in non-Hispanic black women 12–49 years of age.

Source: U.S. Centers for Disease Control and Prevention. 2012. *Second National Report on Biochemical Indicators of Diet and Nutrition in the U.S. Population.* Atlanta: National Center for Environmental Health. www.cdc.gov/nutritionreport.

intestinal iron absorption and deposition of excessive amounts of iron in parenchymal cells with eventual tissue damage. Organs particularly affected by hemochromatosis are the liver, heart, and pancreas, leading to the failure of these organs and possibly death. Iron overload can also result from multiple blood transfusions and the excessive intake of iron from fortified foods and supplements.[16,17,20,27] Among North Americans of European extraction, it is estimated that more than 10% have a mild form of hemochromatosis resulting in a slight to moderate increase in serum ferritin concentration and transferrin saturation, and that 0.3–0.5% have the more severe form causing organ damage and possibly death.[17,27]

The degree of increase in total body iron is an elevated serum ferritin concentration. Figure 9.4 shows age-adjusted prevalence estimates of low (< 15 ng/mL) and high serum ferritin (> 200 ng/mL for men and > 150 ng/mL for women) in U.S. men and women 12–49 years of age, based on data collected by NHANES between 1999 and 2006. As shown in Figure 9.4, women are at risk of iron deficiency while men are at risk of iron excess, and there are marked differences in the prevalence of low and high serum ferritin concentrations between the two sexes.[20,27]

Calcium Status

Calcium is essential for bone and tooth formation, muscle contraction, blood clotting, and cell membrane integrity.[28,29] Of the 1200 g of calcium in the adult body, approximately 99% is contained in the bones. The remaining 1% is found in extracellular fluids, intracellular structures, and cell membranes.[28,29]

Osteoporosis, a calcium-related health condition of concern, is discussed in Chapter 8. Interest in osteoporosis prevention and treatment, coupled with data showing low calcium intakes in certain groups, especially women, has made calcium a current public health issue. This has sparked interest in assessing the body's calcium status.

At the current time, there are no appropriate biochemical indicators for assessing calcium status. This is due in large part to the biological mechanisms that tightly control serum calcium levels despite wide variations in dietary intake and the fact that the skeleton serves as a calcium reserve so large that calcium deficiency at the cellular or tissue level is essentially never encountered, at least for nutritional reasons.[28,31] Potential approaches to assessing calcium status can be categorized in three areas: bone mineral content measurement, biochemical markers, and measures of calcium metabolism.[28] Of these three approaches, measurement of bone mineral content by such methods as quantitative computed tomography, single- and dual-photon absorptiometry, and dual-energy X-ray absorptiometry is currently the most feasible approach to assessing calcium status. These techniques are discussed in Chapter 8. However, fewer biochemical markers and measures of calcium metabolism are available. Attempts to identify a calcium status indicator in blood have been unsuccessful.

Serum Calcium Fractions

Serum calcium exists in three fractions: protein-bound, ionized, and complexed.[28] These and other values for calcium in body fluids are shown in Table 9.7. The protein-bound calcium is considered physiologically inactive, whereas the ionized fraction is considered physiologically active and functions as an intracellular regulator.[30–32] Complexed calcium is complexed with small negative ions, such as citrate, phosphate, and lactate. Its biological role is uncertain. Because the ionized and complexed

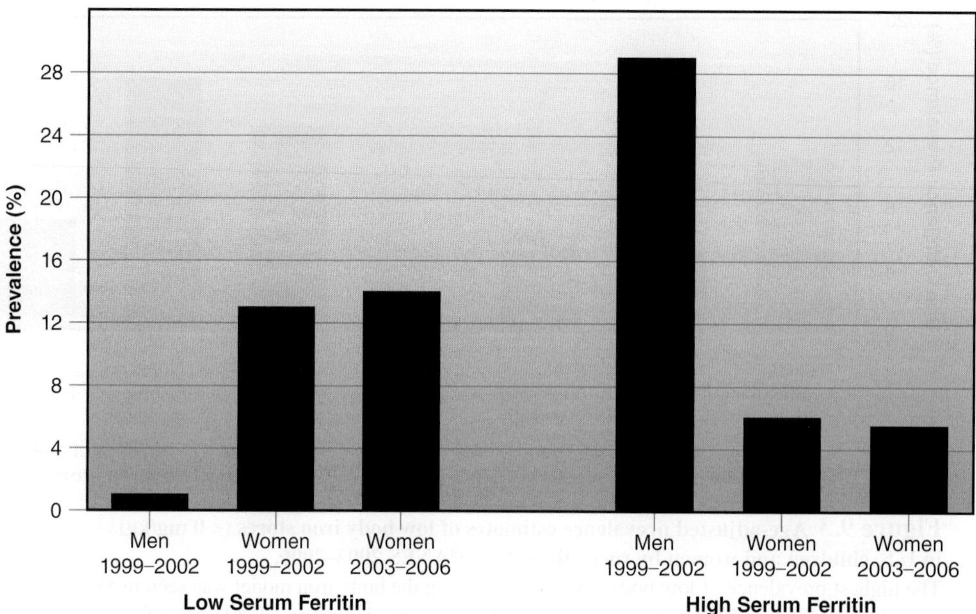

Figure 9.4 Age-adjusted prevalence estimates of low (< 15 ng/mL) and high serum ferritin (> 200 ng/mL for men and > 150 ng/mL for women) in U.S. men and women 12–49 years of age, NHANES 1999–2006.

Women are at risk of iron deficiency while men are at risk of iron excess, as shown by the marked differences in the prevalence of low and high serum ferritin concentrations between the two sexes.

Source: U.S. Centers for Disease Control and Prevention. 2012. *Second National Report on Biochemical Indicators of Diet and Nutrition in the U.S. Population.* Atlanta: National Center for Environmental Health. www.cdc.gov/nutritionreport.

TABLE 9.7 Normal Values for Calcium in Body Fluids

	Mean	Normal Range
Plasma		
Total calcium (mmol/L)	2.5	2.3–2.75
Ionized (mmol/L)	1.18	1.1–1.28
Complexed (mmol/L)		0.15–0.30
Protein-bound (mmol/L)		0.93–1.08
Urine		
24-hour calcium (mmol/L)		
Women	4.55	1.25–10
Men	6.22	1.25–12.5
Fasting calcium: creatinine ratio (molar)		
Postmenopausal women	0.341 ± 0.183*	
Men	0.169 ± 0.099*	

Adapted from Weaver CM. 1990. Assessing calcium status and metabolism. *Journal of Nutrition* 120:1470–1473.

*Mean ± SD.

calcium are diffusible across semipermeable membranes, these two fractions can be collectively referred to as *ultrafilterable calcium.* Serum levels of calcium are so tightly controlled by the body that there is little, if any, association between dietary calcium intake and serum levels.[32] Altered serum calcium levels are rare and indicate serious metabolic problems rather than low or high dietary intakes. Low serum calcium, or hypocalcemia (serum calcium concentration < 2.3 mmol/L), can result from a variety of conditions, including hypoparathyroidism (deficient or absent levels of parathyroid hormone), renal disease, and acute pancreatitis. High serum calcium concentrations, or hypercalcemia (serum calcium > 2.75 mmol/L), can be due to increased intestinal absorption, bone resorption, or renal tubular reabsorption resulting from such conditions as hyperparathyroidism, hyperthyroidism, and hypervitaminosis D (excessive intake of vitamin D).[30,31]

Urinary Calcium

Urinary calcium levels are more responsive to changes in dietary calcium intake than are serum levels.[31] However, urinary calcium is affected by a number of other factors, including those factors leading to hypercalcemia. When serum levels are high, more calcium is available to be excreted through the urine. There is a diurnal variation in urinary calcium, with concentrations higher during the day and lower in the evening.[30] Calcium output tends to be increased when the diet is rich in dietary protein and is low in phosphate and tends to be decreased by high-protein diets rich in phosphate.[30] Urinary calcium losses are increased when the volume of urine output is higher and when the kidneys' ability to reabsorb calcium is impaired.[31,32] Hypocalciuria can result from those factors leading to hypocalcemia as well as from renal failure.[36,37]

Use of the ratio of calcium to creatinine calculated from 2-hour fasting urine samples has been suggested as a possible indicator of calcium status but requires further research. The calcium level in an overnight urine sample shows potential as an indicator of compliance with calcium supplementation.[31]

Zinc Status

Zinc's most important physiologic function is as a component of numerous enzymes.[16,33–35] Consequently, zinc is involved in many metabolic processes, including protein synthesis, wound healing, immune function, and tissue growth and maintenance. Severe zinc deficiency characterized by hypogonadism and dwarfism has been observed in the Middle East. Evidence of milder forms of zinc deficiency (detected by biochemical and clinical measurements) has been found in several population groups in the United States. In humans and laboratory animals, a reduction or cessation of growth is an early response to zinc deficiency, and supplementation in growth-retarded infants and children who are mildly zinc deficient can result in a growth response.[33,34]

Because there is concern about the adequacy of zinc intake among certain groups, especially females, zinc is considered a potential public health issue for which further study is needed. Nutrient intake data and other specific findings suggest that several U.S. population groups may have marginal zinc intakes. According to NHANES data, the average intake of zinc among females ages 20 to 49 years (approximately 9.6 mg/d) is roughly 80% of the RDA. Biochemical and clinical data derived from U.S. government nutritional monitoring activities, however, show no impairment of zinc status.

Plasma Zinc Concentrations

There is currently no specific sensitive biochemical or functional indicator of zinc status.[33] Static measurements of plasma zinc are available, but their use is complicated by the body's homeostatic control of zinc levels and by factors influencing serum zinc levels that are unrelated to nutritional status.[33,34]

There is little, if any, functional reserve of zinc in the body, as there is of some other nutrients (for example, iron, calcium, and vitamin A). The body's zinc levels are maintained by both conservation and redistribution of tissue zinc. In mild zinc deficiency, conservation is manifested by reduction or cessation of growth in growing organisms and by decreased excretion in nongrowing organisms. In most instances of mild deficiency, this appears to be the extent of clinical and biochemical changes. If the deficiency is severe, however, additional clinical signs soon appear.[16,33]

Mature animals and humans have a remarkable capacity to conserve zinc when intakes are low. As a result, inducing zinc deficiency in full-grown animals can be difficult.[33] Several mechanisms are responsible for this. Fecal zinc excretion, for example, can be cut by as much as 60% when dietary intake is low. Not only is the efficiency of intestinal absorption of zinc increased, but losses via the gastrointestinal tract, urine, and sweat are diminished.[33–38]

In laboratory animals, deficiency can lead to selective redistribution of zinc from certain tissues to support other, higher-priority tissues. In mild zinc deficiency, plasma zinc levels apparently can be maintained at the expense of zinc from other tissues.[33,34] Some evidence suggests that redistribution of total body zinc also occurs in humans.

The result of the body's conservation of and ability to redistribute zinc is that measurements of plasma zinc are not a reliable indicator of dietary zinc intake or changes in whole-body zinc status.[38] This is especially the case in mild zinc deficiency. For example, plasma zinc concentrations in growth-retarded children whose growth responded to zinc supplementation were not significantly different from concentrations in normally developed children either before or after supplementation.[38] Despite these limitations, measurement of plasma zinc concentration may be a useful, albeit late, indicator of the size of the body's exchangeable zinc pool. Less than expected values may signal a loss of zinc from bone and liver and increased risk for clinical and metabolic signs of zinc deficiency.[37,38]

Several factors unrelated to nutritional status can influence plasma zinc levels. Decreased levels can result from stress, infection or inflammation, and use of estrogens, oral contraceptives, and corticosteroids.[16,33,34] Plasma zinc can fall by 15% to 20% following a meal.[35] Increased plasma zinc concentrations can result from fasting and red blood cell hemolysis.

Metallothionen and Zinc Status

Metallothionen is a protein found in most tissues but primarily in the liver, pancreas, kidney, and intestinal mucosa. Metallothionen holds promise as a potential indicator of zinc status, particularly when used in conjunction with plasma zinc levels.[35,38] Measurable amounts are found in serum and in red blood cells. Metallothionen has the capacity of binding zinc and copper, and tissue metallothionen concentrations often are proportional to zinc status. In animals, levels are almost undetectable in zinc deficiency and are responsive to zinc supplementation. Whereas plasma zinc levels fall in response to acute stimuli (for example, stress, infection, and inflammation), hepatic and serum metallothionen levels are increased in response to these stimuli. Thus, when plasma levels of zinc fall and of metallothionen rise, it is likely that tissue zinc has been redistributed in response to acute stimuli and that a zinc deficiency is not present because metallothionen is not responsive to acute stimuli in zinc-deficient animals. If plasma zinc and metallothionen are both below expected levels, it is likely that zinc deficiency is present. Erythrocyte metallothionen (which is not affected by stress) also can be used as an indicator of zinc status.[35]

Hair Zinc

Several researchers have investigated the use of zinc in hair as an indicator of body zinc status.[36,38] Decreased concentration of zinc in hair has been reported in zinc-deficient dwarfs, in marginally deficient children and adolescents, and in conditions related to zinc deficiency, such as celiac disease, acrodermatitis enteropathica, and sickle-cell disease. Because hair grows slowly (about 1 cm per month), levels of zinc and other trace elements in hair reflect nutritional status over many months and thus are not affected by diurnal variations or short-term fluctuations in nutritional status. Because of this, hair zinc levels may not be correlated with measurements of zinc in serum or erythrocytes, which reflect shorter-term zinc status.[36,38] Obtaining a sample is noninvasive, and analyzing hair for zinc and other trace elements is relatively easy.

It is important to note that trace elements in hair can come from endogenous sources (those that are ingested or inhaled by the subject and then enter the hair through the hair follicle) and exogenous sources (contamination from trace elements in dust, water, cosmetics, and so on).[39] A major drawback in using hair as an indicator of trace element status is its susceptibility to contamination from these exogenous sources. Some exogenous contaminants can be removed by carefully washing the hair sample before analysis, and several standardized washing procedures have been suggested.[39] However, some contaminants may be difficult or impossible to remove. Selenium, an ingredient in some antidandruff shampoos, is known to increase the selenium content of hair and cannot be removed by the recommended washing procedures.[39]

A variety of other nonnutritional factors may affect the trace element content of hair. Included among these are certain diseases, rate of hair growth, hair color, sex, pregnancy, and age.[39] It has been reported, for example, that higher concentrations of zinc, iron, nickel, and copper can be found in red hair, compared with brown hair, and that iron and manganese are found in higher concentrations in brown hair than in blonde hair.[36,38,39] These factors limit the usefulness of hair as an index of zinc and other trace element status.

Urinary Zinc

Lower than expected concentrations of zinc have been reported in the urine of zinc-depleted persons.[35,36] However, factors other than nutritional status can influence urinary zinc levels, such as liver cirrhosis, viral hepatitis, sickle-cell anemia, surgery, and total parenteral nutrition. Problems associated with obtaining 24-hour urine collections can also complicate use of this indicator. Consequently, urine measurements of zinc are not the preferred approach to assessing zinc status.

Iodine Status

Iodine is a trace element essential for the synthesis of thyroid hormones that regulate metabolic processes related to normal growth and development in humans and animals.[24,40] Inadequate intake of iodine leads to insufficient production of thyroid hormones, resulting in a variety of adverse effects collectively referred to as iodine deficiency disorders. In humans these include mental retardation, hypothyroidism, cretinism, goiter, and varying degrees of other growth and developmental abnormalities (see Box 9.1). Thyroid hormones are particularly important for central nervous system development during uterine development and the first two years of life, making this the most critical period for adequate

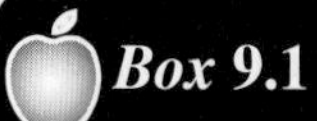

Box 9.1 Manifestations of Iodine Deficiency Disorder Throughout the Lifespan

Fetal Period
Spontaneous abortion
Stillbirth
Congenital anomalies in offspring
Increased perinatal mortality

Neonatal Period
Increased infant mortality
Cretinism

Childhood and Adolescence
Impaired mental function
Cretinism
Delayed physical development

Adulthood
Impaired mental function
Decreased ability to learn
Apathy
Reduced work productivity

All Ages
Goiter
Hypothyroidism
Increased susceptibility of the thyroid gland to nuclear radiation

Source: Adapted from Zimmermann MB, Jooste PL, Pandav CS. 2008. Iodine-deficiency disorders. *Lancet* 372:1251–1262; and Zimmermann MB. 2009. Iodine deficiency. *Endocrine Reviews* 30:376–408.

iodine intake. Deficiency during pregnancy can lead to spontaneous abortion, stillbirth, congenital anomalies in offspring, and increased perinatal and infant mortality. Severe iodine deficiency in utero can result in a condition known as cretinism, which is characterized by gross mental retardation, short stature, deaf-mutism, and spasticity.[41,42] According to the World Health Organization, iodine deficiency is the leading cause of mental retardation in the world. Studies of moderately to severely iodine-deficient populations indicate that chronic iodine deficiency can reduce the intelligence quotient (IQ) by 12.5 to 13.5 points.[24,41] The provision of an iodine supplement to moderately iodine-deficient children has been shown to improve cognitive functioning, suggesting that in some instances cognitive impairment can be at least partly reversed by iodine repletion.[41]

The classic sign of iodine deficiency is thyroid gland enlargement, or goiter, which can occur at any age, including infancy. Goiter is the earliest and most obvious manifestation of iodine deficiency but certainly not its most devastating consequence.[40,41] When iodine intake is insufficient, the anterior pituitary gland increases its secretion of thyroid-stimulating hormone (TSH) in an effort to maximize the thyroid gland's uptake of available iodine, which stimulates thyroid hypertrophy and hyperplasia. Initially goiters are a small, diffuse, and uniform enlargement of the thyroid gland, increasing in size as the iodine deficiency continues. Over time they can develop nodules or lumps and become massive enough to compress neighboring structures, such as the trachea, esophagus, and nerves, as shown in Figure 9.5. In some instances surgical removal is required.[40–42] In younger patients and those with relatively small, diffuse, and soft goiters, iodine repletion can result in a variable degree of shrinkage of the goiter. However, in older patients and those with nodular or fibrotic goiters, fewer than one-third experience any significant shrinkage of the goiter.[43] Paradoxically, excessive iodine intake can cause goiter, as well as hyperthyroidism and hypothyroidism, and increases the risk of thyroid cancer.[20]

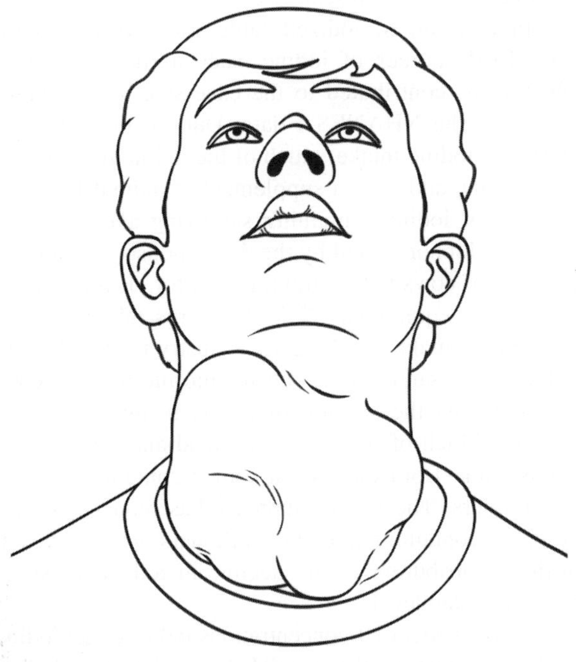

Figure 9.5 **Goiter in the neck of an adolescent.**

Assessing Iodine Status

Because more than 90% of dietary iodine is eventually excreted in the urine, urinary iodine (UI) is the most widely used indicator of recent iodine intake and nutrition status.[24,41,42,44] For individuals, a 24-hour urine collection is necessary to estimate iodine intake using UI concentration. Because 24-hour urine collections are impractical in field studies involving large numbers of subjects, spot urine collections from a representative sample of the target population can be used to calculate median UI in nanograms of iodine per milliliter of urine (ng/mL). Variations in UI concentrations due to differences in hydration among the subjects and the day-to-day variation in iodine intake by individuals will be evened out when a sufficiently large number of spot urine samples are collected from each group or subgroup. The categories for median UI concentrations developed by the World Health Organization (WHO) for assessing iodine status in school-age children and adults (excluding pregnant and lactating women) are shown in Table 9.8. The WHO's categories for median UI concentrations for assessing iodine status in pregnant and lactating women and children less than 2 years of age are shown in Table 9.9. Because of hydration status and day-to-day variation in iodine intake, UI concentrations of spot urine samples are not a reliable indicator of an individual's iodine status. Therefore, it would be a mistake to assume that an individual is iodine deficient based on a UI concentration < 100 ng/mL in a single spot urine sample collected from that individual.[24,45]

In addition to UI concentration, other methods for assessing iodine status include serum thyroglobulin, the goiter rate, and serum concentration of thyroid-stimulating hormone (TSH). While UI concentration is a sensitive indicator of recent iodine intake (days), serum thyroglobulin reflects iodine status over an intermediate period of time spanning weeks to months, and the goiter rate reflects long-term iodine status spanning months to years. TSH is a sensitive indicator of iodine status during the neonatal period. Thyroid hormone concentrations are considered unreliable indicators of iodine status.[41]

Iodine Status in the United States

In the early part of the 20th century, prior to the iodization of table salt, iodine deficiency diseases, particularly goiter, were common and a significant problem. Goiter

TABLE 9.8 World Health Organization Criteria for Assessing Iodine Nutrition Based on Median Urinary Iodine Concentrations of School-age Children (≥ 6 Years of Age) and Adults*

Median Urinary Iodine (ng/mL)	Category of Iodine Intake	Iodine Status
< 20	Insufficient	Severe iodine deficiency
20–49	Insufficient	Moderate iodine deficiency
50–99	Insufficient	Mild iodine deficiency
100–199	Adequate	Adequate iodine nutrition
200–299	Above Requirements	Likely to provide adequate intake for pregnant/lactating women but may pose a slight risk of more than adequate intake in the overall population
≥ 300	Excessive	Risk of adverse health consequences (e.g., iodine-induced hyperthyroidism, autoimmune thyroid disease)

Source: Adapted from U.S. Department of Health and Human Services. 2012. *Second National Report on Biochemical Indicators of Diet and Nutrition in the U.S. Population.* National Center for Environmental Health, Centers for Disease Control and Prevention. www.cdc.gov/nutritionreport.

*These criteria do not apply to pregnant or lactating women or to children less than 2 years of age.

TABLE 9.9 World Health Organization Categories for Median UI Concentrations for Assessing Iodine Status in Pregnant and Lactating Women and Children Less than 2 Years of Age

Population Group	Median Urinary Iodine (ng/mL)	Category of Iodine Intake
Pregnant Women	< 150	Insufficient
	150–249	Adequate
	250–499	More than adequate
	≥ 500	Excessive
Lactating Women	< 100	Insufficient
	≥ 100	Adequate
Children < 2 years of age	< 100	Insufficient
	≥ 100	Adequate

Source: Adapted from Andersson M, de Benoist B, Rogers L. 2010. Epidemiology of iodine deficiency: salt iodisation and iodine status. *Best Practices & Research Clinical Endocrinology & Metabolism* 24:1–11.

was endemic in the United States and Canada, particularly the Great Lakes region, the interior, the U.S. Pacific Northwest, and British Columbia. Voluntary iodization of table salt was introduced in the United States in the 1920s, but it is not mandatory. In Canada, the iodization of table salt is mandatory. The level of iodization is 100 parts per million (PPM), with 1 g of table salt providing 100 μg of iodine. The RDA for adults of 150 μg/d can be met by less than 2 grams of iodized table salt. The RDA for women who are pregnant or lactating, 220 μg/d and 290 μg/d, respectively, can be met by less than 3 g of iodized table salt per day. By the mid-1900s, the iodine status of people in North America dramatically improved, goiter was rare, and iodine deficiency disorders were no long considered a public health problem.[24,46] However, in 1970 the U.S. population was thought to have an excessive iodine intake, with iodine-induced hypothyroidism, autoimmune thyroiditis, and hyperthyroidism becoming more of a problem than iodine deficiency disorders.[46–48] Data from NHANES I, conducted in 1971–1974 found a median UI concentration of 320 ng/mL, representing excessive iodine intake according to WHO criteria shown in Table 9.8. Since then, UI concentrations in Americans have declined and stabilized. Recent data from NHANES shown in Figure 9.6 indicate that iodine intake for the overall U.S. population is adequate with median UI concentrations within the 100 to 200 ng/mL range, indicating adequate iodine intake and with no group with a median UI concentration representing excessive intake.[20]

In addition to iodized table salt, other adventitious food sources of iodine, such as dairy products and breads, contributed to the excessive iodine intake shown by the NHANES I data. During this period of excessive iodine intake, much of the iodine in milk was from iodine added as a supplement to animal feed and residues of iodine-containing sanitizing agents (disinfectant iodophors) used by the dairy industry to sanitize the teats of cows before milking and for cleaning milk-processing equipment.[24,46,48] Concerns about excessive iodine intake led the dairy industry to switch from iodine-based sanitizing agents to chlorine-based agents, thus reducing the amount of iodine in milk in recent decades. Much of the iodine in bread and other baked goods came from the use of iodine-containing dough conditioners. The baking industry has reduced its use of iodine-containing dough conditioners in recent years, further contributing to the decline in iodine intake to more adequate levels.

While median UI concentrations indicate that iodine intake is adequate for the overall U.S. population, including

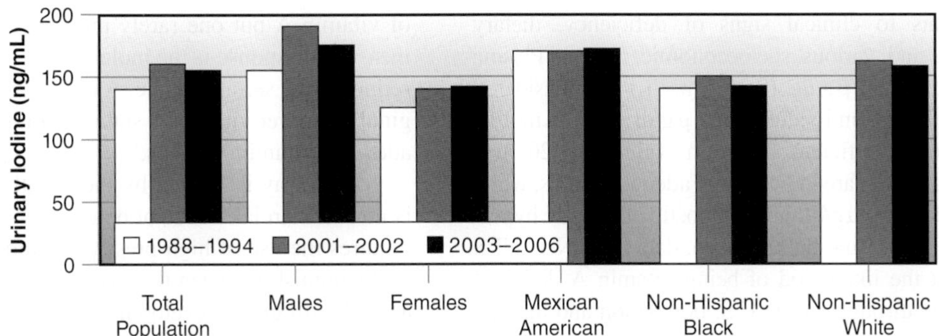

Figure 9.6 Age-adjusted mean concentrations of urinary iodine in the U.S. population aged 6 years and older by sex or race/ethnicity, National Health and Nutrition Examination Survey, 1988–2006.

Between 1988 and 2006, urinary iodine concentrations remained relatively stable and within the range of adequacy, which is 100 to 200 nanograms of iodine per milliliter of urine (ng/mL).

Source: U.S. Department of Health and Human Services. 2012. *Second National Report on Biochemical Indicators of Diet and Nutrition in the U.S. Population.* National Center for Environmental Health, Centers for Disease Control and Prevention. www.cdc.gov/nutritionreport.

children, women 20 to 39 years of age have the lowest UI concentrations, just slightly above the range representing insufficient.[24,47,49] Because requirements increase during pregnancy and lactation, the American Thyroid Association recommends that pregnant women in the United States and Canada take a prenatal supplement containing 150 μg of iodine daily and that all prenatal supplements contain 150 μg of iodine. Approximately half (49%) of commercially available prenatal supplements marketed in the United States contain iodine, and < 20% of women of childbearing age are consuming supplements containing iodine.[24,50] Mandatory iodization of all table salt sold in the United States would also help ensure adequate iodine intakes in women of childbearing age. Iodization of table salt in the United States is voluntary, and iodized salt is chosen by only 50 to 60% of the U.S. population. In addition, approximately 75% of all sodium consumed by Americans is that added in the processing and manufacturing of food, little of which is iodized. Consequently, efforts to reduce the amount of sodium in processed foods will have little, if any, adverse impact on iodine intakes in the United States. In fact, if the amount of sodium added during the manufacturing and processing of foods were reduced as some groups recommend, Americans would increase their use of iodized table salt during cooking and at the table, thus ensuring that more Americans have adequate iodine intakes. Efforts to prevent iodine deficiency and efforts to reduce salt consumption to prevent chronic disease do not conflict. As long as all salt consumed is iodized, adequate iodine intake is certain, even at levels of salt intake currently recommended by the *Dietary Guidelines for Americans* for persons 51 years of age and older and those of any age who are African American, or have hypertension, diabetes, or chronic kidney disease.[48,51,52]

VITAMIN A STATUS

Vitamin A status can be grouped into five categories: deficient, marginal, adequate, excessive, and toxic. In the deficient and toxic states, clinical signs are evident, while biochemical or static tests of vitamin A status must be relied on in the marginal, adequate, and excessive states.[53] Biochemical assessment of vitamin A status generally involves measurements of plasma concentrations of retinol or the vitamin A carrier protein, retinol binding protein (RBP), retinol isotope dilution, and dose-response tests. Used less frequently are examination of epithelial cells of the conjunctiva, assessment of dark adaptation, and liver biopsy.[1,16,53,54] These approaches are best used when assessing the vitamin A status of populations. The approaches for diagnosing vitamin A deficiency in an individual are limited to retinol isotope dilution, assessment of dark adaptation, and liver biopsy.[54] Vitamin A levels in breast milk can also be used as an index of vitamin A status in lactating women and in detecting response to maternal supplementation.[55]

Plasma Levels

Measurement of plasma concentration of retinol is the most common biochemical measure of vitamin A in a population group.[1,16,53,54] Under normal conditions, about 95% of plasma vitamin A is in the form of retinol and bound to retinol-binding protein, and about 5% is unbound and in the form of retinyl esters.[53,54] Serum measurements are predictive of vitamin A status only when the body's reserves are either critically depleted or overfilled. Because plasma concentration of retinol may be within the expected range despite low vitamin A concentrations within the liver, test results should be interpreted with caution.[54] However, data from plasma measurements can be of some value in drawing conclusions about the relationship of plasma measurements to clinical signs of deficiency, dietary intake data, and various socioeconomic factors. Plasma concentrations <10 μg/dL (0.35 μmol/L) are considered severely deficient, and values < 20 μg/dL (0.70 μmol/L) are considered deficient.[20] Serum values > 20 μg/dL (> 0.70 μmol/L) are indicative of adequate status, while serum levels > 300 μg/dL are diagnostic of chronic hypervitaminosis A.[20] Using these criteria, data from NHANES indicate that the likelihood of being vitamin A deficient was very low throughout the U.S. population and that the likelihood of vitamin A excess was also very low, but it increased with increasing age. For the past two decades, more than 95% of the U.S. population have had adequate serum concentrations of vitamin A.[20] The plasma concentration of retinol-binding protein (RBP) can be used as a surrogate measure of plasma retinol, but it is affected by conditions other than vitamin A status. It is likely to be low during conditions of malnutrition and inflammation.[53]

Relative Dose Response

The relative dose-response test (RDR) and modified relative dose-response test (MRDR) are based on the principle that, when stores of retinol are high, plasma retinol concentration is little affected by oral administration of vitamin A. But when reserves are low, the plasma retinol concentration increases markedly, reaching a peak 5 h after an oral dose. As hepatic vitamin A stores become depleted, retinol-binding protein (RBP) accumulates in the liver in an unbound state known as *apo-RBP.* When vitamin A is given to a subject whose stores are depleted, the vitamin A is absorbed from the intestinal tract; is taken up by the liver, where it binds to the apo-RBP; and then is released from the liver in the form of *holo-RBP* (the complex of RBP and vitamin A). In the RDR, a fasting blood sample is taken, followed by oral administration of vitamin A as retinyl palmitate. Another blood sample is drawn 5 hours later. Comparison of the fasting and postdosing holo-RBP measurements represents the extent of apo-RBP accumulation, which is directly related to the shortage of vitamin A.[1,16,53,54]

The RDR is calculated using the following formula:[1]

$$\text{RDR} = \frac{\text{Vit A}_5 - \text{vit A}_0}{\text{Vit A}_5} \times 100$$

where vit A_5 = serum vitamin A level 5 hours after receiving the dose of vitamin A and vit A_0 = fasting serum vitamin A level.

An RDR > 50% is considered indicative of acute deficiency, values between 20% and 50% indicate marginal status, and values < 20% suggest adequate intake.[1] Limitations of the RDR include the 5-hour waiting period and the need to draw two blood samples.[1]

The MRDR is based on the same principle but uses only one blood sample 5 hours after administration of the test dose of dehydroretinol, a naturally occurring form of vitamin A but one rarely present in most diets.[1] The measured response is the molar ratio of dehydroretinol to retinol in the serum sample. A ratio > 0.06 indicates marginal or poorer vitamin A status. A ratio < 0.03 indicates adequate vitamin A status.[1]

The assay is limited by the fact that there currently is no commercial source of dehydroretinol, and the assay requires the use of high-pressure liquid chromatography to distinguish between the two forms of vitamin A. The assay is still under development but does have the advantage of requiring only one blood sample.[1]

Conjunctival Impression Cytology

Vitamin A deficiency can result in morphologic changes in epithelial cells covering the body and lining its cavities. It can result in a decline in the number of mucus-producing goblet cells in the epithelium of the conjunctiva of the eye. The epithelial cells also may take on a more squamous appearance—flatter cells, smaller nuclei, and with the cytoplasm making up a greater proportion of the total cell. The conjunctival impression cytology test involves the microscopic examination of the conjunctival epithelial cells to determine morphologic changes indicative of vitamin A deficiency.[1,16]

A minute sample of epithelial cells can be obtained by touching a strip of cellulose ester filter paper to the outer portion of the conjunctiva for 3 to 5 seconds and then gently removing it. The filter paper with the adherent epithelial cells is placed in a fixative solution, where it can be stored until being stained and examined by ordinary light microscopy.[1]

The test is limited by several factors and is not widely used.[1] It is difficult to get tissue samples from children under 3 years of age, and the cytologists must follow standardized criteria in evaluating samples. The sensitivity of the test is limited by conjunctival and systemic infections and possibly by severe malnutrition.[1,16]

Dark Adaptation

The best-defined function of vitamin A is its role in the visual process. The visual pigment rhodopsin is generated when the protein opsin in the rods of the retina combines with a *cis*-isomer of retinol. When light strikes the eye, rhodopsin is split into opsin and a *trans*-isomer of retinol, generating the visual-response signal. The *trans*-isomer is then converted back to the *cis*-isomer, which then combines with opsin to reform rhodopsin. During this process, some of the retinol isomer is lost and must be replaced by vitamin A present in the retina. Under normal conditions, sufficient retinol is present, and rhodopsin is readily formed. When vitamin A is in short supply, less rhodopsin is formed, and the eye fails to adapt as readily to low light levels after exposure to bright light levels.[1,16]

Tests are available to directly measure the level of rhodopsin and its rate of regeneration. Field tests measuring visual acuity in dim light after exposure to bright light also can be used.[1] However, the relative dose response, when available, is a more specific and objective test of vitamin A status and is preferred over functional tests of dark adaptation.

Direct Measurement of Liver Stores

Direct measurement of hepatic vitamin A stores in liver tissue is considered the "gold standard" of vitamin A status, but its invasive nature limits its usefulness.[53] In many countries, the median vitamin A concentration in liver tissue of well-nourished persons is approximately 100 μg of retinol/g of liver tissue. A concentration > 20 μg of retinol/g of liver tissue is considered adequate for both children and adults of all ages.[53] Concentrations < 5 μg of retinol/g of liver tissue are associated with vitamin A deficiency.

The assay can be done on a very small amount of liver tissue obtained by inserting a biopsy needle through the abdominal wall. Because of the invasiveness of the biopsy procedure, assaying liver tissue for vitamin A is limited to situations when a liver biopsy is necessary for diagnostic purposes or when liver tissue can be obtained from postmortem examinations.[16,53]

Retinol Isotope Dilution

The best way to represent vitamin A status is in terms of total body stores of vitamin A. Approximately 90% of the body's vitamin A stores are in the liver, but direct measurement of vitamin A concentration in the liver is not practical in most instances because a liver biopsy is a highly invasive surgical procedure. A noninvasive, indirect approach to measuring total body stores of vitamin A is retinol isotope dilution, which is considered the best approach currently available for assessing vitamin A status with the least risk to subjects.[1,16,56] The procedure involves administering to a subject a known amount of vitamin A that is labeled with a nonradioactive isotope. This is ingested with an adequate amount of fat to ensure suitable absorption. After a period of approximately two to three weeks, the isotopically labeled vitamin A mixes with the body's existing total pool of unlabeled vitamin A. A sample of blood is then removed from the subject and the plasma concentrations of the labeled and unlabeled vitamin A are measured. Using a mathematical formula, the ratio of the labeled vitamin A to the unlabeled vitamin A is calculated. This ratio is used to estimate the size of the subject's total vitamin A pool.[56,57] Limitations of this method include the high cost of the isotopically labeled vitamin A and the sophisticated laboratory techniques needed to measure the plasma concentrations of the labeled and unlabeled vitamin A. However, it is the only noninvasive method currently available for assessing the full range of vitamin A status, from deficient to toxic (hypervitaminosis A).[1,56,57]

VITAMIN D STATUS

The major physiological function of vitamin D in vertebrates, including humans, is to maintain serum calcium and phosphorus concentrations in a range that supports bone mineralization, neuromuscular function, and various cellular processes. Vitamin D increases serum concentrations of calcium and phosphorus by promoting their absorption by the small intestine, promoting their reabsorption by the kidney, and stimulating bone resorption with the release of calcium and phosphorus from bone.[58] The role of vitamin D in maintaining skeletal health is well established.[30] Deficiency of vitamin D causes growth retardation and rickets in children. In adults vitamin D deficiency causes osteomalacia, and precipitates and exacerbates bone demineralization, leading to osteopenia, osteoporosis, and increased fracture risk.[58] What is less certain and a matter of debate is whether vitamin D exposure at levels sufficient to prevent clinically evident bone disease is optimal in terms of reducing risk of a variety of other conditions not traditionally linked to vitamin D. Research suggests that increasing vitamin D exposure decreases risk of certain types of cancer, type 1 and type 2 diabetes, respiratory tract infections, and influenza and asthma in children.[59–61]

Vitamin D (calciferol) is a fat-soluble sterol found in a limited number of foods, including fish-liver oils, fatty fishes, mushrooms, egg yolks, and liver.[20] The two major forms of vitamin D are cholecalciferol (D_3) and ergocalciferol (D_2). Vitamin D_3 is synthesized in the skin of vertebrates by the action of ultraviolet B (UVB) radiation on 7-dehydrocholesterol present in the skin. Vitamin D_2 is produced by UV irradiation of ergosterol, as sterol occurring in molds, yeast, and higher-order plants. Vitamin D in humans comes from two sources: from that present in the foods we eat and from that synthesized in the body by sun exposure. If sun exposure is sufficient, dietary intake is not necessary. However, cutaneous synthesis of vitamin D_3 is decreased by such factors as living at a higher latitude, older age, darker skin pigmentation, less skin exposed to sunlight, and sunscreen use. Major dietary sources of vitamin D in the United States are foods fortified with vitamin D, including milk products, some citrus juices, and ready-to-eat breakfast cereals.[20] Practically all fortified foods and supplements in the United States use vitamin D_3 instead of vitamin D_2.[62]

Assessing Vitamin D Status

Vitamin D status is best assessed by measuring the serum concentration of 25-hydroxyvitamin D [25(OH)D], the major circulating form of the vitamin, which reflects total vitamin D exposure from food, supplements, and synthesis.[20,30] Although serum concentration of 25(OH)D is not considered a validated health outcome indicator, it is the measure preferred by clinicians to assess total vitamin D exposure and allows comparisons to be made between exposure and health outcomes. What serum concentrations of 25(OH)D represent an optimal vitamin D exposure is a matter of some disagreement. There has been no systematic, evidence-based development process to establish 25(OH)D cutpoints for defining what is indicative of vitamin D deficiency or adequacy.[20,30,62] Based on its review of the available data, the Institute of Medicine's Committee to Review Dietary Reference Intakes for Vitamin D and Calcium concluded that persons are at risk of deficiency relative to bone health when the serum concentration of 25(OH)D is < 30 nmol/L (nanomoles per liter). The Committee concluded that some, but not all, persons are potentially at risk of inadequate vitamin D exposure when their serum 25(OH)D is between 30 and 50 nmol/L. Practically all persons have a sufficient exposure with serum 25(OH)D between 50 and 75 nmol/L. The Committee concluded that serum concentrations between 75 and 125 nmol/L were not consistently associated with increased benefits and that there may be reason for concern at concentrations > 125 nmol/L.[30] The Committee concluded that a serum 25(OH)D of 40 nmol/L represented a vitamin D exposure that met the average requirement and was consistent with the Estimated Average Requirement (EAR). A serum 25(OH)D concentration of approximately 50 nmol/L represented a vitamin D exposure that was associated with benefit for nearly all the population, and was consistent with the Recommended Dietary Allowance (RDA).[30] In marked contrast to these conclusions are those of other researchers who suggest that a serum 25(OH)D concentration of 75 nmol/L is closer to the bottom of the range for acceptable skeletal health and that a serum 25(OH)D concentration < 120 nmol/L is associated with preventable diseases.[60,62]

Beginning with NHANES III in 1988, the vitamin D status of the U.S. population has been monitored. NHANES collects survey information and biological samples during the summer from people living at higher latitudes and in the winter from those living in lower latitudes. Serum 25(OH)D concentration data from NHANES are shown in Figure 9.7. Between 1988 and the periods 2001–2002 and 2003–2006, serum concentration of 25(OH)D in the United States decreased approximately 10%. Factors that could help explain this decrease include increased body mass index (which is associated with a lower serum 25(OH)D concentration), decreased milk intake, and increased use of sunscreen and other sun protection measures. Using the criteria suggested by the Institute of Medicine's Committee to Review Dietary Reference Intakes for Vitamin D and Calcium, serum 25(OH)D concentrations for the total population are within the range consistent with sufficient vitamin D exposure and those for non-Hispanic blacks are at the lower end of the range that is consistent with being potentially at risk of inadequate vitamin D exposure. It is important to note that because the values represented by Figure 9.7 are means, half of the group is above the mean and the other half of the group is below the mean.[20] Data from

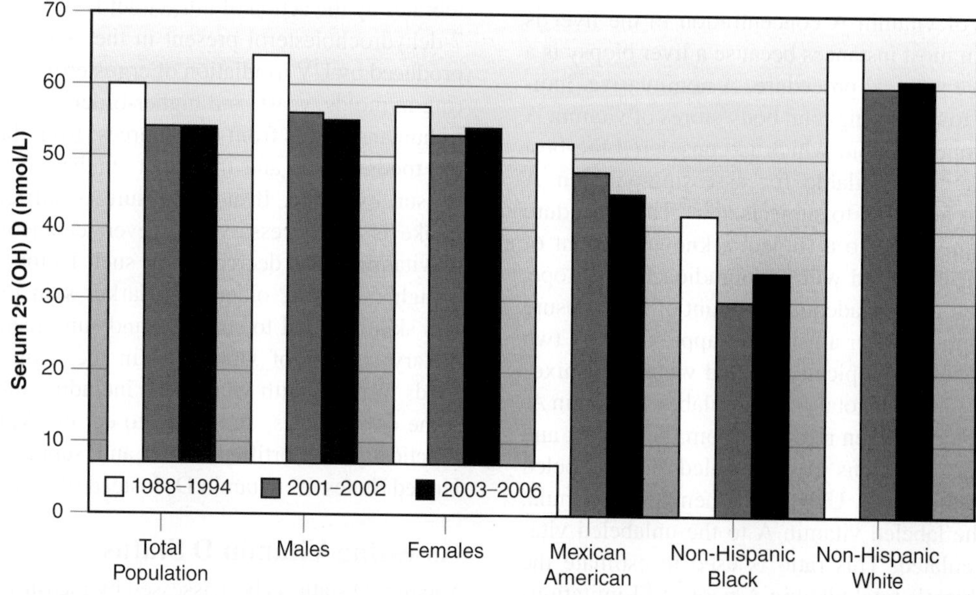

Figure 9.7 Age-adjusted mean concentrations of serum 25-hydroxyvitamin D [25(OH)S] in the U.S. population aged 12 years and older by sex or race/ethnicity, National Health and Nutrition Examination Survey, 1988–2006.

Between 1988 and the periods 2001–2002 and 2003–2006, serum concentration of 25(OH)D in the United States decreased approximately 10%.

Source: U.S. Department of Health and Human Services. 2012. *Second National Report on Biochemical Indicators of Diet and Nutrition in the U.S. Population.* National Center for Environmental Health, Centers for Disease Control and Prevention. www.cdc.gov/nutritionreport.

NHANES show that serum 25(OH)D concentrations decrease with increasing age and that among the three race/ethnic groups, non-Hispanic whites had the highest 25(OH)D concentrations and non-Hispanic blacks had the lowest concentrations.[20] According to data from NHANES 2003–2006 shown in Figure 9.8, non-Hispanic blacks 1 year of age and older had the highest prevalence of serum 25(OH)D concentrations that were < 30 nmol/L (considered consistent with vitamin D deficiency). Non-Hispanic blacks and Mexican Americans had the highest prevalence of serum 25(OH)D concentrations that were 30 to < 50 nmol/L (considered consistent with being at risk of vitamin D deficiency).

Vitamin C Status

Vitamin C is a generic term for compounds exhibiting the biological activity of *ascorbic acid,* the reduced form of vitamin C. The oxidized form of vitamin C is known as *dehydroascorbic acid.* The sum of ascorbic acid and dehydroascorbic acid constitutes all the naturally occurring biologically active vitamin C.[63,64] When used in this chapter, the term *vitamin C* refers to total vitamin C—the sum of ascorbic acid and dehydroascorbic acid.

Vitamin C is necessary for the formation of collagen; the maintenance of capillaries, bone, and teeth; the promotion of iron absorption; and the protection of vitamins and minerals from oxidation. Evidence from several large cohort studies suggest a protective effect against certain cancers and CHD, but these observations are not supported by most randomized clinical trials.[65] Deficiency of vitamin C results in scurvy, a condition characterized by weakness, hemorrhages in the skin and gums, and defects in bone development in children.

Vitamin C status is assessed by measuring total ascorbic acid in serum (or plasma) and in leucocytes (white blood cells). The serum concentration of ascorbic acid is considered an index of the circulating vitamin available to the tissues. The leucocyte concentration is considered an index of tissue stores.[20] Vitamin C deficiency is generally defined as a serum (or plasma) concentration < 11.4 micromoles per liter (μmol/L) or the level at which signs and symptoms of scurvy begin to appear. A low serum (or plasma) concentration is 11.4 to 23.0 μmol/L.[20]

Data collected by NHANES in 2003–2006 show that the prevalence of low serum concentrations among all individuals in the United States 6 years of age and older is

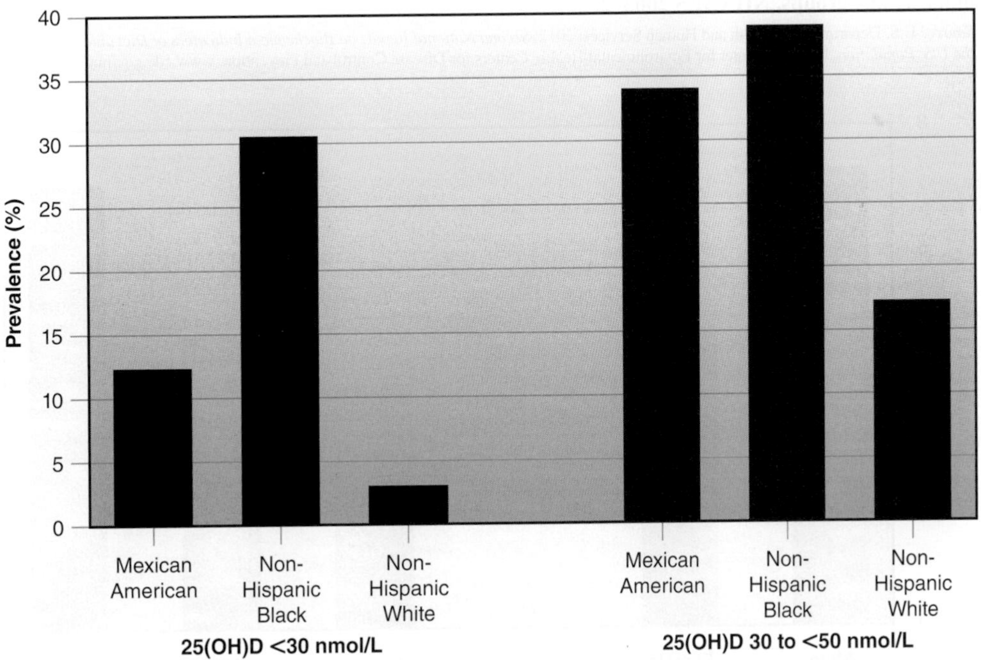

Figure 9.8 Age-adjusted prevalence estimates of serum 25-hydroxyvitamin D [25(OH)D] concentrations less than 30 nmol/L and 30 to less than 50 nmol/L in the U.S. population aged 1 year and older by race/ethnicity, National Health and Nutrition Examination Survey, 2003–2006. Non-Hispanic blacks 1 year of age and older had the highest prevalence of serum 25(OH)D concentrations that were < 30 nmol/L (considered consistent with vitamin D deficiency). Non-Hispanic blacks and Mexican Americans had the highest prevalence of serum 25(OH)D concentrations that were 30 to < 50 nmol/L (considered consistent with at risk of vitamin D deficiency).

Source: U.S. Department of Health and Human Services. 2012. *Second National Report on Biochemical Indicators of Diet and Nutrition in the U.S. Population.* National Center for Environmental Health, Centers for Disease Control and Prevention. www.cdc.gov/nutritionreport.

6%. As shown in Figure 9.9, the prevalence of vitamin C deficiency (serum concentration < 11.4 μmol/L) and low serum vitamin C (serum concentrations 11.4–23.0 μmol/L) are lowest in children and adolescents. As shown in Figure 9.10, U.S. females are at lower risk of vitamin C deficiency than U.S. males, and non-Hispanic whites had a greater prevalence of low vitamin C than non-Hispanic blacks and Mexican Americans.[20]

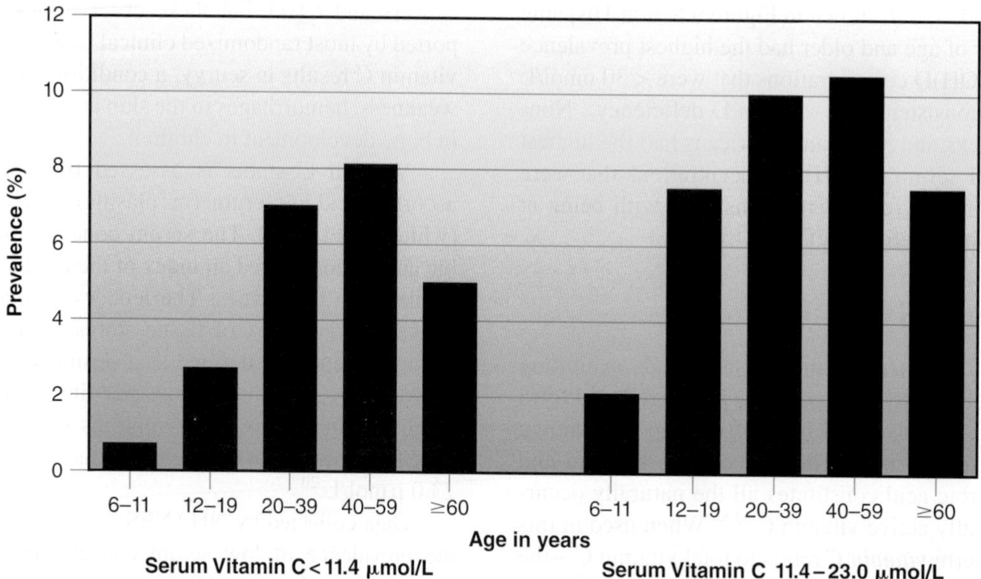

Figure 9.9 Prevalence estimates of vitamin C deficiency (serum concentrations < 11.4 μmol/L) and of low vitamin C concentrations (11.4–23.0 μmol/L) in the U.S. population aged 6 years and older by age groups, NHANES 2003–2006.

Source: U.S. Department of Health and Human Services. 2012. *Second National Report on Biochemical Indicators of Diet and Nutrition in the U.S. Population.* National Center for Environmental Health, Centers for Disease Control and Prevention. www.cdc.gov/nutritionreport.

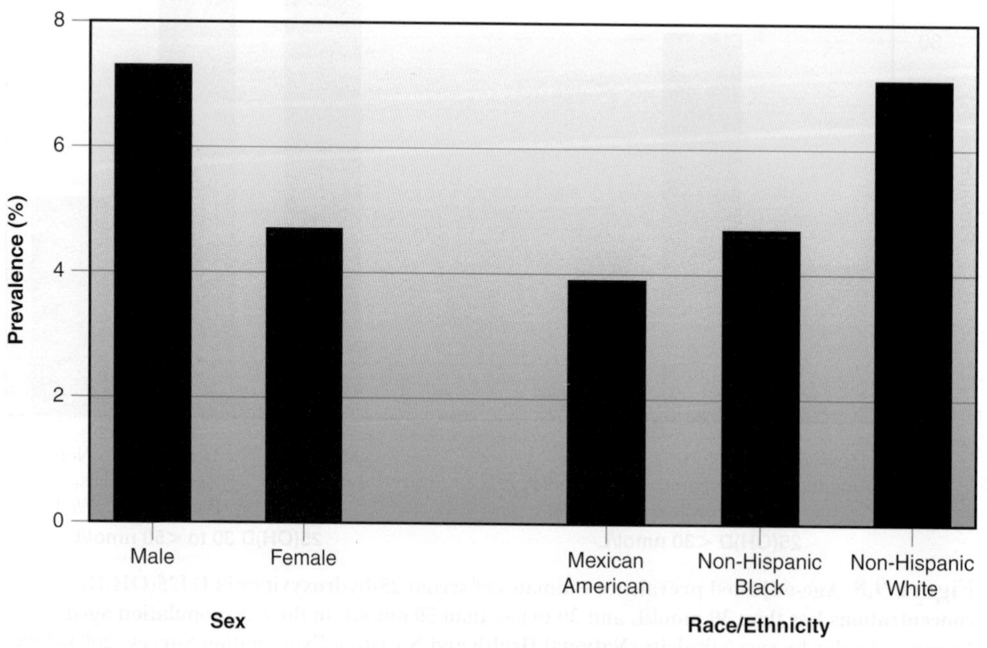

Figure 9.10 Age-adjusted prevalence estimates of vitamin C deficiency (serum concentrations < 11.4 μmol/L) in the U.S. population aged 6 years and older by sex and race/ethnicity, NHANES 2003–2006.

Source: U.S. Department of Health and Human Services. 2012. *Second National Report on Biochemical Indicators of Diet and Nutrition in the U.S. Population.* National Center for Environmental Health, Centers for Disease Control and Prevention. www.cdc.gov/nutritionreport.

Serum and Leukocyte Vitamin C

Measurement of serum (or plasma) vitamin C is the most commonly used biochemical procedure for assessing vitamin C status.[20,64,66,67] However, in recent years, there has been increasing interest in using the level of vitamin C in polymorphonuclear leukocytes (the granular leukocytes: neutrophils, eosinophils, and basophils) and the mononuclear leukocytes (the agranular leukocytes: lymphocytes and monocytes) as indicators of vitamin C status.[63,64] Serum levels of ascorbic acid have been shown to correlate with dietary vitamin C intake and with vitamin C levels in leukocytes (white blood cells).[20] However, research suggests that vitamin C concentration in serum is a better indicator of recent dietary intake of vitamin C than leukocyte levels and that leukocyte vitamin C levels better represent cellular stores and the total body pool of the vitamin.

Factors affecting vitamin C levels in tissues and fluids include cigarette smoking and sex.[66,67] Compared with nonsmokers, cigarette smokers tend to have lower vitamin C levels in serum and leukocytes even after correcting for vitamin C intake.[67] The metabolic turnover of vitamin C in smokers has been estimated to be 35 mg/d greater than that of nonsmokers. However, evidence suggests that smokers may need to ingest > 200 mg of vitamin C daily to achieve serum ascorbic acid levels typically seen in nonsmokers meeting the RDA currently set at 90 mg/d for adult males and 75 mg/d for adult females.[67]

After correcting for vitamin C intakes, females consistently show higher vitamin C levels in tissues and fluids than males.[64,71,75] Age does not appear to influence vitamin C levels in adults.[64,69]

Vitamin B_6 Status

The vitamin B_6 group is composed of three naturally occurring compounds related chemically, metabolically, and functionally: pyridoxine (PN), pyridoxal (PL), and pyridoxamine (PM). Within the liver, erythrocytes, and other tissues of the body, these forms are phosphorylated into pyridoxal 5′-phosphate (PLP) and pyridoxamine phosphate (PMP). PLP and PMP primarily serve as coenzymes in a large variety of reactions.[68,69] Especially important among these are the transamination reactions in protein metabolism. PLP also is involved in other metabolic transformations of amino acids and in the metabolism of carbohydrates, lipids, and nucleic acids.[68,69] Because of its role in protein metabolism, the requirement for vitamin B_6 is directly proportional to protein intake.[70]

Although frank vitamin B_6 deficiency resulting in clinical manifestations is not considered widespread in the general U.S. population, there is evidence of impaired status among certain groups—most notably, the elderly and alcoholic individuals. There is also concern about excessive vitamin B_6 intake and the possibility of resulting peripheral nervous system damage.[70]

Vitamin B_6 status can be assessed by several methods. Static measurements can be made of vitamin B_6 concentrations in blood or urine, and functional tests can measure the activity of several enzymes dependent on vitamin B_6.[68,71,72]

Plasma and Erythrocyte Pyridoxal 5′-Phosphate

The most frequently used biochemical indicator of vitamin B_6 status is plasma PLP.[68,71,72] PLP accounts for approximately 70% to 90% of the total vitamin B_6 present in plasma.[68,72] PL is the next most abundant form in plasma, followed by lower levels of PN and PM.[71]

Fasting measurements of plasma PLP are considered the single most informative indicator of vitamin B_6 status for healthy persons. Use of this single measure is limited by the fact that abnormally low concentrations of plasma PLP may result from asthma, coronary heart disease, and pregnancy and may not reflect a true vitamin B_6 deficiency.[71] Dietary intake of vitamin B_6 and protein can affect plasma PLP concentrations as well. As shown in Table 9.10, increases in dietary vitamin B_6 intake raise plasma PLP, and plasma levels fall in response to increased protein consumption.[70,72] Thus, although plasma PLP is a valuable measure, the assessment of vitamin B_6 status is best accomplished by using several indicators in conjunction with each other—for example, measures of other vitamin B_6 forms and/or functional tests.[70–72] Table 9.11 lists expected biochemical values for adults with adequate vitamin B_6 status for various measures of the vitamin.

Measurement of PLP in erythrocytes has been suggested as another approach to assessing vitamin B_6 status. Certain characteristics of the erythrocyte may make it unrepresentative of other body tissues. The ability of hemoglobin to bind tightly to PLP and PL, along with the relatively long life of red blood cells (about 120 days),

TABLE 9.10 Factors Affecting Plasma PLP* Concentrations

Factors	Effect
Increased vitamin B_6 intake	Increases
Increased protein intake	Decreases
Increased glucose	Decreases (a)†
Increased plasma volume	Decreases
Increased physical activity	Increases (a)
Decreased uptake into nonhepatic tissues	Increases
Increased age	Decreases

Adapted from Leklem JE. 1990. Vitamin B_6: A status report. *Journal of Nutrition* 120:1503–1507.

*PLP = pyridoxal 5′-phosphate.

†(a) indicates that the effect is an acute effect.

TABLE 9.11 Indices for Evaluating Vitamin B_6 Status and Suggested Values for Adequate Status in Adults

Indices	Suggested Values for Adequate Status*
Direct	
Blood	
Plasma pyridoxal 5′-phosphate (PLP)	> 30 nmol/L
Plasma pyridoxal	NV†
Plasma total vitamin B_6	> 40 nmol/L
Erythrocyte PLP	NV
Urine	
4-pyridoxic acid	> 3.0 μmol/day
Indirect	
Urine	
3-g methionine load; cystathionine	< 350 μmol/day
Oxalate excretion	NV
Diet Intake	
Vitamin B_6 intake, weekly average	> 1.2–1.5 mg/day
Vitamin B_6: protein ratio	> 0.020
Other	
Electroencephalogram pattern	NV

Adapted from Leklem JE. 1990. Vitamin B_6: A status report. *Journal of Nutrition* 120:1503–1507.

*These values are dependent on sex, age, and, for most, protein intake.

†NV = no value established; limited data are available.

‡The index value for each transaminase represents the ratio of the enzyme activity with added PLP to the activity without PLP added.

may make red blood cells a significant reservoir for vitamin B_6 and may complicate the use of erythrocyte PLP levels as a useful indicator of vitamin B_6 status.[70–72]

Plasma Pyridoxal

Measurement of plasma PL has been suggested as an additional indicator of B_6 status to use with plasma PLP. PL is the major dietary form of the vitamin, crosses all membranes on absorption from the gastrointestinal tract, and comprises about 8% to 30% of the total plasma vitamin B_6. There are questions about how well plasma PL represents vitamin B_6 status, and further research is needed on this indicator. Despite these questions, plasma PL is recommended in the assessment of B_6 status.[72]

Urinary 4-pyridoxic Acid

4-pyridoxic acid (4-PA) is the major urinary metabolite of vitamin B_6. Urinary excretion of 4-PA has been shown to change rapidly in response to alterations in vitamin B_6 intake and to be indicative of immediate dietary intake. Thus, it is considered useful as a short-term index of vitamin B_6 status. In studies of subjects whose usual dietary intake of vitamin B_6 was known, males had a 4-PA excretion of 3.5 μmol/day, and females had a 4-PA excretion of > 3.2 μmol/day. Urinary excretions of 4-PA of ≥ 3.0 μmol/day appear to be indicative of acceptable vitamin B_6 status.[1] 4-PA is likely to be absent from urine of persons with a marked vitamin B_6 deficiency. The value of this method is limited by the need for a complete 24-hour urine collection.[20,68,72]

Methionine Load Test

The principle of the methionine load test is similar to that of the tryptophan load test. PLP is required in the metabolism of the amino acid methionine. Compared with persons with adequate vitamin B_6 status, those with impaired vitamin B_6 status have higher urine levels of the metabolites cystathionine and cysteine sulfonic acid following consumption of 3 g of methionine.[72]

Use of this test is limited by the required 24-hour urine sample and factors other than vitamin B_6 status that can affect test results (for example, protein intake). Because this test has been used in a limited number of studies, no definitive values for urinary cystathionine are available. The value of < 350 μmol/day given in Table 9.11 is based on three studies.[72]

FOLATE STATUS

Folate, or folacin, is a group of water-soluble compounds with properties and chemical structures similar to those of folic acid, or pteroylglutamic acid. Folate functions as a coenzyme transporting single carbon groups from one compound to another in amino acid metabolism and nucleic acid synthesis. One of the most significant of folate's functions appears to be purine and pyrimidine synthesis. Folate deficiency can lead to inhibition of DNA synthesis, impaired cell division, and alterations in protein synthesis. It is especially important during periods of rapid cell division and growth, such as occurs during pregnancy and infancy.[20,70,73,74] Clinical trials have shown that a marginal folate intake during pregnancy increases the risk of an infant being born with a neural tube defect (i.e., spina bifida, encephalocele, and anencephaly) and that folate supplementation reduces the number of pregnancies affected by neural tube defects (NTDs). This led the U.S. Food and Drug Administration to require the addition of folic acid to enriched cereal products beginning in 1998.[20] Since then, the rate of NTDs has declined by 36%.[75] The *Dietary Guidelines for Americans* has identified folic acid as a nutrient of concern for women capable of becoming pregnant, because many women do not meet the recommended intake. The *Guidelines* advise all women who are capable of becoming pregnant to consume 400 μg of synthetic folic acid daily from fortified foods and/or supplements in addition to the food forms of folate from a varied diet.[51]

The recommended measurements for assessing folate status are serum folate concentration and red blood cell (RBC) folate concentration.[20,73] Serum folate is largely the product of absorbed dietary folate and fluctuates daily. It provides information about recent folate intake and does not necessarily represent tissue stores. Nonnutritional factors that can increase serum folate concentrations include acute renal failure, active liver disease, and hemolysis of red blood cells. Alcohol consumption, cigarette smoking, and oral contraceptive use may lower serum folate levels.[70,73] RBC folate concentration is considered the best clinical index of folate stores in the tissues of the body. RBC folate concentration reflects folate status at the time the erythrocyte was synthesized, because only young cells in the bone marrow take up folate.[70] Unlike serum folate, RBC folate is less subject to transient fluctuations in dietary intake. It decreases after tissue stores are depleted because erythrocytes have a 120-day average life span and reflect folate status at the time of their synthesis. It has been shown to correlate with liver folate stores and to reflect total body stores.[70,73]

The monitoring of serum folate concentration in the U.S. population began with NHANES I (1974–1975). The measurement of RBC folate concentration began with NHANES II (1978–1980). NHANES has continued measuring these biomarkers since then.[74] Figure 9.11 shows the age-adjusted mean concentrations of serum folate in the U.S. population aged 4 years and older by sex or race/ethnicity from 1988 to 2006.[20] Based on the assay method consistently used throughout this time period, a low serum folate concentration is considered < 2 ng/mL. As can be seen in Figure 9.11, serum folate concentrations more than doubled after the FDA required the addition of folic acid to enriched cereal products beginning in 1998.

Figure 9.12 shows the age-adjusted mean concentrations of RBC folate in the U.S. population aged 4 years and older by sex or race/ethnicity from 1988 to 2006.[20] Based on the assay method consistently used throughout this time period, a low RBC folate concentration is considered < 95 ng/mL. The cutoff values for defining low values will vary depending on the assay used to measure folate concentrations.[20,73,74] The plasma concentration of homocysteine, an amino acid naturally found in the blood, can be elevated by folate deficiency, but plasma homocysteine is not specific for folate deficiency because it is also elevated during deficiency of vitamin B_6 and vitamin B_{12}.[20]

VITAMIN B_{12} STATUS

Vitamin B_{12}, or cobalamin, include a group of cobalt-containing molecules that can be converted to methylcobalamin or 5′-deoxyadenosylcobalamin, the two coenzyme forms of vitamin B_{12} that are active in human metabolism.[70,76] Vitamin B_{12} is synthesized by bacteria, fungi, and algae, but not by yeast, plants, and animals. Vitamin B_{12} synthesized by bacteria accumulates in the tissues of animals that are then consumed by humans.

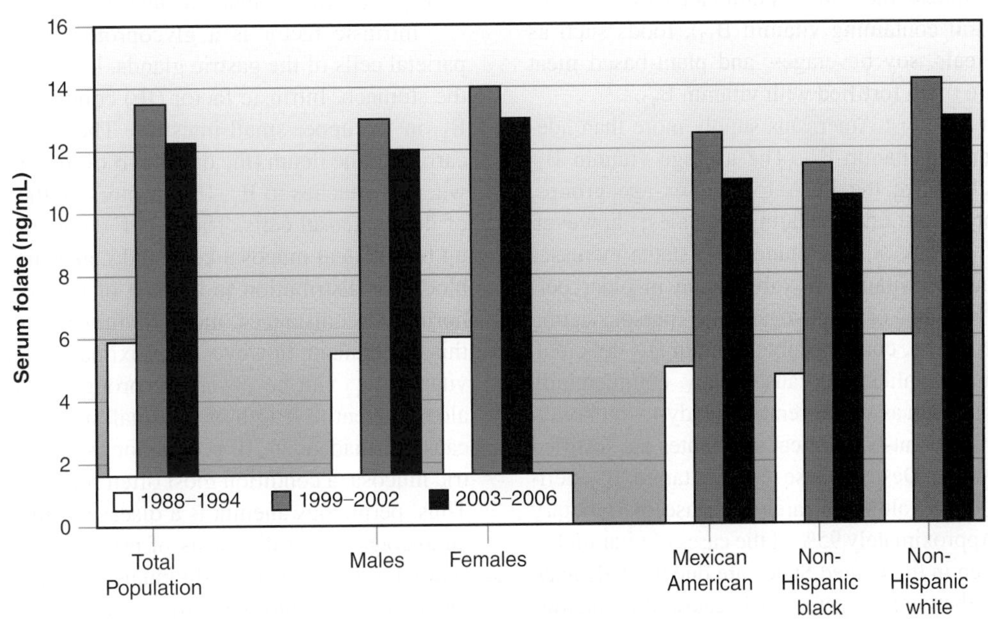

Figure 9.11 Age-adjusted mean concentrations of serum folate in the U.S. population aged 4 years and older by sex or race/ethnicity, NHANES 1988–2006.

Serum folate concentrations more than doubled after the FDA required the addition of folic acid to enriched cereal products beginning in 1998.

Source: U.S. Department of Health and Human Services. 2012. *Second National Report on Biochemical Indicators of Diet and Nutrition in the U.S. Population.* National Center for Environmental Health, Centers for Disease Control and Prevention. www.cdc.gov/nutritionreport.

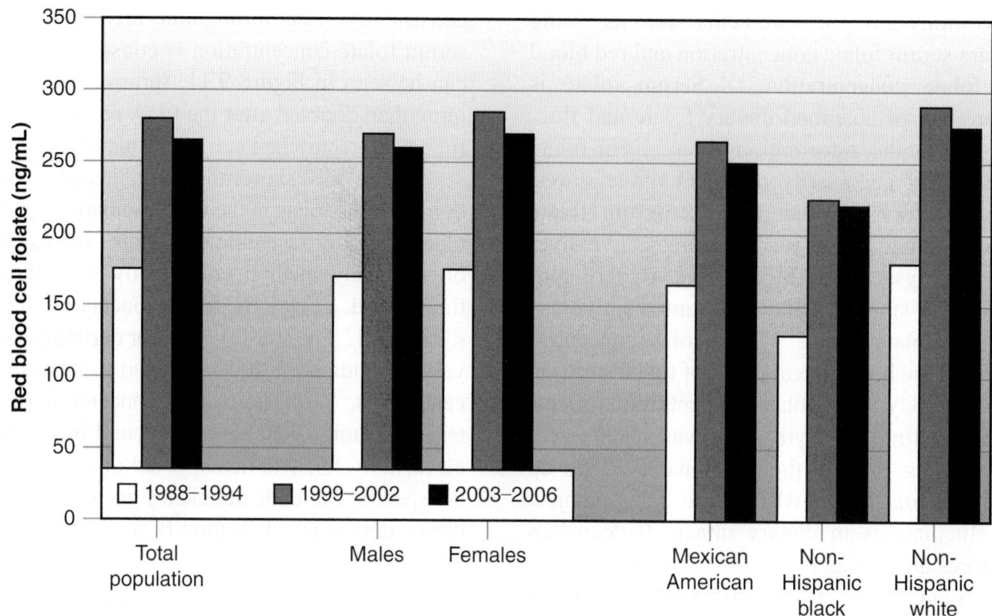

Figure 9.12 Age-adjusted mean concentrations of red blood cell folate in the U.S. population aged 4 years and older by sex or race/ethnicity, NHANES 1988–2006.
Red blood cell folate concentrations increased by approximately 50% after the FDA required the addition of folic acid to enriched cereal products beginning in 1998.

Source: U.S. Department of Health and Human Services. 2012. *Second National Report on Biochemical Indicators of Diet and Nutrition in the U.S. Population.* National Center for Environmental Health, Centers for Disease Control and Prevention. www.cdc.gov/nutritionreport.

Thus, animal products serve as the primary dietary source of vitamin B_{12}. Although plants are essentially devoid of vitamin B_{12} (unless they are contaminated by microorganisms or soil containing vitamin B_{12}), foods such as breakfast cereals, soy beverages, and plant-based meat substitutes are often fortified with vitamin B_{12}.

The diets of most Americans supply more than adequate amounts of vitamin B_{12}. The average vitamin B_{12} intake is well above the RDA for all sex-age groups, including pregnant and lactating females; however, after age 40 the risk of low vitamin B_{12} status increases due to diminished vitamin B_{12} absorption in older persons.[20,70,77,78] Vegans, or strict vegetarians (persons eating no animal products), could become vitamin B_{12} deficient, although this is unlikely because many commercially available foods such as soy beverages, ready-to-eat breakfast cereals, and plant-based meat substitutes are fortified with vitamin B_{12}. Despite these facts, vitamin B_{12} deficiency does occur, although rarely because of a dietary deficiency. Approximately 95% of the cases of vitamin B_{12} deficiency seen in the United States are due to inadequate absorption of the vitamin, generally because of pernicious anemia caused by inadequate production of intrinsic factor. Approximately 2% of elderly people in the United States have clinical vitamin B_{12} deficiency and 10–20% have subclinical deficiency.[78] Because most vitamin B_{12} absorption occurs in the distal ileum, B_{12} malabsorption could also result from surgical resection of the distal ileum, bacterial overgrowth in the small intestine ("blind loop" syndrome), or damage to the ileum from such causes as tropical sprue or regional enteritis.[70,77]

Intrinsic factor is a glycoprotein produced by the parietal cells of the gastric glands, located in the body of the stomach. Intrinsic factor (IF) combines with vitamin B_{12} in the upper small intestine. The B_{12}-IF complex is carried to the ileum (the distal part of the small intestine), where it attaches to B_{12}-IF receptors on the brush border of ileal mucosal cells. The B_{12}-IF complex is then taken up by the ileal mucosal cells and makes its way into the blood for distribution to the rest of the body.[70,77] Under normal circumstances, most vitamin B_{12} is absorbed by this mechanism; however, approximately 1% of ingested vitamin B_{12} can be absorbed through passive diffusion along the entire length of the small intestine.[77] The usual cause of inadequate IF production is atrophy of the gastric mucosa, a condition most often seen in older persons. Thus, pernicious anemia is a disease of the elderly, with an average age at diagnosis of 60 years. Because a substantial proportion of individuals 50 years of age and older have a diminished ability to absorb naturally occurring vitamin B_{12}, the *Dietary Guidelines for Americans* recommend that these individuals include foods fortified with vitamin B_{12} or take supplements.[51] Other causes of inadequate IF production include total gastrectomy and extensive damage to the gastric mucosa caused by ingestion of corrosive agents.[70,77]

Clinical features of vitamin B_{12} deficiency involve the blood, the gastrointestinal tract, and the nervous system. An early feature of vitamin B_{12} deficiency is megaloblastic anemia, which is characterized by the presence of abnormally large cells (megaloblasts) in the peripheral blood and a low hemoglobin level. A mean corpuscular volume (MCV) > 100 fL is suggestive of megaloblastic anemia. The tongue may become sore, smooth, and beefy red. Anorexia with moderate weight loss and diarrhea may also be present. The most troublesome consequences of B_{12} deficiency occur in the nervous system. Neurologic manifestations include demyelination and axonal degeneration of the peripheral nerves, spinal cord, and cerebrum. Eventually, irreversible neuronal death can occur in these areas. The earliest symptoms of these changes are numbness and paresthesias (abnormal sensations, such as burning, prickling, or the feeling that ants are crawling on the skin) in the extremities. This can progress to weakness, muscular incoordination (ataxia), irritability, forgetfulness, severe dementia, and even psychosis.[77]

Biochemical Indicators of B_{12} Status

Currently recommended biomarkers for assessing vitamin B_{12} status are those that directly measure vitamin B_{12} in the blood and functional biomarkers measuring metabolites that accumulate when vitamin B_{12} status is inadequate.[78,79] Direct measures of circulating vitamin B_{12} are serum or plasma total cobalamin and serum holo-transcobalamin II (holo-TC II), the transport protein of absorbed vitamin B_{12}. These measures reflect the broad range of vitamin B_{12} status from severe deficiency to adequacy.[20,78] A functional biomarker specific to vitamin B_{12} status is urinary or serum methylmalonic acid (MMA), which is increased when vitamin B_{12} status is inadequate. Another functional biomarker is the plasma concentration of total homocysteine (tHcy), which increases when vitamin B_{12} status is inadequate, but is also increased during folate and vitamin B_6 deficiency.[20,70,78,79] Both MMA and tHcy reflect early changes in vitamin B_{12} status and are useful for identifying subclinical B_{12} deficiency. But the fact that tHcy is increased by folate deficiency limits its usefulness as a biomarker for vitamin B_{12}.[79]

Factors unrelated to vitamin B_{12} status can potentially affect all four of the biomarkers. MMA and tHcy are increased by impaired renal function, even when it is mild as evidenced by minor changes in creatinine and indices of glomerular filtration, which is common in older persons.[20] Elevation of cobalamin and holo-TC II are generally only seen in advanced renal failure. Genetics can influence serum concentrations, transport, and metabolism. Serum cobalamin concentration is decreased in pregnancy and folate deficiency. There are also concerns about suboptimal laboratory monitoring and proficiency testing.[79] Because there is no single biomarker that is considered a "gold standard" for vitamin B_{12} status assessment, information from two or more tests should be used to assess vitamin B_{12} status.[79]

Data on the age-adjusted mean concentrations of serum vitamin B_{12} in the U.S. population aged 4 years and older collected by NHANES in 1991–2006 are shown in Figure 9.13. In these data, a low serum vitamin B_{12} concentration is defined as < 200 pg/mL, indicating that for all groups, mean serum vitamin B_{12} concentrations were adequate. Figure 9.14 shows prevalence estimates of low serum vitamin B_{12}, high plasma methylmalonic acid (MMA), and high plasma total homocysteine (tHcy) concentrations in persons in the United States 60 years of age and older based on data collected by NHANES in 2003–2006.[20] Assessing the extent of inadequate vitamin B_{12} status is complicated by the fact that serum tHcy is not specific to vitamin B_{12} deficiency (it is also increased by folate deficiency) and tHcy and MMA are both elevated when renal function is impaired, a common condition in elderly people.[20]

BLOOD CHEMISTRY TESTS

Blood chemistry tests include a variety of assays performed on plasma or serum that are useful in the diagnosis and management of disease. They include electrolytes, enzymes, metabolites, and other miscellaneous substances, which are discussed in this section. When run at one time, blood chemistry tests often are known by such names as the *chemistry profile, chemistry panel, chem profile,* and *chem panel.* To perform these tests, clinical laboratories use automated analyzers capable of performing several thousand blood tests per hour. The patient's plasma or serum sample is placed into the analyzer, which performs the desired tests and provides a printout of the patient's results, including reference ranges and flagged abnormal results. A related series of tests, often known as the *coronary risk profile,* measures levels of triglyceride, total cholesterol, and HDL-C (cholesterol carried by high-density lipoproteins) and calculates LDL-C (cholesterol carried by low-density lipoproteins) and, in some instances, the total cholesterol/HDL-C ratio. These are discussed in Chapter 8.

Following is a brief overview of the major blood chemistry tests. Normal adult serum levels (known as reference ranges) are given. These reference ranges vary, depending on the individual biochemical and analytic method used. It is generally best, however, to use reference ranges suggested by the laboratory performing the analyses.

Alanine Aminotransferase

Alanine aminotransferase (ALT), also known as serum glutamic pyruvic transaminase (SGPT), is an enzyme found in large concentrations in the liver and to a lesser extent in the kidneys, skeletal muscles, and myocardium (heart muscle).[94] Injury to the liver caused by such conditions as hepatitis (viral, alcoholic, and so on), cirrhosis, and bile duct obstruction or from drugs toxic to the liver is the

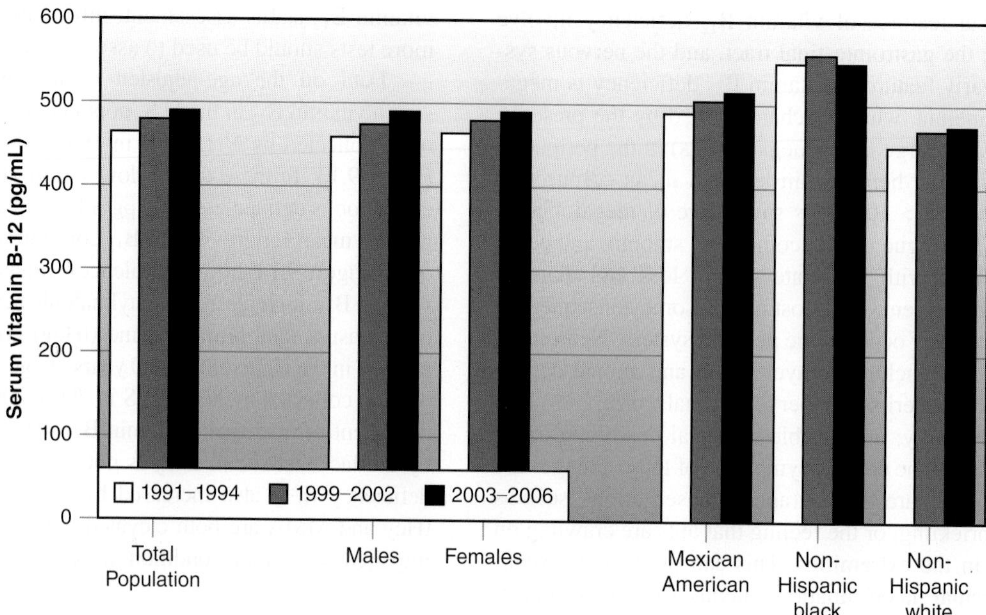

Figure 9.13 Age-adjusted mean concentrations of serum vitamin B_{12} in the U.S. population aged 4 years and older by sex or race/ethnicity, NHANES 1991–2006.

A low serum vitamin B_{12} concentration is defined as < 200 pg/mL, indicating that for all groups, serum vitamin B_{12} concentrations were adequate.

Source: U.S. Department of Health and Human Services. 2012. *Second National Report on Biochemical Indicators of Diet and Nutrition in the U.S. Population.* National Center for Environmental Health, Centers for Disease Control and Prevention. www.cdc.gov/nutritionreport.

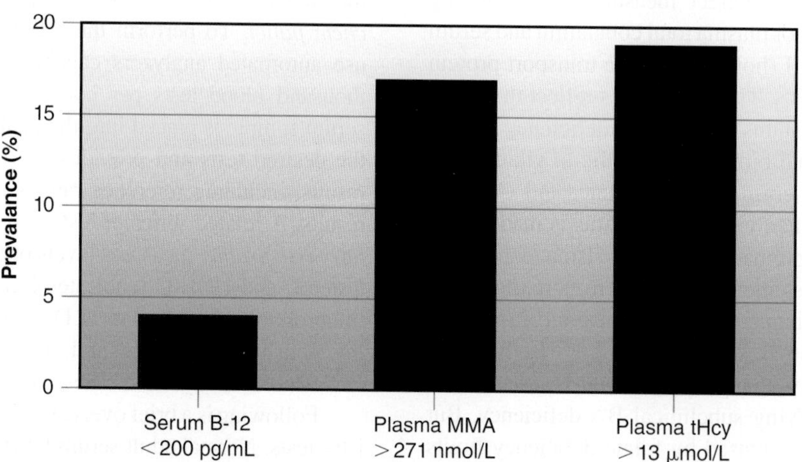

Figure 9.14 Prevalence estimates of low serum vitamin B_{12} (B-12), high plasma methylmalonic acid (MMA), and high plasma total homocysteine (tHcy) concentrations in persons in the United States who were 60 years of age and older, NHANES 2003–2006.

Source: U.S. Department of Health and Human Services. 2012. *Second National Report on Biochemical Indicators of Diet and Nutrition in the U.S. Population.* National Center for Environmental Health, Centers for Disease Control and Prevention. www.cdc.gov/nutritionreport.

usual cause of elevated serum ALT levels. Levels may be elevated to a lesser extent in myocardial infarction, musculoskeletal diseases, and acute pancreatitis. Decreased levels may result from chronic renal dialysis.[12,80] The adult reference range is 4 to 36 IU/L or 4 to 36 U/L.[12]

Albumin and Total Protein

Albumin is a serum protein produced in the liver. Total protein is the sum of all serum proteins, but the vast majority of total protein is composed of albumin and globulin. Once total protein and albumin are known, an estimate of globulin can be calculated. Levels of albumin and total protein reflect nutritional status, and alterations suggest the need for further diagnostic testing. The adult reference range for albumin is 3.5 to 5.0 g/dL or 35 to 50 g/L; for globulin, 2.3 to 3.5 g/dL or 23 to 35 g/L; and for total protein, 6.4 to 8.3 g/dL or 64 to 83 g/L.[12]

Alkaline Phosphatase

Alkaline phosphatase (ALP) is an enzyme found in the liver, bone, placenta, and intestine and is useful in detecting diseases in these organs. Expected values are higher in children, during skeletal growth in adolescents, and during pregnancy.[12] Elevated levels can be seen in conditions involving increased deposition of calcium in bone (hyperparathyroidism, healing fractures, certain bone tumors) and certain liver diseases 30 to 120 U/L or 0.5 to 2.0 μkat/L. Low levels of ALP usually are not clinically significant. The adult reference range is 30 to 120 U/L or 0.5 to 2.0 μkat/L.[12]

Aspartate Aminotransferase

Aspartate aminotransferase (AST), also known as serum glutamic oxaloacetic transaminase (SGOT), is an enzyme found in large concentrations in the myocardium, liver, skeletal muscles, kidneys, and pancreas. Within 8 to 12 hours following injury to these organs, AST is released into the blood. Serum levels peak in 24 to 36 hours and then return to normal in about 4 to 6 days following injury.[12,80] Elevated levels are seen in such conditions as myocardial infarction (blood levels reflect the size of the infarct), liver diseases (for example, acute viral hepatitis), pancreatitis, musculoskeletal injuries, and exposure to drugs toxic to the liver.[93] The adult reference range is 0 to 35 U/L or 0 to 0.58 μkat/L.[12]

Bilirubin

Bilirubin, the major pigment of bile, is produced by the spleen, liver, and bone marrow from the breakdown of the heme portion of hemoglobin and is released into the blood. Most of the bilirubin combines with albumin to form what is called free, or unconjugated, bilirubin. Free bilirubin then is absorbed by the liver, where it is conjugated (joined) to other molecules to form what is called conjugated bilirubin and is then excreted into the bile. Serum bilirubin levels can be reported as direct bilirubin, indirect bilirubin, or total bilirubin. Direct bilirubin is a measure of conjugated bilirubin in serum. Indirect bilirubin is a measure of free, or unconjugated, bilirubin in serum. Total bilirubin is a measure of both direct and indirect bilirubin.[12]

Serum bilirubin rises when the liver is unable to either conjugate or excrete bilirubin. Elevated conjugated (direct) bilirubin suggests obstruction of bile passages within or near the liver. Elevated free, or unconjugated (indirect), bilirubin is indicative of excessive hemolysis (destruction) of red blood cells. Elevated indirect bilirubin also is seen in neonates whose immature livers are unable to adequately conjugate bilirubin. A serum bilirubin concentration greater than about 2 mg/dL results in jaundice. The adult reference ranges for adults are 0.3 to 1.0 mg/dL or 5.1 to 17.0 μmol/L for total bilirubin, 0.1 to 0.3 mg/dL or 1.7 to 5.1 μmol/L for direct (conjugated), and 0.2 to 0.8 mg/dL or 3.4 to 12.0 μmol/L for indirect (unconjugated) bilirubin.[12]

Blood Urea Nitrogen

Urea, the end product of protein metabolism and the primary method of nitrogen excretion, is formed in the liver and excreted by the kidneys in urine. An increased blood urea level usually indicates renal failure, although it may also result from dehydration, gastrointestinal bleeding, congestive heart failure, high protein intake, insufficient renal blood supply, or blockage of the urinary tract.[12,80] Blood urea nitrogen (BUN) is more easily measured than urea and is used as an index of blood urea levels. Elevated BUN is referred to as azotemia. Decreased BUN can result from liver disease, overhydration, malnutrition, or anabolic steroid use. In the absence of other signs elevated BUN is probably insignificant. The adult reference range is 10 to 20 mg/dL or 3.6 to 7.1 mmol/L.[12]

Calcium

Serum levels of calcium, an important cation (positively charged ion), are helpful in detecting disorders of the bones and parathyroid glands, kidney failure, and certain cancers. Calcium is discussed at length in the earlier section "Calcium Status." The adult reference range for total calcium is 9.0 to 10.5 mg/dL or 2.25 to 2.75 mmol/L, and for ionized calcium it is 4.5 to 5.6 mg/dL or 1.05 to 1.30 mmol/L.[12]

Carbon Dioxide

Measurement of carbon dioxide (CO_2) in serum helps assess the body's acid-base balance. Elevated CO_2 is seen in metabolic alkalosis, and decreased levels reflect metabolic acidosis. The adult reference range in serum or plasma is 23 to 30 mEq/L or 23 to 30 mmol/L.[12]

Chloride

Chloride, an electrolyte, is the primary anion (negatively charged ion) within the extracellular fluid. It works in conjunction with sodium to help regulate acid-base balance, osmotic pressure, and fluid distribution within the body. It often is measured along with sodium, potassium, and carbon dioxide. Low serum chloride levels (hypochloremia) are associated with alkalosis and low serum potassium levels (hypokalemia). Hypokalemia may not accompany hypochloremia if the patient receives a potassium supplement that does not contain chloride or takes a potassium-sparing diuretic. Hyperchloremia (elevated serum chloride) may be seen in kidney disease, overactive thyroid, anemia, or heart disease. The adult reference range is 100 to 106 mEq/L or 100 to 106 mmol/L.[12]

Cholesterol

According to the National Cholesterol Education Program, a desirable serum total cholesterol level is < 200 mg/dL (5.17 mmol/L). Chapter 8 discusses recommended levels of serum cholesterol and its relationship to coronary heart disease. Population reference values for serum total cholesterol are shown in Appendix Q.

Creatinine

Measurement of serum creatinine, like measurement of blood urea nitrogen, is used for evaluating renal function. Elevated serum levels are seen when 50% or more of the kidney's nephrons are destroyed. The reference range for adult males is 0.6 to 1.2 mg/dL or 53 to 106 μmol/L, and for adult females it is 0.6 to 1.2 mg/dL or 53 to 106 μmol/L.[12]

Glucose

Measurement of serum glucose is of interest in the diagnosis and management of diabetes mellitus. This is discussed in detail in Chapter 8. Use of serum glucose to diagnose diabetes is discussed at length in Chapter 8. Serum glucose can also be used to diagnose hypoglycemia, or low blood sugar. Glycosylated hemoglobin (HbA_{1C}), an index of long-term blood sugar control, and the oral glucose tolerance test (OGTT) are also discussed in Chapter 8.

Lactic Dehydrogenase

Lactic dehydrogenase (LDH), an enzyme found in the cells of many organs (skeletal muscles, myocardium, liver, pancreas, spleen, and brain), is released into the blood when cellular damage to these organs occurs. Serum levels of LDH rise 12 to 24 hours following a myocardial infarction and are often measured to determine whether an infarction has occurred. Increased LDH may result from a number of other conditions, including hepatitis, cancer, kidney disease, burns, and trauma. Measurement of five forms of LDH, known as isoenzymes, allows a more definitive diagnosis to be made. Low serum LDH is of no clinical significance. The adult reference range for serum LDH is 100 to 190 U/L.[12]

Phosphorus

The serum level of phosphorus (also known as inorganic phosphorus) is closely correlated with serum calcium level. Elevated serum phosphorus (hyperphosphatemia) is seen in renal failure, hypoparathyroidism, hyperthyroidism, and increased phosphate intake (use of phosphate-containing laxatives and enemas). Low serum phosphorus (hypophosphatemia) can be seen in hyperparathyroidism, rickets, osteomalacia, and chronic use of antacids containing aluminum hydroxide or calcium carbonate, which binds phosphorus in the gastrointestinal tract and prevents its absorption. The adult reference range is 3.0 to 4.5 mg/dL or 0.97 to 1.45 mmol/L.[12]

Potassium

Potassium, the major intracellular cation, is involved in the maintenance of acid-base balance, the body's fluid balance, and nerve impulse transmission. Elevated serum potassium (hyperkalemia) is most often due to renal failure but also may result from inadequate adrenal gland function (Addison's disease), severe burns, or crushing injuries. Low serum potassium (hypokalemia) can result from a number of causes, including use of diuretics or intravenous fluid administration without adequate potassium supplementation, vomiting, diarrhea, and eating disorders.[12] The reference range for adults is 3.5 to 5.0 mEq/L or 3.5 to 5.0 mmol/L.[12]

Sodium

Sodium, the major extracellular cation, is primarily involved in the maintenance of fluid balance and acid-base balance. Elevated serum levels (hypernatremia) are most frequently seen in dehydration resulting from insufficient water intake, excessive water output (for example, severe diarrhea or vomiting, profuse sweating, burns), or loss of antidiuretic hormone control. Hypernatremia suggests the need for water. Hyponatremia may be due to conditions resulting in excessive sodium loss from the body (vomiting, diarrhea, gastric suctioning, diuretic use), conditions resulting in fluid retention (congestive heart failure or renal disease), or water intoxication. The adult reference range is 135 to 145 mEq/L or 135 to 145 mmol/L.[12]

Triglyceride

Triglyceride (TG) is a useful indicator of lipid tolerance in patients receiving total parenteral nutrition. Fasting serum TG provides a good estimate of very low-density lipoprotein levels. Factors contributing to increased fasting serum TG include genetic factors, obesity, physical inactivity, cigarette smoking, excess alcohol intake, very-high carbohydrate diets, type 2 diabetes, chronic renal failure, nephrotic syndrome, and use of such drugs as corticosteroids, protease inhibitors, beta-adrenergic blocking agents, and estrogen. Elevated serum TG is now considered a risk factor for coronary heart disease and an indicator of persons needing coronary heart disease risk-reduction intervention. According to the National Cholesterol Education Program, a normal serum TG is < 150 mg/dL (< 1.69 mmol/L).[95] Borderline-high and high TG are 150 to 199 mg/dL (1.69 to 2.25 mmol/L) and 200 to 499 mg/dL (2.26 to 5.63 mmol/L), respectively. Very-high serum TG is considered ≥ 500 mg/dL (5.64 mmol/L). Population reference values for serum TG are shown in Appendix Q.

SUMMARY

1. Biochemical tests to assess nutritional status can be grouped into two general categories: static and functional tests. Static tests are based on measurement of a nutrient or specific metabolite in the blood, urine, or body tissue. Functional tests involve the physiologic processes that rely on the presence of adequate quantities of a nutrient.

2. The value of biochemical tests is limited by nonnutritional factors affecting test results and the occasional inability of tests to identify the nutrient deficiency. Monitoring nutritional status requires the use of several biochemical tests used in conjunction with each other and with data derived from dietary, anthropometric, and clinical methods. Compared with other assessment methods, biochemical tests have the advantage of being somewhat more objective and quantitative.

3. Protein-energy malnutrition can be either primary (insufficient intake of protein and calories) or secondary (resulting from other diseases). When severe, it results in kwashiorkor (principally a protein deficiency), marasmus (predominantly an energy deficiency), or marasmic kwashiorkor (a combination of chronic energy deficit and chronic or acute protein deficiency).

4. Creatinine is a muscle metabolite excreted in urine used to quantitate muscle mass. Creatinine is excreted in a relatively constant proportion to the body's muscle mass. Muscle mass can be estimated by comparing 24-hour urine creatinine excretion with certain standards. The creatinine-height index is a ratio of a patient's measured 24-hour urinary creatinine excretion and the expected excretion by a reference adult of the same sex and stature expressed as a percent of expected value.

5. Included among the serum proteins used to assess protein nutriture are albumin, transferrin, prealbumin, and retinol-binding protein. Considerations in their use include their body pool amount, half-life, and responsiveness to protein and energy depletion and repletion. Other considerations include how serum proteins are affected by nutritional and nonnutritional factors and how they correlate with morbidity and mortality.

6. Iron deficiency is the most common single nutrient deficiency in the United States and the most common cause of anemia. Serum ferritin is the most useful index of the body's iron stores. Hemoglobin is the most widely used screening test for iron-deficiency anemia but is not an early indicator of iron depletion. Hematocrit is defined as the percentage of red blood cells making up the entire volume of whole blood.

7. Models that combine several indicators of iron status are better at predicting the presence of iron deficiency. Among these are the body iron model, the ferritin model, and the MCV model. These models allow better discrimination between iron-deficiency anemias and those caused by infection, inflammation, and chronic disease than do single measurements.

8. Biochemical tests for assessing calcium status are hampered by the body's tight control of serum calcium levels. Measurement of urinary calcium, which is more responsive to dietary calcium change than serum calcium, is limited by the need for 24-hour urine samples and several nonnutritional factors that affect results.

9. Despite changes in dietary intake, the body maintains tight metabolic control of zinc status through conservation and redistribution of tissue zinc. Consequently, there are no sensitive biochemical or functional indicators of zinc status. Serum zinc level is not reflective of dietary changes and is only a late indicator of the body's exchangeable zinc pool size.

10. Iodine is a trace element essential for the synthesis of thyroid hormones, which regulate metabolic processes related to normal growth and development. Although iodine status is adequate in North American populations, it is a significant public health problem in much of the world, resulting in goiter, cretinism, and impaired mental and physical development.

11. Assessing vitamin A status involves measurement of plasma concentrations of retinol or the vitamin A carrier protein, retinol-binding protein (RBP), retinol isotope dilution, and dose-response tests.

12. The major function of vitamin D is to maintain serum calcium and phosphorus concentrations in a range that supports bone mineralization, neuromuscular function, and various cellular processes. Vitamin D status is best assessed by measuring the serum concentration of 25-hydroxyvitamin D [25(OH)D], the major circulating form of the vitamin, which reflects total vitamin D exposure from food, supplements, and synthesis.

13. Measurements of vitamin C in serum and leukocytes can be used for assessing vitamin C

status. Serum vitamin C is a good indicator of recent vitamin C intake, whereas leukocyte vitamin C better represents cellular stores and the total body pool.

14. Assays for assessing vitamin B_6 status include measurement of plasma pyridoxal 5′-phosphate (PLP), plasma pyridoxal, and urine 4-pyridoxic acid. A functional measure is the methionine load test.

15. Plasma PLP appears to be the single most informative indicator of vitamin B_6 status for healthy persons, but results must sometimes be interpreted with caution because values can be affected by several diseases. 4-pyridoxic acid is the major urinary metabolite of vitamin B_6. It is considered a useful indicator of immediate dietary intake and of short-term vitamin B_6 status.

16. Measures for assessing folate status include measurement of serum folate and erythrocyte folate. Serum folate provides information about recent folate intake and does not necessarily represent tissue stores. Erythrocyte folate is considered to be the best clinical index of depleted tissue stores.

17. The primary cause of vitamin B_{12} deficiency is inadequate absorption, usually because of inadequate gastric production of intrinsic factor, although ileal resection or ileal dysfunction can also cause B_{12} malabsorption. Vitamin B_{12} is assessed by directly measuring serum concentrations of vitamin B_{12} or its transport protein, or by measuring metabolites in the blood that are increased when B_{12} status is compromised.

18. Blood chemistry tests are assays performed on the substances in plasma or serum that are useful in diagnosing and managing disease. They include electrolytes, enzymes, metabolites, and other substances present in serum or plasma. These tests usually are performed using an automated chemistry analyzer capable of performing several thousand blood tests per hour.

References

1. Tanumihardjo SA. 2011. Vitamin A: Biomarkers of nutrition for development. *American Journal of Clinical Nutrition* 94:658S–665S.
2. Heimburger DC. 2012. Malnutrition and Nutritional Assessment. In Longo DL, Fauci AS, Kasper DL, Hauser SL, Jameson JL, Loscalzo J (eds.), *Harrison's principles of internal medicine,* 18th ed. New York: McGraw-Hill, 605–612.
3. Bingham SA. 1994. The use of 24-h urine samples and energy expenditure to validate dietary assessments. *American Journal of Clinical Nutrition* 59:S227–S231.
4. Tran KM, Johnson RK, Soultanakis RP, Matthews DE. 2000. In-person vs telephone administered multiple-pass 24-hour recalls in women: Validation with doubly labeled water. *Journal of the American Dietetic Association* 100:777–780, 783.
5. Gibson RS. 2005. *Nutritional Assessment,* 2nd ed. New York: Oxford University Press.
6. Mosby TT, Barr RD, Pencharz PB. 2009. Nutritional assessment of children with cancer. *Journal of Pediatric Oncology Nursing* 26:186–197.
7. Torun B. 2006. Protein-Energy Malnutrition. In Shils ME, Shike M, Ross AC, Cabellero B, Cousins RJ (eds.), *Modern nutrition in health and disease,* 10th ed. Philadelphia: Lippincott Williams & Wilkins, 881–908.
8. Hoffer LJ. 2001. Clinical nutrition: 1. Protein-energy malnutrition in the inpatient. *Canadian Medical Association Journal* 165:1345–1349.
9. McKnight K, Farmer A, Zuberbuhler L, Mger D. 2010. Identification and treatment of protein-energy malnutrition in renal disease. *Canadian Journal of Dietetic Practice and Research* 71:27–32.
10. Panel on Macronutrients, Panel on the Definition of Dietary Fiber, Subcommittee on Upper Reference Levels of Nutrients, Subcommittee on Interpretation and Uses of Dietary Reference Intakes, Standing Committee on the Scientific Evaluation of Dietary Reference Intakes. 2002. *Dietary Reference Intakes for energy, carbohydrate, fiber, fat, fatty acids, cholesterol, protein, and amino acids.* Washington, DC: National Academy Press.
11. Charney P, Malone AM. 2009. *ADA pocket guide to nutrition assessment,* 2nd ed. Chicago: American Dietetic Association.
12. Pagana KD, Pagana TJ. 2010. *Mosby's manual of diagnostic and laboratory tests,* 4th ed. St. Louis: Mosby Elsevier.
13. Ross CA. 2006. Vitamin A and carotenoids. In Shils ME, Shike M, Ross AC, Cabellero B, Cousins RJ (eds.), *Modern nutrition in health and disease,* 10th ed. Philadelphia: Lippincott Williams & Wilkins, 351–375.
14. Mei Z, Cogswell ME, Looker AC, Pfeiffer CM, Cusick SE, Lacher DA, Grummer-Strawn LM. 2011.

Assessment of iron status in US pregnant women from the National Health and Nutrition Examination Survey (NHANES), 1999–2006. *American Journal of Clinical Nutrition* 93:1312–1320.

15. Lynch S. 2011. Improving the assessment of iron status. *American Journal of Clinical Nutrition* 93:1188–1189.
16. Panel on Micronutrients, Subcommittee on Upper Reference Levels of Nutrients and of Interpretation and Uses of Dietary Reference Intakes, Standing Committee on the Scientific Evaluation of Dietary Reference Intakes. 2001. *Dietary Reference Intakes for vitamin A, vitamin K, arsenic, boron, chromium, copper, iodine, iron, manganese, molybdenum, nickel, silicon, vanadium, and zinc.* Washington, DC: National Academy Press.
17. Cook JD, Flowers CH, Skikne BS. 2003. The quantitative assessment of body iron. *Blood* 101:3359–3364.
18. Adamson JW. 2012. Iron deficiency and other hypoproliferative anemias. In Longo DL, Fauci AS, Kasper DL, Hauser SL, Jameson JL, Loscalzo J (eds.), *Harrison's principles of internal medicine,* 18th ed. New York: McGraw-Hill, 844–851.
19. Wood RJ, Ronnenbeg AG. 2006. Iron. In Shils ME, Shike M, Ross AC, Cabellero B, Cousins RJ (eds.), *Modern nutrition in health and disease,* 10th ed. Philadelphia: Lippincott Williams & Wilkins, 248–270.
20. U.S. Centers for Disease Control and Prevention. 2012. *Second national report on biochemical indicators of diet and nutrition in the U.S. population.* Atlanta: National Center for Environmental Health. www.cdc.gov/nutritionreport.
21. Skikne BS, Flowers CH, Cook JD. 1990. Serum transferrin receptor: A quantitative measure of tissue iron deficiency. *Blood* 75:1870–1878.
22. Skikne BS. 2008. Serum transferrin receptor. *American Journal of Hematology* 83:872–875.
23. Cogswell ME, Looker AC, Pfeiffer CM, Cook JD, Lacher DA, Beard JL, Lynch SR, Grummer-Strawn LM. 2009. Assessment of iron deficiency in US preschool children and nonpregnant females of childbearing age: National Health and Nutrition Examination Survey 2003–2006. *American Journal of Clinical Nutrition* 89:1334–1342.
24. U.S. Centers for Disease Control and Prevention. 2008. *National report on biochemical indicators of diet and nutrition in the U.S. population 1999–2002.* Atlanta: National Center for Environmental Health.
25. Expert Scientific Working Group. 1985. Summary of a report on assessment of the iron nutritional status of the United States population. *American Journal of Clinical Nutrition* 42:1318–1330.
26. Life Sciences Research Office, Federation of American Societies for Experimental Biology. 1989. *Nutrition monitoring in the United States: An update report on nutrition monitoring.* Washington, DC: U.S. Department of Health and Human Services, Public Health Service.
27. Powell LW. 2012. Hemochromatosis. In Longo DL, Fauci AS, Kasper DL, Hauser SL, Jameson JL, Loscalzo J (eds.), *Harrison's principles of internal medicine,* 18th ed. New York: McGraw-Hill, 3162–3167.
28. Weaver CM, Heaney RP. 2006. Calcium. In Shils ME, Shike M, Ross AC, Cabellero B, Cousins RJ (eds.), *Modern nutrition in health and disease,* 10th ed. Philadelphia: Lippincott Williams & Wilkins, 194–210.
29. Weaver CM. 2006. Calcium. In Bowman BA, Russell RM (eds.), *Present knowledge in nutrition,* 9th ed. Washington, DC: International Life Sciences Institute, 373–382.
30. Committee to Review Dietary Reference Intakes for Vitamin D and Calcium, Food and Nutrition Board. Ross AC, Taylor CL, Yaktine AL, Del Valle HB (eds.), 2011. *Dietary Reference Intakes for calcium and vitamin D.* Washington, DC: National Academy Press.
31. Weaver CM. 1990. Assessing calcium status and metabolism. *Journal of Nutrition* 120:1470–1473.
32. Nordin BEC, Need AG, Hartley TF, Philcox JC, Wilcox M, Thomas DW. 1989. Improved method for calculating calcium fractions in plasma: Reference values and effects of menopause. *Clinical Chemistry* 35:14–17.
33. King JC, Cousins RJ. 2006. Zinc. In Shils ME, Shike M, Ross AC, Cabellero B, Cousins RJ (eds.), *Modern nutrition in health and disease,* 10th ed. Philadelphia: Lippincott Williams & Wilkins, 271–285.
34. Cousins RJ. 2006. Zinc. In Bowman BA, Russell RM (eds.), *Present knowledge in nutrition,* 9th ed. Washington, DC: International Life Sciences Institute, 445–457.
35. King JC. 2011. Zinc: An essential but elusive nutrient. *American Journal of Clinical Nutrition* 94:679S–684S.
36. Lowe NM, Fekete K, Decsi T. 2009. Methods of assessment of zinc status in humans: A systematic review. *American Journal of Clinical Nutrition* 89:2040S–2051S.
37. Hotz C, Lowe NM, Araya M, Brown KH. 2003. Assessment of the trace element status of individuals and populations: The example of zinc and copper. *Journal of Nutrition* 133:1563S–1568S.
38. Hambidge M. 2003. Biomarkers of trace mineral intake and status. *Journal of Nutrition* 133:948S–955S.
39. Taylor A. 1986. Usefulness of measurements of trace elements in hair. *Annals of Clinical Biochemistry* 23:364–378.
40. Dunn JT. 2006. Iodine. In Shils ME, Shike M, Ross AC, Cabellero B, Cousins RJ (eds.), *Modern nutrition in health and disease,* 10th ed. Philadelphia: Lippincott Williams & Wilkins, 300–310.
41. Zimmermann MB, Jooste PL, Pandav CS. 2008. Iodine-

deficiency disorders. *Lancet* 372:1251–1262.

42. Zimmermann MB. 2009. Iodine deficiency. *Endocrine Reviews* 30:376–408.
43. Jameson JL, Weetman AP. 2012. Disorders of the thyroid gland. In Longo DL, Fauci AS, Kasper DL, Hauser SL, Jameson JL, Loscalzo J (eds.), *Harrison's principles of internal medicine,* 18th ed. New York: McGraw-Hill, 2911–2939.
44. Ristic-Medic D, Piskackova Z, Hooper L, Ruprish J, Casgrain A, Ashton K, Pavlovic M, Glibetic M. 2009. Methods of assessment of iodine status in humans: A systematic review. *American Journal of Clinical Nutrition* 89:2052S–2069S.
45. Zimmermann MB. 2006. Iodine and the iodine deficiency disorders. In Bowman BA, Russell RM (eds.), *Present knowledge in nutrition,* 9th ed. Washington, DC: International Life Science Institute, 471–479.
46. Lee K, Bradley R, Dwyer J, Lee SL. 1999. Too much versus too little: The implication of current iodine intake in the United States. *Nutrition Reviews* 57:177–181.
47. Hollowell JG, Haddow JE. 2007. The prevalence of iodine deficiency in women of reproductive age in the United States of America. *Public Health Nutrition* 10:1532–1539.
48. Zimmermann MB. 2011. Iodine deficiency in industrialized countries. *Clinical Endocrinology* 75:287–288.
49. Zimmerman MB. 2007. The impact of iodised salt or iodine supplements on iodine status during pregnancy, lactation and infancy. *Public Health Nutrition* 10:1584–1595.
50. Perrine CG, Kerrick K, Serdula MK, Sullivan KM. 2010. Some subgroups of reproductive age women in the United States may be at risk for iodine deficiency. *Journal of Nutrition* 140:1489–1494.
51. U.S. Department of Health and Human Services and U.S. Department of Agriculture. 2010. *Dietary Guidelines for Americans, 2010.* Washington, DC: U.S. Government Printing Office. www.dietaryguidelines.gov.
52. Appel LJ, Frohlich ED, Hgall JE, Pearson TA, Sacco RL, et al. 2011. The importance of population-wide sodium reduction as a means to prevent cardiovascular disease and stroke: A call to action from the American Heart Association. *Circulation* 123:1138–1143.
53. Ross AC. 2006. Vitamin A and carotenoids. In Shils ME, Shike M, Ross AC, Cabellero B, Cousins RJ (eds.), *Modern nutrition in health and disease,* 10th ed. Philadelphia: Lippincott Williams & Wilkins, 351–375.
54. Solomons NW. 2006. Vitamin A. In Bowman BA, Russell RM (eds.), *Present knowledge in nutrition,* 9th ed. Washington, DC: International Life Sciences Institute, 157–183.
55. Rice AL, Stoltzfus RJ, de Francisco A, Kjolhede CL. 2000. Evaluation of serum retinol, the modified-relative-dose-response ratio, and breast-milk vitamin A as indicators of response postpartum maternal vitamin A supplementation. *American Journal of Clinical Nutrition* 71:799–806.
56. Furr HC, Green MH, Haskell M, Mokhtar N, Nestel P, Newton S, Ribaya-Mercado JD, Tang G, Tanumihardjo S, Wasantwisut E. 2005. Stable isotope dilution techniques for assessing vitamin A status and bioavailability of provitamin A carotenoids in humans. *Public Health Nutrition* 8:596–607.
57. Olson JA. Isotope-dilution techniques: A wave of the future in human nutrition. *American Journal of Clinical Nutrition* 66:186–187.
58. Holick MF. 2006. Vitamin D. In Shils ME, Shike M, Ross AC, Cabellero B, Cousins RJ (eds.), *Modern nutrition in health and disease,* 10th ed. Philadelphia: Lippincott Williams & Wilkins, 376–395.
59. Holick MF. 2011. Health benefits of vitamin D and sunlight: A D-bate. *Nature Reviews Endocrinology* 7:73–75.
60. Heaney RP, Holick MF. 2011. Why the IOM recommendations for vitamin D are deficient. *Journal of Bone and Mineral Research* 26:455–457.
61. Holick MF, Chen TC. 2008. Vitamin D deficiency: A worldwide problem with health consequences. *American Journal of Clinical Nutrition* 87:1080S–1086S.
62. Heaney RP. 2011. Assessing vitamin D status. *Current Opinion in Clinical Nutrition and Metabolic Care* 14:440–444.
63. Levine M, Katz A, Padayatty SJ. 2006. Vitamin C. In Shils ME, Shike M, Ross AC, Cabellero B, Cousins RJ (eds.), *Modern nutrition in health and disease,* 10th ed. Philadelphia: Lippincott Williams & Wilkins, 507–524.
64. Jacob RA. 1990. Assessment of human vitamin C status. *Journal of Nutrition* 120:1480–1485.
65. Lykkesfeldt J, Poulsen HE. 2010. Is vitamin C supplementation beneficial? Lessons learned from randomised controlled trials. *British Journal of Nutrition* 103:1251–1259.
66. Johnston CS. 2006. Vitamin C. In Bowman BA, Russell RM (eds.), *Present knowledge in nutrition,* 9th ed. Washington, DC: International Life Sciences Institute, 233–241.
67. Standing Committee on the Scientific Evaluation of Dietary Reference Intakes, Food and Nutrition Board, Institute of Medicine. 2000. *Dietary Reference Intakes for vitamin C, vitamin E, selenium, and carotenoids.* Washington, DC: National Academy Press.
68. Mackey AD, Davis SR, Gregory JF. 2006. Vitamin B_6. In Shils ME, Shike M, Ross AC, Cabellero B, Cousins RJ (eds.), *Modern nutrition in health and disease,* 10th ed. Philadelphia: Lippincott Williams & Wilkins, 452–461.
69. McCormick DB. 2006. Vitamin B_6. In Bowman BA, Russell RM (eds.), *Present knowledge in nutrition,* 9th ed. Washington, DC: International Life Sciences Institute, 269–277.
70. Standing Committee on the Scientific Evaluation of Dietary Reference Intakes, Food and

Nutrition Board, Institute of Medicine. 1998. *Dietary Reference Intakes for thiamin, riboflavin, niacin, vitamin B6, folate, vitamin B12, pantothenic acid, biotin, and choline.* Washington, DC: National Academy Press.

71. Leklem JE. 1988. Vitamin B_6 metabolism and function in humans. In Leklem JE, Reynolds RD (eds.), *Clinical and physiological applications of vitamin B_6*. New York: Alan R. Liss.
72. Leklem JE. 1990. Vitamin B_6: A status report. *Journal of Nutrition* 120:1503–1507.
73. Carmel R. 2006. Folic acid. In Shils ME, Shike M, Ross AC, Cabellero B, Cousins RJ (eds.), *Modern nutrition in health and disease,* 10th ed. Philadelphia: Lippincott Williams & Wilkins, 470–481.
74. Yetley EA, Pfeiffer CM, Phinney KW, et al. 2011. Biomarkers of folate status in NHANES: A roundtable summary. *American Journal of Clinical Nutrition* 94:303S–312S.
75. U.S. Centers for Disease Control and Prevention. 2010. CDC grand rounds: Additional opportunities to prevent neural tube defects with folic acid fortification. *Morbidity and Mortality Weekly Report* 59:980–984.
76. Carmel R. 2006. Cobalamin (vitamin B_{12}). In Shils ME, Shike M, Ross AC, Cabellero B, Cousins RJ (eds.), *Modern nutrition in health and disease,* 10th ed. Philadelphia: Lippincott Williams & Wilkins, 482–497.
77. Hofafbrand AV. 2012. Megaloblastic anemias. In Longo DL, Fauci AS, Kasper DL, Hauser SL, Jameson JL, Loscalzo J (eds.), *Harrison's principles of internal medicine,* 18th ed. New York: McGraw-Hill, 862–872.
78. Yetley EA, Pfeiffer CM, Phinney KW, et al. 2011. Biomarkers of vitamin B-12 status in NHANES: A roundtable summary. *American Journal of Clinical Nutrition* 94:313S–321S.
79. Carmel R. 2011. Biomarkers of cobalamin (vitamin B-12) status in the epidemiologic setting: a critical overview of context, applications, and performance characteristics of cobalamin, methylmalonic acid, and holotranscobalamin II. *American Journal of Clinical Nutrition* 94:348S–358S.
80. Malarkey LM, McMorrow ME. 2012. *Saunders nursing guide to laboratory and diagnostic tests,* 2nd ed. St. Louis: Elsevier/Saunders.

ASSESSMENT ACTIVITY 9.1

Visiting a Clinical Laboratory

Every hospital or clinic has a clinical laboratory where at least some of the facility's biochemical tests are performed. Specimens are sometimes sent to an outside clinical laboratory because it has specialized instruments and expertise or because its automated analyzers allow certain tests to be performed more economically. However, all hospitals have facilities for performing certain basic tests, especially those required in emergency situations. Among these are tests for electrolytes, blood gases, enzymes diagnostic of cardiac or liver disease, and glucose.

Your class can arrange to visit a clinical laboratory to see how some of these tests are performed. You may be surprised by the capability of various automated instruments used to perform the chemistry profile and complete blood count on a single specimen of serum or whole blood.

ASSESSMENT ACTIVITY 9.2

Chemistry Profile, Complete Blood Count, and Coronary Risk Profile

The chemistry profile, complete blood count (CBC), and coronary risk profile are among the most basic series of tests performed by clinical laboratories. Generally included in the chemistry profile are those tests listed in the section entitled "Blood Chemistry Tests." Included in the CBC are the red blood cell count, white blood cell count, and measurements of hemoglobin, hematocrit, mean corpuscular volume, mean corpuscular hemoglobin, and mean corpuscular hemoglobin concentration. The coronary risk profile measures levels of triglyceride, total cholesterol, and HDL-C (cholesterol carried by high-density lipoproteins) and calculates LDL-C (cholesterol carried by low-density lipoproteins) and the total cholesterol/HDL-C ratio. These tests are discussed in Chapter 8. These measurements are routinely performed using automated instruments capable of performing several thousand tests per hour.

Members of your class may want to have their blood drawn by a qualified venipuncturist and have the samples sent to a clinical laboratory for analysis. Tests that might be performed include the CBC, chemistry profile, and coronary risk profile.

Another example of a simple test that can be done in the classroom is the hematocrit. The necessary equipment includes a centrifuge, capillary tubes, lancets, alcohol wipes, gloves, and some way of comparing the volume of whole blood in the capillary tube with the volume of packed cells after the tube is spun down. Whatever approach your class takes, compare your test results with the reference values given in this chapter and Chapter 8. Obtain an average value for the class and compare this with the reference values.

Remember, in handling blood specimens or any bodily fluid, precautions must be taken to protect patients and laboratory staff from infectious agents, especially those causing hepatitis as well as the human immunodeficiency virus (HIV). All bodily fluids must be regarded as being infectious and handled with the utmost care. All syringes, lancets, needles, tubes, and other materials that have come in contact with blood or other bodily fluids must be handled safely and disposed of properly. Gloves should be worn whenever drawing blood or handling other bodily fluids.

CHAPTER

Clinical Assessment of Nutritional Status 10

Outline

Introduction
Medical History
Dietary History
Subjective Global Assessment
Protein-Energy Malnutrition
HIV Infection
Eating Disorders
Mini Nutritional Assessment
Summary
References
Assessment Activity 10.1: Using Subjective Global Assessment

Student Learning Outcomes

After studying this chapter, the student will be able to:

1. Name the components of a patient's medical history that are relevant to nutritional assessment.
2. Explain the advantages and limitations of Subjective Global Assessment.
3. Use Subjective Global Assessment to assess a patient's nutritional status.
4. Differentiate between kwashiorkor and marasmus.
5. Calculate and interpret percent weight for height.
6. Calculate and interpret percent height for age.
7. Describe the body composition changes that result from lipodystrophy in HIV patients.
8. Discuss the American Psychiatric Association's diagnostic criteria for anorexia nervosa and bulimia.

Introduction

Clinical assessment of nutritional status involves a detailed history, a thorough physical examination, and the interpretation of the signs and symptoms associated with malnutrition. It can be an efficient and effective way for an experienced and astute clinician to evaluate a patient's nutritional status without having to depend entirely on laboratory and diagnostic tests that may delay initiation of nutritional support and increase the time and cost of hospitalization. **Signs** are defined as observations, made by a qualified examiner, of which the patient is usually unaware. **Symptoms** are clinical manifestations reported by the patient. This chapter discusses clinical assessment of nutritional status and gives examples of clinical indicators of impaired nutritional status. As a dietitian or nutritionist, you will likely see some of the conditions discussed and illustrated in this chapter. For example, protein-energy malnutrition and severe wasting are common features of certain cancers, acquired immunodeficiency syndrome (AIDS), and advanced disease of the gastrointestinal tract. However, some of the other conditions discussed in this chapter, such as clinical signs of advanced nutrient deficiency, are not often seen in developed countries but occur more frequently in less industrialized nations. But given the global nature of the work of health care professionals, understanding how to evaluate advanced malnutrition and starvation will be of interest to students and practitioners of nutrition. Because many of the clinical findings are not specific for a particular nutrient deficiency, they often must be integrated with anthropometric, biochemical, and dietary data before arriving at a definitive diagnosis.

Medical History

Obtaining a patient's history is the first step in the clinical assessment of nutritional status.[1] A good way to begin is by reviewing the patient's medical record, giving careful attention to the patient's medical history.[2,3] Components from the medical history to consider in nutritional assessment are shown in Box 10.1.

Essential components of a patient's history include pertinent facts about past and current health and use of medications, as well as personal and household information.[1,2] A variety of diseases can affect nutritional status. Among these are diabetes, kidney disease, various cancers, coronary heart disease, stroke, liver disease (e.g., hepatitis and cirrhosis), gallbladder disease, AIDS, ulcers, and colitis, as well as recent or past surgical procedures. Other conditions affecting nutritional status also should be explored: the ability to chew and swallow; appetite; and the presence of vomiting, diarrhea, constipation, flatulence, belching, or indigestion. An inquiry should be made about the patient's usual weight and any recent changes (gains or losses) in weight. A systematic approach to the detection of deficiency syndromes based on findings from the history is shown in Table 10.1.

Information on the use of medications will provide clues about the patient's actual or perceived medical condition. This will include prescription and over-the-counter medications, vitamin and mineral supplements, and nontraditional medications, such as herbal and folk remedies. This information can also be helpful in identifying drug-nutrient interactions potentially having an adverse effect on the patient's nutritional status.[3]

Psychosocial factors include the patient's age; occupation; educational level; marital status; income; living arrangements; number of dependents; use of alcohol, tobacco, and illicit drugs; degree of social and emotional support; and access to and ability to pay for health care. These factors are summarized in Box 10.2.

The necessary detail of the history will vary depending on circumstances and will be influenced by the patient's ability to respond to questioning. In some instances, the necessary information might need to be obtained from

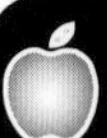

Box 10.1 Components of the Medical History to Consider in Nutritional Assessment

- Past and current diagnoses of nutritional consequence
- Diagnostic procedures
- Surgeries
- Chemotherapy and radiation therapy
- History of nutrition-related problems
- Existing nutrient deficiencies
- Medications and their nutrient interactions
- Psychosocial history—alcohol, smoking, finances, social support
- Signs or symptoms suggestive of vitamin deficiency
- Signs or symptoms suggestive of mineral deficiency

Adapted from Phinney SD. 1981. The assessment of protein nutrition in the hospitalized patient. *Clinics in Laboratory Medicine* 1:767–774; McLaren DS. 1992. *A colour atlas and text of diet-related disorders,* 2nd ed. London: Mosby Europe; Jeejeebhoy KN. 1994. Clinical and functional assessments. In Shils ME, Olson JA, Shike M (eds.), *Modern nutrition in health and disease,* 8th ed. Philadelphia: Lea & Febiger.

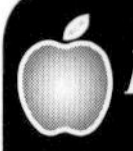

Box 10.2 Factors to Consider in Taking a Patient's Dietary History

- Weight changes
- Usual meal pattern
- Appetite
- Satiety
- Discomfort after eating
- Chewing/swallowing ability
- Likes/dislikes
- Taste changes/aversions
- Allergies
- Nausea/vomiting
- Bowel habits—diarrhea, constipation, steatorrhea
- Living conditions
- Snack consumption
- Vitamin/mineral supplement use
- Alcohol/drug use
- Previous diet restrictions
- Surgery/chronic diseases
- Ability to purchase and prepare food
- Access to and ability to pay for health care

TABLE 10.1 Nutritional History Screens—a Systematic Approach to the Detection of Deficiency Syndromes

Mechanism of Deficiency	If History Of	Suspect Deficiency Of
Inadequate intake	Alcoholism	Energy, protein, thiamin, niacin, folate, pyridoxine, riboflavin
	Avoidance of fruit, vegetables, grains	Vitamin C, thiamin, niacin, folate
	Avoidance of meat, dairy products, eggs	Protein, vitamin B_{12}
	Constipation, hemorrhoids, diverticulosis	Dietary fiber
	Isolation, poverty, dental disease, food idiosyncrasies	Various nutrients
	Weight loss	Energy, other nutrients
Inadequate absorption	Drugs (especially antacids, anticonvulsants, cholestyramine, laxatives, neomycin, alcohol)	Various nutrients, depending on drug/nutrient interaction
	Malabsorption (diarrhea, weight loss, steatorrhea)	Vitamins A, D, K; energy; protein; calcium; magnesium; zinc
	Parasites	Iron, vitamin B_{12} (fish tapeworm)
	Pernicious anemia	Vitamin B_{12}
	Surgery	
	Gastrectomy	Vitamin B_{12}, iron
	Small bowel resection	Vitamin B_{12}, (if distal ileum), others as in malabsorption
Decreased utilization	Drugs (especially anticonvulsants, antimetabolites, oral contraceptives, isoniazid, alcohol)	Various nutrients, depending on drug/nutrient interaction
	Inborn errors of metabolism (by family history)	Various nutrients
Increased losses	Alcohol abuse	Magnesium, zinc
	Blood loss	Iron
	Centesis (ascitic, pleural taps)	Protein
	Diabetes, uncontrolled	Energy
	Diarrhea	Protein, zinc, electrolytes
	Draining abscesses, wounds	Protein, zinc
	Nephrotic syndrome	Protein, zinc
	Peritoneal dialysis or hemodialysis	Protein, water-soluble vitamins, zinc
Increased requirements	Fever	Energy
	Hyperthyroidism	Energy
	Physiologic demands (infancy, adolescence, pregnancy, lactation)	Various nutrients
	Surgery, trauma, burns, infection	Energy, protein, vitamin C, zinc
	Tissue hypoxia	Energy (inefficient utilization)
	Cigarette smoking	Vitamin C, folic acid

a surrogate (a parent, a companion, a sibling, or another person knowledgeable about the patient's life habits). Much of this information can be obtained from the history and physical examination performed by the admitting physician, from the notes of nurses or social workers, and from previous medical records. Remember that this and all information about the patient should be dealt with in a confidential and strictly professional manner.

DIETARY HISTORY

Included with the dietary history is information about the patient's eating practices. This includes a wide range of information about usual eating patterns (timing and location of meals and snacks), food preferences and aversions, intolerances and allergies, amount of money available for purchasing food, ability to obtain and prepare food, eligibility for and access to food assistance programs, and use of vitamin, mineral, and other supplements. These and other factors are included in Box 10.2.

For example, when inquiring about appetite, satiety, or discomfort, it is important to ask if the patient has experienced any changes in desire for food, if he or she experiences satiety earlier or later than usual, and if there is any pain or discomfort associated with eating. Questions about the ability to chew and swallow food are important. Are there dental or oral problems making it difficult to chew certain foods or to consume adequate energy to support normal body weight? If the patient wears dentures, are they well fitting? If swallowing is painful or difficult, for what foods?

Questioning the patient about bowel habits can often provide information pertinent to the diagnosis of gastrointestinal disease. The patient should be asked about changes in bowel habits, such as constipation, diarrhea, or unusual amounts of flatus (gas), and about stool consistency and color. Obviously, the presence of bright red blood in the stool is an important finding. Stools containing digested blood (e.g., from a bleeding peptic ulcer) may appear black or tarry. The finding of frothy, watery, and foul-smelling stools suggests the possibility of fat malabsorption. Table 10.2 gives a listing of clinical findings and links their presence with either an excess or a deficiency of various nutrients.

Subjective Global Assessment

Subjective Global Assessment (SGA) is a clinical technique for assessing the nutritional status of a patient based on features of the patient's history and physical examination.[4] Unlike traditional methods that rely heavily on objective anthropometric and biochemical data, SGA is based on four elements of the patient's history (recent loss of body weight, changes in usual diet, presence of significant gastrointestinal symptoms, and the patient's functional capacity) and three elements of the physical examination (loss of subcutaneous fat, muscle wasting, and presence of edema or ascites).[4] Information obtained from the history and physical examination can be entered into a form, such as the one shown in Figure 10.1, to arrive at an SGA rating of nutritional status.

Elements of the History

The first of the four elements of the SGA history is the percent and pattern of weight loss within 6 months prior to examination. A weight loss < 5% is considered small. A 5% to 10% weight loss is considered potentially significant. A weight loss > 10% is considered definitely significant. The pattern of weight loss is also important. A patient who has lost 12% of his or her weight in the past 6 months but has recently gained 6% of it back is considered better nourished than a patient who has lost 6% of his or her weight in the past 6 months and continues to lose weight. Information about the patient's maximum weight and what it was 6 months ago can be compared with the patient's current weight. Questions about changes in the way clothing fits may confirm reports of weight change. Information about changes in body weight in the past 2 weeks (increase, no change, decrease) should be elicited as well. These data can be entered or noted in the appropriate places in Figure 10.1.

Dietary intake, the second element of the history, is classified as either normal (i.e., what the patient usually eats) or abnormal (i.e., a change from the patient's usual diet). If intake is abnormal, the duration in weeks is entered, and the appropriate box is checked to indicate the type of dietary intake abnormality (i.e., increased intake, suboptimal solid, full-liquid, IV or hypocaloric liquids, or starvation). The patient can be asked if the amount of food consumed has changed and, if so, by how much and why. If the patient is eating less, it would be valuable to know what happens when he or she tries to eat more. Ask for a description of a typical breakfast, lunch, and dinner and how that compares with what the patient typically ate 6 or 12 months ago.

Information about any gastrointestinal symptoms persisting more than 2 weeks (the third history element) should be elicited and noted on the form. Diarrhea or occasional vomiting lasting only a few days is not considered significant. The presence or absence of any dysfunction in the patient's ability to attend to activities of daily living (the last history element) should also be noted on the form. If a dysfunction is present, its duration and type should be noted.

Elements of the Physical Examination

The first of the three elements of the physical examination is loss of subcutaneous fat. The four anatomic areas listed in Figure 10.1 (shoulders, triceps, chest, and hands) should be checked for loss of fullness or loose-fitting skin, although the latter may appear in older persons who are not malnourished. Illustrations of subcutaneous fat loss in the arm, chest wall, and hands are shown in Figure 10.2 and Figure 10.3. Loss of subcutaneous fat should be noted as normal (0), mild loss (1+), moderate loss (2+), or severe loss (3+).

According to Detsky, the presence of muscle wasting (the second element of the physical examination) is best assessed by examining the deltoid muscles (located at the sides of the shoulders) and the quadriceps femoris muscles (the muscles of the anterior thigh).[4] Loss of subcutaneous fat in the shoulders and deltoid muscle wasting gives the shoulders a squared-off appearance, similar to that shown in Figure 10.4. These areas can be assessed as being normal or mildly, moderately, or severely wasted.

The presence of edema at the ankle or sacrum can also be assessed as absent, mild, moderate, or severe. The presence of "pitting" edema can be checked by momentarily pressing the area with a finger and then looking for a persistent depression (more than 5 seconds) where the finger was. Ankle edema and ascites can be assessed as absent, mild, moderate, or severe. When considerable edema or ascites are present, weight loss is a less important variable.

The final step in SGA is arriving at a rating of nutritional assessment. Instead of an explicit numerical weighting scheme SGA depends on the clinician's subjectively combining the various elements to arrive at an overall, or global, assessment. Patients with weight loss > 10% that is continuing, poor dietary intake, and severe loss of subcutaneous fat and muscle wasting fall within the severely malnourished category (class C rank). Patients with at least a 5% weight loss, reduced dietary intake, and mild to moderate loss of subcutaneous fat and muscle wasting fall within the moderately malnourished category (class B rank). Patients are generally ranked as well nourished when they have had a recent improvement in appetite or the other historical features of SGA. A class A rank would be given to patients having a recent

TABLE 10.2 Clinical Nutrition Examination

Clinical Findings	Consider Deficiency Of	Consider Excess Of	Frequency
Hair, Nails			
Flag sign (traverse depigmentation of hair)	Protein		Rare
Easily pluckable hair	Protein		Common
Sparse hair	Protein, biotin, zinc	Vitamin A	Occasional
Corkscrew hairs and unemerged coiled hairs	Vitamin C		Common
Traverse ridging of nails	Protein		Occasional
Skin			
Scaling	Vitamin A, zinc, essential fatty acids	Vitamin A	Occasional
Cellophane appearance	Protein		Occasional
Cracking (flaky paint or crazy pavement dermatosis)	Protein		Rare
Follicular hyperkeratosis	Vitamins A, C		Occasional
Petechiae (especially perifollicular)	Vitamin C		Occasional
Purpura	Vitamins C, K		Common
Pigmentation, desquamation of sun-exposed areas	Niacin		Rare
Yellow pigmentation-sparing sclerae (benign)		Carotene	Common
Eyes			
Papilledema		Vitamin A	Rare
Night blindness	Vitamin A		Rare
Perioral			
Angular stomatitis	Riboflavin, pyridoxine, niacin		Occasional
Cheilosis (dry, cracking, ulcerated lips)	Riboflavin, pyridoxine, niacin		Rare
Oral			
Atrophic lingual papillae (slick tongue)	Riboflavin, niacin, folate, vitamin B_{12}, protein, iron		Common
Glossitis (scarlet, raw tongue)	Riboflavin, niacin, pyridoxine, folate, vitamin B_{12}		Occasional
Hypogeusesthesia, hyposmia	Zinc		Occasional
Swollen, retracted, bleeding gums (if teeth are present)	Vitamin C		Occasional
Bones, Joints			
Beading of ribs, epiphyseal swelling, bowlegs	Vitamin D		Rare
Tenderness (subperiosteal hemorrhage in child)	Vitamin C		Rare
Neurologic			
Headache		Vitamin A	Rare
Drowsiness, lethargy, vomiting		Vitamins A, D	Rare
Dementia	Niacin, vitamin B_{12}		Rare
Confabulation, disorientation	Thiamin (Korsakoff's psychosis)		Occasional
Ophthalmoplegia	Thiamin, phosphorus		Occasional
Peripheral neuropathy (e.g., weakness; paresthesia; ataxia; decreased tendon reflexes; fine tactile sense, vibratory sense, and position sense)	Thiamin, pyridoxine, vitamin B_{12}	Pyridoxine	Occasional
Tetany	Calcium, magnesium		Occasional
Other			
Parotid enlargement	Protein (also consider bulimia)		Occasional
Heart failure	Thiamin (wet beriberi), phosphorus		Occasional
Sudden heart failure, death	Vitamin C		Rare
Hepatomegaly	Protein	Vitamin A	Rare
Edema	Protein, thiamin		Common
Poor wound healing, pressure ulcers	Protein, vitamin C, zinc		Common

HISTORY

1. Weight Change

$$\% \text{ Wt change} = \frac{\text{wt 6 months ago} - \text{current wt}}{\text{wt 6 mos ago}} \times 100$$

Maximum body weight ________
Weight 6 months ago ________
Current weight ________
Overall weight loss in past 6 months ________
Percent weight loss in past 6 months ________
Change in 2 past weeks: _____ increase _____ no change _____ decrease

2. Dietary Intake (relative to normal)

_______ No change
_______ Change Duration: _______ Weeks
Type: _______ Increased intake
_______ Suboptimal solid diet
_______ Full liquid diet
_______ IV or hypocaloric liquids
_______ Starvation

3. Gastrointestinal Symptoms (lasting > 2 weeks)

_______ None
_______ Nausea _______ Vomiting _______ Diarrhea _______ Anorexia

4. Functional Capacity

_______ No dysfunction
_______ Dysfunction Duration: _______ weeks
Type: _______ Works suboptimally
_______ Ambulatory
_______ Bedridden

PHYSICAL EXAMINATION

(For each trait specify: 0 = normal; 1+ = mild; 2+ = moderate; 3+ = severe)

_______ Loss of subcutaneous fat (shoulders, triceps, chest, hands)
_______ Muscle wasting (quadriceps, deltoids)
_______ Ankle edema
_______ Ascites

Subjective Global Assessment Rating (select one)

_______ A = well nourished
_______ B = moderately (or suspected of being) malnourished
_______ C = severely malnourished

Figure 10.1 Form for rating nutritional status based on Subjective Global Assessment.

Source: Adapted from Detsky AS, McLaughlin JR, Baker JP, Johnston N, Whittaker S, Mendelson RA, Jeejeebhoy KN. 1987. What is Subjective Global Assessment of nutritional status? *Journal of Parenteral and Enteral Nutrition* 11:8–13; Detsky AS, Smalley PS, Change J. 1994. Is this patient malnourished? *Journal of the American Medical Association* 271:54–58.

increase in weight (that is not fluid retention), even if their net loss for the past 6 months was between 5% and 10%. Using this approach, very few well-nourished patients are classified as malnourished, but some patients with mild malnutrition may be missed.[4]

Despite this subjective nature, clinicians (nurses and residents) trained to use SGA were shown to have arrived at very similar rankings when comparing their evaluations of a series of 109 patients.[4] The method has also been shown to be a powerful predictor of postoperative complications.[4,5] SGA has been shown to be a simple, safe, effective, and inexpensive tool for clinicians to identify patients who are malnourished or at risk of malnutrition. It is regarded by many as the most reliable and efficient method to assess nutritional status at the bedside and is considered the gold standard for bedside assessment tools.[6,7]

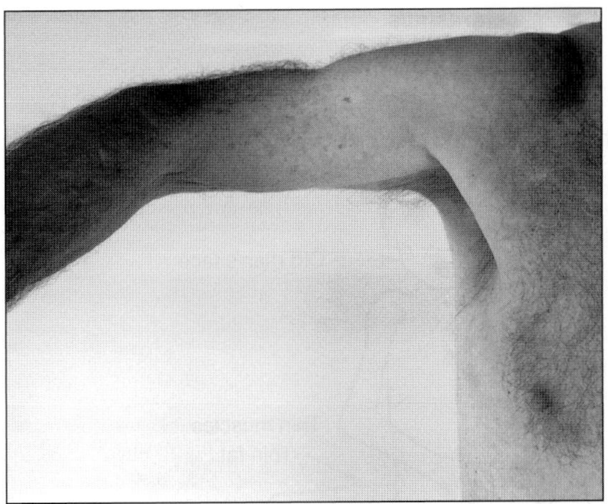

Figure 10.2 Subcutaneous tissue loss from the arm and chest wall.

Source: The McGraw-Hill Companies, Inc./Mark Dierker, photographer.

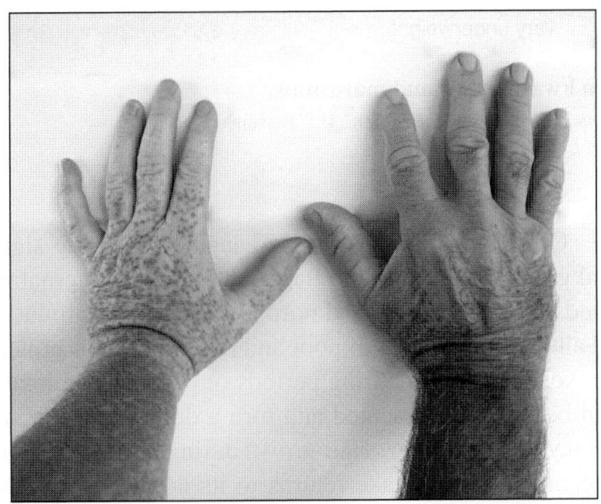

Figure 10.3

Loss of subcutaneous tissue can be clearly seen in the hand on the left, compared with the hand of a healthy person on the right.

Source: The McGraw-Hill Companies, Inc./Mark Dierker, photographer.

PROTEIN-ENERGY MALNUTRITION

Clinical Signs

In its most severe states, protein-energy malnutrition (PEM) takes the form of kwashiorkor or marasmus. Kwashiorkor is predominantly a protein deficiency, whereas marasmus is mainly an energy deficiency.[8] Kwashiorkor (Figure 10.5) is characterized by a relatively normal weight, generally intact skeletal musculature, and decreased concentrations of serum proteins.[8–10] A common feature is soft, pitting, painless edema in the feet and legs, extending into the perineum, upper extremities,

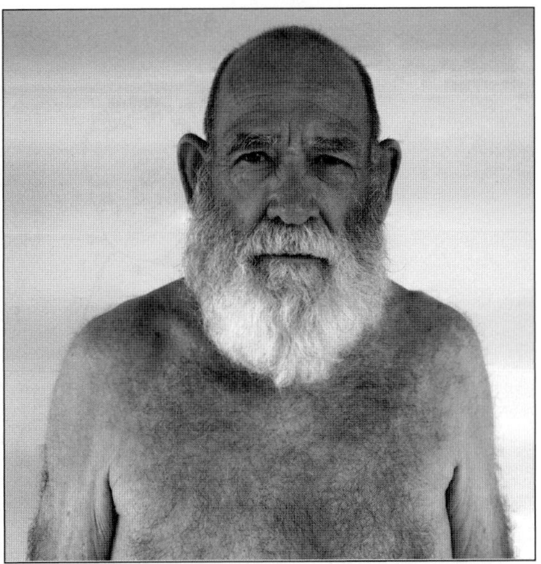

Figure 10.4

The squared-off appearance of the shoulders indicates the loss of subcutaneous tissue and wasting of the deltoid muscle. Loss of subcutaneous fat and muscle wasting is also apparent in the upper arms.

Source: The McGraw-Hill Companies, Inc./Mark Dierker, photographer.

and face in severe cases. The hair can become dry, brittle, dull, and easily pulled out without pain. The marasmic patient typically presents with significant loss of body weight, skeletal muscle, and adipose tissue mass but with serum protein concentrations relatively intact. Patients are often seen at 60% or less of their expected weight for height, and marasmic children have a marked reduction in their longitudinal growth. Patients are described as having a "skin and bones" appearance. General characteristics of kwashiorkor and marasmus are outlined in Table 10.3.

Although such obvious cases of kwashiorkor and marasmus as illustrated in Figure 10.5 will not often be seen in developed countries, severe cases of protein-energy malnutrition and wasting still occur, especially as a result of AIDS, certain cancers, some gastrointestinal diseases, and alcoholism and other instances of substance abuse. The emaciated condition of the body and general ill health resulting from these and other diseases is also called **cachexia.** Many patients presenting with protein-energy malnutrition and wasting will have diagnostic features in common with either marasmus or kwashiorkor. For example, Figure 10.6 illustrates a case of severe protein-energy malnutrition having several diagnostic features common to marasmus. When this 29-year-old male presented for treatment (A and B), he had lost considerable skeletal muscle, adipose tissue, and body weight. There was no edema present. The wasting is particularly apparent in the neck, shoulders, and upper arm in A and B. After 3 months

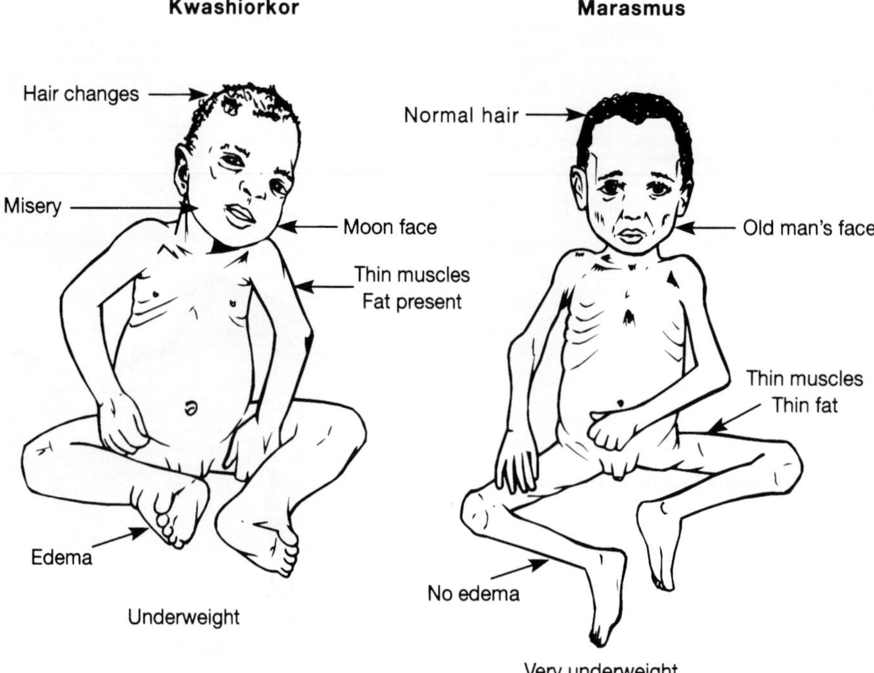

Figure 10.5 Differences in clinical signs between kwashiorkor and marasmus.

Source: Adapted from Jellife DB. 1968. *Clinical nutrition in developing countries.* Washington, DC: U.S. Department of Health and Human Services.

of nutritional support (C and D), there was an obvious increase in skeletal muscle, adipose tissue, and body weight. The face became fuller and there was considerably less wasting apparent in the neck, shoulders, and upper arm.

An example of severe protein-energy malnutrition is illustrated in Figure 10.7. As is the case with kwashiorkor, edema can be clearly seen, especially in the legs and feet of this 46-year-old male (A and B). Some wasting can also be seen in the neck, shoulders, and upper arms. After 3 months of treatment (C and D), there was a fuller appearance to the face, neck, shoulders, and upper arms and no apparent edema.

TABLE 10.3 Characteristics of Kwashiorkor and Marasmus

Variable	Kwashiorkor	Marasmus
Skeletal muscle	No major losses	Significant losses
Serum proteins	Significantly decreased	Relatively normal
Adipose tissue	Preserved	Significant loss
Body weight	Relatively normal	Significant loss
Edema	Pitting edema common	Absent
Predisposing factors	Ample energy with little or no protein	Starvation, lack of both protein and total energy

Other clinical signs of PEM include the "flag sign" and growth failure. In the flag sign, there are alternating bands of depigmented and normal-colored hair produced by alternating periods of poor and relatively good protein intake. Hair grown during periods of poor protein intake can become depigmented and turn a dull brown, red, or even yellowish white. Hair grown during periods of more adequate protein intake returns to its normal color. The flag sign is especially noticeable in persons with long, dark-colored hair. An example of the flag sign is shown Figure 10.8.

Growth failure (or failure to thrive) is the most common sign of malnutrition in children. It is a failure to gain weight and height at the expected rate. Growth failure can result from one or any combination of factors, such as inadequate nutrient intake, nutrient malabsorption, failure to utilize nutrients, increased nutrient losses, and increased nutrient requirements. Major contributing factors to growth failure include poverty, inadequate emotional and social nurturing, and infections, especially parasitic gut infestations. Figure 10.9 illustrates growth failure. The ages of the children in this picture are, from left to right, 2, 4.5, and 5.5 years. The child on the left and the child in the center are of normal size for their age. However, the child on the right has a markedly reduced height for age and weight for age, although his weight-to-height ratio is normal and there appear to be no other signs of clinical malnutrition. Although he is 3.5 years older than the child on the left, he is less than 5 cm taller.

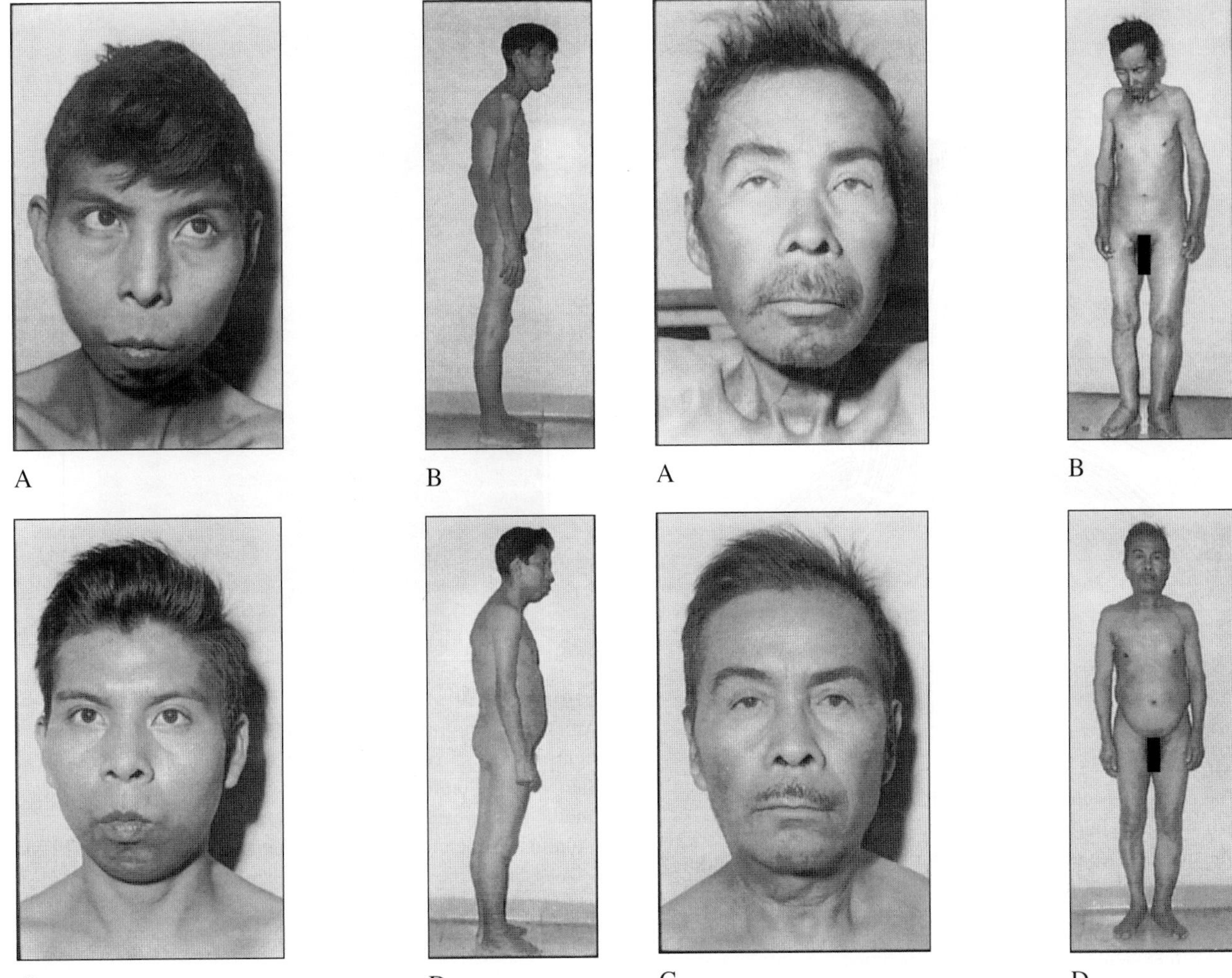

Figure 10.6 Marasmic-like severe protein-energy malnutrition in a 29-year-old male before treatment (A and B) and after 3 months of nutritional support (C and D).

Source: From McLaren DS. 1992. *A colour atlas and text of diet-related disorders,* 2nd ed. London: Mosby Europe.

Figure 10.7 Kwashiorkor-like protein-energy malnutrition in a 46-year-old male before treatment (A and B) and after 3 months of nutritional support (C and D).

Source: From McLaren DS. 1992. *A colour atlas and text of diet-related disorders,* 2nd ed. London: Mosby Europe.

Classifying Protein-Energy Malnutrition

The severity of PEM in children and adolescents can be classified using records of age and measurements of weight and height or length.[8] From these, weight for height (or length) and height for age can be calculated. Weight for height is a convenient index of current nutritional status, while height for age better represents past nutritional status. In this context of classifying the severity of PEM, **wasting** has been suggested as a term for a deficit in weight for height, and the term **stunting** has been suggested for a deficit in height for age. Patients with PEM can be placed in one of four categories: normal; wasted but not stunted (indicating acute PEM); wasted and stunted (indicating acute and chronic PEM); or stunted but not wasted (indicating past PEM with adequate nutrition at present).[6] The severity of wasting can be determined by calculating weight as a percentage of the reference median weight for height using the following equation:

$$\%\text{ weight for height} = \frac{\text{Actual body weight}}{\text{Reference weight for height}} \times 100$$

where reference weight for height = the median (or 50th percentile) weight for height for the subject's age and sex. To determine the severity of stunting, calculate the height as a percentage of the reference height for age using the following equation:

$$\%\text{ height for age} = \frac{\text{Actual height or length}}{\text{Reference height for age}} \times 100$$

where reference height for age = the median (or 50th percentile) height for the subject's age and sex. The values

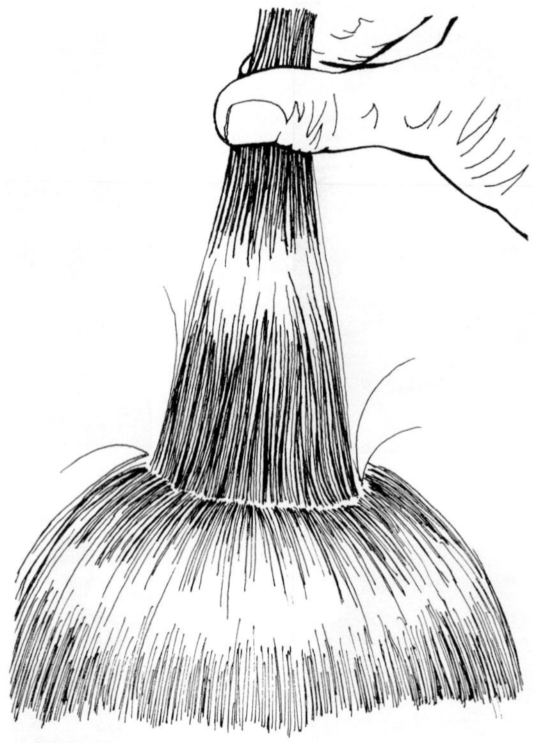

Figure 10.8
The flag sign is characterized by bands of depigmented hair that grew during periods of inadequate protein intake. The normally colored hair grew during periods of relatively adequate protein intake.

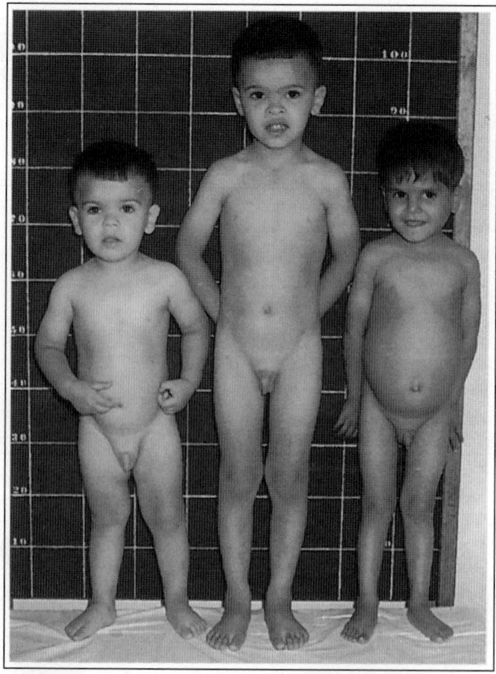

Figure 10.9
An example of growth failure can be seen in the child to the right, who is 5.5 years old and yet no more than 5 cm taller than the child on the left, who is 2 years old. The child in the middle is 4.5 years old. Less than expected height for age (stunting) is the most common evidence of chronic, mild PEM.
Source: From McLaren DS. 1992. *A colour atlas and text of diet-related disorders,* 2nd ed. London: Mosby Europe.

derived from these equations can then be compared with the reference values shown in Table 10.4 to classify the severity of wasting or stunting.

A simple approach to assessing the severity of PEM in an adult is to compare his or her body mass index (kg/m^2) (see Chapter 6) with the reference values shown in Table 10.5. The table also gives values for determining the presence of PEM in adolescents but does not allow the severity of PEM in this age group to be assessed.[8] These values can be used for either males or females.

HIV Infection

Nutritional alterations are common in persons infected with the human immunodeficiency virus (HIV), the cause of acquired immunodeficiency syndrome, or AIDS. Before the development of HIV antiretroviral drugs for treating HIV infection, a common feature of patients with AIDS was PEM characterized by marked weight loss and depletion of body cell mass, a condition known as HIV wasting syndrome.[11–13] During this era, more than 60% of HIV-positive patients presented with PEM, and, in roughly 80% of deaths attributed to AIDS, protein-energy malnutrition was considered a concurrent cause of death.[13] Since AIDS was first recognized in 1981, remarkable progress has been made in developing antiretroviral agents for treating HIV infection and AIDS. These drugs have improved the quality and duration of life of HIV-infected persons in the industrialized world and have led to decreased incidence of the severe malnutrition characteristic of HIV wasting syndrome, although altered body fat distribution, loss of lean body mass or fat-free mass, and metabolic alterations are still common in these HIV patients. In some older HIV-infected patients, overweight and obesity with loss of fat-free mass occurs.[11–15]

HIV wasting syndrome is typically characterized by the disproportionate loss of lean body mass and muscle wasting with relative preservation of fat mass.[15,16] The U.S. Centers for Disease Control and Prevention's definition of HIV wasting syndrome is shown in Box 10.3. Wasting is of considerable concern because it is associated with increased morbidity in people with AIDS.[12] It results in physical impairment, psychologic stress, decreased tolerance of therapeutic agents, increased susceptibility to infection, and overall diminished quality of life. The known adverse effects of malnutrition on immune function also suggest that wasting may independently affect the progression of AIDS. Prevention of HIV wasting and preservation of body weight (both adipose tissue and lean tissue mass) may enhance survival,

TABLE 10.4 Reference Values for Classifying Deficits in Weight for Height and Height for Age*

Classification	Weight for Height† (Deficit = Wasting)	Height for Age† (Deficit = Stunting)
Normal	90% to 110%	95% to 105%
Mild deficit	80% to 89%	90% to 94%
Moderate deficit	75% to 79%	85% to 89%
Severe deficit	< 75% or with edema	< 85%

Adapted from Torun B. 2006. Protein-energy malnutrition. In Shils ME, Shike M, Ross AC, Cabellero B, Cousins RJ (eds.), *Modern nutrition in health and disease,* 10th ed. Philadelphia: Lippincott Williams & Wilkins, 881–908.

*Reference values for classifying the severity of deficits in weight for height (wasting) are derived using the percentage of reference median weight for height, and deficits in height for age (stunting) are derived using the percentage of reference median height for age. Median weight for height and median height for age are derived from the CDC growth charts (see Chapter 6).

†Percentage calculated from equations discussed in the text.

TABLE 10.5 Reference Values for Classifying the Severity of Protein-Energy Malnutrition (PEM) in Adult Males and Females and the Presence of PEM in Adolescent Males and Females

Subject Age	Body Mass Index	PEM
18 years and older	< 16.0	Severe
	16.0–16.9	Moderate
	17.0–18.4	Mild
	≥ 18.5	Not Present
14–17 years old	14.5– < 16.5	Present
	< 14.5	Severe
11–13 years old	13.5– < 15.0	Present
	< 13.5	Severe

Adapted from Torun B. 2006. Protein-energy malnutrition. In Shils ME, Shike M, Ross AC, Cabellero B, Cousins RJ (eds.), *Modern nutrition in health and disease,* 10th ed. Philadelphia: Lippincott Williams & Wilkins, 881–908.

enhance physical and social functioning, and enrich the quality of life of people with AIDS.[11,12,14] Although HIV wasting is a multifactorial condition, the causes can be categorized under three general headings: decreased food intake, increased nutrient requirements, and nutrient malabsorption. These are outlined in Table 10.6.

With the introduction of protease inhibitors in 1996 and even newer antiretroviral therapies in more recent years, the number of patients dying from AIDS in developed countries has decreased by 67%, the prognosis of HIV-infected patients in these countries has dramatically improved, and HIV wasting syndrome is no longer the AIDS terminal phase.[13] Despite these dramatic improvements, some people with AIDS experience marked changes in body fat distribution (referred to as lipodystrophy) and certain metabolic alterations, such as hyperlipidemia, insulin resistance, and diabetes mellitus.[13,15,16] These changes in body fat distribution include fat accumulation (lipohypertrophy) in the abdominal region (truncal and visceral obesity), in the axillary pads (bilateral symmetric lipomatosis), and in the dorsocervical pads at the posterior base of the neck (referred to by some as "buffalo hump" or "bull neck") and loss of fat (lipoatrophy) in the arms, legs, and nasolabial and cheek pads (peripheral lipodystrophy).[13] An example of increased adiposity in the dorsocervical pads of a patient receiving protease inhibitor therapy for AIDS is shown in Figure 10.10. It appears that these alterations in body fat distribution are due, at least in part, to certain metabolic changes brought about by the multiple drugs used to treat HIV infection.[13–18] The so-called buffalo hump is also a clinical feature of Cushing's syndrome, a combination of symptoms and signs resulting from a persistent elevation of serum glucocorticosteroids. Unlike the loss of facial fat seen in patients presenting with peripheral lipodystrophy, a characteristic feature of Cushing's syndrome is a fullness or roundness of the face, which is referred to as "moon face."

Because changes in the distribution of body fat and increased adiposity can occur at the same time as decreased fat-free mass in patients with HIV/AIDS, changes in weight and BMI alone may not be suitable indicators of nutritional status. Approaches to assessing body fat distribution, somatic muscle status, and body composition will be required in some instances to evaluate a patient's nutritional status and response to HIV/AIDS therapy and nutritional support.[15,16,19] Approaches that can be used to monitor changes in body fat distribution include waist circumference, waist-to-hip ratio, skinfold measurements, dual-energy X-ray absorptiometry (DXA), and computed tomography. Somatic or skeletal muscle status can be assessed using mid-arm circumference, arm muscle area,

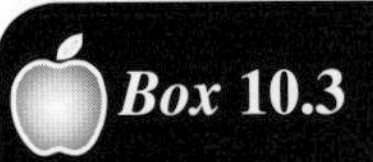

Box 10.3 HIV Wasting Syndrome as Defined by the U.S. Centers for Disease Control and Prevention

1. Involuntary weight loss of more than 10% of weight
2. Chronic diarrhea (at least two loose stools a day for 30 days or more) or chronic weakness
3. Constant or intermittent fever for 30 days or more
4. Absence of a condition or an illness other than HIV infection that might cause symptoms

Adapted from Kurtzweil P. 1995. Warding off HIV wasting syndrome. *FDA Consumer* 29(3):16–20.

TABLE 10.6 Causes of and Contributing Factors for HIV Wasting Syndrome

Causes	Contributing Factors
Decreased Food Intake	
Loss of appetite	Nausea, vomiting, medications, altered taste; anorexia caused by the effects of cytokines, such as tissue necrosis factor, interleukin-1, and interferon; the presence of undigested micronutrients in ileum and colon may also depress appetite
Difficulty chewing and swallowing	Mouth and throat sores from Kaposi's sarcoma and opportunistic infections, such as candidiasis and herpes simplex; esophageal ulcers of viral, mycobacterial, and neoplastic origin; neurologic disease
Decreased interest in eating	Depression, ostracism, isolation, loneliness
Inability to prepare meals	Lack of access to food, poverty, profound weakness, AIDS-induced dementia
Increased Nutrient Requirements	
Hypermetabolism	Resting metabolic rate is generally increased in persons with AIDS unless severe wasting is present; loss of adipose tissue and negative nitrogen balance are exacerbated by near-normal serum levels of the thyroid hormone triiodothyronine (T_3) that ordinarily fall below normal in the presence of malnutrition and wasting
Fever	Opportunistic infections of viral, mycobacterial, and neoplastic origin
Nutrient Malabsorption	
Diarrhea	Occurs in > 50% of persons with AIDS; many cases apparently caused by protozoal infections
Inflammation of bowel mucosa	Protozoal infections (cryptosporidiosis and microsporidiosis) appear to result in malabsorption apart from diarrhea; deficiency of lactase and disaccharidase activity seen; HIV alone may affect the structure and function of the small bowel

Data from Oster MH, Enders SR, Samuels SJ, Cone LA, Hooton TM, Browder HP, Flynn NM. 1994. Megestrol acetate in patients with AIDS and cachexia. *Annals of Internal Medicine* 121:400–408; Von Roenn JH, Armstrong D, Kotler DP, Cohn DL, Klimas NG, Tchekmedyian NS, Cone L, Brennan PJ, Weitzman SA. 1994. Megestrol acetate in patients with AIDS-related cachexia. *Annals of Internal Medicine* 121:393–399; Hecker LM, Kotler DP. 1990. Malnutrition in patients with AIDS. *Nutrition Reviews* 48:393–401; Singer P, Katz DP, Dillon L, Kirvelä O, Lazarus T, Askanazi J. 1992. Nutritional aspects of the acquired immunodeficiency syndrome. *American Journal of Gastroenterology* 87:265–273.

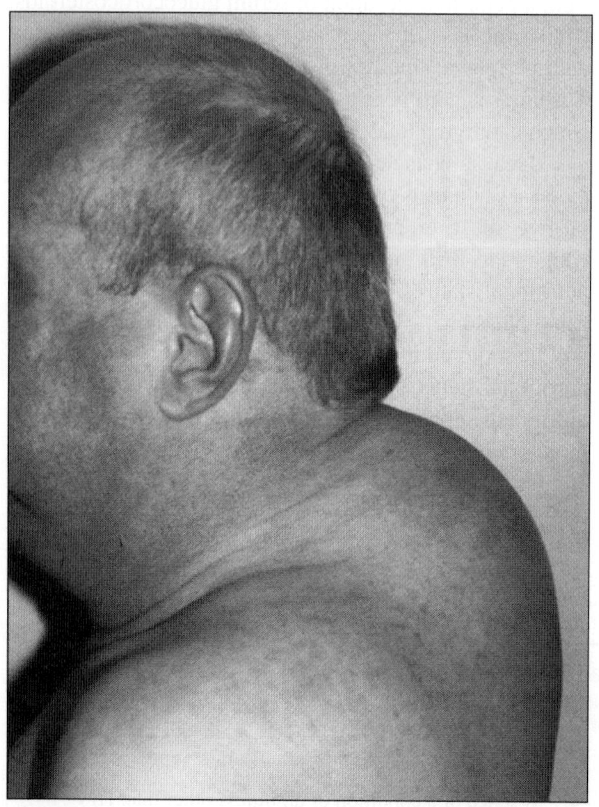

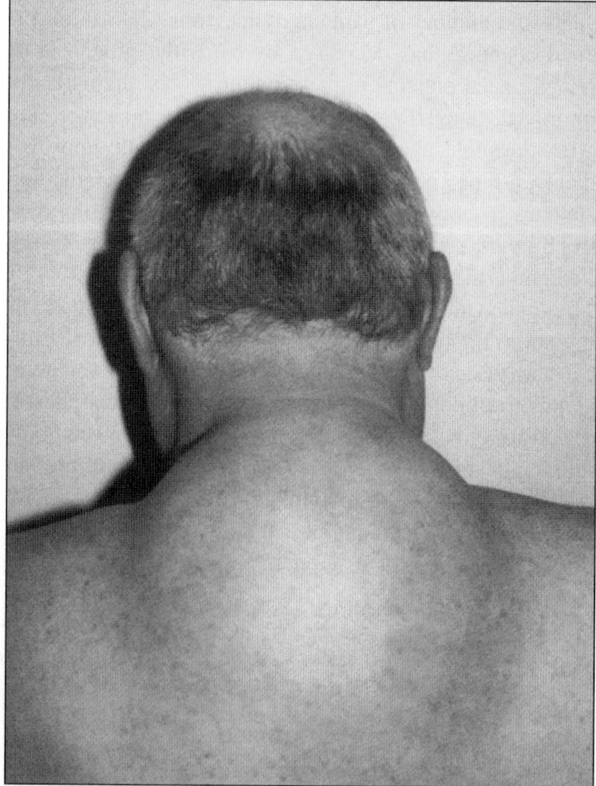

Figure 10.10 Increased adiposity in the dorsocervical fat pads of a patient receiving protease inhibitor therapy for AIDS. This is referred to by some as "buffalo hump" or "bull neck" and is one of the alterations in body fat distribution seen in AIDS patients presenting with lipodystrophy syndrome.

Source: Reproduced with permission of *Canadian Journal of Plastic Surgery*. 1999; 7:129–131.

the creatinine-height index, and computed tomography. Changes in body composition can be assessed using skinfold measurements, bioelectrical impedance analysis, DXA, and computed tomography.[15,16,19]

EATING DISORDERS

Anorexia nervosa and bulimia nervosa are conditions in which a disturbance in eating behavior is seen. Both have clinical signs aiding in their diagnosis. Anorexia nervosa is characterized by a refusal to maintain a minimally normal body weight, an intense fear of gaining weight that is not alleviated by losing weight, and a distorted perception of body shape or size in which a person feels overweight (either globally or in certain body areas) despite being markedly underweight.[20] The American Psychiatric Association's diagnostic criteria for anorexia nervosa are shown in Box 10.4. A prominent clinical feature of persons with anorexia nervosa is marked weight loss, which in some instances can become extreme and life threatening. Figure 10.11 gives an example of the severe wasting commonly seen in persons with anorexia nervosa.

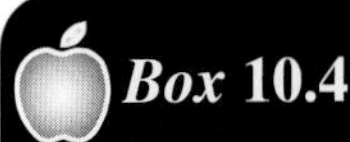

Box 10.4 The American Psychiatric Association's Diagnostic Criteria for Anorexia Nervosa

A. Refusal to maintain body weight at or above a minimally normal weight for age and height (e.g., weight loss leading to maintenance of body weight less than 85% of that expected or failure to make expected weight gain during period of growth, leading to body weight less than 85% of that expected)

B. Intense fear of gaining weight or becoming fat, even though underweight

C. Disturbance in the way in which one's body weight or shape is experienced, undue influence of body weight or shape on self-evaluation, or denial of the seriousness of the current low body weight

D. In postmenarcheal females, amenorrhea—i.e., the absence of at least three consecutive menstrual cycles (a woman is considered to have amenorrhea if her periods occur only following hormone administration—e.g., estrogen)

TYPES OF ANOREXIA NERVOSA

Restricting type: During the current episode of anorexia nervosa, the person has not regularly engaged in binge-eating or purging behavior (i.e., self-induced vomiting or the misuse of laxatives, diuretics, or enemas)

Binge-eating/purging type: During the current episode of anorexia nervosa, the person has regularly engaged in binge-eating or purging behavior (i.e., self-induced vomiting or the misuse of laxatives, diuretics, or enemas)

Reprinted with permission from the *Diagnostic and Statistical Manual of Mental Disorders*, Fourth Edition, Text Revision, (Copyright 2000). American Psychiatric Association.

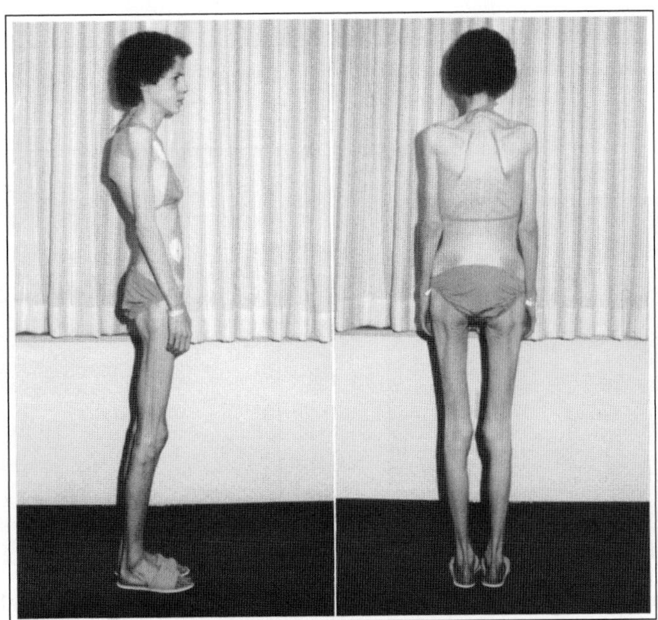

Figure 10.11 **Severe wasting seen in a person with anorexia nervosa.**

Source: From McLaren DS. 1992. *A colour atlas and text of diet-related disorders*, 2nd ed. London: Mosby Europe.

Bulimia nervosa is characterized by episodes of binging (eating unusually large amounts of food in a discrete period of time), followed by some behavior to prevent weight gain, such as purging (usually self-induced vomiting but also including misuse of laxatives, diuretics, enemas, or other medications), fasting, or excessive exercise.[20–23] The American Psychiatric Association's diagnostic criteria for bulimia nervosa are shown in Box 10.5. Persons with bulimia nervosa are usually within the normal weight range, although some may be slightly underweight or overweight. Recurrent vomiting may erode the teeth, especially the lingual surfaces of the front teeth, and increase the incidence of dental caries. An example of dental erosion in an 18-year-old female who had, from age 15 years, used vomiting as a purging method is shown in Figure 10.12. There may also be noticeable enlargement of the salivary glands, particularly the parotid glands. An example of asymmetrical hypertrophy of the parotid gland in a 20-year-old female who developed bulimia nervosa at age 17 years is shown in Figure 10.13.

A third category of disordered eating recognized by the American Psychiatric Association is called eating disorder not otherwise specified. This category is for eating disorders that fail to meet the criteria for either anorexia nervosa or bulimia nervosa.[16,17] Examples of disordered eating that fall under this category are outlined in Box 10.6.

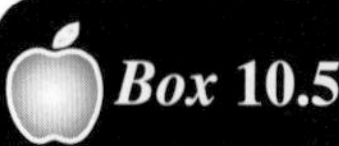

Box 10.5 The American Psychiatric Association's Diagnostic Criteria for Bulimia Nervosa

A. Recurrent episodes of binge eating. An episode of binge eating is characterized by both of the following:
   (1) Eating, in a discrete period (e.g., within any 2-hour period), an amount of food that is definitely larger than most people would eat during a similar period of time and under similar circumstances
   (2) A sense of lack of control over eating during the episode (e.g., a feeling that one cannot stop eating or control what or how much one is eating)

B. Recurrent inappropriate compensatory behavior in order to prevent weight gain, such as self-induced vomiting; misuse of laxatives, diuretics, enemas, or other medications; fasting; or excessive exercise

C. The binge eating and inappropriate compensatory behaviors both occur, on average, at least twice a week for 3 months

D. Self-evaluation is unduly influenced by body shape and weight

E. The disturbance does not occur exclusively during episodes of anorexia nervosa

Types of Bulimia Nervosa

Purging type: During the current episode of bulimia nervosa, the person has regularly engaged in self-induced vomiting or the misuse of laxatives, diuretics, or enemas

Nonpurging type: During the current episode of bulimia nervosa, the person has used other inappropriate compensatory behaviors, such as fasting or excessive exercise, but has not regularly engaged in self-induced vomiting or the misuse of laxatives, diuretics, or enemas

Reprinted with permission from the *Diagnostic and Statistical Manual of Mental Disorders*, Fourth Edition, Text Revision, (Copyright 2000). American Psychiatric Association.

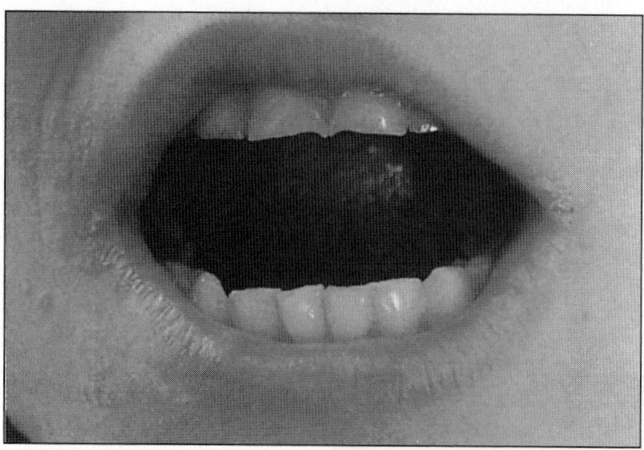

Figure 10.12 **Dental erosion in an 18-year-old female who had been vomiting to control her weight from the age of 15 years; note that her top incisors are markedly eroded.**

Source: From McLaren DS. 1992. *A colour atlas and text of diet-related disorders,* 2nd ed. London: Mosby Europe.

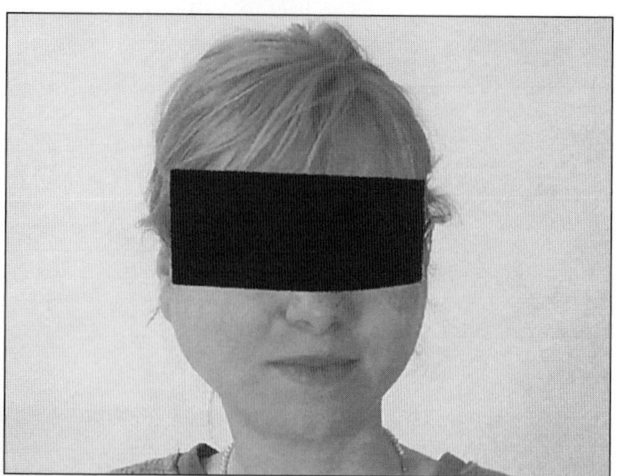

Figure 10.13 **Asymmetrical parotid gland enlargement in a 20-year-old female who developed bulimia nervosa at the age of 17 years; she was vomiting four times each day.**

Source: From McLaren DS. 1992. *A colour atlas and text of diet-related disorders,* 2nd ed. London: Mosby Europe.

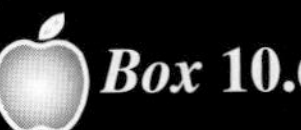

Box 10.6 Eating Disorder Not Otherwise Specified

1. For females, all of the criteria for anorexia nervosa are met except that the individual has regular menses
2. All of the criteria for anorexia nervosa are met except that, despite significant weight loss, the individual's current weight is in the normal range
3. All of the criteria for bulimia nervosa are met except that the binge eating and inappropriate compensatory mechanisms occur at a frequency of less than twice a week or for a duration of less than 3 months
4. The regular use of inappropriate compensatory behavior by an individual of normal body weight after eating small amounts of food (e.g., self-induced vomiting after the consumption of two cookies)
5. Repeatedly chewing and spitting out, but not swallowing, large amounts of food
6. Binge-eating disorder: recurrent episodes of binge eating in the absence of the regular use of inappropriate compensatory behaviors characteristic of bulimia nervosa

SUMMARY

1. The first step in the clinical assessment of nutritional status is obtaining a patient's history. This includes pertinent facts about past and current health and use of medications, as well as personal and household information. Sources include the patient's medical record and data obtained directly from the patient or those familiar with the patient.
2. A diet history is valuable in understanding a patient's nutritional status. This includes information about a patient's usual eating pattern, food likes and dislikes, and intolerances and allergies, as well as money available for purchasing food, ability to obtain and prepare food, eligibility for and access to food assistance programs, and use of vitamin, mineral, and other supplements.
3. Subjective Global Assessment is a clinical technique for assessing the nutritional status of a patient based on features of the patient's history and physical examination, rather than relying on more objective measures of nutritional status, such as anthropometric and biochemical data.
4. In severe PEM, the conditions known as kwashiorkor and marasmus are seen. Kwashiorkor is predominantly a protein deficiency characterized by a relatively normal weight, generally intact skeletal musculature, decreased concentrations of serum proteins, and edema. Marasmus is mainly an energy deficiency characterized by significant loss of body weight, skeletal muscle, and adipose tissue mass, but with serum protein concentrations relatively intact and no edema.
5. Severe cases of PEM and wasting can result from AIDS, certain cancers, some gastrointestinal diseases, and alcoholism and other drug abuse. The emaciation and general ill health seen in these diseases is sometimes called cachexia.
6. Growth failure and flag sign are two conditions seen in severe PEM. The flag sign is characterized by alternating bands of depigmented and normal-colored hair produced by alternating periods of poor and relatively good protein intake. Growth failure, a failure to gain weight and height at the expected rate, is the most common sign of malnutrition in children.
7. The severity of PEM in children and adolescents can be assessed by calculating weight as a percentage of reference median weight for height and by calculating height as a percentage of reference height for age. These two values can then be compared with published guidelines. The severity of PEM in an adult can be assessed by comparing body mass index (kg/m^2) with the reference values.
8. Prior to the development of HIV antiretroviral drugs for treating HIV infection, HIV wasting was a common feature of patients with AIDS. Although advances in HIV/AIDS drug treatment have led to decreased incidence of HIV wasting syndrome, altered metabolism and body fat distribution remain common in HIV patients, particularly those treated with protease inhibitors. Metabolic alterations include hyperlipidemia, insulin resistance, and diabetes mellitus. Changes in body fat distribution include fat accumulation in the abdominal region (truncal and visceral obesity) and in the dorsocervical

pads of the neck ("buffalo hump" or "bull neck") and loss of fat in the arms, legs, and nasolabial and cheek pads (peripheral lipodystrophy).

9. Anorexia nervosa is characterized by a refusal to maintain a minimally normal body weight, an intense fear of gaining weight, and a distorted perception of body shape or size. Bulimia nervosa is characterized by episodes of binging, followed by some behavior to prevent weight gain, such as purging, fasting, or exercising excessively.

References

1. Corish CA, Kennedy NP. 2000. Protein-energy undernutrition in hospital in-patients. *British Journal of Nutrition* 83:575–591.
2. Dwyer J. 2012. Nutrient requirements and dietary assessment. In Longo DL, Fauci AS, Kasper DL, Hauser SL, Jameson JL, Loscalzo J (eds.), *Harrison's principles of internal medicine,* 18th ed. New York: McGraw-Hill, 588–593.
3. Charney P, Malone AM. 2009. *ADA pocket guide to nutrition assessment,* 2nd ed. Chicago: American Dietetic Association.
4. Detsky AS, Smalley PS, Change J. 1994. Is this patient malnourished? *Journal of the American Medical Association* 271:54–58.
5. Gupta D, Lammersfeld CA, Vashi PG, Burrows J, Lis CG, Grutsch JF. 2005. Prognostic significance of Subjective Global Assessment (SGA) in advanced colorectal cancer. *European Journal of Clinical Nutrition* 59:35–40.
6. Makhija S, Baker J. 2008. The subjective global assessment: A review of its use in clinical practice. *Nutrition in Clinical Practice* 23:405–409.
7. Keith JN. 2008. Bedside nutrition assessment past, present, and future: A review of the subjective global assessment. *Nutrition in Clinical Practice* 23:410–416.
8. Torun B. 2006. Protein-energy malnutrition. In Shils ME, Shike M, Ross AC, Cabellero B, Cousins RJ (eds.), *Modern nutrition in health and disease,* 10th ed. Philadelphia: Lippincott Williams & Wilkins, 881–908.
9. Heimburger DC. 2012. Malnutrition and nutritional assessment. In Longo DL, Fauci AS, Kasper DL, Hauser SL, Jameson JL, Loscalzo J (eds.), *Harrison's principles of internal medicine,* 18th ed. New York: McGraw-Hill, 605–612.
10. McLaren DS. 1992. *A colour atlas and text of diet-related disorders,* 2nd ed. London: Mosby Europe.
11. Kotler DP. 2000. Nutritional alterations associated with HIV infection. *Journal of Acquired Immune Deficiency Syndromes* 25:S81–S87.
12. Semba RD. 2006. Nutrition and infection. In Shils ME, Shike M, Ross AC, Cabellero B, Cousins RJ (eds.), *Modern nutrition in health and disease,* 10th ed. Philadelphia: Lippincott Williams & Wilkins, 1401–1413.
13. Scevola D, DiMatteo A, Uberti F, Minoia G, Poletti F, Faga A. 2000. Reversal of cachexia in patients treated with potent antiretroviral therapy. *AIDS Reader* 10:365–369.
14. Fauci AS, Lane HC. 2012. Human immunodeficiency virus disease: AIDS and related disorders. In Longo DL, Fauci AS, Kasper DL, Hauser SL, Jameson JL, Loscalzo J (eds.), *Harrison's principles of internal medicine,* 18th ed. New York: McGraw-Hill, 1506–1587.
15. Thibault R, Cano N, Pichard C. 2011. Quantification of lean tissue losses during cancer and HIV infection/AIDS. *Current Opinion in Clinical Nutrition and Metabolic Care* 14:261–267.
16. Moreno S, Miralles C, Negredo E, Domingo P, Estrada V, Gutierrez F, Lozano F, Martinez E. 2009. Disorders of body fat distribution in HIV-1-infected patients. *AIDS Reviews* 11:126–134.
17. Engleson ES, Kotler DP, Tan YX, Agin D, Wang J, Pierson RN, Heymsfield SB. 1999. Fat distribution in HIV-infected patients reporting truncal enlargement quantified by whole-body magnetic resonance imaging. *American Journal of Clinical Nutrition* 69:1162–1169.
18. Peters W, Phillips A. 1999. Buffalo hump and HIV-1 infection: Current concepts and treatment of a patient with the use of suction-assisted lipectomy. *Canadian Journal of Plastic Surgery* 7:129–131.
19. Ruiz M, Kamerman LA. 2010. Nutritional screening tools for HIV-infected patients: Implications for elderly patients. *Journal of the International Association of Physicians in AIDS Care* 9:362–367.
20. American Psychiatric Association. 2000. *Diagnostic and statistical manual of mental disorders,* 4th ed., text rev. Washington, DC: American Psychiatric Association.
21. American Psychiatric Association. 2006. *Practice guideline for the treatment of patients with eating disorders,* 3rd ed. Washington, DC: American Psychiatric Association.
22. Williams PM, Goodie J, Motsinger CD. 2008. Treating eating disorders in primary care. *American Family Physician* 77:187–195.
23. Weaver L, Liebman R. 2011. Assessment of anorexia nervosa in children and adolescents. *Current Psychiatry Reports* 13:93–98.

ASSESSMENT ACTIVITY 10.1

Using Subjective Global Assessment

This assessment activity gives you an opportunity to practice using Subjective Global Assessment (SGA), a clinical technique for assessing nutritional status using data from a patient's history and physical examination, both of which can be found in a patient's medical record. Begin by making two photocopies of the SGA rating form found in Figure 10.1. Then, using the information from each of the following two cases, complete the chart and arrive at an SGA rating of each patient's nutritional status. You may find it helpful to review the section "Subjective Global Assessment," which explains SGA.

The following cases are straightforward; you and your classmates should arrive at the same rating for each case. However, because of the subjective nature of this approach, there may be an occasional instance when two or more health professionals do not arrive at the same rating of one patient's nutritional status. This should not detract from the usefulness of SGA because clinicians generally arrive at decisions by carefully evaluating the available evidence in light of professional knowledge and past experiences. Thus, health care is not only a science but also an art.

Case 1

A 73-year-old female is admitted to the hospital complaining of loss of appetite and rapid onset of satiety for 6 weeks. For the past 3 days, she has vomited practically all food and beverages consumed. She is ambulatory but has felt weak and has been unable to carry out her activities of daily living for the past 2 weeks. On physical examination, the woman looks somewhat wasted with moderate loss of subcutaneous tissue in the upper arms, shoulders, and thoracic regions. There is moderate edema in the ankles but no ascites present. For the past 10 years or so, her body weight has been stable at approximately 147 lb (66.8 kg). However, in the past 4 months or so, she has steadily lost weight. Her current weight is 123 lb (55.9 kg). Using SGA, how would you rate her nutritional status?

Case 2

A 61-year-old male is admitted to the hospital for resection of his sigmoid colon and rectum, following discovery of a mass in the sigmoid colon by his physician during a flexible sigmoidoscopy. The patient originally complained of bright red blood in his bowel movements. He reported no significant gastrointestinal symptoms other than the bleeding. He denies any change in his functional capacity. His maximum weight was 167 lb (75.9 kg) at age 46 years. In his late 40s, he lost about 15 lb (6.8 kg) and for the past 12 years has maintained his weight at about 152 lb (69.1 kg). Between 2 and 6 months before admission, his appetite was less than normal and he gradually lost 13 lb (5.9 kg). In the past 2 months before admission, his appetite improved and he gained 5 lb (2.3 kg). On physical examination, there is no evidence of subcutaneous tissue loss, muscle wasting, edema, or ascites.

CHAPTER

11 Counseling Theory and Technique

Outline

Introduction
Communication
Interviewing
Counseling Theories
Initiating and Maintaining Dietary Change
Knowing One's Limits
Summary
References
Assessment Activity 11.1: Counseling Practice

Student Learning Outcomes

After studying this chapter, the student will be able to:

1. Describe the communication model.
2. Name the six steps of listening.
3. Differentiate between open questions and closed questions.
4. Discuss the key concepts of the major counseling theories.
5. Name the characteristics of effective counselors.
6. Identify instances when a patient should be referred to someone else for counseling.

Introduction

Awareness of nutritional status and dietary practices obtained through nutritional assessment often is followed by attempts to change dietary behavior. This chapter provides a brief introduction to several counseling theories that provide a variety of useful techniques for initiating and maintaining dietary change.

The purpose of this chapter is *not* to teach you how to be a therapist. It is intended to briefly introduce you to those theories that are most pertinent to nutritional counseling and to acquaint you with some fundamental approaches to counseling your clients. The most effective counselors are those who adapt techniques from several counseling theories to suit their needs and those of their individual clients. As you study this chapter, note the different counseling theories and techniques. Then, based on your professional judgment, use those techniques you feel are best suited to you and the needs of your clients.

Because communication lies at the foundation of interviewing and counseling, the first part of this chapter deals with fundamentals of communication theory and basic skills necessary for effective listening and interviewing. The chapter ends with a practical plan for initiating and maintaining dietary change.

Finally, as important as good nutrition is to health, do not lose sight of the fact that other practices, such as cigarette smoking, physical inactivity, and excessive alcohol use, have a profound impact on health. Cigarette smoking, for example, has been called the "leading cause of preventable death in the United States" and is responsible for more than 440,000 deaths every year in the United States.[1] You should be a model of good health habits, not only those relating to diet but in all areas. By so doing, you will be most effective in helping your clients achieve better health.

COMMUNICATION

Communication is the process of sending and receiving messages. It lies at the foundation of all efforts to interview, counsel, educate, and change behavior. Although we all communicate (or at least attempt to) and have a basic idea of what it involves, communication is a complex process and is not easily defined. The simplified communication model in Figure 11.1 shows the major components of human communication: sender, receiver, message, and feedback.

The *sender* is the one initiating the communication, the first person to speak. The *message* is the communication. It contains components that are both verbal (what is spoken) and nonverbal (what is implied by the emotional tone of the sender's voice, facial expression, posture, diction, pronunciation, choice of words, dress, and the environment in which the communication occurs).[2] Verbal and nonverbal communication occur simultaneously. The *receiver* is the listener, the one to whom the message is sent. *Feedback* is the response the receiver gives to messages after interpreting them. Feedback distinguishes one-way communication

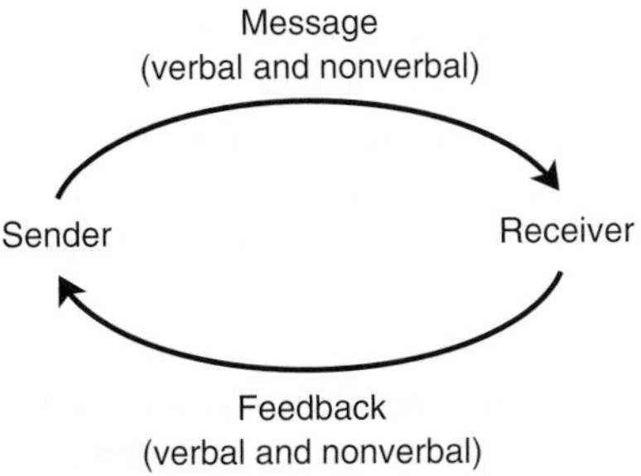

Figure 11.1 **A communication model.**

from two-way communication.[2] The absence of feedback or making no provision for it will likely result in distorted communication because the sender is unable to determine how the message was received. As with the message, feedback is both verbal and nonverbal.

Interference is anything adversely affecting transmission or interpretation of the message. It can arise from the environment or the emotional or physiologic state of either the sender or the receiver. Noise, lack of privacy, interruptions, an office that is too hot or too cold, and uncomfortable seating are examples of environmental factors that may cause interference. Emotional factors leading to interference include fear of disease or death, loneliness, grief, prejudice, and bias. Physiologic factors such as pain, deficits of hearing or vision, and difficulty in speaking can often be sources of interference.

Verbal Communication

Dietary counseling generally involves some type of behavioral change on the receiver's part. The receiver may perceive attempts to change lifelong habits or practices he or she enjoys as a potential threat. Thus, the receiver may become defensive, which interferes with good communication. The receiver's defensive reactions can be prevented or minimized through the use of the guidelines to supportive communication outlined in Box 11.1 and the following paragraphs. The more supportive communication is, the less the receiver perceives it as a threat and the more he or she is able to concentrate on the structure, content, and meaning of the message.[2]

Describe behavior rather than evaluate it. Discussing a client's behavior in a judgmental or evaluative way will likely cause the client to become defensive. The client will then be thinking of ways to defend himself or herself rather than concentrating on the counselor's message. Evaluating or judging behavior can lead to an argument. Instead, the counselor can present the facts or seek information in objective, nonjudgmental ways that do not imply guilt or ask the client to change his or her behavior.

For example, in an attempt to raise awareness of the seriousness of the problem at hand, a counselor may accuse a client with poorly controlled diabetes of being "irresponsible" or "committing suicide." A better approach would be to objectively discuss the client's blood sugar levels and nonjudgmentally discuss factors that may be affecting them.

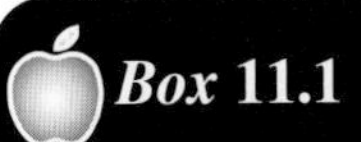

Box 11.1 **Guidelines to More Supportive Communication**

Description rather than evaluation
Problem orientation rather than manipulation
Equality rather than superiority
Empathy rather than neutrality
Provisionalism rather than certainty

Use problem orientation rather than manipulation. Much of our speech is an attempt to persuade others to alter their behavior, attitudes, or activities. Often, when we want people to see things our way, we lead them through a series of questions until they arrive at the "correct conclusion." This is a form of manipulation and implies that the person being directed is inadequate or inferior. This is likely to result in a defensive response that interferes with communication. Problem orientation, on the other hand, is the antithesis of persuasion. The sender communicates a desire to work with the receiver in defining a mutual problem and seeking a workable solution. The sender implies that he or she has no prearranged answer or viewpoint and no hidden agenda to exert control over the receiver. Thus, the receiver arrives at his or her own conclusions and establishes goals and objectives to which there will be greater adherence.

Communicate equality rather than superiority. A sender can promote supportive communication by considering himself or herself a collaborator with or an equal to the receiver. When treated with respect and trust and involved in participative problem solving, the receiver will feel more obligated to the success of any agreed-on solution. If the sender communicates superiority, the receiver will likely become defensive. Although clients often need and appreciate the reassurance of a dietitian's nutritional expertise, dietitians should avoid urging a particular plan of action based primarily on their superior knowledge or ability.

Empathize rather than remain neutral. Communication conveying compassion and respect for others is supportive and defense-reducing. Particularly reassuring is a sender who identifies with the problems and shares in the feelings of the receiver. Communication conveying neutrality may indicate a lack of concern for the receiver's welfare. Attempts to reassure the receiver that he or she is overly anxious or need not feel rejected or bad deny the legitimacy of the receiver's emotions and suggest a lack of acceptance.

Be receptive rather than dogmatic. A willingness to hold one's own attitudes as provisional, to examine other ideas rather than take sides, and to solve problems rather than debate issues gives listeners a sense of participation in and control over the problem-solving process. On the other hand, persons who seem to know all the answers or who regard themselves as teachers rather than team players tend to put others on guard and stifle supportive communication.

Nonverbal Communication

As was shown in Figure 11.1, communication occurs simultaneously on two levels—verbal and nonverbal. Sometimes referred to as *body language,* nonverbal communication in the form of gestures, posture, facial expressions, and tone of voice is sometimes a more reliable indicator of the client's feelings and attitudes than are his or her words.[3] Verbal communication is generally under conscious control and is subject to censorship. It can be used to persuade, mislead, or cover facts a client wishes to hide. Nonverbal communication, on the other hand, is not as easily controlled by conscious thought and often can be a more reliable indicator of a person's dominant emotions than are his or her words.[2,4] Lack of congruence, or agreement, between verbal and nonverbal communication can be an important indicator that a client is consciously or unconsciously omitting something.

Facial expressions are an important source of nonverbal communication. Sadness often can be seen in the face of a distressed client through a downturned mouth or quivering lip. Unusually prolonged and intense eye contact may indicate anger. Guilt, insecurity, or fear may be indicated by failure to maintain eye contact, especially when this occurs during discussion of a particularly sensitive topic.[4]

Posture may indicate a person's feelings. A client seated with arms relaxed at the sides and slightly slouched in the chair can communicate openness, whereas a client may communicate a distrustful, defensive attitude by sitting up very straight with arms tightly crossed over the chest. A client who leans away from the counselor or moves her chair to distance herself may indicate defensiveness or distrust. One leaning closer to the counselor may express a desire for greater intimacy.[3,4] Cultural differences exist in what is considered to be a comfortable distance between two communicating persons. In general, people from Latin cultures prefer being closer, whereas those from North America and parts of Europe favor a somewhat greater distance.[4]

The tone of voice is an important indicator, as well. A client asked about his diet may warmly and pleasantly respond, "It's going well," and mean just that. The same words uttered in a mechanistic and toneless way may indicate a problem with the diet.

Nonverbal communication also facilitates the dietitian's communication to clients. Appropriate eye contact, gestures, facial expressions, and posture assure the client of the dietitian's attention, interest, acceptance, and support. The astute dietitian should carefully note the client's nonverbal cues and their possible significance and use nonverbal communication to respond to the client in a supportive way.[2]

Effective Communication

Effective communication requires consideration of several factors. It is important that messages and feedback be transmitted in ways that are understandable to both sender and receiver. When talking with clients or providing instruction, health professionals should use understandable language and minimize use of medical terminology. Feedback should be encouraged, and the receiver should be given ample opportunity to ask questions and clarify any potential misunderstandings. Both sender and receiver should be aware of their nonverbal communication, so that it supports, rather than interferes with, effective communication.

The environment in which communication takes place should be comfortable, conducive to good communication, and as free as possible of interferences that can adversely affect communication. Adequate time for counseling and client instruction is necessary before clients can even begin to change lifelong habits and adopt new ones. Awareness of the client's abilities, concerns, and fears is also important to effective communication. The dietitian also should be aware of his or her own concerns and limitations and should avoid allowing these to interfere with the communication process.

Consider a dietitian seated at the bedside of a patient in whom diabetes has been recently diagnosed. The dietitian is giving the patient some last-minute instructions on the diabetic exchange system before the patient is discharged. Environmental interference can come from the roommate's television, interruptions from a nurse or physician, a phone call, or the arrival of a visitor. The patient's fear about having diabetes, concerns about being able to manage a new diet, worries about hospitalization costs, and thoughts about what the future holds may preoccupy her mind and interfere with the instruction. The dietitian also may be preoccupied with concerns of his own, such as other patients needing assessment and instruction, and these can interfere with the communication process. This is obviously not an ideal situation for communication or instruction, but, unfortunately, it is one commonly encountered in real life. Awareness of these and other impediments to good communication, however, is necessary before they can be addressed and effectively dealt with.

Listening

Communication is a two-way process. It involves not only *sending* messages but *receiving* them as well. Listening, therefore, is essential to the interviewing and counseling process. In some instances, the best help a counselor can give a client is to simply listen attentively and nonjudgmentally. It is also an excellent way to establish good rapport with a client.[2,4] As important as listening is, most of us are not very good at it.[4] Listening is a highly active process demanding concentration and attention. It involves six steps (Table 11.1).[4]

A number of misconceptions exist about listening.[4] For example, some people believe that *hearing* and *listening* are the same activity. Listening is a process involving much more than simply hearing sounds, such as music or voices. It is mistakenly assumed that, when several people hear the same sound (for example, a person talking), they all receive the same message. Quite the opposite is true. Listening is a highly subjective experience, and the interpretations placed on what is heard can vary widely from person to person.

TABLE 11.1 The Six Steps of Listening

1. Hearing: Receiving sound waves by the ear
2. Attending: Mentally focusing on a specific sound
3. Understanding: Interpreting the message and assignment of meaning by the brain
4. Remembering: Storing the message for later use
5. Evaluating: Making an evaluative judgment about the message
6. Responding: Making a verbal and/or nonverbal response to the message

Adapted from Samovar LA. 2000. *Oral communication: Speaking across cultures,* 11th ed. Los Angeles: Roxbury Publishing Company.

Some people believe that listening is a passive activity, when in reality it is an active process requiring concentration and specific skills that can be learned if one wants to be a better listener.[4,5] Listening skills can be grouped under four categories: openness, concentration, attention, and comprehension.[3,4]

Openness, or objectivity, involves a willingness to investigate new ideas and to interact with others with minimal internal distortion from personal prejudices. Openness does not necessarily mean acceptance or approval of another's ideas but simply a willingness to "hear a person out." It requires the listener to set aside his or her personal biases, which may interfere with effective listening.[4]

Concentration entails focusing the mind on what the speaker is saying. It is made easier when environmental distractions and interferences are minimized. Counseling should take place in a room that is quiet, comfortable, and private.

It is estimated that people with normal intelligence think about five times faster than they talk.[2] Thus, while listening to another person talk, our minds can simultaneously be thinking other things. Unfortunately, many people have allowed this to become a major barrier to effective listening. Rather than focusing the mind on critical and careful listening, we often take mental excursions ranging from thinking about the speaker's hair style to daydreaming.[4] A good listener uses this extra mental capacity to analyze and understand the speaker's verbal and nonverbal messages.

The counselor should indicate that the client has his or her full attention and acceptance by maintaining good eye contact with the client and having an empathic facial expression and relaxed posture. The counselor should give the client ample opportunity for expression without interruption while providing occasional, brief verbal and nonverbal responses indicating reception of the message. Appropriately timed nods or verbal responses such as "I understand" or "I see" will help assure the client of the counselor's attentive listening.

Comprehension involves not only attaching meaning to information but also correctly interpreting the meaning of the client's communication. The counselor's comprehension of the client's message can be enhanced through use of such techniques as reflection, paraphrasing, clarification, and probing. Reflection is restating the affective, or emotional, part of the client's words. This gives the client an opportunity to hear what she has just said and to elaborate on her emotions. A client may say, "I feel depressed about my lack of progress." The affective part of this message is the statement "I feel depressed." In reflection, the counselor simply restates the client's words: "You say you feel depressed." This gives the client an opportunity to elaborate on her feelings. In paraphrasing, the client's message is restated, or rephrased, in the counselor's own words. This helps ensure that the counselor has correctly interpreted the client's message. Clarification is simply asking the client to repeat or restate what was just said. Probing is asking the client to provide greater detail on some specific point. It is often used when collecting a 24-hour dietary recall.

Interviewing

Interviewing can be defined as a guided communication process between two persons or parties with the predetermined purpose of obtaining or exchanging specific information through the asking and answering of questions.[2,5] The goal of the interview is obtaining specific information from the client while maintaining an interpersonal environment conducive to disclosure by the client.[2] Of the several types of interviews that exist, the nutrition counselor is primarily concerned with interviews to gather information from clients, give information to clients, and deal with client problems.[5]

Interviewing Skills

As in communication, there are several basic conditions or skills that increase a person's effectiveness as an interviewer. Among these are physical surroundings, freedom from interruption and interference, privacy, good rapport, attentiveness, openness, and the client's context.[2] Factors to consider in the physical surroundings are the comfort of both the client and the interviewer, the seating arrangement, the distance between the interviewer and client, and the presence of physical barriers separating them.

It is best to conduct an interview in a location free of interruptions and interferences. In an office setting, the counselor should arrange to have phone calls held. In a hospital, interviews should not be scheduled during the time of physicians' rounds, nursing or other care, or visiting hours. A convenient time should be arranged with nursing and other staff. When held in the patient's room, arrangements can be made with nursing staff to avoid unnecessary interruptions, the patient's door can be closed, televisions and radios can be turned down or off, and visitors can be kindly asked to step outside.[2,3,5] However, parents, spouses, partners, and siblings can be important sources of information about the patient. The counselor may want to have them present during the interview or available for questions later.

Early establishment of good rapport is essential to an effective interview. Establishing good client rapport will place the client at ease and make him or her more willing to share important information.[2] A counselor should begin the interview with a pleasant greeting. She should introduce herself and briefly give the reason for the interview. If the counselor is late, she should apologize for any inconvenience and explain why.[5]

Attentiveness, as in the context of listening, is also an important interviewing skill. Nonverbal and verbal expressions of attention, such as appropriate eye contact, posture, facial expressions, well-timed nods, or relevant verbal responses, will help assure the client of the counselor's interest and attention. Openness, or interviewer objectivity, as in listening, is an important interviewing skill.

The client's emotional context—his or her beliefs, attitudes, feelings, and values—is also an important consideration when interviewing. Fears about health, concerns about death, feelings of loneliness, or grief may preoccupy a client's thoughts and interfere with his or her ability to participate in the interview. Putting apprehensive clients at ease and allowing them to express their feelings can help alleviate their fears and facilitate the interviewing process.

Obtaining Information

Before the interview, the counselor should review the client's medical record for pertinent information. This provides the counselor with considerable background information on the client and allows the interview to be more directed and concise. Using the "funnel sequence" is suggested. This begins with more general, open questions and gradually narrows to more specific inquiries using closed questions.[5]

Open questions invite rather than demand answers and provide clients substantial freedom in determining the amount and type of information to give.[2,5] Open questions let the client talk and offer information that he or she feels is important. They are generally easy to answer and pose little threat to the client. They give the counselor the opportunity to listen and observe. However, they have the disadvantage of consuming large amounts of time if clients dwell on irrelevant information.[5] Examples of open questions are given in Box 11.2.

Closed questions, on the other hand, are restrictive; they allow the counselor to control answers and to ask for specific information. They often provide too little information and fail to reveal why a client has a particular attitude.[5] Examples of closed questions are given in Box 11.2.

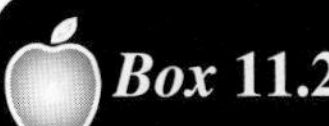

Box 11.2 Examples of Different Types of Questions

OPEN QUESTIONS

"Tell me about yourself."

"Tell me about your eating habits."

"What have you been doing to lower your blood cholesterol level?"

CLOSED QUESTIONS

"Do you smoke?"

"Do you salt your food at the table?"

"Do you eat chicken with or without the skin?"

NEUTRAL QUESTIONS

"What is the first thing you have to eat or drink after waking up in the morning?"

"What kind of milk do you drink?"

"How many times a week do you eat ice cream?"

LEADING QUESTIONS

"What do you eat for breakfast?"

"You don't use whole milk, do you?"

"Do you eat ice cream *every* evening?"

Questions also can be classified as neutral or leading (Box 11.2).[5] *Neutral questions* allow the client to answer without pressure or direction from the counselor. In *leading questions,* the counselor makes implicit or explicit suggestions about the expected or desired answer. In answering leading questions, the client merely agrees with what the counselor is apparently suggesting. Counselors should avoid leading clients either by verbal or nonverbal means. When clients respond to their questions, counselors must avoid such expressions as surprise, agreement, disagreement, or disgust, which can suggest expected or desired answers.[2]

When information is sought from or provided to clients, counselors should use understandable language. Health care professionals often make the mistake of assuming that clients understand the technical language used daily in hospitals and other health care organizations. Or they assume that if a client does not understand something, he or she will simply ask what a word means. Many clients are so overwhelmed by the unfamiliar or intimidated by the authority of health care professionals that they fail to seek answers to their questions. Thus, a counselor should avoid using technical language with clients and should not assume that clients will understand medical terminology even if it is explained to them.

COUNSELING THEORIES

Several counseling theories and techniques have been developed and are currently in use today. The purpose of this section is not to teach you how to be a therapist; that takes considerable professional training and practice. Rather, the purpose is to briefly introduce you to those theories that are most pertinent to nutritional counseling and to acquaint you with some fundamental approaches to counseling your clients.

Each counseling theory discussed in the following pages has something of value to offer the dietetic practitioner. Each also has certain limitations or drawbacks. An awareness of these theories and an ability to adapt their more fundamental and benign counseling techniques to suit each unique counseling situation will greatly enhance your ability as a helping professional.

Person-Centered Approach

The person-centered approach to counseling is based primarily on the work of psychologist Carl Rogers.[6–8] Rogers taught that, if people could experience human relationships characterized by respect and trust, they would develop in a positive and constructive manner. He objected to the idea that people need to be instructed, punished, rewarded, and managed by others who are in a superior and "expert" position. He believed that people possess an innate ability to move away from maladjustment to psychologic health. The primary responsibility for this rests with the client, rather than with an authority who directs a passive client.[9]

Rogers advocated three qualities of counselors that create a growth-promoting climate in which persons advance to become what they are capable of becoming. These counselor qualities are genuineness, or realness; unconditional positive regard and acceptance of the client; and deep understanding of the client's feelings. According to Rogers, if a counselor communicates these attitudes, clients will become less defensive, more open to experiences within themselves and the world, and able to relate to others in social and constructive ways.[9] Rogers wrote, "If I can provide a certain type of relationship, the other person will discover within himself the capacity to use that relationship for growth and change, and personal development will occur."[6]

The client's personality change is brought about by the counselor's attitudes instead of by certain techniques, theories, or knowledge. The counselor's primary task is providing a therapeutic climate in which the client feels free to explore areas of his or her life that are currently distorted or denied to awareness. Within this climate, the client is then able to lose his or her "defenses and rigid perceptions and move to a higher level of personal functioning."[9]

The counselor's genuineness, or realness, is the congruence between what is expressed to the client and what is experienced within the counselor's mind. Through genuineness, the counselor serves as a model of a human struggling toward greater awareness and personal functioning.[9]

Unconditional positive regard and acceptance allow the client to be accepted as he or she is and to express feelings and attitudes without risk of losing the counselor's acceptance. Although the client's *feelings* are accepted, not all *overt behavior* is approved or accepted. According to Rogers, the greater the counselor's degree of positive regard and acceptance of the client, the greater will be the success of therapy.[9]

As the counselor develops a deep understanding of the client's feelings and experiences, he or she is able to sense the client's feelings as if they were his or her own. This permits the counselor to expand the client's awareness and understanding of these feelings and to help the client resolve internal conflicts and become more the person the client wishes to become.[9]

The person-centered approach has the advantage of being a safer approach to counseling than other models that place the counselor in a directive position of making interpretations, forming diagnoses, and attempting more drastic personality changes. Its core skills of listening, understanding, caring, and acceptance are needed by all counselors. No matter what counseling approach they use, counselors lacking in these core skills will not be effective in carrying out their treatment. These skills are also valuable for others in the helping professions. Although people in crisis do not necessarily need answers, they do need someone willing to really listen, care, and understand and on whom they can unload their feelings and experiences without fear of rejection. The presence of a caring, listening, understanding person can do much to promote healing.[9]

Counselors using the person-centered approach have been criticized for merely giving support to clients without challenging them. Rogers has suggested, therefore, that counselors include more "caring confrontations." Counselors using caring confrontation are more active in suggesting topics for exploration, interpreting behavior, helping clients set goals, and giving advice.[9]

Behavior Modification

Behavior modification (also known as behavior therapy) attempts to alter previously learned human behavior or to encourage the development of new behavior through a variety of action-oriented methods, as opposed to changing feelings or thoughts.[2,9,10] A major premise of behavior modification is that "all behavior, normal or abnormal, is acquired and maintained according to certain definable principles."[11] Behaviors resulting in positive consequences tend to be repeated, and those behaviors not followed by favorable consequences tend not to be repeated.

Early, or "radical," behaviorists viewed human behavior as almost totally the result of positive reinforcements (the addition of something, such as praise or money, as a consequence of behavior) or negative reinforcements (the removal of unpleasant stimuli once a certain behavior is performed). Currently, behaviorists view humans as both the *product* of environmental influences and the *producer* of their environment. Early behaviorists viewed humans as lacking freedom and self-determination. Modern behaviorists, on the other hand, acknowledge the presence of freedom and self-determination. They attempt to increase clients' freedom and control by assisting them in overcoming crippling behaviors and becoming freer to choose from options that were previously not available to them.[9]

Antecedents and Consequences

Behaviorists view actions as being preceded by antecedents and followed by consequences.[10,12] For example, eating is generally preceded by some antecedent or stimulus, such as smelling or seeing food, coming home from work or school, sitting down to study or watch television, seeing an advertisement for food on television or in a magazine, or experiencing anxiety, boredom, or loneliness. Behavior modification holds that, when antecedents to behaviors are recognized, they can be modified or controlled to decrease the occurrence of negative behaviors and increase the occurrence of positive behaviors. This is referred to as stimulus control. Examples of stimulus control include eating before grocery shopping, preparing a shopping list and purchasing only the items on the list, storing food out of sight, and avoiding the purchase of ready-to-eat foods.

Consequences reinforce the behavior they follow. They may be positive, negative, or neutral. When consequences are positive, behavior is more likely to be repeated. Behavior followed by negative consequences is less likely to be repeated. The delicious tastes and feelings of satiety accompanying a meal are examples of positive consequences that reinforce, or reward, the practice of eating. Behaviorists also believe that positive consequences are more effective in promoting behavioral change than are negative consequences.[10]

Self-monitoring

A valuable behavior modification technique is self-monitoring, or recordkeeping—the careful observation and accurate recording of the behavior to be controlled.[9,11,13] If the behavior is eating, for example, clients carefully observe their eating and record its occurrence, along with comments about relevant antecedents and consequences related to their eating. Self-monitoring has several functions:[13]

- It provides information about eating habits and the factors influencing them.
- It involves clients in observing and analyzing their dietary habits.
- It increases clients' awareness of their diets and behavior as it happens.
- It gives the counselor and client something to review objectively and impartially. For example, they focus on specific problem behaviors in the record, not in the client.
- It increases the clients' skills in manipulating their diets to achieve desired results (for example, finding suitable low-fat entrees to replace others that are high in total fat and saturated fat or finding acceptable low-calorie snack foods to replace high-calorie snacks).
- It increases counselor-client interaction.
- It allows client and counselor to monitor behavior over time and track client progress.

Various forms have been developed for self-monitoring.[13] One example is shown in Appendix R. In general, forms for self-monitoring eating behavior should allow the recording of such information as the food eaten, how food was prepared, the amount eaten, where and when the food was eaten, what happened or how the client felt before eating, what happened or how the client felt after eating, and whether the food was eaten alone or with someone else and with whom.

For monitoring behaviors related to a specific goal (for example, substitution of high-calorie snacks with low-calorie snacks), the client can record the day, time, type of snack eaten, and amount eaten on a pocket-sized card, which he or she can carry.

To be successful, the self-monitoring method ought to be easy to use, convenient, and readily available when the behavior occurs; be clearly understood by the client; be relevant to the dietary problem; and be used for observational purposes rather than to judge the problem.

Goals and Self-contracts

Behaviorists believe that feelings result from behavior.[9] Consequently, the focus of attention in counseling is changing behavior, not altering feelings or delving into past experiences. Goals are of central importance in behavior modification and are expressed in terms of altering overt behavior in ways that are both specific and measurable. Therefore, the goals of therapy must be clear, specific, measurable, attainable, and agreed on by both the client and the counselor. The client selects counseling goals at the beginning of the counseling process.

For example, a client may want to decrease his elevated total cholesterol level to less than 200 mg/dL. Having been taught by the counselor that total cholesterol levels are related to saturated fat intake, the client, with the counselor's assistance, may decide to use soft tub margarine instead of butter at home and to remove the skin from chicken before eating it. The client's progress then can be evaluated objectively in terms of goal attainment and other measurable ways. For example, the client's self-monitoring records can demonstrate adherence to the goals, and measurements of total serum cholesterol may indicate overall progress in lowering serum cholesterol.

Once goals are identified, the counselor can help the client write a self-contract. This is an agreement the client enters into with himself or herself to help build commitment to the goal for change.[12,13] The contract should clearly state the goal in terms of a specific time frame and detail the reward for successfully achieving the goal. As an option, it may state the punishment, if any, for not reaching the goal. An example of a self-contract is shown in Figure 11.2.

Modeling

In addition to believing that learning occurs through positive or negative reinforcements, behaviorists hold that people learn through the process of modeling.[9,10,12,13] Also known as observational learning or imitation, modeling is "the process by which the behavior of an individual or a group (the model) acts as a stimulus for similar thoughts, attitudes, and behaviors on the part of observers."[9] Through modeling, clients develop new behaviors without trial-and-error learning. Clients, for example, can learn new behaviors by observing the success of other

Self-contract

____
Name

____
Period of time

____
Specific behavior goal

____
Reward when successful

____________ ________
Signature Date

____________ ________
Signature Date

Figure 11.2 A self-contract.

group members or through others' success stories shared by the counselor.[10]

Modeling can take place by observing a live model (for example, counselors demonstrate the behavior they hope clients will acquire), symbolic models (the client observes the desired behavior performed on videotape or film), or multiple models (new skills are learned as successful peers within the group demonstrate the desired behavior).[9] Modeling is more likely to be successful when the model is similar to the client in age, sex, race, and attitudes than when the model is unlike the client. The likelihood that behaviors will be imitated by clients is increased when models are competent in performing the behavior, exhibit warmth, and possess a realistic degree of prestige and status.

Reinforcers

According to behavior modification, behavior is maintained and strengthened when followed by positive reinforcers.[9,11,12] Thus, a positive reinforcer is any consequence that maintains and strengthens behavior by its presence; in other words, the positive reinforcer makes the behavior more likely to recur.[12] A negative reinforcer is an unpleasant consequence that maintains and strengthens behavior by its being removed from the situation.[12] Reinforcers are often referred to as rewards. Rewards that are effective in reinforcing behavior can take many forms and vary from client to client.

If rewards are used, the counselor must identify rewards likely to effectively reinforce desired behaviors and set up a reinforcement system. As an example, consider a client on a weight control program. The counselor and client can set up a system that allows the client to receive a reward for having lost a certain amount of weight. The weight loss goal may be set rather low to make it easily attainable at the beginning of counseling. As counseling progresses and the client develops skill in managing his behavior, successive goals can be somewhat more difficult to attain. Rewards can include money or material items (an amount of money or a certain purchase for each goal reached), activities (doing something the client especially enjoys each time a goal is reached), or social interaction (visiting someone special or making a phone call when a goal is attained).[10,12] Examples of rewards are shown in Box 11.3.

Behavior Modification Techniques Summarized

Behavior modification uses a number of techniques. The major ones employed in weight management are outlined in Table 11.2.[11] Some of these techniques were not originally developed by behaviorists but were adapted from other approaches or disciplines and incorporated into behavior modification programs to increase the success of behavioral change. Among these are nutrition education, physical activity, and cognitive restructuring. Cognitive restructuring will be discussed in the section "Rational-Emotive Therapy."

Behavior modification has contributed a variety of specific behavioral techniques to nutritional counseling and the treatment of diet-related problems. Its emphasis on changing problem behaviors rather than merely talking about problems and gathering insights allows counselors to focus on assisting clients in formulating a specific plan of action. However, in its attempt to deal with problem solving and the changing of certain behaviors, it has been criticized for deemphasizing the role of feelings and emotions in counseling.[9]

Rational-Emotive Therapy

Unlike behavior modification, which primarily focuses on the relationship between our environment and behavior, rational-emotive therapy (RET) deals with the effects that our thoughts have on our behavior.[2] The major premise of RET is that emotional disturbances are largely the product of irrational thinking.[9] RET holds that our emotions are mainly the product of our beliefs, evaluations, interpretations, and reactions to life situations.[9]

RET views humans as having the potential for both rational thinking and irrational thinking. It views humans as engaging in considerable self-talk and self-evaluation, much of which is irrational and self-denigrating and can result in emotional disturbances. Rather than factors outside of ourselves being the main determinants of behavior, RET holds that our irrational beliefs about ourselves primarily determine our behavior, emotions, and the resulting consequences. In other words, people "are disturbed not by things, but by the view which they take of them."[9] Thus, RET focuses on disputing irrational beliefs and helping people change the irrational beliefs that directly result in disturbed emotions and dysfunctional behavior.[9]

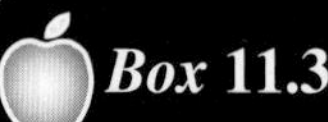

Box 11.3 **Examples of Rewards Used in Behavior Modification**

Spending money on appropriate things	Taking an afternoon or day off
Reading a book	Visiting a friend
Watching television	Spending time at a favorite hobby
Making a long-distance call	Relaxing or taking a nap

TABLE 11.2 Examples of Behavior Modification Techniques Used in Weight Control Programs

Stimulus Control

Shopping

Shop for food after eating.
Shop from a list.
Avoid ready-to-eat foods.
Do not carry more cash than needed for shopping.

Plans

Plan to limit food intake.
Substitute exercise for snacking.
Eat meals and snacks at scheduled times.
Do not accept food offered by others.

Activities

Store food out of sight.
Eat all food in the same place.
Remove food from inappropriate storage areas in the house.
Keep serving dishes off the table.
Use smaller dishes and utensils.
Avoid being the food server.
Leave the table immediately after eating.
Do not save leftovers.

Holidays and Parties

Drink fewer alcoholic beverages.
Plan eating habits before parties.
Eat a low-calorie snack before parties.
Practice polite ways to decline food.
Do not get discouraged by an occasional setback.

Eating Behavior

Put the fork down between mouthfuls.
Chew thoroughly before swallowing.
Prepare foods one portion at a time.
Leave some food on the plate.
Pause in the middle of the meal.
Do nothing else while eating (read, watch television).
Solicit help from family and friends.
Have family and friends provide help in the form of praise and material reward.
Use self-monitoring records as basis for rewards.
Plan specific rewards for specific behaviors (behavioral contracts).

Self-monitoring

Keep diet diary that includes time and place of eating, type and amount of food, who is present, and how you feel.

Nutrition Education

Use diet diary to identify problem areas.
Make small changes that you can continue.
Learn nutritional values of foods.
Decrease fat intake; increase intake of complex carbohydrates.

Physical Activity

Routine activity: increase routine activity, increase use of stairs, and keep record of distance walked daily.
Exercise: begin a very mild exercise program, keep a record of daily exercise, and increase the exercise very gradually.

Cognitive Restructuring

Avoid setting unreasonable goals.
Think about progress, not shortcomings.
Avoid imperatives, such as "always" and "never."
Counter negative thoughts with rational statements.
Set weight goals.

Adapted from Stunkard AJ, Berthold HC. 1985. What is behavior therapy? A very short description of behavioral weight control. *American Journal of Clinical Nutrition* 41:821–823.

A client's self-talk can be viewed as positive, neutral, or negative. Positive self-talk supports behavioral change, whereas negative self-talk opposes change. Consider a client beginning a weight management program. An example of positive self-talk is the client's silently observing, "I'm going to like this program." Negative self-talk is the thought "I don't think I can handle this" or "I'm no good at dieting; I'll never succeed at this program." According to RET, the likelihood of successful behavioral change is considerably less when people view themselves as failing, as compared with when they see themselves succeeding. In addition, persons viewing themselves as failing at weight management are less likely to begin addressing their behavioral problems, and, when faced with difficult challenges (for example, the urging of friends to eat fattening food at a party), they are more likely to slip from their program and to give it up altogether.[9,10]

Although our irrational beliefs may have begun through early indoctrination by our parents or significant others ("You're never going to amount to anything!"), it is primarily our own repetition of these irrational thoughts that keeps these dysfunctional attitudes alive and operative within us. Thus, RET teaches that we are largely responsible for creating our own problems, that we have the ability to change, that we must identify our irrational beliefs, and that we must dispute these irrational beliefs using the process of cognitive restructuring.[9]

The first step in cognitive restructuring is becoming aware of negative self-talk.[2,9,14,15] One approach is asking the client to record his or her irrational and destructive internal messages on a form similar to the one shown in Table 11.3.[15] Once an irrational internal message is identified, it can be disputed by substituting it with a rational, self-defensive statement.

Clients can be led to dispute their irrational self-talk and beliefs by encouraging them to ask such questions as "What is the factual evidence in support of my thoughts?" "Why do I assume I am a rotten person because of the way I behave?" "Would it really be catastrophic if my worst fears were to come true?" and "What can I say in defense of myself?"[9,14] As clients learn to recognize and dispute their irrational self-criticisms, they then can be encouraged to substitute negative self-talk with positive, self-affirming statements.

Other RET techniques include the changing of one's language, cognitive rehearsal, and thought stopping.[2,9,12,14,15] An example of changing one's language is avoiding negative self-fulfilling statements ("I will fail, I will look like a pig, and no one will like me"). People telling themselves that they will fail may actually increase the probability of failure. Cognitive rehearsal (also known as rational-emotive imagery) involves clients' thinking, feeling, and behaving the way they would like to in real life. As clients see themselves overcoming in their thoughts, the likelihood of them overcoming in real life is increased. Thought stopping is a two-step process. First, whenever a negative thought enters the client's mind, he or she says, "Stop!" either out loud or very clearly within the mind. This is followed by substituting a positive, rational thought for the negative, irrational thought. Again, the basis of these exercises is that our language (either audible or silent) influences our thoughts, which in turn influence our emotions and behavior.

Reality Therapy

The central premises of reality therapy are that individuals are responsible for their behavior and that, if a person's current behavior is not meeting his or her needs, steps can be taken to change behavior so that personal needs are met.[9,16] Reality therapy is based primarily on the work of psychiatrist William Glasser, who abandoned traditional psychoanalysis early in his career and went on to develop his own counseling approach. According to Glasser, every person's behavior is an attempt to fulfill his or her basic human needs. "It is always what we want at the time that causes our behavior."[17] According to Glasser, rather than being determined by outside forces (as is taught by behaviorists), behavior is completely driven from within the person by the necessity to fulfill five innate needs: survival, love, power, fun, and freedom.[17] "All of our lives we must attempt to live in a way that will best satisfy one or more of these needs."[17]

Glasser teaches that each of us creates our own inner world from which we view the world outside of ourselves.

TABLE 11.3 Identifying and Disputing Irrational and Destructive Thoughts

Irrational Thought	Rational, Self-defensive Statement
"I can't believe I ate six of those cookies! I've blown it. Oh well, I may as well go ahead and finish the rest of the bag."	"I *did* slip by eating those six cookies, but I *did not* blow my program. The best thing for me to do now is to stop eating them. I *can* do better."
"I ate half a bag of potato chips! I'm an absolute failure."	"My success or failure at anything is not based on one incident. I'm human. It's okay to make mistakes once in awhile. I don't have to be perfect."
"The way she's looking at me, she must think my idea is stupid."	"I can't read other people's minds. The way to find out what she thinks is to just ask. Besides, not everyone has to like my idea."

Each person is responsible for the kind of inner world he or she creates. Instead of external factors depressing or angering us, we anger or depress ourselves. "Neurotic" and "psychotic" behavior does not just happen to us; it is something we choose in an attempt to control our world. If a client complains of anxiety, the counselor may ask what behavior is causing the anxiety. The focus is not on the anxiety but on whatever behavior is causing the anxiety. According to Glasser, once people acknowledge and act on the reality that their behavior is the result of their choices, change occurs.[9]

Reality therapy begins by the counselor's establishing an accepting and supportive relationship with the client. The client is then led to examine and evaluate his own behavior to determine if it is contributing to his problems. Once the client acknowledges he is not getting what he wants from his behavior, the counselor helps the client develop an action plan for changing his behavior so that it contributes to his success. The plan should have goals that are simple, specific, clear, and attainable and that involve something the client will do soon and on a daily basis. The counselor then helps the client make a commitment to follow through with the plan and to refuse to give up. The counselor makes it clear to the client that he will neither accept excuses nor use punishment to coerce the client.

Many people tend to blame other individuals or circumstances for their problems. Reality therapy asserts that people are responsible for their own behavior and attacks the excuses many people make for their actions in an attempt to evade responsibility.[18] A client who runs to the refrigerator every time she feels anxious, for example, may benefit from acknowledging that her behavior does not depend on an outside stimulus (in this case, the "anxiety") but on her own conscious choice. The client should be helped to recognize that she has a variety of options for dealing with her anxiety. Then, under the guidance of a counselor, the client can select from her options and develop a plan to deal with her problematic behavior in positive ways.[18]

Initiating and Maintaining Dietary Change: A Practical Plan

A number of counselor characteristics and behavioral change techniques can be identified. These characteristics and techniques are effective in initiating and maintaining nutrition behavior, but their use does not guarantee success. Each nutrition counselor will want to integrate them into a total program with which he or she feels comfortable. The counselor will also want to consider clients' needs, resources, and social support, as well as the skill level of support staff.

No single counseling approach can be recommended for all clients. Rather, counselors are encouraged to use an eclectic approach—that is, one composed of elements drawn from a variety of approaches. An effective behavioral change program would selectively incorporate several techniques into a multicomponent program that is suitable to both the counselor and the client. However, it is neither necessary nor wise to use all the counseling techniques at one's disposal.

Motivation

No counselor can motivate a client. Motivation comes only from within the client. A counselor can only create a climate that will help clients motivate themselves. People tend to be motivated by challenge, growth, achievement, promotion, and recognition. Emphasis should be placed on providing a proper environment for self-growth by challenging clients, giving them responsibility and encouragement, and giving full range to individual strength.

Characteristics of Effective Counselors

From this discussion of counseling theories, it is possible to identify several characteristics of effective counselors. By practicing good communication, listening, and counseling skills, one of the first steps in initiating behavioral change can take place—establishing good rapport with the client. The following are characteristics of effective counselors:

- Empathy—the ability to climb into the world of the client and communicate back feelings of understanding
- Respect—a deep and genuine appreciation for the worth of a client, separate and apart from his or her behavior; the strength and ability of the client to overcome and adjust is appreciated
- Warmth—communication of concern and appropriate affection
- Genuineness—being freely and deeply oneself; one is congruent and not just playing a role
- Concreteness—essential ideas and elements are ferreted out
- Self-disclosure—information about self is revealed for the benefit of the client at the appropriate time
- Potency and self-actualization—one is dynamic, is in command, conveys feelings of trust and warmth, is competent, is inner-directed, is creative, is sensitive, is nonjudgmental, is productive, is serene, and is satisfied; this comes across to the client in a helpful way.[19]

Initial Assessment

The initial assessment of the client serves several important functions:

- It makes the counselor and client aware of the client's dietary habits and health history, as well as related factors.

- It provides baseline information from which to gauge progress.
- It alerts the counselor and client to the various demands being placed on the client, so that realistic priorities can be set.
- It gives the counselor and client ideas for making dietary changes.
- It gives the counselor an opportunity to develop rapport and a sense of partnership with the client.
- It enables the counselor to develop a plan of gradual change suitable to the client's way of living.[13]

As discussed in Chapters 3 and 8, a variety of techniques can be used for obtaining dietary information. In addition to these data, however, information should be collected on the client's current health status, health history, and past and present health habits.

Initiating Dietary Change

Counselors and clients should have reasonable expectations about what changes should be undertaken, the extent of change, and the rate at which change is made. Clients should be carefully guided in what benefits they can reasonably expect from dietary change and the amount of change necessary to realize those benefits.[13,20,21]

Goals can be set by the client under the guidance of the counselor. Goals should be specific, measurable, reasonable, and attainable. Whatever the final behavioral goal is, most people will not be able to master it at the first effort or in one step. Behavioral change should be approached gradually, with a number of small, easily attained goals that collectively lead to the final goal. A client can never begin too low and the steps upward can never be too small.[12] Short-term goals spanning 1 to 2 weeks are more effective than long-term goals covering months.[20] Because obstacles and setbacks will be encountered, goals should have some flexibility. One approach to building a client's commitment to attaining goals can be through a written self-contract.

Reinforcers, or rewards, can help promote maintenance of behavioral change, especially at the beginning of a program. If they are used, counselors will need to work with each client (and possibly with a key individual providing social support for the client) to identify reinforcers providing ample incentive to goal attainment. At this time, the use of other behavior modification strategies can be discussed with the client. Serious consideration should be given to using stimulus control, self-monitoring, and cognitive restructuring in ways suitable to both counselor and client.

Maintaining Dietary Change

Although counselors can assist clients in making dietary changes (for example, in learning about nutrition, setting realistic goals, and managing the antecedents to behaviors), it is ultimately the client's responsibility to change dietary habits. To be permanently successful, clients will need to be guided toward self-sufficiency.[13]

A key element in self-sufficiency is the client's involvement in the change process.[13] The client should be asked, "What changes can *you* make?" "What can *you* say when someone offers you another serving of dessert?" "What steps can *you* take to avoid overeating at a party?" The more the client "owns" the program, the more successful he or she will be at maintaining dietary change.

Four areas where counselors can help clients increase self-control over eating habits are maintenance of commitment, recordkeeping, environmental restructuring, and use of rewards.[13] At first, most clients are enthusiastic about behavioral change. After several days or weeks, however, this enthusiasm begins to wane. Some suggestions for strengthening commitment to dietary change include the following:

- Praise the client for his or her successful experiences and attribute success to the client's abilities.
- Encourage the client to tell family members and friends about his or her dietary goals. After making a public commitment to dietary change, adherence to the program is more likely.
- Ask the client to state the kinds of problems he or she will likely encounter. Problems will occur, but they will be less likely to derail the client's progress when they are anticipated and planned for.
- Concentrate on foods the client can eat, rather than those to be avoided. Help clients realize that healthy eating is not synonymous with deprivation.[13]

Recordkeeping provides information on the client's performance, aids the client in observing and analyzing his or her environment, and helps in recognizing the antecedents to eating behavior. Recordkeeping can range from marking a 3 × 5-inch card every time a between-meal snack is declined to keeping elaborate food records.[13]

Some researchers think that restructuring the environment is the most important technique in maintaining change. Counselors can ask clients to identify specific changes that can be made in their physical, social, and cognitive (mental) environments to promote long-term dietary change.

A client may associate an event—such as sitting in a favorite chair, reading the newspaper or watching television—with eating high-calorie foods. The presence of inappropriate foods at home also can be a deterrent to successful change. Altering the arrangement of furniture in the room where television is watched or the newspaper is read can help promote and maintain change. Purchasing healthful foods to substitute for inappropriate items can be helpful as well.

The counselor should ask the client to identify social situations that promote poor eating habits. How is the client's eating behavior affected by various social functions or what family and friends say to the client? The counselor should explore with the client ways that social interactions can be supportive of dietary change. What could family and friends say to promote the client's success? Through role playing, the client can develop skill in asking for support from others.[13] In dealing with the mental environment, the client should be encouraged to use some of the cognitive restructuring techniques discussed in the "Rational-Emotive Therapy" section.

Relapse Prevention

For the purposes of behavioral change, a relapse can be defined as the resumption of an unwanted habit or behavior that one has, for a period of time, overcome or turned from.[12,22] Consider a man with the habit of eating a half-pint of premium butter-pecan ice cream every evening. For several weeks he has limited himself to only 1 cup of nonfat frozen dessert four evenings a week. When he returns to 2 cups of butter-pecan ice cream every evening for several weeks, he has relapsed. However, if he merely indulges once or twice in butter-pecan ice cream while spending a weekend with relatives and then returns to 1 cup of the nonfat variety four evenings a week, he has only experienced a lapse. A lapse can be defined as "a single event, a reemergence of a previous habit, which may or may not lead to a state of relapse."[21] Thus, a lapse is a temporary fall, a slip, or a mistake. When a lapse occurs, corrective action can be taken to prevent a relapse—a total loss of control—from occurring.[21]

A key to relapse prevention is to prepare clients for the occurrence of lapses and to help them cope in ways that prevent a relapse.[20] If counselors and clients have previously discussed the likelihood of lapses' occurring, clients will be better prepared when they do occur, and the risk of lapses' leading to full-blown relapses will be minimized. Clients should be taught to anticipate situations likely to produce lapses, such as illness, travel, live-in visitors, overwork, emotional distress, and schedule changes.[20]

Counselors should help clients view lapses for what they really are—merely a temporary fall. A counselor and client can discuss what corrective actions the client can take to recover from the lapse and to prevent a relapse from occurring. Techniques such as modeling, role playing, cognitive rehearsal, and direct instruction can help in this.[2] A client needs to be assured that, if a relapse does occur, it is not the end of the world. The client has suffered a setback, but prompt action can limit the lapse to a temporary setback.

KNOWING ONE'S LIMITS

When working with clients, it is important that counselors know the limits of their abilities to help people and when they need to refer a client to more experienced help. Emotional problems are common, and from time to time nutrition counselors encounter individuals needing psychologic counseling. If a client indicates that she is having emotional problems, a nutrition counselor may very gently and tactfully ask if she would like assistance in getting psychologic counseling from a local mental health clinic or professional. The counselor may help her in calling and making an appointment with an appropriate agency or person.[9,20]

Some individuals may not be ready or willing to change certain habits. Circumstances in a person's life may not be conducive to change at the particular time he is seeing a counselor. It may be necessary to suggest that a client postpone weight loss or control of mildly elevated serum cholesterol until *after* he deals with a more pressing problem, such as separation, divorce, bankruptcy, or substance abuse.

This chapter has offered a very brief overview of dietary counseling. It is meant to be only an introduction to the topic. Readers interested in developing the skill of nutritional counseling are encouraged to take coursework and to study other sources for further information. Other excellent resources include the following:

Bauer KD, Liou D, Sokolik CA. 2012. *Nutrition counseling and education skill development,* 2nd ed. Belmont, CA: Wadsworth, Cengage Learning.

Holli BB, Maillet J, Beto JA, Calabrese RJ. 2009. *Communication and education skills for dietetics professionals,* 5th ed. Philadelphia: Wolters Kluwer Health/Lippincott Williams & Wilkins.

Watson DL, Tharp RG. 2007. *Self-directed behavior: Self-modification for personal adjustment,* 9th ed. Belmont, CA: Wadsworth/Thomson Learning.

SUMMARY

1. Communication, the process of sending and receiving messages, lies at the foundation of all efforts to interview, counsel, educate, and change diet. The basic components of human communication are the sender, receiver, message, feedback, and interference.

2. A counselor's attempts to help bring about dietary change may elicit a defensive reaction from the receiver or client. When this occurs, the receiver fails to concentrate on the structure, content, and meaning of the message. This is one source of interference to communication. When communication is supportive of the receiver, this defensive reaction can be prevented, and the interference to communication can be minimized.

3. Communication occurs simultaneously at both the verbal and nonverbal levels. Nonverbal communication involves gestures, posture, facial expressions, and tone of voice. It is sometimes a more reliable indicator of a person's true feelings than are words. Unlike verbal communication, which is generally under conscious control and subject to censorship, nonverbal communication is not as easily controlled by conscious thought. It is also an effective way for the counselor to communicate to the client.
4. Effective communication is promoted by proper use of feedback, language that is understandable to both counselor and client, an environment that is conducive to good communication, and awareness of the physical and psychologic barriers to communication.
5. Listening is an important part of interviewing and counseling and an excellent way to establish rapport. Despite its importance, most people are not good listeners. Listening involves six steps: hearing, attending, understanding, remembering, evaluating, and responding.
6. Rather than being a passive activity, listening is a highly active process demanding concentration and attention. It is also a skill that can be learned. Listening skills can be grouped under four categories: openness, concentration, attention, and comprehension.
7. Interviewing is a guided communication process between two persons for the purpose of obtaining or exchanging specific information through the asking and answering of questions. The goal of the interview is obtaining specific information from the client while maintaining an interpersonal environment conducive to disclosure by the client. Conditions that increase interviewing effectiveness include comfortable physical surroundings, freedom from interruption and interference, and privacy. Counselor qualities that contribute to a successful interview include the ability to establish good rapport, attentiveness, openness, and an understanding of the client's situation.
8. Several types of questions can be used in the interview. Open questions invite rather than demand answers and give the client substantial freedom in determining the amount and type of information to give. Closed questions are restrictive and allow the counselor to control answers and ask for specific information. Neutral questions allow the client to answer without pressure or direction from the counselor. Leading questions contain implicit or explicit suggestions about the expected or desired answer.
9. The person-centered approach to counseling is largely based on the idea that, if people experience human relationships characterized by respect and trust, they will develop in a positive and constructive manner. Three counselor qualities that create a growth-promoting climate for the client are genuineness, or realness; unconditional positive regard and acceptance of the client; and deep understanding of the client's feelings. Within this climate, the client is then able to lose his or her "defenses and rigid perceptions and move to a higher level of personal functioning."[10]
10. The main contribution of person-centered therapy is its core skills: listening, understanding, caring, and acceptance. Regardless of the approach used, counselors deficient in these skills will lack efficiency in carrying out their treatment. The presence of a caring, listening, understanding person can do much to promote healing in a person experiencing a crisis.
11. Behavior modification attempts to alter previously learned human behavior or encourage the learning of new behavior through a variety of action-oriented methods, as opposed to changing feelings or thoughts. Although early behaviorists viewed human behavior as almost totally the result of reinforcements, modern behaviorists view humans as both the product of environmental influences and the producer of their environment.
12. Behaviorists view actions as being preceded by antecedents and followed by consequences. The modification or control of antecedents to decrease the occurrence of negative behaviors and increase the occurrence of positive behaviors is referred to as stimulus control. Other techniques of behavior modification include self-monitoring, or recordkeeping; modeling; cognitive restructuring; education; physical activity; and the use of goals, self-contracts, and reinforcers.
13. The major premise of rational-emotive therapy (RET) is that emotional disturbances are largely the product of irrational thinking. RET holds that our emotions are mainly the product of our beliefs, evaluations, interpretations, and reactions to life situations. Rather than factors outside of ourselves being the main determinants of behavior, RET holds that our irrational beliefs about ourselves primarily determine our behavior, emotions, and the resulting consequences.
14. A major technique of RET is cognitive restructuring, which focuses on helping people dispute their irrational beliefs and change the thoughts that directly

result in disturbed emotions and dysfunctional behavior. RET also uses such techniques as cognitive rehearsal and thought stopping.

15. Reality therapy views every person's behavior as an attempt to fulfill his or her basic human needs. Reality therapy views behavior as being driven not by outside forces but from within the person by the necessity to fulfill the need for survival, love, power, fun, and freedom. Each individual is responsible for his or her behavior, and, if current behavior is not meeting a person's needs, he or she can take steps to change behavior so that personal needs are met.
16. In reality therapy, the counselor begins by establishing an accepting and supportive relationship with a client. The client is then led to examine and evaluate his behavior to determine if it is contributing to his problems. Once the client acknowledges he is not getting what he wants from his behavior, the counselor helps the client develop an action plan for changing his behavior, so that it contributes to his success.
17. No single counseling approach can be recommended for all clients. Counselors are encouraged to use an eclectic approach—one composed of elements drawn from a variety of methods. An effective behavioral change program would selectively incorporate several techniques into a multicomponent program that is suitable to both the counselor and the client.
18. In addition to having good communication and listening skills, effective counselors convey empathy, respect, warmth, genuineness, concreteness, openness, potency, and self-actualization.
19. It is important for counselors and clients to have reasonable expectations about what changes should be undertaken, the extent of change, and the rate at which change is made. Goals set by the client under the guidance of the counselor should be specific, measurable, reasonable, and attainable. Behavioral change will be more successful when achieved through a number of small steps. Short-term goals spanning 1 to 2 weeks are more effective than long-term goals covering months.
20. If rewards are used, counselors will need to work with each client to identify those providing ample incentive to goal attainment. Serious consideration also should be given to using stimulus control, self-monitoring, and cognitive restructuring in ways suitable to both counselor and client.
21. It is ultimately the client's responsibility to change dietary habits. To be permanently successful, clients need to be guided toward self-sufficiency. Four areas where counselors can help clients develop self-sufficiency in dietary change are maintenance of commitment, recordkeeping, environmental restructuring, and use of reinforcers.
22. A relapse can be defined as the resumption of an unwanted habit or behavior that one has, for a period of time, overcome or turned from. A lapse can be defined as a temporary fall, or a reemergence of a previous habit, which may or may not lead to a state of relapse. Counselors should prepare clients for the occurrence of lapses and help them cope in ways that will prevent a relapse. Clients should be taught to anticipate situations likely to produce lapses, such as illness, travel, live-in visitors, overwork, emotional distress, and schedule changes.
23. Counselors should know the limits of their abilities and when they need to refer clients needing psychologic counseling to more experienced help. Some individuals may not be ready or willing to change certain habits. It may be necessary to suggest that a client postpone dietary change until after his or her more pressing problems have been resolved.

REFERENCES

1. Institute of Medicine. 2007. *Ending the tobacco problem: A blueprint for the nation.* Washington, DC: National Academies Press.
2. Holli BB, Maillet J, Beto JA, Calabrese RJ. 2009. *Communication and education skills for dietetics professionals,* 5th ed. Philadelphia: Wolters Kluwer Health/Lippincott Williams & Wilkins.
3. Bauer KD, Liou D, Sokolik CA. 2012. *Nutrition counseling and education skill development,* 2nd ed. Belmont, CA: Wadsworth, Cengage Learning.
4. Samovar LA. 2000. *Oral communication: Speaking across cultures,* 11th ed. Los Angeles: Roxbury.
5. Stewart CJ, Cash WB. 2006. *Interviewing: Principles and practices,* 11th ed. Boston: McGraw-Hill.
6. Rogers C. 1961. *On becoming a person.* Boston: Houghton Mifflin.

7. Rogers C. 1970. *Carl Rogers on encounter groups.* New York: Harper & Row.
8. Rogers C. 1977. *Carl Rogers on personal power: Inner strength and its revolutionary impact.* New York: Delacorte.
9. Corey G. 2009. *Theory and practice of counseling and psychotherapy,* 8th ed. Belmont, CA: Thomson Brooks/Cole.
10. Elder JA, Ayala GX, Harris S. 1999. Theories and intervention approaches to health-behavior change in primary care. *American Journal of Preventive Medicine* 17:275–284.
11. Stunkard AJ, Berthold HC. 1985. What is behavior therapy? A very short description of behavioral weight control. *American Journal of Clinical Nutrition* 41:821–823.
12. Watson DL, Tharp RG. 2007. *Self-directed behavior: Self-modification for personal adjustment,* 9th ed. Belmont, CA: Wadsworth/Thomson Learning.
13. Raab C, Tillotson JL. 1985. *Heart to heart: A manual on nutrition counseling for the reduction of cardiovascular disease risk factors.* Bethesda, MD: U.S. Department of Health and Human Services, Public Health Service; National Institutes of Health.
14. Bandura A. 1997. *Self-efficacy: The exercise of control.* New York: W. H. Freeman.
15. Burns DD. 2000. *Feeling good: The new mood therapy.* New York: Quill.
16. Burns DD. 1999. *The feeling good handbook.* New York: Plume.
17. Glasser W. 2001. *Reality therapy in action.* New York: Harper-Collins.
18. Glasser W. 1998. *The quality school: Managing students without coercion.* New York: Harper-Perennial.
19. Hoeltzel KE. 1986. Counseling methods for dietitians. *Topics in Clinical Nutrition* 1:33–42.
20. Nieman DC. 2011. *Exercise testing and prescription: A health-related approach,* 7th ed. New York: McGraw-Hill.
21. Thompson WR, Gordon NF, Pescatello LS. 2010. *ASCM's guidelines for exercise testing and prescription,* 8th ed. Philadelphia: Lippincott Williams & Wilkins.
22. Brownell KD, Marlatt GA, Lichtenstein E, Wilson GT. 1986. Understanding and preventing relapse. *American Psychologist* 41:765–782.

Assessment Activity 11.1

Counseling Practice

Becoming an effective counselor requires considerable skill and practice. This assessment activity is designed to help you get your feet wet.

Members of your class should divide into groups of two students each. You should take the 3-day food record that you completed in Assessment Activity 3.2 and the result of the computerized analysis of that food record and give these to your partner.

Review your partner's food record and computerized analysis. Study the Competency Checklist for Nutrition Counselors shown in Appendix S. Use this as a guide for your counseling session and to evaluate yourself after you have counseled your partner.

Using techniques discussed in this chapter, assist your partner in identifying one specific, measurable, and attainable goal that will improve his or her diet. Guide your partner in developing a simple action plan for attaining the goal he or she has decided on.

Videotape (or audiotape) the counseling session and view (or listen to) it alone later to see how you did. Look for what you did right and note improvements you can make next time. Use the Competency Checklist for Nutrition Counselors in Appendix S to evaluate your counseling skills.

If time allows, repeat this exercise.

APPENDIX

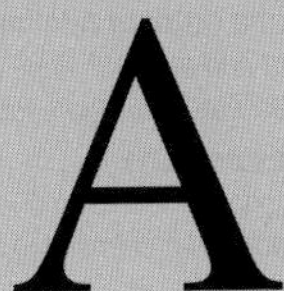

Nutrition Assessment and Monitoring and Evaluation Terminology

This is a combined list of Nutrition Assessment and Monitoring and Evaluation terms. Indicators that are shaded are used ONLY for nutrition assessment. The rest of the indicators are used for assessment and monitoring and evaluation.

FOOD/NUTRITION-RELATED HISTORY (FH)

Food and nutrient intake, food and nutrient administration, medication/herbal supplement use, knowledge/beliefs/attitudes, behavior, food and supply availability, physical activity and function, nutrition-related patient/client-centered measures.

Food and Nutrient Intake (1)

Composition and adequacy of food and nutrient intake and meal and snack patterns.

Energy Intake (1.1)

Total energy intake from all sources, including food, beverages, supplements, and via enteral and parenteral routes.

Energy intake (1.1.1)

❑ Total energy intake	FH-1.1.1.1

Food and Beverage Intake (1.2)

Type, amount, and pattern of intake of foods and food groups, indices of diet quality, intake of fluids, breast milk and infant formula.

Fluid/beverage intake (1.2.1)

❑ Oral fluids	FH-1.2.1.1
❑ Food-derived fluids	FH-1.2.1.2
❑ Liquid meal replacement or supplement	FH-1.2.1.3

Food intake (1.2.2)

❑ Amount of food	FH-1.2.2.1
❑ Types of food/meals	FH-1.2.2.2
❑ Meal/snack pattern	FH-1.2.2.3
❑ Diet quality index	FH-1.2.2.4
❑ Food variety	FH-1.2.2.5

Breast milk/infant formula intake (1.2.3)

❑ Breast milk intake	FH-1.2.3.1
❑ Infant formula intake	FH-1.2.3.2

Enteral and Parenteral Nutrition Intake (1.3)

Specialized nutrition support intake from all sources, e.g., enteral and parenteral routes.

Enteral nutrition intake (1.3.1)

❑ Formula/solution	FH-1.3.1.1
❑ Feeding tube flush	FH-1.3.1.2

Parenteral nutrition intake (1.3.2)

❑ Formula/solution	FH-1.3.2.1
❑ IV fluids	FH-1.3.2.2

Bioactive Substance Intake (1.4)

Alcohol, plant stanol and sterol esters, soy protein, psyllium and β-glucan, and caffeine intake from all sources, e.g., food, beverages, supplements, and via enteral and parenteral routes.

Alcohol intake (1.4.1)

❑ Drink size/volume	FH-1.4.1.1
❑ Frequency	FH-1.4.1.2
❑ Pattern of alcohol consumption	FH-1.4.1.3

Bioactive substance intake (1.4.2)

❑ Plant sterol and stanol esters	FH-1.4.2.1
❑ Soy protein	FH-1.4.2.2
❑ Psyllium and β-glucan	FH-1.4.2.3
❑ Food additives *(specify)*	FH-1.4.2.4
❑ Other *(specify)*	FH-1.4.2.5

Caffeine intake (1.4.3)

❑ Total caffeine	FH-1.4.3.1

Macronutrient Intake (1.5)

Fat and cholesterol, protein, carbohydrate, and fiber intake from all sources including food, beverages, supplements, and via enteral and parenteral routes.

Fat and cholesterol intake (1.5.1)

❑ Total fat	FH-1.5.1.1
❑ Saturated fat	FH-1.5.1.2
❑ Trans fatty acids	FH-1.5.1.3
❑ Polyunsaturated fat	FH-1.5.1.4
❑ Monounsaturated fat	FH-1.5.1.5
❑ Omega-3 fatty acids	FH-1.5.1.6
❑ Dietary cholesterol	FH-1.5.1.7
❑ Essential fatty acids	FH-1.5.1.8

Protein intake (1.5.2)

❑ Total protein	FH-1.5.2.1
❑ High biological value protein	FH-1.5.2.2
❑ Casein	FH-1.5.2.3
❑ Whey	FH-1.5.2.4
❑ Amino acids	FH-1.5.2.5
❑ Essential amino acids	FH-1.5.2.6

Carbohydrate intake (1.5.3)

❑ Total carbohydrate	FH-1.5.3.1
❑ Sugar	FH-1.5.3.2
❑ Starch	FH-1.5.3.3
❑ Glycemic index	FH-1.5.3.4
❑ Glycemic load	FH-1.5.3.5
❑ Source of carbohydrate	FH-1.5.3.6
❑ Insulin-to-carbohydrate ratio	FH-1.5.3.7

Fiber intake (1.5.4)

❑ Total fiber	FH-1.5.4.1
❑ Soluble fiber	FH-1.5.4.2
❑ Insoluble fiber	FH-1.5.4.3

Micronutrient Intake (1.6)

Vitamin and mineral intake from all sources, e.g., food, beverages, supplements, and via enteral and parenteral routes.

Vitamin intake (1.6.1)

❑ A (1)	❑ Riboflavin (7)
❑ C (2)	❑ Niacin (8)
❑ D (3)	❑ Folate (9)
❑ E (4)	❑ B6 (10)
❑ K (5)	❑ B12 (11)
❑ Thiamin (6)	❑ Multivitamin (12)

❑ Other *(specify)* ________________ (13)

Mineral/element intake (1.6.2)

❑ Calcium (1)	❑ Potassium (5)
❑ Chloride (2)	❑ Phosphorus (6)
❑ Iron (3)	❑ Sodium (7)

Mineral/element intake (1.6.2), ***(cont'd)***

❑ Magnesium (4) ❑ Zinc (8)
❑ Multi-mineral (9)
❑ Multi-trace element (10)
❑ Other, *(specify)* ______________ (11)

Food and Nutrient Administration (2)

Current and previous diets and/or food modifications, eating environment, and enteral and parenteral nutrition administration.

Diet History (2.1)

Description of food and drink regularly provided or consumed, past diets followed or prescribed and counseling received, and the eating environment.

Diet order (2.1.1)

❑ General, healthful diet	FH-2.1.1.1
❑ Modified diet *(specify)* ______________	FH-2.1.1.2
❑ Enteral nutrition order *(specify)* ______________	FH-2.1.1.3
❑ Parenteral nutrition order *(specify)* ______________	FH-2.1.1.4

Diet experience (2.1.2)

❑ Previously prescribed diets	FH-2.1.2.1
❑ Previous diet/nutrition education/counseling	FH-2.1.2.2
❑ Self-selected diet/s followed	FH-2.1.2.3
❑ Dieting attempts	FH-2.1.2.4

Eating environment (2.1.3)

❑ Location	FH-2.1.3.1
❑ Atmosphere	FH-2.1.3.2
❑ Caregiver/companion	FH-2.1.3.3
❑ Appropriate breastfeeding accommodations/facility	FH-2.1.3.4
❑ Eats alone	FH-2.1.3.5

Enteral and parenteral nutrition administration (2.1.4)

❑ Enteral access	FH-2.1.4.1
❑ Parenteral access	FH-2.1.4.2

Medication and Herbal Supplement Use (3)

Prescription and over-the-counter medications, including herbal preparations and complementary medicine products used.

Medication and herbal supplements (3.1)

❑ Medications, specify prescription or OTC	FH-3.1.1
❑ Herbal/complementary products *(specify)*	FH-3.1.2
❑ Misuse of medication *(specify)*	FH-3.1.3

Knowledge/Beliefs/Attitudes (4)

Understanding of nutrition-related concepts and conviction of the truth and feelings/emotions toward some nutrition-related statement or phenomenon, along with readiness to change nutrition-related behaviors.

Food and nutrition knowledge (4.1)

❑ Area(s) and level of knowledge	FH-4.1.1
❑ Diagnosis specific or global nutrition-related knowledge score	FH-4.1.2

Beliefs and attitudes (4.2)

❑ Conflict with personal/family value system	FH-4.2.1
❑ Distorted body image	FH-4.2.2
❑ End-of-life decisions	FH-4.2.3
❑ Motivation	FH-4.2.4
❑ Preoccupation with food/nutrients	FH-4.2.5
❑ Preoccupation with weight	FH-4.2.6
❑ Readiness to change nutrition-related behaviors	FH-4.2.7
❑ Self-efficacy	FH-4.2.8
❑ Self-talk/cognitions	FH-4.2.9
❑ Unrealistic nutrition-related goals	FH-4.2.10
❑ Unscientific beliefs/attitudes	FH-4.2.11
❑ Food preferences *(specify)*	FH-4.2.12
❑ Emotions *(specify)*	FH-4.2.13

Behavior (5)

Patient/client activities and actions, which influence achievement of nutrition-related goals.

Adherence (5.1)

❑ Self-reported adherence score	FH-5.1.1
❑ Nutrition visit attendance	FH-5.1.2
❑ Ability to recall nutrition goals	FH-5.1.3
❑ Self-monitoring at agreed upon rate	FH-5.1.4
❑ Self-management as agreed upon	FH-5.1.5

Avoidance behavior (5.2)

❑ Avoidance	FH-5.2.1
❑ Restrictive eating	FH-5.2.2
❑ Cause of avoidance behavior	FH-5.2.3

Bingeing and purging behavior (5.3)

❑ Binge eating behavior	FH-5.3.1
❑ Purging behavior	FH-5.3.2

Mealtime behavior (5.4)

❑ Meal duration	FH-5.4.1
❑ Percent of meal time spent eating	FH-5.4.2
❑ Preference to drink rather than eat	FH-5.4.3
❑ Refusal to eat/chew	FH-5.4.4
❑ Spitting food out	FH-5.4.5
❑ Rumination	FH-5.4.6
❑ Patient/client/caregiver fatigue during feeding process resulting in inadequate intake	FH-5.4.7
❑ Willingness to try new foods	FH-5.4.8
❑ Limited number of accepted foods	FH-5.4.9
❑ Rigid sensory preferences	FH-5.4.10

Social network (5.5)

❑ Ability to build and utilize social network	FH-5.5.1

Factors Affecting Access to Food and Food/Nutrition-Related Supplies (6)

Factors that affect intake and availability of a sufficient quantity of safe, healthful food as well as food/nutrition-related supplies.

Food/nutrition program participation (6.1)

❑ Eligibility for government programs	FH-6.1.1
❑ Participation in government programs	FH-6.1.2
❑ Eligibility for community programs	FH-6.1.3
❑ Participation in community programs	FH-6.1.4

Safe food/meal availability (6.2)

❑ Availability of shopping facilities	FH-6.2.1
❑ Procurement, identification of safe food	FH-6.2.2
❑ Appropriate meal preparation facilities	FH-6.2.3
❑ Availability of safe food storage	FH-6.2.4
❑ Appropriate storage technique	FH-6.2.5

Safe water availability (6.3)

❑ Availability of potable water	FH-6.3.1
❑ Appropriate water decontamination	FH-6.3.2

Food and nutrition-related supplies availability (6.4)

❑ Access to food and nutrition-related supplies	FH-6.4.1
❑ Access to assistive eating devices	FH-6.4.2
❑ Access to assistive food preparation devices	FH 6.4.3

Physical Activity and Function (7)

Physical activity, cognitive and physical ability to engage in specific tasks, e.g., breastfeeding, self-feeding.

Breastfeeding (7.1)

❑ Initiation of breastfeeding	FH-7.1.1
❑ Duration of breastfeeding	FH-7.1.2
❑ Exclusive breastfeeding	FH-7.1.3
❑ Breastfeeding problems	FH-7.1.4

Nutrition-related ADLs and IADLs (7.2)

❑ Physical ability to complete tasks for meal preparation	FH-7.2.1
❑ Physical ability to self-feed	FH-7.2.2
❑ Ability to position self in relation to plate	FH-7.2.3
❑ Receives assistance with intake	FH 7.2.4
❑ Ability to use adaptive eating devices	FH 7.2.5
❑ Cognitive ability to complete tasks for meal preparation	FH-7.2.6
❑ Remembers to eat, recalls eating	FH-7.2.7
❑ Mini Mental State Examination Score	FH-7.2.8
❑ Nutrition-related activities of daily living (ADL) score	FH-7.2.9
❑ Nutrition-related instrumental activities of daily living (IADL) score	FH-7.2.10

Physical activity (7.3)

❑ Physical activity history	FH-7.3.1
❑ Consistency	FH-7.3.2
❑ Frequency	FH-7.3.3
❑ Duration	FH-7.3.4
❑ Intensity	FH-7.3.5
❑ Type of physical activity	FH-7.3.6
❑ Strength	FH-7.3.7
❑ TV/screen time	FH-7.3.8
❑ Other sedentary activity time	FH-7.3.9
❑ Involuntary physical movement	FH-7.3.10
❑ NEAT	FH-7.3.11

Nutrition-Related Patient/Client-Centered Measures (8)

Patient/client's perception of his or her nutrition intervention and its impact on life.

Nutrition quality of life (8.1)

❑ Nutrition quality of life responses	FH-8.1.1

ANTHROPOMETRIC MEASUREMENTS (AD)

Height, weight, body mass index (BMI), growth pattern indices/percentile ranks, and weight history.

Body composition/growth/weight history (1.1)

❑ Height/length	AD-1.1.1
❑ Weight	AD-1.1.2

Body composition/growth/weight history (1.1), ***(cont'd)***

❑ Frame size	AD-1.1.3
❑ Weight change	AD-1.1.4
❑ Body mass index	AD-1.1.5
❑ Growth pattern indices/percentile ranks	AD-1.1.6
❑ Body compartment estimates	AD-1.1.7

BIOCHEMICAL DATA, MEDICAL TESTS AND PROCEDURES (BD)

Laboratory data, (e.g., electrolytes, glucose, and lipid panel) and tests (e.g., gastric emptying time, resting metabolic rate).

Acid-base balance (1.1)

❑ Arterial pH	BD-1.1.1
❑ Arterial bicarbonate	BD-1.1.2
❑ Partial pressure of carbon dioxide in arterial blood, $PaCO_2$	BD-1.1.3
❑ Partial pressure of oxygen in arterial blood, PaO_2	BD-1.1.4
❑ Venous pH	BD-1.1.5
❑ Venous bicarbonate	BD-1.1.6

Electrolyte and renal profile (1.2)

❑ BUN	BD-1.2.1
❑ Creatinine	BD-1.2.2
❑ BUN:creatinine ratio	BD-1.2.3
❑ Glomerular filtration rate	BD-1.2.4
❑ Sodium	BD-1.2.5
❑ Chloride	BD-1.2.6
❑ Potassium	BD-1.2.7
❑ Magnesium	BD-1.2.8
❑ Calcium, serum	BD-1.2.9
❑ Calcium, ionized	BD-1.2.10
❑ Phosphorus	BD-1.2.11
❑ Serum osmolality	BD-1.2.12
❑ Parathyroid hormone	BD-1.2.13

Essential fatty acid profile (1.3)

❑ Triene:Tetraene ratio	BD-1.3.1

Gastrointestinal profile (1.4)

❑ Alkaline phophatase	BD-1.4.1
❑ Alanine aminotransferase, ALT	BD-1.4.2
❑ Aspartate aminotransferase, AST	BD-1.4.3
❑ Gamma glutamyl transferase, GGT	BD-1.4.4
❑ Gastric residual volume	BD-1.4.5
❑ Bilirubin, total	BD-1.4.6
❑ Ammonia, serum	BD-1.4.7
❑ Toxicology report, including alcohol	BD-1.4.8
❑ Prothrombin time, PT	BD-1.4.9
❑ Partial thromboplastin time, PTT	BD-1.4.10
❑ INR (ratio)	BD-1.4.11
❑ Fecal fat	BD-1.4.12
❑ Amylase	BD-1.4.13
❑ Lipase	BD-1.4.14
❑ Other digestive enzymes *(specify)*	BD-1.4.15
❑ D-xylose	BD-1.4.16
❑ Hydrogen breath test	BD-1.4.17
❑ Intestinal biopsy	BD-1.4.18
❑ Stool culture	BD-1.4.19
❑ Gastric emptying time	BD-1.4.20
❑ Small bowel transit time	BD-1.4.21
❑ Abdominal films	BD-1.4.22
❑ Swallow study	BD-1.4.23

Glucose/endocrine profile (1.5)

❑ Glucose, fasting	BD-1.5.1
❑ Glucose, casual	BD-1.5.2
❑ HgbA1c	BD-1.5.3
❑ Preprandial capillary plasma glucose	BD-1.5.4
❑ Peak postprandial capillary plasma glucose	BD-1.5.5
❑ Glucose tolerance test	BD-1.5.6
❑ Cortisol level	BD-1.5.7
❑ IGF-binding protein	BD-1.5.8
❑ Thyroid function tests (TSH, T4, T3)	BD-1.5.9

Inflammatory profile (1.6)

❑ C-reactive protein	BD-1.6.1

Lipid profile (1.7)

❑ Cholesterol, serum	BD-1.7.1
❑ Cholesterol, HDL	BD-1.7.2
❑ Cholesterol, LDL	BD-1.7.3
❑ Cholesterol, non-HDL	BD-1.7.4
❑ Total cholesterol:HDL cholesterol	BD-1.7.5
❑ LDL:HDL	BD-1.7.6
❑ Triglycerides, serum	BD-1.7.7

Metabolic rate profile (1.8)

❑ Resting metabolic rate, measured	BD-1.8.1
❑ RQ	BD-1.8.2

Mineral profile (1.9)

❑ Copper, serum or plasma	BD-1.9.1
❑ Iodine, urinary excretion	BD-1.9.2
❑ Zinc, serum or plasma	BD-1.9.3
❑ Other	BD-1.9.4

Nutritional anemia profile (1.10)

❑ Hemoglobin	BD-1.10.1
❑ Hematocrit	BD-1.10.2
❑ Mean corpuscular volume	BD-1.10.3
❑ Red blood cell folate	BD-1.10.4
❑ Red cell distribution width	BD-1.10.5
❑ B12, serum	BD-1.10.6
❑ Methylmalonic acid, serum	BD-1.10.7
❑ Folate, serum	BD-1.10.8
❑ Homocysteine, serum	BD-1.10.9
❑ Ferritin, serum	BD-1.10.10
❑ Iron, serum	BD-1.10.11
❑ Total iron-binding capacity	BD-1.10.12
❑ Transferrin saturation	BD-1.10.13

Protein profile (1.11)

❑ Albumin	BD-1.11.1
❑ Prealbumin	BD-1.11.2
❑ Transferrin	BD-1.11.3
❑ Phenylalanine, plasma	BD-1.11.4
❑ Tyrosine, plasma	BD-1.11.5
❑ Amino acid, other, specify	BD-1.11.6
❑ Antibody level, specify	BD-1.11.7

Urine profile (1.12)

❑ Urine color	BD-1.12.1
❑ Urine osmolality	BD-1.12.2
❑ Urine specific gravity	BD-1.12.3
❑ Urine test, specify	BD-1.12.4
❑ Urine volume	BD-1.12.5

Vitamin profile (1.13)

❑ Vitamin A, serum or plasma retinol	BD-1.13.1
❑ Vitamin C, plasma or serum	BD-1.13.2
❑ Vitamin D, 25-hydroxy	BD-1.13.3
❑ Vitamin E, plasma alpha-tocopherol	BD-1.13.4
❑ Thiamin, activity coefficient for erythrocyte transketolase activity	BD-1.13.5
❑ Riboflavin, activity coefficient for erythrocyte glutathionereductase activity	BD-1.13.6
❑ Niacin, urinary N'methyl-nicotinamide concentration	BD-1.13.7
❑ Vitamin B6, plasma or serum pyridoxal 5'phosphate concentration	BD-1.13.8
❑ Other	BD-1.13.9

NUTRITION-FOCUSED PHYSICAL FINDINGS (PD)

Findings from an evaluation of body systems, muscle and subcutaneous fat wasting, oral health, suck/swallow/breathe ability, appetite, and affect.

Nutrition-focused physical findings (1.1)

❑ Overall appearance *(specify)* ______	PD-1.1.1
❑ Body language *(specify)* ______	PD-1.1.2
❑ Cardiovascular-pulmonary *(specify)* ______	PD-1.1.3
❑ Extremities, muscles and bones *(specify)* ______	PD-1.1.4
❑ Digestive system (mouth to rectum) *(specify)* ______	PD-1.1.5
❑ Head and eyes *(specify)* ______	PD-1.1.6
❑ Nerves and cognition *(specify)* ______	PD-1.1.7
❑ Skin *(specify)* ______	PD-1.1.8
❑ Vital signs *(specify)* ______	PD-1.1.9

CLIENT HISTORY (CH)

Current and past information related to personal, medical, family, and social history.

Personal History (1)

General patient/client information such as age, gender, race/ethnicity, language, education, and role in family.

Personal data (1.1)

❑ Age	CH-1.1.1
❑ Gender	CH-1.1.2
❑ Race/Ethnicity	CH-1.1.3
❑ Language	CH-1.1.4
❑ Literacy factors	CH-1.1.5
❑ Education	CH-1.1.6

Personal data (1.1), *(cont'd)*

- ❑ Role in family CH-1.1.7
- ❑ Tobacco use CH-1.1.8
- ❑ Physical disability CH-1.1.9
- ❑ Mobility CH-1.1.10

Patient/Client/Family Medical/Health History (2)

Patient/client or family disease states, conditions, and illnesses that may have nutritional impact.

Patient/client OR family nutrition-oriented medical/health history (2.1)

Specify issue(s) and whether it is patient/client history (P) or family history (F)

- ❑ Patient/client chief nutrition complaint CH-2.1.1
  (specify) ________ P or F
- ❑ Cardiovascular CH-2.1.2
  (specify) ________ P or F
- ❑ Endocrine/metabolism CH-2.1.3
  (specify) ________ P or F
- ❑ Excretory CH-2.1.4
  (specify) ________ P or F
- ❑ Gastrointestinal CH-2.1.5
  (specify) ________ P or F
- ❑ Gynecological CH-2.1.6
  (specify) ________ P or F
- ❑ Hematology/oncology CH-2.1.7
  (specify) ________ P or F
- ❑ Immune (e.g., food allergies) CH-2.1.8
  (specify) ________ P or F
- ❑ Integumentary CH-2.1.9
  (specify) ________ P or F
- ❑ Musculoskeletal CH-2.1.10
  (specify) ________ P or F
- ❑ Neurological CH-2.1.11
  (specify) ________ P or F
- ❑ Psychological CH-2.1.12
  (specify) ________ P or F
- ❑ Respiratory CH-2.1.13
  (specify) ________ P or F
- ❑ Other CH-2.1.14
  (specify) ________ P or F

Treatments/therapy/complementary/alternative medicine (2.2)

Documented medical or surgical treatments, complementary and alternative medicine that may impact nutritional status of the patient

- ❑ Medical treatment/therapy CH-2.2.1
  (specify) ________
- ❑ Surgical treatment CH-2.2.2
  (specify) ________
- ❑ Complementary/alternative medicine CH-2.2.3
  (specify) ________
- ❑ Palliative/end-of-life care CH-2.2.4
  (specify) ________

Social History (3)

Patient/client socioeconomic status, housing situation, medical care support and involvement in social groups.

Social history (3.1)

- ❑ Socioeconomic factors CH-3.1.1
  (specify) ________
- ❑ Living/housing situation CH-3.1.2
  (specify) ________
- ❑ Domestic issues CH-3.1.3
  (specify) ________
- ❑ Social and medical support CH-3.1.4
  (specify) ________
- ❑ Geographic location of home CH-3.1.5
  (specify) ________
- ❑ Occupation CH-3.1.6
  (specify) ________
- ❑ Religion CH-3.1.7
  (specify) ________
- ❑ History of recent crisis CH-3.1.8
  (specify) ________
- ❑ Daily stress level CH-3.1.9

COMPARATIVE STANDARDS (CS)

Energy Needs (1)

Estimated energy needs (1.1)

- ❑ Total energy estimated needs CS-1.1.1
- ❑ Method for estimating needs CS-1.1.2

Macronutrient Needs (2)

Estimated fat needs (2.1)

- ❑ Total fat estimated needs CS-2.1.1
- ❑ Type of fat needed CS-2.1.2
- ❑ Method for estimating needs CS-2.1.3

Estimated protein needs (2.2)

- ❑ Total protein estimated needs CS-2.2.1
- ❑ Type of protein needed CS-2.2.2
- ❑ Method for estimating needs CS-2.2.3

Estimated carbohydrate needs (2.3)

- ❑ Total carbohydrate estimated needs CS-2.3.1
- ❑ Type of carbohydrate needed CS-2.3.2
- ❑ Method for estimating needs CS-2.3.3

Estimated fiber needs (2.4)

- ❑ Total fiber estimated needs CS-2.4.1
- ❑ Type of fiber needed CS-2.4.2
- ❑ Method for estimating needs CS-2.4.3

Fluid Needs (3)

Estimated fluid needs (3.1)

- ❑ Total fluid estimated needs CS-3.1.1
- ❑ Method for estimating needs CS-3.1.2

Micronutrient Needs (4)

Estimated vitamin needs (4.1)

- ❑ A (1) ❑ Riboflavin (7)
- ❑ C (2) ❑ Niacin (8)
- ❑ D (3) ❑ Folate (9)
- ❑ E (4) ❑ B6 (10)
- ❑ K (5) ❑ B12 (11)
- ❑ Thiamin (6)
- ❑ Other *(specify)* (12)
- ❑ Method for estimating needs (13)

Estimated mineral needs (4.2)

- ❑ Calcium (1) ❑ Potassium (5)
- ❑ Chloride (2) ❑ Phosphorus (6)
- ❑ Iron (3) ❑ Sodium (7)
- ❑ Magnesium (4) ❑ Zinc (8)
- ❑ Other *(specify)* (9)
- ❑ Method for estimating needs (10)

Weight and Growth Recommendation (5)

Recommended body weight/body mass index/growth (5.1)

- ❑ Ideal/reference body weight (IBW) CS-5.1.1
- ❑ Recommended body mass index (BMI) CS-5.1.2
- ❑ Desired growth pattern CS-5.1.3

APPENDIX B

Nutrition Diagnostic Terminology

INTAKE — NI

Defined as "actual problems related to intake of energy, nutrients, fluids, bioactive substances through oral diet or nutrition support"

Energy Balance (1)

Defined as "actual or estimated changes in energy (kcal) balance"

- ❑ Unused — NI-1.1
- ❑ Increased energy expenditure — NI-1.2
- ❑ Unused — NI-1.3
- ❑ Inadequate energy intake — NI-1.4
- ❑ Excessive energy intake — NI-1.5
- ❑ Predicted suboptimal energy intake — NI-1.6
- ❑ Predicted excessive energy intake — NI-1.7

Oral or Nutrition Support Intake (2)

Defined as "actual or estimated food and beverage intake from oral diet or nutrition support compared with patient goal"

- ❑ Inadequate oral intake — NI-2.1
- ❑ Excessive oral intake — NI-2.2
- ❑ Inadequate enteral nutrition infusion — NI-2.3
- ❑ Excessive enteral nutrition infusion — NI-2.4
- ❑ Less than optimal enteral nutrition — NI-2.5
- ❑ Inadequate parenteral nutrition infusion — NI-2.6
- ❑ Excessive parenteral nutrition infusion — NI-2.7
- ❑ Less than optimal parenteral nutrition — NI-2.8
- ❑ Limited food acceptance — NI-2.9

Fluid Intake (3)

Defined as "actual or estimated fluid intake compared with patient goal"

- ❑ Inadequate fluid intake — NI-3.1
- ❑ Excessive fluid intake — NI-3.2

Bioactive Substances (4)

Defined as "actual or observed intake of bioactive substances, including single or multiple functional food components, ingredients, dietary supplements, alcohol"

- ❑ Inadequate bioactive substance intake — NI-4.1
- ❑ Excessive bioactive substance intake — NI-4.2
- ❑ Excessive alcohol intake — NI-4.3

Nutrient (5)

Defined as "actual or estimated intake of specific nutrient groups or single nutrients as compared with desired levels"

- ❑ Increased nutrient needs — NI-5.1
  (specify) ____________
- ❑ Malnutrition — NI-5.2
- ❑ Inadequate protein-energy intake — NI-5.3
- ❑ Decreased nutrient needs — NI-5.4
  (specify) ____________
- ❑ Imbalance of nutrients — NI-5.5

Fat and Cholesterol (5.6)

- ❑ Inadequate fat intake — NI-5.6.1
- ❑ Excessive fat intake — NI-5.6.2
- ❑ Inappropriate intake of fats — NI-5.6.3
  (specify) ____________

Protein (5.7)

- ❑ Inadequate protein intake — NI-5.7.1
- ❑ Excessive protein intake — NI-5.7.2
- ❑ Inappropriate intake of protein or amino acids — NI-5.7.3
  (specify) ____________

Carbohydrate and Fiber (5.8)

- ❑ Inadequate carbohydrate intake — NI-5.8.1
- ❑ Excessive carbohydrate intake — NI-5.8.2
- ❑ Inappropriate intake of types of carbohydrate — NI-5.8.3
  (specify) ____________
- ❑ Inconsistent carbohydrate intake — NI-5.8.4
- ❑ Inadequate fiber intake — NI-5.8.5
- ❑ Excessive fiber intake — NI-5.8.6

Vitamin (5.9)

- ❑ Inadequate vitamin intake — NI-5.9.1
  (specify) ____________
  - ❑ A (1) ❑ Riboflavin (7)
  - ❑ C (2) ❑ Niacin (8)
  - ❑ D (3) ❑ Folate (9)
  - ❑ E (4) ❑ B6 (10)
  - ❑ K (5) ❑ B12 (11)
  - ❑ Thiamin (6)
  - ❑ Other *(specify)* ____________ (12)
- ❑ Excessive vitamin intake — NI-5.9.2
  (specify) ____________
  - ❑ A (1) ❑ Riboflavin (7)
  - ❑ C (2) ❑ Niacin (8)
  - ❑ D (3) ❑ Folate (9)
  - ❑ E (4) ❑ B6 (10)
  - ❑ K (5) ❑ B12 (11)
  - ❑ Thiamin (6)
  - ❑ Other *(specify)* ____________ (12)

Mineral (5.10)

- ❑ Inadequate mineral intake — NI-5.10.1
  (specify) ____________
  - ❑ Calcium (1) ❑ Potassium (5)
  - ❑ Chloride (2) ❑ Phosphorus (6)
  - ❑ Iron (3) ❑ Sodium (7)
  - ❑ Magnesium (4) ❑ Zinc (8)
  - ❑ Other *(specify)* ____________ (9)
- ❑ Excessive mineral intake — NI-5.10.2
  (specify) ____________
  - ❑ Calcium (1) ❑ Potassium (5)
  - ❑ Chloride (2) ❑ Phosphorus (6)
  - ❑ Iron (3) ❑ Sodium (7)
  - ❑ Magnesium (4) ❑ Zinc (8)
  - ❑ Other *(specify)* ____________ (9)

Multi-nutrient (5.11)

- ❑ Predicted suboptimal nutrient intake — NI-5.11.1
- ❑ Predicted excessive nutrient intake — NI-5.11.2

CLINICAL — NC

Defined as "nutritional findings/problems identified that relate to medical or physical conditions"

Functional (1)

Defined as "change in physical or mechanical functioning that interferes with or prevents desired nutritional consequences"

- ❑ Swallowing difficulty — NC-1.1
- ❑ Biting/Chewing (masticatory) difficulty — NC-1.2

Functional (1), ***(cont'd)***

❑ Breastfeeding difficulty	NC-1.3
❑ Altered GI function	NC-1.4

Biochemical (2)

Defined as "change in capacity to metabolize nutrients as a result of medications, surgery, or as indicated by altered lab values"

❑ Impaired nutrient utilization	NC-2.1
❑ Altered nutrition-related laboratory values (specify) ________	NC-2.2
❑ Food-medication interaction	NC-2.3
❑ Predicted food-medication interaction	NC-2.4

Weight (3)

Defined as "chronic weight or changed weight status when compared with usual or desired body weight"

❑ Underweight	NC-3.1
❑ Unintended weight loss	NC-3.2
❑ Overweight/obesity	NC-3.3
❑ Unintended weight gain	NC-3.4

BEHAVIORAL-ENVIRONMENTAL NB

Defined as "nutritional findings/problems identified that relate to knowledge, attitudes/beliefs, physical environment, access to food, or food safety"

Knowledge and Beliefs (1)

Defined as "actual knowledge and beliefs as related, observed, or documented"

❑ Food- and nutrition-related knowledge deficit	NB-1.1
❑ Harmful beliefs/attitudes about food- or nutrition-related topics (use with caution)	NB-1.2
❑ Not ready for diet/lifestyle change	NB-1.3
❑ Self-monitoring deficit	NB-1.4
❑ Disordered eating pattern	NB-1.5
❑ Limited adherence to nutrition-related recommendations	NB-1.6
❑ Undesirable food choices	NB-1.7

Physical Activity and Function (2)

Defined as "actual physical activity, self-care, and quality-of-life problems as reported, observed, or documented"

❑ Physical inactivity	NB-2.1
❑ Excessive physical activity	NB-2.2
❑ Inability or lack of desire to manage self-care	NB-2.3
❑ Impaired ability to prepare foods/meals	NB-2.4
❑ Poor nutrition quality of life	NB-2.5
❑ Self-feeding difficulty	NB-2.6

Food Safety and Access (3)

Defined as "actual problems with food safety or access to food, water, or nutrition-related supplies"

❑ Intake of unsafe food	NB-3.1
❑ Limited access to food or water	NB-3.2
❑ Limited access to nutrition-related supplies	NB-3.3

APPENDIX C

Nutrition Intervention Terminology

NUTRITION PRESCRIPTION

The patient/client's individualized recommended dietary intake of energy and/or selected foods or nutrients based on current reference standards and dietary guidelines and the patient/client's health condition and nutrition diagnosis (*specify*).

____

____

____

FOOD AND/OR NUTRIENT DELIVERY — ND

Meal and Snacks (1)
Regular eating event (meal); food served between regular meals (snack).

- ❑ General/healthful diet — ND-1.1
- ❑ Modify distribution, type, or amount of food and nutrients within meals or at specified time — ND-1.2
- ❑ Specific foods/beverages or groups — ND-1.3
- ❑ Other — ND-1.4
  (specify) ______________

Enteral and Parenteral Nutrition (2)
Nutrition provided through the GI tract via tube, catheter, or stoma (enteral) or intravenously (centrally or peripherally) (parenteral).

Enteral Nutrition (2.1)
Nutrition provided through the GI tract.

- ❑ Formula/solution — ND-2.1.1
- ❑ Insert enteral feeding tube — ND-2.1.2
- ❑ Site care — ND-2.1.3
- ❑ Feeding tube flush — ND-2.1.4

Parenteral Nutrition/IV Fluids (2.2)
Nutrition and fluids provided intravenously.

- ❑ Formula/solution — ND-2.2.1
- ❑ Site care — ND-2.2.2
- ❑ IV fluids — ND-2.2.3

Supplements (3)

Medical Food Supplements (3.1)
Commercial or prepared foods or beverages that supplement energy, protein, carbohydrate, fiber, fat intake.

Type

- ❑ Commercial beverage — ND-3.1.1
- ❑ Commercial food — ND-3.1.2
- ❑ Modified beverage — ND-3.1.3
- ❑ Modified food — ND-3.1.4
- ❑ Purpose — ND-3.1.5
  (specify) ______________

Vitamin and Mineral Supplements (3.2)
Supplemental vitamins or minerals.

- ❑ Multivitamin/mineral — ND-3.2.1
- ❑ Multi-trace elements — ND-3.2.2
- ❑ Vitamin — ND-3.2.3
  - ❑ A (1) ❑ Riboflavin (7)
  - ❑ C (2) ❑ Niacin (8)
  - ❑ D (3) ❑ Folate (9)
  - ❑ E (4) ❑ B6 (10)
  - ❑ K (5) ❑ B12 (11)
  - ❑ Thiamin (6)
  - ❑ Other *(specify)* ______________ (12)
- ❑ Mineral — ND-3.2.4
  - ❑ Calcium (1) ❑ Potassium (5)
  - ❑ Chloride (2) ❑ Phosphorus (6)
  - ❑ Iron (3) ❑ Sodium (7)
  - ❑ Magnesium (4) ❑ Zinc (8)
  - ❑ Other *(specify)* ______________ (9)

Bioactive Substance Management (3.3)
Addition or change in provision of bioactive substances.

- ❑ Plant sterol and stanol esters — ND-3.3.1
- ❑ Soy protein — ND-3.3.2
- ❑ Psyllium and β-glucan — ND-3.3.3
- ❑ Food additives — ND-3.3.4
- ❑ Other — ND-3.3.5
  (specify) ______________

Feeding Assistance (4)
Accommodation or assistance in eating.

- ❑ Adaptive equipment — ND-4.1
- ❑ Feeding position — ND-4.2
- ❑ Meal set-up — ND-4.3
- ❑ Mouth care — ND-4.4
- ❑ Other — ND-4.5
  (specify) ______________

Feeding Environment (5)
Adjustment of the factors where food is served that impact food consumption.

- ❑ Lighting — ND-5.1
- ❑ Odors — ND-5.2
- ❑ Distractions — ND-5.3
- ❑ Table height — ND-5.4
- ❑ Table service/set up — ND-5.5
- ❑ Room temperature — ND-5.6
- ❑ Other — ND-5.7
  (specify) ______________

Nutrition-Related Medication Management (6)
Modification of a medication or herbal to optimize patient/client nutritional or health status.
❑ Medications ND-6.1
(specify prescription or OTC) ____
❑ Herbal/complementary products ND-6.2
(specify) ____

NUTRITION EDUCATION **E**

Nutrition Education-Content (1)
Instruction or training intended to lead to nutrition-related knowledge.
❑ Purpose of the nutrition education E-1.1
❑ Priority modifications E-1.2
❑ Survival information E-1.3
❑ Nutrition relationship to health/disease E-1.4
❑ Recommended modifications E-1.5
❑ Other or related topics E-1.6
❑ Other E-1.7
(specify) ____

Nutrition Education-Application (2)
Instruction or training leading to nutrition-related result interpretation or skills.
❑ Result interpretation E-2.1
❑ Skill development E-2.2
❑ Other E-2.3
(specify) ____

NUTRITION COUNSELING C

Theoretical Basis/Approach (1)
The theories or models used to design and implement an intervention.
❑ Cognitive-Behavioral Theory C-1.1
❑ Health Belief Model C-1.2
❑ Social Learning Theory C-1.3
❑ Transtheoretical Model/Stages of Change C-1.4
❑ Other C-1.5
(specify) ____

Strategies (2)
Selectively applied evidence-based methods or plans of action designed to achieve a particular goal.
❑ Motivational interviewing C-2.1
❑ Goal setting C-2.2
❑ Self-monitoring C-2.3
❑ Problem solving C-2.4
❑ Social support C-2.5
❑ Stress management C-2.6
❑ Stimulus control C-2.7
❑ Cognitive restructuring C-2.8
❑ Relapse prevention C-2.9
❑ Rewards/contingency management C-2.10
❑ Other C-2.11
(specify) ____

COORDINATION OF NUTRITION CARE RC

Coordination of Other Care During Nutrition Care (1)
Facilitating services with other professionals, institutions, or agencies during nutrition care.
❑ Team meeting RC-1.1
❑ Referral to RD with different expertise RC-1.2
❑ Collaboration/referral to other providers RC-1.3
❑ Referral to community agencies/ programs RC-1.4
(specify) ____

Discharge and Transfer of Nutrition Care to New Setting or Provider (2)
Discharge planning and transfer of nutrition care from one level or location of care to another.
❑ Collaboration/referral to other providers RC-2.1
❑ Referral to community agencies/ programs RC-2.2
(specify) ____

APPENDIX

D

Food Record Recording Form

7 - Day Food Diary

Name ______________________ Age ________

Address ______________________ City ________

State ______________ Zip ________ Phone ________

Height ____________ Weight ____________ Sex ________

Physician/Dietitian ______________________ Phone ________

For Females Only: Are you pregnant? ____________

Are you breast-feeding? ____________

Directions for Using the Food Diary

1. Keep your food diary current. List foods immediately after they are eaten. **Please print all entries**.
2. Record only one food item per line in this record booklet.
3. Be as specific as possible when describing the food item eaten: the way it was cooked (if it was cooked) and the amount that was eaten.
4. Include brand names whenever possible.
5. Report only the food portion that was actually eaten — for example: **T-bone steak, 4-oz broiled.** (Do not include the bones.)
6. Record amounts in household measures — for example: **ounces, tablespoons, cups, slices** or **units**, as in 1 cup nonfat milk, two slices of wheat toast, or one raw apple.
7. Include method that was used to prepare food item — for example: **fresh, frozen, stewed, fried, baked, canned, broiled, raw**, or **braised**.
8. For canned foods, include the liquid in which it was canned — for example: **sliced peaches in heavy syrup, fruit cocktail in light syrup,** or **tuna in water**.
9. Food items listed without specific amounts eaten will be analyzed using portion sizes.
10. Do not alter your normal diet during the period you keep this diary.
11. Remember to record the amounts of visible fats (oils, butter, salad dressings, margarine, and so on) you eat or use in cooking.

Time	Food Item and Method of Preparation	Amount Eaten
7 am	Apple, raw, fresh	1 medium
12 pm	Beef Stew	10 oz portion
12 pm	Bread, whole wheat, fresh	2 Slices
3 pm	Cereal, Corn Flakes	2 Cups
	with sugar	2 Tbs.
	with milk, non fat	½ cup
7 pm	Chicken, Fried	2 legs
7 pm	Coleslaw, with mayo	1 cup
7 pm	Eggs, Chicken (fried in butter)	2 large
7 pm	Fish, salmon, baked	10 oz

Name ______________________________ Date ______________

Time	Food Item and Method of Preparation	Amount Eaten

APPENDIX

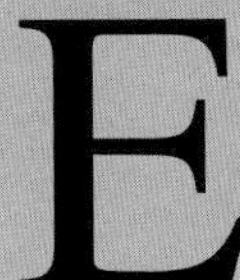

Fruit and Vegetable Screener Developed by the U.S. National Cancer Institute

From Risk Factor Monitoring and Methods Branch, National Cancer Institute, National Institutes for Health, U.S. Department of Health and Human Services.

NATIONAL INSTITUTES OF HEALTH
EATING AT AMERICA'S TABLE STUDY
QUICK FOOD SCAN

- The person who completed the telephone interviews for the Eating at America's Table Study should fill out this questionnaire.
- Use only a No. 2 pencil.
- Be certain to completely blacken in each of the answers, and erase completely if you make any changes.
- Do not make any stray marks on this form.
- When you complete this questionnaire, please return it in the postage-paid envelope to:

  National Cancer Institute
  EPN, Room 313
  6130 Executive Blvd., MSC 7344
  Bethesda, MD 20892-7344

BAR

CODE

LABEL

HERE

NOTIFICATION TO RESPONDENT OF ESTIMATED BURDEN

Public reporting burden for this collection of information is estimated to average 15 minutes per response, including the time for reviewing instructions, searching existing data sources, gathering and maintaining the data needed, and completing and reviewing the collection of information. An agency may not conduct or sponsor, and a person is not required to respond to, a collection of information unless it displays a currently valid OMB control number. Send comments regarding this burden estimate or any other aspect of this collection of information, including suggestions for reducing this burden, to: NIH, Project Clearance Office, 6701 Rockledge Drive, MSC 7730, Bethesda, MD 20892-7730, ATTN: PRA (0925-0450). Do not return the completed form to this address.

PLEASE DO NOT WRITE IN THIS AREA

SERIAL

INSTRUCTIONS

- **Think about what you usually ate last month.**
- **Please think about all the fruits and vegetables that you ate last month. Include those that were:**
  - **raw and cooked,**
  - **eaten as snacks and at meals,**
  - **eaten at home and away from home (restaurants, friends, take-out), and**
  - **eaten alone and mixed with other foods.**
- **Report how many times per month, week, or day you ate each food, and if you ate it, how much you usually had.**
- **If you mark "Never" for a question, follow the "Go to" instruction.**
- **Choose the best answer for each question. Mark only one response for each question.**

1. Over the last month, how many times per month, week, or day did you drink **100% juice** such as orange, apple, grape, or grapefruit juice? **Do not count** fruit drinks like Kool-Aid, lemonade, Hi-C, cranberry juice drink, Tang, and Twister. Include juice you drank at all mealtimes and between meals.

○	○	○	○	○	○	○	○	○	○
Never (Go to Question 2)	1-3 times last month	1-2 times per week	3-4 times per week	5-6 times per week	1 time per day	2 times per day	3 times per day	4 times per day	5 or more times per day

1a. Each time you drank **100% juice**, how much did you usually drink?

○	○	○	○
Less than ¾ cup (less than 6 ounces)	¾ to 1¼ cup (6 to 10 ounces)	1¼ to 2 cups (10 to 16 ounces)	More than 2 cups (more than 16 ounces)

2. Over the last month, how many times per month, week, or day did you eat **fruit**? Count any kind of fruit—fresh, canned, and frozen. **Do not count** juices. Include fruit you ate at all mealtimes and for snacks.

○	○	○	○	○	○	○	○	○	○
Never (Go to Question 3)	1-3 times last month	1-2 times per week	3-4 times per week	5-6 times per week	1 time per day	2 times per day	3 times per day	4 times per day	5 or more times per day

2a. Each time you ate **fruit**, how much did you usually eat?

○	○	○	○
Less than 1 medium fruit	1 medium fruit	2 medium fruits	More than 2 medium fruits

OR

○	○	○	○
Less than ½ cup	About ½ cup	About 1 cup	More than 1 cup

3. Over the last month, how often did you eat **lettuce salad (with or without other vegetables)**?

○ Never (Go to Question 4) ○ 1-3 times last month ○ 1-2 times per week ○ 3-4 times per week ○ 5-6 times per week ○ 1 time per day ○ 2 times per day ○ 3 times per day ○ 4 times per day ○ 5 or more times per day

3a. Each time you ate **lettuce salad**, how much did you usually eat?

○ About ½ cup ○ About 1 cup ○ About 2 cups ○ More than 2 cups

4. Over the last month, how often did you eat **French fries** or **fried potatoes**?

○ Never (Go to Question 5) ○ 1-3 times last month ○ 1-2 times per week ○ 3-4 times per week ○ 5-6 times per week ○ 1 time per day ○ 2 times per day ○ 3 times per day ○ 4 times per day ○ 5 or more times per day

4a. Each time you ate **French fries** or **fried potatoes**, how much did you usually eat?

○ Small order or less (About 1 cup or less) ○ Medium order (About 1½ cups) ○ Large order (About 2 cups) ○ Super Size order or more (About 3 cups or more)

5. Over the last month, how often did you eat **other white potatoes**? Count **baked, boiled**, and **mashed potatoes, potato salad,** and **white potatoes that were not fried.**

○ Never (Go to Question 6) ○ 1-3 times last month ○ 1-2 times per week ○ 3-4 times per week ○ 5-6 times per week ○ 1 time per day ○ 2 times per day ○ 3 times per day ○ 4 times per day ○ 5 or more times per day

5a. Each time you ate **these potatoes**, how much did you usually eat?

○ 1 small potato or less (½ cup or less) ○ 1 medium potato (½ to 1 cup) ○ 1 large potato (1 to 1½ cups) ○ 2 medium potatoes or more (1½ cups or more)

6. Over the last month, how often did you eat **cooked dried beans**? Count **baked beans, bean soup, refried beans, pork and beans** and **other bean dishes.**

○ Never (Go to Question 7) ○ 1-3 times last month ○ 1-2 times per week ○ 3-4 times per week ○ 5-6 times per week ○ 1 time per day ○ 2 times per day ○ 3 times per day ○ 4 times per day ○ 5 or more times per day

6a. Each time you ate **these beans**, how much did you usually eat?

○ Less than ½ cup ○ ½ to 1 cup ○ 1 to 1½ cups ○ More than 1½ cups

7. Over the last month, how often did you eat **other vegetables**?

DO NOT COUNT:
- Lettuce salads
- White potatoes
- Cooked dried beans
- Vegetables in mixtures, such as in sandwiches, omelets, casseroles, Mexican dishes, stews, stir-fry, soups, etc.
- Rice

COUNT:
- All other vegetables—raw, cooked, canned, and frozen

○ Never (Go to Question 8) ○ 1-3 times last month ○ 1-2 times per week ○ 3-4 times per week ○ 5-6 times per week ○ 1 time per day ○ 2 times per day ○ 3 times per day ○ 4 times per day ○ 5 or more times per day

7a. Each of these times that you ate **other vegetables**, how much did you usually eat?

○ Less than ½ cup ○ ½ to 1 cup ○ 1 to 2 cups ○ More than 2 cups

8. Over the last month, how often did you eat **tomato sauce**? Include tomato sauce on pasta or macaroni, rice, pizza and other dishes.

○ Never (Go to Question 9) ○ 1-3 times last month ○ 1-2 times per week ○ 3-4 times per week ○ 5-6 times per week ○ 1 time per day ○ 2 times per day ○ 3 times per day ○ 4 times per day ○ 5 or more times per day

8a. Each time you ate **tomato sauce**, how much did you usually eat?

○ About ¼ cup ○ About ½ cup ○ About 1 cup ○ More than 1 cup

9. Over the last month, how often did you eat **vegetable soups**? Include tomato soup, gazpacho, beef with vegetable soup, minestrone soup, and other soups made with vegetables.

○ Never (Go to Question 10) ○ 1-3 times last month ○ 1-2 times per week ○ 3-4 times per week ○ 5-6 times per week ○ 1 time per day ○ 2 times per day ○ 3 times per day ○ 4 times per day ○ 5 or more times per day

9a. Each time you ate **vegetable soup**, how much did you usually eat?

○ Less than 1 cup ○ 1 to 2 cups ○ 2 to 3 cups ○ More than 3 cups

10. Over the last month, how often did you eat **mixtures that included vegetables**? Count such foods as sandwiches, casseroles, stews, stir-fry, omelets, and tacos.

○ Never ○ 1-3 times last month ○ 1-2 times per week ○ 3-4 times per week ○ 5-6 times per week ○ 1 time per day ○ 2 times per day ○ 3 times per day ○ 4 times per day ○ 5 or more times per day

DesignExpert™ by NCS Printed in U.S.A. Mark Reflex® EW-226427-1:654321 HC03

Thank you very much for completing this questionnaire. Please return it in the enclosed, postage-paid envelope or to the address listed on the front page.

APPENDIX

MEDFICTS* Dietary Assessment Questionnaire

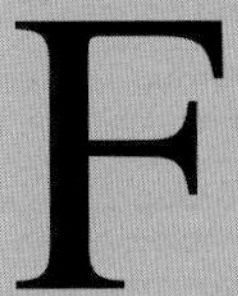

In each food category for both Group 1 and Group 2 foods check one box from the "Weekly Consumption" column (number of servings eaten per week) and then check one box from the "Serving Size" column. If you check Rarely/Never, do not check a serving size box. See next page for score.

Food Category	Weekly Consumption			Serving Size			Score
	Rarely/ never	3 or less	4 or more	Small <5 oz/d 1 pt	Average 5 oz/d 2 pts	Large >5 oz/d 3 pts	
Meats • Recommended amount per day: ≤5 oz (equal in size to 2 decks of playing cards) • Base your estimate on the food you consume most often. • Beef and lamb selections are trimmed to 1/8" fat.							
Group 1. 10 gm or more total fat in 3 oz cooked portion **Beef –** Ground beef, Ribs, Steak (T-bone, Flank, Porterhouse, Tenderloin), Chuck blade roast, Brisket, Meatloaf (w/ground beef), Corned beef **Processed meats –** ¼ lb burger or lg. sandwich, Bacon, Lunch meat, Sausage/knockwurst, Hot dogs, Ham (bone-end), Ground turkey **Other meats, Poultry, Seafood**—Pork chops (center loin), Pork roast (Blade, Boston, Sirloin), Pork spareribs, Ground pork, Lamb chops, Lamb (ribs), Organ meats[†], Chicken w/skin, Eel, Mackerel, Pompano	☐	☐ 3 pts	☐ 7pts x	☐ 1 pt	☐ 2 pts	☐ 3 pts	____
Group 2. Less than 10 gm total fat in 3 oz cooked portion **Lean beef –** Round steak (Eye of round, Top round), Sirloin[‡], Tip & bottom round[‡], Chuck arm pot roast[‡], Top Loin[‡] **Low-fat processed meats –** Low-fat lunch meat, Canadian bacon, "Lean" fast food sandwich, Boneless ham **Other meats, Poultry, Seafood –** Chicken, Turkey (w/o skin)[§], most Seafood[†], Lamb leg shank, Pork tenderloin, Sirloin top loin, Veal cutlets, Sirloin, Shoulder, Ground veal, Venison, Veal chops and ribs[‡], Lamb (whole leg, loin, fore-shank, sirloin)[‡]	☐	☐	☐	☐	☐	☐[¥] 6 pts	____
Eggs – Weekly consumption is the number of times you eat eggs each week				Check the number of eggs eaten each time			
Group 1. Whole eggs, Yolks	☐	☐ 3 pts	☐ 7 pts x	≤1 ☐ 1 pt	2 ☐ 2 pts	≥3 ☐ 3 pts	____
Group 2. Egg whites, Egg substitutes (½ cup)	☐	☐	☐	☐	☐	☐	____
Dairy							
Milk – Average serving 1 cup **Group 1.** Whole milk, 2% milk, 2% buttermilk, Yogurt (whole milk)	☐	☐ 3 pts	☐ 7 pts x	☐ 1 pt	☐ 2 pts	☐ 3 pts	____
Group 2. Fat-free milk, 1% milk, Fat-free buttermilk, Yogurt (Fat-free, 1% low fat)	☐	☐	☐	☐	☐	☐	____
Cheese – Average serving 1 oz **Group 1.** Cream cheese, Cheddar, Monterey Jack, Colby, Swiss, American processed, Blue cheese, Regular cottage cheese (½ cup), and Ricotta (¼ cup)	☐	☐ 3 pts	☐ 7 pts x	☐ 1 pt	☐ 2 pts	☐ 3 pts	____
Group 2. Low-fat & fat-free cheeses, Fat-free milk mozzarella, String cheese, Low-fat, Fat-free milk & Fat-free cottage cheese (½ cup) and Ricotta (¼ cup)	☐	☐	☐	☐	☐	☐	____
Frozen Desserts – Average serving ½ cup **Group 1.** Ice cream, Milk shakes	☐	☐ 3 pts	☐ 7 pts x	☐ 1 pt	☐ 2 pts	☐ 3 pts	____
Group 2. Low-fat ice cream, Frozen yogurt	☐	☐	☐	☐	☐	☐	____

Food Category	Weekly Consumption: Rarely/ never	Weekly Consumption: 3 or less	Weekly Consumption: 4 or more	Serving Size: Small <5 oz/d 1 pt	Serving Size: Average 5 oz/d 2 pts	Serving Size: Large >5 oz/d 3 pts	Score
Frying Foods – Average servings: see below. This section refers to method of prepartion for vegetables and meat.							
Group 1. French fries, Fried vegetables (½ cup), Fried chicken, fish, meat (3 oz)	☐	☐ 3 pts	☐ 7 pts	x ☐ 1 pt	☐ 2 pts	☐ 3 pts	____
Group 2. Vegetables, not deep fried (½ cup), Meat, poultry, or fish—prepared by baking, broiling, grilling, poaching, roasting, stewing: (3 oz)	☐	☐	☐	☐	☐	☐	____
In Baked Goods – 1 Average serving							
Group 1. Doughnuts, Biscuits, Butter rolls, Muffins, Croissants, Sweet rolls, Danish, Cakes, Pies, Coffee cakes, Cookies	☐	☐ 3 pts	☐ 7 pts	x ☐ 1 pt	☐ 2 pts	☐ 3 pts	____
Group 2. Fruit bars, Low-fat cookies/cakes/pastries, Angel food cake, Homemade baked goods with vegetable oils, breads, bagels	☐	☐	☐	☐	☐	☐	____
Convenience Foods							
Group 1. Canned, Packaged, or Frozen dinners: e.g., Pizza (1 slice), Macaroni & cheese (1 cup), Pot pie (1), Cream soups (1 cup), Potato, rice & pasta dishes with cream/cheese sauces (½ cup)	☐	☐ 3 pts	☐ 7 pts	x ☐ 1 pt	☐ 2 pts	☐ 3 pts	____
Group 2. Diet/Reduced calorie or reduced fat dinners (1), Potato, rice & pasta dishes without cream/cheese sauces (½ cup)	☐	☐	☐	☐	☐	☐	____
Table Fats – Average serving: 1 Tbsp							
Group 1. Butter, Stick margarine, Regular salad dressing, Mayonnaise, Sour cream (2 Tbsp)	☐	☐ 3 pts	☐ 7 pts	x ☐ 1 pt	☐ 2 pts	☐ 3 pts	____
Group 2. Diet and tub margarine, Low-fat & fat-free salad dressing, Low-fat & fat-free mayonnaise	☐	☐	☐	☐	☐	☐	____
Snacks							
Group 1. Chips (potato, corn, taco), Cheese puffs, Snack mix, Nuts (1 oz), Regular crackers (½ oz), Candy (milk chocolate, caramel, coconut) (about 1½ oz), Regular popcorn (3 cups)	☐	☐ 3 pts	☐ 7 pts	x ☐ 1 pt	☐ 2 pts	☐ 3 pts	____
Group 2. Pretzels, Fat-free chips (1 oz), Low-fat crackers (1/2 oz), Fruit, Fruit rolls, Licorice, Hard candy (1 med piece), Bread sticks (1–2 pcs), Air-popped or low-fat popcorn (3 cups)	☐	☐	☐	☐	☐	☐	____

† Organ meats, shrimp, abalone, and squid are low in fat but high in cholesterol.
‡ Only lean cuts with all visible fat trimmed. If not trimmed of all visible fat, score as if in Group 1.
¥ Score 6 pts if this box is checked.
§ All parts not listed in group 1 have <10 gm total fat.

Total from page 1 _____

Total from page 2 _____

FINAL SCORE _____

To Score: For each food category, multiply points in weekly consumption box by points in serving size box and record total in score column. If Group 2 foods checked, no points are scored (except for Group 2 meats, large serving = 6 pts).

Example:

☐	☐ 3 pts	☑ 7 pts	x ☐ 1 pt	☐ 2 pts	☑ 3 pts	21

Add score on page 1 and page 2 to get final score.

Key:
≥70 Need to make some dietary changes
40–70 Heart-Healthy Diet
<40 TLC Diet

From National Cholesterol Education Program. 2001. *Third report of the Expert Panel on Detection, Evaluation, and Treatment of High Blood Cholesterol in Adults.* Bethesda, MD: U.S. Department of Health and Human Services.

*MEDFICTS = **M**eats, **E**ggs, **D**airy, **F**rying Foods, **I**n baked goods, **C**onvenience foods, **T**able fats, **S**nacks.

APPENDIX

G

The National Institute of Health's The Diet History Questionnaire II

From the Risk Factor Monitoring and Methods Branch, Division of Cancer Control and Population Sciences, National Cancer Institute, National Institutes of Health, U.S. Department of Health and Human Services. http://www.riskfactor.cancer.gov/dhq2/.

*This appendix contains the first eight pages of the Diet History Questionnaire II. For the complete questionnaire, visit the *Nutritional Assessment* website at www.mhhe.com/lee-nieman6.

NATIONAL INSTITUTES OF HEALTH

Diet History Questionnaire II

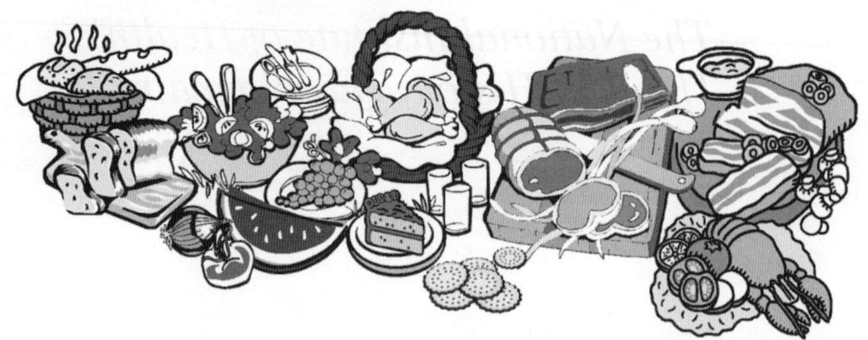

GENERAL INSTRUCTIONS

- Answer each question as best you can. Estimate if you are not sure. A guess is better than leaving a blank.
- Use only a black ball-point pen. Do not use a pencil or felt-tip pen. Do not fold, staple, or tear the pages.
- Put an X in the box next to your answer.
- If you make any changes, cross out the incorrect answer and put an X in the box next to the correct answer. Also draw a circle around the correct answer.
- If you mark NEVER, NO, or DON'T KNOW for a question, please follow any arrows or instructions that direct you to the next question.

BEFORE TURNING THE PAGE, PLEASE COMPLETE THE FOLLOWING QUESTIONS.

Today's date:

MONTH	DAY		YEAR
☐ Jan	☐0	☐0	☐ 2010
☐ Feb	☐1	☐1	☐ 2011
☐ Mar	☐2	☐2	☐ 2012
☐ Apr	☐3	☐3	☐ 2013
☐ May		☐4	☐ 2014
☐ Jun		☐5	☐ 2015
☐ Jul		☐6	☐ 2016
☐ Aug		☐7	☐ 2017
☐ Sep		☐8	☐ 2018
☐ Oct		☐9	☐ 2019
☐ Nov			☐ 2020
☐ Dec			

In what month were you born?

☐ Jan
☐ Feb
☐ Mar
☐ Apr
☐ May
☐ Jun
☐ Jul
☐ Aug
☐ Sep
☐ Oct
☐ Nov
☐ Dec

In what year were you born?

19 |___|___|

☐0	☐0
☐1	☐1
☐2	☐2
☐3	☐3
☐4	☐4
☐5	☐5
☐6	☐6
☐7	☐7
☐8	☐8
☐9	☐9

Are you male or female?

☐Male
☐Female

BAR CODE LABEL OR SUBJECT ID HERE

|___|___|___|___|___|___|___|___|

DHQ II PastYear

1. Over the past 12 months, how often did you drink **carrot juice**?

- ☐ NEVER (GO TO QUESTION 2)

- ☐ 1 time per month or less
- ☐ 2–3 times per month
- ☐ 1–2 times per week
- ☐ 3–4 times per week
- ☐ 5–6 times per week
- ☐ 1 time per day
- ☐ 2–3 times per day
- ☐ 4–5 times per day
- ☐ 6 or more times per day

1a. Each time you drank **carrot juice**, how much did you usually drink?

- ☐ Less than ½ cup (4 ounces)
- ☐ ½ to 1¼ cups (4 to 10 ounces)
- ☐ More than 1¼ cups (10 ounces)

2. Over the past 12 months, how often did you drink **tomato juice** or **other vegetable juice**? *(Please do not include carrot juice.)*

- ☐ NEVER (GO TO QUESTION 3)

- ☐ 1 time per month or less
- ☐ 2–3 times per month
- ☐ 1–2 times per week
- ☐ 3–4 times per week
- ☐ 5–6 times per week
- ☐ 1 time per day
- ☐ 2–3 times per day
- ☐ 4–5 times per day
- ☐ 6 or more times per day

2a. Each time you drank **tomato juice** or **other vegetable juice**, how much did you usually drink?

- ☐ Less than ¾ cup (6 ounces)
- ☐ ¾ to 1¼ cups (6 to 10 ounces)
- ☐ More than 1¼ cups (10 ounces)

3. Over the past 12 months, how often did you drink **orange juice** or **grapefruit juice?**

- ☐ NEVER (GO TO QUESTION 4)

- ☐ 1 time per month or less
- ☐ 2–3 times per month
- ☐ 1–2 times per week
- ☐ 3–4 times per week
- ☐ 5–6 times per week
- ☐ 1 time per day
- ☐ 2–3 times per day
- ☐ 4–5 times per day
- ☐ 6 or more times per day

3a. Each time you drank **orange juice** or **grapefruit juice**, how much did you usually drink?

- ☐ Less than ¾ cup (6 ounces)
- ☐ ¾ to 1¼ cups (6 to 10 ounces)
- ☐ More than 1¼ cups (10 ounces)

Question 4 appears in the next column

3b. How often was the orange juice or grapefruit juice you drank **calcium-fortified**?

- ☐ Almost never or never
- ☐ About ¼ of the time
- ☐ About ½ of the time
- ☐ About ¾ of the time
- ☐ Almost always or always

4. Over the past 12 months, how often did you drink **other 100% fruit juice** or **100% fruit juice mixtures** (such as apple, grape, pineapple, or others)?

- ☐ NEVER (GO TO QUESTION 5)

- ☐ 1 time per month or less
- ☐ 2–3 times per month
- ☐ 1–2 times per week
- ☐ 3–4 times per week
- ☐ 5–6 times per week
- ☐ 1 time per day
- ☐ 2–3 times per day
- ☐ 4–5 times per day
- ☐ 6 or more times per day

4a. Each time you drank **other 100% fruit juice** or **100% fruit juice mixtures**, how much did you usually drink?

- ☐ Less than ¾ cup (6 ounces)
- ☐ ¾ to 1½ cups (6 to 12 ounces)
- ☐ More than 1½ cups (12 ounces)

4b. How often were the other 100% fruit juice or 100% fruit juice mixtures you drank **calcium-fortified**?

- ☐ Almost never or never
- ☐ About ¼ of the time
- ☐ About ½ of the time
- ☐ About ¾ of the time
- ☐ Almost always or always

5. How often did you drink **other fruit drinks** (such as cranberry cocktail, Hi-C, lemonade, or Kool-Aid, diet or regular)?

- ☐ NEVER (GO TO QUESTION 6)

- ☐ 1 time per month or less
- ☐ 2–3 times per month
- ☐ 1–2 times per week
- ☐ 3–4 times per week
- ☐ 5–6 times per week
- ☐ 1 time per day
- ☐ 2–3 times per day
- ☐ 4–5 times per day
- ☐ 6 or more times per day

Question 6 appears on the next page

Over the past 12 months…

5a. Each time you drank **fruit drinks**, how much did you usually drink?

- ☐ Less than 1 cup (8 ounces)
- ☐ 1 to 2 cups (8 to 16 ounces)
- ☐ More than 2 cups (16 ounces)

5b. How often were your fruit drinks **diet** or **sugar-free**?

- ☐ Almost never or never
- ☐ About ¼ of the time
- ☐ About ½ of the time
- ☐ About ¾ of the time
- ☐ Almost always or always

6. How often did you drink **milk as a beverage** (NOT in coffee, NOT in cereal)? *(Please do not include chocolate milk and hot chocolate.)*

- ☐ NEVER (GO TO QUESTION 7)

- ☐ 1 time per month or less
- ☐ 2–3 times per month
- ☐ 1–2 times per week
- ☐ 3–4 times per week
- ☐ 5–6 times per week
- ☐ 1 time per day
- ☐ 2–3 times per day
- ☐ 4–5 times per day
- ☐ 6 or more times per day

6a. Each time you drank **milk as a beverage**, how much did you usually drink?

- ☐ Less than 1 cup (8 ounces)
- ☐ 1 to 1½ cups (8 to 12 ounces)
- ☐ More than 1½ cups (12 ounces)

6b. What kind of **milk** did you usually drink?

- ☐ Whole milk
- ☐ 2% fat milk
- ☐ 1 % fat milk
- ☐ Skim, nonfat, or ½% fat milk
- ☐ Soy milk
- ☐ Rice milk
- ☐ Other

7. How often did you drink **chocolate milk** (including hot chocolate)?

- ☐ NEVER (GO TO QUESTION 8)

- ☐ 1 time per month or less
- ☐ 2–3 times per month
- ☐ 1–2 times per week
- ☐ 3–4 times per week
- ☐ 5–6 times per week
- ☐ 1 time per day
- ☐ 2–3 times per day
- ☐ 4–5 times per day
- ☐ 6 or more times per day

Question 8 appears in the next column

7a. Each time you drank **chocolate milk**, how much did you usually drink?

- ☐ Less than 1 cup (8 ounces)
- ☐ 1 to 1½ cups (8 to 12 ounces)
- ☐ More than 1½ cups (12 ounces)

7b. How often was the chocolate milk **reduced-fat** or **fat-free**?

- ☐ Almost never or never
- ☐ About ¼ of the time
- ☐ About ½ of the time
- ☐ About ¾ of the time
- ☐ Almost always or always

8. How often did you drink **meal replacement** or **high-protein beverages** (such as Instant Breakfast, Ensure, Slimfast, Sustacal or others)?

- ☐ NEVER (GO TO QUESTION 9)

- ☐ 1 time per month or less
- ☐ 2–3 times per month
- ☐ 1–2 times per week
- ☐ 3–4 times per week
- ☐ 5–6 times per week
- ☐ 1 time per day
- ☐ 2–3 times per day
- ☐ 4–5 times per day
- ☐ 6 or more times per day

8a. Each time you drank **meal replacement** or **high-protein beverages**, how much did you usually drink?

- ☐ Less than 1 cup (8 ounces)
- ☐ 1 to 1½ cups (8 to 12 ounces)
- ☐ More than 1½ cups (12 ounces)

9. Over the past 12 months, did you drink **soda** or **pop**?

- ☐ NO (GO TO QUESTION 10)
- ☐ YES

9a. How often did you drink **soda** or **pop IN THE SUMMER**?

- ☐ NEVER

- ☐ 1 time per month or less
- ☐ 2–3 times per month
- ☐ 1–2 times per week
- ☐ 3–4 times per week
- ☐ 5–6 times per week
- ☐ 1 time per day
- ☐ 2–3 times per day
- ☐ 4–5 times per day
- ☐ 6 or more times per day

Question 10 appears on the next page

Over the past 12 months...

9b. How often did you drink **soda** or **pop DURING THE REST OF THE YEAR**?

☐ NEVER

☐ 1 time per month or less
☐ 2–3 times per month
☐ 1–2 times per week
☐ 3–4 times per week
☐ 5–6 times per week
☐ 1 time per day
☐ 2–3 times per day
☐ 4–5 times per day
☐ 6 or more times per day

9c. Each time you drank **soda** or **pop,** how much did you usually drink?

☐ Less than 12 ounces or less than 1 can or bottle
☐ 12 to 16 ounces or 1 can or bottle
☐ More than 16 ounces or more than 1 can or bottle

9d. How often were these sodas or pop **diet** or **sugar-free**?

☐ Almost never or never
☐ About ¼ of the time
☐ About ½ of the time
☐ About ¾ of the time
☐ Almost always or always

9e. How often were these sodas or pop **caffeine-free**?

☐ Almost never or never
☐ About ¼ of the time
☐ About ½ of the time
☐ About ¾ of the time
☐ Almost always or always

10. Over the past 12 months, did you drink **sports drinks** (such as Propel, PowerAde, or Gatorade)?

☐ NO (GO TO QUESTION 11)

☐ YES

10a. How often did you drink **sports drinks IN THE SUMMER**?

☐ NEVER

☐ 1 time per month or less
☐ 2–3 times per month
☐ 1–2 times per week
☐ 3–4 times per week
☐ 5–6 times per week
☐ 1 time per day
☐ 2–3 times per day
☐ 4–5 times per day
☐ 6 or more times per day

Question 11 appears in the next column

10b. How often did you drink **sports drinks DURING THE REST OF THE YEAR**?

☐ NEVER

☐ 1 time per month or less
☐ 2–3 times per month
☐ 1–2 times per week
☐ 3–4 times per week
☐ 5–6 times per week
☐ 1 time per day
☐ 2–3 times per day
☐ 4–5 times per day
☐ 6 or more times per day

10c. Each time you drank **sports drinks**, how much did you usually drink?

☐ Less than 12 ounces or less than 1 bottle
☐ 12 to 24 ounces or 1 to 2 bottles
☐ More than 24 ounces or more than 2 bottles

11. Over the past 12 months, did you drink **energy drinks** (such as Red Bull or Jolt)?

☐ NO (GO TO QUESTION 12)

☐ YES

11a. How often did you drink **energy drinks IN THE SUMMER**?

☐ NEVER

☐ 1 time per month or less
☐ 2–3 times per month
☐ 1–2 times per week
☐ 3–4 times per week
☐ 5–6 times per week
☐ 1 time per day
☐ 2–3 times per day
☐ 4–5 times per day
☐ 6 or more times per day

11b. How often did you drink **energy drinks DURING THE REST OF THE YEAR**?

☐ NEVER

☐ 1 time per month or less
☐ 2–3 times per month
☐ 1–2 times per week
☐ 3–4 times per week
☐ 5–6 times per week
☐ 1 time per day
☐ 2–3 times per day
☐ 4–5 times per day
☐ 6 or more times per day

11c. Each time you drank **energy drinks**, how much did you usually drink?

☐ Less than 8 ounces or less than 1 cup
☐ 8 to 16 ounces or 1 to 2 cups
☐ More than 16 ounces or more than 2 cups

Question 12 appears on the next page

Over the past 12 months…

12. Over the past 12 months, did you drink **beer**?

☐ NO (GO TO QUESTION 13)

☐ YES

12a. How often did you drink **beer IN THE SUMMER**?

☐ NEVER

☐ 1 time per month or less
☐ 2–3 times per month
☐ 1–2 times per week
☐ 3–4 times per week
☐ 5–6 times per week
☐ 1 time per day
☐ 2–3 times per day
☐ 4–5 times per day
☐ 6 or more times per day

12b. How often did you drink **beer DURING THE REST OF THE YEAR**?

☐ NEVER

☐ 1 time per month or less
☐ 2–3 times per month
☐ 1–2 times per week
☐ 3–4 times per week
☐ 5–6 times per week
☐ 1 time per day
☐ 2–3 times per day
☐ 4–5 times per day
☐ 6 or more times per day

12c. Each time you drank **beer**, how much did you usually drink?

☐ Less than a 12-ounce can or bottle
☐ 1 to 3 12-ounce cans or bottles
☐ More than 3 12-ounce cans or bottles

13. Over the past 12 months, did you drink **water** (including tap, bottled, and carbonated water)?

☐ NO (GO TO QUESTION 14)

☐ YES

13a. How often did you drink **water** (including tap, bottled, and carbonated water) **IN THE SUMMER**?

☐ NEVER

☐ 1 time per month or less
☐ 2–3 times per month
☐ 1–2 times per week
☐ 3–4 times per week
☐ 5–6 times per week
☐ 1 time per day
☐ 2–3 times per day
☐ 4–5 times per day
☐ 6 or more times per day

Question 14 appears in the next column

13b. How often did you drink **water** (including tap, bottled, and carbonated water) **DURING THE REST OF THE YEAR**?

☐ NEVER

☐ 1 time per month or less
☐ 2–3 times per month
☐ 1–2 times per week
☐ 3–4 times per week
☐ 5–6 times per week
☐ 1 time per day
☐ 2–3 times per day
☐ 4–5 times per day
☐ 6 or more times per day

13c. Each time you drank **water**, how much did you usually drink?

☐ Less than 12 ounces or less than 1 bottle
☐ 12 to 24 ounces or 1 to 2 bottles
☐ More than 24 ounces or more than 2 bottles

13d. How often was the water you drank **tap water**?

☐ Almost never or never
☐ About ¼ of the time
☐ About ½ of the time
☐ About ¾ of the time
☐ Almost always or always

13e. How often was the water you drank **bottled, sweetened water** (with low or no-calorie sweetener, including carbonated water)?

☐ Almost never or never
☐ About ¼ of the time
☐ About ½ of the time
☐ About ¾ of the time
☐ Almost always or always

13f. How often was the water you drank **bottled, unsweetened water** (including carbonated water)?

☐ Almost never or never
☐ About ¼ of the time
☐ About ½ of the time
☐ About ¾ of the time
☐ Almost always or always

14. How often did you drink **wine** or **wine coolers**?

☐ NEVER (GO TO QUESTION 15)

☐ 1 time per month or less
☐ 2–3 times per month
☐ 1–2 times per week
☐ 3–4 times per week
☐ 5–6 times per week
☐ 1 time per day
☐ 2–3 times per day
☐ 4–5 times per day
☐ 6 or more times per day

Question 15 appears on the next page

Over the past 12 months...

14a. Each time you drank **wine** or **wine coolers**, how much did you usually drink?

- ☐ Less than 5 ounces or less than 1 glass
- ☐ 5 to 12 ounces or 1 to 2 glasses
- ☐ More than 12 ounces or more than 2 glasses

15. How often did you drink **liquor** or **mixed drinks**?

- ☐ NEVER (GO TO QUESTION 16)

- ☐ 1 time per month or less
- ☐ 2–3 times per month
- ☐ 1–2 times per week
- ☐ 3–4 times per week
- ☐ 5–6 times per week
- ☐ 1 time per day
- ☐ 2–3 times per day
- ☐ 4–5 times per day
- ☐ 6 or more times per day

15a. Each time you drank **liquor** or **mixed drinks**, how much did you usually drink?

- ☐ Less than 1 shot of liquor
- ☐ 1 to 3 shots of liquor
- ☐ More than 3 shots of liquor

16. Over the past 12 months, did you eat **oatmeal, grits,** or **other cooked cereal?**

- ☐ NO (GO TO QUESTION 17)
- ☐ YES

16a. How often did you eat **oatmeal**, **grits**, or **other cooked cereal IN THE WINTER**?

- ☐ NEVER

- ☐ 1–6 times per winter
- ☐ 7–11 times per winter
- ☐ 1 time per month
- ☐ 2–3 times per month
- ☐ 1 time per week
- ☐ 2 times per week
- ☐ 3–4 times per week
- ☐ 5–6 times per week
- ☐ 1 time per day
- ☐ 2 or more times per day

16b. How often did you eat **oatmeal**, **grits**, or **other cooked cereal DURING THE REST OF THE YEAR**?

- ☐ NEVER

- ☐ 1–6 times per year
- ☐ 7–11 times per year
- ☐ 1 time per month
- ☐ 2–3 times per month
- ☐ 1 time per week
- ☐ 2 times per week
- ☐ 3–4 times per week
- ☐ 5–6 times per week
- ☐ 1 time per day
- ☐ 2 or more times per day

Question 17 appears in the next column

16c. Each time you ate **oatmeal, grits,** or **other cooked cereal,** how much did you usually eat?

- ☐ Less than ¾ cup
- ☐ ¾ to 1¼ cups
- ☐ More than 1¼ cups

16d. How often was **butter** or **margarine** added to your oatmeal, grits or other cooked cereal?

- ☐ Almost never or never
- ☐ About ¼ of the time
- ☐ About ½ of the time
- ☐ About ¾ of the time
- ☐ Almost always or always

17. How often did you eat **cold cereal**?

- ☐ NEVER (GO TO QUESTION 18)

- ☐ 1–6 times per year
- ☐ 7–11 times per year
- ☐ 1 time per month
- ☐ 2–3 times per month
- ☐ 1 time per week
- ☐ 2 times per week
- ☐ 3–4 times per week
- ☐ 5–6 times per week
- ☐ 1 time per day
- ☐ 2 or more times per day

17a. Each time you ate **cold cereal**, how much did you usually eat?

- ☐ Less than 1 cup
- ☐ 1 to 2½ cups
- ☐ More than 2½ cups

17b. How often was the cold cereal you ate **Total Raisin Bran**, **Total Cereal**, or **Product 19**?

- ☐ Almost never or never
- ☐ About ¼ of the time
- ☐ About ½ of the time
- ☐ About ¾ of the time
- ☐ Almost always or always

17c. How often was the cold cereal you ate **All Bran**, **Fiber One**, **100% Bran**, or **All-Bran Bran Buds**?

- ☐ Almost never or never
- ☐ About ¼ of the time
- ☐ About ½ of the time
- ☐ About ¾ of the time
- ☐ Almost always or always

Question 18 appears on the next page

Over the <u>past 12 months</u>...

17d. How often was the cold cereal you ate **some other bran** or **fiber cereal** (such as Cheerios, Shredded Wheat, Raisin Bran, Bran Flakes, Grape-Nuts, Granola, Wheaties, or Healthy Choice)?

- ☐ Almost never or never
- ☐ About ¼ of the time
- ☐ About ½ of the time
- ☐ About ¾ of the time
- ☐ Almost always or always

17e. How often was the cold cereal you ate any **other type of cold cereal** (such as Corn Flakes, Rice Krispies, Frosted Flakes, Special K, Froot Loops, Cap'n Crunch, or others)?

- ☐ Almost never or never
- ☐ About ¼ of the time
- ☐ About ½ of the time
- ☐ About ¾ of the time
- ☐ Almost always or always

17f. Was **milk** added to your cold cereal?

- ☐ NO (GO TO QUESTION 18)
- ☐ YES

17g. What kind of **milk** was usually added?

- ☐ Whole milk
- ☐ 2% fat milk
- ☐ 1% fat milk
- ☐ Skim, nonfat, or ½% fat milk
- ☐ Soy milk
- ☐ Rice milk
- ☐ Other

17h. Each time **milk was added to your cold cereal**, how much was usually added?

- ☐ Less than ½ cup
- ☐ ½ to 1 cup
- ☐ More than 1 cup

18. How often did you eat **applesauce**?

- ☐ NEVER (GO TO QUESTION 19)

☐ 1–6 times per year	☐ 2 times per week
☐ 7–11 times per year	☐ 3–4 times per week
☐ 1 time per month	☐ 5–6 times per week
☐ 2–3 times per month	☐ 1 time per day
☐ 1 time per week	☐ 2 or more times per day

Question 19 appears in the next column

18a. Each time you ate **applesauce**, how much did you usually eat?

- ☐ Less than ½ cup
- ☐ ½ to 1 cup
- ☐ More than 1 cup

19. How often did you eat **apples**?

- ☐ NEVER (GO TO QUESTION 20)

☐ 1–6 times per year	☐ 2 times per week
☐ 7–11 times per year	☐ 3–4 times per week
☐ 1 time per month	☐ 5–6 times per week
☐ 2–3 times per month	☐ 1 time per day
☐ 1 time per week	☐ 2 or more times per day

19a. Each time you ate **apples**, how many did you usually eat?

- ☐ Less than 1 apple
- ☐ 1 apple
- ☐ More than 1 apple

20. How often did you eat **pears** (fresh, canned, or frozen)?

- ☐ NEVER (GO TO QUESTION 21)

☐ 1–6 times per year	☐ 2 times per week
☐ 7–11 times per year	☐ 3–4 times per week
☐ 1 time per month	☐ 5–6 times per week
☐ 2–3 times per month	☐ 1 time per day
☐ 1 time per week	☐ 2 or more times per day

20a. Each time you ate **pears**, how many did you usually eat?

- ☐ Less than 1 pear
- ☐ 1 pear
- ☐ More than 1 pear

21. How often did you eat **bananas?**

- ☐ NEVER (GO TO QUESTION 22)

☐ 1–6 times per year	☐ 2 times per week
☐ 7–11 times per year	☐ 3–4 times per week
☐ 1 time per month	☐ 5–6 times per week
☐ 2–3 times per month	☐ 1 time per day
☐ 1 time per week	☐ 2 or more times per day

Question 22 appears on the next page

Over the past 12 months…

21a. Each time you ate **bananas**, how many did you usually eat?

- ☐ Less than 1 banana
- ☐ 1 banana
- ☐ More than 1 banana

22. How often did you eat **dried fruit** (such as prunes or raisins)? *(Please do not include dried apricots.)*

- ☐ NEVER (GO TO QUESTION 23)

- ☐ 1–6 times per year
- ☐ 7–11 times per year
- ☐ 1 time per month
- ☐ 2–3 times per month
- ☐ 1 time per week
- ☐ 2 times per week
- ☐ 3–4 times per week
- ☐ 5–6 times per week
- ☐ 1 time per day
- ☐ 2 or more times per day

22a. Each time you ate **dried fruit**, how much did you usually eat?

- ☐ Less than 2 tablespoons
- ☐ 2 to 5 tablespoons
- ☐ More than 5 tablespoons

23. Over the past 12 months, did you eat **peaches, nectarines,** or **plums**?

- ☐ NO (GO TO QUESTION 24)
- ☐ YES

23a. How often did you eat **fresh peaches, nectarines**, or **plums WHEN IN SEASON**?

- ☐ NEVER

- ☐ 1–6 times per season
- ☐ 7–11 times per season
- ☐ 1 time per month
- ☐ 2–3 times per month
- ☐ 1 time per week
- ☐ 2 times per week
- ☐ 3–4 times per week
- ☐ 5–6 times per week
- ☐ 1 time per day
- ☐ 2 or more times per day

23b. How often did you eat **peaches, nectarines,** or **plums** (fresh, canned, or frozen) **DURING THE REST OF THE YEAR**?

- ☐ NEVER

- ☐ 1–6 times per year
- ☐ 7–11 times per year
- ☐ 1 time per month
- ☐ 2–3 times per month
- ☐ 1 time per week
- ☐ 2 times per week
- ☐ 3–4 times per week
- ☐ 5–6 times per week
- ☐ 1 time per day
- ☐ 2 or more times per day

Question 24 appears in the next column

23c. Each time you ate **peaches, nectarines,** or **plums,** how much did you usually eat?

- ☐ Less than 1 fruit or less than ½ cup
- ☐ 1 to 2 fruits or ½ to ¾ cup
- ☐ More than 2 fruits or more than ¾ cup

24. How often did you eat **grapes**?

- ☐ NEVER (GO TO QUESTION 25)

- ☐ 1–6 times per year
- ☐ 7–11 times per year
- ☐ 1 time per month
- ☐ 2–3 times per month
- ☐ 1 time per week
- ☐ 2 times per week
- ☐ 3–4 times per week
- ☐ 5–6 times per week
- ☐ 1 time per day
- ☐ 2 or more times per day

24a. Each time you ate **grapes**, how much did you usually eat?

- ☐ Less than ½ cup or less than 10 grapes
- ☐ ½ to 1 cup or 10 to 30 grapes
- ☐ More than 1 cup or more than 30 grapes

25. Over the past 12 months, did you eat **cantaloupe**?

- ☐ NO (GO TO QUESTION 26)
- ☐ YES

25a. How often did you eat **fresh cantaloupe WHEN IN SEASON**?

- ☐ NEVER

- ☐ 1–6 times per season
- ☐ 7–11 times per season
- ☐ 1 time per month
- ☐ 2–3 times per month
- ☐ 1 time per week
- ☐ 2 times per week
- ☐ 3–4 times per week
- ☐ 5–6 times per week
- ☐ 1 time per day
- ☐ 2 or more times per day

25b. How often did you eat **cantaloupe** (fresh or frozen) **DURING THE REST OF THE YEAR**?

- ☐ NEVER

- ☐ 1–6 times per year
- ☐ 7–11 times per year
- ☐ 1 time per month
- ☐ 2–3 times per month
- ☐ 1 time per week
- ☐ 2 times per week
- ☐ 3–4 times per week
- ☐ 5–6 times per week
- ☐ 1 time per day
- ☐ 2 or more times per day

Question 26 appears on the next page

APPENDIX

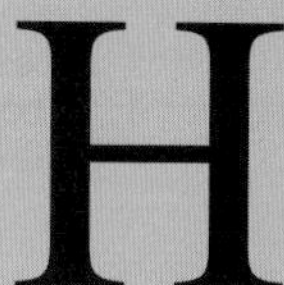

The NHANES Food Frequency Questionnaire

From the Risk Factor Monitoring and Methods Branch, Division of Cancer Control and Population Sciences, National Cancer Institute, National Institutes of Health, U.S. Department of Health and Human Services. http://www.riskfactor.cancer.gov/dhq2/.

*This appendix contains the first eight pages of the NHANES Food Frequency Questionnaire. For the complete questionnaire, visit the *Nutritional Assessment* website at www.mhhe.com/lee-nieman6.

NHANES Food Questionnaire

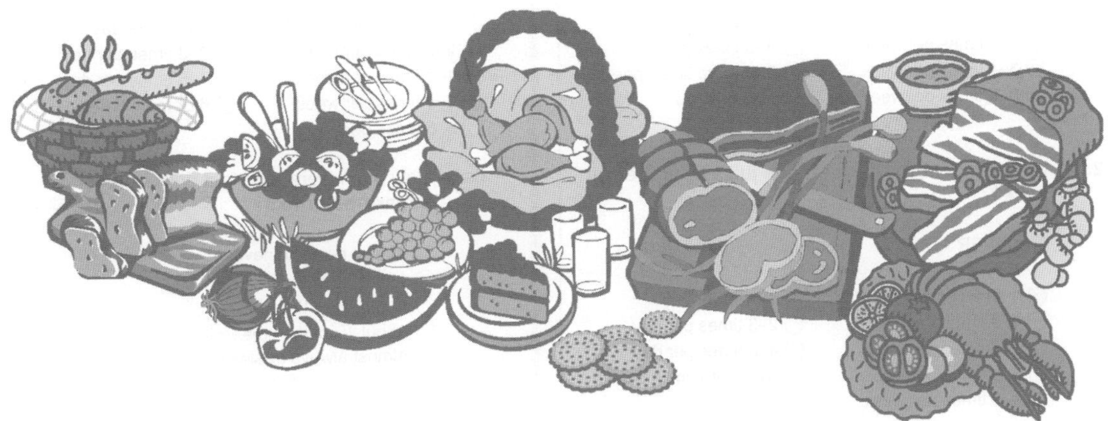

3/8" SPINE PERF

More than one member of your household may have received a questionnaire. Please make sure this is your booklet before answering any questions.

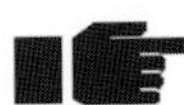

LABEL HERE

GENERAL INSTRUCTIONS

- **Answer each question as best you can. Estimate if you are not sure. A guess is better than leaving a blank.**
- **Use only a No. 2 pencil.**
- **Be certain to completely blacken in each of the answers.**
- **Erase completely if you make any changes.**
- **Do not make any stray marks on this form.**
- **If you blacken NEVER or NO for a question, please follow any arrows or instructions that direct you to the next question.**

PLEASE DO NOT WRITE IN THIS AREA

SERIAL #

1. Over the <u>past 12 months</u>, how often did you drink **tomato juice** or **vegetable juice**?

- ◯ NEVER

- ◯ 1 time per month or less
- ◯ 2–3 times per month
- ◯ 1–2 times per week
- ◯ 3–4 times per week
- ◯ 5–6 times per week
- ◯ 1 time per day
- ◯ 2–3 times per day
- ◯ 4–5 times per day
- ◯ 6 or more times per day

2. How often did you drink **orange juice** or **grapefruit juice?**

- ◯ NEVER

- ◯ 1 time per month or less
- ◯ 2–3 times per month
- ◯ 1–2 times per week
- ◯ 3–4 times per week
- ◯ 5–6 times per week
- ◯ 1 time per day
- ◯ 2–3 times per day
- ◯ 4–5 times per day
- ◯ 6 or more times per day

3. How often did you drink **apple juice?**

- ◯ NEVER

- ◯ 1 time per month or less
- ◯ 2–3 times per month
- ◯ 1–2 times per week
- ◯ 3–4 times per week
- ◯ 5–6 times per week
- ◯ 1 time per day
- ◯ 2–3 times per day
- ◯ 4–5 times per day
- ◯ 6 or more times per day

4. How often did you drink **grape juice?**

- ◯ NEVER

- ◯ 1 time per month or less
- ◯ 2–3 times per month
- ◯ 1–2 times per week
- ◯ 3–4 times per week
- ◯ 5–6 times per week
- ◯ 1 time per day
- ◯ 2–3 times per day
- ◯ 4–5 times per day
- ◯ 6 or more times per day

5. How often did you drink **other 100% fruit juice** or **100% fruit juice mixtures** (such as pineapple, prune, or others)?

- ◯ NEVER

- ◯ 1 time per month or less
- ◯ 2–3 times per month
- ◯ 1–2 times per week
- ◯ 3–4 times per week
- ◯ 5–6 times per week
- ◯ 1 time per day
- ◯ 2–3 times per day
- ◯ 4–5 times per day
- ◯ 6 or more times per day

3/8" SPINE PERF

6. How often did you drink other **fruit drinks** (such as cranberry cocktail, Hi-C, lemonade, or Kool-Aid, diet or regular)?

- ◯ NEVER (GO TO QUESTION 7)

- ◯ 1 time per month or less
- ◯ 2–3 times per month
- ◯ 1–2 times per week
- ◯ 3–4 times per week
- ◯ 5–6 times per week
- ◯ 1 time per day
- ◯ 2–3 times per day
- ◯ 4–5 times per day
- ◯ 6 or more times per day

6a. How often were your fruit drinks **diet** or **sugar-free drinks**?

- ◯ Almost never or never
- ◯ About 1/4 of the time
- ◯ About 1/2 of the time
- ◯ About 3/4 of the time
- ◯ Almost always or always

7. How often did you drink **milk as a beverage** (NOT in coffee, NOT in cereal)? (Please include chocolate milk and hot chocolate.)

- ◯ NEVER (GO TO QUESTION 8)

- ◯ 1 time per month or less
- ◯ 2–3 times per month
- ◯ 1–2 times per week
- ◯ 3–4 times per week
- ◯ 5–6 times per week
- ◯ 1 time per day
- ◯ 2–3 times per day
- ◯ 4–5 times per day
- ◯ 6 or more times per day

7a. What kind of **milk** did you usually drink?

- ◯ Whole milk
- ◯ 2% fat milk
- ◯ 1% fat milk
- ◯ Skim, nonfat, or 1/2% fat milk
- ◯ Soy milk
- ◯ Rice milk
- ◯ Raw, unpasteurized milk
- ◯ Other

BAR CODE LABEL HERE

Question 8 appears on the next page.

Over the past 12 months...

8. How often did you drink **meal replacement, energy, or high-protein beverages** such as Instant Breakfast, Ensure, Slimfast, Sustacal or others?

○ NEVER

○ 1 time per month or less
○ 2–3 times per month
○ 1–2 times per week
○ 3–4 times per week
○ 5–6 times per week
○ 1 time per day
○ 2–3 times per day
○ 4–5 times per day
○ 6 or more times per day

9. Over the past 12 months, did you drink **soft drinks, soda,** or **pop**?

○ NO (GO TO QUESTION 10)

○ YES

9a. How often did you drink **soft drinks, soda,** or **pop IN THE SUMMER**?

○ NEVER

○ 1 time per month or less
○ 2–3 times per month
○ 1–2 times per week
○ 3–4 times per week
○ 5–6 times per week
○ 1 time per day
○ 2–3 times per day
○ 4–5 times per day
○ 6 or more times per day

9b. How often did you drink **soft drinks, soda,** or **pop DURING THE REST OF THE YEAR**?

○ NEVER

○ 1 time per month or less
○ 2–3 times per month
○ 1–2 times per week
○ 3–4 times per week
○ 5–6 times per week
○ 1 time per day
○ 2–3 times per day
○ 4–5 times per day
○ 6 or more times per day

9c. How often were these soft drinks, soda, or pop **diet** or **sugar-free**?

○ Almost never or never
○ About 1/4 of the time
○ About 1/2 of the time
○ About 3/4 of the time
○ Almost always or always

9d. How often were these soft drinks, soda, or pop **caffeine-free**?

○ Almost never or never
○ About 1/4 of the time
○ About 1/2 of the time
○ About 3/4 of the time
○ Almost always or always

Question 10 appears in the next column.

10. Over the past 12 months, did you drink **beer**?

○ NO (GO TO QUESTION 11)

○ YES

10a. How often did you drink **beer IN THE SUMMER**?

○ NEVER

○ 1 time per month or less
○ 2–3 times per month
○ 1–2 times per week
○ 3–4 times per week
○ 5–6 times per week
○ 1 time per day
○ 2–3 times per day
○ 4–5 times per day
○ 6 or more times per day

10b. How often did you drink **beer DURING THE REST OF THE YEAR**?

○ NEVER

○ 1 time per month or less
○ 2–3 times per month
○ 1–2 times per week
○ 3–4 times per week
○ 5–6 times per week
○ 1 time per day
○ 2–3 times per day
○ 4–5 times per day
○ 6 or more times per day

11. How often did you drink **wine** or **wine coolers**?

○ NEVER

○ 1 time per month or less
○ 2–3 times per month
○ 1–2 times per week
○ 3–4 times per week
○ 5–6 times per week
○ 1 time per day
○ 2–3 times per day
○ 4–5 times per day
○ 6 or more times per day

12. How often did you drink **liquor** or **mixed drinks**?

○ NEVER

○ 1 time per month or less
○ 2–3 times per month
○ 1–2 times per week
○ 3–4 times per week
○ 5–6 times per week
○ 1 time per day
○ 2–3 times per day
○ 4–5 times per day
○ 6 or more times per day

244004 - 2/6

Over the past 12 months...

13. Did you eat **oatmeal, grits,** or **other cooked cereal?**

○ NO (GO TO QUESTION 14)

○ YES

13a. How often did you eat **oatmeal, grits,** or **other cooked cereal IN THE WINTER**?

○ NEVER

○ 1–6 times per winter
○ 7–11 times per winter
○ 1 time per month
○ 2–3 times per month
○ 1 time per week
○ 2 times per week
○ 3–4 times per week
○ 5–6 times per week
○ 1 time per day
○ 2 or more times per day

13b. How often did you eat **oatmeal, grits,** or **other cooked cereal DURING THE REST OF THE YEAR?**

○ NEVER

○ 1–6 times per year
○ 7–11 times per year
○ 1 time per month
○ 2–3 times per month
○ 1 time per week
○ 2 times per week
○ 3–4 times per week
○ 5–6 times per week
○ 1 time per day
○ 2 or more times per day

13c. How often was the cooked cereal you ate **oatmeal**?

○ Almost never or never
○ About 1/4 of the time
○ About 1/2 of the time
○ About 3/4 of the time
○ Almost always or always

14. How often did you eat **cold cereal**?

○ NEVER (GO TO QUESTION 15)

○ 1–6 times per year
○ 7–11 times per year
○ 1 time per month
○ 2–3 times per month
○ 1 time per week
○ 2 times per week
○ 3–4 times per week
○ 5–6 times per week
○ 1 time per day
○ 2 or more times per day

Question 15 appears in the next column.

14a. How often was the cold cereal you ate a **whole grain type** (such as shredded wheat, Wheaties, Cheerios, Raisin Bran or other bran, oat, or whole wheat cereal)?

○ Almost never or never
○ About 1/4 of the time
○ About 1/2 of the time
○ About 3/4 of the time
○ Almost always or always

14b. Was **milk** added to your cold cereal?

○ NO (GO TO QUESTION 15)

○ YES

14c. What kind of **milk** was usually added?

○ Whole milk
○ 2% fat milk
○ 1% fat milk
○ Skim, nonfat, or 1/2% fat milk
○ Soy milk
○ Rice milk
○ Raw, unpasteurized milk
○ Other

15. How often did you eat **applesauce**?

○ NEVER

○ 1–6 times per year
○ 7–11 times per year
○ 1 time per month
○ 2–3 times per month
○ 1 time per week
○ 2 times per week
○ 3–4 times per week
○ 5–6 times per week
○ 1 time per day
○ 2 or more times per day

16. How often did you eat **apples**?

○ NEVER

○ 1–6 times per year
○ 7–11 times per year
○ 1 time per month
○ 2–3 times per month
○ 1 time per week
○ 2 times per week
○ 3–4 times per week
○ 5–6 times per week
○ 1 time per day
○ 2 or more times per day

17. How often did you eat **pears** (fresh, canned, or frozen)?

○ NEVER

○ 1–6 times per year
○ 7–11 times per year
○ 1 time per month
○ 2–3 times per month
○ 1 time per week
○ 2 times per week
○ 3–4 times per week
○ 5–6 times per week
○ 1 time per day
○ 2 or more times per day

Over the past 12 months...

18. How often did you eat **bananas** ?

○ NEVER

○ 1–6 times per year
○ 7–11 times per year
○ 1 time per month
○ 2–3 times per month
○ 1 time per week
○ 2 times per week
○ 3–4 times per week
○ 5–6 times per week
○ 1 time per day
○ 2 or more times per day

19. How often did you eat **pineapple**?

○ NEVER

○ 1–6 times per year
○ 7–11 times per year
○ 1 time per month
○ 2–3 times per month
○ 1 time per week
○ 2 times per week
○ 3–4 times per week
○ 5–6 times per week
○ 1 time per day
○ 2 or more times per day

20. How often did you eat **dried fruit**, such as prunes or raisins?

○ NEVER

○ 1–6 times per year
○ 7–11 times per year
○ 1 time per month
○ 2–3 times per month
○ 1 time per week
○ 2 times per week
○ 3–4 times per week
○ 5–6 times per week
○ 1 time per day
○ 2 or more times per day

21. Over the past 12 months, did you eat **peaches, nectarines,** or **plums**?

○ NO (GO TO QUESTION 22)

○ YES

21a. How often did you eat **fresh peaches, nectarines**, or **plums WHEN IN SEASON**?

○ NEVER

○ 1–6 times per season
○ 7–11 times per season
○ 1 time per month
○ 2–3 times per month
○ 1 time per week
○ 2 times per week
○ 3–4 times per week
○ 5–6 times per week
○ 1 time per day
○ 2 or more times per day

Question 22 appears in the next column.

21b. How often did you eat **peaches, nectarines,** or **plums** (fresh, canned, or frozen) **DURING THE REST OF THE YEAR**?

○ NEVER

○ 1–6 times per year
○ 7–11 times per year
○ 1 time per month
○ 2–3 times per month
○ 1 time per week
○ 2 times per week
○ 3–4 times per week
○ 5–6 times per week
○ 1 time per day
○ 2 or more times per day

22. How often did you eat **grapes**?

○ NEVER

○ 1–6 times per year
○ 7–11 times per year
○ 1 time per month
○ 2–3 times per month
○ 1 time per week
○ 2 times per week
○ 3–4 times per week
○ 5–6 times per week
○ 1 time per day
○ 2 or more times per day

23. Over the past 12 months, did you eat **melons** (such as cantaloupe, watermelon, or honeydew)?

○ NO (GO TO QUESTION 24)

○ YES

23a. How often did you eat **fresh melons** (such as cantaloupe, watermelon, or honeydew) **WHEN IN SEASON**?

○ NEVER

○ 1–6 times per season
○ 7–11 times per season
○ 1 time per month
○ 2–3 times per month
○ 1 time per week
○ 2 times per week
○ 3–4 times per week
○ 5–6 times per week
○ 1 time per day
○ 2 or more times per day

23b. How often did you eat **fresh or frozen melons** (such as cantaloupe, watermelon, or honeydew) **DURING THE REST OF THE YEAR**?

○ NEVER

○ 1–6 times per year
○ 7–11 times per year
○ 1 time per month
○ 2–3 times per month
○ 1 time per week
○ 2 times per week
○ 3–4 times per week
○ 5–6 times per week
○ 1 time per day
○ 2 or more times per day

Question 24 appears on the next page.

244004 - 3/6

Over the past 12 months...

24. Did you eat **strawberries**?

○ NO **(GO TO QUESTION 25)**

○ YES

24a. How often did you eat **fresh strawberries WHEN IN SEASON**?

○ NEVER

○ 1–6 times per season
○ 7–11 times per season
○ 1 time per month
○ 2–3 times per month
○ 1 time per week
○ 2 times per week
○ 3–4 times per week
○ 5–6 times per week
○ 1 time per day
○ 2 or more times per day

24b. How often did you eat **fresh** or **frozen strawberries DURING THE REST OF THE YEAR**?

○ NEVER

○ 1–6 times per year
○ 7–11 times per year
○ 1 time per month
○ 2–3 times per month
○ 1 time per week
○ 2 times per week
○ 3–4 times per week
○ 5–6 times per week
○ 1 time per day
○ 2 or more times per day

25. Over the past 12 months, did you eat **oranges, tangerines, clementines,** or **tangelos**?

○ NO **(GO TO QUESTION 26)**

○ YES

25a. How often did you eat **fresh oranges, tangerines, clementines,** or **tangelos WHEN IN SEASON**?

○ NEVER

○ 1–6 times per season
○ 7–11 times per season
○ 1 time per month
○ 2–3 times per month
○ 1 time per week
○ 2 times per week
○ 3–4 times per week
○ 5–6 times per week
○ 1 time per day
○ 2 or more times per day

Question 26 appears in the next column.

25b. How often did you eat **oranges, tangerines, clementines,** or **tangelos** (fresh or canned) **DURING THE REST OF THE YEAR**?

○ NEVER

○ 1–6 times per year
○ 7–11 times per year
○ 1 time per month
○ 2–3 times per month
○ 1 time per week
○ 2 times per week
○ 3–4 times per week
○ 5–6 times per week
○ 1 time per day
○ 2 or more times per day

26. Over the past 12 months, did you eat **grapefruit**?

○ NO **(GO TO QUESTION 27)**

○ YES

26a. How often did you eat **fresh grapefruit WHEN IN SEASON**?

○ NEVER

○ 1–6 times per season
○ 7–11 times per season
○ 1 time per month
○ 2–3 times per month
○ 1 time per week
○ 2 times per week
○ 3–4 times per week
○ 5–6 times per week
○ 1 time per day
○ 2 or more times per day

26b. How often did you eat **grapefruit** (fresh or canned) **DURING THE REST OF THE YEAR?**

○ NEVER

○ 1–6 times per year
○ 7–11 times per year
○ 1 time per month
○ 2–3 times per month
○ 1 time per week
○ 2 times per week
○ 3–4 times per week
○ 5–6 times per week
○ 1 time per day
○ 2 or more times per day

27. How often did you eat **other kinds of fruit**?

○ NEVER

○ 1–6 times per year
○ 7–11 times per year
○ 1 time per month
○ 2–3 times per month
○ 1 time per week
○ 2 times per week
○ 3–4 times per week
○ 5–6 times per week
○ 1 time per day
○ 2 or more times per day

3/8" SPINE PERF

Over the past 12 months...

28. How often did you eat **COOKED greens** (such as spinach, turnip, collard, mustard, chard, or kale)?

○ NEVER

○ 1–6 times per year
○ 7–11 times per year
○ 1 time per month
○ 2–3 times per month
○ 1 time per week
○ 2 times per week
○ 3–4 times per week
○ 5–6 times per week
○ 1 time per day
○ 2 or more times per day

29. How often did you eat **RAW greens** (such as spinach, turnip, collard, mustard, chard, or kale)? (*We will ask about lettuce later.*)

○ NEVER

○ 1–6 times per year
○ 7–11 times per year
○ 1 time per month
○ 2–3 times per month
○ 1 time per week
○ 2 times per week
○ 3–4 times per week
○ 5–6 times per week
○ 1 time per day
○ 2 or more times per day

30. How often did you eat **coleslaw**?

○ NEVER

○ 1–6 times per year
○ 7–11 times per year
○ 1 time per month
○ 2–3 times per month
○ 1 time per week
○ 2 times per week
○ 3–4 times per week
○ 5–6 times per week
○ 1 time per day
○ 2 or more times per day

31. How often did you eat **sauerkraut** or **cabbage** (other than coleslaw)?

○ NEVER

○ 1–6 times per year
○ 7–11 times per year
○ 1 time per month
○ 2–3 times per month
○ 1 time per week
○ 2 times per week
○ 3–4 times per week
○ 5–6 times per week
○ 1 time per day
○ 2 or more times per day

32. How often did you eat **carrots** (fresh, canned, or frozen)?

○ NEVER

○ 1–6 times per year
○ 7–11 times per year
○ 1 time per month
○ 2–3 times per month
○ 1 time per week
○ 2 times per week
○ 3–4 times per week
○ 5–6 times per week
○ 1 time per day
○ 2 or more times per day

33. How often did you eat **string beans** or **green beans** (fresh, canned, or frozen)?

○ NEVER

○ 1–6 times per year
○ 7–11 times per year
○ 1 time per month
○ 2–3 times per month
○ 1 time per week
○ 2 times per week
○ 3–4 times per week
○ 5–6 times per week
○ 1 time per day
○ 2 or more times per day

34. How often did you eat **peas** (fresh, canned, or frozen)?

○ NEVER

○ 1–6 times per year
○ 7–11 times per year
○ 1 time per month
○ 2–3 times per month
○ 1 time per week
○ 2 times per week
○ 3–4 times per week
○ 5–6 times per week
○ 1 time per day
○ 2 or more times per day

35. Over the past 12 months, did you eat **corn**?

○ NO **(GO TO QUESTION 36)**

○ YES

35a. How often did you eat **corn** (fresh, canned, or frozen) **WHEN IN SEASON**?

○ NEVER

○ 1–6 times per season
○ 7–11 times per season
○ 1 time per month
○ 2–3 times per month
○ 1 time per week
○ 2 times per week
○ 3–4 times per week
○ 5–6 times per week
○ 1 time per day
○ 2 or more times per day

35b. How often did you eat **corn** (fresh, canned, or frozen) **DURING THE REST OF THE YEAR**?

○ NEVER

○ 1–6 times per year
○ 7–11 times per year
○ 1 time per month
○ 2–3 times per month
○ 1 time per week
○ 2 times per week
○ 3–4 times per week
○ 5–6 times per week
○ 1 time per day
○ 2 or more times per day

Question 36 appears on the next page.

244004 - 4/6

APPENDIX I

2011 Behavioral Risk Factor Surveillance System Questionnaire

The Behavioral Risk Factor Surveillance System (BRFSS) questionnaire is composed of three sections: the core component, the optional modules, and state-added questions. All health departments must ask the core component questions without modification in wording; however, the modules are optional, and states may add their own questions. The core component consists of a fixed core of questions, a rotating core of questions, and an emerging core of questions. The fixed core includes questions about current behaviors that affect health (e.g., tobacco use, women's health) and questions on demographic characteristics. The rotating core is made up of two distinct sets of questions, each asked in alternating years by all states, addressing different topics. In the years when rotating topics are not used in the core, they are supported as optional modules. The emerging core is a set of up to five questions that focus on issues of a late-breaking nature and do not necessarily receive the same scrutiny that other questions receive before being added to the instrument. These questions are part of the core for one year and are evaluated during or soon after the year concludes to determine their potential value in future surveys.

Core Sections

- Section 1: Health Status
- Section 2: Healthy Days — Health-Related Quality of Life
- Section 3: Health Care Access
- Section 4: Hypertension Awareness
- Section 5: Cholesterol Awareness
- Section 6: Chronic Health Conditions
- Section 7: Tobacco Use
- Section 8: Demographics
- Section 9: Fruits and Vegetables
- Section 10: Exercise (Physical Activity)
- Section 11: Disability
- Section 12: Arthritis Burden
- Section 13: Seatbelt Use
- Section 14: Immunization
- Section 15: Alcohol Consumption
- Section 16: HIV/AIDS

Optional Modules

- Module 1: Pre-Diabetes
- Module 2: Diabetes
- Module 3: Healthy Days (Symptoms)
- Module 4: Sugar Sweetened Beverages and Menu Labeling
- Module 5: Preconception Health/Family Planning
- Module 6: Visual Impairment and Access to Eye Care
- Module 7: Inadequate Sleep
- Module 8: High Risk/Health Care Worker
- Module 9: Cardiovascular Health
- Module 10: Actions to Control High Blood Pressure
- Module 11: Heart Attack and Stroke
- Module 12: Breast/Cervical Cancer Screening
- Module 13: Prostate Cancer Screening
- Module 14: Colorectal Cancer Screening
- Module 15: Smoking Cessation

Module 16: Secondhand Smoke
Module 17: Adult Asthma History
Module 18: Arthritis Management
Module 19: Tetanus Diphtheria (Adults)
Module 20: Adult Human Papilloma Virus (HPV)
Module 21: Shingles
Module 22: Chronic Obstructive Pulmonary Disease (COPD)
Module 23: General Preparedness
Module 24: Veterans' Health
Module 25: Reactions to Race
Module 26: Anxiety and Depression
Module 27: Cognitive Impairment
Module 28: Social Context
Module 29: HIV/AIDS
Module 30: Emotional Support and Life Satisfaction
Module 31: Adverse Childhood Experience
Module 32: Random Child Selection
Module 33: Childhood Asthma Prevalence
Module 34: Child Immunization (Influenza)

This appendix includes questions from only the following core sections and option modules:

Section 4: Hypertension Awareness
Section 5: Cholesterol Awareness
Section 6: Chronic Health Conditions
Section 10: Exercise (Physical Activity)
Section 15: Alcohol Consumption
Module 1: Pre-Diabetes
Module 2: Diabetes
Module 4: Sugar Sweetened Beverages and Menu Labeling
Module 9: Cardiovascular Health

For the complete BRFSS questionnaire and for additional links regarding the BRFSS, visit the *Nutritional Assessment* website at www.mhhe.com/lee-nieman6.

Source: From the National Center for Chronic Disease Prevention and Health Promotion, Centers for Disease Control and Prevention, U.S. Department of Health and Human Services. http://www.cdc.gov/brfss/.

Section 4: Hypertension Awareness

4.1 Have you EVER been told by a doctor, nurse, or other health professional that you have high blood pressure? (84)

Read only if necessary: By "other health professional" we mean a nurse practitioner, a physician's assistant, or some other licensed healths professional.

1 Yes **If "Yes" and respondent is female, ask: "Was this only when you were pregnant?"**
2 Yes, but female told only during pregnancy [Go to next section]
3 No [Go to next section]
4 Told borderline high or pre-hypertensive [Go to next section]
7 Don't know / Not sure (Go to next section)
9 Refused [Go to next section]

4.2 Are you currently taking medicine for your high blood pressure? (85)

1 Yes
2 No
7 Don't know / Not sure
9 Refused

Section 5: Cholesterol Awareness

5.1 Blood cholesterol is a fatty substance found in the blood. Have you EVER had your blood cholesterol checked? (86)

1 Yes
2 No [Go to next section]
7 Don't know / Not sure [Go to next section]
9 Refused [Go to next section]

5.2 About how long has it been since you last had your blood cholesterol checked? (87)

Read only if necessary:
1 Within the past year (anytime less than 12 months ago)
2 Within the past 2 years (1 year but less than 2 years ago)
3 Within the past 5 years (2 years but less than 5 years ago)
4 5 or more years ago
Do not read:
7 Don't know / Not sure
9 Refused

5.3 Have you EVER been told by a doctor, nurse or other health professional that your blood cholesterol is high? (88)

1 Yes
2 No
7 Don't know / Not sure
9 Refused

Section 9: Fruits and Vegetables

These next questions are about the fruits and vegetables you ate or drank during the past 30 days. Please think about all forms of fruits and vegetables including cooked or raw, fresh, frozen, or canned. Please think about all meals, snacks, and food consumed at home and away from home.

I will be asking how often you ate or drank each one: for example, once a day, twice a week, three times a month, and so forth.

INTERVIEWER NOTE: If respondent responds less than once per month, put "0" times per month. If respondent gives a number without a time frame, ask: "Was that per day, week, or month?"

9.1 During the past month, how many times per day, week or month did you drink 100% PURE fruit juices? Do not include fruit-flavored drinks with added sugar or fruit juice you made at home and added sugar to. Only include 100% juice. (153–155)

1 _ _ Per day
2 _ _ Per week
3 _ _ Per month
5 5 5 Never
7 7 7 Don't know / Not sure
9 9 9 Refused

INTERVIEWER NOTE: Do not include fruit drinks with added sugar or other added sweeteners like Kool-aid, Hi-C, lemonade, cranberry cocktail, Tampico, Sunny Delight, Snapple, Fruitopia, Gatorade, Power-Ade, or yogurt drinks.

Do not include fruit juice drinks that provide 100% daily vitamin C but include added sugar.

Do not include vegetable juices such as tomato and VB if respondent provides but include in "other vegetables" question 9.6.

DO include 100% pure juices including orange, mango, papaya, pineapple, apple, grape (white or red), or grapefruit. Only count cranberry juice if the R perception is that it is 100% juice with no sugar or artificial sweetener added. 100% juice blends such as orange-pineapple, orange-tangerine, cranberry-grape are also acceptable as are fruit-vegetable 100% blends. 100% pure juice from concentrate (i.e., reconstituted) is counted.

9.2 During the past month, not counting juice, how many times per day, week, or month did you eat fruit? Count fresh, frozen, or canned fruit. (156–158)

1 _ _ Per day
2 _ _ Per week
3 _ _ Per month
5 5 5 Never
7 7 7 Don't know / Not sure
9 9 9 Refused

Read only if necessary: "Your best guess is fine. Include apples, bananas, applesauce, oranges, grapefruit, fruit salad, watermelon, cantaloupe or musk melon, papaya, lychees, star fruit, pomegranates, mangos, grapes, and berries such as blueberries and strawberries."

INTERVIEWER NOTE: Do not count fruit jam, jelly, or fruit preserves.

Do not include dried fruit in ready-to-eat cereals.

Do include dried raisins, cran-raisins if respondent tells you—*but due to their small serving size they* are *not included in the prompt.*

Do include cut up fresh, frozen, or canned fruit added to yogurt, cereal, jello, and other meal items.

Include culturally and geographically appropriate fruits that are not mentioned (e.g. genip, soursop, sugar apple, figs, tamarind, bread fruit, sea grapes, carambola, longans, lychees, akee, rambutan, etc.).

9.3 During the past month, how many times per day, week, or month did you eat cooked or canned beans, such as refried, baked, black, garbanzo beans, beans in soup, soybeans, edamame, tofu or lentils. Do NOT include long green beans. (159–161)

1 _ _ Per day
2 _ _ Per week
3 _ _ Per month
5 5 5 Never
7 7 7 Don't know / Not sure
9 9 9 Refused

Read only if necessary: "Include round or oval beans or peas such as navy, pinto, split peas, cow peas, hummus, lentils, soy beans and tofu. Do NOT include long green beans such as string beans, broad or winged beans, or pole beans."

INTERVIEWER NOTE: Include soybeans also called edamame, tofu (bean curd made from soybeans), kidney, pinto, hummus, lentils, black, black-eyed peas, cow peas, lima beans, and white beans.

Include bean burgers including garden burgers and veggie burgers.

Include falafel and tempeh.

9.4 During the past month, how many times per day, week, or month did you eat dark green vegetables for example broccoli or dark leafy greens including romaine, chard, collard greens or spinach? (162–164)

1 _ _ Per day
2 _ _ Per week
3 _ _ Per month
5 5 5 Never
7 7 7 Don't know / Not sure
9 9 9 Refused

INTERVIEWER NOTE: Each time a vegetable is eaten it counts as one time.

INTERVIEWER NOTE: Include all raw leafy green salads including spinach, mesclun, romaine lettuce, bok choy, dark green leafy lettuce, dandelions, komatsuna, watercress, and arugula.

Do not include iceberg (head) lettuce if specifically told type of lettuce. Include all cooked greens including kale, collard greens, choys, turnip greens, mustard greens.

9.5 During the past month, how many times per day, week, or month did you eat orange-colored vegetables such as sweet potatoes, pumpkin, winter squash, or carrots? (165–167)

1 _ _ Per day
2 _ _ Per week
3 _ _ Per month
5 5 5 Never
7 7 7 Don't know / Not sure
9 9 9 Refused

Read only if needed: "Winter squash have hard, thick skins and deep yellow to orange flesh. They include acorn, buttercup, and spaghetti squash."

FOR INTERVIEWER: Include all forms of carrots including long or baby-cut.

Include carrot-slaw (e.g. shredded carrots with or without other vegetables or fruit).

Include all forms of sweet potatoes including baked, mashed, casserole, pie, or sweet potatoes fries.

Include all hard-winter squash varieties including acorn, autumn cup, banana, buttercup, delicate, hubbard, kabocha (Also known as an Ebisu, Delica, Hoka, Hokkaido, or Japanese Pumpkin: blue kuri), and spaghetti squash. Include all forms including soup.

Include pumpkin, including pumpkin soup and pie. Do not include pumpkin bars, cake, bread or other grain-based desert-type food containing pumpkin (i.e. similar to banana bars, zucchini bars we do not include).

9.6 Not counting what you just told me about, during the past month, about how many times per day, week, or month did you eat OTHER vegetables? Examples of other vegetables include tomatoes, tomato juice or V-8 juice, corn, eggplant, peas, lettuce, cabbage, and white potatoes that are not fried such as baked or mashed potatoes. (168–170)

1 _ _ Per day
2 _ _ Per week
3 _ _ Per month
5 5 5 Never
7 7 7 Don't know / Not sure
9 9 9 Refused

Read only if needed: "Do not count vegetables you have already counted and do not include fried potatoes."

INTERVIEWER NOTE: Include corn, peas, tomatoes, okra, beets, cauliflower, bean sprouts, avocado, cucumber, onions, peppers (red, green, yellow, orange); all cabbage including American-style cole-slaw; mushrooms, snow peas, snap peas, broad beans, string, wax-, or pole-beans.

Include any form of the vegetable (raw, cooked, canned, or frozen).

Do not include products consumed usually as condiments including ketchup, catsup, salsa, chutney, relish.

Do include tomato juice if respondent did not count in fruit juice.

Include culturally and geographically appropriate vegetables that are not mentioned (e.g. daikon, jicama, oriental cucumber, etc.).

Do not include rice or other grains.

SECTION 10: EXERCISE (PHYSICAL ACTIVITY)

The next few questions are about exercise, recreation, or physical activities other than your regular job duties.

INTERVIEWER INSTRUCTION: If respondent does not have a "regular job duty" or is retired, they may count the physical activity or exercise they spend the most time doing in a regular month.

10.1 During the past month, other than your regular job, did you participate in any physical activities or exercises such as running, calisthenics, golf, gardening, or walking for exercise? (171)

1 Yes
2 No [Go to Q10.8]
7 Don't know / Not sure [Go to Q10.8]
9 Refused [Go to Q10.8]

10.2 What type of physical activity or exercise did you spend the most time doing during the past month? (172–173)

_ _ (Specify) [See Coding List A]
7 7 Don't know / Not Sure [Go to Q10.8]
9 9 Refused [Go to Q10.8]

INTERVIEWER INSTRUCTION: If the respondent's activity is not included in the Coding List A, choose the option listed as "Other".

INTERVIEWER NOTE: Housework may be included as a physical activity or exercise spent and can be coded as "Other".

10.3 How many times per week or per month did you take part in this activity during the past month? (174–176)

1 _ _ Times per week
2 _ _ Times per month
7 7 7 Don't know / Not sure
9 9 9 Refused

10.4 And when you took part in this activity, for how many minutes or hours did you usually keep at it? (177–179)

_: _ _ Hours and minutes
7 7 7 Don't know/Not sure
9 9 9 Refused

10.5 What other type of physical activity gave you the next most exercise during the past month? (160–181)

_ _ (Specify) [See Coding List A]
8 8 No other activity [Go to Q10.8]
7 7 Don't know / Not Sure [Go to Q10.8]
9 9 Refused [Go to Q10.8]

INTERVIEWER INSTRUCTION: If the respondent's activity is not included in the Coding List A, choose the option listed as "Other".

INTERVIEWER NOTE: Housework may be included as a physical activity or exercise spent and can be coded as "Other".

10.6 How many times per week or per month did you take part in this activity during the past month? (182–184)

1 _ _ Times per week
2 _ _ Times per month
7 7 7 Don't know / Not sure
9 9 9 Refused

10.7 And when you took part in this activity, for how many minutes or hours did you usually keep at it? (185–187)

_: _ _ Hours and minutes
7 7 7 Don't know / Not sure
9 9 9 Refused

10.8 During the past month, how many times per week or per month did you do physical activities or exercises to STRENGTHEN your muscles? Do NOT count aerobic activities like walking, running, or bicycling. Count activities using your own body weight like yoga, sit-ups or push-ups and those using weight machines, free weights, or elastic bands. (188–190)

1 _ _ Times per week
2 _ _ Times per month
8 8 8 Never
7 7 7 Don't know / Not sure
9 9 9 Refused

Section 15: Alcohol Consumption

15.1 During the past 30 days, how many days per week or per month did you have at least one drink of any alcoholic beverage such as beer, wine, a malt beverage or liquor? (209–211)

1 _ _ Days per week
2 _ _ Days in past 30 days
8 8 8 No drinks in past 30 days [Go to next section]
7 7 7 Don't know / Not sure [Go to next section]
9 9 9 Refused [Go to next section]

15.2 One drink is equivalent to a 12-ounce beer, a 5-ounce glass of wine, or a drink with one shot of liquor. During the past 30 days, on the days when you drank, about how many drinks did you drink on the average? (212–213)

NOTE: A 40 ounce beer would count as 3 drinks, or a cocktail drink with 2 shots would count as 2 drinks.

_ _ Number of drinks
7 7 Don't know / Not sure
9 9 Refused

15.3 Considering all types of alcoholic beverages, how many times during the past 30 days did you have X [CATI $X = 5$ for men, $X = 4$ for women] or more drinks on an occasion? (214–215)

_ _	Number of times
8 8	None
7 7	Don't know / Not sure
9 9	Refused

15.4 During the past 30 days, what is the largest number of drinks you had on any occasion? (216–217)

_ _	Number of drinks
7 7	Don't know / Not sure
9 9	Refused

MODULE 1: PRE-DIABETES

NOTE: Only asked of those not responding "Yes" (code = 1) to Core Q6.13 (Diabetes awareness question).

1. Have you had a test for high blood sugar or diabetes within the past three years? (245)

1	Yes
2	No
7	Don't know / Not sure
9	Refused

CATI NOTE: If Core Q6.13 = 4 (No, pre-diabetes or borderline diabetes); answer Q2 "Yes" (code = 1)

2. Have you ever been told by a doctor or other health professional that you have pre-diabetes or borderline diabetes?

1	Yes	**If "Yes" and respondent is female, ask: "Was this only when you were pregnant?" (246)**
2	Yes, during pregnancy	
3	No	
7	Don't know / Not sure	
9	Refused	

MODULE 2: DIABETES

To be asked following Core Q6.13; if response is "Yes" (code = 1)

1. How old were you when you were told you have diabetes? (247–248)

_ _	Code age in years [97 = 97 and older]
9 8	Don't know / Not sure
9 9	Refused

2. Are you now taking insulin? (249)

1	Yes
2	No
9	Refused

3. About how often do you check your blood for glucose or sugar? Include times when checked by a family member or friend, but do NOT include times when checked by a health professional. (250–252)

1 _ _	Times per day
2 _ _	Times per week
3 _ _	Times per month
4 _ _	Times per year
8 8 8	Never
7 7 7	Don't know / Not sure
9 9 9	Refused

4. About how often do you check your feet for any sores or irritations? Include times when checked by a family member or friend, but do NOT include times when checked by a health professional. (253–255)

1 _ _	Times per day
2 _ _	Times per week
3 _ _	Times per month
4 _ _	Times per year
5 5 5	No feet
8 8 8	Never
7 7 7	Don't know / Not sure
9 9 9	Refused

5. About how many times in the past 12 months have you seen a doctor, nurse, or other health professional for your diabetes? (256–257)

_ _	Number of times [76 = 76 or more]
8 8	None
7 7	Don't know / Not sure
9 9	Refused

6. A test for "A one C" measures the average level of blood sugar over the past three months. About how many times in the past 12 months has a doctor, nurse, or other health professional checked you for "A one C"? (258–259)

_ _	Number of times [76 = 76 or more]
8 8	None
9 8	Never heard of "A one C" test
7 7	Don't know / Not sure
9 9	Refused

CATI NOTE: If Q4 = 5 5 5 "No feet". go to Q8.

7. About how many times in the past 12 months has a health professional checked your feet for any sores or irritations? (260–261)

_ _	Number of times [76 = 76 or more]
8 8	None
7 7	Don't know / Not sure
9 9	Refused

8. When was the last time you had an eye exam in which the pupils were dilated? This would have made you temporarily sensitive to bright light. (262)

	Read only if necessary:
1	Within the past month (anytime less than 1 month ago)
2	Within the past year (1 month but less than 12 months ago)
3	Within the past 2 years (1 year but less than 2 years ago)
4	2 or more years ago
	Do not read:
7	Don't know / Not sure
6	Never
9	Refused

9. Has a doctor ever told you that diabetes has affected your eyes or that you had retinopathy? (263)

1	Yes
2	No
7	Don't know / Not sure
9	Refused

10. Have you ever taken a course or class in how to manage your diabetes yourself? (264)

1	Yes
2	No
7	Don't know / Not sure
9	Refused

Module 4: Sugar Sweetened Beverages and Menu Labeling

1. About how often do you drink regular soda or pop that contains sugar? Do not include diet soda or diet pop. (273–275)

1 _ _	Times per day
2 _ _	Times per week
3 _ _	Times per month
8 8 8	Never
7 7 7	Don't know / Not sure
9 9 9	Refused

2. About how often do you drink sweetened fruit drinks, such as Kool-aid, cranberry, and lemonade? Include fruit drinks you made at home and added sugar to. (276–278)

1 _ _	Times per day
2 _ _	Times per week
3 _ _	Times per month
8 8 8	Never
7 7 7	Don't know / Not sure
9 9 9	Refused

3. The next question is about eating out at fast food and chain restaurants. When calorie information is available in the restaurant, how often does this information help you decide what to order? (279–280)

	Please read:
01	Always
02	Most of the time
03	About half the time
04	Sometimes
05	Never
	Do not read:
06	Never noticed or never looked for calorie information
08	Usually cannot find calorie information
55	Do not eat at fast food or chain restaurants
77	Don't know / Not sure
99	Refused

Module 9: Cardiovascular Health

I would like to ask you a few more questions about your cardiovascular or heart health.

CATI NOTE: If Core Q6.1 = 1 (Yes), continue, If Core Q6.1 = 2, 7, or 9 (No, Don't know, or Refused), skip Q1.

1. Following your heart attack, did you go to any kind of outpatient rehabilitation? This is sometimes called "rehab." (312)

1	Yes
2	No
7	Don't know / Not sure
9	Refused

CATI NOTE: If Core Q6.3 = 1 (Yes), ask Q2. If Core Q6.3 = 2, 7, or 9 (No, Don't know, or Refused), skip Q2.

2. Following your stroke, did you go to any kind of outpatient rehabilitation? This is sometimes called "rehab." (312)

   1 Yes

   2 No

   7 Don't know / Not sure

   9 Refused

[Question 3 is asked of all respondents.]

3. Do you take aspirin daily or every other day? (314)

   1 Yes [Go to next module]

   2 No

   7 Don't know / Not sure

   9 Refused

4. Do you have a health problem or condition that makes taking aspirin unsafe for you? (315)

   If "Yes", ask "Is this a stomach condition?" Code upset stomach as stomach problems.

   1 Yes, not stomach related

   2 Yes, stomach problems

   3 No

   7 Don't know / Not sure

   9 Refused

APPENDIX

J Suppliers of Nutritional Assessment Equipment

SUPPLIERS

Beta Technology, Inc.
831-426-0882
800-858-2382
www.beta-technology.com

Biodynamics Corporation
800-869-6987
206-526-0205
www.biodyncorp.com

Cosmed
925-676-6002
800-426-3763
www.cosmed.com

Country Technology, Inc.
608-735-4718
www.fitnessmart.com

Creative Health Products, Inc.
800-742-4478
734-996-5900
www.chponline.com

Davco Weight Scales Inc.
250-747-8371
877-747-8371
www.davco.bc.ca

Detecto Scales
800-641-2008
www.detectoscale.com

Novel Products, Inc.
800-323-5143
815-624-4888
www.novelproductsinc.com

Ontario Association of Sport and Exercise Sciences
519-942-2620
www.oases.on.ca

RJL Systems, Inc.
800-528-4513
586-790-0200
www.rjlsystems.com

Seca Corporation
800-542-7322
888-705-7397
www.seca.com

Seritex, Inc.
973-472-4200
www.seritex.com

Stadiometer.com
866-500-9808
www.stadiometer.com

Tanita Corporation
847-640-9241
www.tanita.com

Valhalla Scientific
(858) 457-5576
www.valhallascientific.com

EQUIPMENT

Anthropometric Tapes

Country Technology, Inc.
Creative Health Products, Inc.
Novel Products, Inc.
Ontario Association of Sport and Exercise Sciences
Seca Corporation
Seritex, Inc.

Bioelectrical Impedance Instruments

Biodynamics Corporation
Country Technology, Inc.
Creative Health Products
RJL Systems, Inc.
Tanita Corporation of America, Inc.
Valhalla Scientific

Knee Height & Sliding Calipers

Creative Health Products, Inc.
Seritex, Inc.

Recumbent Length Measurement Equipment

Novel Products, Inc.
Seca Corporation
Seritex, Inc.
Stadiometer.com

Skinfold Calipers

Beta Technology
Country Technology, Inc.
Creative Health Products, Inc.
Novel Products, Inc.
Ontario Association of Sport and Exercise Sciences
Seca Corporation
Seritex, Inc.

Stadiometers

Country Technology, Inc.
Creative Health Products, Inc.
Novel Products, Inc.

Seca Corporation
Seritex, Inc.
Stadiometer.com

Strength Testing

Country Technology, Inc.
Creative Health Products, Inc.
Novel Products, Inc.

Weight Scales

Country Technology, Inc.
Creative Health Products, Inc.
Davco Weight Scales, Inc.
Detecto Scales
Novel Products, Inc.
Ontario Association of Sport and Exercise Sciences
Seca Corporation
Tanita Corporation of America, Inc.

Whole-Body Plethysmography

Cosmed

APPENDIX

K

*CDC Clinical Growth Charts**

From National Center for Health Statistics, Centers for Disease Control and Prevention, U.S. Department of Health and Human Services.
*For additional information relating to the CDC Growth Charts, visit the *Nutritional Assessment* website at www.mhhe.com/lee-nieman6.

Birth to 24 months: Boys
Length-for-age and Weight-for-age percentiles

NAME ______________________

RECORD # ______

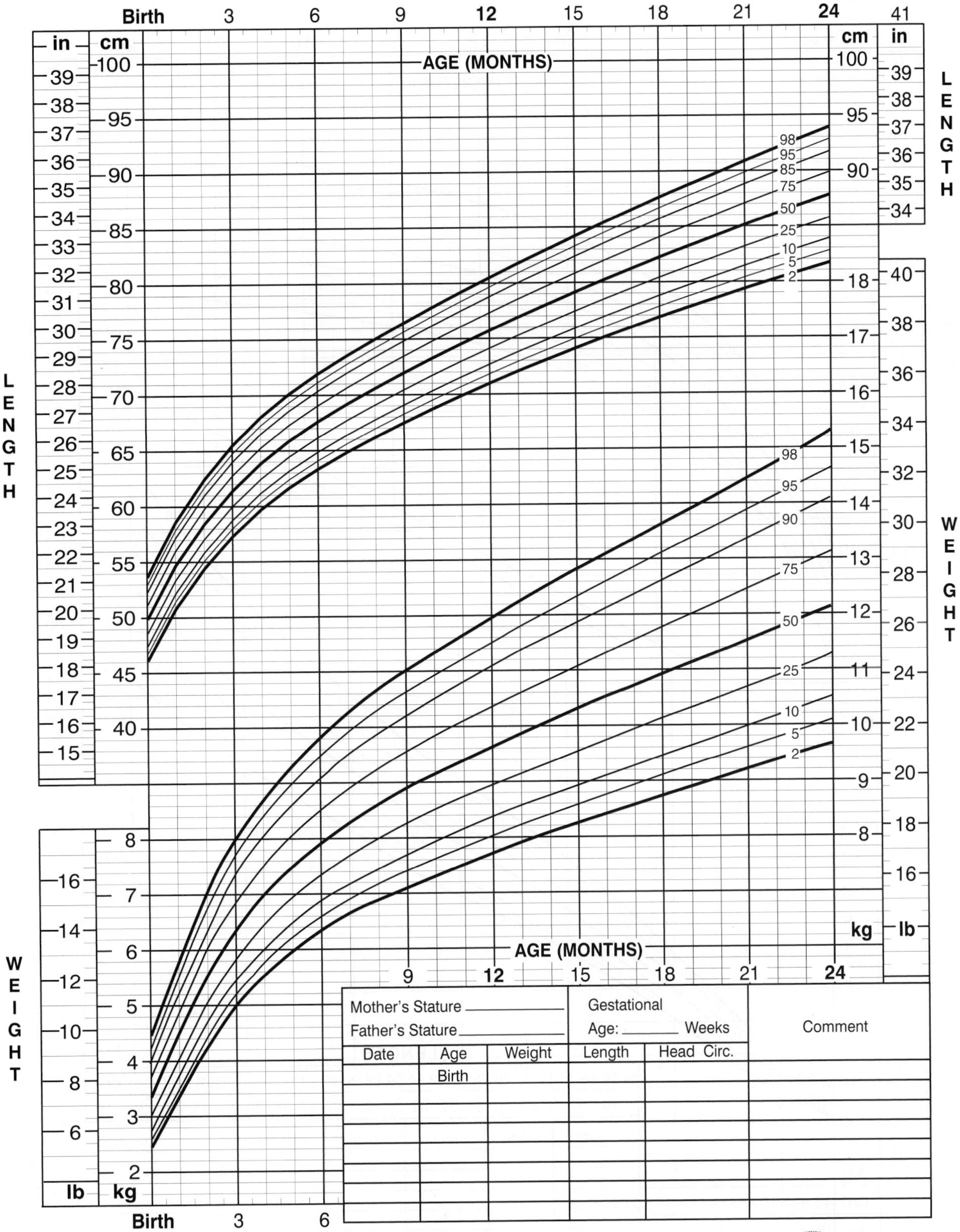

Mother's Stature ______ Father's Stature ______			Gestational Age: ______ Weeks		Comment
Date	Age	Weight	Length	Head Circ.	
	Birth				

Published by the Centers for Disease Control and Prevention, November 1, 2009

SOURCE: WHO Child Growth Standards (http://www.who.int/childgrowth/en)

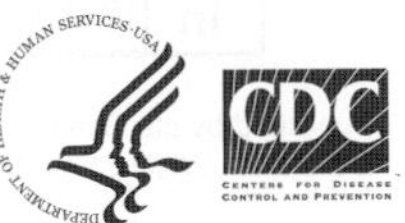

Birth to 24 months: Boys
Head circumference-for-age and Weight-for-length percentiles

NAME ____________________

RECORD # ____________

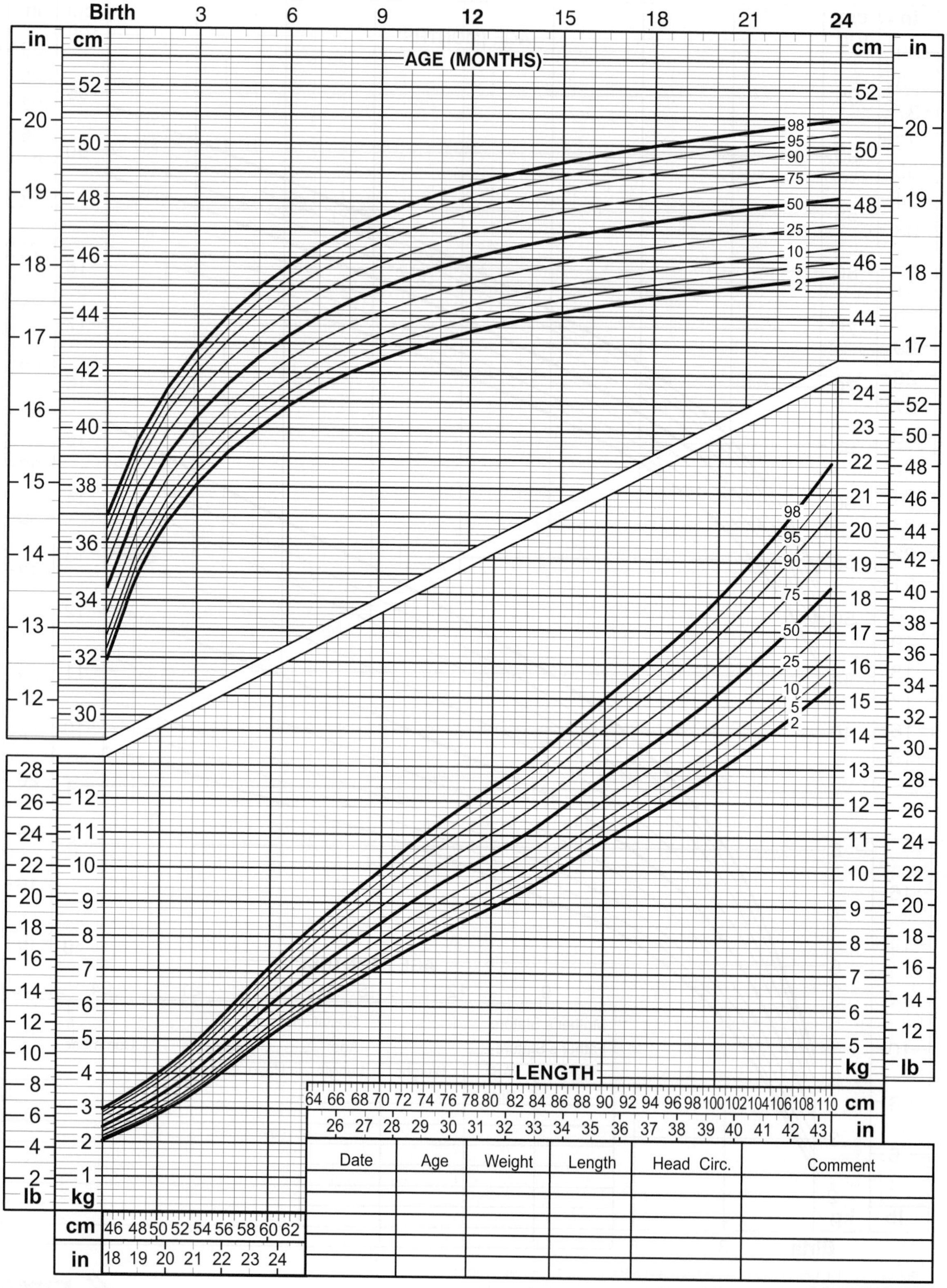

AGE (MONTHS)

HEAD CIRCUMFERENCE

WEIGHT

LENGTH

Date	Age	Weight	Length	Head Circ.	Comment

Published by the Centers for Disease Control and Prevention, November 1, 2009
SOURCE: WHO Child Growth Standards (http://www.who.int/childgrowth/en)

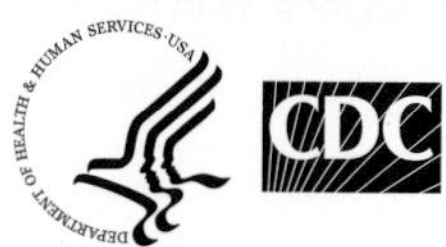

Birth to 24 months: Girls
Length-for-age and Weight-for-age percentiles

NAME ____________________

RECORD # ____________

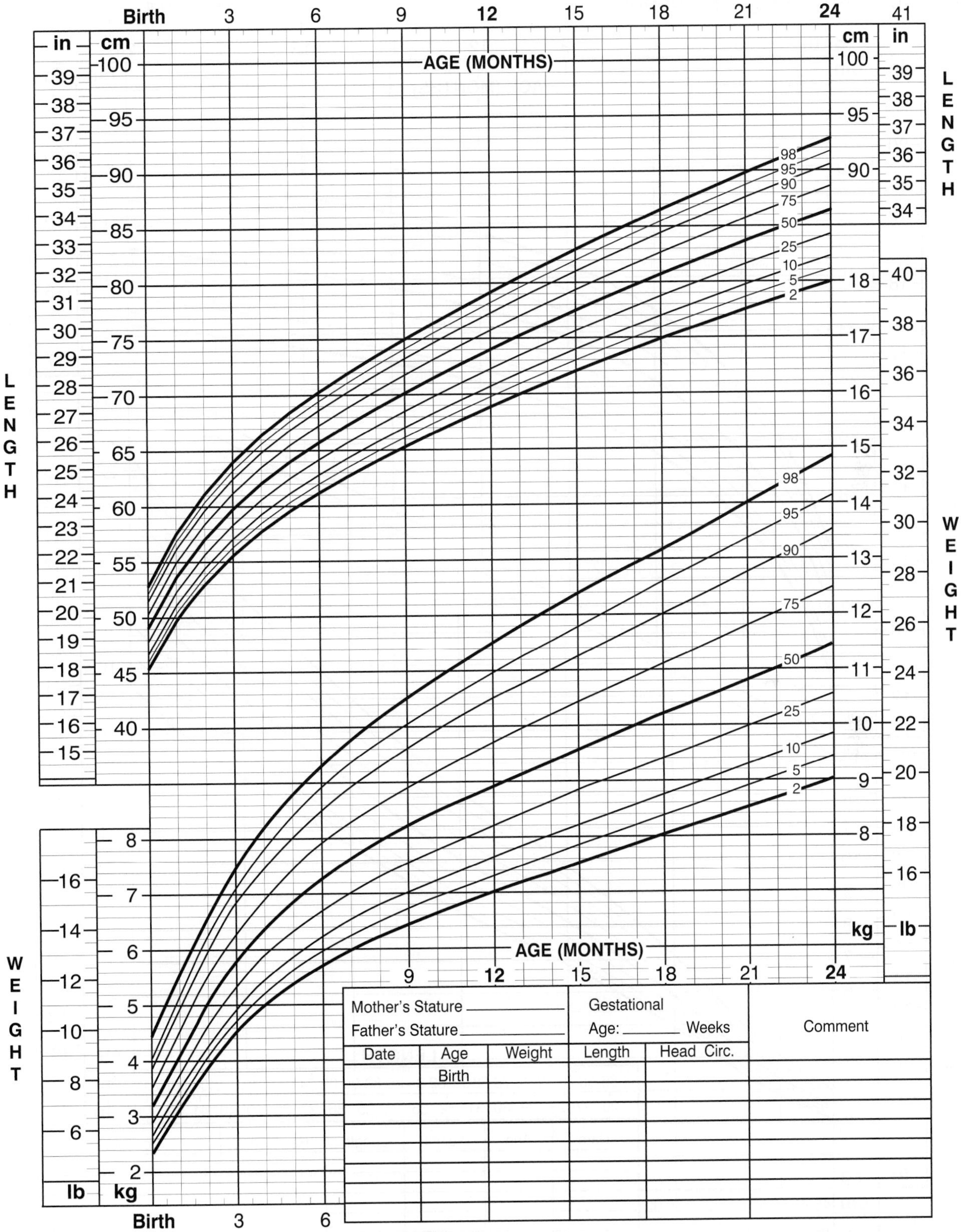

Mother's Stature ______ Father's Stature ______			Gestational Age: ______ Weeks		Comment
Date	Age	Weight	Length	Head Circ.	
	Birth				

Published by the Centers for Disease Control and Prevention, November 1, 2009
SOURCE: WHO Child Growth Standards (http://www.who.int/childgrowth/en)

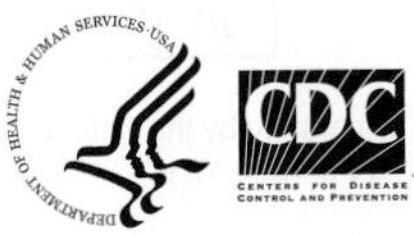

Birth to 24 months: Girls
Head circumference-for-age and Weight-for-length percentiles

NAME ____________________

RECORD # ____________

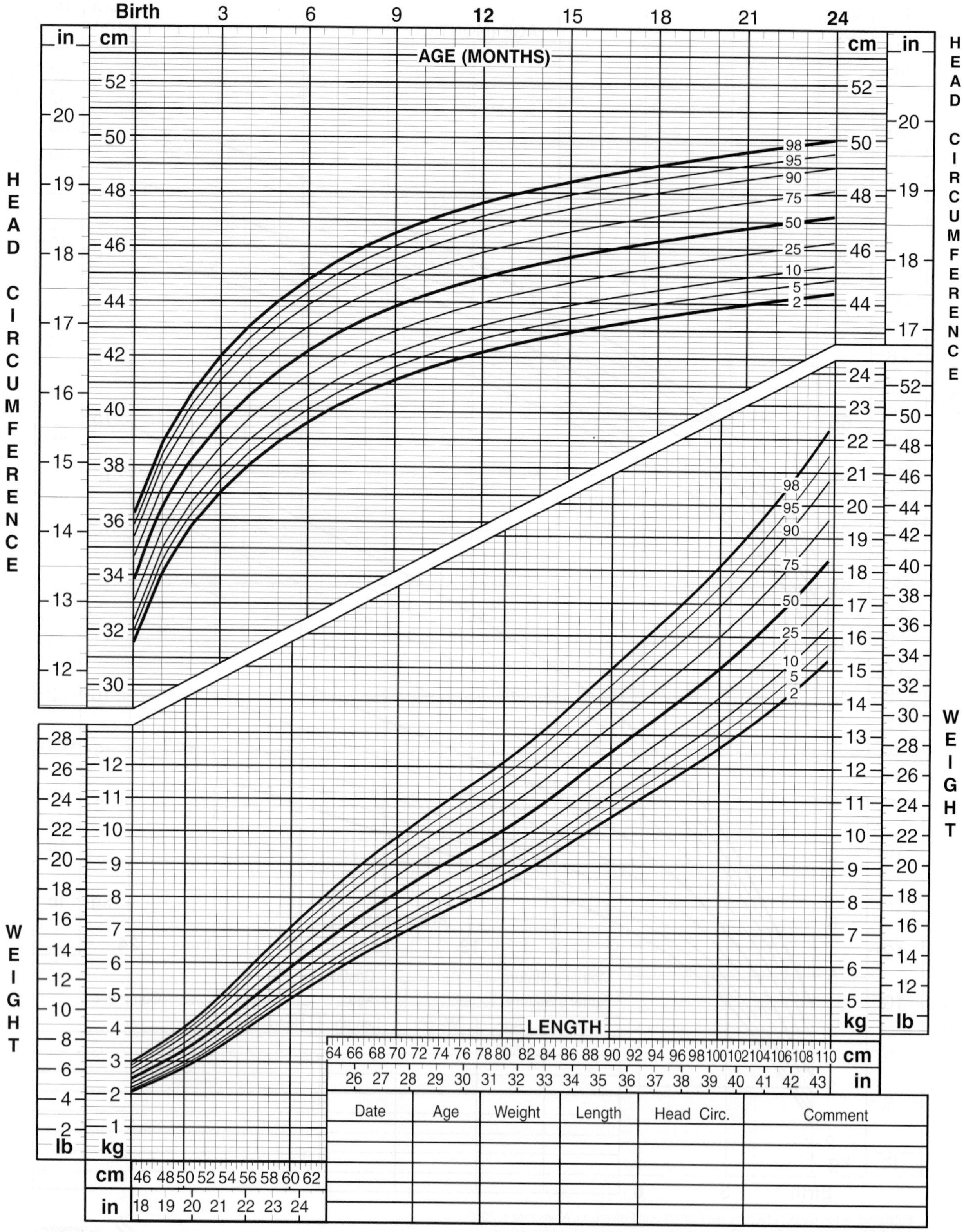

Date	Age	Weight	Length	Head Circ.	Comment

Published by the Centers for Disease Control and Prevention, November 1, 2009
SOURCE: WHO Child Growth Standards (http://www.who.int/childgrowth/en)

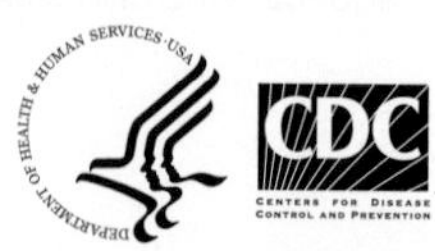

2 to 20 years: Boys
Stature-for-age and Weight-for-age percentiles

NAME ______________________

RECORD # ______________

Mother's Stature ____________ Father's Stature ____________

Date	Age	Weight	Stature	BMI*

***To Calculate BMI**: Weight (kg) ÷ Stature (cm) ÷ Stature (cm) x 10,000
or Weight (lb) ÷ Stature (in) ÷ Stature (in) x 703

Revised and corrected November 21, 2000.
SOURCE: Developed by the National Center for Health Statistics in collaboration with the National Center for Chronic Disease Prevention and Health Promotion (2000).
http://www.cdc.gov/growthcharts

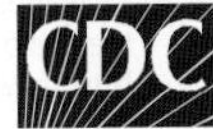

2 to 20 years: Boys
Body mass index-for-age percentiles

NAME ______________________

RECORD # ____________

Date	Age	Weight	Stature	BMI*	Comments

***To Calculate BMI**: Weight (kg) ÷ Stature (cm) ÷ Stature (cm) x 10,000
or Weight (lb) ÷ Stature (in) ÷ Stature (in) x 703

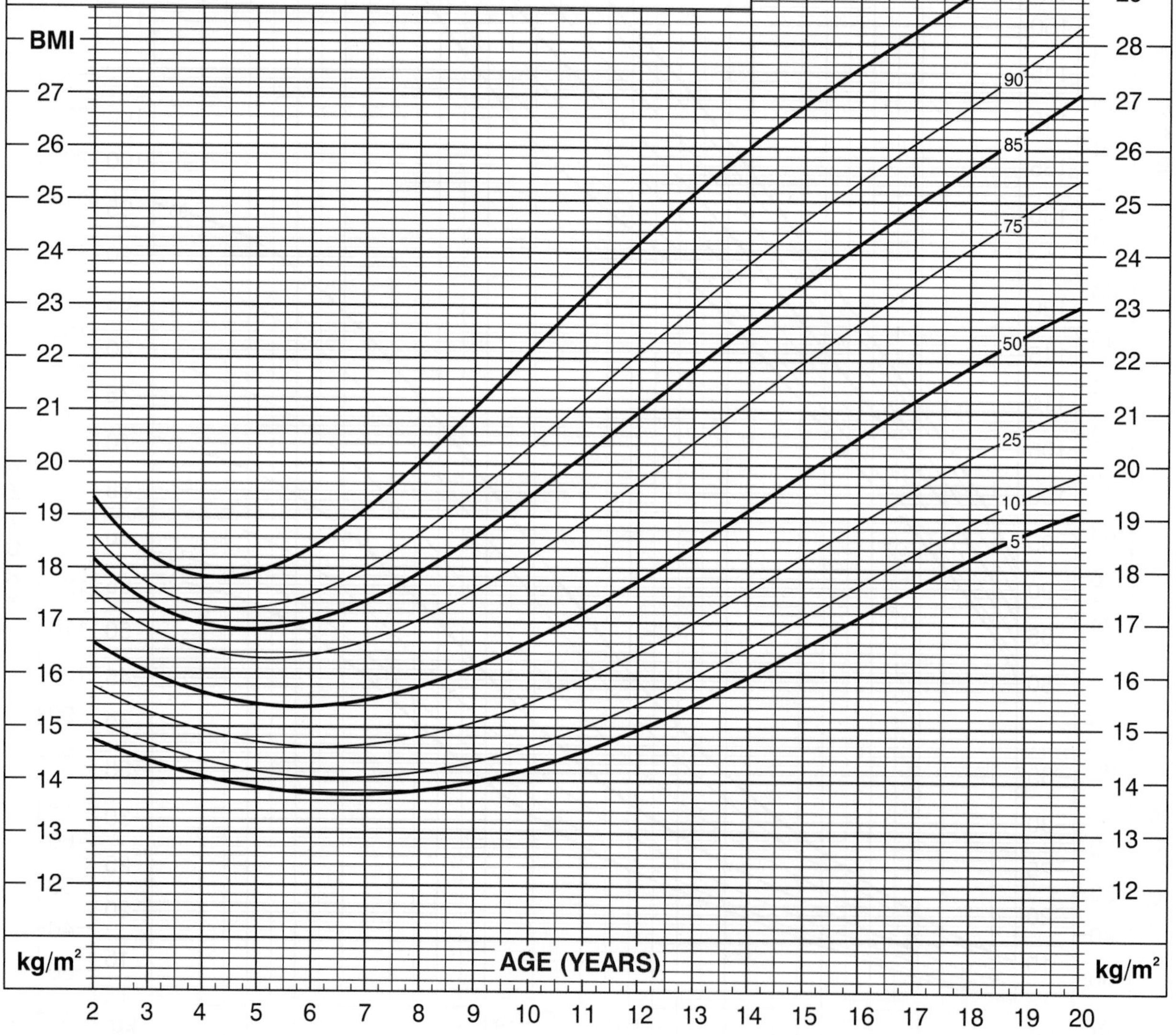

BMI

35 34 33 32 31 30 29 28 27 26 25 24 23 22 21 20 19 18 17 16 15 14 13 12

95 90 85 75 50 25 10 5

kg/m²

AGE (YEARS)

2 3 4 5 6 7 8 9 10 11 12 13 14 15 16 17 18 19 20

SOURCE: Developed by the National Center for Health Statistics in collaboration with the National Center for Chronic Disease Prevention and Health Promotion (2000).
http://www.cdc.gov/growthcharts

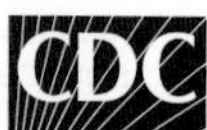

2 to 20 years: Girls
Stature-for-age and Weight-for-age percentiles

NAME ______________________

RECORD # ______________

Mother's Stature		Father's Stature		
Date	Age	Weight	Stature	BMI*

***To Calculate BMI**: Weight (kg) ÷ Stature (cm) ÷ Stature (cm) x 10,000
or Weight (lb) ÷ Stature (in) ÷ Stature (in) x 703

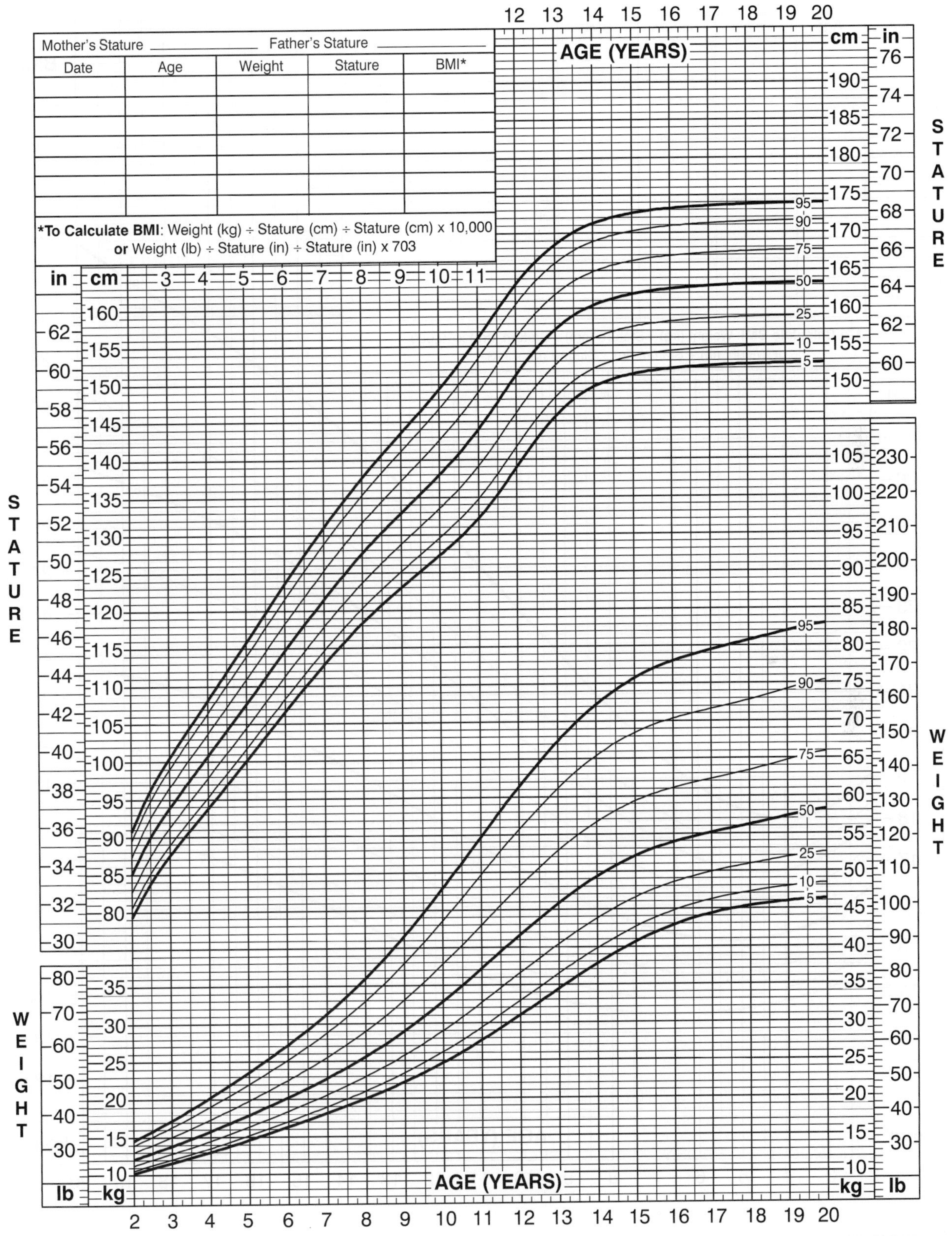

Revised and corrected November 21, 2000.
SOURCE: Developed by the National Center for Health Statistics in collaboration with the National Center for Chronic Disease Prevention and Health Promotion (2000).
http://www.cdc.gov/growthcharts

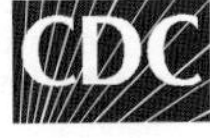

2 to 20 years: Girls
Body mass index-for-age percentiles

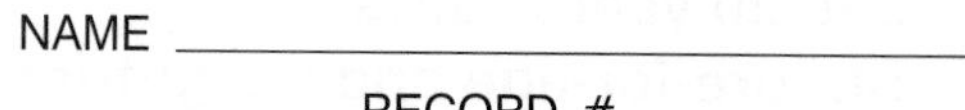

Date	Age	Weight	Stature	BMI*	Comments

***To Calculate BMI**: Weight (kg) ÷ Stature (cm) ÷ Stature (cm) x 10,000
or Weight (lb) ÷ Stature (in) ÷ Stature (in) x 703

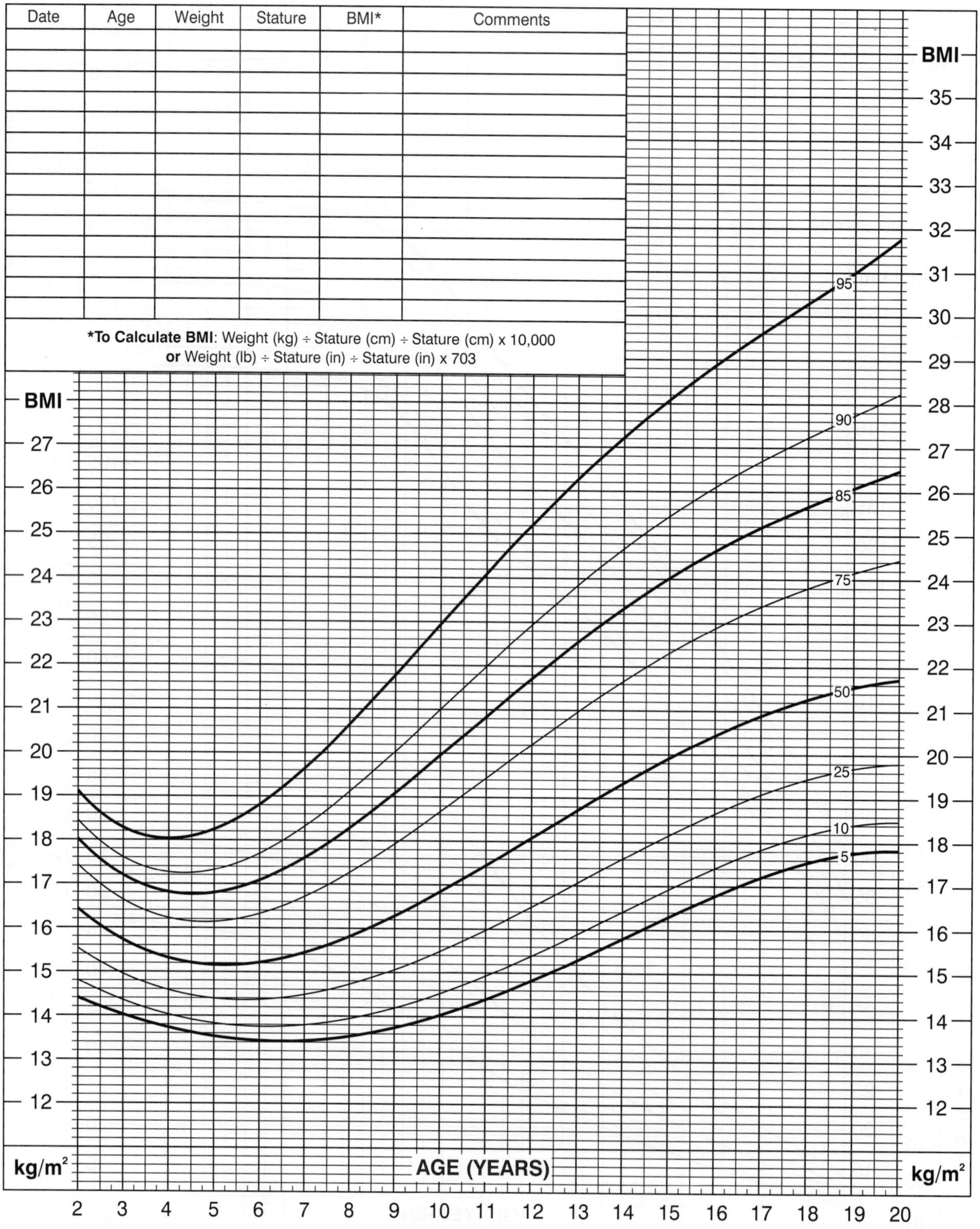

BMI
35
34
33
32
31
30
29
28
27
26
25
24
23
22
21
20
19
18
17
16
15
14
13
12
kg/m²

95
90
85
75
50
25
10
5

AGE (YEARS)
2 3 4 5 6 7 8 9 10 11 12 13 14 15 16 17 18 19 20

SOURCE: Developed by the National Center for Health Statistics in collaboration with the National Center for Chronic Disease Prevention and Health Promotion (2000).
http://www.cdc.gov/growthcharts

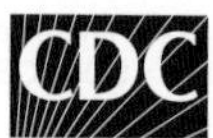

NAME ______________________

RECORD # ______________

Weight-for-stature percentiles: Boys

Date	Age	Weight	Stature	Comments

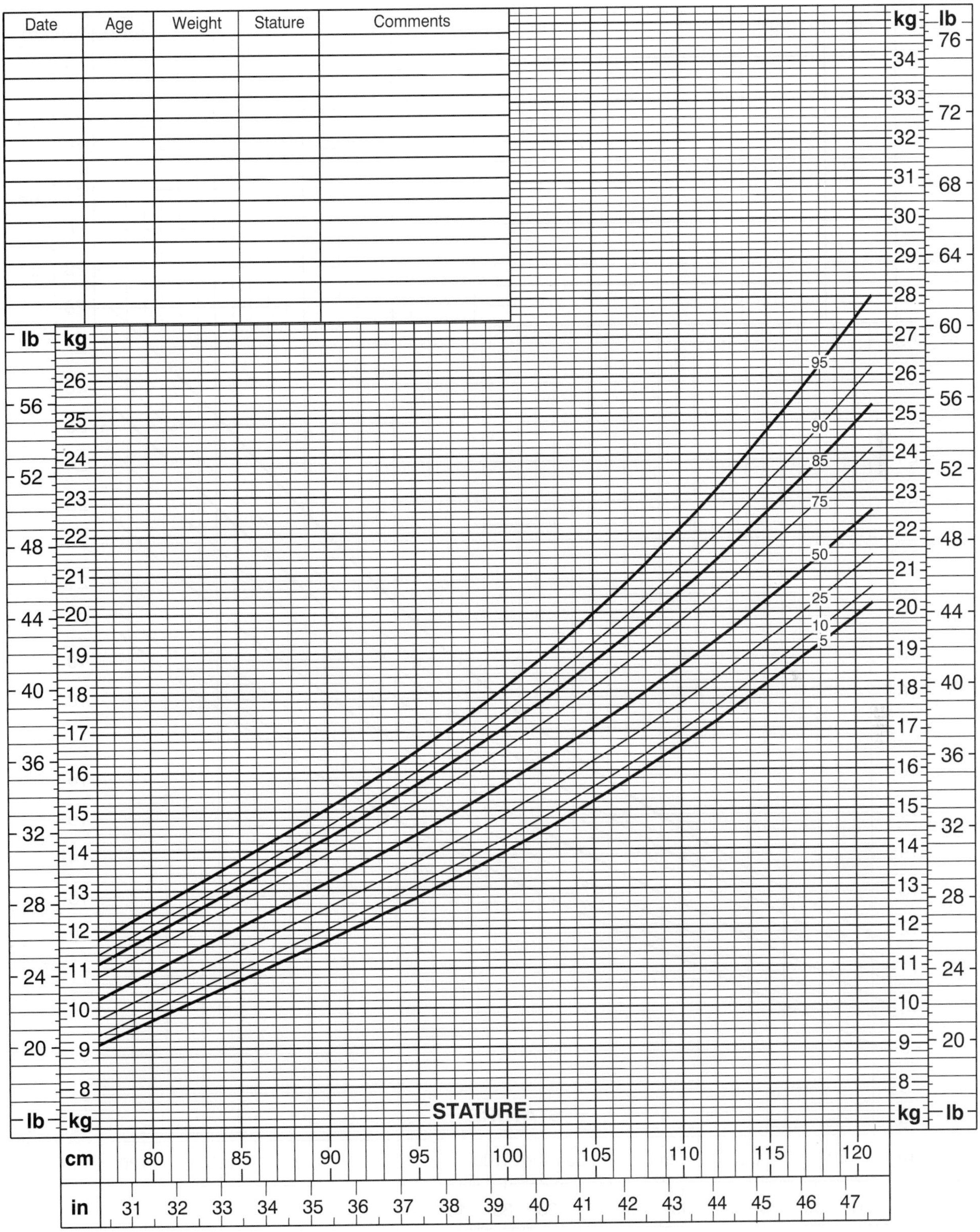

lb kg 26 56 25 24 52 23 22 48 21 44 20 19 40 18 17 36 16 15 32 14 13 28 12 11 24 10 20 9 8 lb kg

95 90 85 75 50 25 10 5

kg lb 76 34 33 72 32 31 68 30 29 64 28 60 27 26 56 25 24 52 23 22 48 21 20 44 19 18 40 17 16 36 15 32 14 13 28 12 11 24 10 9 20 8 kg lb

STATURE

cm 80 85 90 95 100 105 110 115 120

in 31 32 33 34 35 36 37 38 39 40 41 42 43 44 45 46 47

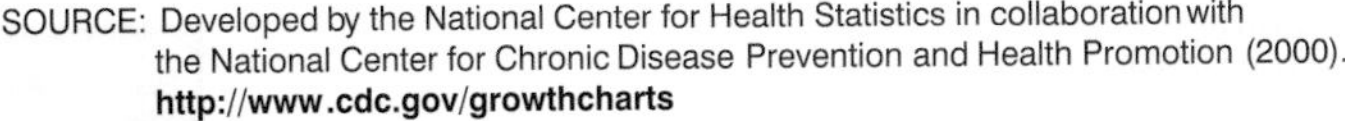
SOURCE: Developed by the National Center for Health Statistics in collaboration with the National Center for Chronic Disease Prevention and Health Promotion (2000).
http://www.cdc.gov/growthcharts

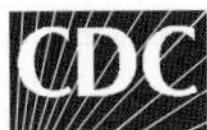

NAME ______________________________

Weight-for-stature percentiles: Girls

RECORD # ______________

Date	Age	Weight	Stature	Comments

kg 34 33 32 31 30 29 28 27 26 25 24 23 22 21 20 19 18 17 16 15 14 13 12 11 10 9 8 kg

lb 76 72 68 64 60 56 52 48 44 40 36 32 28 24 20 lb

95 90 85 75 50 25 10 5

STATURE

cm 80 85 90 95 100 105 110 115 120

in 31 32 33 34 35 36 37 38 39 40 41 42 43 44 45 46 47

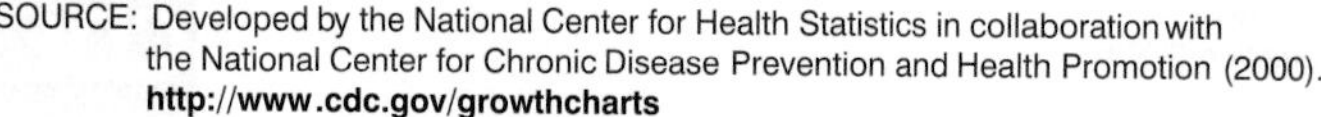

SOURCE: Developed by the National Center for Health Statistics in collaboration with the National Center for Chronic Disease Prevention and Health Promotion (2000).
http://www.cdc.gov/growthcharts

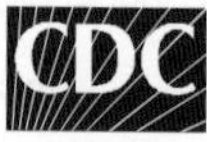

APPENDIX

L

Mean Body Weight, Height, and Body Mass Index, United States, 1960–2006

From National Center for Health Statistics, Centers for Disease Control and Prevention, U.S. Department of Health and Human Services.

TABLE 1 Mean Weight (Pounds) by Survey, Sex, and Age; Children: United States

Sex and Age	NHES II, 1963–65 Sample Size	NHES II, 1963–65 Mean	NHES II, 1963–65 Standard Error of the Mean	NHANES I, 1971–74 Sample Size	NHANES I, 1971–74 Mean	NHANES I, 1971–74 Standard Error of the Mean	NHANES II, 1976–80 Sample Size	NHANES II, 1976–80 Mean	NHANES II, 1976–80 Standard Error of the Mean
Male									
2 years	—	—	—	298	29.8	0.4	370	29.5	0.2
3 years	—	—	—	308	34.3	0.3	421	34.2	0.3
4 years	—	—	—	304	39.0	0.3	405	38.8	0.3
5 years	—	—	—	273	44.4	0.4	393	43.4	0.3
6 years	575	48.4	0.3	179	48.5	0.7	146	50.2	0.8
7 years	632	54.3	0.4	164	54.8	0.9	150	54.8	0.8
8 years	618	61.1	0.5	152	58.1	0.7	145	61.6	1.4
9 years	603	68.5	0.9	169	69.5	1.7	141	67.6	1.4
10 years	576	74.2	0.6	184	75.3	1.2	165	79.7	1.6
11 years	595	84.1	0.7	178	85.4	1.8	153	87.4	2.0
12 years	—	—	—	200	96.8	1.8	147	96.9	2.2
13 years	—	—	—	174	109.9	2.1	165	108.9	2.6
14 years	—	—	—	174	123.8	2.1	188	124.0	1.9
15 years	—	—	—	171	132.6	2.7	180	134.7	2.2
16 years	—	—	—	169	147.2	2.8	180	146.3	2.6
17 years	—	—	—	176	151.0	2.4	183	146.6	1.7
18 years	—	—	—	124	163.4	2.8	156	156.4	2.6
19 years	—	—	—	136	159.7	2.8	150	158.0	1.9
Female									
2 years	—	—	—	272	28.5	0.3	330	28.2	0.1
3 years	—	—	—	292	33.1	0.4	367	32.5	0.2
4 years	—	—	—	281	37.0	0.4	388	37.0	0.3
5 years	—	—	—	314	43.3	0.6	369	42.7	0.6
6 years	536	47.4	0.5	176	47.5	0.7	150	48.1	0.8
7 years	609	53.2	0.4	169	53.4	0.9	154	54.2	1.0
8 years	613	60.6	0.5	152	60.5	1.1	125	60.6	0.9
9 years	581	69.1	0.8	171	70.3	1.2	154	69.7	1.6
10 years	584	77.4	0.9	197	74.4	1.3	128	78.6	1.4
11 years	525	87.6	1.0	166	90.7	1.8	143	91.1	1.9
12 years	—	—	—	177	102.8	2.3	146	101.3	2.0
13 years	—	—	—	198	113.9	2.3	155	112.0	2.6
14 years	—	—	—	184	120.2	2.2	181	119.5	2.3
15 years	—	—	—	167	124.6	2.0	144	121.1	1.9
16 years	—	—	—	171	124.9	2.3	167	126.9	1.9
17 years	—	—	—	150	130.8	3.6	134	131.1	2.1
18 years	—	—	—	141	128.1	2.4	156	129.9	2.2
19 years	—	—	—	130	131.0	3.2	158	131.5	2.1

Sex and Age	NHANES III, 1988–94 Sample Size	NHANES III, 1988–94 Mean	NHANES III, 1988–94 Standard Error of the Mean	NHANES 1999–2002 Sample Size	NHANES 1999–2002 Mean	NHANES 1999–2002 Standard Error of the Mean	NHANES 2003–2006 Sample Size	NHANES 2003–2006 Mean	NHANES 2003–2006 Standard Error of the Mean
Male									
2 years	644	29.9	0.2	262	30.2	0.2	292	31.1	0.31
3 years	516	34.7	0.4	216	35.0	0.4	210	34.8	0.35
4 years	549	38.8	0.4	179	40.8	0.5	208	40.9	0.68
5 years	497	44.1	0.4	147	46.9	1.1	202	48.7	1.07
6 years	283	51.1	1.2	182	51.7	0.9	176	53.3	0.72
7 years	269	57.8	1.0	185	59.8	1.0	181	58.7	1.28
8 years	266	66.5	1.9	214	72.0	2.1	151	69.3	1.99
9 years	281	75.7	2.1	174	79.2	1.5	176	76.3	1.57
10 years	297	82.1	1.9	187	84.9	1.8	172	88.3	1.89
11 years	281	93.5	2.0	182	96.2	2.4	158	103.2	3.58
12 years	203	108.0	2.4	299	110.9	2.8	275	112.0	2.71
13 years	187	118.8	2.2	298	118.6	4.1	284	127.4	3.03
14 years	188	141.0	7.9	266	140.5	3.6	260	139.1	3.81
15 years	187	147.2	4.2	283	150.3	2.5	270	154.9	2.99
16 years	194	151.2	3.6	306	163.7	3.0	308	167.7	3.31
17 years	196	160.3	2.9	313	166.3	3.0	279	165.4	2.86
18 years	176	156.8	3.7	284	166.4	2.5	283	170.2	3.68
19 years	168	160.6	4.7	270	172.1	2.8	271	176.8	3.54
Female									
2 years	624	29.0	0.2	248	29.2	0.3	335	29.5	0.29
3 years	587	33.9	0.3	178	33.4	0.5	191	34.8	0.45
4 years	537	39.3	0.8	191	39.5	0.7	226	39.4	0.46
5 years	554	44.3	0.5	186	45.3	1.3	199	45.3	0.82
6 years	272	49.7	1.3	171	49.2	1.1	193	51.5	1.08
7 years	274	58.1	1.7	196	56.9	1.0	157	60.2	1.37
8 years	248	65.7	1.4	184	70.1	2.6	184	67.7	2.07
9 years	280	75.6	2.7	183	78.0	1.6	185	81.0	2.18
10 years	258	83.4	2.7	164	87.9	2.3	189	93.5	2.35
11 years	275	97.1	2.4	194	105.4	2.9	175	108.4	2.88
12 years	236	107.8	2.6	316	114.3	2.3	249	116.7	2.88
13 years	220	122.8	3.5	321	127.0	3.0	292	126.4	2.15
14 years	218	128.6	3.0	324	131.7	2.2	269	129.6	3.85
15 years	191	127.8	2.3	266	134.4	3.7	248	134.2	1.67
16 years	208	134.9	3.0	273	138.5	2.6	253	135.6	2.10
17 years	201	137.3	2.6	256	135.8	2.7	252	145.6	3.65
18 years	175	134.6	4.1	243	143.5	3.3	272	149.0	4.75
19 years	177	138.9	4.2	225	149.3	2.7	239	148.6	3.95

—Data not available.

NOTE: NHES II: National Health Examination Survey, Cycle II, ages 6–11 years: NHES III: National Health Examination Survey, Cycle III, ages 12–17 years; and NHANES: National Health and Nutrition Examination Survey.

TABLE 2 Mean Weight (Kilograms) by Survey, Sex, and Age; Children: United States

Sex and Age	NHES II, 1963–65			NHANES I, 1971–74			NHANES II, 1976–80			NHANES III, 1988–94			NHANES 1999–2002			NHANES 2003–2006		
	Sample Size	Mean	Standard Error of the Mean	Sample Size	Mean	Standard Error of the Mean	Sample Size	Mean	Standard Error of the Mean	Sample Size	Mean	Standard Error of the Mean	Sample Size	Mean	Standard Error of the Mean	Sample Size	Mean	Standard Error of the Mean
Male																		
2 years	—	—	—	298	13.6	0.2	370	13.4	0.1	644	13.6	0.1	262	13.7	0.1	292	14.1	0.14
3 years	—	—	—	308	15.6	0.1	421	15.5	0.1	516	15.8	0.2	216	15.9	0.2	210	15.8	0.16
4 years	—	—	—	304	17.7	0.1	405	17.6	0.1	549	17.6	0.2	179	18.5	0.2	208	18.6	0.31
5 years	—	—	—	273	20.2	0.2	393	19.7	0.1	497	20.1	0.2	147	21.3	0.5	202	22.1	0.49
6 years	575	22.0	0.1	179	22.0	0.3	146	22.8	0.4	283	23.2	0.6	182	23.5	0.4	176	24.2	0.33
7 years	632	24.7	0.2	164	24.9	0.4	150	24.9	0.4	269	26.3	0.4	185	27.2	0.4	181	26.6	0.58
8 years	618	27.8	0.2	152	26.4	0.3	145	28.0	0.6	266	30.2	0.8	214	32.7	1.0	151	31.4	0.90
9 years	603	31.2	0.4	169	31.6	0.8	141	30.7	0.6	281	34.4	1.0	174	36.0	0.7	176	34.6	0.71
10 years	576	33.7	0.3	184	34.2	0.6	165	36.2	0.7	297	37.3	0.9	187	38.6	0.8	172	40.1	0.86
11 years	595	38.2	0.3	178	38.8	0.8	153	39.7	0.9	281	42.5	0.9	182	43.7	1.1	158	46.8	1.62
12 years	—	—	—	200	44.0	0.8	147	44.1	1.0	203	49.1	1.1	299	50.4	1.3	275	50.8	1.23
13 years	—	—	—	174	49.9	1.0	165	49.5	1.2	187	54.0	1.0	298	53.9	1.9	284	57.8	1.37
14 years	—	—	—	174	56.3	0.9	188	56.4	0.9	188	64.1	3.6	266	63.9	1.6	260	63.1	1.73
15 years	—	—	—	171	60.3	1.2	180	61.2	1.0	187	66.9	1.9	283	68.3	1.1	270	70.2	1.36
16 years	—	—	—	169	66.9	1.3	180	66.5	1.2	194	68.7	1.6	306	74.4	1.4	308	76.1	1.50
17 years	—	—	—	176	68.6	1.1	183	66.7	0.8	196	72.9	1.3	313	75.6	1.4	279	75.0	1.30
18 years	—	—	—	124	74.3	1.3	156	71.1	1.2	176	71.3	1.7	284	75.6	1.1	283	77.2	1.67
19 years	—	—	—	136	72.6	1.3	150	71.8	0.8	168	73.0	2.2	270	78.2	1.3	271	80.2	1.60
Female																		
2 years	—	—	—	272	13.0	0.1	330	12.8	0.1	624	13.2	0.1	248	13.3	0.1	335	13.4	0.13
3 years	—	—	—	292	15.0	0.2	367	14.8	0.1	587	15.4	0.1	178	15.2	0.2	191	15.8	0.20
4 years	—	—	—	281	16.8	0.2	388	16.8	0.2	537	17.9	0.3	191	17.9	0.3	226	17.9	0.21
5 years	—	—	—	314	19.7	0.3	369	19.4	0.3	554	20.2	0.2	186	20.6	0.6	199	20.5	0.37
6 years	536	21.5	0.2	176	21.6	0.3	150	21.9	0.4	272	22.6	0.6	171	22.4	0.5	193	23.4	0.49
7 years	609	24.2	0.2	169	24.3	0.4	154	24.6	0.5	274	26.4	0.8	196	25.9	0.5	157	27.3	0.62
8 years	613	27.5	0.2	152	27.5	0.5	125	27.5	0.4	248	29.9	0.6	184	31.9	1.2	184	30.7	0.94
9 years	581	31.4	0.4	171	32.0	0.6	154	31.7	0.7	280	34.4	1.2	183	35.4	0.7	185	36.7	0.99
10 years	584	35.2	0.4	197	33.8	0.6	128	35.7	0.6	258	37.9	1.2	164	40.0	1.0	189	42.4	1.07
11 years	525	39.8	0.4	166	41.2	0.8	143	41.4	0.9	275	44.1	1.1	194	47.9	1.3	175	49.2	1.31
12 years	—	—	—	177	46.7	1.0	146	46.1	0.9	236	49.0	1.2	316	52.0	1.1	249	52.9	1.31
13 years	—	—	—	198	51.8	1.0	155	50.9	1.2	220	55.8	1.6	321	57.7	1.4	292	57.4	0.98
14 years	—	—	—	184	54.6	1.0	181	54.3	1.0	218	58.5	1.4	324	59.9	1.0	269	58.8	1.75
15 years	—	—	—	167	56.6	0.9	144	55.0	0.8	191	58.1	1.1	266	61.1	1.7	248	60.9	0.76
16 years	—	—	—	171	56.8	1.1	167	57.7	0.9	208	61.3	1.4	273	63.0	1.2	253	61.5	0.95
17 years	—	—	—	150	59.5	1.6	134	59.6	1.0	201	62.4	1.2	256	64.7	1.2	252	66.0	1.66
18 years	—	—	—	141	58.2	1.1	156	59.0	1.0	175	61.2	1.9	243	65.2	1.5	272	67.6	2.15
19 years	—	—	—	130	59.5	1.4	158	59.8	1.0	177	63.2	1.9	225	67.9	1.2	239	67.4	1.79

—Data not available.
NOTE: NHES II: National Health Examination Survey, Cycle II, ages 6–11 years; NHES III: National Health Examination Survey, Cycle III, ages 12–17 years; and NHANES: National Health and Nutrition Examination Survey.

TABLE 3 Mean Height (Inches) by Survey, Sex, and Age; Children: United States

Sex and Age	NHES II, 1963–65 Sample Size	NHES II, 1963–65 Mean	NHES II, 1963–65 Standard Error of the Mean	NHANES I, 1971–74 Sample Size	NHANES I, 1971–74 Mean	NHANES I, 1971–74 Standard Error of the Mean	NHANES II, 1976–80 Sample Size	NHANES II, 1976–80 Mean	NHANES II, 1976–80 Standard Error of the Mean	NHANES III, 1988–94 Sample Size	NHANES III, 1988–94 Mean	NHANES III, 1988–94 Standard Error of the Mean	NHANES 1999–2002 Sample Size	NHANES 1999–2002 Mean	NHANES 1999–2002 Standard Error of the Mean	NHANES 2003–2006 Sample Size	NHANES 2003–2006 Mean	NHANES 2003–2006 Standard Error of the Mean
Male																		
2 years	—	—	—	298	35.9	0.2	350	35.8	0.1	589	35.8	0.1	254	35.9	0.1	258	36.2	0.09
3 years	—	—	—	308	38.8	0.1	421	38.9	0.1	513	38.9	0.1	222	38.8	0.1	209	38.8	0.17
4 years	—	—	—	304	41.8	0.1	405	41.5	0.1	551	41.4	0.1	183	41.9	0.2	206	42.2	0.17
5 years	—	—	—	273	44.4	0.1	393	44.2	0.1	497	44.2	0.1	156	44.5	0.2	202	45.0	0.20
6 years	575	46.7	0.1	179	46.5	0.2	146	46.9	0.2	283	46.8	0.3	188	46.9	0.2	176	47.5	0.19
7 years	632	49.0	0.1	164	49.2	0.2	150	49.0	0.2	270	49.6	0.2	187	49.7	0.2	181	49.1	0.29
8 years	618	51.2	0.1	152	50.8	0.2	145	51.0	0.3	269	51.7	0.2	217	52.2	0.3	152	51.6	0.27
9 years	603	53.3	0.2	169	53.2	0.3	141	53.1	0.2	280	54.2	0.3	177	54.4	0.2	176	53.9	0.19
10 years	576	55.2	0.1	184	55.1	0.2	165	55.6	0.2	297	55.9	0.4	188	55.7	0.2	171	56.0	0.30
11 years	595	57.3	0.1	178	57.6	0.3	153	57.3	0.2	285	58.0	0.3	187	58.5	0.4	158	59.1	0.46
12 years	—	—	—	200	60.2	0.3	147	60.0	0.3	207	61.2	0.4	301	60.9	0.3	275	60.9	0.21
13 years	—	—	—	174	62.7	0.3	165	62.3	0.3	190	63.6	0.3	298	63.1	0.3	284	63.7	0.34
14 years	—	—	—	174	65.6	0.2	188	65.7	0.3	191	66.5	0.3	267	66.3	0.4	260	66.4	0.28
15 years	—	—	—	171	67.2	0.3	180	67.4	0.3	188	68.0	0.4	287	68.4	0.2	270	68.3	0.24
16 years	—	—	—	169	68.9	0.3	180	68.3	0.2	197	68.9	0.4	310	69.0	0.2	308	69.2	0.26
17 years	—	—	—	176	69.6	0.2	183	68.8	0.2	196	69.5	0.4	317	69.0	0.2	278	69.5	0.19
18 years	—	—	—	124	69.5	0.3	156	69.8	0.2	176	69.8	0.4	289	69.5	0.3	284	69.6	0.21
19 years	—	—	—	136	69.5	0.3	150	69.3	0.2	169	69.1	0.2	275	69.6	0.3	271	69.6	0.36
Female																		
2 years	—	—	—	272	35.5	0.1	314	35.2	0.1	564	35.3	0.1	233	35.5	0.1	285	35.5	0.15
3 years	—	—	—	292	38.4	0.1	367	38.2	0.1	590	38.7	0.1	187	38.4	0.2	187	38.7	0.14
4 years	—	—	—	281	41.0	0.1	388	41.0	0.1	535	41.4	0.1	195	41.7	0.2	225	41.4	0.16
5 years	—	—	—	314	44.2	0.1	369	43.8	0.2	557	44.2	0.2	190	44.3	0.3	199	44.2	0.21
6 years	536	46.39	0.11	176	46.5	0.2	150	46.4	0.2	274	46.4	0.3	172	46.1	0.3	193	46.9	0.21
7 years	609	48.63	0.07	169	49.0	0.3	154	48.6	0.3	275	49.0	0.3	200	49.0	0.2	157	49.5	0.30
8 years	613	50.93	0.12	152	50.9	0.2	125	51.0	0.2	247	51.6	0.2	184	51.5	0.2	184	51.7	0.21
9 years	581	53.34	0.13	171	53.5	0.2	154	52.8	0.2	282	53.8	0.3	189	53.9	0.3	185	54.5	0.28
10 years	584	55.48	0.12	197	55.2	0.3	128	55.8	0.2	262	56.2	0.2	164	56.4	0.3	189	56.8	0.29
11 years	525	57.99	0.11	166	58.3	0.3	143	58.0	0.3	275	59.1	0.3	194	59.6	0.3	174	59.6	0.27
12 years	—	—	—	177	60.8	0.2	146	60.6	0.3	239	61.2	0.3	318	61.4	0.3	249	61.7	0.22
13 years	—	—	—	198	62.6	0.2	155	62.5	0.2	225	63.0	0.3	324	62.6	0.3	292	62.4	0.24
14 years	—	—	—	184	63.3	0.2	181	63.3	0.3	224	63.5	0.3	326	63.7	0.2	270	63.2	0.23
15 years	—	—	—	167	64.4	0.2	144	64.3	0.2	195	64.1	0.3	271	63.8	0.3	254	63.8	0.24
16 years	—	—	—	171	63.7	0.2	167	64.1	0.2	214	64.2	0.3	275	63.8	0.2	261	64.1	0.23
17 years	—	—	—	150	63.8	0.3	134	64.4	0.2	201	64.4	0.2	258	64.2	0.2	275	63.9	0.16
18 years	—	—	—	141	64.8	0.2	156	64.1	0.2	175	64.2	0.3	249	64.2	0.2	304	64.2	0.19
19 years	—	—	—	130	64.2	0.2	158	64.3	0.2	178	64.3	0.3	231	64.2	0.3	267	64.2	0.23

—Data not available.

NOTE: NHES II: National Health Examination Survey, Cycle II, ages 6–11 years; NHES III: National Health Examination Survey, Cycle III, ages 12–17 years; and NHANES: National Health and Nutrition Examination Survey.

TABLE 4 Mean Height (Centimeters) by Survey, Sex, and Age; Children: United States

Sex and Age	NHES II, 1963–65			NHANES I, 1971–74			NHANES II, 1976–80			NHANES III, 1988–94			NHANES 1999–2002			NHANES 2003–2006		
	Sample Size	Mean	Standard Error of the Mean	Sample Size	Mean	Standard Error of the Mean	Sample Size	Mean	Standard Error of the Mean	Sample Size	Mean	Standard Error of the Mean	Sample Size	Mean	Standard Error of the Mean	Sample Size	Mean	Standard Error of the Mean
Male																		
2 years	—	—	—	298	91.1	0.4	350	91.1	0.2	589	90.9	0.2	254	91.2	0.3	258	91.9	0.22
3 years	—	—	—	308	98.5	0.3	421	98.7	0.3	513	98.8	0.3	222	98.6	0.3	209	98.5	0.44
4 years	—	—	—	304	106.0	0.3	405	105.5	0.4	551	105.2	0.4	183	106.5	0.4	206	107.1	0.44
5 years	—	—	—	273	112.8	0.3	393	112.3	0.3	497	112.3	0.3	156	113.0	0.5	202	114.4	0.52
6 years	575	118.6	0.2	179	118.1	0.6	146	119.1	0.5	283	118.9	1.7	188	119.2	0.5	176	120.6	0.47
7 years	632	124.5	0.3	164	125.0	0.5	150	124.5	0.5	270	125.9	0.6	187	126.2	0.6	181	124.7	0.75
8 years	618	130.0	0.3	152	129.0	0.5	145	129.6	0.7	269	131.3	1.6	217	132.5	0.7	152	131.1	0.68
9 years	603	135.5	0.4	169	135.2	0.6	141	135.0	0.6	280	137.7	0.7	177	138.1	0.4	176	136.8	0.49
10 years	576	140.2	0.3	184	140.0	0.5	165	141.3	0.6	297	142.0	1.1	188	141.4	0.6	171	142.3	0.77
11 years	595	145.5	0.3	178	146.3	0.7	153	145.5	0.6	285	147.4	0.7	187	148.7	0.9	158	150.0	1.16
12 years	—	—	—	200	152.8	0.7	147	152.5	1.7	207	155.5	1.1	301	154.8	0.7	275	154.7	0.54
13 years	—	—	—	174	159.3	0.8	165	158.3	0.8	190	161.6	0.8	298	160.1	0.8	284	161.9	0.87
14 years	—	—	—	174	166.7	0.6	188	166.8	0.6	191	169.0	0.9	267	168.5	0.9	260	168.7	0.70
15 years	—	—	—	171	170.8	0.9	180	171.2	0.7	188	172.8	1.0	287	173.8	0.6	270	173.3	0.61
16 years	—	—	—	169	175.0	0.8	180	173.4	0.5	197	175.0	0.9	310	175.3	0.6	308	175.9	0.66
17 years	—	—	—	176	176.9	0.5	183	174.8	0.5	196	176.5	0.9	317	175.3	0.6	278	176.6	0.49
18 years	—	—	—	124	176.6	0.7	156	177.3	0.6	176	177.3	1.0	289	176.4	0.7	284	176.8	0.54
19 years	—	—	—	136	176.5	0.9	150	176.1	0.5	169	175.5	0.6	275	176.7	0.6	271	176.7	0.91
Female																		
2 years	—	—	—	272	90.1	0.3	314	89.4	0.3	564	89.7	0.2	233	90.1	0.4	285	90.2	0.39
3 years	—	—	—	292	97.7	0.3	367	97.1	0.2	590	98.2	0.2	187	97.6	0.5	187	98.3	0.35
4 years	—	—	—	281	104.2	0.4	388	104.2	0.4	535	105.1	0.3	195	105.9	0.5	225	105.2	0.40
5 years	—	—	—	314	112.2	0.4	369	111.2	0.4	557	112.2	0.5	190	112.4	0.7	199	112.2	0.54
6 years	536	117.8	0.3	176	118.2	0.5	150	117.9	0.6	274	117.9	0.6	172	117.1	0.7	193	119.0	0.53
7 years	609	123.5	0.2	169	124.6	0.7	154	123.4	0.7	275	124.3	0.7	200	124.4	0.5	157	125.8	0.77
8 years	613	129.4	0.3	152	129.2	0.6	125	129.5	0.5	247	131.1	0.6	184	130.9	0.6	184	131.3	0.54
9 years	581	135.5	0.3	171	135.9	0.5	154	134.1	0.5	282	136.6	0.7	189	136.9	0.7	185	138.6	0.70
10 years	584	140.9	0.3	197	140.1	0.8	128	141.7	0.6	262	142.7	0.6	164	143.3	0.9	189	144.2	0.73
11 years	525	147.3	0.3	166	148.2	0.8	143	147.4	0.7	275	150.2	0.7	194	151.4	0.7	174	151.3	0.69
12 years	—	—	—	177	154.6	0.6	146	153.8	0.6	239	155.5	0.7	318	156.0	0.7	249	156.7	0.55
13 years	—	—	—	198	158.9	0.5	155	158.7	0.5	225	159.9	0.9	324	159.1	0.6	292	158.6	0.62
14 years	—	—	—	184	160.8	0.6	181	160.7	0.7	224	161.2	0.7	326	161.8	0.6	270	160.5	0.58
15 years	—	—	—	167	163.6	0.6	144	163.3	0.5	195	162.8	0.6	271	162.0	0.6	254	162.1	0.60
16 years	—	—	—	171	161.7	0.5	167	162.8	0.5	214	163.0	0.7	275	161.9	0.5	261	162.9	0.58
17 years	—	—	—	150	162.1	0.9	134	163.5	0.6	201	163.6	0.6	258	163.2	0.6	275	162.2	0.41
18 years	—	—	—	141	164.7	0.5	156	162.8	0.5	175	163.2	0.9	249	163.0	0.5	304	163.0	0.49
19 years	—	—	—	130	163.1	0.5	158	163.2	0.4	178	163.4	0.7	231	163.1	0.7	267	163.1	0.58

—Data not available.

NOTE: NHES II: National Health Examination Survey, Cycle II, ages 6–11 years; NHES III: National Health Examination Survey, Cycle III, ages 12–17 years; and NHANES: National Health and Nutrition Examination Survey.

TABLE 5 Mean Body Mass Index (BMI) by Survey, Sex, and Age; Children: United States

Sex and Age	NHES II, 1963–65			NHANES I, 1971–74			NHANES II, 1976–80			NHANES III, 1988–94			NHANES 1999–2002			NHANES 2003–2006		
	Sample Size	Mean	Standard Error of the Mean	Sample Size	Mean	Standard Error of the Mean	Sample Size	Mean	Standard Error of the Mean	Sample Size	Mean	Standard Error of the Mean	Sample Size	Mean	Standard Error of the Mean	Sample Size	Mean	Standard Error of the Mean
Male																		
2 years	—	—	—	298	16.3	0.1	350	16.2	0.1	588	16.5	0.1	225	16.6	0.1	258	16.8	0.10
3 years	—	—	—	308	16.0	0.1	421	15.9	0.1	512	16.1	0.2	209	16.2	0.1	209	16.2	0.11
4 years	—	—	—	304	15.7	0.1	405	15.8	0.1	547	15.9	0.1	178	16.3	0.2	206	16.2	0.14
5 years	—	—	—	273	15.8	0.1	393	15.6	0.1	495	15.9	0.1	147	16.5	0.3	202	16.8	0.25
6 years	575	15.6	0.1	179	15.7	0.2	146	16.0	0.2	282	16.3	0.3	182	16.4	0.2	176	16.5	0.15
7 years	632	15.9	0.1	164	15.8	0.2	150	16.0	0.2	269	16.5	0.2	185	17.0	0.2	181	16.9	0.24
8 years	618	16.3	0.1	152	15.8	0.2	145	16.5	0.2	266	17.3	0.4	214	18.4	0.4	151	18.1	0.35
9 years	603	16.9	0.2	169	17.1	0.3	141	16.8	0.2	279	18.0	0.4	174	18.7	0.3	176	18.4	0.34
10 years	576	17.1	0.1	184	17.3	0.2	165	18.0	0.3	297	18.4	0.3	187	19.1	0.3	171	19.6	0.33
11 years	595	17.9	0.1	178	18.0	0.3	153	18.6	0.3	280	19.4	0.3	182	19.6	0.4	158	20.5	0.54
12 years	—	—	—	200	18.7	0.2	147	18.8	0.3	203	20.1	0.3	299	20.7	0.4	275	21.0	0.44
13 years	—	—	—	174	19.6	0.3	165	19.5	0.4	187	20.5	0.3	298	20.7	0.5	284	21.8	0.40
14 years	—	—	—	174	20.2	0.3	188	20.2	0.2	188	22.3	1.1	266	22.3	0.4	260	22.0	0.51
15 years	—	—	—	171	20.5	0.3	180	20.8	0.3	187	22.3	0.5	283	22.5	0.3	270	23.2	0.36
16 years	—	—	—	169	21.8	0.3	180	22.0	0.3	194	22.3	0.5	306	24.1	0.4	308	24.5	0.43
17 years	—	—	—	176	21.9	0.3	183	21.8	0.2	196	23.4	0.4	313	24.5	0.4	278	24.0	0.45
18 years	—	—	—	124	23.7	0.3	156	22.6	0.4	176	22.6	0.5	284	24.2	0.3	283	24.6	0.54
19 years	—	—	—	136	23.3	0.5	150	23.1	0.3	168	23.7	0.6	269	24.9	0.4	271	25.6	0.53
Female																		
2 years	—	—	—	272	15.9	0.1	314	16.1	0.1	562	16.5	0.1	214	16.4	0.1	285	16.6	0.11
3 years	—	—	—	292	15.7	0.1	367	15.6	0.1	582	15.9	0.1	173	16.0	0.1	187	16.3	0.18
4 years	—	—	—	281	15.5	0.1	388	15.5	0.1	533	16.0	0.2	190	15.9	0.2	224	16.1	0.14
5 years	—	—	—	314	15.5	0.1	369	15.6	0.1	554	15.9	0.1	186	16.1	0.3	199	16.2	0.19
6 years	536	15.4	0.1	176	15.4	0.1	150	15.6	0.2	272	16.1	0.3	170	16.2	0.2	193	16.4	0.21
7 years	609	15.8	0.1	169	15.6	0.2	154	16.1	0.2	274	16.9	0.3	196	16.6	0.2	157	17.1	0.26
8 years	613	16.4	0.1	152	16.4	0.2	125	16.3	0.2	247	17.3	0.3	184	18.3	0.5	184	17.6	0.42
9 years	581	17.0	0.1	171	17.2	0.2	154	17.5	0.3	280	18.2	0.5	183	18.7	0.3	185	18.9	0.36
10 years	584	17.6	0.2	197	17.1	0.2	128	17.7	0.3	258	18.4	0.4	163	19.3	0.3	189	20.2	0.40
11 years	525	18.2	0.2	166	18.6	0.3	143	18.9	0.3	275	19.4	0.4	194	20.7	0.4	174	21.3	0.47
12 years	—	—	—	177	19.5	0.4	146	19.3	0.3	236	20.2	0.5	315	21.2	0.4	249	21.4	0.45
13 years	—	—	—	198	20.4	0.3	155	20.1	0.4	220	21.8	0.6	321	22.6	0.4	292	22.7	0.35
14 years	—	—	—	184	21.1	0.3	181	21.0	0.3	218	22.4	0.5	324	22.9	0.4	269	22.8	0.62
15 years	—	—	—	167	21.1	0.3	144	20.6	0.3	191	21.9	0.4	266	23.2	0.5	247	23.2	0.28
16 years	—	—	—	171	21.7	0.3	167	21.8	0.3	208	23.0	0.5	273	24.0	0.4	253	23.2	0.39
17 years	—	—	—	150	22.6	0.5	134	22.3	0.4	201	23.3	0.5	255	23.1	0.4	252	25.0	0.60
18 years	—	—	—	141	21.5	0.3	156	22.3	0.4	175	22.9	0.6	243	24.4	0.5	271	25.4	0.80
19 years	—	—	—	130	22.5	0.6	158	22.4	0.3	177	23.7	0.8	225	25.5	0.4	238	25.3	0.64

—Data not available.

NOTES: BMI is calculated as weight in kilograms divided by square of height in meters. NHES II: National Health Examination Survey, Cycle II, ages 6–11 years; NHES III: National Health Examination survey, Cycle III, ages 12–17 years; NHANES: National Health and Nutrition Examination Survey.

TABLE 6 Mean Weight (Pounds) by Survey, Sex, and Age Group; Adults: United States

Sex and Age	NHES I, 1960–62			NHANES I, 1971–74			NHANES II, 1976–80			NHANES III, 1988–94			NHANES 1992–2002			NHANES 2003–2006		
	Sample Size	Mean	Standard Error of the Mean	Sample Size	Mean	Standard Error of the Mean	Sample Size	Mean	Standard Error of the Mean	Sample Size	Mean	Standard Error of the Mean	Sample Size	Mean	Standard Error of the Mean	Sample Size	Mean	Standard Error of the Mean
Male																		
20 years and over	—	—	—	—	—	—	—	—	—	7,755	181.3	0.8	4,314	189.8	0.9	4,489	194.7	1.02
20–74 years	2,895	166.3	0.7	4,992	173.4	0.6	5,604	173.8	0.4	6,860	182.4	0.8	3,791	191.0	1.0	—	—	—
20–29 years	585	163.9	1.6	986	169.6	1.3	1,261	167.9	1.0	1,638	172.5	1.4	712	183.4	1.5	811	188.3	2.33
30–39 years	714	169.9	1.4	654	178.1	1.7	871	175.5	0.9	1,468	182.3	2.0	704	189.1	2.0	741	194.1	1.77
40–49 years	649	169.1	1.4	715	177.6	1.2	695	179.7	1.0	1,220	187.3	1.7	776	196.0	1.6	769	202.3	1.88
50–59 years	487	167.7	1.3	717	173.2	1.1	691	176.0	1.3	851	189.2	1.2	598	195.4	2.1	591	198.8	2.10
60–74 years	460	158.9	1.5	1,920	165.4	1.0	2,086	167.5	1.0	1,683	180.8	1.1	1,001	191.5	1.4	—	—	—
75 years and over	—	—	—	—	—	—	—	—	—	895	166.0	1.5	523	172.7	1.4	—	—	—
60–69																669	198.3	2.16
70–79																555	187.4	2.03
80 years and over																353	168.1	1.36
Female																		
20 years and over	—	—	—	—	—	—	—	—	—	8,483	153.0	0.9	4,299	162.9	1.0	4,330	164.7	1.17
20–74 years	3,231	140.2	0.5	7,919	144.2	0.6	6,161	145.4	0.6	7,461	154.1	0.9	3,745	164.3	1.1	—	—	—
20–29 years	672	127.7	0.9	2,122	133.9	0.8	1,290	135.7	1.0	1,663	141.7	1.4	656	156.5	2.0	706	155.9	2.27
30–39 years	749	138.8	1.2	1,654	144.4	1.1	964	145.5	1.4	1,773	154.4	1.8	699	163.0	2.0	663	164.7	2.34
40–49 years	759	142.8	1.1	1,232	148.7	1.3	765	148.8	1.4	1,355	157.5	1.8	787	168.2	2.4	779	171.3	2.27
50–59 years	554	146.5	1.3	780	148.2	1.4	793	150.4	1.3	996	163.4	1.8	593	169.2	2.5	602	172.1	2.53
60–74 years	497	147.3	1.2	2,131	146.3	1.0	2,349	146.9	0.8	1,674	154.2	1.0	1,010	164.7	1.2	—	—	—
75 years and over	—	—	—	—	—	—	—	—	—	1,022	139.4	1.3	554	146.6	2.1	—	—	—
60–69																694	170.5	2.02
70–79																468	155.6	2.35
80 years and over																418	142.2	1.53

—Data not available.

NOTE: NHES I: National Health Examination Survey, Cycle I, ages 20–74 years; and NHANES: National Health and Nutrition Examination Survey.

TABLE 7 Mean Weight (Kilograms) by Survey, Sex, and Age Group; Adults: United States

Sex and Age	NHES I, 1960–62			NHANES I, 1971–74			NHANES II, 1976–80			NHANES III, 1988–94			NHANES 1992–2002			NHANES 2003–2006		
	Sample Size	Mean	Standard Error of the Mean	Sample Size	Mean	Standard Error of the Mean	Sample Size	Mean	Standard Error of the Mean	Sample Size	Mean	Standard Error of the Mean	Sample Size	Mean	Standard Error of the Mean	Sample Size	Mean	Standard Error of the Mean
Male																		
20 years and over	—	—	—	—	—	—	—	—	—	7,755	82.3	0.3	4,314	86.1	0.4	4,489	88.3	0.46
20–74 years	2,895	75.6	0.3	4,992	78.8	0.3	5,604	79.0	0.2	6,860	82.9	0.4	3,791	86.8	0.5	—	—	—
20–29 years	585	74.5	0.7	986	77.1	0.6	1,261	76.3	0.5	1,638	78.4	0.6	712	83.4	0.7	811	85.4	1.06
30–39 years	714	77.2	0.6	654	81.0	0.8	871	79.8	0.4	1,468	82.9	0.9	704	86.0	0.9	741	88.1	0.80
40–49 years	649	76.9	0.6	715	80.7	0.5	695	81.7	0.5	1,220	85.1	0.8	776	89.1	0.7	769	91.8	0.83
50–59 years	487	76.2	0.6	717	78.7	0.5	691	80.0	0.6	851	86.0	0.5	598	88.8	0.9	591	90.2	0.95
60–74 years	460	72.2	0.7	1,920	75.2	0.4	2,086	76.1	0.5	1,683	82.2	0.5	1,001	87.1	0.6	—	—	—
75 years and over	—	—	—	—	—	—	—	—	—	895	75.4	0.7	523	78.5	0.6	—	—	—
60–69																669	90.0	0.98
70–79																555	85.0	0.92
80 years and over																353	76.3	0.62
Female																		
20 years and over	—	—	—	—	—	—	—	—	—	8,483	69.5	0.4	4,299	74.0	0.5	4,330	74.7	0.53
20–74 years	3,231	63.7	0.2	7,919	65.6	0.3	6,161	66.1	0.3	7,461	70.0	0.4	3,745	74.7	0.5	—	—	—
20–29 years	672	58.0	0.4	2,122	60.9	0.4	1,290	61.7	0.5	1,663	64.4	0.6	656	71.1	0.9	706	70.7	1.03
30–39 years	749	63.1	0.5	1,654	65.6	0.5	964	66.1	0.6	1,773	70.2	0.8	699	74.1	0.9	663	74.7	1.06
40–49 years	759	64.9	0.5	1,232	67.6	0.6	765	67.6	0.6	1,355	71.6	0.8	787	76.5	1.1	779	77.7	1.03
50–59 years	554	66.6	0.6	780	67.4	0.6	793	68.4	0.6	996	74.3	0.8	593	76.9	1.1	602	78.0	1.15
60–74 years	497	67.0	0.6	2,131	66.5	0.4	2,349	66.8	0.4	1,674	70.1	0.5	1,010	74.9	0.9	—	—	—
75 years and over	—	—	—	—	—	—	—	—	—	1,022	63.4	0.6	554	66.6	0.9	—	—	—
60–69																694	77.3	0.91
70–79																468	70.6	1.07
80 years and over																418	64.5	0.69

—Data not available.

NOTE: NHES I: National Health Examination Survey, Cycle I, ages 20–74 years; and NHANES: National Health and Nutrition Examination Survey.

TABLE 8 Mean Height (Inches) by Survey, Sex, and Age Group; Adults: United States

Sex and Age	NHES I, 1960–62			NHANES I, 1971–74			NHANES II, 1976–80			NHANES III, 1988–94			NHANES 1992–2002			NHANES 2003–2006		
	Sample Size	Mean	Standard Error of the Mean	Sample Size	Mean	Standard Error of the Mean	Sample Size	Mean	Standard Error of the Mean	Sample Size	Mean	Standard Error of the Mean	Sample Size	Mean	Standard Error of the Mean	Sample Size	Mean	Standard Error of the Mean
Male																		
20 years and over	—	—	—	—	—	—	—	—	—	7,757	69.0	0.1	4,341	69.2	0.1	4,482	69.4	0.07
20–74 years	2,895	68.3	0.1	4,992	68.9	0.1	5,604	69.1	0.1	6,862	69.2	0.1	3,836	69.4	0.1	—	—	—
20–29 years	585	68.9	0.1	986	69.7	0.2	1,261	69.7	0.1	1,639	69.3	0.1	724	69.6	0.1	808	69.9	0.13
30–39 years	714	68.9	0.1	654	69.3	0.1	871	69.4	0.1	1,468	69.5	0.1	717	69.5	0.1	742	96.4	0.13
40–49 years	649	68.3	0.1	715	69.1	0.1	695	69.3	0.1	1,220	69.4	0.1	784	69.7	0.1	769	69.7	0.11
50–59 years	487	67.8	0.1	717	68.5	0.2	691	68.8	0.1	851	69.2	0.1	601	69.2	0.1	591	69.5	0.15
60–74 years	460	67.0	0.2	1,920	67.6	0.1	2,086	67.8	0.1	1,684	68.3	0.1	1,010	68.6	0.1	—	—	—
75 years and over	—	—	—	—	—	—	—	—	—	895	67.2	0.1	505	67.4	0.2	—	—	—
60–69																668	69.0	0.11
70–79																555	68.4	0.16
80 years and over																349	67.2	0.14
Female																		
20 years and over	—	—	—	—	—	—	—	—	—	8,498	63.7	0.1	4,308	63.8	0.1	4,857	63.8	0.06
20–74 years	3,231	63.1	0.1	7,919	63.6	0.0	6,161	63.7	0.0	7,473	63.9	0.1	3,770	64.0	0.1	—	—	—
20–29 years	672	63.7	0.1	2,122	64.1	0.1	1,290	64.3	0.1	1,665	64.1	0.1	663	64.1	0.1	1,061	64.3	0.12
30–39 years	749	63.7	0.1	1,654	64.1	0.1	964	64.2	0.1	1,776	64.3	0.1	708	64.2	0.1	842	64.3	0.13
40–49 years	759	63.2	0.1	1,232	63.9	0.1	765	63.9	0.1	1,354	64.1	0.1	794	64.3	0.1	784	64.2	0.12
50–59 years	554	62.6	0.1	780	63.2	0.1	793	63.2	0.1	998	63.7	0.1	601	63.9	0.1	604	63.9	0.13
60–74 years	497	61.8	0.1	2,131	63.4	0.1	2,349	62.5	0.1	1,680	62.9	0.1	1,004	63.0	0.1	—	—	—
75 years and over	—	—	—	—	—	—	—	—	—	1,025	61.5	0.1	538	62.0	0.1	—	—	—
60–69																691	63.7	0.13
70–79																463	62.7	0.13
80 years and over																412	61.4	0.15

—Data not available.

NOTE: NHES I: National Health Examination Survey, Cycle I, ages 20–74 years; and NHANES: National Health and Nutrition Examination Survey.

Table 9 Mean Height (Centimeters) by Survey, Sex, and Age Group; Adults: United States

Sex and Age	NHES I, 1960–62			NHANES I, 1971–74			NHANES II, 1976–80			NHANES III, 1988–94			NHANES 1992–2002			NHANES 2003–2006		
	Sample Size	Mean	Standard Error of the Mean	Sample Size	Mean	Standard Error of the Mean	Sample Size	Mean	Standard Error of the Mean	Sample Size	Mean	Standard Error of the Mean	Sample Size	Mean	Standard Error of the Mean	Sample Size	Mean	Standard Error of the Mean
Male																		
20 years and over	—	—	—	—	—	—	—	—	—	7,757	175.4	0.1	4,341	175.8	0.1	4,482	176.3	0.17
20–74 years	2,895	173.4	0.2	4,992	175.1	0.2	5,604	175.4	0.2	6,862	175.8	0.1	3,836	176.2	0.2	—	—	—
20–29 years	585	175.0	0.3	986	177.1	0.4	1,261	177.1	0.3	1,639	176.1	0.3	724	176.7	0.3	808	177.6	0.34
30–39 years	714	174.9	0.3	654	176.1	0.3	871	176.3	0.3	1,468	176.6	0.3	717	176.4	0.3	742	176.4	0.33
40–49 years	649	173.4	0.4	715	175.5	0.3	695	175.9	0.3	1,220	176.3	0.3	784	177.2	0.3	769	117.1	0.28
50–59 years	487	172.3	0.4	717	174.0	0.4	691	174.7	0.3	851	175.8	0.3	601	175.8	0.3	591	176.6	0.38
60–74 years	460	170.2	0.4	1,920	171.8	0.3	2,086	172.1	0.2	1,684	173.6	0.2	1,010	174.4	0.3	—	—	—
75 years and over	—	—	—	—	—	—	—	—	—	895	170.7	0.3	505	171.3	0.4	—	—	—
60–69																668	175.4	0.28
70–79																555	173.8	0.41
80 years and over																349	170.7	0.36
Female																		
20 years and over	—	—	—	—	—	—	—	—	—	8,498	161.8	0.1	4,308	162.0	0.1	4,857	162.2	0.16
20–74 years	3,231	160.2	0.2	7,919	161.6	0.1	6,161	161.8	0.1	7,473	162.3	0.1	3,770	162.5	0.1	—	—	—
20–29 years	672	161.8	0.3	2,122	162.8	0.1	1,290	163.3	0.2	1,665	162.8	0.2	663	162.8	0.3	1,061	163.2	0.31
30–39 years	749	161.8	0.3	1,654	162.9	0.2	964	163.1	0.2	1,776	163.4	0.3	708	163.0	0.3	842	163.2	0.32
40–49 years	759	160.5	0.2	1,232	162.3	0.3	765	162.3	0.3	1,354	162.8	0.3	794	163.4	0.2	784	163.1	0.29
50–59 years	554	158.9	0.3	780	160.4	0.2	793	160.5	0.3	998	161.8	0.3	601	162.3	0.3	604	162.2	0.34
60–74 years	497	157.1	0.3	2,131	158.6	0.2	2,349	158.8	0.2	1,680	159.8	0.2	1,004	160.0	0.2	—	—	—
75 years and over	—	—	—	—	—	—	—	—	—	1,025	156.2	0.4	538	157.4	0.3	—	—	—
60–69																691	161.8	0.33
70–79																463	159.2	0.34
80 years and over																412	156.0	0.37

—Data not available.

NOTE: NHES I: National Health Examination Survey, Cycle I, ages 20–74 years; and NHANES: National Health and Nutrition Examination Survey.

TABLE 10 Mean Body Mass Index (BMI) by Survey, Sex, and Age Group; Adults: United States

Sex and Age	NHES I, 1960–62			NHANES I, 1971–74			NHANES II, 1976–80			NHANES III, 1988–94			NHANES 1992–2002			NHANES 2003–2006		
	Sample Size	Mean	Standard Error of the Mean	Sample Size	Mean	Standard Error of the Mean	Sample Size	Mean	Standard Error of the Mean	Sample Size	Mean	Standard Error of the Mean	Sample Size	Mean	Standard Error of the Mean	Sample Size	Mean	Standard Error of the Mean
Male																		
20 years and over	—	—	—	—	—	—	—	—	—	7,755	26.7	0.1	4,262	27.8	0.1	4,474	28.4	0.14
20–74 years	2,895	25.1	0.1	4,992	25.7	0.1	5,604	25.6	0.1	6,860	26.8	0.1	3,775	27.9	0.1	—	—	—
20–29 years	585	24.3	0.2	986	24.5	0.1	1,261	24.3	0.1	1,638	25.2	0.2	712	26.6	0.2	808	27.0	0.31
30–39 years	714	25.2	0.2	654	26.1	0.2	871	25.6	0.1	1,468	26.5	0.2	704	27.5	0.3	741	28.2	0.23
40–49 years	649	25.6	0.2	715	26.2	0.2	695	26.4	0.2	1,220	27.3	0.2	774	28.4	0.3	768	29.2	0.26
50–59 years	487	25.6	0.2	717	26.0	0.2	691	26.2	0.2	851	27.8	0.2	594	28.7	0.3	590	28.9	0.27
60–74 years	460	24.9	0.2	1,920	25.4	0.1	2,086	25.7	0.1	1,683	27.2	0.2	991	28.6	0.2	—	—	—
75 years and over	—	—	—	—	—	—	—	—	—	895	25.9	0.2	487	26.8	0.2	—	—	—
60–69																665	29.2	0.29
70–79																554	28.1	0.25
80 years and over																348	26.2	0.19
Female																		
20 years and over	—	—	—	—	—	—	—	—	—	8,480.0	26.5	0.1	4,243	28.1	0.2	4,313	28.4	0.19
20–74 years	3,231	24.9	0.1	7,919	25.1	0.1	6,161	25.3	0.1	7,459.0	26.6	0.2	3,719	28.2	0.2	—	—	—
20–29 years	672	22.2	0.2	2,122	23.0	0.1	1,290	23.1	0.2	1,663.0	24.3	0.2	654	26.8	0.3	705	26.5	0.36
30–39 years	749	24.1	0.2	1,654	24.7	0.2	964	24.9	0.2	1,773.0	26.3	0.3	698	27.9	0.3	663	28.1	0.38
40–49 years	759	25.2	0.2	1,232	25.7	0.2	765	25.7	0.2	1,354.0	27.1	0.3	783	28.6	0.4	778	29.2	0.39
50–59 years	554	26.4	0.2	780	26.2	0.2	793	26.5	0.2	996.0	28.4	0.3	591	29.2	0.4	602	29.6	0.39
60–74 years	497	27.2	0.2	2,131	26.5	0.2	2,349	26.5	0.1	1,673.0	27.4	0.2	993	29.2	0.2	—	—	—
75 years and over	—	—	—	—	—	—	—	—	—	1,021.0	25.9	0.2	524	26.8	0.4	—	—	—
60–69																691	29.5	0.33
70–79																463	27.8	0.40
80 years and over																411	264	0.27

—Data not available.

NOTES: BMI is calculated as weight in kilograms divided by square of height in meters. NHES I: National Health Examination Survey, Cycle I, ages 20–74 years; and NHANES: National Health and Nutrition Examination Survey.

Table 11 Mean Weight (Pounds) by Survey, Sex, Race/Ethnicity, and Age Group; Adults: United States

Sex, Race/Ethnicity, and Age	HHANES, 1982–84			NHANES III, 1988–94			NHANES 1999–2002			NHANES 2003–2006		
	Sample Size	Mean	Standard Error of the Mean	Sample Size	Mean	Standard Error of the Mean	Sample Size	Mean	Standard Error of the Mean	Sample Size	Mean	Standard Error of the Mean
Male												
Non-Hispanic white:												
20 years and over	—	—	—	3,152	183.7	0.9	2,149	193.1	1.0	2,339	197.4	1.05
20–39 years	—	—	—	846	180.2	1.5	607	189.7	1.8	666	193.5	1.98
40–59 years	—	—	—	842	190.3	1.4	676	199.5	1.5	709	203.8	1.88
60 years and over	—	—	—	1,464	179.0	0.9	866	188.8	1.0	964	192.3	1.27
Non-Hispanic black:												
20 years and over	—	—	—	2,091	181.2	0.9	824	189.2	1.3	941	199.8	2.19
20–39 years	—	—	—	985	182.0	1.2	279	189.1	2.7	361	202.4	3.31
40–59 years	—	—	—	583	185.4	1.7	289	191.1	2.6	316	201.0	2.56
60 years and over	—	—	—	523	173.1	1.8	256	186.5	2.3	264	189.0	2.66
Mexican American:												
20 years and over	—	—	—	2,229	172.3	0.9	1,027	177.3	1.1	903	180.5	1.88
20–74 years	2,273	166.9	0.8	2,127	173.3	0.9	961	178.3	1.2	—	—	—
20–39 years	1,133	165.4	1.7	1,143	166.9	1.5	399	172.5	2.2	375	181.1	2.89
40–59 years	856	170.8	0.7	558	181.6	1.5	310	183.6	2.0	247	180.7	2.03
60–74 years	284	161.2	1.3	426	170.0	1.8	252	180.3	2.6	—	—	—
60 years and over										281	175.9	2.55
75 years and over	—	—	—	528	166.6	1.9	318	175.7	2.4	—	—	—
Female												
Non-Hispanic white:												
20 years and over	—	—	—	3,554	151.4	1.0	2,063	161.7	1.2	2,233	163.7	1.26
20–39 years	—	—	—	1,030	146.4	1.4	569	158.4	2.0	615	158.9	2.17
40–59 years	—	—	—	950	158.5	1.5	632	167.6	2.2	674	171.0	2.01
60 years and over	—	—	—	1,574	148.5	1.1	862	158.0	1.2	944	158.8	1.32
Non-Hispanic black:												
20 years and over	—	—	—	2,452	169.7	1.2	870	182.4	1.5	959	184.8	1.56
20–39 years	—	—	—	1,191	162.8	1.7	298	179.2	3.0	329	181.6	2.94
40–59 years	—	—	—	721	179.3	2.3	297	189.3	2.7	355	190.1	1.61
60 years and over	—	—	—	540	166.2	2.3	275	176.6	3.3	275	180.8	2.94
Mexican American:												
20 years and over	—	—	—	2,108	152.6	1.0	1,019	157.1	1.6	817	162.2	2.07
20–74 years	3,039	145.8	0.8	2,014	153.8	1.1	964	158.4	1.5	—	—	—
20–39 years	1,482	140.5	0.8	1,063	148.1	1.5	358	152.9	2.2	300	160.5	2.73
40–59 years	1,159	151.1	1.2	558	160.4	1.5	332	165.5	2.6	234	168.4	2.68
60–74 years	398	146.8	1.9	393	152.5	2.4	274	155.0	2.2	—	—	—
60 years and over										283	153.0	2.22
75 years and over	—	—	—	487	147.9	2.0	329	150.7	2.6	—	—	—

—Data not available.

NOTE: HHANES: Hispanic Health and Nutrition Examination Survey; and NHANES: National Health and Nutrition Examination Survey.

TABLE 12 Mean Weight (Kilograms) by Survey, Sex, Race/Ethnicity, and Age Group; Adults: United States

Sex, Race/Ethnicity, and Age	HHANES, 1982–84 Sample Size	HHANES, 1982–84 Mean	HHANES, 1982–84 Standard Error of the Mean	NHANES III, 1988–94 Sample Size	NHANES III, 1988–94 Mean	NHANES III, 1988–94 Standard Error of the Mean	NHANES 1999–2002 Sample Size	NHANES 1999–2002 Mean	NHANES 1999–2002 Standard Error of the Mean	NHANES 2003–2006 Sample Size	NHANES 2003–2006 Mean	NHANES 2003–2006 Standard Error of the Mean
Male												
Non-Hispanic white:												
20 years and over	—	—	—	3,152	83.5	0.4	2,149	87.8	0.5	2,339	89.6	0.48
20–39 years	—	—	—	846	81.9	0.7	607	86.2	0.8	666	87.7	0.90
40–59 years	—	—	—	842	86.5	0.6	676	90.7	0.7	709	92.5	0.85
60 years and over	—	—	—	1,464	81.4	0.4	866	85.8	0.4	964	87.2	0.58
Non-Hispanic black:												
20 years and over	—	—	—	2,091	82.4	0.4	824	86.0	0.6	941	90.6	0.99
20–39 years	—	—	—	985	82.7	0.6	279	85.9	1.2	361	91.8	1.50
40–59 years	—	—	—	583	84.3	0.8	289	86.8	1.2	316	91.2	1.16
60 years and over	—	—	—	523	78.7	0.8	256	84.8	1.1	264	85.7	1.21
Mexican American:												
20 years and over	—	—	—	2,229	78.3	0.4	1,027	80.6	0.5	903	81.9	0.85
20–74 years	2,273	75.9	0.4	2,127	78.8	0.4	961	81.0	0.5	—	—	—
20–39 years	1,133	75.2	0.8	1,143	75.9	0.7	399	78.4	1.0	375	82.1	1.31
40–59 years	856	77.6	0.3	558	82.5	0.7	310	83.4	0.9	247	82.0	0.92
60–74 years	284	73.3	0.6	426	77.3	0.8	252	82.0	1.2	—	—	—
60 years and over										281	79.8	1.15
75 years and over	—	—	—	528	75.7	0.9	318	79.8	1.1	—	—	—
Female												
Non-Hispanic white:												
20 years and over	—	—	—	3,554	68.8	0.5	2,063	73.5	0.6	2,233	74.3	0.57
20–39 years	—	—	—	1,030	66.6	0.6	569	72.0	0.9	615	72.1	0.99
40–59 years	—	—	—	950	72.1	0.7	632	76.2	1.0	574	77.6	0.91
60 years and over	—	—	—	1,574	67.5	0.5	862	71.8	0.5	944	72.0	0.60
Non-Hispanic black:												
20 years and over	—	—	—	2,452	77.2	0.6	870	82.9	0.7	959	83.8	0.71
20–39 years	—	—	—	1,191	74.0	0.8	298	81.5	1.4	329	82.4	1.33
40–59 years	—	—	—	721	81.5	1.1	297	86.0	1.2	355	86.2	0.73
60 years and over	—	—	—	540	75.5	1.0	275	80.3	1.5	275	82.0	1.33
Mexican American:												
20 years and over	—	—	—	2,108	69.4	0.5	1,019	71.4	0.7	817	73.6	0.94
20–74 years	3,039	66.3	0.4	2,014	69.9	0.5	964	72.0	0.7	—	—	—
20–39 years	1,482	63.9	0.4	1,063	67.3	0.7	358	69.5	1.0	300	72.8	1.24
40–59 years	1,159	68.7	0.6	558	72.9	0.7	332	75.2	1.2	234	76.4	1.22
60–74 years	398	66.7	0.9	393	69.3	1.1	274	70.5	1.0	—	—	—
60 years and over										283	69.4	1.01
75 years and over	—	—	—	487	67.2	0.9	329	68.5	1.2	—	—	—

—Data not available.

NOTE: HHANES: Hispanic Health and Nutrition Examination Survey; and NHANES: National Health and Nutrition Examination Survey.

TABLE 13 Mean Height (Inches) by Survey, Sex, Race/Ethnicity, and Age Group; Adults: United States

Sex, Race/Ethnicity, and Age	HHANES, 1982–84			NHANES III, 1988–94			NHANES 1999–2002			NHANES 2003–2006		
	Sample Size	Mean	Standard Error of the Mean	Sample Size	Mean	Standard Error of the Mean	Sample Size	Mean	Standard Error of the Mean	Sample Size	Mean	Standard Error of the Mean
Male												
Non-Hispanic white:												
20 years and over	—	—	—	3,152	69.5	0.1	2,149	69.7	0.1	2,331	69.9	0.08
20–39 years	—	—	—	846	69.9	0.1	613	70.2	0.1	664	70.4	0.10
40–59 years	—	—	—	842	69.7	0.1	681	70.0	0.1	710	70.1	0.14
60 years and over	—	—	—	1,464	68.3	0.1	855	68.6	0.1	957	68.8	0.08
Non-Hispanic black:												
20 years and over	—	—	—	2,091	69.2	0.1	837	69.5	0.1	943	69.8	0.08
20–39 years	—	—	—	985	69.7	0.1	284	70.0	0.1	361	70.1	0.14
40–59 years	—	—	—	583	69.4	0.1	294	69.6	0.1	316	69.8	0.13
60 years and over	—	—	—	523	68.0	0.1	259	68.5	0.2	266	68.6	0.20
Mexican American:												
20 years and over	—	—	—	2,231	66.6	0.1	1,039	66.7	0.1	902	67.0	0.13
20–74 years	2,273	66.9	0.1	2,129	66.8	0.1	980	66.8	0.1	—	—	—
20–39 years	1,133	67.4	0.2	1,144	67.0	0.1	409	66.8	0.2	375	67.2	0.18
40–59 years	856	66.8	0.1	558	66.8	0.1	313	66.9	0.2	246	67.0	0.16
60–74 years	284	65.7	0.1	427	66.1	0.2	258	66.5	0.2	—	—	—
60 years and over										281	66.1	0.17
75 years and over	—	—	—	529	65.8	0.2	317	66.3	0.2	—	—	—
Female												
Non-Hispanic white:												
20 years and over	—	—	—	3,557	64.0	0.1	2,056	64.2	0.1	2,477	64.2	0.06
20–39 years	—	—	—	1,030	64.6	0.1	573	64.6	0.1	866	64.9	0.09
40–59 years	—	—	—	950	64.2	0.1	638	64.6	0.1	677	64.4	0.11
60 years and over	—	—	—	1,577	62.6	0.1	845	62.8	0.1	934	63.1	0.11
Non-Hispanic black:												
20 years and over	—	—	—	2,453	64.1	0.1	881	64.2	0.1	1,035	64.1	0.10
20–39 years	—	—	—	1,191	64.4	0.1	304	64.6	0.1	407	64.3	0.17
40–59 years	—	—	—	721	64.4	0.1	299	64.3	0.1	355	64.3	0.16
60 years and over	—	—	—	541	63.0	0.1	278	63.2	0.1	273	63.2	0.12
Mexican American:												
20 years and over	—	—	—	2,119	61.5	0.1	1,020	61.8	0.1	975	62.1	0.10
20–74 years	3,039	61.6	0.1	2,025	61.6	0.1	967	61.9	0.1	—	—	—
20–39 years	1,482	62.1	0.1	1,068	61.9	0.1	361	62.3	0.2	455	62.5	0.13
40–59 years	1,159	61.5	0.1	559	61.7	0.1	335	61.9	0.2	238	62.1	0.19
60–74 years	398	60.6	0.2	398	60.6	0.1	271	60.9	0.1	—	—	—
60 years and over										282	60.6	0.19
75 years and over	—	—	—	492	60.3	0.1	324	60.7	0.1	—	—	—

—Data not available.

NOTE: HHANES: Hispanic Health and Nutrition Examination Survey; and NHANES: National Health and Nutrition Examination Survey.

TABLE 14 Mean Height (Centimeters) by Survey, Sex, Race/Ethnicity, and Age Group; Adults: United States

Sex, Race/Ethnicity, and Age	HHANES, 1982–84			NHANES III, 1988–94			NHANES 1999–2002			NHANES 2003–2006		
	Sample Size	Mean	Standard Error of the Mean	Sample Size	Mean	Standard Error of the Mean	Sample Size	Mean	Standard Error of the Mean	Sample Size	Mean	Standard Error of the Mean
Male												
Non-Hispanic white:												
20 years and over	—	—	—	3,152	176.4	0.1	2,149	177.2	0.2	2,331	177.5	0.20
20–39 years	—	—	—	846	177.7	0.2	613	178.2	0.2	664	178.9	0.25
40–59 years	—	—	—	842	177.0	0.3	681	177.8	0.3	710	178.0	0.35
60 years and over	—	—	—	1,464	173.5	0.2	855	174.3	0.2	957	174.6	0.20
Non-Hispanic black:												
20 years and over	—	—	—	2,091	175.8	0.2	837	176.6	0.2	943	177.2	0.20
20–39 years	—	—	—	985	177.1	0.2	284	177.8	0.4	361	178.0	0.35
40–59 years	—	—	—	583	176.2	0.3	294	176.8	0.4	316	177.4	0.33
60 years and over	—	—	—	523	172.7	0.2	259	174.1	0.4	266	174.3	0.52
Mexican American:												
20 years and over	—	—	—	2,231	169.2	0.1	1,039	169.4	0.3	902	170.3	0.34
20–74 years	2,273	169.9	0.3	2,129	169.6	0.2	980	169.6	0.3	—	—	—
20–39 years	1,133	171.1	0.5	1,144	170.1	0.2	409	169.7	0.4	375	170.6	0.46
40–59 years	856	169.8	0.3	558	169.6	0.3	313	169.8	0.5	246	170.2	0.40
60–74 years	284	166.8	0.3	427	167.8	0.4	258	169.0	0.4	—	—	—
60 years and over										281	167.8	0.42
75 years and over	—	—	—	529	167.0	0.4	317	168.5	0.4	—	—	—
Female												
Non-Hispanic white:												
20 years and over	—	—	—	3,557	162.5	0.2	2,056	163.0	0.1	2,477	163.0	0.15
20–39 years	—	—	—	1,030	164.1	0.2	573	164.1	0.3	866	164.8	0.22
40–59 years	—	—	—	950	163.0	0.3	638	164.0	0.2	677	163.6	0.27
60 years and over	—	—	—	1,577	159.0	0.3	845	159.6	0.2	934	160.2	0.27
Non-Hispanic black:												
20 years and over	—	—	—	2,453	162.8	0.2	881	163.0	0.2	1,035	162.7	0.26
20–39 years	—	—	—	1,191	163.7	0.2	304	164.0	0.4	407	163.2	0.43
40–59 years	—	—	—	721	163.6	0.3	299	163.4	0.3	355	163.2	0.40
60 years and over	—	—	—	541	160.1	0.2	278	160.6	0.3	273	160.6	0.32
Mexican American:												
20 years and over	—	—	—	2,119	156.1	0.2	1,020	156.9	0.3	975	157.8	0.24
20–74 years	3,039	156.5	0.3	2,025	156.6	0.2	967	157.3	0.3	—	—	—
20–39 years	1,482	157.8	0.3	1,068	157.3	0.3	361	158.1	0.5	455	158.7	0.32
40–59 years	1,159	156.1	0.3	559	156.8	0.3	335	157.3	0.4	238	157.7	0.48
60–74 years	398	154.0	0.5	398	153.9	0.3	271	154.8	0.4	—	—	—
60 years and over										282	153.9	0.48
75 years and over	—	—	—	492	153.1	0.3	324	154.1	0.3	—	—	—

—Data not available.

NOTE: HHANES: Hispanic Health and Nutrition Examination Survey; and NHANES: National Health and Nutrition Examination Survey.

Table 15 Mean Body Mass Index (BMI) by Survey, Sex, Race/Ethnicity, and Age Group; Adults: United States

	HHANES, 1982–84			NHANES III, 1988–94			NHANES 1999–2002			NHANES 2003–2006		
Sex, Race/Ethnicity, and Age	Sample Size	Mean	Standard Error of the Mean	Sample Size	Mean	Standard Error of the Mean	Sample Size	Mean	Standard Error of the Mean	Sample Size	Mean	Standard Error of the Mean
Male												
Non-Hispanic white:												
20 years and over	—	—	—	3,152	26.8	0.1	2,116	27.9	0.2	2,328	28.4	0.16
20–39 years	—	—	—	846	25.9	0.2	607	27.1	0.2	664	27.4	0.26
40–59 years	—	—	—	842	27.6	0.2	673	28.7	0.3	708	29.4	0.26
60 years and over	—	—	—	1,464	27.0	0.1	836	28.3	0.1	956	28.6	0.16
Non-Hispanic black:												
20 years and over	—	—	—	2,091	26.6	0.1	820	27.5	0.2	939	28.8	0.30
20–39 years	—	—	—	985	26.3	0.2	279	27.1	0.3	360	28.9	0.45
40–59 years	—	—	—	583	27.1	0.2	289	27.7	0.4	316	28.9	0.37
60 years and over	—	—	—	523	26.4	0.3	252	28.0	0.3	263	28.1	0.30
Mexican American:												
20 years and over	—	—	—	2,229	27.3	0.1	1,018	28.0	0.2	901	28.2	0.26
20–74 years	2,273	26.2	0.2	2,127	27.3	0.1	959	28.1	0.2	—	—	—
20–39 years	1,133	25.6	0.3	1,143	26.1	0.2	399	27.1	0.3	375	28.1	0.36
40–59 years	856	26.9	0.1	558	28.6	0.2	309	28.9	0.3	246	28.3	0.31
60–74 years	284	26.3	0.2	426	27.4	0.3	251	28.6	0.3	—	—	—
60 years and over										280	28.2	0.33
75 years and over	—	—	—	528	27.1	0.3	310	28.1	0.3	—	—	—
Female												
Non-Hispanic white:												
20 years and over	—	—	—	3,554	26.1	0.2	2,026	27.6	0.2	2,222	27.9	0.22
20–39 years	—	—	—	1,030	24.7	0.2	567	26.7	0.3	615	26.5	0.36
40–59 years	—	—	—	950	27.2	0.3	629	28.3	0.4	673	29.0	0.35
60 years and over	—	—	—	1,574	26.7	0.2	830	28.2	0.2	934	28.0	0.21
Non-Hispanic black:												
20 years and over	—	—	—	2,451	29.1	0.2	863	31.1	0.3	956	31.6	0.28
20–39 years	—	—	—	1,191	27.6	0.3	298	30.2	0.5	328	30.8	0.46
40–59 years	—	—	—	721	30.4	0.3	294	32.1	0.5	355	32.4	0.33
60 years and over	—	—	—	539	29.4	0.4	271	31.1	0.6	273	31.8	0.44
Mexican American:												
20 years and over	—	—	—	2,106	28.4	0.2	1,012	29.0	0.3	815	29.5	03.7
20–74 years	3,039	27.1	0.1	2,013	28.5	0.2	960	29.1	0.3	—	—	—
20–39 years	1,482	25.6	0.2	1,063	27.2	0.2	358	27.8	0.4	300	28.8	0.47
40–59 years	1,159	28.2	0.2	557	29.7	0.3	332	30.4	0.5	234	30.7	0.50
60–74 years	398	28.1	0.3	393	29.2	0.4	270	29.5	0.3	—	—	—
60 years and over										281	29.2	0.44
75 years and over	—	—	—	486	28.7	0.4	322	28.9	0.4	—	—	—

—Data not available.

NOTES: BMI is calculated as weight in kilograms divided by square of height in meters. HHANES: Hispanic Health and Nutrition Examination Survey; and NHANES: National Health and Nutrition Examination Survey.

APPENDIX

M

Triceps Skinfold Norms from NHANES 2003–2006

From National Center for Health Statistics, Centers for Disease Control and Prevention, U.S. Department of Health and Human Services.

Triceps skinfold thickness in millimeters for children and adolescents aged 2 months–19 years by sex and age, by mean, standard error of the mean, and selected percentiles: United States 2003–2006.

Sex and age†	Number examined	Mean	Standard error	Percentile								
				5th	10th	15th	25th	50th	75th	85th	90th	95th
Male				Millimeters								
2 months	11	*	*	*	*	*	*	*	*	*	*	*
3–5 months	128	11.0	0.25	*	8.4	8.7	9.0	10.5	12.0	13.9	14.5	*
6–8 months	128	10.6	0.26	*	7.3	8.0	8.9	10.1	12.3	13.0	13.4	*
9–11 months	122	10.2	0.30	*	*	7.7	8.1	9.7	11.9	12.9	*	*
1 year	336	9.8	0.19	6.4	7.2	7.4	8.0	9.4	11.0	12.0	12.5	14.3
2 years	260	9.6	0.13	6.3	6.8	7.2	8.0	9.5	11.1	12.0	12.7	13.2
3 years	195	9.3	0.21	*	6.4	6.9	7.3	9.0	10.7	11.4	12.0	*
4 years	199	9.1	0.26	*	6.2	6.5	7.0	8.3	10.4	11.5	12.3	*
5 years	197	10.0	0.32	*	6.1	6.5	7.2	8.7	11.0	12.9	15.8	*
6 years	173	9.8	0.25	*	6.0	6.3	7.1	8.9	11.9	13.0	14.6	*
7 years	176	10.5	0.53	*	6.2	6.6	7.4	8.9	12.1	13.7	15.4	*
8 years	146	11.7	0.69	*	6.2	6.4	7.2	10.0	14.5	17.7	20.6	*
9 years	173	12.6	0.51	*	6.4	6.9	7.6	11.4	16.2	19.3	20.3	*
10 years	169	14.4	0.54	*	7.4	8.1	8.8	12.2	18.9	21.2	24.1	*
11 years	147	15.3	0.93	*	7.6	8.0	9.3	13.1	19.3	24.2	26.6	*
12 years	265	15.4	0.56	6.1	7.4	8.4	9.5	12.9	20.4	23.4	26.5	28.9
13 years	277	14.6	0.58	6.3	6.8	7.4	8.2	12.3	18.7	23.9	26.2	28.7
14 years	253	13.4	0.62	*	6.4	6.8	7.8	10.4	17.7	22.6	24.9	*
15 years	263	12.6	0.45	6.4	6.7	7.3	8.0	9.9	15.4	19.2	22.4	26.4
16 years	290	13.6	0.47	5.8	6.2	6.8	7.4	9.9	19.1	24.5	26.3	29.1
17 years	259	12.7	0.56	5.2	6.0	6.5	7.3	10.1	17.2	19.8	22.4	26.4
18 years	266	13.1	0.88	5.4	6.2	6.5	7.2	9.9	17.8	20.8	24.7	28.7
19 years	254	13.6	0.72	*	5.9	6.9	7.9	11.0	16.2	22.9	26.6	*
Female												
2 months	9	*	*	*	*	*	*	*	*	*	*	*
3–5 months	91	10.8	0.31	*	*	8.0	8.9	10.6	11.9	13.4	*	*
6–8 months	120	11.1	0.30	*	*	7.6	8.8	11.3	12.8	13.9	*	*
9–11 months	118	10.8	0.24	*	*	8.0	8.9	10.9	12.3	12.9	*	*
1 year	316	10.1	0.19	6.5	7.2	7.5	8.3	9.7	11.4	12.7	13.2	14.6
2 years	299	10.5	0.21	6.3	7.0	7.7	8.4	10.1	12.4	13.2	14.2	15.3
3 years	174	10.2	0.28	*	6.7	7.0	7.6	9.4	11.9	13.2	14.8	*
4 years	220	10.6	0.23	*	7.1	7.4	8.2	10.3	12.1	13.2	14.2	*
5 years	194	10.7	0.32	*	7.2	7.6	8.4	9.9	12.1	13.3	14.9	*
6 years	188	10.8	0.30	*	6.2	6.9	8.0	10.0	12.9	14.7	15.1	*
7 years	153	12.7	0.38	*	7.7	8.0	8.8	11.0	15.0	18.4	19.8	*
8 years	176	12.6	0.48	*	7.4	7.8	8.7	11.0	15.3	17.7	20.1	*
9 years	182	15.5	0.59	*	8.4	9.2	10.7	14.1	18.4	22.2	24.6	*
10 years	176	16.4	0.60	*	8.3	9.6	11.3	15.1	19.9	22.8	26.6	*
11 years	167	17.6	0.72	*	8.8	9.3	11.2	16.0	22.9	26.0	28.5	*
12 years	231	16.0	0.52	*	8.9	9.2	11.1	14.6	19.8	22.8	25.5	*
13 years	274	18.8	0.49	9.2	10.2	10.8	12.9	18.3	23.2	26.0	29.2	32.1
14 years	252	18.3	0.84	*	10.1	11.1	12.9	16.2	23.9	26.4	27.6	*
15 years	226	19.7	0.65	*	11.0	11.9	13.8	18.5	23.8	26.4	30.0	*
16 years	236	18.8	0.72	*	10.5	11.2	13.2	17.1	23.3	27.0	29.3	*
17 years	227	20.3	0.56	*	11.3	13.1	14.6	18.7	25.1	28.0	29.7	*
18 years	246	21.0	0.76	*	11.1	12.8	14.8	20.1	26.2	29.9	33.2	*
19 years	208	20.5	0.80	*	11.2	12.3	14.2	19.9	25.2	27.1	29.5	*

*Figure does not meet standards of reliability or precision.

†Age shown is age at time of examination.

NOTE: Pregnant females were excluded.

Triceps skinfold thickness in millimeters for females 20 years of age and older by race and ethnicity and age, by mean, standard error of the mean, and selected percentiles: United States 2003–2006.

Race and ethnicity and age	Number examined	Mean	Standard error	Percentile								
				5th	10th	15th	25th	50th	75th	85th	90th	95th
				Millimeters								
All race and ethnicity groups†												
20 years and over	3552	24.1	0.22	11.6	13.9	15.5	18.3	24.0	29.9	32.4	34.2	36.4
20–29 years	599	21.8	0.44	10.4	11.9	13.2	15.5	21.1	27.3	30.3	32.4	34.7
30–39 years	538	24.3	0.54	12.1	14.7	15.8	18.2	23.9	30.2	32.9	35.3	37.4
40–49 years	617	25.1	0.44	12.1	14.1	15.9	19.5	25.6	30.9	33.6	35.2	36.9
50–59 years	477	25.6	0.36	13.3	16.1	17.5	20.5	25.9	31.0	33.2	34.9	36.5
60–69 years	570	25.3	0.42	13.4	16.6	18.1	20.3	25.4	30.2	32.8	34.2	36.0
70–79 years	408	23.2	0.41	11.2	14.2	15.7	17.9	22.9	28.7	31.1	32.7	36.0
80 years and over	343	20.2	0.41	10.1	11.3	12.7	14.7	19.0	25.0	28.5	30.1	32.7
Non-Hispanic white												
20 years and over	1909	23.9	0.26	11.6	13.7	15.3	18.0	23.8	29.8	32.3	34.0	36.1
20–39 years	540	22.8	0.50	11.1	13.1	14.1	16.8	22.1	28.5	31.6	33.2	36.4
40–59 years	565	25.1	0.40	12.3	14.7	16.3	19.8	25.5	31.0	33.1	34.4	36.7
60 years and over	804	23.5	0.34	11.2	13.9	15.6	18.0	23.5	28.8	31.8	32.9	35.2
Non-Hispanic black												
20 years and over	686	25.4	0.37	10.6	14.1	16.0	19.5	25.9	31.6	34.5	35.9	37.3
20–39 years	242	24.1	0.61	10.1	12.4	14.4	18.1	24.2	30.0	33.1	35.0	37.2
40–59 years	231	27.1	0.45	10.6	16.1	18.2	22.0	28.0	33.8	35.7	36.8	38.2
60 years and over	213	24.9	0.44	11.2	14.4	16.3	18.9	25.1	30.8	33.1	34.7	36.2
Mexican American												
20 years and over	676	24.9	0.53	13.3	15.9	17.2	19.9	24.3	30.1	32.6	34.6	36.3
20–39 years	244	24.6	0.62	13.0	14.8	16.8	19.2	23.5	30.2	32.5	34.7	36.3
40–59 years	196	26.0	0.64	*	17.0	18.6	21.2	26.1	30.1	33.5	34.9	*
60 years and over	236	23.0	0.35	*	14.4	15.6	18.9	22.2	27.3	30.4	32.3	*

*Figure does not meet standards of reliability or precision.

†Persons of other races and unknown race and ethnicity are included.

NOTE: Pregnant females were excluded.

Triceps skinfold thickness in millimeters for males 20 years of age and older by race and ethnicity and age, by mean, standard error of the mean, and selected percentiles: United States 2003–2006.

Race and ethnicity and age	Number examined	Mean	Standard error	Percentile 5th	10th	15th	25th	50th	75th	85th	90th	95th
				Millimeters								
All race and ethnicity groups†												
20 years and over	4152	15.0	0.19	6.1	7.3	8.3	10.1	13.8	18.8	21.9	24.2	28.1
20–29 years	755	14.3	0.35	5.0	6.2	7.1	8.8	12.7	18.9	21.7	25.4	29.4
30–39 years	690	14.7	0.28	5.8	7.1	8.2	10.0	13.6	18.3	21.4	23.4	27.0
40–49 years	705	15.3	0.35	6.6	7.6	8.7	10.4	13.9	19.2	22.3	24.1	27.9
50–59 years	542	15.1	0.41	6.2	7.4	8.9	10.8	14.1	18.5	21.5	23.2	26.7
60–69 years	618	16.1	0.43	7.3	8.3	9.4	11.2	14.9	19.7	22.5	25.2	30.3
70–79 years	520	15.6	0.33	7.1	8.7	9.5	11.0	14.0	19.2	22.5	25.0	29.1
80 years and over	322	13.9	0.26	6.8	7.6	8.3	9.7	12.7	16.2	19.8	21.6	24.4
Non-Hispanic white												
20 years and over	2177	15.2	0.21	6.1	7.4	8.6	10.3	13.9	19.1	22.1	24.4	28.5
20–39 years	639	14.5	0.33	5.4	6.4	7.5	9.2	13.1	18.7	21.4	24.0	28.5
40–59 years	651	15.5	0.38	6.4	7.6	9.1	10.9	14.1	19.3	22.5	24.3	28.0
60 years and over	887	15.9	0.31	7.3	8.6	9.4	11.1	14.4	19.1	22.4	24.9	29.7
Non-Hispanic black												
20 years and over	838	14.3	0.22	4.9	6.1	7.0	8.7	12.8	18.4	21.8	24.1	28.1
20–39 years	318	14.4	0.39	4.7	5.3	6.3	8.4	12.8	18.9	22.4	24.8	30.8
40–59 years	274	13.7	0.36	5.4	6.5	7.1	8.7	12.2	17.4	20.3	22.0	24.7
60 years and over	246	15.5	0.42	4.8	6.9	7.9	10.0	14.0	20.4	24.0	26.2	29.9
Mexican American												
20 years and over	848	14.2	0.40	6.2	7.4	8.5	9.8	13.0	17.1	20.1	22.9	26.3
20–39 years	348	14.8	0.59	6.0	7.2	8.5	10.0	13.4	18.0	21.8	24.4	27.3
40–59 years	238	13.3	0.33	*	7.7	8.2	9.1	12.0	15.9	18.0	19.7	*
60 years and over	262	13.7	0.45	*	8.1	8.6	9.7	12.5	16.0	19.6	21.1	*

* Figure does not meet standards of reliability or precision.

† Persons of other races and unknown race and ethnicity are included.

APPENDIX

N

Subscapular Skinfold Norms from NHANES 2003–2006

From National Center for Health Statistics, Centers for Disease Control and Prevention, U.S. Department of Health and Human Services.

Subscapular skinfold thickness in millimeters for children and adolescents aged 2 months–19 years by sex and age, by mean, standard error of the mean, and selected percentiles: United States 2003–2006.

Sex and age†	Number examined	Mean	Standard error	Percentile								
				5th	10th	15th	25th	50th	75th	85th	90th	95th
				Millimeters								
Male												
2 months	12	*	*	*	*	*	*	*	*	*	*	*
3–5 months	126	8.3	0.20	*	*	6.5	7.0	7.9	9.2	10.6	*	*
6–8 months	126	7.6	0.18	*	*	5.8	6.2	7.3	8.4	9.2	*	*
9–11 months	121	7.6	0.26	*	*	5.6	5.9	7.1	9.0	9.5	*	*
1 year	333	6.8	0.11	4.8	5.0	5.2	5.7	6.5	7.5	8.2	8.5	9.7
2 years	255	6.5	0.10	*	4.8	4.9	5.2	6.0	7.1	8.2	8.5	*
3 years	196	6.7	0.18	*	4.4	4.7	5.2	6.2	7.7	8.4	9.1	*
4 years	197	6.1	0.19	*	4.1	4.3	4.8	5.4	6.3	7.3	8.4	*
5 years	196	7.3	0.46	*	4.3	4.5	4.9	5.9	7.3	9.1	11.9	*
6 years	170	7.0	0.20	*	4.3	4.5	4.9	5.9	7.9	9.2	10.5	*
7 years	174	7.1	0.35	*	4.3	4.5	4.9	5.9	7.5	9.0	10.4	*
8 years	140	7.9	0.53	*	4.2	4.4	4.8	5.9	8.7	11.3	15.0	*
9 years	164	8.8	0.50	*	4.4	4.9	5.4	6.7	9.7	14.3	16.5	*
10 years	165	10.4	0.65	*	4.9	5.1	5.9	7.4	13.4	17.1	20.4	*
11 years	141	10.7	0.59	*	5.2	5.4	5.9	7.8	14.8	17.3	20.5	*
12 years	258	11.5	0.61	4.9	5.1	5.5	6.0	8.5	14.6	18.1	21.9	29.3
13 years	272	12.0	0.64	5.0	5.6	6.1	6.6	9.3	15.2	19.8	22.4	25.8
14 years	242	10.6	0.46	*	5.7	6.1	6.7	8.5	13.4	15.8	19.3	*
15 years	257	11.2	0.41	6.0	6.5	6.9	7.2	9.0	12.9	15.2	20.1	24.5
16 years	285	12.7	0.38	6.4	6.7	7.2	7.8	9.6	16.3	20.8	23.6	26.5
17 years	256	12.7	0.60	6.2	7.1	7.5	8.2	10.0	14.4	20.5	24.2	27.8
18 years	257	13.9	0.69	7.1	7.4	8.0	8.7	10.5	17.4	21.7	24.5	28.4
19 years	240	14.5	0.62	*	7.8	8.2	9.1	12.4	18.0	21.4	26.1	*
Female												
2 months	10	*	*	*	*	*	*	*	*	*	*	*
3–5 months	92	8.4	0.26	*	*	5.9	6.4	8.1	9.6	10.4	*	*
6–8 months	116	8.4	0.37	*	*	5.9	6.3	7.8	9.6	10.8	*	*
9–11 months	120	8.3	0.16	*	5.9	6.1	6.6	7.9	9.2	10.4	11.0	*
1 year	310	7.3	0.12	4.9	5.1	5.3	5.9	6.9	8.3	8.9	9.3	10.5
2 years	292	7.0	0.16	4.5	4.9	5.0	5.4	6.3	7.9	9.0	9.8	10.7
3 years	173	7.2	0.23	*	4.6	4.9	5.3	6.5	8.0	9.1	11.0	*
4 years	216	7.2	0.21	*	4.9	5.0	5.2	6.3	7.9	9.5	10.4	*
5 years	191	7.8	0.40	*	4.9	5.2	5.4	6.3	8.2	9.9	12.1	*
6 years	185	7.5	0.24	*	4.5	4.8	5.3	6.5	8.4	10.3	11.8	*
7 years	148	8.5	0.40	*	4.6	5.0	5.4	7.3	9.8	11.9	12.9	*
8 years	174	9.1	0.53	*	4.7	5.0	5.5	6.8	10.1	13.4	17.9	*
9 years	174	11.1	0.50	*	5.4	6.1	6.7	9.4	13.7	17.6	19.0	*
10 years	168	12.1	0.44	*	5.7	6.1	7.4	10.1	16.1	19.1	20.2	*
11 years	158	13.5	0.61	*	6.3	6.8	8.0	11.5	17.9	21.0	23.2	*
12 years	225	12.4	0.61	*	6.1	6.9	7.9	10.6	15.3	19.0	20.6	*
13 years	268	14.6	0.65	6.0	7.1	7.7	8.7	12.7	18.3	23.9	26.3	28.9
14 years	240	14.0	0.72	6.9	7.6	8.1	9.0	11.7	16.3	20.8	24.1	29.8
15 years	220	15.7	0.49	*	7.9	8.6	9.9	13.9	20.2	22.8	24.4	*
16 years	226	14.8	0.52	*	8.1	8.6	9.3	12.9	17.5	20.7	24.9	*
17 years	213	16.2	0.56	*	8.3	9.0	10.5	14.2	19.6	24.6	27.3	*
18 years	226	16.7	0.62	*	8.4	9.3	10.8	15.0	20.9	24.2	25.8	*
19 years	192	18.2	0.78	*	8.5	9.0	10.7	16.5	24.4	25.9	28.1	*

* Figure does not meet standards of reliability or precision.

† Age shown is age at time of examination.

NOTE: Pregnant females were excluded.

Subscapular skinfold thickness in millimeters for females 20 years of age and older by race and ethnicity and age, by mean, standard error of the mean, and selected percentiles: United States 2003–2006.

Race and ethnicity and age	Number examined	Mean	Standard error	Percentile 5th	10th	15th	25th	50th	75th	85th	90th	95th
				Millimeters								
All race and ethnicity groups†												
20 years and over	3186	20.8	0.24	8.4	10.0	11.3	13.9	20.3	26.8	30.4	32.6	35.1
20–29 years	526	18.3	0.49	7.6	8.9	10.0	11.7	16.3	24.1	27.3	30.5	33.9
30–39 years	492	21.1	0.50	9.2	10.6	11.8	14.3	20.2	27.4	30.9	32.2	35.3
40–49 years	521	22.2	0.46	9.1	10.7	12.3	15.2	22.7	28.5	31.8	33.9	35.6
50–59 years	406	22.6	0.41	8.8	11.6	13.0	16.5	22.6	28.9	31.7	34.1	36.2
60–69 years	534	22.3	0.41	9.1	10.9	13.5	16.7	21.8	28.0	32.0	33.0	34.9
70–79 years	375	19.3	0.54	7.4	9.3	10.5	13.8	19.3	23.9	27.0	29.5	32.4
80 years and over	333	16.1	0.36	6.9	8.1	8.8	10.4	14.4	21.3	24.4	25.4	28.2
Non-Hispanic white												
20 years and over	1904	20.1	0.26	8.1	9.6	10.8	13.2	19.4	25.8	29.9	31.7	34.8
20–39 years	516	18.8	0.45	7.8	9.2	10.3	12.1	16.8	24.4	28.5	31.0	33.8
40–59 years	513	21.7	0.39	8.7	10.4	12.1	14.8	21.9	28.3	30.9	33.3	35.6
60 years and over	775	19.4	0.37	7.6	9.2	10.2	12.9	19.3	24.8	27.8	30.2	33.0
Non-Hispanic black												
20 years and over	571	24.0	0.54	9.5	12.0	13.4	17.5	24.3	30.8	33.8	34.6	36.8
20–39 years	210	22.4	0.81	*	10.7	12.0	15.0	22.4	29.4	32.5	34.0	*
40–59 years	182	26.1	0.66	*	15.1	17.0	20.6	26.5	32.6	34.2	35.3	*
60 years and over	179	24.0	0.71	*	12.6	13.9	17.6	23.6	30.2	32.5	35.1	*
Mexican American												
20 years and over	569	23.2	0.59	10.9	13.6	14.6	17.2	23.2	28.2	31.2	33.5	35.7
20–39 years	200	23.0	0.99	*	11.9	13.9	16.3	23.2	28.7	31.9	34.0	*
40–59 years	145	24.1	0.50	*	15.1	16.2	18.8	24.0	28.3	31.14	33.2	*
60 years and over	224	21.6	0.50	*	13.2	14.1	17.1	20.6	25.7	29.4	31.2	*

* Figure does not meet standards of reliability or precision.

† Persons of other races and unknown race and ethnicity are included.

NOTE: Pregnant females were excluded.

Subscapular skinfold thickness in millimeters for males 20 years of age and older by race and ethnicity and age, by mean, standard error of the mean, and selected percentiles: United States 2003–2006.

Race and ethnicity and age	Number examined	Mean	Standard error	Percentile								
				5th	10th	15th	25th	50th	75th	85th	90th	95th
				Millimeters								
All race and ethnicity groups												
20 years and over	3529	19.3	0.17	8.9	10.2	11.5	13.9	18.6	24.1	26.9	29.1	32.1
20–29 years	688	16.8	0.34	7.8	8.8	9.4	11.1	15.7	20.9	23.9	26.0	29.6
30–39 years	583	19.1	0.31	8.8	10.3	11.9	13.2	18.5	24.0	26.7	28.2	31.1
40–49 years	576	20.7	0.34	9.4	11.1	12.8	15.6	20.2	25.7	28.7	30.3	32.4
50–59 years	442	20.2	0.40	9.4	11.3	12.9	14.9	19.9	24.9	27.4	29.7	32.4
60–69 years	493	21.1	0.38	10.9	12.1	14.2	16.4	20.5	24.9	27.9	30.4	34.4
70–79 years	455	19.8	0.32	9.9	12.1	13.2	15.5	18.9	23.5	26.7	29.2	32.6
80 years and over	292	17.0	0.36	8.3	9.2	10.4	11.9	16.4	20.7	23.1	25.7	27.1
Non-Hispanic white												
20 years and over	1900	19.1	0.18	8.9	10.1	11.4	13.7	18.4	23.9	26.6	28.7	32.0
20–39 years	575	17.3	0.35	8.0	9.0	9.8	11.8	16.3	21.4	24.8	26.8	29.5
40–59 years	554	20.5	0.32	9.5	11.2	12.9	15.1	20.1	25.2	28.0	30.0	32.6
60 years and over	771	19.8	0.23	10.1	11.5	12.7	15.2	19.2	23.4	26.7	28.7	32.1
Non-Hispanic black												
20 years and over	664	19.3	0.35	8.0	9.1	10.2	12.8	18.6	24.8	28.4	30.9	33.8
20–39 years	271	18.5	0.51	7.9	8.6	10.0	11.9	17.2	23.8	26.8	29.2	34.0
40–59 years	204	19.6	0.60	8.4	9.2	10.4	13.4	18.9	25.8	28.7	30.7	33.0
60 years and over	189	21.1	0.49	7.1	8.7	12.1	15.3	21.0	26.1	30.4	32.8	35.7
Mexican American												
20 years and over	720	19.7	0.50	9.7	10.8	12.5	14.9	19.4	23.8	26.3	28.2	31.4
20–39 years	301	19.4	0.67	*	10.4	12.0	14.1	19.2	23.7	26.4	28.2	*
40–59 years	194	20.2	0.48	*	12.2	13.6	16.3	20.1	24.2	26.3	27.9	*
60 years and over	225	19.6	0.62	*	10.4	12.5	15.2	19.0	22.9	25.8	29.3	*

* Figure does not meet standards of reliability or precision.

APPENDIX

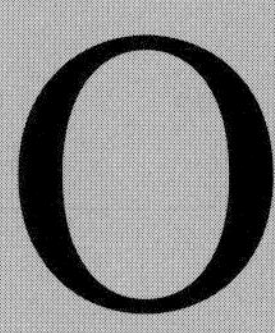

Means, Standard Deviations, and Percentiles of Sum of Triceps and Subscapular Skinfold Thickness (mm) by Age for Males and Females of 2 to 90 Years (See Table 7.2 for Interpretation Guidelines)

Frisancho AR. 2008. *Anthropometric Standards: An Interactive Nutritional Reference of Body Size and Body Composition for Children and Adults.* Ann Arbor: University of Michigan Press. Copyright by the University of Michigan, 2008. Reprinted with permission of the University of Michigan Press.

Mean (M), standard deviation (SD), and percentiles of sum of triceps and subscapular skinfold thickness (mm) by age for males and females of 2 to 90 years

					Percentiles								
Age Group (years)	**Mean Age (years)**	**N**	**M**	**SD**	**5th**	**10th**	**15th**	**25th**	**50th**	**75th**	**85th**	**90th**	**95th**
					Males								
2.0–2.9	2.46	544	14.8	4.0	9.4	10.4	11.1	12.3	14.8	17.7	19.5	20.8	22.8
3.0–3.9	3.45	482	14.2	3.8	9.0	10.0	10.7	11.7	14.1	16.8	18.4	19.6	21.5
4.0–4.9	4.47	540	14.4	3.9	8.6	9.6	10.3	11.4	13.7	16.4	18.0	19.3	21.2
5.0–5.9	5.43	490	14.8	4.4	8.1	9.1	9.8	10.9	13.4	16.4	18.2	19.5	21.7
6.0–6.9	6.45	258	15.4	6.1	6.8	7.9	8.7	10.1	13.3	17.3	19.9	21.8	25.0
7.0–7.9	7.47	270	16.0	7.1	6.4	7.5	8.5	10.0	13.5	18.1	21.1	23.4	27.2
8.0–8.9	8.46	258	16.7	7.4	6.7	7.9	8.9	10.5	14.2	19.1	22.3	24.7	28.8
9.0–9.9	9.50	276	17.3	7.7	7.3	8.7	9.7	11.5	15.5	20.8	24.3	26.9	31.3
10.0–10.9	10.45	287	17.9	7.9	7.9	9.4	10.5	12.4	16.8	22.5	26.3	29.2	33.9
11.0–11.9	11.44	271	18.5	8.2	8.3	9.8	11.0	13.1	17.7	23.8	27.7	30.8	35.8
12.0–12.9	12.47	199	19.1	8.5	8.3	9.9	11.1	13.1	17.8	24.0	28.0	31.0	36.1
13.0–13.9	13.47	187	19.7	9.7	7.4	8.9	10.2	12.3	17.2	23.9	28.4	31.8	37.6
14.0–14.9	14.49	177	20.2	10.6	6.6	8.2	9.4	11.5	16.5	23.3	28.0	31.6	37.7
15.0–15.9	15.45	177	20.6	10.3	6.9	8.4	9.6	11.6	16.3	22.7	27.0	30.2	35.7
16.0–16.9	16.45	188	21.1	10.0	7.6	9.2	10.4	12.5	17.3	23.7	27.9	31.1	36.6
17.0–17.9	17.45	186	21.5	9.9	8.6	10.4	11.7	13.9	19.0	25.8	30.2	33.6	39.2
18.0–18.9	18.45	167	22.0	9.5	9.7	11.5	12.8	15.1	20.3	27.0	31.4	34.7	40.2
19.0–19.9	19.43	153	22.4	9.4	10.1	12.0	13.3	15.6	20.9	27.6	32.0	35.3	40.7
20.0–29.9	24.96	1537	25.0	9.8	11.7	14.2	16.1	19.0	25.2	32.3	36.5	39.5	44.1
30.0–39.9	34.72	1355	30.0	10.9	13.2	16.5	18.8	22.3	29.2	36.5	40.7	43.5	47.8
40.0–49.9	44.35	1095	31.7	10.5	15.4	18.6	20.8	24.2	30.9	38.0	41.9	44.7	48.9
50.0–59.9	54.89	768	31.9	10.1	16.3	19.5	21.8	25.1	31.8	38.7	42.6	45.3	49.3
60.0–69.9	64.83	1059	31.8	10.1	16.4	19.6	21.9	25.3	32.0	39.0	42.8	45.5	49.6
70.0–79.9	74.16	753	30.9	9.9	15.5	18.7	20.8	24.2	30.6	37.3	41.0	43.6	47.5
80.0–90.9	84.09	535	27.5	8.6	14.0	16.8	18.7	21.6	27.2	32.9	36.1	38.3	41.6

continued

Mean (M), standard deviation (SD), and percentiles of sum of triceps and subscapular skinfold thickness (mm) by age for males and females of 2 to 90 years—*continued*

Age Group (years)	Mean Age (years)	N	M	SD	Percentiles								
					5th	10th	15th	25th	50th	75th	85th	90th	95th
Females													
2.0–2.9	2.45	533	16.8	4.9	9.7	10.8	11.6	12.9	15.8	19.2	21.4	22.9	25.5
3.0–3.9	3.46	554	15.5	4.7	9.3	10.4	11.2	12.6	15.5	19.0	21.1	22.8	25.4
4.0–4.9	4.43	525	15.3	5.7	8.2	9.4	10.4	11.9	15.4	19.7	22.6	24.7	28.2
5.0–5.9	5.46	541	15.9	6.9	7.4	8.7	9.7	11.4	15.3	20.5	23.9	26.6	30.9
6.0–6.9	6.47	272	17.1	8.1	7.1	8.5	9.6	11.4	15.7	21.5	25.4	28.5	33.6
7.0–7.9	7.44	260	18.6	9.2	7.1	8.6	9.8	11.7	16.4	22.9	27.3	30.7	36.6
8.0–8.9	8.47	243	20.4	10.5	7.5	9.1	10.3	12.4	17.6	24.8	29.8	33.6	40.3
9.0–9.9	9.43	264	22.2	11.5	8.0	9.7	11.1	13.4	19.1	27.0	32.4	36.7	43.9
10.0–10.9	10.43	252	24.2	12.3	8.9	10.8	12.3	14.9	21.0	29.6	35.4	40.0	47.9
11.0–11.9	11.46	276	26.1	12.9	10.2	12.3	13.9	16.7	23.4	32.5	38.7	43.6	51.8
12.0–12.9	12.46	214	27.9	13.1	11.8	14.1	15.9	18.9	25.9	35.5	42.0	47.0	55.4
13.0–13.9	13.45	222	29.5	13.1	13.5	15.9	17.8	21.0	28.4	38.3	44.8	49.9	58.4
14.0–14.9	14.47	214	31.0	13.2	15.0	17.5	19.5	22.8	30.4	40.4	47.0	52.0	60.4
15.0–15.9	15.47	181	32.4	13.2	15.7	18.4	20.5	23.9	31.6	41.4	47.7	52.5	60.3
16.0–16.9	16.46	212	33.6	13.4	16.3	19.1	21.2	24.6	32.4	42.2	48.4	53.1	60.8
17.0–17.9	17.45	193	34.6	13.6	16.5	19.5	21.7	25.4	33.4	43.2	49.3	53.8	60.9
18.0–18.9	18.43	173	35.5	14.0	16.4	19.7	22.1	26.0	34.4	44.4	50.4	54.8	61.6
19.0–19.9	19.48	178	36.4	14.4	16.4	19.7	22.1	26.1	34.5	44.6	50.7	55.1	62.0
20.0–29.9	24.91	1671	39.6	15.1	19.1	22.8	25.5	29.8	39.1	50.0	56.6	61.4	68.9
30.0–39.9	34.85	1578	45.4	15.4	24.0	27.8	30.7	35.2	44.7	55.7	62.2	66.9	74.2
40.0–49.9	44.28	1137	50.6	15.5	25.9	31.2	34.8	40.3	50.6	61.2	66.9	70.9	76.7
50.0–59.9	54.83	856	50.6	15.4	25.7	31.1	34.8	40.3	50.7	61.2	66.8	70.7	76.4
60.0–69.9	64.82	1010	47.2	14.4	23.9	29.0	32.4	37.6	47.2	57.0	62.3	65.9	71.3
70.0–79.9	74.46	831	42.1	14.0	19.3	24.2	27.5	32.5	41.8	51.3	56.4	59.9	65.1
80.0–90.9	84.45	554	33.8	12.4	13.4	17.5	20.4	24.6	32.6	40.7	45.1	48.1	52.5

APPENDIX

P

Means, Standard Deviations, and Percentiles of Upper-Arm Muscle Area (cm^2) by Age for Males and Females of 2 to 90 Years (See Table 7.6 for Interpretation Guidelines)

Frisancho AR. 2008. *Anthropometric Standards: An Interactive Nutritional Reference of Body Size and Body Composition for Children and Adults.* Ann Arbor: University of Michigan Press.

Mean (M), standard deviation (SD), and percentiles of mid-upper arm muscle area (cm^2) by age for males and females of 2 to 90 years

Age Group (years)	Mean Age (years)	N	M	SD	Percentiles 5th	10th	15th	25th	50th	75th	85th	90th	95th
					Males								
2.0–2.9	2.46	548	14.7	2.2	11.4	12.0	12.5	13.2	14.5	16.0	16.9	17.5	18.5
3.0–3.9	3.45	481	16.4	2.5	12.4	13.1	13.7	14.5	16.1	17.9	18.9	19.6	20.7
4.0–4.9	4.47	542	17.4	2.8	13.0	13.8	14.3	15.2	16.9	18.8	19.9	20.7	21.9
5.0–5.9	5.43	492	18.2	3.1	13.6	14.5	15.1	16.1	18.1	20.3	21.6	22.5	23.9
6.0–6.9	6.45	258	19.3	3.6	14.6	15.6	16.3	17.4	19.8	22.4	23.9	25.0	26.7
7.0–7.9	7.47	271	20.8	3.9	15.8	16.9	17.7	19.0	21.5	24.4	26.2	27.4	29.3
8.0–8.9	8.46	257	22.8	4.3	17.0	18.2	19.1	20.5	23.2	26.4	28.2	29.5	31.6
9.0–9.9	9.50	282	25.6	5.0	18.2	19.6	20.5	22.0	25.1	28.6	30.7	32.2	34.5
10.0–10.9	10.45	287	28.6	5.9	19.3	20.9	22.0	23.7	27.2	31.3	33.7	35.5	38.2
11.0–11.9	11.44	272	32.1	7.2	20.8	22.6	23.9	25.9	30.2	35.0	38.0	40.1	43.4
12.0–12.9	12.47	201	36.1	8.0	23.1	25.2	26.7	29.1	34.1	40.0	43.5	46.0	50.1
13.0–13.9	13.47	188	40.0	9.4	26.3	28.6	30.3	33.0	38.7	45.3	49.2	52.1	56.6
14.0–14.9	14.49	179	44.1	9.8	30.3	32.9	34.7	37.7	43.7	50.7	54.9	58.0	62.7
15.0–15.9	15.45	177	47.9	9.5	34.3	37.0	38.9	42.0	48.3	55.6	59.9	63.0	67.8
16.0–16.9	16.45	191	51.6	10.4	37.6	40.5	42.6	45.8	52.5	60.1	64.6	67.9	72.9
17.0–17.9	17.45	188	55.0	11.2	40.0	43.1	45.3	48.8	56.0	64.2	69.0	72.5	78.0
18.0–18.9	18.45	167	58.0	11.7	42.0	45.2	47.5	51.2	58.6	67.1	72.2	75.8	81.5
19.0–19.9	19.43	154	60.6	12.2	42.6	45.8	48.2	51.8	59.4	68.0	73.1	76.7	82.5
20.0–29.9	24.96	1564	64.5	13.4	45.2	48.8	51.4	55.4	63.8	73.4	79.1	83.2	89.6
30.0–39.9	34.72	1405	66.6	13.5	48.7	52.4	55.2	59.4	68.1	78.1	84.0	88.3	95.0
40.0–49.9	44.35	1158	69.9	12.8	49.8	53.5	56.2	60.5	69.1	79.0	84.8	89.0	95.6
50.0–59.9	54.89	815	67.4	12.6	49.7	53.3	55.8	59.7	67.8	76.9	82.3	86.1	92.1
60.0–69.9	64.83	1122	64.8	12.4	46.8	50.2	52.7	56.5	64.4	73.3	78.6	82.4	88.3
70.0–79.9	74.16	820	59.5	11.1	43.5	46.5	48.8	52.2	59.2	67.2	71.8	75.2	80.4
80.0–90.9	84.09	635	52.7	10.1	38.1	40.9	42.9	46.0	52.4	59.6	63.9	66.9	71.7

continued

Mean (M), standard deviation (SD), and percentiles of mid-upper arm muscle area (cm^2) by age for males and females of 2 to 90 years—*continued*

Age Group (years)	Mean Age (years)	N	M	SD	Percentiles								
					5th	10th	15th	25th	50th	75th	85th	90th	95th
Females													
2.0–2.9	2.45	534	15.0	2.2	10.9	11.5	12.0	12.6	14.0	15.5	16.4	17.0	18.0
3.0–3.9	3.46	554	14.7	2.4	11.9	12.6	13.1	13.9	15.5	17.2	18.3	19.0	20.1
4.0–4.9	4.43	526	15.3	2.6	12.7	13.5	14.1	15.0	16.8	18.9	20.1	20.9	22.2
5.0–5.9	5.46	540	10.8	3.1	13.2	14.1	14.7	15.7	17.8	20.1	21.5	22.5	24.0
6.0–6.9	6.47	272	18.8	3.6	13.6	14.6	15.4	16.5	18.8	21.4	22.9	24.0	25.8
7.0–7.9	7.44	263	20.9	4.2	14.0	15.1	15.8	17.1	19.6	22.4	24.1	25.3	27.3
8.0–8.9	8.47	245	23.2	4.5	14.6	15.7	16.6	17.9	20.7	23.8	25.7	27.1	29.2
9.0–9.9	9.43	266	25.4	5.6	15.7	17.0	17.9	19.4	22.5	26.1	28.2	29.7	32.2
10.0–10.9	10.43	254	27.6	5.5	17.7	19.2	20.3	21.9	25.5	29.5	32.0	33.7	36.5
11.0–11.9	11.46	281	29.7	6.5	20.2	21.9	23.2	25.1	29.1	33.8	36.6	38.6	41.8
12.0–12.9	12.46	216	31.5	6.9	22.6	24.5	25.9	28.0	32.5	37.7	40.8	43.1	46.6
13.0–13.9	13.45	224	33.1	7.3	24.3	26.3	27.8	30.1	35.0	40.5	43.9	46.3	50.1
14.0–14.9	14.47	218	34.5	7.6	25.1	27.2	28.7	31.1	36.1	41.9	45.3	47.8	51.8
15.0–15.9	15.47	187	35.6	8.0	25.1	27.2	28.7	31.2	36.2	42.1	45.6	48.2	52.2
16.0–16.9	16.46	216	36.6	8.2	24.9	27.1	28.6	31.0	36.1	41.9	45.4	48.0	52.0
17.0–17.9	17.45	202	37.4	8.6	24.7	26.8	28.4	30.9	36.1	42.1	45.8	48.4	52.6
18.0–18.9	18.43	178	38.0	8.7	24.9	27.0	28.6	31.1	36.3	42.4	46.0	48.7	52.9
19.0–19.9	19.48	182	38.5	8.8	25.3	27.5	29.1	31.6	36.9	43.0	46.7	49.4	53.6
20.0–29.9	24.91	1766	39.9	9.1	26.4	28.7	30.3	32.9	38.4	44.7	48.6	51.3	55.7
30.0–39.9	34.85	1698	42.3	10.5	27.4	30.0	31.9	34.9	41.3	48.8	53.4	56.7	62.0
40.0–49.9	44.28	1227	44.8	11.3	29.0	31.8	33.9	37.1	44.1	52.2	57.2	60.9	66.7
50.0–59.9	54.83	928	45.7	11.7	28.8	31.7	33.7	37.0	44.1	52.4	57.4	61.2	67.1
60.0–69.9	64.82	1092	45.1	11.7	28.1	30.9	32.9	36.2	43.1	51.2	56.2	59.9	65.7
70.0–79.9	74.46	899	43.7	11.3	27.5	30.2	32.2	35.3	42.1	50.1	54.9	58.5	64.2
80.0–90.9	84.45	696	41.0	10.5	26.2	28.8	30.7	33.7	40.1	47.6	52.2	55.6	61.0

APPENDIX

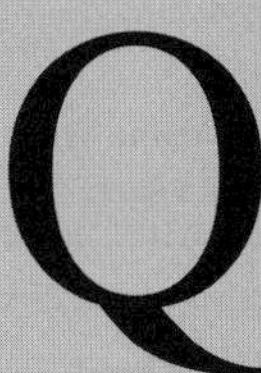

Reference Values for Serum Total Cholesterol and Serum High-Density Lipoprotein, by Sex, Age, Race/Ethnicity, 1988–1994

Data from the National Center for Health Statistics, Centers for Disease Control and Prevention, U.S. Department of Health and Human Services.

Serum Total Cholesterol of Males 4 Years of Age and Older by Age: Mean and Selected Percentiles, United States, 1988–94

Age in Years	Number of Examined Persons	Mean	Standard Deviation	Standard Error of the Mean	Selected Percentiles								
					5th	10th	15th	25th	50th	75th	85th	90th	95th
4 years and older, crude	11,200	192	41.9	0.63	131	142	149	162	189	220	237	248	266
4 years and older, age adjusted		191											
4–5 years	846	161	24.3	1.33	123	133	136	144	159	175	185	192	203
6–8 years	695	166	26.4	1.59	127	135	140	147	165	183	191	203	212
9–11 years	757	172	28.4	1.64	135	140	145	153	171	189	196	209	227
12–15 years	703	158	27.5	1.65	117	124	130	140	158	174	184	192	203
16–19 years	668	158	29.7	1.82	117	123	127	138	156	175	190	200	214
20 years and older, crude	7531	202	41.0	0.75	139	151	160	173	200	228	244	255	273
20 years and older, age adjusted		202											
20–74 years	6587	202	41.0	0.80	139	151	160	173	200	228	244	255	273
20–74 years, age adjusted		201											
20–29 years	1551	180	36.2	1.46	127	137	145	155	177	200	216	225	242
30–39 years	1389	201	39.3	1.68	139	153	162	171	199	228	244	253	267
40–49 years	1169	211	39.2	1.82	147	164	173	186	209	236	249	261	275
50–59 years	829	216	40.8	2.25	154	166	177	191	214	240	257	270	286
60–69 years	1137	217	39.2	1.85	152	169	177	190	215	241	256	270	285
70–79 years	812	208	39.2	2.18	148	159	169	180	205	233	248	256	275
80+ years	644	201	41.0	2.56	140	152	158	170	198	226	244	253	270

Serum Total Cholesterol of Males 4 Years of Age and Older by Race/Ethnicity and Age: Mean and Selected Percentiles, United States, 1988–94

Non-Hispanic White, Age in Years	Number of Examined Persons	Mean	Standard Deviation	Standard Error of the Mean	Selected Percentiles								
					5th	10th	15th	25th	50th	75th	85th	90th	95th
4 years and older, crude	4097	194	41.7	0.8	132	143	150	164	191	222	238	248	267
4 years and older, age adjusted		190											
4–5 years	210	160	22.4	1.8	130	134	140	144	159	174	181	186	197
6–11 years	387	169	26.0	1.5	128	139	144	151	167	184	193	200	216
12–19 years	339	157	28.3	1.8	116	120	126	137	155	173	184	195	205
20 years and older, crude	3161	203	40.4	0.8	141	153	162	174	201	229	244	256	272
20 years and older, age adjusted		201											
20–74 years	2449	203	40.5	1.0	141	153	162	174	201	229	244	256	272
20–74 years, age adjusted		201											
20–29 years	381	179	35.9	2.2	125	137	144	154	175	198	215	224	239
30–39 years	434	201	38.5	2.2	142	156	163	171	199	228	244	253	267
40–49 years	421	212	38.5	2.2	152	166	175	187	209	237	249	261	275
50–59 years	411	216	39.8	2.3	155	166	176	193	213	238	259	272	286
60–69 years	499	217	37.6	2.0	157	171	178	192	215	241	253	267	283
70+ years	1015	206	39.3	1.4	146	155	165	177	203	230	246	255	273

Serum Total Cholesterol of Males 4 Years of Age and Older by Race/Ethnicity and Age: Mean and Selected Percentiles, United States, 1988–94

Non-Hispanic Black, Age in Years	Number of Examined Persons	Mean	Standard Deviation	Standard Error of the Mean	Selected Percentiles								
					5th	10th	15th	25th	50th	75th	85th	90th	95th
4 years and older, crude	3154	188	41.5	0.8	131	140	148	159	184	212	228	240	264
4 years and older, age adjusted		191											
4–5 years	275	164	26.9	1.8	122	127	135	148	164	181	192	200	211
6–11 years	480	172	30.0	1.5	128	137	143	153	169	190	200	207	224
12–19 years	476	166	30.6	1.6	119	131	136	147	163	185	193	201	220
20 years and older, crude	1923	198	42.8	1.1	136	147	155	169	195	222	239	251	275
20 years and older, age adjusted		200											
20–74 years	1813	198	42.7	1.1	136	147	155	169	195	222	238	251	274
20–74 years, age adjusted	1813	200											
20–29 years	456	185	35.6	1.8	133	141	149	161	181	207	221	232	249
30–39 years	451	193	40.1	2.1	134	142	153	162	191	216	227	236	262
40–49 years	333	206	43.2	2.6	143	152	165	178	202	228	249	265	285
50–59 years	203	213	48.4	3.8	136	154	165	180	211	239	255	277	309
60–69 years	268	215	47.8	3.2	148	166	173	181	211	244	263	274	294
70+ years	212	207	42.3	3.2	141	155	159	178	206	233	249	257	289

Serum Total Cholesterol of Males 4 Years of Age and Older by Race/Ethnicity and Age: Mean and Selected Percentiles, United States, 1988–94

Mexican Americans, Age in Years	Number of Examined Persons	Mean	Standard Deviation	Standard Error of the Mean	Selected Percentiles								
					5th	10th	15th	25th	50th	75th	85th	90th	95th
4 years and older, crude	3499	187	42.5	0.9	129	139	146	157	182	212	228	242	260
4 years and older, age adjusted		192											
4–5 years	316	158	26.3	1.9	119	127	133	140	156	172	185	195	204
6–11 years	515	168	26.8	1.5	128	136	139	149	166	185	196	205	215
12–19 years	493	161	30.3	1.8	119	126	132	141	157	177	191	200	213
20 years and older, crude		199	43.1	1.2	137	150	157	171	197	224	241	253	272
20 years and older, age adjusted		203											
20–74 years	2073	200	43.2	1.2	138	150	158	171	197	224	241	253	273
20–74 years, age adjusted	2073	204											
20–29 years	644	184	38.3	1.9	130	142	149	157	177	205	219	232	250
30–39 years	449	205	41.6	2.5	141	157	168	179	200	227	247	257	274
40–49 years	370	212	42.2	2.8	150	163	172	186	210	233	249	266	290
50–59 years	176	215	50.3	4.9	146*	167	179	189	218	235	256	269	279*
60–69 years	337	219	40.6	2.9	160	175	181	188	219	245	258	267	285
70+ years	199	203	41.1	3.7	144*	153	158	173	202	232	241	254	273*

* Value based on a limited number of observations.

Serum Total Cholesterol of Females 4 Years of Age and Older by Age: Mean and Selected Percentiles, United States, 1988–94

Age in Years	Number of Examined Persons	Mean	Standard Deviation	Standard Error of the Mean	Selected Percentiles								
					5th	10th	15th	25th	50th	75th	85th	90th	95th
4 years and older, crude	12,361	197	45.1	0.61	135	145	153	165	191	224	244	257	278
4 years and older, age adjusted		195											
4–5 years	861	164	25.9	1.32	126	134	140	146	163	179	190	197	206
6–8 years	672	166	26.5	1.53	127	136	143	150	165	181	190	196	203
9–11 years	731	169	26.7	1.48	131	137	143	149	167	185	196	205	219
12–15 years	799	164	29.8	1.58	123	130	135	143	160	182	192	201	218
16–19 years	767	171	39.8	2.16	118	128	136	145	164	189	203	217	238
20 years and older, crude	8531	206	44.7	0.73	143	153	161	175	201	233	251	265	284
20 years and older, age adjusted		206											
20–74 years	7429	204	44.2	0.77	142	152	160	173	199	231	249	262	282
20–74 years, age adjusted		204											
20–29 years	1760	183	37.2	1.33	131	141	147	157	179	205	217	229	244
30–39 years	1750	189	34.7	1.24	138	147	153	166	186	209	226	234	250
40–49 years	1300	204	38.2	1.59	150	158	164	177	201	225	245	254	277
50–59 years	962	228	43.8	2.12	166	177	184	199	224	255	273	284	304
60–69 years	1109	235	45.5	2.05	170	183	193	205	230	258	278	290	309
70–79 years	934	233	44.8	2.20	164	177	188	200	233	262	277	287	309
80+ years	716	228	43.3	2.43	165	177	183	196	224	254	270	285	305

Serum Total Cholesterol of Females 4 Years of Age and Older by Race/Ethnicity and Age: Mean and Selected Percentiles, United States, 1988–94

Non-Hispanic White, Age in Years	Number of Examined Persons	Mean	Standard Deviation	Standard Error of the Mean	Selected Percentiles								
					5th	10th	15th	25th	50th	75th	85th	90th	95th
4 years and older, crude	4661	200	45.4	0.8	137	147	154	167	194	227	246	259	280
4 years and older, age adjusted		195											
4–5 years	226	163	23.9	1.8	128	137	140	146	162	177	184	195	208
6–11 years	366	167	25.6	1.6	128	135	143	150	167	183	194	198	212
12–19 years	424	166	36.8	2.1	118	128	134	142	160	185	196	203	227
20 years and older, crude	3645	208	44.6	0.9	144	155	163	177	203	235	252	267	284
20 years and older, age adjusted		206											
20–74 years	2818	206	44.1	1.0	143	153	162	175	201	233	250	263	282
20–74 years, age adjusted		205											
20–29 years	480	183	37.0	2.0	133	141	148	156	182	206	217	229	243
30–39 years	570	188	33.7	1.6	139	147	154	166	185	209	225	233	249
40–49 years	464	205	37.3	2.0	150	158	167	178	202	226	245	253	274
50–59 years	466	230	43.5	2.3	171	179	187	200	226	256	275	285	304
60–69 years	477	234	44.9	2.4	173	184	193	205	229	257	276	288	309
70+ years	1188	232	43.9	1.5	166	178	187	199	232	259	274	285	308

Serum Total Cholesterol of Females 4 Years of Age and Older by Race/Ethnicity and Age: Mean and Selected Percentiles, United States, 1988–94

Non-Hispanic Black, Age in Years	Number of Examined Persons	Mean	Standard Deviation	Standard Error of the Mean	Selected Percentiles								
					5th	10th	15th	25th	50th	75th	85th	90th	95th
4 years and older, crude	3638	193	44.2	0.9	131	142	150	162	187	217	236	251	273
4 years and older, age adjusted		195											
4–5 years	270	167	30.1	2.2	121	131	141	148	165	184	191	201	220
6–11 years	461	173	31.4	1.7	131	141	144	150	169	192	206	213	227
12–19 years	547	170	33.4	1.7	120	130	137	148	167	190	208	216	229
20 years and older, crude	2360	201	45.3	1.1	136	148	157	170	196	226	246	261	284
20 years and older, age adjusted		205											
20–74 years	2209	200	44.7	1.1	136	147	157	169	195	224	244	259	281
20–74 years, age adjusted	2209	203											
20–29 years	577	184	38.2	1.9	129	139	148	158	181	204	216	227	253
30–39 years	596	187	35.4	1.7	132	142	151	164	184	209	221	230	248
40–49 years	420	203	39.5	2.3	141	155	165	177	201	225	241	251	269
50–59 years	255	224	47.2	3.5	152	167	175	193	218	257	272	281	302
60–69 years	270	238	50.2	3.6	170	180	192	207	234	262	284	295	322
70+ years	242	227	48.1	3.7	156	171	178	195	224	257	275	291	304

Serum Total Cholesterol of Females 4 Years of Age and Older by Race/Ethnicity and Age: Mean and Selected Percentiles, United States, 1988–94

Mexican Americans, Age in Years	Number of Examined Persons	Mean	Standard Deviation	Standard Error of the Mean	Selected Percentiles 5th	10th	15th	25th	50th	75th	85th	90th	95th
4 years and older, crude	3517	186	42.6	0.9	129	140	145	156	182	210	228	239	261
4 years and older, age adjusted		193											
4–5 years	321	163	28.3	2.0	121	129	138	147	163	183	191	198	206
6–11 years	522	165	30.6	1.7	126	135	141	146	162	180	188	199	209
12–19 years	509	166	33.6	1.9	120	126	133	143	160	185	199	209	224
20 years and older, crude		198	43.3	1.2	139	148	156	167	193	223	238	249	274
20 years and older, age adjusted		204											
20–74 years	2070	197	43.1	1.2	138	147	155	166	192	222	237	249	274
20–74 years, age adjusted	2070	202											
20–29 years	631	183	40.2	2.0	132	140	144	156	177	203	220	232	245
30–39 years	506	191	39.1	2.2	136	146	153	164	187	213	231	238	266
40–49 years	352	205	41.6	2.8	149	158	163	177	202	225	242	254	282
50–59 years	186	222	40.7	3.7	158*	182	186	196	218	240	255	268	294*
60–69 years	318	229	39.9	2.8	165	180	188	203	230	256	267	282	297
70+ years	172	221	43.1	4.1	153*	167	184	198	219	241	262	283	295*

* Value based on a limited number of observations.

Serum High-Density Lipoprotein (HDL) Cholesterol of Males 4 Years of Age and Older by Age: Mean and Selected Percentiles, United States, 1988–94

Age in Years	Number of Examined Persons	Mean	Standard Deviation	Standard Error of the Mean	Selected Percentiles 5th	10th	15th	25th	50th	75th	85th	90th	95th
4 years and older, crude	11,123	47	13.4	0.21	28	32	34	38	45	54	60	64	72
4 years and older, age adjusted		47											
4–5 years	845	50	11.9	0.69	31	36	38	42	49	56	63	66	72
6–8 years	692	53	12.3	0.78	33	38	40	44	52	61	65	68	74
9–11 years	752	54	12.7	0.77	37	39	42	44	53	62	67	71	76
12–15 years	697	48	11.3	0.71	33	36	37	40	47	55	60	63	68
16–19 years	664	46	11.1	0.72	30	33	36	38	45	52	57	61	67
20 years and older, crude	7473	46	13.7	0.26	28	31	34	37	44	53	58	63	72
20 years and older, age adjusted		46											
20–74 years	6535	46	13.6	0.28	28	30	33	37	44	53	58	62	72
20–74 years, age adjusted		46											
20–29 years	1541	47	12.5	0.53	29	33	35	39	45	54	60	63	69
30–39 years	1379	46	13.3	0.60	27	32	34	37	44	52	58	61	70
40–49 years	1152	45	14.8	0.73	26	30	32	36	43	51	58	64	74
50–59 years	823	44	13.9	0.81	27	30	32	36	42	51	56	61	75
60–69 years	1130	46	13.7	0.68	28	31	32	36	43	53	58	63	72
70–79 years	808	46	14.9	0.87	28	31	33	36	44	53	59	63	74
80+ years	640	47	14.2	0.94	29	31	34	38	44	55	63	66	74

Serum High-Density Lipoprotein (HDL) Cholesterol of Males 4 Years of Age and Older by Race/Ethnicity and Age: Mean and Selected Percentiles, United States, 1988–94

Non-Hispanic White, Age in Years	Number of Examined Persons	Mean	Standard Deviation	Standard Error of the Mean	Selected Percentiles 5th	10th	15th	25th	50th	75th	85th	90th	95th
4 years and older, crude	4069	46	12.9	0.3	28	31	34	37	44	53	58	62	69
4 years and older, age adjusted		46											
4–5 years	210	49	11.8	1.0	30	35	36	41	48	54	62	64	66
6–11 years	386	52	12.0	0.8	34	38	40	44	51	61	65	68	73
12–19 years	335	45	10.1	0.7	31	34	36	38	44	52	55	59	63
20 years and older, crude	3138	45	13.2	0.3	27	30	33	36	43	52	57	61	71
20 years and older, age adjusted		45											
20–74 years	2431	45	13.1	0.3	27	30	33	36	43	51	57	61	70
20–74 years, age adjusted		45											
20–29 years	378	46	12.1	0.8	28	31	34	38	44	53	59	62	69
30–39 years	431	45	12.7	0.8	26	31	34	37	43	51	55	61	68
40–49 years	416	44	14.1	0.9	26	29	31	35	42	50	54	61	72
50–59 years	409	44	13.6	0.9	26	30	31	35	42	50	55	61	74
60–69 years	495	45	13.3	0.8	28	30	32	36	42	53	58	62	71
70+ years	1009	46	13.6	0.6	28	31	33	36	43	53	59	63	72

Serum High-Density Lipoprotein (HDL) Cholesterol of Males 4 Years of Age and Older by Race/Ethnicity and Age: Mean and Selected Percentiles, United States, 1988–94

Non-Hispanic Black, Age in Years	Number of Examined Persons	Mean	Standard Deviation	Standard Error of the Mean	Selected Percentiles 5th	10th	15th	25th	50th	75th	85th	90th	95th
4 years and older, crude	3137	53	15.7	0.3	33	36	38	42	51	61	69	73	83
4 years and older, age adjusted		53											
4–5 years	274	53	11.6	0.8	36	39	42	46	52	59	65	69	75
6–11 years	475	59	14.0	0.7	40	42	44	50	58	68	74	77	86
12–19 years	472	53	12.0	0.6	36	38	42	45	52	60	66	68	73
20 years and older, crude	1916	52	16.7	0.4	32	35	37	41	50	60	68	74	85
20 years and older, age adjusted		52											
20–74 years	1807	52	16.6	0.4	32	35	37	41	49	60	68	74	85
20–74 years, age adjusted	1807	52											
20–29 years	455	53	14.7	0.8	35	37	38	42	51	59	68	73	82
30–39 years	450	52	16.2	0.9	32	35	37	41	49	61	68	73	83
40–49 years	330	53	18.7	1.2	30	34	36	40	48	62	70	80	91
50–59 years	202	51	17.6	1.4	29	33	36	39	47	56	67	77	86
60–69 years	268	51	17.1	1.2	30	34	36	38	48	61	70	74	80
70+ years	211	54	18.4	1.4	33	38	40	43	51	60	67	74	95

Serum High-Density Lipoprotein (HDL) Cholesterol of Males 4 Years of Age and Older by Race/Ethnicity and Age: Mean and Selected Percentiles, United States, 1988–94

Mexican Americans, Age in Years	Number of Examined Persons	Mean	Standard Deviation	Standard Error of the Mean	Selected Percentiles								
					5th	10th	15th	25th	50th	75th	85th	90th	95th
4 years and older, crude	3471	47	12.7	0.3	30	33	35	38	46	54	60	64	70
4 years and older, age adjusted		47											
4–5 years	316	50	12.9	0.9	29	34	38	41	49	58	63	65	72
6–11 years	513	54	12.9	0.7	35	38	41	44	53	63	67	70	75
12–19 years	491	48	11.4	0.6	31	34	37	40	47	54	60	63	67
20 years and older, crude		46	12.5	0.3	28	32	34	37	44	52	58	61	67
20 years and older, age adjusted		45											
20–74 years	2049	46	12.5	0.3	28	32	34	37	44	53	58	61	67
20–74 years, age adjusted	2049	46											
20–29 years	640	46	11.0	0.5	30	33	36	39	45	53	57	61	66
30–39 years	444	46	13.9	0.8	27	31	34	37	44	52	58	64	74
40–49 years	361	44	12.3	0.8	28	30	32	35	41	50	57	60	66
50–59 years	173	46	14.1	1.3	28*	30	33	36	43	54	60	63	80*
60–69 years	335	45	12.8	0.9	30	32	34	37	43	51	57	61	66
70+ years	198	44	12.9	1.1	28*	30	33	37	41	50	57	63	67*

* Value based on a limited number of observations.

Serum High-Density Lipoprotein (HDL) Cholesterol of Females 4 Years of Age and Older by Age: Mean and Selected Percentiles, United States, 1988–94

Age in Years	Number of Examined Persons	Mean	Standard Deviation	Standard Error of the Mean	Selected Percentiles								
					5th	10th	15th	25th	50th	75th	85th	90th	95th
4 years and older, crude	12,286	54	14.8	0.20	34	38	40	44	53	63	68	73	80
4 years and older, age adjusted		54											
4–5 years	852	48	11.3	0.58	30	35	37	40	47	55	59	62	68
6–8 years	670	50	11.2	0.65	33	38	40	43	49	58	61	65	70
9–11 years	727	51	11.3	0.63	33	38	40	42	50	58	61	66	70
12–15 years	797	51	11.6	0.61	34	37	40	43	50	59	63	66	70
16–19 years	762	52	12.0	0.66	34	38	40	44	52	60	63	67	73
20 years and older, crude	8478	55	15.5	0.25	34	38	41	44	54	64	70	75	83
20 years and older, age adjusted		55											
20–74 years	7382	55	15.4	0.27	34	38	41	45	53	64	70	75	83
20–74 years, age adjusted		55											
20–29 years	1751	55	14.8	0.53	35	38	41	45	53	64	70	75	84
30–39 years	1744	54	15.0	0.54	33	37	40	44	53	64	69	74	81
40–49 years	1282	55	14.0	0.59	36	38	41	45	53	64	68	72	79
50–59 years	955	57	17.2	0.83	34	38	41	45	54	65	73	78	87
60–69 years	1104	56	17.2	0.78	32	37	40	44	53	65	72	78	87
70–79 years	929	56	16.4	0.81	32	36	40	45	55	64	71	75	84
80+ years	713	56	15.9	0.89	33	37	40	44	54	65	71	76	85

Serum High-Density Lipoprotein (HDL) Cholesterol of Females 4 Years of Age and Older by Race/Ethnicity and Age: Mean and Selected Percentiles, United States, 1988–94

Non-Hispanic White, Age in Years	Number of Examined Persons	Mean	Standard Deviation	Standard Error of the Mean	Selected Percentiles								
					5th	10th	15th	25th	50th	75th	85th	90th	95th
4 years and older, crude	4625	54	15.0	0.3	34	38	40	44	53	63	69	73	81
4 years and older, age adjusted		54											
4–5 years	224	46	11.0	0.8	30	34	36	39	46	52	57	61	68
6–11 years	363	49	10.5	0.6	32	38	39	42	48	55	60	62	68
12–19 years	423	51	11.1	0.6	32	37	39	42	51	58	61	64	70
20 years and older, crude	3615	56	15.6	0.3	34	38	41	45	54	64	70	76	84
20 years and older, age adjusted		56											
20–74 years	2793	56	15.6	0.3	34	38	41	45	54	64	70	76	84
20–74 years, age adjusted		56											
20–29 years	475	55	15.2	0.8	36	38	41	44	53	64	71	76	86
30–39 years	566	55	15.1	0.7	33	37	40	44	54	64	69	74	82
40–49 years	456	56	13.7	0.7	37	39	42	46	54	65	69	72	79
50–59 years	464	57	17.7	1.0	34	38	41	45	54	66	75	79	87
60–69 years	473	56	17.1	0.9	31	37	40	44	53	65	72	78	86
70+ years	1181	55	16.0	0.5	32	36	40	44	54	64	71	75	83

Serum High-Density Lipoprotein (HDL) Cholesterol of Females 4 Years of Age and Older by Race/Ethnicity and Age: Mean and Selected Percentiles, United States, 1988–94

Non-Hispanic Black, Age in Years	Number of Examined Persons	Mean	Standard Deviation	Standard Error of the Mean	Selected Percentiles								
					5th	10th	15th	25th	50th	75th	85th	90th	95th
4 years and older, crude	3614	57	15.6	0.3	36	39	42	46	55	65	72	77	85
4 years and older, age adjusted		57											
4–5 years	263	53	11.7	0.9	35	38	42	45	52	59	64	69	76
6–11 years	460	56	12.9	0.7	36	41	44	47	56	65	70	72	78
12–19 years	543	56	13.5	0.7	36	40	43	46	54	62	70	73	80
20 years and older, crude	2348	57	16.4	0.4	35	39	42	46	55	66	73	79	86
20 years and older, age adjusted		58											
20–74 years	2198	57	16.2	0.4	35	39	42	46	55	66	73	78	85
20–74 years, age adjusted	2198	57											
20–29 years	576	58	14.6	0.7	37	41	44	48	57	66	72	77	84
30–39 years	595	57	15.7	0.8	36	39	42	46	54	66	72	78	85
40–49 years	415	55	17.3	1.0	34	37	40	43	52	63	71	77	86
50–59 years	252	57	15.5	1.2	35	39	41	46	55	67	73	77	85
60–69 years	269	60	19.2	1.4	34	39	42	47	57	70	77	82	89
70+ years	241	61	18.9	1.4	35	40	42	47	58	72	80	86	92

Serum High-Density Lipoprotein (HDL) Cholesterol of Females 4 Years of Age and Older by Race/Ethnicity and Age: Mean and Selected Percentiles, United States, 1988–94

Mexican Americans, Age in Years	Number of Examined Persons	Mean	Standard Deviation	Standard Error of the Mean	Selected Percentiles								
					5th	10th	15th	25th	50th	75th	85th	90th	95th
4 years and older, crude	3504	52	13.2	0.3	33	37	39	43	51	59	65	69	77
4 years and older, age adjusted		52											
4–5 years	321	49	11.0	0.8	32	36	38	41	49	56	60	62	65
6–11 years	520	51	11.7	0.6	34	38	40	43	50	58	63	67	73
12–19 years	507	53	12.4	0.7	35	38	40	44	52	59	64	69	76
20 years and older, crude		52	13.8	0.4	33	36	38	42	51	60	66	71	77
20 years and older, age adjusted		53											
20–74 years	2061	52	13.8	0.4	33	36	38	42	50	59	66	71	77
20–74 years, age adjusted	2061	52											
20–29 years	628	53	13.4	0.7	34	37	39	44	51	59	66	71	77
30–39 years	506	51	13.7	0.8	31	36	38	42	50	59	65	70	77
40–49 years	348	50	12.7	0.8	32	35	37	41	49	57	62	65	70
50–59 years	184	55	15.4	1.4	34*	38	42	45	52	63	71	77	87*
60–69 years	318	54	14.7	1.0	32	36	40	44	52	63	69	73	81
70+ years	172	55	16.1	1.5	34*	36	39	44	54	65	71	76	80*

* Value based on a limited number of observations.

APPENDIX

R

Example of a Form That Can Be Used for Self-Monitoring Eating Behavior

Food Record

Name ______________________ Day of week ______________ Date ______________

Time	Time Spent	Food Eaten—How Prepared	Amount	Place, Person(s) with Whom Food Was Eaten, Other Activities, Mood/Feelings

Remember: Do not alter your normal diet while keeping this record. For the requested information, provide responses that are as accurate as possible.

APPENDIX

S Competency Checklist for Nutrition Counselors

This can be used by counselors to identify the competencies they already possess and those they want to develop.

From Raab C, and Tillotson JL. 1985. *Heart to heart: A manual on nutrition counseling for the reduction of cardiovascular disease risk factors.* Bethesda, MD: U.S. Department of Health and Human Services: Public Health Service; National Institutes of Health.

Nutrition Information for Particular Patient	Performance Objectives	Needs More Work	Not Attempted Yet	Good
1. Counselor knows the essential elements and rationale behind patient's prescribed diet (e.g., low-fat, low-sodium, etc.).	1a. Is familiar with all the food categories of the diet	______	______	______
	1b. Is comfortable with substitutions and rationale for selection of food	______	______	______
	1c. Is prepared to help patient adapt diet to his or her needs	______	______	______
2. Counselor has knowledge of local eating patterns.	2a. Has some grasp of regional customs and of what foods are available in area	______	______	______
	2b. Is familiar with frequently patronized restaurants and food chains and will ask patient his or her favorites	______	______	______
3. At the outset, counselor makes reasonably sure that patient's knowledge of prescribed diet is adequate.	3a. Takes a history to find out patient's dietary background	______	______	______
	3b. At first session, discusses long-term goals and explains diet thoroughly, making sure patient understands	______	______	______
	3c. Eliminates patient's knowledge gaps (by discussing diet further, giving examples, using visuals, etc.) so following sessions can concentrate on goal setting	______	______	______
	3d. Initially, asks patient for food diary; analyzes with patient to assess current diet and eating behavior	______	______	______
Communication Skills				
4. Counselor sets appropriate tone for counseling sessions through preparation, manner, and physical setting.	4a. Makes appointment with patient, allowing enough time for comfortable, thorough discussion	______	______	______
	4b. Arranges for private, quiet setting	______	______	______

continued

Nutrition Information for Particular Patient	Performance Objectives	Needs More Work	Not Attempted Yet	Good
Communication Skills—(cont'd)				
	4c. Establishes patient's ability to see and to read and speak English; adapts counseling if necessary	____	____	____
	4d. Shows interest in patient as an individual, looks for his or her particular needs and preferences	____	____	____
	4e. Maintains relaxed, comfortable manner; makes patient feel at ease	____	____	____
	4f. Indicates intentions to talk and to listen	____	____	____
5. Counselor prepares self and patient for continuing relationship over a specified period.	5a. Explains initially the necessity of follow-up over time	____	____	____
	5b. Outlines plans for working with patient—a certain number of sessions over a certain period of time with occasional contact by phone and mail	____	____	____
6. Counselor uses principles of good communication.	6a. Uses primarily open-ended questions (rather than those answered by yes or no)	____	____	____
	6b. Guards against doing most of the talking; shows ability to listen	____	____	____
	6c. Is able to tolerate periods of silence	____	____	____
	6d. Shows nonjudgmental, noncritical attitude toward patient's eating pattern and chosen lifestyle	____	____	____
	6e. Uses words patient can understand	____	____	____
7. Counselor communicates interest and confidence both nonverbally and verbally.	7a. Shows poise and interest through posture and "body language"	____	____	____
	7b. Has frequent eye contact with patient	____	____	____
	7c. Uses gestures and words to encourage patient to communicate freely, without putting words in patient's mouth	____	____	____
Counseling Approaches		____	____	____
8. Counselor is aware that the change process is the responsibility of the patient.	8a. Does not assume responsibility for changes or consequences	____	____	____
	8b. Does not become too ego-involved in patient's eventual success or failure	____	____	____
9. Counselor is aware of need for patient to recognize manageable goals.	9a. Helps patient choose an initial goal that is easily achieved	____	____	____
	9b. Helps patient set specific and short-term goals that are progressively more challenging	____	____	____
	9c. Is able to help patient evaluate goals	____	____	____
	9d. Helps patient avoid failure through too large or too many goals	____	____	____
10. Counselor is able to help patient set up recordkeeping and/or tally systems.	10a. Can help patient verbalize a method appropriate to the task	____	____	____
	10b. Can suggest alternate methods for patient's consideration without dictating choice	____	____	____
	10c. Emphasizes need for accurate records	____	____	____

Nutrition Information for Particular Patient	Performance Objectives	Needs More Work	Not Attempted Yet	Good
Counseling Approaches—(cont'd)				
	10d. Is able to help patient review food records patient can understand	______	______	______
11. Counselor is aware of the need to examine and anticipate obstacles that will interfere with progress.	11a. Can review with patient potential obstacles in social, personal, and physical environments	______	______	______
	11b. Can help patient identify actual or potential problems and deal with these by encouraging patient to restructure environment and by role playing problem situations with him or her	______	______	______
	11c. Discusses how patient will deal with possible failure	______	______	______
12. Counselor is able to define own role in giving support and feedback.	12a. Can avoid taking the major responsibility	______	______	______
	12b. Can place the responsibility for change on patient	______	______	______
	12c. Is aware of own biases and belief systems and is able to ignore them	______	______	______
13. Counselor is able to evaluate progress toward the stated goal.	13a. Is able to give patient feedback about progress	______	______	______
	13b. Keeps notes in sufficient detail to depict patient's responsibilities and progress	______	______	______
	13c. Measures progress by a combination of biological measures, food intake evaluation, and subjective judgments, with an emphasis on changing behavior	______	______	______
14. Counselor encourages patient to get family and friends involved.	14a. Helps patient recognize their strong influence on him or her, suggests that patient ask openly for their support	______	______	______
	14b. Suggests that patient ask them to participate in some way: sharing new tastes and habits, helping with food selection, limiting inappropriate foods	______	______	______
	14c. Can help patient cope with negative feedback through anticipating and rehearsing problem situations	______	______	______
	14d. Can evaluate whether they are potentially supportive or destructive	______	______	______
	14e. Can utilize them as a support without losing sight of the primary responsibility resting with patient	______	______	______
15. Counselor is able to understand that his or her role is not simply that of information-giver or instructor.	15a. Acts as facilitator for patient	______	______	______
	15b. Is appropriately assertive	______	______	______
	15c. Is able to resist "lecturing"	______	______	______
16. Counselor is aware of the need to keep patient task-oriented.	16a. Recognizes delaying tactics and distractions	______	______	______
	16b. Is able to redirect the session toward specifics	______	______	______
	16c. Responds pleasantly but professionally to patient's attempts at humor	______	______	______

Glossary

absorptiometry A measurement approach based on the uptake of energy from radiation (e.g., photons or X rays) by the tissue or medium being measured (e.g., bone mineral content).

Acceptable Macronutrient Distribution Ranges Recommended levels of intake for total fat, *n*-6 polyunsaturated fatty acids (linolenic acid), *n*-3 polyunsaturated fatty acids (α-linolenic acid), carbohydrate, and protein to ensure adequate intake and to decrease risk of chronic disease.

accuracy The degree to which a measured value represents the real, or true, value.

acromion process The spine of the scapula (shoulder blade) extending toward the outside of the body. The acromion process, or tip, is used as an anatomic landmark in arm anthropometric measurements (e.g., midarm circumference and triceps skinfold measurement).

actuarial data Statistical information relating to life expectancy, collected by the insurance industry and used, for example, to develop height-weight charts.

Adequate Intake The recommended daily dietary intake level assumed to be adequate and based on experimentally determined approximations of nutrient intake by a group of healthy people. It is an observational standard used when there are insufficient data available to determine a Recommended Dietary Allowance. One of four nutrient reference intakes included in the Dietary Reference Intakes.

age-adjusted death rate The number of deaths in a specific age group for a given calendar year, divided by the population of the same age group as of July 1 of that year. (The quotient being multiplied by 1000.) Also known as "age-specific" death rate.

air displacement plethysmography An approach to measuring body volume that is based on the difference between the volume of air within an empty chamber of known volume and the volume of air when a subject is inside the chamber. The volume of air the subject displaces when inside the chamber is equivalent to the subject's volume, from which body density and percent body fat can then be calculated.

albumin A serum protein, produced by the liver, used as an indicator of nutritional status.

AMDR see Acceptable Macronutrient Distribution Ranges.

anabolism The process by which body cells convert simple biological substances into more complex compounds.

android obesity Excess body fat that is predominantly within the abdomen and upper body, as opposed to the hips and thighs. This is the typical pattern of male obesity.

anemia A hemoglobin level below the normal reference range for individuals of the same sex and age.

anergy A less than expected or absent immune reaction in response to the injection of antigens within the skin.

angina pectoris Chest pain caused by lack of oxygen supply (known as ischemia) within the heart muscle or myocardium.

anorexia nervosa A condition of disturbed or disordered eating behavior characterized by a refusal to maintain a minimally normal body weight, an intense fear of gaining weight (not alleviated by losing weight), and a distorted perception of body shape or size in which a person feels overweight (either globally or in certain body areas), despite being markedly underweight.

antecedent A preceding event, condition, or cause. Behaviorists regard an action as being preceded by an antecedent. Behavior modification theory holds that, when antecedents to behaviors are recognized, the antecedents can be modified or controlled to decrease the occurrence of negative behaviors and increase the occurrence of positive behaviors. This is referred to as stimulus control.

anthropometry Measurement of the body (stature, weight, circumferences, and skinfold thickness).

apoproteins Special proteins, found in lipoproteins, that control the interaction and metabolic fate of lipoproteins. Apoproteins activate enzymes that modify the composition and structure of lipoproteins, are involved in the binding and ingestion of lipoproteins by cells, and participate in the exchange of lipids between lipoproteins of different classes.

appendicular skeleton The portion of the skeleton that contains the bones of the limbs, pelvis, clavicles, and scapulae.

Archimedes' principle The fact that an object's volume, when submerged in water, equals the volume of water the object displaces. Thus, if the mass and the volume of a body are known, the density of that body can be calculated.

This principle is used to determine whole-body density in hydrostatic weighing.

arm muscle area An indicator of total body muscle calculated from the triceps skinfold thickness and midarm circumference.

arteriography A radiographic study of an artery or arterial system in which contrast medium is injected into an artery to determine the condition of the artery (e.g., narrowing due to atherosclerosis).

atherogenic Atherosclerosis-producing.

atherosclerosis A progressive disorder beginning in childhood with the appearance of lesions in the form of fatty streaks in the lining of the coronary arteries or aorta. These may eventually progress to fatty and fibrous plaques or even larger, more complicated lesions. As the lesions develop, the progressive narrowing of the vessels reduces blood flow to the tissues supplied by the affected vessels.

attenuate To decrease the amount, force, or value of something. In dual-energy X-ray absorptiometry (DXA), for example, minerals in bone oppose the transmission of X rays through bones, thus attenuating X rays. The degree to which bones attenuate (i.e., oppose the transmission of) X rays is used to determine bone mineral density in DXA.

auscultation The act of listening for sounds arising from organs (e.g., heart and lungs), typically using a stethoscope.

axial skeleton The part of the skeleton composed of the skull, vertebral column, sternum, and ribs.

balance sheet approach The most common method of estimating per capita food availability at the national level. Food exports, nonfood use (e.g., livestock feed, seed, and industrial use), and year-end inventories are subtracted from data on beginning-year inventories, total food production, and imports to arrive at an estimate of per capita food availability.

balloon angioplasty A surgical procedure in which a balloon catheter is inserted through the skin into a narrowed blood vessel and inflated to enlarge its interior opening, or lumen, in order to increase blood flow through the affected vessel.

basal metabolic rate (BMR) An individual's energy expenditure measured in the postabsorptive state (no food consumed during the previous 12 hours) after resting quietly for 30 minutes in a thermally neutral environment. (Room temperature is perceived as neither hot nor cold.)

behavior modification A behavioral change theory that attempts to alter previously learned behavior or to encourage the learning of new behavior through a variety of action-oriented methods, as opposed to changing feelings or thoughts.

Behavior Risk Factor Surveillance System An ongoing data-collection program administered by the U.S. Centers for Disease Control and Prevention to monitor state-level prevalence of the major behavioral risks associated with the leading causes of premature morbidity and mortality. It provides state-specific data on personal health behavior and disease risk factors, which allow states to better target their resources for disease risk factor intervention and health promotion activities.

beriberi A disease resulting from thiamin deficiency and characterized by nervous tingling throughout the body, poor arm-leg coordination, deep calf muscle pain, heart enlargement, and occasional edema.

bias A measure of inaccuracy or departure from accuracy.

binge eating The practice of eating an unusually large amount of food in a discrete period of time.

bioelectrical impedance The measure of resistance to an alternating current in an organism. Used to estimate total body water from which percent body fat and lean body mass can be calculated using various equations.

biological marker A nutrient, food component, or metabolite that can be objectively measured and used to represent dietary or nutrient intake.

biopsy The removal and examination of tissue samples to determine the presence or concentration of certain nutrients (or the presence or absence of disease).

BMI Body mass index. *See* Quetelet's index.

body cell mass The metabolically active, energy-requiring mass of the body.

body composition The proportions of various tissues (fat, muscle, and bone) or elements (e.g., hydrogen, potassium, carbon, calcium, nitrogen) making up the body, usually expressed as percent body fat and percent lean body mass.

body density The mass of the body per unit volume, generally measured by hydrostatic weighing. Percent body fat can then be estimated from body density using the Siri or Brozek equations.

body mass index *See* Quetelet's index.

bone mineral density The amount of mineral (primarily calcium and phosphorus) in bone per volume or per area. For example, dual-energy X-ray absorptiometry (DXA) provides an areal measurement of bone mineral density (BMD) in grams of bone mineral per cubic centimeter (g/cm^2).

bulimia nervosa An eating disorder characterized by episodes of binge eating followed by some behavior to prevent weight gain, such as purging, fasting, or exercising excessively.

bypass surgery A surgical procedure creating an auxiliary flow, a shunt, or a pathway around a diseased or malfunctioning body area to restore normal or nearly normal body function (e.g., coronary bypass, intestinal bypass).

cachexia Profound physical wasting and malnutrition usually associated with chronic disease, advanced acquired immune deficiency syndrome, alcoholism, or drug abuse.

cadaver A dead body used for anatomic, anthropometric, or other study. Only by analyzing cadavers can direct measurement of human body composition be made.

calorie count Calculation of the energy and nutrient value of foods eaten by a subject, such as a hospitalized patient.

calorimetry Measurement of a subject's energy expenditure.

cancer A group of diseases characterized by abnormal growth of cells that, when uncontrolled, invade other tissues or organs, interfering with their normal function and nutrition.

cardiovascular disease A variety of pathologic processes pertaining to the heart and blood vessels (coronary artery disease and hypertension).

case-control study Comparison of current disease status with the level of past exposure to some factor of interest (e.g., some nutrient or dietary component) in two groups of subjects (cases and controls), in an attempt to determine how past exposure to the factor relates to currently existing disease.

catabolism The breaking down of more complex compounds into simple biological substances, generally resulting in energy release.

cerebrovascular disease A group of disorders, characterized by decreased blood supply to the brain, resulting from hemorrhage of or atherosclerosis within the cerebral arteries.

CHD Coronary heart disease.

CHI Creatinine-height index.

cholesterol A fatlike sterol found in animal products and normally produced by the body. It serves as a precursor for bile acids and steroid hormones and is an essential component of the plasma membrane and the myelin sheaths of nerves. Serum cholesterol levels are causally related to risk for coronary artery disease.

chronic disease A disease progressing over a long period of time, such as coronary heart disease, certain cancers, stroke, diabetes mellitus, and atherosclerosis.

chylomicrons Lipoproteins synthesized in the small intestine that transport dietary triglycerides from the small intestine to adipose tissue, muscle, and the liver. They are 90% triglyceride by weight and are naturally found in serum shortly after meals, but they are not normally present in fasting serum.

cirrhosis Inflammation of the interstitial tissue of an organ, especially the liver.

closed questions Questions that are restrictive and allow an interviewer to control answers and ask for specific information. They are often answered by a simple yes or no response.

coding Assigning a number to each food item recorded in a 24-hour recall or food record that identifies the food for purposes of computerized nutrient analysis.

coefficient of variation (CV) A measure of precision calculated by dividing the standard deviation by the mean and multiplying by 100 (CV = SD ÷ mean × 100).

cognitive restructuring Elimination of negative, irrational thoughts through increasing awareness of one's self-talk, disputing and changing negative self-talk, and using cognitive rehearsal and thought stopping.

cohort study *See* longitudinal study.

computed tomography (CT) An imaging technique producing highly detailed cross-sectional body images from computerized processing of X-ray beam transmission through body tissues of differing density.

computer hardware The physical components of a computer (e.g., the monitor, disc drives, central processing unit, and keyboard).

conjunctival impression cytology Microscopic examination of the conjunctival epithelial cells used to detect early morphologic changes indicative of vitamin A deficiency.

consequences Events that follow and are causally linked to certain behaviors. Consequences reinforce, or reward, the behavior they follow, and they may be positive, negative, or neutral. When consequences are positive, behavior is more likely to be repeated. Behavior followed by negative consequences is less likely to be repeated.

Continuing Survey of Food Intakes by Individuals (CSFII) A nationally representative survey of individual dietary intake by Americans that was conducted periodically by the U.S. Department of Agriculture between 1985 and 1998.

coronary heart disease (CHD) A disease of the heart resulting from inadequate circulation of blood to local areas of the heart muscle. The disease is almost always a consequence of focal narrowing of the coronary arteries by atherosclerosis and is known as ischemic heart disease or coronary artery disease.

correlational study A research design in which the occurrence of one variable is compared with the occurrence of another variable within the same population. The study is useful for generating hypotheses regarding the associations between suspected risk factors and disease risk.

creatine A nitrogen-containing compound, 98% of which is found in muscle in the form of creatine phosphate. Creatine spontaneously dehydrates to form creatinine, which is then excreted unaltered in the urine.

creatinine The end product of creatine metabolism. Twenty-four-hour urinary creatinine excretion is used as an index of body muscle mass.

creatinine-height index (CHI) An index or a ratio sometimes used to assess body protein status. CHI = 24-hour urinary creatinine excretion ÷ expected creatinine excretion of a reference adult of the same sex and stature × 100.

cross-sectional survey A study design in which disease and various factors of interest are simultaneously examined in groups at a specific period of time.

CSFII Continuing Survey of Food Intakes by Individuals.

CT Computed tomography.

CV Coefficient of variation.

Daily Reference Value (DRV) A dietary reference value serving as a basis for the Daily Values. DRVs are for nutrients (e.g., total fat, cholesterol, total carbohydrate, and dietary fiber) for which no set of standards existed before passage of the Nutrition Labeling and Education Act of 1990.

Daily Value (DV) A dietary reference value appearing on the nutrition labels of foods regulated by the FDA and the USDA as part of the Nutrition Labeling and Education Act of 1990. It is derived from the Daily Reference Values (DRVs) and the Reference Daily Intakes (RDIs). The daily value on food labels shows the percent of the DRVs or RDIs that a serving of food provides.

deciliter (dL) A unit of volume in the metric system. One deciliter equals 10^{-1} liter, 1/10 of a liter, or 100 milliliters.

deficiency diseases Diseases caused by a lack of adequate dietary nutrients, vitamins, or minerals (e.g., rickets, pellagra, beriberi, xerophthalmia, and goiter).

densitometry Measurement of body density.

density *See* body density.

deuterium A radioactive hydrogen isotope having twice the mass of common light hydrogen atoms. Known as "heavy hydrogen."

deuterium oxide "Heavy water" composed of oxygen and deuterium (D_2O or ^2H_2O). Used in the determination of total body water.

DHHS United States Department of Health and Human Services.

diabetes mellitus A metabolic disorder characterized by inadequate insulin secretion by the pancreas or the inability of certain cells to use insulin and resulting in abnormally high serum glucose levels. Diabetes mellitus can be classified as type 1 diabetes, type 2 diabetes, or gestational diabetes mellitus (GDM).

dietary fiber Nondigestible carbohydrates and lignin that are naturally present in plant foods and that are consumed in their natural, intact state as part of an unrefined food.

Dietary Goals for the United States Seven dietary goals established by the U.S. Senate Select Committee on Nutrition and Human Needs in 1977 for improving the quality of the American diet.

Dietary Reference Intakes Reference values that are quantitative estimates of nutrient intakes to be used for planning and assessing diets for apparently healthy people in various life-stage and gender groups in the United States and Canada. The Dietary Reference Intakes include the Estimated Average Requirement, the Recommended Dietary Allowance, the Adequate Intake, and the Tolerable Upper Intake Level.

diet history An approach to assessing an individual's usual dietary intake over an extended period of time (e.g., past month or year). This typically involves Burke's four assessment steps: collecting general information about the subject's health habits, questioning the subject about his or her usual eating pattern, performing a "cross check" on the data given in step 2, and having the subject complete a 3-day food record.

dilution techniques An approach to indirectly measure total body water (TBW). A known concentration and volume of a tracer is given to a subject orally or parenterally, time is allowed for the tracer to equilibrate with the subject's body water, and the concentration of the tracer is analyzed in a sample of the subject's blood, urine, or saliva.

direct calorimetry Measurement of the body's heat output using an airtight, thermally insulated living chamber.

distal Away from the center of the body.

diurnal variations Cyclical changes occurring throughout the day.

dL Deciliter.

DPA Dual-photon absorptiometry.

DRV Daily Reference Value.

dual-energy X-ray absorptiometry (DXA) An approach for measuring bone mineral content in the appendicular skeleton, axial skeleton, or whole body using an X-ray source operating at two energy levels.

dual-photon absorptiometry (DPA) An approach for measuring bone mineral content using photons at two different energy levels derived from a radioisotopic source (gadolinium-153).

duplicate food collections A direct method of calculating nutrient intake in which subjects place an identical portion of all foods and beverages consumed during a specified period in collection containers. This is then chemically analyzed at a laboratory for nutrient content, which provides a potentially more accurate determination of actual nutrient intake; it is compared with calculations based on food composition data.

DV Daily Value.

DXA Dual-energy X-ray absorptiometry.

electrolyte An electrically charged particle (anion or cation), present in solution within the body, that is capable of conducting an electrical charge. Sodium, chloride, potassium, and bicarbonate are electrolytes commonly found in the body.

endemic In epidemiology, a disease or condition that persistently occurs at low to moderate levels over a relatively long period of time.

enrichment The addition of certain nutrients lost in food during processing according to some standard stipulated by law.

enteral nutrition The delivery of food or nutrients into the esophagus, stomach, or small intestine through tubes to improve nutritional status.

epidemic In epidemiology, a disease or condition that occurs at a higher rate than is normally expected based on past experience.

epidemiology The study of the distribution and determinants of disease and health outcomes in human populations in order to generate evidence that contributes to the prevention of disease and adverse health outcomes and the promotion of health.

erythrocyte Red blood cell, or RBC.

essential lipid The small amount of lipid (constituting about 1.5% to 3% of lean body weight), serving as a structural component of cell membranes and the nervous system, that is necessary for life.

Estimated Average Requirement The daily dietary intake level estimated to meet the nutrient requirement of 50% of healthy individuals in a particular life stage and gender group. One of four nutrient reference intakes included in the Dietary Reference Intakes.

estimated food record A method of recording individual food intake in which the amounts and types of all food and beverages are recorded for a specific period of time, usually ranging from 1 to 7 days. Portion sizes are estimated using household measures (e.g., cups, tablespoons, teaspoons), a ruler, or containers (e.g., coffee cups, bowls, glasses). Certain items (e.g., eggs, apples, 12-ounce cans of soda) are counted as units.

Estimated Energy Requirement The average dietary energy intake that is predicted to maintain energy balance in a healthy adult of a defined age, gender, weight, height, and level of physical activity, consistent with good health. In children and pregnant and lactating women, it includes the needs associated with the deposition of tissues or the secretion of milk consistent with good health.

etiology The cause of a disease or an abnormal condition.

euglycemia A condition in which the plasma glucose level is considered within normal limits.

false negative Nutrient intake misclassified as adequate when it is actually inadequate.

false positive Nutrient intake misclassified as inadequate when it is actually adequate.

fatty streak The initial step of atherosclerosis, usually beginning in childhood, in which lipids (primarily cholesterol and its esters) become deposited in macrophages and smooth muscle cells within the inner lining of large elastic and muscular arteries.

FDA Food and Drug Administration.

femtoliter (fL) A unit of volume in the metric system. One femtoliter equals 10^{-15} liter.

ferritin The combination of the protein apoferritin and iron that functions as the primary storage form for body iron. It is primarily found in the liver, spleen, and bone marrow.

ferritin model A model for assessing the prevalence of iron deficiency, requiring abnormal values for at least two of the following measurements: serum ferritin level, transferrin saturation, and erythrocyte protoporphyrin level.

fibrous plaque A collection of lipids within the arterial walls during adolescence and early adulthood, creating a projection into the channel, or lumen, of the artery, resulting in impaired blood flow and oxygen delivery to a tissue or an organ.

fL Femtoliter.

flag sign Alternating bands of depigmented and normal-colored hair produced by alternating periods of poor and relatively good nutritional status.

food balance sheet *See* balance sheet approach.

food exchange system A meal planning method, originally developed for the diabetic diet, that simplifies control of energy consumption, helps ensure adequate nutrient intake, and allows considerable variety in food selection.

food frequency questionnaire A questionnaire listing foods on which individuals indicate how often they consume each listed item during certain time intervals (daily, weekly, or monthly). Standard portion sizes are used and an estimate of nutrient intake is provided on the questionnaire. Sometimes referred to as the semi-quantitative food frequency or list-based diet history approach.

food inventory record An approach to household food consumption measurement in which total household food use is calculated by subtracting food on hand at the end of the survey period (ending inventory) from the sum of food on hand at the start of the survey period (beginning inventory) and food brought into the household during the survey.

food list-recall approach A method of measuring household food consumption in which an interviewer, using a detailed listing of foods, asks the respondent to recall the amount of food used by the household during the preceding week and the amount paid for purchased items. This approach has been used in the Nationwide Food Consumption Survey (NFCS).

food propensity questionnaire A questionnaire similar to a food frequency questionnaire that determines the probability that a person will consume a specific food or beverage on any given day over a designated time, usually the previous year.

fortification The addition of nutrients to food at a nutrient concentration greater than originally present and/or the addition of nutrients not initially existing in food.

four-compartment model A body composition model viewing the body as being composed of four chemical groups: water, protein, mineral, and fat.

Frankfort horizontal plane An imaginary plane intersecting the lowest point on the margin of the orbit (the bony socket of the eye) and the tragion (the notch above the tragus, the cartilaginous projection just anterior to the external opening of the ear). This plane should be horizontal with the head and in line with the spine.

Friedewald equation An equation that can be used to calculate the concentration of serum low-density lipoprotein cholesterol (LDL-C) when total cholesterol (TC), high-density lipoprotein cholesterol (HDL-C), and triglyceride (TG) are known. When solving for LDL-C the equation is: $\text{LDL-C} = \text{TC} - \text{HDL-C} - (\text{TG} \div 5)$. It was named for William T. Friedewald, M.D. who developed it.

functional fiber Nondigestible carbohydrates that have beneficial physiological effects in humans but that have been isolated or extracted from foods and then added as an ingredient to food or taken as a dietary supplement.

g Abbreviation for gram.

generalized equations Regression equations for estimating body density or percent body fat from anthropometric measures that are applicable to population groups varying widely in adiposity and age.

globesity A term coined by the World Health Organization to describe the global epidemic of obesity.

glycated hemoglobin Hemoglobin that has glucose bound to it. Also referred to as hemoglobin A_{1C} or simply as an A1C test, it reflects average blood glucose levels during the past 8 to 12 weeks.

goiter Thyroid gland enlargement caused by dietary iodine deficiency.

gram A unit of mass in the metric system. One gram equals 10^{-3} kilogram, 1 pound equals 453.5924 grams, and 1 ounce equals 28.350 grams.

gynoid obesity Excess body fat that is predominantly within the hips and thighs, as opposed to within the abdomen and upper body. This is the usual pattern of female obesity.

HANES Health and Nutrition Examination Survey.

HDL High-density lipoprotein.

Healthy Eating Index An instrument developed by the U.S. Department of Agriculture to provide a single summary measure of overall dietary quality.

height-weight indices Various ratios or indices expressing body weight in terms of height. Among these are Quetelet's index and Benn's index.

hemoglobin The iron-containing protein pigment of red blood cells that carries oxygen to body cells. Blood hemoglobin levels can reflect iron status (e.g., abnormally low hemoglobin may mean anemia).

hemoglobin A_{1C} *See* glycated hemoglobin.

HHANES Hispanic Health and Nutrition Examination Survey.

high-density lipoprotein (HDL) A serum lipoprotein synthesized by the liver and intestine that transports cholesterol within the bloodstream. As the serum level of HDL increases, risk of coronary artery disease decreases.

hydrostatic weighing Underwater weighing. The most widely used technique of determining whole-body density, based on Archimedes' principle.

hydroxyapatite Calcium and phosphate crystals providing rigidity to teeth and bones.

hyperlipidemia Excessively high levels of lipids in the blood.

hypermetabolism An increased rate of energy and protein metabolism accompanying trauma, infection, burns, or surgery.

hypertension Persistently elevated arterial blood pressure.

hypervitaminosis A An excessive consumption of vitamin A.

IDL Intermediate-density lipoproteins.

iliac crest The crest, or top, of the ilium (the largest of three bones making up the outer half of the pelvis). The crest is the bony spine located just below the waist. Used as an anatomic landmark in skinfold measurement sites.

impedance The opposition to an alternating current, composed of two elements: resistance and reactance.

imputed data Data used by compilers of food composition tables when certain nutrient data are unavailable. These data are obtained from similar foods or ingredients for which data are more complete.

incidence The number of new cases of a disease divided by the total number of persons at risk of the disease within a specific time period, usually one year. It indicates a person's risk or chances of developing the disease per year.

index of nutritional quality (INQ) A concept related to nutrient density that allows the quantity of a nutrient per 1000 kcal in a food, meal, or diet to be compared with a nutrient standard.

indirect colorimetry The determination of energy expenditure by measuring the body's oxygen consumption and carbon dioxide production.

infarction Death of tissue (necrosis) due to the upstream obstruction of the tissue's arterial blood supply. Infarction, which can occur in any organ, generally results from atherosclerosis. When it occurs in the heart, it is referred to as a myocardial infarction.

infectious disease Any disease caused by the invasion and multiplication of microorganisms, such as bacteria, fungi, or viruses.

infrared interactance When infrared light is projected through the skin, some of the energy is reflected from the skin and underlying tissues. Estimates of body composition are made by analyzing certain characteristics of this reflected energy.

INQ Index of nutritional quality.

intermediate-density lipoproteins (IDL) Lipoprotein particles created by the removal of triglycerides from VLDL. IDL is a midway product in the conversion of VLDL to LDL.

International Unit (IU) An amount defined by the International Conference for Unification of Formulae and used to express the quantity of certain substances.

International System of Units A system of measurement that is the most widely used internationally and that is almost universally used in science. It is abbreviated SI from the French term *Système International d'Unités.* It is derived and extended from the metric system; however, not all metric units of measurement are accepted as SI units.

intraindividual variability Change in an individual's nutrient intake from day to day.

in vivo neutron activation analysis *See* neutron activation analysis.

iron deficiency The depletion of body iron stores, corresponding to the second and third stages in the development of iron deficiency.

iron-deficiency anemia A low hemoglobin value found in association with iron deficiency. Theoretically, anemia corresponds to the third stage of iron deficiency.

iron overload An excessive accumulation of iron storage in tissues.

ischemia Impaired blood flow, causing oxygen-nutrition deprivation to associated tissues, resulting in pain (e.g., angina pectoris) or, if severe enough, tissue death, as in heart attack.

IU International Unit.

joule An SI unit of work or energy. The amount of work done by a force of 1 newton acting over the distance of 1 meter. One joule = 0.239 kcal. *See also* kilojoule.

kat/L The SI unit of enzyme activity. One katal per liter is the amount of enzyme necessary to catalyze a reaction at the rate of 1 mole of substrate per second per liter (mol · s−1 · L−1).

kcal Kilocalorie.

kg Kilogram.

kilocalorie (kcal) The amount of energy required to raise the temperature of 1 liter of water 1°C. A unit of heat equal to 1000 calories. Also known as a large calorie. One kcal equals 0.239 kilojoule.

kilogram (kg) A unit of mass in the metric system. One kilogram equals 1000 grams, or 2.2046 pounds.

kilojoule (kj) An SI unit of work or energy. A kilojoule equals 1000 joules. A kilojoule is equivalent to 4.18 kcal. *See also* joule.

kj Kilojoule.

kwashiorkor A protein deficiency, generally seen in children, characterized by edema, growth failure, and muscle wasting.

lapse A single or temporary recurrence of an unwanted habit or behavior that one has overcome or has turned from for a period of time.

LDL Low-density lipoprotein.

LDL receptors Molecules on the surface of plasma membranes of hepatic and peripheral cells that recognize and remove low-density lipoprotein from the blood.

leading question A question that contains an implicit or explicit suggestion about the expected desired answer.

life expectancy The average number of years of life remaining for a person of a given age and sex. In most countries, improvements in nutrition, public health, and medicine have resulted in more people, on average, living longer, thus increasing life expectancy.

lipoproteins Spherical macromolecular complexes of lipids (triglycerides, cholesterol, cholesterol esters, and phospholipids) and special proteins known as apoproteins that transport lipids from sites of absorption or synthesis to sites of storage or metabolism via the blood. They include chylomicrons, LDL, IDL, VLDL, and HDL.

list-based diet history *See* food frequency questionnaire.

longitudinal study Cohort study. A study design comparing future exposure to various factors in a group (cohort) of subjects in an attempt to determine how exposure with the factors relates to diseases that may develop.

low-density lipoprotein (LDL) A serum lipoprotein whose primary role is transporting cholesterol to the various cells of the body. LDL contains approximately 70% of the serum's total cholesterol, is considered the most atherogenic (atherosclerosis-producing) lipoprotein, and is the prime target of attempts to lower serum cholesterol. Low serum levels of LDL cholesterol are desirable.

μ The Greek letter mu, used as a prefix in such instances as μg (microgram) and μL (microliter), where it indicates 10^{-6}, or one-millionth.

m Meter.

magnetic resonance imaging (MRI) A technology allowing both imaging of the body and *in vivo* chemical analysis without radiation hazard to the subject.

malnutrition This can mean any nutrition disorder but usually refers to failing health caused by long-term nutritional inadequacies.

marasmic kwashiorkor A combination of chronic energy deficiency and chronic or acute protein deficiency.

marasmus Predominantly an energy (kilocalorie) deficiency presenting with significant loss of body weight, skeletal muscle, and adipose tissue mass, but with serum protein concentrations relatively intact.

MCV Mean corpuscular (red blood cell) volume.

MCV model A model for assessing the prevalence of iron deficiency that requires abnormal values for at least two of the following measurements: mean corpuscular volume, transferrin saturation, or erythrocyte protoporphyrin level.

mean A value calculated by summing all the observations in a sample and dividing the sum by the number of observations. Also referred to as the arithmetic mean or, simply, average. One of three measures of central tendency, along with median and mode.

median The observation that divides the distribution into equal halves, with 50% of the observations above and 50% of the observations below this point. Also known as the 50th percentile. One of the three measures of central tendency, along with mean and mode.

menopause The cessation of monthly menses.

meter (m) A unit of distance in the metric system. One meter equals 100 centimeters, 1000 millimeters, and 39.37 inches.

Metropolitan relative weight An individual's actual body weight divided by the midpoint value of weight range for a given height (obtained from a Metropolitan Life Insurance Company height-weight table) and then multiplied by 100. *See also* relative weight.

mg Milligram.

MI Myocardial infarction.

midaxillary line An imaginary line running vertically through the middle of the axilla, used as an anatomic landmark in skinfold measurements.

milligram (mg) A unit of mass in the metric system. 10^{-3} gram, or one-thousandth of a gram.

millimeter (mm) A unit of distance in the metric system. 10^{-3} meter, or 1/1000 of a meter.

millimole (mmol) 10^{-3} mole, or 1/1000 of a gram.

missing foods Foods eaten but not reported by participants of nutritional surveys.

mm Millimeter.

mmol Millimole.

mode The observation that occurs most frequently. One of the three measures of central tendency, along with mean and median.

modeling Observational learning, or imitation. A learning process in behavior modification in which observers learn new behaviors by watching the actions of a model.

morbidity Illness or sickness.

morphology The study of the shape and structure of organisms, organs, or parts.

mortality Death.

myocardial infarction (MI) Heart attack. The death of an area of heart tissue caused by blockage of the coronary artery feeding that area.

myocardium Heart muscle.

National Health and Nutrition Examination Survey (NHANES) A continuous, annual cross-sectional survey, conducted by the U.S. Department of Health and Human Services, that assesses food intake, height, weight, blood pressure, vitamin and mineral levels, and a number of other health parameters in a statistically selected group of Americans.

National Nutrition Monitoring System (NNMS) A congressionally mandated system in which the USDA and USDHHS are to work cooperatively in collecting data relating to health and nutritional status measurements, food composition measurements, dietary knowledge, attitude assessment, and surveillance of the food supply.

Nationwide Food Consumption Survey (NFCS) A periodic survey of food consumption at the household and individual levels, conducted by the USDA from 1977 to 1988.

NCEP National Cholesterol Education Program.

NCHS National Center for Health Statistics.

negative nitrogen balance A condition in which nitrogen loss from the body exceeds nitrogen intake. Negative nitrogen balance is often seen in the case of illness, trauma, burns, or recovery from major surgery.

negative reinforcer An unpleasant consequence of a behavior that maintains and strengthens the behavior by the negative reinforcer's being removed from the situation.

neutral questions Questions that allow a client to respond without pressure or direction from the interviewer.

neutron activation analysis A technology allowing in vivo measurement of the body's content of calcium, iodine, hydrogen, sodium, chloride, phosphorus, carbon, and other elements. A neutron beam is directed to the subject, and the response of various elements within the body allows estimation of the quantities of these elements.

NFCS Nationwide Food Consumption Survey.

NHANES National Health and Nutrition Examination Survey.

NHANES I The first National Health and Nutrition Examination Survey.

NHANES II The second National Health and Nutrition Examination Survey.

NHANES III The third National Health and Nutrition Examination Survey.

NHES National Health Examination Survey.

nitrogen balance A condition in which nitrogen losses from the body are equal to nitrogen intake. Nitrogen balance is the expected state of the healthy adult.

NLEA Nutrition Labeling and Education Act.

NMR Nuclear magnetic resonance.

nomogram A graphic device with several vertical scales allowing calculation of certain values when a straightedge is connected between two scales and the desired value is read from a third scale.

nonambulatory Unable to walk (ambulate).

nonquantitative food frequency questionnaire A food frequency questionnaire assessing frequency of food consumption but not the size of food servings.

nuclear magnetic resonance (NMR) Earlier name for magnetic resonance imaging (MRI).

nutrient database A compilation of data on the nutrient content of various foods. The database may exist in book form or as an electronic file accessible by computer.

nutrient density The nutritional composition of foods expressed in terms of nutrient quantity per 1000 kcal. If the quantity of nutrients per 1000 kcal is great enough, then the nutrient needs of a person will be met when his or her energy needs are met.

nutritional assessment The measurement of indicators of dietary status and nutrition-related health status of individuals or populations to identify the possible occurrence, nature, and extent of impaired nutritional status (ranging from deficiency to toxicity).

nutritional epidemiology The application of epidemiologic principles to the study of how diet and nutrition influence the occurrence of disease.

nutritional monitoring The assessment of dietary or nutritional status at intermittent times with the aim of detecting changes in the dietary or nutritional status of a population.

nutritional screening The process of identifying characteristics known to be associated with nutrition problems in order to pinpoint individuals who are malnourished or at risk for malnutrition.

nutritional surveillance Continuous assessment of nutritional status for the purpose of detecting changes in trend or distribution in order to initiate corrective measures.

Nutrition Labeling and Education Act (NLEA) A law passed by the U.S. Congress in 1990, mandating nutrition labeling for virtually all processed foods regulated by the U.S. Food and Drug Administration, authorizing appropriate health claims on food labels, and calling for activities to educate consumers about food labels.

obesity An excessive accumulation of body fat.

observational standards A dietary standard based on clinical observation, as opposed to scientific measurement of actual need.

olecranon process The bony projection of the distal ulna at the elbow. Used as an anatomic landmark in upper-arm anthropometric measurements.

open questions Questions providing individuals with considerable freedom in deciding the amount and type of information to give in answering an interviewer's questions.

osteopenia A condition in which bone mineral density is decreased but not to the point that a diagnosis of osteoporosis can be made. According to World Health Organization criteria, osteopenia occurs when the T-score is between −1.0 and −2.5.

osteoporosis A condition in which there is a marked decrease in bone mineral density and deterioration of bone microarchitecture, compromised bone strength, and an increased susceptibility to fracture and painful morbidity. According to World Health Organization criteria, osteoporosis occurs when the T-score is less than −2.5.

overnutrition The condition resulting from the excessive intake of foods in general or particular food components.

overweight Body weight in excess of a particular standard and sometimes used as an index of obesity.

parallax The apparent difference in the reading of a measurement scale (e.g., a skinfold caliper's needle) when viewed from various points not in a straight line with the eye.

parenteral nutrition The process of administering nutrients directly into veins to improve nutritional status.

pellagra A niacin deficiency syndrome characterized by inflamed mucous membranes, mental deterioration, diarrhea, and eruptions in skin areas exposed to light or injury.

PEM Protein-energy malnutrition.

percentiles Divisions of a distribution into equal, ordered subgroups of hundredths. The 50th percentile is the median. The 90th percentile, for example, is an observation whose value exceeds 90% of the set of observations and is exceeded by only 10%.

peripheral vascular disease Atherosclerotic changes within the aorta, iliac, and femoral arteries, affecting blood flow in the body's periphery.

pg Picograms.

phantom foods Foods not eaten but reported as having been eaten by participants of nutrition surveys.

picograms (pg) A unit of mass in the metric system. One picogram equals 10^{-12} gram, or one-trillionth of a gram.

plasma The liquid component of blood that has not clotted. An anticoagulant added to the glass tube used to draw blood from a subject's vein prevents clotting of the blood. This tube is then centrifuged, leaving the blood cells at the bottom of the tube and the plasma at the top. Unlike serum, plasma contains the clotting factors.

plethysmography *See* air displacement plethysmography.

population-specific equations Regression equations for estimating body density or percent body fat from anthropometric measures that can be applied only to population groups sharing certain features, such as sex, age, and adiposity.

positive nitrogen balance Nitrogen intake exceeds nitrogen loss from the body. This is commonly seen during growth, pregnancy, and recovery from trauma, surgery, or illness.

positive reinforcer Any consequence (reward) that maintains and strengthens behavior by its presence. (The positive reinforcer makes the behavior more likely to recur.)

postprandial After a meal.

power-type indices Indices such as Quetelet's index and Benn's index.

precision The difference in results when the same measurement is repeatedly performed on the same sample.

prediabetes A term used to represent impaired fasting glucose (IFG) or impaired glucose tolerance (IGT) based on the observation that most people have either IFG or IGT before they are diagnosed with type 2 diabetes.

prevalence The number of existing cases of a disease or condition divided by the total number of people in a given population at a designated time. It indicates the burden of a disease or how common it is.

propensity The probability that a person will consume a specific food or beverage on any given day over a designated time, usually the previous year.

protein-energy malnutrition (PEM) An inadequate consumption of protein and energy, resulting in a gradual body wasting and increased susceptibility to infection.

provisional tables Provisional data supplied by the United States Department of Agriculture for special nutrients or foods, such as dietary fiber, bakery foods, vitamin K, fatty acids, and sugar, that are often released years before more complete data are available.

proximal Toward the center of the body.

QCT Quantitative computed tomography.

quantitative computed tomography (QCT) An imaging technique consisting of an array of X-ray sources and radiation detectors aligned opposite each other. As the X-ray beams pass through the subject, they are weakened, or attenuated, by the body's tissues and eventually picked up by the detectors. Data from the detectors are then transmitted to a computer, which reconstructs the subject's cross-sectional anatomy, using mathematic equations adapted for computer processing.

quantitative food frequency questionnaire *See* semi-quantitative food frequency questionnaire.

quantitative ultrasound The transmission of high-frequency sound waves through bone to determine its fracture risk.

Quetelet's index Weight in kilograms divided by height in meters squared (kg/m^2). The most widely used weight-height or power-type index.

rational-emotive therapy (RET) A counseling approach based on the premise that emotional disturbances are a product of irrational thinking. RET holds that emotions are primarily the result of our beliefs, evaluations, interpretations, and reactions to life situations, which in turn determine our behavior. Behavior is altered by correcting the thought process using methods such as cognitive restructuring, language changing, cognitive rehearsal, and thought stopping.

RDA Recommended Dietary Allowance.

RDIs Reference Daily Intakes.

reality therapy A therapy based primarily on the work of psychiatrist William Glasser and his premise that every person's behavior is an attempt to fulfill his or her basic human needs (behavior driven completely from within). Emphasis is placed on individual responsibility for actions and client participation in decision making.

Recommended Dietary Allowance The average daily dietary intake level sufficient to meet the nutrient requirement of nearly all (97% to 98%) healthy individuals in a particular life stage or gender group. One of four nutrient reference intakes included in the Dietary Reference Intakes.

recumbent The position of lying down. Recumbent length, for example, is obtained with the subject lying down and is generally reserved for children younger than 24 months of age or for children between 24 and 36 months who cannot stand erect without assistance.

REE Resting energy expenditure.

reference amount The amount of a food typically consumed per eating occasion as determined by food consumption surveys and which is used when determining the serving size listed on that food's Nutrition Facts label. The serving size listed on the food's Nutrition Facts label is the amount in common household measures closest to the reference amount.

Reference Daily Intakes (RDIs) A set of dietary references that serves as the basis for the Daily Values and are based on the Recommended Dietary Allowances (RDAs) for essential vitamins and minerals and, in selected groups, protein. The RDIs replace the U.S. Recommended Daily Allowances (U.S. RDAs).

regression equations Equations developed by comparing a variety of anthropometric measures with measurements of body density (usually by hydrostatic weighing) to see which anthropometric measures are best at predicting body density. A statistical process called multiple-regression analysis is used to develop the equations.

relapse The resumption of an unwanted habit or behavior that one has, for a period of time, overcome or turned from.

relative weight A subject's actual body weight divided by the midpoint value of weight range for a given height and then multiplied by 100. *See also* Metropolitan relative weight.

reliability *See* reproducibility.

remodeling The dynamic process of skeletal change in which bones are constantly undergoing resorption and reformation.

reproducibility Also known as reliability. The ability of a method to yield the same measurement value on two or more different occasions, assuming that nothing has changed in the interim.

resting energy expenditure (REE) Also known as resting metabolic rate. This term is used for metabolic rate or energy expenditure in the awake, resting, and postabsorptive individual.

RET Rational-emotive therapy.

rickets A condition, especially found in infants and children, characterized by malformed bones, delayed fontanel closure, and muscle pain, due to a deficiency of vitamin D.

scurvy An ascorbic acid (vitamin C) deficiency disease characterized by anemia, spongy and bleeding gums, and capillary hemorrhages.

secular trend In epidemiology, changes in prevalence of a disease or condition over time.

self-contract An agreement an individual makes with himself or herself to help build commitment to behaviorial change.

semiquantitative food frequency questionnaire A food frequency questionnaire that assesses both frequency and portion size of food consumption. *See also* food frequency questionnaire.

sensitivity A test's ability to indicate an abnormality where there is one.

serum The liquid component of blood that has clotted. A plain glass tube is used to draw blood from a subject's vein, and after several minutes the blood clots. This tube is then centrifuged, leaving the blood cells at the bottom of the tube and the serum at the top. Unlike plasma, serum does not contain the clotting factors.

serum proteins Proteins present in serum (the liquid portion of clotted blood) that are often regarded as indicators of the body's visceral protein status (e.g., albumin).

shortfall nutrients Nutrients whose intakes are below recommended levels among a significant part of the population.

SI The abbreviation for the International System of Units, derived from the French term *Système International d'Unités*. *See* International System of Units.

signs Observations made by a qualified examiner during a physical examination.

single-photon absorptiometry (SPA) An approach for measuring bone mineral content using photons at a single energy level derived from a radioisotopic source (iodine-125).

skinfold thickness A double fold of skin that is measured with skinfold calipers at various body sites.

software program The entire set of programs, procedures, and related documentation associated with computer programs. The list of program commands that operate a particular program on the computer.

somatic protein Protein contained in the body's skeletal muscles.

SPA Single-photon absorptiometry.

specificity A test's ability to indicate normalcy where there is no abnormality.

stadiometer A device capable of measuring stature in children over 2 years of age and in adults. This measure is taken in a standing position.

standard deviation (SD) A measure of how much a frequency distribution varies from the mean.

stature Standing height.

stimulus control A behavior modification technique in which behavioral antecedents are recognized and modified or controlled to decrease the occurrence of negative behaviors and to increase the occurrence of positive behaviors.

stroke A blockage or rupture of a blood vessel supplying the brain, with resulting loss of consciousness, paralysis, or other symptoms.

stunting A decreased height-for-age. It is generally seen in long-term, mild to moderate protein-energy malnutrition.

Subjective Global Assessment A clinical approach to assessing the nutritional status of a patient using information gained from the patient's history and physical examination.

supine The position in which one is lying on his or her back.

surrogate source A source of information about a subject's behavior (e.g., dietary practices) from a source other than the subject. Typical surrogate sources include a spouse, child, close relative, and friend of the subject.

symptoms Disease manifestations that the patient is usually aware of and often complains of.

Système International d'Unités A French translation of International System of Units. *See* International System of Units.

TEF Thermal effect of food.

thermic effect of exercise Energy expenditure resulting from physical activity.

thermic effect of food (TEF) Also known as diet-induced thermogenesis or the specific dynamic action of food. TEF is the increased energy expenditure following food consumption or administration of parenteral or enteral nutrition caused by absorption and metabolism of food and nutrients.

TOBEC Total body electrical conductivity.

Tolerable Upper Intake Level The highest level of daily nutrient intake likely to pose no risk for adverse health effects for almost all apparently healthy individuals in the general population. As intake increases above this level, risk for adverse (toxic) effects increases. One of four nutrient reference intakes included in the Dietary Reference Intakes.

total body electrical conductivity (TOBEC) A method of assessing body composition in which a subject is placed in an electromagnetic field (EMF). Since electrolytes within the fat-free mass are capable of conducting electricity, the degree to which the EMF is disrupted is related to the amount of fat-free mass within the subject's body.

total fiber The sum of dietary fiber and functional fiber. *See* dietary fiber and functional fiber.

total water The total amount of water a person consumes which includes drinking water, water in other beverages, and water or moisture in food.

transferrin The form in which iron is transported within the blood.

tritium An isotope of hydrogen having three times the mass of ordinary hydrogen. It is commonly used as a tracer in the determination of total body water.

T-score A representation of the number of standard deviations above or below the mean value of a reference population. When used in evaluating bone mineral density (BMD), the T-score is the number of standard deviations above or below the mean BMD of the reference population, which is a large group of healthy young adults of the same sex. According to the World Health Organization, an adult can be diagnosed with osteoporosis if his or her bone mineral density corresponds to a T-score at or below −2.5.

24-hour recall A method of dietary recall in which a trained interviewer asks the subject to remember in detail all foods and beverages consumed during the past 24 hours. This information is recorded by the interviewer for later coding and analysis.

two-compartment model A body composition model that views the body as being composed of two compartments: fat mass and fat-free mass, or, according to an alternative approach, adipose tissue and lean body mass.

triglyceride A lipid composed of a glycerol molecule to which are attached three fatty acid molecules and the chemical form of most fat in food and in the body. Triglyceride is also found in the blood, primarily in very low-density lipoprotein particles and chylomicrons.

ulna The larger, inner bone of the forearm. Used as an anatomic landmark in arm anthropometry.

ultrasound A diagnostic method used for imaging internal organs and estimating the thickness of subcutaneous adipose tissue. High-frequency sound waves are transmitted into the body from a transducer (sound transmitter) applied to the skin surface. As ultrasound strikes the interface between two tissues differing in density (e.g., adipose tissue and muscle), some of it is reflected back and received by the transducer. Alterations between the signal as it is transmitted and received are used to image internal organs and to determine subcutaneous tissue thickness.

undernutrition A condition resulting from the inadequate intake of food in general or particular food components.

underwater weighing *See* hydrostatic weighing.

USDA United States Department of Agriculture.

USRDA U.S. Recommended Daily Allowances.

U.S. Recommended Daily Allowances (USRDA) A set of nutrition standards developed by the FDA for use in regulating the nutrition labeling of food. They were replaced by the Reference Daily Intakes.

validity The ability of an instrument to measure what it is intended to measure. Validating a method of measuring dietary intake, for example, involves comparing measurements of intake obtained by that method with intake measurements obtained by some other accepted approach.

very low-density lipoprotein (VLDL) A lipoprotein, present in blood, that is synthesized by the liver and primarily carries triglyceride to cells for storage and metabolism.

viscera Organs of the body (such as liver, kidneys, heart).

visceral protein Protein found in the body's organs or viscera, as well as that in the serum and in blood cells.

VLDL Very low-density lipoprotein.

waist circumference The distance around the horizontal plane through the abdomen at the level of the iliac crest of a standing subject. This measurement is used as an index of abdominal fat content.

wasting A decreased weight-for-age. It is generally seen in severe protein-energy malnutrition.

weighed food record A method of recording individual food intake in which the amounts and types of all food and beverages are recorded for a specific period of time, usually ranging from 1 to 7 days. Portion sizes are determined by accurate weighing.

weight-height indices *See* height-weight indices.

WIC Special Supplemental Nutrition Program for Women, Infants, and Children.

xerophthalmia An eye disease caused by vitamin A deficiency in which the conjunctiva and cornea dry and thicken, in part because of decreased mucus production. If not treated in earlier stages with vitamin A supplements, permanent damage may ensue, with softening of the cornea and subsequent blindness.

Index

3-Methylhistidine, 206
24-hour recall, 78, 79–81, 82, 92–93, 101, 105–107, 108, 123, 133, 146, 225
Abdominal fat, 15–16, 185–186, 285–286, 301–302
Abdominal skinfold measurements, 193, 194
Academy of Nutrition and Dietetics, 64–67
  domains for nutrition terms, 8, 9, 10
  "Nutrition Assessment and Nutrition Monitoring and Evaluation Reference Sheets," 11
  standardized terminology for nutritional assessment, 3, 4, 7–11
Acceptable Macronutrient Distribution Ranges (AMDRs), 37–38
Accuracy, in measuring lipids and lipoproteins, 279, 280–281
Acute infections, in cholesterol measurement, 282
Adequate Intake (AI), 26, 29, 30, 33–34, 36–38, 39
Adipose tissue samples, 97
Adolescents
  blood pressure evaluation, 288–293, 314–315
  body mass index (BMI), 173, 175, 271–272, 436, 438, 446
  bone health and, 301
  CDC growth charts, 171–176, 288, 435–438
  cholesterol levels, 262, 469–473
  coronary heart disease risk, 262, 271–276
  mean body mass index (BMI) in U.S., 446
  mean height in U.S., 444–445
  mean weight in U.S., 442–446
  prevalence of obesity, 15
  serum folate levels, 341
  serum vitamin B_{12}, 344
  vitamin C status, 338
  vitamin D status, 336
Adult Nutrition Surveillance System, 119
Adults
  bone health and, 301. *See also* Osteoporosis
  CDC growth charts, 171–176
  cholesterol levels, 469–473
  estimating risk of coronary heart disease, 264, 265
  hypertension classification and prevalence, 283–284
  iron status, 327, 328
  mean body mass index in U.S., 3, 452, 456
  mean height in U.S., 444–445, 449–450, 454–455
  mean weight in U.S., 447–448, 453
  serum folate levels, 341
  serum vitamin B_{12}, 344
  vitamin C status, 338
  vitamin D status, 336
  weight measurement, 170–171
Adverse health effects, 34–35, 38
African Americans. *See* Race/ethnicity
Age-adjusted death rate, 16
Agricultural Research Service (ARS), 150
Air-displacement plethysmography, 3, 202–204
Alanine aminotransferase (ALT), 343–344
Albumin, 3, 320–321, 344–345
Alcohol
  bone health and, 300
  diabetes and, 306
  hypertension risk and, 287
  vitamin B_6 status and, 339
Alkaline phosphatase (ALP), 345
Allard equations, 243–244
ALP (alkaline phosphatase), 345
ALT (alanine aminotransferase), 343–344
Ambulatory blood pressure monitoring (ABPM), 283, 288
American Academy of Family Physicians, 273–274
American Academy of Pediatrics, 174, 273–274
American Cancer Society, 16, 17, 51
American Diabetes Association, 6, 13, 51, 64–67, 302–303, 305, 306
American Dietetic Association, 4, 24, 64–67, 160, 161
American Health Foundation, 46
American Heart Association, 6, 15, 46, 257, 260, 276–279
American Institute for Cancer Research (AICR), 61–64
American Medical Association (AMA), 46, 287
American Psychiatric Association (APA), 365–367
American Society for Parenteral and Enteral Nutrition, 3
American Thyroid Association, 333
Anabolism, 320
Android obesity, 185
Anemia, 322–324
Angina pectoris, 257
Anorexia nervosa, 365
Anthropometric assessment, 6, 7, 15, 124, 125, 166–212, 388–389
  anthropometry, defined, 3, 167
  body composition measures. *See* Body composition
  body fat distribution, 3, 185–186, 188–199, 285–286, 363–365
  cadaveric studies, 187–188, 271
  CDC growth charts, 171–176, 288, 430–440
  frame size measurement, 179–180
  head circumference measurement, 169, 432, 434
  height-weight indices, 177, 180–185
  length measurement, 167–168, 171–172
  stature measurement, 168–169
  weight measurement, 170–171
  weight standards, 176–179
Anticoagulants, in cholesterol measurement, 282
Apoproteins, 259
Archimedes' principle, 199–200
Arm muscle area (AMA), 226, 228, 233–234, 235, 255, 467–468
ASA24 (automated, self-administered 24-hour dietary recall), 78, 81, 93, 108
Asians. *See* Race/ethnicity
Aspartate aminotransferase (AST), 345
Assessment. *See* Measuring diet; Nutritional assessment
Atherosclerosis, 260, 271
Atwater, Wilber Olin, 22
Audio computer-assisted personal self-interview (ACASI), 124
Automated, self-administered 24-hour dietary recall (ASA24), 78, 81, 93, 108
Automated Multiple-Pass Method (AMPM) of collecting 24-hour recall, 78, 81, 93, 101, 123, 133

Balance sheet approach, 91–92, 110, 113–114
Basal metabolic rate (BMR), 235
Basic Four foundation diet, 58, 59
Basic Seven foundation diet, 58, 59
Behavior modification, 376–378
  antecedents and consequences, 376
  goals and self-contracts, 377
  modeling, 377–378
  reinforcers, 378
  self-monitoring, 376–377
  in weight control programs, 379
Behavioral Risk Factor Surveillance System (BRFSS), 16, 78, 119, 125, 129–130, 144, 420–427
Beriberi, 2
Beverages, trends, 138
Bias, in measuring lipids and lipoproteins, 279, 280–281
Bicarbonate-urea method, 238
Bilirubin, 345
Biochemical assessment, 3, 6, 7, 95–97, 317–348, 389
  blood chemistry tests, 343–346, 351–352
  of calcium status, 327–329
  of diabetes mellitus, 302–305
  of folate status, 340–341
  of iodine status, 330–333
  of iron status, 322–327
  of protein status, 222, 244–245, 318–322, 344–345
  of serum lipids, 258–263, 279–282
  use of biochemical measures, 318
  of vitamin A status, 333–335
  of vitamin B_6 status, 339–340

Biochemical assessment—*Cont.*
of vitamin B_{12} status, 341–343
of vitamin C status, 337–339
of vitamin D status, 335–337
of zinc status, 329–330
Bioelectrical impedance, 3, 207
Biomarkers. *See* Biochemical assessment
Blacks. *See* Race/ethnicity
"Blind loop" syndrome, 342
Block, Gladys, 86, 162
Block Health Habits and History Questionnaire (HHHQ), 86, 162
Block questionnaires, 86, 88–89, 162
Blood chemistry tests, 343–346, 351–352
Blood pressure. *See* Hypertension
Blood samples, 97
Blood urea nitrogen (BUN), 345
Body composition, 176, 186–210
3-methylhistidine as index of muscle and fat-free mass, 206
Body Composition Worksheet, 201
cadaveric studies, 187–188
computed tomography (CT), 208–209
creatinine excretion in estimating body muscle mass, 206
densitometry, 3, 199–204
dual-energy X-ray absorbancy, 209–210, 295–296, 298–299
electrical conductance of fat and fat-free tissue, 206–207
HIV-related alterations in body fat distribution, 363, 364
infrared interactance analysis, 208
magnetic resonance imaging (MRI), 209
neutron activation analysis for bone mineral content, 205–206
skinfold measurements, 3, 188–199, 220, 457–468
total body potassium to estimate body fat, 205
total body water to estimate body fat, 204–205
ultrasound, 208, 296–299
Body density, 3, 199–204
Body fat distribution, 185–186
HIV-related changes in, 363, 364
skinfold measurements, 3, 188–199, 285–286
Body language, 372
Body mass index (BMI), 13–14, 225–226
in adults, 3, 452, 456
body mass index-for-age, 175–176
CDC growth charts, 172–174, 430–440
in children and adolescents, 173, 175, 271–272, 436, 438, 446
death and, 176–177
development of, 181–184
hypertension risk and, 285–286
Body muscle mass
3-Methylhistidine analysis and, 206
arm muscle area (AMA), 226, 228, 233–234, 235, 255, 467–468
creatinine excretion and, 206, 233
Body weight. *See also* Obesity; Overweight
assessment and classification, 218–219
CDC growth charts, 171–176, 430–440
computational formulas, 171, 225–226, 228–229, 231–234, 255
eating disorders, 3, 295, 365–367
energy expenditure and, 97–98
estimating, 225–226, 228–229, 231–233, 254
height-weight indices, 177, 180–185
height-weight tables, 177–179
of hospitalized patients, 225–226, 228–229, 231–233, 254
hypertension risk and, 285–286
maintaining, 97–98
mean weight in U.S. by sex and age group, 442–446, 447–448, 453
measuring, 170–171
protein status and, 319
relative weight, 177, 180–181
weight management, 13–15, 97–98, 379, 381–383
weight standards, 176–179
Bogalusa Heart Study, 271
Bone mineral density (BMD), 293–300, 301
dual-energy X-ray absorptiometry (DXA) and, 209–210, 295–296, 298–299
neutron activation analysis for, 205–206
quantitative ultrasound and, 296–299
Bone remodeling, 294
Boys. *See* Males
BRFSS (Behavioral Risk Factor Surveillance System), 16, 78, 119, 125, 129–130, 144, 420–427
British Association for Parenteral and Enteral Nutrition, 250
British Heart Foundation, 6
Broadband ultrasound attenuation (BUA), 298
Brussels Cadaver Analysis Study (CAS), 187–188
Bulimia nervosa, 4, 366
Burke, B. S., 89
Burns, energy requirements, 242–244

C-reactive protein (hs-CRP), 260, 267
Cachexia, 359
Cadaveric studies, 187–188, 271
Calcium, 327–329
bone health and, 299–301
estimating intake, 315–316
serum calcium fractions, 327–328
serum calcium levels, 345
urinary calcium, 328–329
Calf circumference, 228–229
Calipers, 189–190, 191
Calorimetry
bicarbonate-urea method, 238
defined, 235
direct, 235–236
doubly labeled water method, 237–238
Estimated Average Requirement (EAR), 26–27, 28, 38–39
Estimated Energy Requirement (EER), 26, 27, 35, 38–39, 235–238, 240–243, 274–275
indirect, 236–237
nutrient density, 39–41
resting energy expenditure (REE), 98, 234–235, 238–244
Canadian Diabetes Association, 6
Canadian Diet and Breast Cancer Prevention Trial, 97
Canadian Heart and Stroke Foundation, 6
Canadian Recommended Nutrient Intakes (RNIs), 159
Canadian Total Diet Study, 127
Cancer, 2, 3, 4, 16, 17, 61–64
Carbohydrates
in coronary heart disease treatment, 278–279
in diabetes treatment, 306
Dietary Reference Intakes (DRIs), 36–38
trends, 134
Carbon dioxide, 345
Cardiovascular disease. *See* Coronary heart disease (CHD)
Cardiovascular Health Integrated Lifestyle Diet (CHILD 1), 273–274
Case-control studies, 78
Catabolism, 320
Causative risk factors, 15, 16
CDC. *See* U.S. Centers for Disease Control and Prevention (CDC)
CHD. *See* Coronary heart disease (CHD)
CHILD 1 (Cardiovascular Health Integrated Lifestyle Diet), 273–274
Child and Adult Care Food Program, 47
Children
blood pressure evaluation, 288–293, 314–315
blood pressure levels, 289–290, 291–292
body mass index (BMI), 173, 175, 271–272, 436, 438, 446
bone health and, 301
CDC growth charts, 171–176, 288, 435–438
cholesterol levels, 262, 469–473
coronary heart disease risk, 262, 273–275
iron status, 327, 328
length measurement, 167–168, 171–172
mean height in U.S., 444–445
mean weight in U.S., 442–446
prevalence of obesity, 15
serum folate levels, 341
serum vitamin B_{12}, 344
vitamin C status, 338
weight measurement, 170–171
Chitin, 37
Chitosan, 37
Chloride, 345–346
Cholesterol
blood chemistry tests, 346
in coronary heart disease (CHD), 258–271
dietary, 277–278
issues in measuring, 279–282
lowering in population, 270–271
total cholesterol levels, 260–263, 469–473
Cholesterol Reference Method Laboratory Network, 280–281
Choose My Plate SuperTracker, 61, 161, 162
Chronic diseases, 1–3, 4, 15, 24, 41, 50. *See also specific diseases*
Chylomicrons, 259
Cigarette smoking, 263, 300, 371
Client history, 7, 225, 354–356, 389–390
Clinical assessment, 6, 353–368
dietary history, 89–90, 355–356
eating disorders, 365–367
HIV infection, 353, 362–365
in hypertension prevention, 284–285
medical history, 354–355
protein-energy malnutrition (PEM), 13, 222, 319, 320, 359–362
signs and symptoms in, 3–4, 8–10, 353
Subjective Global Assessment (SGA), 4, 356–359, 369
Clinical NutriBase System, 160–161
Closed circuit calorimetry, 236
Closed questions, 374–375
Coefficient of variation (CV), 33
Cognitive rehearsal, 380
Cohort studies, 78–79
Communication, 371–374
communication model, 371
defined, 371
effective, 372–373
listening, 373–374
nonverbal, 372, 373
verbal, 371–372
Complete blood count (CBC), 351–352
Computed tomography (CT), in determining body composition, 208–209
Computer-assisted personal interviewer (CAPI) technology, 124, 131
Computerized metabolic monitor, 237
Computers in nutritional assessment, 146–163
ASA24 (automated, self-administered 24-hour dietary recall; National Cancer Institute), 78, 81, 93, 108

Automated Multiple-Pass Method (AMPM) of collecting 24-hour recall (USDA), 78, 81, 93, 101, 123, 133
computer-assisted personal interviewer (CAPI) technology, 124, 131
DHQ*Web, 86, 93, 107–108
digital imaging technology, 93–94
examples of computerized dietary analysis systems, 160–161
factors in selecting dietary analysis systems, 147–161
Internet sources and tools, 86, 88–89, 93, 107–108, 161–162
nutrient databases, 81, 114, 147–158
program operation, 157, 158–159
system output, 157, 159–160
Conditional risk factors, 15, 16
Congregate Nutrition Services, 47
Conjunctival impression cytology, 334
Consolidation, 294
Continuing Survey of Food Intakes by Individuals (CSFII; USDA), 83, 111, 112, 114–115, 121
Coronary artery disease. *See* Coronary heart disease (CHD)
Coronary heart disease (CHD), 2–4, 77, 257–282
coronary heart disease in youth, 262, 271–276
death rates, 257–258
defined, 257
dietary treatment, 276–279
heart attack warning signs, 257
lipids and lipoproteins in, 258–263, 279–282, 313–314, 346
prevention, 258, 266–276
risk factors, 15, 16, 257, 258, 260–267, 271–276, 313–314, 346, 351–352
Coronary risk profile, 351–352
Correlational studies, 75–77
Counseling theory and technique, 370–385
behavior modification, 376–378
characteristics of effective counselors, 381
communication, 371–374
competency checklist for nutrition counselors, 479–481
interviewing, 374–375
person-centered approach, 375–376
practical plan for dietary change, 381–383
rational-emotive therapy (RET), 378–380
reality therapy, 380–381
Creatinine excretion, 206, 233, 319–320, 346
Creatinine-height index (CHI), 319–320
Cretinism, 2
Criterion validity, 95
Critical-thinking skills, 7–8
Cross-sectional studies, 77–78, 120
Current Population Survey (CPS), 116
Curreri equations, 242–243
Cushing's syndrome, 363
Cutpoint approach, 38
Cyberdiet, 161

Daily Reference Values (DRVs), 55–57
Daily Values, 55–57
Dairy products, trends, 136–137
Dark adaptation, 334–335
DASH-type diet, 273–274, 286–288, 306
Death
body mass index (BMI) and, 176–177
coronary heart disease and, 257–258
leading causes, 2–3
mortality, 4, 284
Deficiency diseases, 23. *See also* Malnutrition
anemia, 322–324
iodine, 2, 330–332
kwashiorkor, 359–361
marasmus, 359–361
protein-energy malnutrition (PEM), 13, 222, 319, 320, 359–362
vitamin C, 2, 22, 337–338
vitamin D, 2, 335
Demonstrated/face validity, 95
Densitometry, 199–204
air-displacement plethysmography, 3, 202–204
defined, 199
underwater weighing, 199–202
Deuterium, in total body water (TBW) measurement, 204–205, 207
DHHS. *See* U.S. Department of Health and Human Services (DHHS)
DHQ*Web, 86, 93, 107–108
Diabetes mellitus, 2–4, 13, 130, 300–306
diagnosing, 302–305
medical nutrition therapy, 305–306
types of, 50, 301–302
Diabetes UK, 6
Diagnosis. *See* Nutrition diagnosis
Diastolic blood pressure (DBP), 282–283, 287, 288
Diet and Health: Implications for Reducing Chronic Disease Risk, 41, 50, 51, 183
Diet and Health Knowledge Survey (USDA), 78, 112, 115
Diet history, 89–90, 355–356
Diet History Questionnaire (DHQ), 86, 87, 88, 107–108, 162, 403–411
Diet Quality Index/Revised, 41–42, 79
Dietary Approaches to Stop Hypertension (DASH), 273–274, 286–288, 306
Dietary change plan, 381–383
characteristics of effective counselors, 381
initial assessment, 381–382
initiating dietary change, 382
maintaining dietary change, 382–383
motivation, 381
relapse prevention, 383
Dietary fiber, 36–37, 278–279, 306
Dietary Goals for the United States, 46–47, 50, 51, 59
Dietary guidelines, 44–50
compared with Dietary Reference Intakes (DRIs), 45
early guidelines, 44–46
U.S. dietary goals, 46–50
Dietary Guidelines for Americans, 6, 8, 10, 13–14, 40–44, 47–50, 51, 59, 60, 110, 114, 133, 134, 159, 241, 268, 273–274, 333, 340, 342
Dietary methods of assessment. *See* Nutritional assessment
Dietary Reference Intakes (DRIs), 3, 24–39, 41–42, 133, 159
Adequate Intake (AI), 26, 29, 30, 33–34, 36–38, 39
compared with dietary guidelines, 45
Estimated Average Requirement (EAR), 26–27, 28, 38–39
Estimated Energy Requirement (EER), 26, 27, 35, 39, 235–238, 240–243, 274–275
recommendations for macronutrients, 36–38
Recommended Dietary Allowances (RDAs), 6, 23–24, 26, 27–33, 35, 36–38, 39, 336
Tolerable Upper Intake Level (UL), 26, 31, 32, 34–35, 39
uses of, 38–39
Dietary Reference Values for Food and Energy (UK), 6
Dietary Standard for Canada, 23
Dietary standards, 21–69
dietary guidelines, 44–50
Dietary Reference Intakes (DRIs), 3, 6, 24–39, 41–42, 133, 159
early standards and recommendations, 22–23
to evaluate nutrient intake, 71–72
food exchange system, 64–67, 72–73
food guides, 57–64
indices of diet quality, 41–44, 79
nutrient density, 39–41
nutrition labeling of food, 50–57
Recommended Dietary Allowances (RDAs), 6, 23–24, 26, 27–33, 35, 36–38, 39, 336
Dietary treatment. *See* Medical nutrition therapy
Dietary trends, 131–140
beverages, 138
carbohydrates, 134
dairy products, 136–137
dietary fats and oils, 136
food energy sources, 131–134
fruits and vegetables, 138–139
red meat, poultry, and fish, 138
sweeteners, 134–136
total calories, 139–140
Digital imaging methods, 93–94
Dilution techniques, 204–205, 207
Direct calorimetry, 235–236
Disease prevention, 256–358
coronary heart disease (CHD), 258, 266–276
diabetes mellitus, 300–306
hypertension, 284–285
osteoporosis, 299–300
primary, 266, 273, 285
secondary, 266
Distal measures, 189
Diurnal variations, 171
Doubly labeled water (DLW), 237–238
Douglas bag method, 237
DRIs. *See* Dietary Reference Intakes (DRIs)
Dual-energy X-ray absorptiometry (DXA), 209–210, 295–296, 298–299
Duplicate food collections, 90
DXA (dual-energy X-ray absorptiometry), 209–210, 295–296, 298–299
Dysgeusia, 9

Early and Periodic Screening, Diagnosis, and Treatment (EPSDT) Program, 128
Eating disorders, 3, 295, 365–367
Ecological studies, 75–77
Electrical conductance tests, 206–207
bioelectrical impedance, 3, 207
total body electrical conductivity (TOBEC), 207
Energy expenditure, 26, 35, 97–98, 234–244
formula for, 234–235
measuring, 235–238
Enrichment, 2
Enteral nutrition, 3, 4, 250
Environmental factors, 6, 9
Epidemic, of chronic diseases, 2–3, 15
Erythrocyte protoporphyrin, 322–323, 324–325
ESHA Research, 160–161
Estimated Average Requirement (EAR), 26–27, 28, 38–39
Estimated Energy Requirement (EER), 26, 27, 35, 39, 240–243
by age, gender, and activity level, 274, 275
for hospitalized patients, 234–238
Estimated food records, 81–83
Estrogen, 294–295
Ethnicity. *See* Race/ethnicity
Etiology, 50
Evidence-based practice, 5
Exercise. *See* Physical activity
Experimental studies, 78
Expert Panel on Integrated Guidelines for Cardiovascular Health and Risk Reduction in Children and Adolescents, 272–277

Face validity, 95
Facial expression, in communication process, 372
Fasting, in cholesterol measurement, 282
Fasting plasma glucose (FPG), 303
Fat-free mass, 206–207, 239
Fats and oils, 97
  in coronary heart disease (CHD) treatment, 276–278
  Dietary Reference Intakes (DRIs), 36–38
  trends, 136
FDA. *See* U.S. Food and Drug Administration (FDA)
Federal Citizen Information Center, 161
Federation of American Societies for Experimental Biology, 111
Feedback, in communication process, 371, 372–373
Females. *See also* Osteoporosis
  blood pressure levels, 291–292
  body composition equations, 197, 198, 199
  CDC growth charts, 171–174, 433–434, 437–438
  estimating body weight, 232
  estimating risk of coronary heart disease, 265
  hypertension among, 283–284
  iron status, 327, 328
  mean body mass index in U.S., 452, 456
  mean height in U.S., 444–445, 449–450, 454–455
  mean weight in U.S., 442–443, 447–448, 453
  relationship between BMI and death, 176–177
  serum folate levels, 341, 342
  serum vitamin B_{12}, 344
  vitamin C status, 338
  vitamin D status, 336
Fiber, 36–37
  in coronary heart disease treatment, 278–279
  in diabetes treatment, 306
Fiducial markers, 94
Flag sign, 360, 362
Folate, 79, 322, 340–341, 342
Folic acid supplementation, 260
Food, Nutrition, and the Prevention of Cancer, 61–64
Food accounts, 90–91
Food and Nutrient Database for Dietary Studies (FNDDS; USDA), 81, 114, 150–152, 158
Food and Nutrition Board (FNB), 23–26
Food and Nutrition News, 160
Food balance sheets, 91–92, 110, 113–114
Food disappearance/availability, 46, 75–76, 91–92, 110–111, 112–114
Food energy sources, trends, 131–134
Food exchange systems, 64–67, 72–73
Food frequency questionnaires, 83–89
  Block questionnaires, 86, 88–89, 162
  Continuing Survey of Food Intakes by Individuals (CSFII; USDA), 83, 111, 112, 114–115, 121
  defined, 83
  Diet History Questionnaire (DHQ), 86, 87, 88, 107–108, 162, 403–411
  formats of, 83, 84
  MEDFICTS Dietary Assessment Questionnaire, 79, 84–85, 269, 401–402
  National Cancer Institute, 83–88, 397–400
  NHANES Food Frequency Questionnaire, 86–88, 89, 92–93, 412–419
  strengths and limitations, 88–89, 318
  validity of, 95
  Willett questionnaire, 85–86, 88–89
Food Guide Pyramid, 41, 42, 57, 58, 59–60, 86, 159
Food guides, 57–64
Food insecurity and hunger, 115–118, 119
Food Label and Package Survey, 119
Food/nutrition-related history (FH), 7–9, 225, 355–356, 387–388
Food Processor SQL, 160
Food Quality Protection Act of 1996, 115
Food records/diaries, 79–80, 81–83, 107, 382, 395–396, 478
Food Stamp Program, 24, 110
FoodWorks, 160, 161
Fortification, 2, 342
Frame size measurement, 179–180
Framingham Heart Study, 79, 262, 263
Frankfort horizontal plane, 167–169
Front-of-package labeling systems, 41, 54–55
Fruits
  National Cancer Institute fruit and vegetable screener, 397–400
  trends, 138–139
Functional fiber, 37

Gama, Vasco da, 2
"Generally recognized as safe" (GRAS) status, 287
Gestational diabetes mellitus (GDM), 302
Girls. *See* Females
Glasser, William, 380–381
Globesity, 15
Glucose, 302–304, 346
Glycated hemoglobin, 304–305
Glycosylated hemoglobin, 346
Goals
  in behavior modification, 377
  in dietary change plan, 382
Goiter, 2, 331–332
GRAS ("generally recognized as safe") status, 287
Great Depression, 57, 113
Growth references
  CDC growth charts, 173, 175–176, 277, 430–440
  nature of, 174
Growth standards
  CDC growth charts, 6, 172, 174–175, 277, 430–440
  nature of, 174
Gynoid obesity, 185

Hair zinc, 330
Hamwi, George J., 176–177
Hamwi equations, 176–177, 180
Handheld calorimeters, 237
Harpenden stadiometer, 168
Harris-Benedict equations, 238–239, 242, 243
Harvard University, 85–86, 88–89, 263
Hassle-Free foundation diet, 58, 59
Head circumference
  CDC growth charts, 432, 434
  measuring, 169
Head Start, 128
Health: United States, 112
Health and Diet Survey, 119, 125, 129
Health Canada, 23, 24, 127
Health-care organizations, 13
Health claims, 52–53
Health Professionals Follow-up Study, 86, 263
Healthfinder, 161
Healthy Eating Index (HEI), 42–44, 45
Healthy People 2020, 11, 12, 15, 110, 287, 322
Hearing, listening versus, 373
Heart attack
  in cholesterol measurement, 282
  warning signs, 257
Heart disease. *See* Coronary heart disease (CHD)
Height. *See also* Stature
  CDC growth charts, 171–176, 430–440
  creatinine-height index, 319–320
  height-weight indices, 177, 180–185
  height-weight tables, 177–179
  mean height in U.S., 444–445, 449–450, 454–455
Height-weight indices, 177, 180–185
Height-weight tables, 177–179
Hematochromatosis, 326–327
Hematocrit, 325
Hemoglobin, 3, 302–305, 322, 325
Hemoglobin A1C, 302–305
High blood pressure. *See* Hypertension
High-density lipoprotein (HDL), 258–263, 266, 267, 275, 279–282, 474–477
High-sensitivity C-reactive protein (hs-CRP), 260, 267
Hispanic Americans. *See* Race/ethnicity
Hispanic Health and Nutrition Examination Survey (HHANES), 118–119, 120
HIV infection, 353, 362–365
Home-Delivered Nutrition Services, 47
Homocysteine, 260
Hospitalized patients, 221–251, 254
  determining energy requirements, 234–244
  energy expenditure in disease and injury, 241–244
  Malnutrition Universal Screening Tool (MUST), 248–250
  Mini Nutritional Assessment (MNA), 246–247, 248
  nutritional assessment, 224–234, 246–250
  nutritional screening, 222–224
  protein requirements, 244–245
Household Food Consumption Survey (HFCS; USDA), 112
Human milk, 33, 37
Hunger and food insecurity, 115–118, 119
Hunt, Caroline, 57, 58, 59
Hydrostatic weighing, 199
Hydroxyapatite, 294
Hyperglycemia, 301–304
Hyperkalemia, 346
Hypernatremia, 346
Hypertension, 2, 3, 77–78, 263, 282–293
  ambulatory blood pressure monitoring (ABPM), 283, 288
  evaluating children and adolescents, 288–293, 314–315
  measuring blood pressure, 282–283, 293
  prevention methods, 284–285
  risk factors, 283–288
Hypertriglyceridemia, 306
Hypochronic anemia, 322
Hypoglycemia, 304
Hypokalemia, 346
Hyponatremia, 346

Impaired fasting glucose (IFG), 302
Impaired glucose tolerance (IGT), 302
Incidence, 1
Indian Health Service, Navajo Health and Nutrition Survey, 125, 127
Indirect calorimetry, 236–237
Infant Formula Act of 1980, 53
Infants
  blood pressure levels, 289, 291
  bone health and, 301
  CDC growth charts, 171–175, 277, 431–434
  coronary heart disease risk, 273
  length measurement, 167–168
  weight measurement, 170
Infarction, 257
Infectious disease, 1, 2
Infrared interactance, 208
Initial assessment, in dietary change plan, 381–382

Insoluble fiber, 278–279
Institute of Medicine, 238
Insulin resistance, 301
Interference, in communication process, 371
Intermediate-density lipoprotein (IDL), 259
International Food Information Council, 161
International Network of Food Data Systems (INFOODS), 147
International System of Units (SI), 261
Internet sources and tools, 86, 88–89, 93, 107–108, 161–162
Intervention studies, 78
Interviewing
  computer-assisted, 124, 131
  obtaining information, 374–375
  skills in, 374
  telephone, 92–93
Intraindividual variability, 81
Intrinsic factor, 342
Iodine, 330–333
  assessing iodine status, 331–333
  deficiency disease, 2, 330–332
Iowa Women's Health Study, 86
Iron, 322–327
  assessing iron status, 326
  erythrocyte protoporphyrin, 322–323, 324–325
  hematocrit, 325
  hemoglobin, 3, 302–305, 322, 325
  iron depletion, 322–324
  iron overload, 326–327
  mean corpuscular hemoglobin (MCH), 325, 326
  mean corpuscular volume (MCV), 325–326, 343
  models for assessing iron status, 326
  serum ferritin, 322, 324, 326, 327, 328
  soluble transferrin receptor (sTfR), 324, 326
  total iron-binding capacity (TIBC), 321, 324
Iron-deficient erythropoeisis, 324

Joint Commission on the Accreditation of Health Care Organizations (JCAHCO), 222
Joinville, 2
Journal of Food Composition, 158
Journal of Food Sciences, 158
Journal of Nutrition Education, 160
Journal of the American Dietetic Association, 24, 160

Ketoacidosis, 302
Kidney Foundation of Canada, 6
Kilocalories (kcal), 22
Kilograms (kg), 22
Knee height, 226–227, 228, 232
Kwashiorkor, 359–361

Lactic dehydrogenase (LDH), 346
Lactose malabsorption, 60
Leading questions, 375
Length
  CDC growth charts, 431, 433
  measuring, 167–168, 171–172
Life expectancy, 1
Lifestyle. *See* Therapeutic lifestyle changes (TLC)
Lind, James, 2, 22
Linoleic acid, 36, 37, 97
Lipids
  measurement issues, 279–282
  serum, 258–263, 279–282, 306, 313–314, 469–477
Lipoprotein(a) [Lp(a)], 260
Lipoproteins, 279–282, 306, 313–314
  coronary heart disease and, 260–262, 276
  lipoprotein ratios, 262–263
  measurement issues, 279–282
  serum lipids and, 258–263, 474–477

Listening, 373–374
Louis IX, 2
Low-density-lipoprotein (LDL), 258, 259, 261–263, 266–269, 279–282
Lusk, Graham, 23

Macrocytic anemia, 322
Macronutrients, 22, 23. *See also* Carbohydrates; Fats and oils; Protein
  Acceptable Macronutrient Distribution Ranges (AMDRs), 37–38
  Dietary Reference Intakes (DRIs), 36–38
Magnetic resonance imaging (MRI), 3, 209
Males
  blood pressure levels, 289–290
  body composition equations, 197, 198, 199
  CDC growth charts, 431–432, 435–436
  estimating body weight, 232
  estimating risk of coronary heart disease, 264
  hypertension among, 283–284
  iron status, 328
  mean body mass index in U.S., 452, 456
  mean height in U.S., 444–445, 449–450, 454–455
  mean weight in U.S., 442–443, 447–448, 453
  relationship between BMI and death, 176–177
  serum folate levels, 341, 342
  serum vitamin B_{12}, 344
  vitamin C status, 338
  vitamin D status, 336
Malnutrition, 1, 2, 13. *See also* Deficiency diseases
  Malnutrition Universal Screening Tool (MUST), 248–250
  signs and symptoms of, 3–4
Marasmus, 359–361
Market Basket Study/Total Diet Study, 119, 125, 126–127
Mayo Clinic, 161
McCollum, E. V., 23
Meal planning, 62–63, 65–67
Meals for You (My Menus), 161
Meals on Wheels, 123
Mean corpuscular hemoglobin (MCH), 325, 326
Mean corpuscular volume (MCV), 325–326, 343
Measuring diet, 74–102. *See also* Nutritional assessment
  approaches to, 75–80
  considerations for certain groups, 79, 95, 96
  issues in dietary measurement, 95–101
  reasons for, 75, 76
  research design considerations for, 75–79, 95–98
  techniques in, 80–94. *See also* National dietary and nutrition surveys
  technological innovations in. *See* Computers in nutritional assessment
MEDFICTS Dietary Assessment Questionnaire, 79, 84–85, 269, 401–402
Medial calf skinfold measurements, 194, 195, 196
Median, 175
Medical history, 354–355
Medical nutrition therapy. *See also* Therapeutic lifestyle changes (TLC)
  for coronary heart disease (CHD), 269, 276–279
  for diabetes mellitus, 305–306
  dietary change plan in, 381–383
Medicines, in medical history, 354
Men. *See* Males
Message, in communication process, 371
Metabolic acidosis, 345
Metabolic alkalosis, 345
Metabolic syndrome, 267, 269
Metallothionen, 329
Methionine load test, 340
Metropolitan Life Insurance Company, 177–179

Microcytic anemia, 322
Midarm circumference (MAC), 228, 232, 233, 319
Midaxillary skinfold measurements, 192, 193
Mini Nutritional Assessment (MNA), 246–247, 248
Missing foods, 80
Mobile examination centers (MECs), 121–125
Modeling, in behavior modification, 377–378
Modified relative dose-response test (MRDR), 334
Monitoring nutrition. *See* National dietary and nutrition surveys
Morbidity, 4, 284
Mortality, 4, 284
Motivation, in dietary change plan, 381
Myocardial infarction, 257, 282
MyPlate, 60–64, 159–160, 161
MyPyramid, 60, 114, 162

National Academy of Sciences, 41, 115, 116, 240–241
National Cancer Institute (NCI), 79, 162
  ASA24 (automated, self-administered 24-hour dietary recall), 78, 81, 93, 108
  fruit and vegetable screener, 397–400
  Risk Factor Monitoring and Methods Branch, 83–88
National Center for Health Statistics, 13, 98, 112, 115, 119, 121, 122
National Cholesterol Education Program (NCEP), 51, 84–85, 110, 121, 129, 258, 261–263, 266, 271, 279–282, 314, 346
National dietary and nutrition surveys, 109–142
  dietary trends, 131–140
  examples of, 111
  importance of, 110
  nutritional monitoring and research, 110–112
  role of DHHS, 111, 112, 118–131
  role of USDA, 111, 112–118
  uses of, 111
National Food and Nutrient Analysis Program (NFNAP), 150
National Health and Nutrition Examination Surveys (NHANES), 16, 38, 44, 77–78, 81, 98, 101, 111, 115, 118–119, 120–125, 132, 442–456
  First National Health and Nutrition Examination Survey (NHANES I), 120, 175, 178, 184, 332, 341, 442–451
  Food Frequency Questionnaire (NHANES FFQ), 86–88, 89, 92–93, 412–419
  height-weight tables versus, 177–179
  Hispanic Health and Nutrition Examination Survey (HHANES), 118–119, 120
  mobile examination centers (MECs), 121–125
  Second National Health and Nutrition Examination Survey (NHANES II), 120, 133, 175, 178, 184, 284, 326, 442–451
  Third National Health and Nutrition Examination Survey (NHANES III), 120–121, 175, 183, 184, 261–262, 263, 284, 326, 336, 442–451
  What We Eat in America-NHANES, 121, 131, 133, 134, 135, 150, 152
National Health Examination Surveys (NHES), 118, 119, 124, 175, 270, 442–451
National Health Interview Survey (NHIS), 78, 119, 125, 130–131
National Health Survey Act of 1956, 118
National Heart, Lung and Blood Institute (NHLB), 6, 160, 266, 272, 287
National High Blood Pressure Education Program, 121, 274, 283, 287, 288–293
National Institutes of Health (NIH), 150, 181, 186, 218
National Kidney Foundation, 6

National Nutrition Monitoring and Related Research Act of 1990, 16, 112, 121
National Nutrition Monitoring and Related Research Program (NNMRRP), 16, 111–112, 115
National Research Council, 50, 111, 183
National School Lunch Program, 24, 44, 47
Nationwide Food Consumption Survey (NFCS; USDA), 112
Navajo Health and Nutrition Survey, 125, 127
Nephelometry, 321
Nestlé, 246–247, 248
Neural tube defects (NTDs), 79, 340
Neutral questions, 375
Neutron activation analysis, 205–206
New American Plate, 61–64
NHANES. *See* National Health and Nutrition Examination Surveys (NHANES)
NHES (National Health Examination Surveys), 118, 119, 124, 175, 270, 442–451
NHIS (National Health Interview Survey), 78, 119, 125, 130–131
Niacin, deficiency disease, 2
NIH (National Institutes of Health), 150, 181, 186, 218
Nitrogen
  blood urea nitrogen (BUN), 345
  nitrogen balance, 245, 320
  total urinary nitrogen (TUN), 245
  urea urinary nitrogen (UUN), 245, 320
Nomograms, 181–183, 198
Nonambulatory persons
  length measurement, 167–168
  recumbent skinfold measurements, 229–231
  stature measurement, 169, 227–228
  weight measurement, 171, 226, 228, 229–231
Nonverbal communication, 372, 373
Nurses' Health Study, 86
Nutrient content claims, 52
Nutrient Data Laboratory (NDL), 147–150, 162
Nutrient Databank System (USDA), 147–150
Nutrient Database for Standard Reference (SR), 147–150, 152–156
Nutrient databases, 147–158
  criteria for developing high-quality, 152–158
  United Nations, 147
  USDA, 81, 114, 147–150, 152–158
Nutrient density, 39–41
Nutrient profiling, 41
Nutrition Analysis Tool, 162
Nutrition care criteria, 6
Nutrition care indicators, 5
Nutrition Care Process (NCP), 4–11
  defined, 4
  Nutrition Care Process Model, 5–6
  nutrition diagnosis in, 5, 8–9
  nutrition intervention in, 5, 9–10
  nutritional assessment in, 5–8. *See also* Nutritional assessment
  nutritional monitoring and evaluation in, 5, 10–11
  overview of, 5
  standardized phrases or terms for, 4, 7–10
Nutrition Coordinating Center (NCC), 160
Nutrition Data System for Research (NDS-R), 160
Nutrition diagnosis
  domains of, 9
  in Nutrition Care Process (NCP), 5, 8–9
  PES statement in, 9
  terminology of, 391–392
Nutrition Evaluation Scale System, 93
Nutrition Facts labels, 53, 55, 56
Nutrition intervention
  in Nutrition Care Process (NCP), 5, 9–10
  terminology of, 393–394
Nutrition labeling, 50–57
  Daily Values, 55–57
  front-of-package labeling systems, 41, 54–55
  Nutrition Facts labels, 53, 55, 56
Nutrition Labeling and Education Act (NLEA), 50–55
Nutrition prescription/goal, 6
Nutrition Today, 47, 160
Nutritional analysis software, 4, 147–161
  examples of computerized dietary analysis systems, 160–161
  nutrient databases, 147–158
  program operation, 157, 158–159
  system output, 157, 159–160
Nutritional assessment. *See also* Measuring diet
  client history in, 7, 225, 354–356, 389–390
  clinical practice guidelines for specific conditions, 6, 9
  defined, 3
  in disease prevention. *See* Disease prevention
  equipment suppliers, 428–429
  food frequency questionnaires in. *See* Food frequency questionnaires
  food/nutrition-related history (FH), 7–9, 225, 355–356, 387–388
  of hospitalized patients. *See* Hospitalized patients
  importance of, 4
  methods of, 3–4, 6–7, 8. *See also* Anthropometric assessment; Biochemical assessment; Clinical assessment; Computers in nutritional assessment
  in Nutrition Care Process (NCP), 5, 6–7, 8
  nutrition-focused physical findings in, 7, 389
  opportunities to apply skills in, 11–17
  physical examination in, 225–226, 356–359
  standardized terminology in, 3, 4, 7–8, 9, 10, 11, 387–390
  Subjective Global Assessment (SGA), 4, 356–359, 369
Nutritional epidemiology, 17
Nutritional monitoring and evaluation, 110–111. *See also* National dietary and nutrition surveys
  in Nutrition Care Process (NCP), 5, 10–11
  nutritional monitoring, defined, 110
  research programs, 111–112
  types of, 110–111
Nutritional risk, 224
Nutritional screening
  defined, 3, 6
  as external supportive system, 3, 6
  of hospitalized patients, 222–224
  Nutritional Screening Form, 223–224
NutritionCalc Plus, 160, 161
Nutritionist Pro, 160
NutritionQuest, 86, 162

Obesity. *See also* Overweight; Weight management
  android versus gynoid, 185
  BMI in classifying, 183, 184
  chronic disease and, 3
  defined, 3, 14, 176
  prevalence of, 14–15, 130, 187
Observational standards, 22
OGTT (oral glucose tolerance test), 303, 346
Open circuit calorimetry, 236–237
Open questions, 374
Oral glucose tolerance test (OGTT), 303, 346
Osteopenia, 295–296, 335
Osteoporosis, 17, 293–300, 327, 335
  bone structuring and remodeling, 294
  classification, 294
  defined, 257
  diagnosing, 205–206, 209–210, 295–299
  dual-energy X-ray absorptiometry (DXA) and, 209–210, 295–296, 298–299
  prevention, 299–300
  risk factors, 293, 294–295, 299
Outcomes management system, 6
Overweight. *See also* Obesity; Weight management
  BMI in classifying, 183, 184
  chronic disease and, 3
  defined, 3, 14, 176
  prevalence of, 14–15, 129, 130, 187

Parallax, 168
Parenteral nutrition, 3, 4, 244, 250
Pathobiological Determinants of Atherosclerosis in Youth (PDAY), 271
Peak bone mass, 294, 295
Pectoral skinfold measurements, 190
Pediatric Nutrition Surveillance System (PedNSS), 119, 125, 128
Pellagra, 2
Percentile curves, 171
Peripheral vascular disease, 257
Person-centered approach, 375–376
PES (problem/etiology/signs and symptoms) statement, 9
Phantom foods, 80
Phosphorus, blood chemistry tests, 346
Physical activity
  bone health and, 299–300, 301
  Estimated Energy Requirement (EER) and, 274, 275
  hypertension risk and, 287
  thermic effect of exercise (TEE), 234–235, 239
Physical examination, 225–226, 356–359
Plasma-based markers/biomarkers, 260
Plasma levels, 97
  fasting plasma glucose (FPG), 303
  of vitamin A, 333–334
  of vitamin B_6, 339–340
  of vitamin C, 339
  of zinc, 329
Portion/serving sizes, 52, 98–101
Postprandial measures, 200, 306
Posture
  in cholesterol measurement, 282
  in communication process, 372
Potassium
  blood chemistry tests, 346
  in determining body composition, 205
  urinary, 97
Power-type indices, 181–184
Prealbumin, 321–322
Preanalytical factors, 281
Precision, in measuring lipids and lipoproteins, 279–280
Prediabetes, 302
Predisposing risk factors, 15, 16
Pregnancy
  in cholesterol measurement, 282
  folate status, 79, 340
  gestational diabetes mellitus (GDM), 302
  metabolic rate, 241
Pregnancy Nutrition Surveillance System (PNSS), 125, 127–128
Prehypertension, 3, 283, 288
President's Council on Fitness, Sports & Nutrition, 161
Prevalence, 1
  of overweight and obesity, 14–15, 129, 130, 187
Prevention. *See* Disease prevention
Primary prevention

coronary heart disease (CHD), 266, 273
of hypertension, 285
Primordial prevention, 273
Prospective cohort studies, 78–79
Protease inhibitor therapy, 363
Protective foods, 23
Protein
biochemical measures of, 222, 245, 318–322, 344–345
in coronary heart disease treatment, 278–279
creatinine excretion, 206, 233, 319–320, 346
Dietary Reference Intakes (DRIs), 36–38
estimating needs for, 244–245
losses in disease and injury, 244
nitrogen balance, 245, 320
protein-energy malnutrition (PEM), 13, 222, 319, 320, 359–362
serum proteins, 3, 320–322
trends, 138
Protein degradation, 320
Protein-energy malnutrition (PEM), 13, 222, 319, 320, 359–362
classifying, 361–362
kwashiorkor, 359–361
marasmus, 359–361
Protein synthesis, 320
Proximal measures, 189
Psychosocial factors, 354
Public health approach
to cholesterol reduction, 270–271
to hypertension prevention, 284–285

Quantitative ultrasound (QUS), 296–299
Quetelet's index (BMI). *See* Body mass index (BMI)

Race/ethnicity
Hispanic Health and Nutrition Examination Survey (HHANES), 118–119, 120
hypertension risk, 283–284
iron status, 327
mean body mass index in U.S., 456
mean height in U.S., 455
Navajo Health and Nutrition Survey, 125, 127
serum folate levels, 341, 342
serum vitamin B_{12}, 344
vitamin C status, 338
vitamin D status, 336
Radial immunodiffusion, 321
Rational-emotive therapy (RET), 378–380
RDAs (Recommended Dietary Allowances), 6, 23–24, 26, 27–33, 35, 36–38, 39, 336
RDIs (Reference Daily Intakes), 55, 57
Reality therapy, 380–381
Receiver, in communication process, 371, 373
Recommended Dietary Allowances (RDAs), 6, 23–24, 26, 27–33, 35, 36–38, 39, 336
Recommended Nutrient Intakes (RNIs) for Canadians, 23
Recordkeeping
in dietary change plan, 382
food records/diaries, 79–80, 81–83, 107, 382, 395–396, 478
Recumbent length measurement, 167–168
Recumbent skinfold measurements, 229–231
Red blood cell (RBC) folate concentration, 341
Reference amounts, 52
Reference Daily Intakes (RDIs), 55, 57
Reinforcers
in behavior modification, 378
in dietary change plan, 382
Relapse prevention, 383
Relative/criterion validity, 95
Relative dose-response test (RDR), 334
Relative weight, 177, 180–181
Reliability, 98
Report of the Expert Panel on Population Strategies for Blood Cholesterol Reduction, 270–271
Reproducibility, 98
Resting energy expenditure (REE), 98, 234–235, 238–244
Retinol-binding protein (RBP), 321, 322, 333, 334
Rickets, 2, 335
Rogers, Carl, 375–376

Saturated fatty acids (SFA), 276–277
Scales, 170–171, 200
Screeners. *See* Food frequency questionnaires
Scurvy, 2, 22
Secondary prevention, coronary heart disease (CHD), 266
Self-contracts, 377
Self-monitoring
in behavior modification, 376–377
of blood glucose (SMBG), 303–304
food records/diaries in, 79–80, 81–83, 107, 382, 395–396, 478
Sender, in communication process, 371, 373
Serum calcium fractions, 327–328
Serum calcium levels, 345
Serum creatinine, 346
Serum ferritin, 322, 324, 326, 327, 328
Serum glutamic oxaloacetic transaminase (SGOT), 345
Serum glutamic pyruvic transminase (SGPT), 343–344
Serum iron, 324
Serum lipids, 258–263, 279–282, 306, 313–314, 469–477
Serum methylmalonic acid (MMA), 343
Serum proteins, 3, 320–322
Serum total cholesterol, 260–262, 469–473
Serum (leukocyte) vitamin C, 339
Serving/portion sizes, 52, 98–101
Shortfall nutrients, 59
Signs. *See also* Clinical assessment
defined, 353
of malnutrition, 3–4
in nutrition diagnosis, 8–10
Skinfold calipers, 189–190, 191, 208
Skinfold measurements, 3, 188–199, 208, 220, 226
assumptions, 188, 189
desirable level of fatness, 198–199
measurement techniques, 188–190
multiple-site, 197–198, 465–466
recumbent, 229–231
single-site, 195, 457–464, 467–468
site selection, 190–195
two-site, 195–197
Smith, Edward, 22
Smoking, 263, 300, 371
Sodium
blood chemistry tests, 346
bone health and, 300
diabetes and, 306
hypertension risk and, 286–287
iodized, 333
urinary, 97
SoFAS (solid fats and added sugars), 133–134
Soluble fiber, 278–279
Soluble transferrin receptor (sTfR), 324, 326
Sonometers, 298
Special Supplemental Food Program for Women, Infants, and Children (WIC), 24, 110, 123, 128
Speed of sound (SOS), 298
Sphygmomanometer, 282–283
Stadiometer, 168
Standard deviation (SD), 33
Stature, 168–169. *See also* Height
CDC growth charts, 435, 437, 439, 440
estimating stature of hospitalized patients, 225–228, 254
knee height, 227–228
Stiebeling, Hazel Katherine, 23, 57, 58, 59
Stroke, 257, 282
Stunting, 361
Subjective Global Assessment (SGA), 4, 356–359, 369
Subscapular skinfold measurements, 192, 193, 196, 229–231, 461–466
SuperTracker, 61, 161, 162
Supplemental Children's Survey (USDA), 112, 115
Supplemental Nutrition Assistance Program (SNAP), 24
Suprailiac skinfold measurements, 193, 194
Surgeon General's Report on Nutrition and Health, 50, 51, 183
Surrogate sources, 79, 94
Sweeteners
in diabetes treatment, 306
trends, 134–136
Symptoms. *See also* Clinical assessment
defined, 353
of malnutrition, 3–4
in nutrition diagnosis, 8–10
Systolic blood pressure (SBP), 263, 282–283, 287, 288

T-scores, 295–296, 297
Telephone interviews, 92–93
Ten-State Nutrition Survey, 118, 119–120, 128
Therapeutic lifestyle changes (TLC). *See also* Medical nutrition therapy
for coronary heart disease (CHD), 267–270, 276–279
for hypertension, 283
Therapy. *See* Counseling theory and technique
Thermic effect of disease or injury (TED), 234–235, 241–244
Thermic effect of exercise (TEE), 234–235, 239
Thermic effect of food (TEF), 234–235, 239
Thiamin, deficiency disease, 2
Thigh skinfold measurements, 193–194, 195
Third Report of the Expert Panel on Detection, Evaluation, and Treatment of High Blood Cholesterol in Adults (Adult Treatment Panel III; ATP III), 266–271, 276, 278, 279
Thoracic kyphosis (dowager's hump), 294
Thrombosis, 260
Thyroid-stimulating hormone (TSH), 331
Title V Maternal and Child Health Program, 128
Tolerable Upper Intake Level (UL), 26, 31, 32, 34–35, 39
Tone of voice, in communication process, 372
Toronto formula, 243–244
Total abdominal fat, 185–186
Total analytical error, in measuring lipids and lipoproteins, 279, 281
Total body electrical conductivity (TOBEC), 207
Total body potassium (TBK), 205
Total body water (TBW), 204–205, 207
Total calories
in coronary heart disease treatment, 278
trends, 139–140
Total cholesterol, 260–263, 469–473
Total Diet Study (TDS), 119, 125, 126–127
Total energy expenditure (TEE), 35, 241, 242
Total fat, 37, 38
in coronary heart disease treatment, 278
Total fiber, 36–37
Total iron-binding capacity (TIBC), 321, 324

Total parenteral nutrition (TPN), 244
Total water, 36
Trans fatty acids, 277
Transferrin, 321, 324
Trauma, in cholesterol measurement, 282
Trends. *See* Dietary trends
Tricep skinfold measurements, 190–192, 196, 226, 229–231, 233, 457–460
Triglycerides (TG), 259, 263, 346
Tritium, in total body water (TBW) measurement, 204–205
Type 1 diabetes mellitus, 301–302
Type 2 diabetes mellitus, 50, 301–302

Ultrasound
- in determining body composition, 208
- in diagnosing osteoporosis, 296–299

Underwater weighing, 199–202
United Nations
- Food and Agriculture Organization (FAO), 147
- University Food and Nutrition Program, 147

U.S. Bureau of the Census, 116, 130–131
U.S. Centers for Disease Control and Prevention (CDC)
- Behavioral Risk Factor Surveillance System (BRFSS), 16, 78, 119, 125, 129–130, 144, 420–427
- definition of HIV wasting syndrome, 362–363
- growth charts, 14, 171–176, 277, 288, 430–440
- high-sensitivity C-reactive protein (hs-CRP) analysis, 260, 267
- measuring lipids and lipoproteins, 280–281
- Pediatric Nutrition Surveillance System (PedNSS), 119, 125, 128
- Pregnancy Nutrition Surveillance System (PNSS), 125, 127–128

U.S. Department of Agriculture (USDA), 23
- Automated Multiple-Pass Method (AMPM) of collecting 24-hour recall, 78, 81, 93, 101, 123, 133
- Center for Nutrition Policy and Promotion, 114, 161
- Continuing Survey of Food Intakes by Individuals (CSFII), 83, 111, 112, 114–115, 121
- Diet and Health Knowledge Survey, 78, 112, 115
- *Dietary Guidelines for Americans*, 6, 8, 10, 13–14, 40–44, 47–50, 51, 59, 60, 110, 114, 133, 134, 159, 241, 268, 273–274, 333, 340, 342
- Economic Research Service (ERS) Food Availability (Per Capita) Data System, 114, 131, 134
- Food and Nutrient Database for Dietary Studies (FNDDS), 81, 114, 150–152, 158
- Food and Nutrition Information Center (FNIC), 161
- Food and Nutrition Service, 115, 145
- food guides and pyramids, 41, 42, 57–64, 86, 114, 159, 162
- food insecurity and hunger, 115–118, 119
- *Food Model Booklet*, 99–101
- Food Safety and Inspection Service, 52
- Food Surveys Research Group, 112, 145, 150
- Healthy Eating Index (HEI), 42–44, 45
- Human Nutrition Research Center, 90, 235–236
- meal planning guide, 62–63
- National Nutrition Monitoring and Related Research Program (NNMRRP), 16, 111–112, 115
- Nutrient Data Laboratory (NDL), 147–150, 162
- nutrient databases, 81, 114, 147–150, 152–158
- role in national dietary and nutrition surveys, 111, 112–118
- Supplemental Children's Survey, 112, 115
- surveys of food disappearance/availability, 46, 75–76, 91–92, 110–111, 112–114
- Western Human Nutrition Research Center, 93, 98

U.S. Department of Health and Human Services (DHHS)
- *Dietary Guidelines for Americans*, 6, 8, 10, 13–14, 40–44, 47–50, 51, 59, 60, 110, 114, 133, 159, 241, 268, 273–274, 333, 340, 342
- National Center for Health Statistics, 13, 98, 112, 115, 119, 121, 122
- National Health and Nutrition Examination Surveys (NHANES). *See* National Health and Nutrition Examination Surveys (NHANES)
- National Health Examination Surveys (NHES), 118, 119, 124, 175, 270, 442–451
- National Nutrition Monitoring and Related Research Program (NNMRRP), 16, 111–112, 115
- role in national dietary and nutrition surveys, 111, 112, 118–131
- Ten-State Nutrition Survey, 118, 119–120, 128

U.S. Environmental Protection Agency (EPA), 115
U.S. Food and Drug Administration (FDA), 50, 55, 121, 287, 306, 340
- Center for Food Safety and Applied Nutrition, 129, 161
- Health and Diet Survey, 119, 125, 129
- health claim regulation, 52–53
- Total Diet Study (TDS), 119, 125, 126–127

U.S. Government Accountability Office (GAO), 110, 111
U.S. Public Health Service, 64–67
U.S. Recommended Daily Allowances (U.S. RDAs), 50–51
Unsaturated fat, in coronary heart disease treatment, 278
Urinary methylmalonic acid (MMA), 343
Urine
- creatinine excretion, 319–320
- urea urinary nitrogen (UUN), 245, 320
- urinary 4-pyridoxic acid, 340
- urinary calcium, 328–329
- urinary iodine (UI), 331–333
- urinary nitrogen, 97, 245, 318, 320
- urinary potassium, 97
- urinary sodium, 97
- urinary zinc, 330
- urine samples, 96–97

USDA. *See* U.S. Department of Agriculture (USDA)

Validity, 95–98
- of biological markers, 95–97
- of energy expenditure measures, 97–98
- of food frequency questionnaires, 95
- types, 95

Vegetables
- National Cancer Institute fruit and vegetable screener, 397–400
- trends, 138–139

Vegetarian Resource Group, 161
Venous occlusion, in cholesterol measurement, 282
Verbal communication, 371–372
Very low-density lipoprotein (VLDL), 258–259, 263
Vision, dark adaptation, 334–335
Vitamin A, 333–335
- conjunctival impression cytology, 334
- dark adaptation, 334–335
- deficiency disease, 2
- direct measurement of liver stores, 335
- plasma levels, 333–334
- relative dose-response test (RDR), 334
- retinol isotope dilution, 335

Vitamin B_6
- methionine load test, 340
- plasma PLP, 339–340
- plasma pyridoxal, 340
- urinary 4-pyridoxic acid, 340

Vitamin B_{12}, 322, 341–343, 344
- biochemical indicators, 343
- deficiency disease, 322, 342

Vitamin C, 337–339
- deficiency disease, 2, 22, 337–338
- serum and leukocyte, 339

Vitamin D
- assessing status, 335–337
- deficiency disease, 2, 335
- osteoporosis and, 294, 299

Voit, Carl, 22

Waist-to-hip ratio (WHR), 185–186
Wasting, 361, 362–367
Water, 36
- in determining body composition, 204–205, 207
- doubly labeled water method of calorimetry, 237–238
- underwater weighing, 199–202

Weighed food records, 82–83
Weight. *See* Body weight
Weight management, 13–15, 97–98, 379, 381–382
What We Eat in America-NHANES, 121, 131, 133, 134, 135, 150, 152
WIC (Special Supplemental Food Program for Women, Infants, and Children), 24, 110, 123, 128
Willett, Walter, 85–86, 88–89
Willett questionnaire, 85–86, 88–89
Women. *See* Females
Women's Health Study, 183
World Cancer Research Fund, 61–64
World Health Organization (WHO), 2, 15, 287
- equations for energy requirements, 234–235, 238–239, 239, 242, 243
- iodine status, 331, 332
- Multicentre Growth Reference Study (MGRS), 174
- osteoporosis and, 293, 295–296

World War I, 23, 113
World War II, 113

Xerophthalmia, 2

Youth/Adolescent Questionnaire (YAQ), 86

Zinc, 329–330
- hair zinc, 330
- metallothionen, 329
- plasma zinc concentrations, 329
- urinary zinc, 330